Clinical Pediatric Neurology

Clinical Pediatric Neurology

Edited by
Ronald B. David, MD
Attending Physician
Department of Pediatrics
St. Mary's Hospital
Associate Clinical Professor
Department of Pediatrics
Virginia Commonwealth University School of Medicine
Richmond, Virginia

With Section Editors

John B. Bodensteiner, MD
William Pilcher Chair of Pediatric Neurology
Barrow Neurologic Institute of St. Joseph's Hospital and Medical Center
Phoenix, Arizona

David E. Mandelbaum, MD, PhD
Professor
Department of Clinical Neurosciences and Pediatrics
Alpert Medical School of Brown University
Providence, Rhode Island

Barbara J. Olson, MD
Private Practice
Pediatric Neurology Associates
Assistant Clinical Professor
Department of Pediatrics and Neurology
Vanderbilt University
Nashville, Tennessee

demosMEDICAL
New York

Acquisitions Editor: Beth Barry
Cover Design: Steve Pisano
Copyeditor: Joann Woy
Compositor: Patricia Wallenburg
Printer: Bang Printing

Visit our website at www.demosmedpub.com

Library of Congress Cataloging-in-Publication Data

Clinical pediatric neurology / edited by Ronald B. David. — 3rd ed.
p. ; cm.
Rev. ed. of: Child and adolescent neurology / edited by Ronald B. David. 2nd ed. 2005.
Includes bibliographical references and index.
ISBN-13: 978-1-933864-22-8 (hardcover : alk. paper)
ISBN-10: 1-933864-22-2 (hardcover : alk. paper)
1. Pediatric neurology. I. David, Ronald B. II. Child and adolescent neurology.
[DNLM: 1. Nervous System Diseases—diagnosis. 2. Adolescent. 3. Child. 4. Diagnostic Techniques, Neurological. 5. Infant. 6. Nervous System Diseases—therapy. 7. Neurologic Examination. WS 340 C6415 2009]
RJ486.5.C45 2009
618.92'8—dc22

2008047998

Made in the United States of America

09 10 11 12 5 4 3 2 1

To my children and grandchildren.
To all children . . . but particularly
To the children for whom we care . . .
those whose lives have been touched by the
misfortune of neurologic disorders.

Contents

Preface

Traditional textbooks convey knowledge. It is the goal of this text to convey not only essential knowledge but also the collected wisdom of its many highly regarded contributors. To achieve the goal of conveying not only knowledge but wisdom, each book in this series is built on a structural framework that was well received by critics and readers alike in previous editions. Our text is divided into three sections:

- Tools for diagnosis
- Diseases and disorders
- Common problems

Also included to facilitate a physician's use of this book are:

- Nosologic diagnosis tables,
- "Pearls and Perils" boxes,
- "Consider Consultation When..." boxes,
- Selected annotated bibliographies,
- A complete bibliography,
- And (new in this edition) Key Clinical Questions.

The Nosologic Diagnosis tables are based on a discriminator model to promote clearer understanding and are superior to a criterion-based model and others that lack similar specificity. (See the Appendix for complete description of how this system was developed.)

> Whoever having undertaken to speak or write hath first laid for themselves some [basis] to their argument such as hot or cold or moist or dry or whatever else they choose, thus reducing their subject within a narrow compass.
>
> *Hippocrates*

As Hippocrates has suggested, structure is the key to learning. Unless there is a structure onto which knowledge can be built, confusion and disorganization are the inevitable consequences.

Classification systems induce orderliness in thinking and enhance our ability to communicate effectively. A review of the most enduring hierarchical classification systems, particularly that of Linnaeus (that is, phyla, genera, species), makes clear the value of grouping according to discriminating features, as well as the value of simplicity, expandability, and dynamism.

The goal, whatever the classification system, is to seek the most powerful discriminating features that will produce the greatest diagnostic clarity. Discriminating features should avoid crossing domains. Much of the confusion that arises in diagnosis may be the result of the clinician who unwittingly crosses the anatomic, pathologic, pathophysiologic, phenomenologic, and etiologic classification domains used in medicine (for example, the inclusion of anatomically oriented "temporal lobe seizures" in a phenomenologically based classification system that includes complex partial seizures). Some conditions, such as brain tumors, are classified according to their histopathology and lend themselves well to this classification system. Others, such as headaches and movement disorders, are classified phenomenologically and are therefore much less easily classified. In other cases, discriminators must encompass inclusionary as well as exclusionary features. At times, we can only use a criterion-based system or construct tables to compare features.

Arbitrarily, we label as consistent those features that occur more than 75% of the time; features are considered variable when they occur less than 75% of the time. The diagnostic tables should be viewed, therefore, only as a beginning in the extremely difficult effort to make diagnosis more precise and biologically based. How well this book accomplishes the goals of identifying the most powerful discrimination features for maximum diagnostic clarity is limited by the current state of the art in child and adolescent neurology. In some areas, several features, when clustered together, serve to discriminate.

This text is designed to be pithy, not exhaustive, many other books of that ilk are already available. Each text in this series reflects appropriate stylistic differences among content editors. However, each is built upon the same structural framework; hence the value of this text to the users.

Chapter 16 on "Order and Disorders of Nervous System Development" is particularly noteworthy because of its unique treatment of this very important and timely subject matter.

Acknowledgment

I would like to acknowledge some of the people who have made key contributions to this effort. They include Craig Percy, who initially saw the potential of this effort and headed the team at Demos; the National Institute of Neurological Disorders and Stroke (NINDS)* for its support in nosologic research; and the investigators who were involved with this NINDS project; Dr. Grover Robinson, a long-time friend (who suggested the "Consider Consultation When..." boxes); and Ms. Laura DeYoung a long-time publishing friend. I am also particularly grateful to my associate editor colleagues, Drs. John Bodensteiner, David Mandelbaum, and Barbara Olson, for their extensive and hands-on contribution to this edition. Their help is reflected, I feel, in the extraordinary quality of the present effort. Lastly, I would thank Dr. Susan Pillsbury, a close friend and trusted colleague, whose advice is always cogent and whose personal support is most appreciated.

This text is therefore in no way a singular effort but rather reflects the expertise of all who contributed in so many different ways. It is my hope that this is reflected in the quality of the effort. It is therefore my fondest wish that this text resides on your desk, rather than on your bookshelf.

Ronald B. David, MD

*NINDS 1PO1NS20189–01A1 (Nosology, Higher Cortical Function Disorders in Children).

Contributors

Kevin M. Antshel, PhD
Assistant Professor of Psychiatry
Department of Psychiatry and Behavioral Sciences
State University of New York Upstate Medical University
Syracuse, New York

Jennifer Armstrong-Wells, MD, MPH
Resident Physician
Department of Neurology
University of California San Francisco
San Francisco, California

James F. Bale, Jr., MD
Professor and Associate Chair
Department of Pediatrics
University of Utah School of Medicine
Salt Lake City, Utah

Russell A. Barkley, PhD
Clinical Professor of Psychiatry
Department of Psychiatry
Medical University of South Carolina
Charleston, South Carolina

William E. Bell, MD
Professor Emeritus
Department of Pediatrics and Neurology
The University of Iowa Hospitals
Iowa City, Iowa

Warren T. Blume, MD, CM, FRCP(C)
Professor of Neurology and Pediatrics
Department of Neurology
University Hospital
University of Western Ontario
London, Ontario
Canada

John B. Bodensteiner, MD
William Pilcher Chair of Pediatric Neurology
Barrow Neurologic Institute of St. Joseph's Hospital
and Medical Center
Phoenix, Arizona

Russell J. Butterfield, MD, PhD
Fellow
Department of Neurology
University of Utah School of Medicine
Salt Lake City, Utah

Donna Kathryn Daily, MD, MA
Associate Professor of Pediatrics
Department of Pediatrics
Vanderbilt University Medical School
Nashville, Tennessee

Ronald B. David, MD
Attending Physician
Department of Pediatrics
St. Mary's Hospital
Associate Clinical Professor
Department of Pediatrics
Virginia Commonwealth University School of Medicine
Richmond, Virginia

O'Neill F. D'Cruz, MD, MBA
Clinical Research Physician
Department of Clinical Science
Actelion Parmaceuticals Ltd.
Cherry Hill, New Jersey

Ruthmary K. Deuel, MD
Professor Emeritus
Department of Pediatrics and Neurology
Washington University School of Medicine
St. Louis, Missouri

Emanuel DiCicco-Bloom, MD
Professor
Departments of Neuroscience and Cell Biology and Pediatrics (Neurology)
Robert Wood Johnson School of Medicine
Piscataway, New Jersey

Patricia H. Ellison, MD
Adjunct Professor, Retired
Department of Pediatrics
University of Colorado School of Medicine
Denver, Colorado

Michael Flink, DO, PhD
Assistant Professor
Department of Neurosciences
University of California San Diego School of Medicine
La Jolla, California

John N. Gaitanis, MD
Assistant Professor of Clinical Neurosciences and Pediatrics
Department of Neurology
Warren Alpert School of Medicine at Brown University
Providence, Rhode Island

Laurie Gutmann, MD
Professor of Neurology and Exercise Physiology
Department of Neurology
West Virginia University
Morgantown, West Virginia

Richard H. Haas, MB, B Chir
Professor
Department of Neurosciences and Pediatrics
University of California San Diego
La Jolla, California

Stavros M. Hadjiloizou, MD
Child Neurologist
Department of Epilepsy and Clinical Neurophysiology
Cyprus Paediatric Neurology Institute
The Cyprus Institute of Neurology and Genetics
Nicosia, Cyprus

Gary Hedlund, DO
Adjunct Professor Radiology
Department of Medical Imaging
University of Utah School of Medicine
Salt Lake City, Utah

Frederick W. Henderson, MD
Distinguished Professor of Pediatrics
Department of Pediatrics
University of North Carolina
Chapel Hill, North Carolina

Andrew D. Hershey, MD, PhD, FAHS
Professor of Pediatrics and Neurology
Department of Pediatrics
Cincinnati Children's Hospital Medical Center
University of Cincinnati College of Medicine
Cincinnati, Ohio

Deborah G. Hirtz, MD
Program Director
Office of Clinical Trials
National Institute of Neurological Disorders and Stroke
National Institutes of Health
Rockville, Maryland

H. Terry Hutchinson, MD, PhD
Clinical Professor
Department of Child Neurology
University of California San Francisco
San Francisco, California

Robert A Keating, MD
Chief
Department of Pediatric Neurosurgery
Children's National Medical Center
Professor
Department of Neurosurgery
The George Washington University
Washington, DC

John F. Kerrigan, MD
Director
Pediatric Epilepsy Program
Co-Director
Hypothalamic Hamartoma Program
Barrow Neurologic Institute of St. Joseph's Hospital and Medical Center
Assistant Professor
Department of Clinical Pediatrics and Neurology
University of Arizona College of Medicine Phoenix
Phoenix, Arizona

Paul C. Lebby, PhD
Clinical Neuropsychologist
Department of Neuropsychology and Medical Rehabilitation
Children's Hospital Central California
Madera, California

Tobey J. MacDonald, MD
Director
Department of Hematology/Oncology
Center for Cancer and Blood Disorders
Children's National Medical Center
Associate Professor
Department of Neurology and Pediatrics
The George Washington University
Washington, DC

Michelle M. Macias, MD
Associate Professor of Pediatrics
Department of Pediatrics
Medical University of South Carolina
Charleston, South Carolina

Kenneth J. Mack, MD, PhD
Medical Director
Departments of Neurology and Pediatrics
Mayo Clinic Pediatric Center
Rochester, Minnesota

Paul Maertens, MD
Associate Professor Child Neurology
Department of Neurology and Pediatrics
University of South Alabama
Mobile, Alabama

Amisha Malhotra, MD
Assistant Professor of Pediatrics
Department of Pediatrics
Robert Wood Johnson School of Medicine
University of Medicine and Dentistry of New Jersey
New Brunswick, New Jersey

David E. Mandelbaum, MD, PhD
Professor
Department of Clinical Neurosciences and Pediatrics
Alpert Medical School of Brown University
Providence, Rhode Island

Ruth D. Nass, MD
Professor of Clinical Neurology (Pediatrics)
Department of Neurology
New York University School of Medicine
New York, New York

Karin B. Nelson, MD
Scientist Emeritus
National Institute of Neurological Disorders and Stroke
National Institutes of Health
Bethesda, Maryland

William L. Nyhan, MD, PhD
Professor of Pediatrics
Department of Pediatrics
University of California San Diego
San Diego, California

Barbara J. Olson, MD
Private Practice
Pediatric Neurology Associates
Assistant Clinical Professor
Department of Pediatrics and Neurology
Vanderbilt University
Nashville, Tennessee

Roger J. Packer, MD
Executive Director
Department of Neuroscience and Behavioral Medicine
Director
Brain Tumor Institute
Children's National Medical Center
Professor
Department of Neurology and Pediatrics
The George Washington University
Washington, DC

Amy C. Rauchway, DO
Assistant Professor of Neurology
Departments of Neurology and Psychiatry
Saint Louis University School of Medicine
St. Louis, Missouri

Jack E. Riggs, MD
Professor of Neurology
Department of Neurology
West Virginia University
Morgantown, West Virginia

James J. Riviello, Jr., MD
George Peterkin Endowed Chair in Pediatrics
Professor of Pediatrics and Neurology/Neurophysiology
Departments of Pediatrics and Neurology
Texas Children's Hospital
Houston, Texas

Brian R. Rood, MD
Attending Physician
Department of Hematology/Oncology
Children's National Medical Center
Assistant Professor
Department of Pediatrics
The George Washington University
Washington, DC

Gail Ross, PhD
Associate Professor of Psychology
Departments of Pediatrics and Psychiatry
Weill Medical Center of Cornell University
New York, New York

Barry S. Russman, MD
Professor Pediatrics and Neurology
Oregon Health & Science University
Portland, Oregon

Debora L. Scheffel, PhD
Academic Dean
Jones International University
Centennial, Colorado

John T. Sladky, MD
Chief
Department of Pediatric Neurology
Children's Healthcare of Atlanta at Egleston
Chief
Department of Pediatric Neurology
Emory University School of Medicine
Atlanta, Georgia

Carl E. Stafstrom, MD, PhD
Professor of Neurology and Pediatrics
Department of Neurology
University of Wisconsin
Madison, Wisconsin

Doris A. Trauner, MD
Professor and Chief, Pediatric Neurology
Department of Neurosciences and Pediatrics
Rady Children's Hospital
University of California San Diego School of Medicine
La Jolla, California

Bradley V. Vaughn, MD
Professor of Neurology and Biomedical Engineering
Department of Neurology
University of North Carolina
Chapel Hill, North Carolina

Gilbert Vezina, MD
Chief
Department of Neuroradiology
Children's National Medical Center
Professor
Department of Radiology
The George Washington University
Washington, DC

Max Wiznitzer, MD
Division Of Pediatric Neurology
Rainbow Babies & Children's Hospital
Associate Professor of Pediatrics and Neurology
Case Western Reserve University
Cleveland, Ohio

Clinical Pediatric Neurology

SECTION 1

PEDIATRIC NEUROLOGIC EVALUATION

John B. Bodensteiner

CHAPTER 1

Neurologic History

John B. Bodensteiner and Ronald B. David

Some clinicians have suggested that the taking of the neurologic history is as important as, or potentially more important than, the neurologic examination itself. Other clinicians have suggested that the neurologic history identifies the nature of the disorder or disease, and the neurologic examination confirms or pinpoints its location. The history itself may be a narrative recapitulation of information provided by a child's primary caregiver(s), or it may be generated in response to a questionnaire or checklist. Experienced clinicians realize that the key to making a successful diagnosis often lies in asking the right questions and listening carefully to the answers. Responses to questionnaires or checklists can be used as part of a formal structured interview. Diagnostically, they can be both reliable and valid. For example, a patient may be asked the following questions with respect to headaches: Are your headaches confined to one side of your head? Are your headaches associated with vomiting or a desire to sleep? Do you have visual symptoms, such as dancing lights or other phenomena? An affirmative response to all three questions would permit accuracy of close to 100% for the diagnosis of migraine. No other questions or laboratory investigations may be necessary. Other questions provide clinical rather than diagnostic information, useful in practicing the art as well as the science of medicine.

The reliability of the information gained from a questionnaire depends to some extent on the ability of the respondent to understand the questions being asked. The questions that follow are those used by many clinicians to accomplish this end. Some are also valuable in answering research questions. They are all designed to be useful in the practice of pediatric neurology. Note: This form may be reproduced for clinical use without further permission from the author or publisher. In order to make the questions more useful, we have collected them into groups based on the three most common presenting complaints in the pediatric neurology outpatient setting, namely seizures, headache, and developmental delay. This is not a copyrighted section of this text and clinicians should feel free to lift any or all questions or formats for reproduction and clinical use.

Pearls and Perils

- The diagnosis can often be determined or inferred from one or two key questions.
- Willingness to comply with treatment can be probed by use of key questions.
- Willingness to accept diagnosis can be probed through key questions.

A. Demographic data

1. Name ______________________________
2. Child's date of birth ____________ /____________ /____________
3. Child's age ____________ /____________
4. Child's sex
   a. Male ____________
   b. Female ____________
5. Child's race
   a. Caucasian ____________
   b. African American ____________
   c. Latino ____________
   d. Asian ____________
   e. Other ____________
6. Birthplace ______________________________
7. Name of hospital ______________________________
8. Child's siblings (please list oldest first)

	Age		Sex		Relation to this child			
Initials	Years	Months	M	F	Full	Half	Adopted	Step

9. Marital status of parents
   a. Married ____________
   b. Single ____________
   c. Separated ____________
   d. Divorced ____________
10. Relationship of caregiver to child
    a. Natural parent ____________
    b. Adoptive parent ____________
    c. Stepparent ____________
    d. Foster parent ____________
    e. Grandparent ____________
    f. Aunt or uncle ____________
    g. Brother or sister ____________
    h. Other ____________
11. Parents' educational experience

	Father	Mother
a. Eighth grade or less	____________	____________
b. Attended high school	____________	____________
c. High school graduate	____________	____________
d. Attended college	____________	____________
e. Two-year degree	____________	____________
f. Four-year degree	____________	____________
g. Master's degree	____________	____________
h. Doctorate	____________	____________

12. Handedness of parents

	Father	Mother
a. Right	____________	____________
b. Left	____________	____________
c. Ambidextrous	____________	____________

13. Please check if the parent was or is considered to have difficulty with any of the following:

		Father	Mother
a.	Speech	______	______
b.	Confusion of left and right hands	______	______
c.	Overactivity, restlessness, hyperactivity	______	______
d.	Being clumsy or awkward	______	______
e.	Walking	______	______
f.	Math	______	______
g.	Spelling	______	______
h.	Reading	______	______
i.	Delayed or unintelligible language	______	______
j.	Seizures or convulsions	______	______
k.	Nerves or nervous breakdown	______	______
l.	Mental retardation	______	______

B. Medical information/history

		Yes	No
1.	Please check if your child has ever experienced any of the following:		
a.	More than two episodes of otitis media	______	______
b.	Tubes in ears (myringotomy)	______	______
c.	Visual difficulty requiring either glasses or visual training	______	______
d.	Hearing difficulty requiring the use of a hearing aid	______	______
e.	Movement problems requiring the use of special shoes, splints, braces, or a wheelchair or a specialized program of motor training	______	______
f.	Failure to thrive	______	______
g.	Poisoning or drug overdose	______	______
h.	Eating unusual substances (e.g. paint, plaster)	______	______
i.	Unconscious spells, fainting	______	______
j.	Convulsions, seizures, epilepsy	______	______
k.	Bedwetting beyond the age of 5 years	______	______
l.	Soiling beyond the age of 3 years	______	______
m.	Sleeping problems	______	______
n.	Poor growth or poor weight gain	______	______
o.	Unusual reactions to baby shots	______	______
p.	Toe walking	______	______
q.	Ran or walked more awkwardly than other children	______	______
r.	Ran or walked more slowly than other children	______	______
s.	Picked last or close to last in games where children pick sides	______	______
t.	Tics or unusual movements	______	______
u.	Headaches not relieved by nonprescription pain medicine	______	______
v.	Headaches not relieved by prescription pain medicine	______	______
w.	Headaches occurring in the middle of the night or upon awakening	______	______
x.	Production of unusual odors	______	______
y.	Unusual habits	______	______
z.	Difficulty swallowing	______	______
aa.	Excessive drooling	______	______
bb.	Poor sucking or feeding as an infant	______	______
cc.	Lost once-attained skills (speech, language, or motor)	______	______
dd.	Seemed to be in a world of his own	______	______
ee.	Had difficulty with taking turns	______	______
ff.	Became upset if lined-up toys were disturbed	______	______
2.	Has your child ever been diagnosed as		
a.	Hyperactive (hyperkinetic)	______	______
b.	Brain-damaged	______	______

		Yes	No
c.	Retarded	______	______
d.	Developmentally delayed or disabled	______	______
e.	Having epileptic seizures (including febrile)	______	______
f.	Motor-delayed	______	______
g.	Cerebral-palsied	______	______
h.	Language-delayed	______	______
i.	Immature	______	______
j.	Hearing-impaired or deaf	______	______
k.	Blind or partially sighted	______	______
l.	Emotionally disturbed	______	______
m.	Hypotonic	______	______
n.	Spastic	______	______
o.	Attention deficit-disordered	______	______
p.	Learning-disabled	______	______
q.	Autistic or demonstrating autistic-like behavior	______	______
3.	Has your child ever		
a.	Had a special diet	______	______
b.	Received speech therapy	______	______
c.	Attended a preschool special education program	______	______
d.	Received counseling (family or individual)	______	______
e.	Received special education services, grades K through 12	______	______
f.	Been hospitalized	______	______
g.	Been suspended or discharged from day care, kindergarten or school	______	______

C. Treatment information

		Yes	No
1.	Has your child ever been evaluated by a		
a.	(1) Neurologist (child or general)	______	______
	(2) Pediatrician	______	______
	(3) Family doctor	______	______
	(4) Psychiatrist	______	______
	(5) Physiatrist (physical medicine or rehabilitation specialist)	______	______
b.	School psychologist	______	______
c.	Teacher	______	______
d.	Special education placement committee	______	______
e.	Child development specialist	______	______
f.	Physical or occupational therapist	______	______
g.	Speech/language pathologist	______	______
2.	Has your child ever taken		
a.	Phenobarbital	______	______
b.	Dilantin (phenytoin)	______	______
c.	Mysoline (primidone)	______	______
d.	Depakene, Depakote (valproic acid)	______	______
e.	Tegretol (carbamazepine)	______	______
f.	Zarontin (ethosuximide)	______	______
g.	Valium (diazepam)	______	______
h.	Haldol (haloperidol)	______	______
i.	Klonopin or Clonopin (clonazepam)	______	______
j.	Neurontin (gabapentin)	______	______
k.	Felbatol (felbamate)	______	______
l.	Lamictal (lamotrigine)	______	______
m.	Trileptal (oxcarbazepine)	______	______
n.	Zonegran (zonisamide)	______	______

		Yes	No
o.	Keppra (levetiracetam)	________	________
p.	Topamax (topiramate)	________	________
q.	Gabitril (tiagabine)	________	________
r.	Carbatrol (carbamazepine)	________	________
s.	Ativan (lorazepam)	________	________
t.	Mellaril (thioridazine)	________	________
u.	Dexedrine (dextroamphetamine) or Adderall (mixed amphetamine salts)	________	________
v.	Ritalin (methylphenidate)	________	________
w.	Cylert (pemoline)	________	________
x.	Asthma medication(s)	________	________
y.	Antihistamine(s)	________	________
z.	Decongestants	________	________
aa.	Prozac	________	________
bb.	Zoloft	________	________
cc.	Paxil	________	________
dd.	Lexapro	________	________
ee.	Celexa	________	________
ff.	Wellbutrin	________	________
gg.	Effexor	________	________
hh.	Abilify	________	________
ii.	Geodon	________	________
jj.	Risperdal	________	________
kk.	Seroquel	________	________
ll.	Herbs and complementary medicine	________	________
mm.	Zyprexa	________	________

3. Has your child ever had any unusual reaction to any of the medications listed above? Please list and describe reaction

____

____

____

4. Describe each of your child's emergency room visits or hospitalizations. Begin with the most recent

Age	(Years/Months)	Reason
________	________ / ________	________________________
________	________ / ________	________________________
________	________ / ________	________________________
________	________ / ________	________________________

D. Pregnancy, birth, and development information/history

1. How many pregnancies did the child's mother have?
2. Did you (she) have any

		Yes	No
a.	Miscarriages	________	________
b.	Abortions	________	________
c.	Tubal pregnancies	________	________
d.	Stillbirths	________	________

3. Were any medicines prescribed during your (her) pregnancy with this child, such as

		Yes	No
a.	Pills for nausea	________	________
b.	Antibiotics	________	________
c.	Water pills	________	________
d.	Pain pills	________	________
e.	Thyroid medicine	________	________
f.	Medicine to prevent miscarriage	________	________
g.	Medicine to suppress appetite	________	________

		Yes	No
h.	Sedatives	______	______
i.	Tranquilizers	______	______
j.	Sleeping pills	______	______
k.	Blood pressure pills	______	______
l.	Other (name if known ____________)	______	______

4. Were any of the following used during this child's pregnancy?

		Yes	No
a.	Cigarettes	______	______
b.	Alcohol (beer, wine, or hard liquor)	______	______
c.	Coffee	______	______
d.	Medicine that you bought at the drug store	______	______

5. Did you (she) have any of the following complications during this pregnancy?

		Yes	No
a.	Significant abdominal injury	______	______
b.	Any illness with fever and rashes	______	______
c.	Diabetes	______	______
d.	Operation	______	______
e.	Emotional upset	______	______
f.	Morning sickness	______	______
	(1) Requiring special attention	______	______
	(2) Requiring hospitalization	______	______
g.	Rh incompatibility	______	______
h.	Bleeding from the vagina	______	______
i.	Staining	______	______
j.	Anemia	______	______
k.	Swollen ankles	______	______
l.	Heart disease	______	______
m.	Toxemia, eclampsia, preeclampsia	______	______
n.	High blood pressure	______	______
o.	Kidney disease	______	______
p.	German measles	______	______

6. How much weight was gained during pregnancy? ______ lbs
7. How long was the total period of labor? ______ h
8. How long was the period of hard labor? ______ h
9. How long was it from the time your (her) water broke until the baby was delivered? ______ h
10. During this pregnancy

		Yes	No
a.	Were you (she) confined to bed for more than 1 day?	______	______
b.	Was an ultrasound performed?	______	______
c.	Were there any abnormalities in the ultrasound?	______	______
d.	Were the baby's movements before birth	______	______
	(1) Normal	______	______
	(2) Increased	______	______
	(3) Decreased	______	______
e.	Was amniocentesis performed?	______	______
f.	If so, were there any abnormalities in the amniocentesis?		
g.	Was the placenta examined? If so, was it normal?	______	______

		Yes	No
11.	Was the baby considered premature?	______	______
12.	Was the baby overdue by more than 2 weeks?	______	______
13.	Was there internal manipulation of the baby?	______	______
14.	Was a caesarean birth performed?	______	______
	a. If performed, was it an emergency?	______	______
	b. Was a general anesthetic used?	______	______
15.	Was the baby head first?	______	______

		Yes	No
16.	Were forceps used?	________	________
17.	Did the baby have any bruises?	________	________
18.	Did the baby have any birthmarks?	________	________
19.	Did the baby have breathing problems?	________	________
20.	Was the cord wrapped around the baby's neck?	________	________
21.	If so, was the cord wrapped more than once around the baby's neck or was there a true knot in the cord?	________	________
22.	Did the baby cry quickly?	________	________
23.	Was the baby's color normal?	________	________
24.	Was the baby blue?	________	________
25.	Was the baby yellow (jaundiced)?	________	________
26.	Did the baby require transfusions?	________	________
27.	Did the baby require phototherapy (lights)?	________	________
28.	Was the baby placed in an isolette, incubator, or intensive special care unit?	________	________
29.	Did the baby have seizures or convulsions?	________	________
30.	Did the baby require oxygen?	________	________
31.	Was the baby placed on a respirator (breathing machine)?	________	________
32.	Were there concerns about the baby's heart rate?	________	________
33.	Was the fluid stained with the baby's meconium (bowel movement)?	________	________
34.	Were there other complications? List if known ______________________________	________	________
35.	Did the baby have physical features that were unusual or very much unlike baby's relatives?	________	________
36.	Do you remember the baby's Apgar score?	________	________
	a. Apgar score of 1 minute	________	________
	b. Apgar score of 3 minutes	________	________
	c. Apgar score of 5 minutes	________	________
37.	How long after birth did the parents take the baby home? ________days		
38.	During the first 2 weeks after the birth of the baby		
	a. Was the baby considered to be limp?	________	________
	b. Was the baby considered to be stiff?	________	________
	c. Did the baby have feeding or sucking problems?	________	________
39.	During the first year of life, did the baby		
	a. Have difficulty sleeping?	________	________
	b. Fail to grow or gain weight?	________	________
	c. Show any unusual trembling or unusual movements of arms, legs, or head?	________	________

Questions 40 to 50 should be considered in the evaluation of the complaint of developmental abnormalities. Section E could be added to further assess children somewhat older, such as school-age children.

40. How old was the baby (your best guess) when he or she first

	< 6 mo	6–12 mo	12–18 mo	18–24 mo	24–36 mo	36–48 mo	48+ mo
a. Sat alone	______	______	______	______	______	______	______
b. Crawled	______	______	______	______	______	______	______
c. Stood alone	______	______	______	______	______	______	______
d. Walked with assistance	______	______	______	______	______	______	______
e. Walked without assistance	______	______	______	______	______	______	______
f. Showed hand preference	______	______	______	______	______	______	______
g. Was toilet trained–bowel	______	______	______	______	______	______	______
h. Was toilet trained–urine	______	______	______	______	______	______	______
i. Began to vocalize (babble)	______	______	______	______	______	______	______
j. Began to use words	______	______	______	______	______	______	______
k. Began to talk in sentences	______	______	______	______	______	______	______

	Left	Right	Both
41. Which hand does your child prefer?	________	________	________

	Yes	No
42. Does your child		
a. Cry excessively?	______	______
b. Rarely or never attempt to communicate?	______	______
c. Use mainly gestures to communicate?	______	______
d. Have a hearing problem?	______	______
e. Turn head to distinguish from where a sound is coming?	______	______
43. General language skills		
a. Does your child		
(1) Have difficulty learning new vocabulary words?	______	______
(2) Omit words from sentences (i.e., do his sentences sound telegraphic)?	______	______
(3) Speak in short, incomplete sentences?	______	______
(4) Have trouble with verbs, such as is, am, was, and were?	______	______
(5) Have difficulty following directions?	______	______
(6) Have difficulty understanding long sentences?	______	______
(7) Have difficulty responding appropriately to questions?	______	______
(8) Have problems asking questions beginning with who, what, where, and why?	______	______
(9) Have trouble using present and past tense verbs correctly?	______	______
(10) Show little or no progress in speech and language in the last 6 to 12 months?	______	______
(11) Omit sounds from words?	______	______
(12) Do you feel your child's speech is more difficult to understand than it should be in view of his or her age?	______	______
(13) Does it seem that your child uses t, d, k or g in place of most other consonants when speaking?	______	______
44. Receptive language skills		
a. Does your child		
(1) Understand "where is mother?"	______	______
(2) Point to one body part on request?	______	______
(3) Follow two-step commands two times out of three?	______	______
(4) Know six body parts?	______	______
(5) Understand the concept of "one"?	______	______
(6) Point to spoon and ball and show how a cup is used?	______	______
(7) Recognize day and night?	______	______
(8) Know three out of four prepositions (on, under, in front, behind, etc.)?	______	______
(9) Understand the concept of "three"?	______	______
(10) Identify right and left on self?	______	______
45. Expressive language skills		
a. Does your child		
(1) Know two to four single words?	______	______
(2) Use two-word sentences?	______	______
(3) Refer to self by own name?	______	______
(4) Use plurals?	______	______
(5) Converse in sentences?	______	______
(6) Give full name?	______	______
(7) Comprehend "tired," "cold," and "hungry"?	______	______
(8) Name opposite analogies two times out of three (up/down, mother/father, in/out)?	______	
(9) Comprehend senses (taste, feel, smell, see, hear)?	______	______
(10) Define words correctly six out of nine times (ball, desk, house, banana, curtain, ceiling, bush, sidewalk)?	______	______
46. Other language skills		
a. Does your child		
(1) Have difficulty finding the correct words in conversation?	______	______

	Yes	No
(2) Have difficulty in getting the correct word out to use in conversation?	________	________
(3) Put words in the wrong order?	________	________
(4) Confuse words that have similar sounds?	________	________
(5) Have difficulty pronouncing words or sounds?	________	________
(6) Hesitate or stop before he or she completes sentences?	________	________
(7) Stutter or stammer?	________	________
(8) Respond inconsistently to sound and speech?	________	________
(9) Understand what is said to him or her?	________	________
(10) Label objects (house, tree, car, ball)?	________	________
(11) Label actions (walk, run, sleep, ride, jump, read, write)?	________	________
(12) Understand stories read to him or her?	________	________
(13) Tell about events happening during the day?	________	________
(14) Comment on what he or she is doing?	________	________
(15) Relay a short message?	________	________
47. Is your child		
a. Understood by parents and family?	________	________
b. Understood by other adults?	________	________
c. Understood by other children?	________	________
d. Teased by children about his or her voice?	________	________
e. Teased by children about his or her speech?	________	________
48. Social skill development and idiosyncratic behaviors:		
a. Does your child		
(1) Exhibit affection spontaneously?	________	________
(2) Like to be held or played with as much as other children?	________	________
(3) Share or take turns with other children readily?	________	________
(4) Tend to be bossy or attempt to dominate other children?	________	________
(5) When compared with other children, show decreased eye contact?	________	________
(6) When with a group of children his or her age, stand outside or apart frequently?	________	________
(7) Appear to be in a world of his or her own?	________	________
(8) Walk on his or her tiptoes?	________	________
(9) Flap his hands or arms when excited or stressed?	________	________
(10) Exhibit other repetitive movements when excited or stressed?	________	________
50. Basic educational skills:		
a. Can your child		
(1) Count from 1 to 10?	________	________
Count from 10 to 20?	________	________
(2) Count 1 to 10 objects?	________	________
Count 10 to 20 objects?	________	________
(3) Identify the numbers 1 to 10?	________	________
Identify the numbers 10 to 20?	________	________
(4) Recognize his or her name in print?	________	________
(5) Name letters in his or her name?	________	________
(6) Identify other lctters in the alphabet?	________	________
(7) Print his or her first name correctly?	________	________
(8) Point to basic colors (red, green, blue, yellow, black, white)?	________	________
(9) Understand the concept of money?	________	________
(10) Identify coins (penny, nickel, dime, quarter)?	________	________
(11) Print the numbers 1 to 10?	________	________
(12) Print all the letters of the alphabet?	________	________
(13) Include at least six body parts (head, arms, body, legs, eyes, ears, nose, fingers, hair) when drawing a person?	________	________
(14) Understand the concept of "same or different"?	________	________
(15) Repeat a short sentence?	________	________

	Yes	No
(16) Recognize similar letters?	______	______
Recognize similar words?	______	______
Recognize similar numbers?	______	______
b. Does your child have problems in		
(1) Reading		
Word identification?	______	______
Comprehension?	______	______
Phonics?	______	______
(2) Spelling		
Oral?	______	______
Written?	______	______
(3) Writing		
Legibility?	______	______
Slow speed?	______	______
Sentence construction?	______	______
Basic grammar?	______	______
(4) Math		
Memory of basic facts (addition, subtraction, multiplication, division)?	______	______
Operations (addition, subtraction, multiplication, division)?	______	______
Word problems?	______	______
(5) Organization		
Completing classroom assignments?	______	______
Completing and turning in homework?	______	______
Planning study time or morning routine?	______	______
(6) Reasoning and problem solving (personal or in school)?	______	______
(7) Science, social studies, humanities, foreign languages?	______	______

E. Attention/activity/behavior/habits

	Yes	No
1. Does your child		
a. Sit still for a fascinating activity, such as television or being read to		
(1) For under 5 minutes?	______	______
(2) For 5 to 10 minutes?	______	______
(3) For 10 to 15 minutes?	______	______
(4) For more than 15 minutes	______	______
b. Sit and listen to a story when being read to individually?	______	______
c. Sit and listen to a story as part of a group?	______	______
d. Seem attentive?	______	______
e. Seem to daydream?	______	______
f. Seem to be easily distracted?	______	______
g. Go quickly from one task to another?	______	______
h. Perform better in a calm, nondistracting setting?	______	______
i. Hear, but not appear to listen?	______	______
j. Appear overly frightened or anxious about new experiences?	______	______
k. Avoid written work, such as printing or coloring?	______	______
l. Produce sloppy work, even though he or she tries hard?	______	______
m. Desire friends, but frequently makes them angry?	______	______
n. Insist on being in charge or he or she will not play?	______	______
o. Have verbal fights with children?	______	______
p. Have physical fights with children?	______	______
q. Have a violent temper?	______	______
r. Have temper tantrums?	______	______
s. Steal?	______	______

		Yes	No
t.	Swear or use vulgar language?	______	______
u.	Act verbally abusive to parents?	______	______
v.	Act verbally abusive to other adults?	______	______
w.	Act physically abusive to parents?	______	______
x.	Act physically abusive to other adults?	______	______
y.	Cheat in order to be the winner?	______	______
z.	Lose his or her temper quickly?	______	______
aa.	Allow his or her feelings to be hurt easily?	______	______
bb.	Engage in		
	(1) Head banging?	______	______
	(2) Bed rocking?	______	______
	(3) Hand flapping?	______	______
	(4) Walking on tiptoes?	______	______
cc.	Frequently place his or her hands over ears to block out sound?	______	______
dd.	Show a lack of interest in people?	______	______
ee.	Speak in a mechanical, machine-like voice?	______	______
ff.	Speak in a whisper?	______	______
gg.	Seem preoccupied with strange creatures or monsters?	______	______
hh.	Avoid affection?	______	______
ii.	Avoid eye contact or looking at people?	______	______
jj.	Frequently appear to be in his or her own world?	______	______
kk.	When observed with a group of children, seem to be apart or alone frequently?	______	______
ll.	Seem impulsive?	______	______
mm.	Seem explosive?	______	______
nn.	Change moods quickly?	______	______
oo.	Have difficulty in appreciating danger?	______	______
pp.	Seem easily frustrated?	______	______
qq.	Have trouble waiting his or her turn?	______	______
rr.	Seem extremely talkative?	______	______
ss.	Show shame or remorse?	______	______

2. What type of school does your child attend? Public ______ Private ______
3. At what age did your child begin preschool or day care? ______
4. At what age did your child begin kindergarten? ______
5. What grade does your child attend now? ______

		Yes	No
6.	If in a regular grade (class), does your child receive special help?	______	______
7.	Has your child ever been absent from school for 2 weeks or longer at one time?	______	______
8.	Has your child had frequent short absences from school, resulting in absences of more than 30 days in the school year?	______	______
9.	Has your child ever been suspended from school?	______	______
10.	Has your child ever been retained by either your decision or the school's?	______	______
11.	Was your child ever elected to an honor society?	______	______

F. Skills or abilities

1. Sports

a.	Baseball or softball	______	______
b.	Tennis	______	______
c.	Swimming	______	______
d.	Football	______	______
e.	Soccer	______	______
f.	Basketball	______	______

	Yes	No
g. Computer or video games	________	________
h. Other	________	________
2. Music		
a. Singing	________	________
b. Dancing (including ballet)	________	________
c. Instruments	________	________
Specify ________ ________ ________ ________		
3. Art		
a. Drawing	________	________
b. Copying	________	________
c. Other	________	________
4. Academic		
a. Reading	________	________
b. Creative writing	________	________
c. Math	________	________
d. Computer literate	________	________
e. Typing (keyboarding)	________	________
5. Is your child a member of a		
a. Club	________	________
b. Other student organization	________	________
Specify ________ ________ ________ ________		
6. Has your child ever been elected to an office?	________	________

7. In what skill or ability area(s) does your child seem to excel over most children his or her age?

____

____

G. Signs and symptoms

	Yes	No
1. Seizures:		
a. Has your child had convulsions?	________	________
b. Does your child have staring spells or spells where you cannot get their attention just by calling their name?	________	________
c. Do the convulsions occur only when the child is ill? Or febrile?	________	________
d. Does your child have convulsions (seizures) without fever?	________	________
e. Has your doctor ever used the term epilepsy to refer to your child?	________	________
f. How often do the seizures occur?	________	________
g. Can you tell before the event that it is imminent?	________	________
h. Is the child aware at all before the seizure, during the seizure or immediately after the seizure?	________	________
i. How long is it before the child returns to normal after the seizure/convulsion?	________	________
j. Have the spells changed since they started or are they all the same?	________	________
k. Has the child had an electroencephalogram (EEG) to evaluate the spells?	________	________
l. Has the child had an imaging study of the brain to evaluate the seizures? (MRI, CT)	________	________
m. Has your child taken any medications to prevent seizures?	________	________
n. Do you have medications you are to administer when a seizure occurs?	________	________
o. Has your child had side effects from the medications?	________	________
p. Which medications have been used? Please list them and doses if possible.	________	________
q. Have you had blood levels of the antiepileptic medications (AEDs) measured?	________	________
r. Have you discussed therapies other than AEDs with your doctor?	________	________

	Yes	No
s. Have you considered dietary therapies for the prevention of seizures?	______	______
t. Have you considered surgical therapy for the prevention of seizures?	______	______
2. Headaches		
a. Does your child have or complain of head pain?	______	______
b. How often does this occur?	______	______
c. Are there more than one kind of headache episode?	______	______
d. Do you recognize any stress or environmental factor that will precipitate headache in your child?	______	______
e. Where is the pain located?	______	______
f. Is the pain on one or both sides of the head?	______	______
g. Is the pain in the front or back of the head or both?	______	______
h. Is the child able to describe the pain?	______	______
i. What does the child do when they have a headache?		
(1) Continue playing	______	______
(2) Stop playing and watch TV or listen to music	______	______
(3) Lay in a quiet room	______	______
(4) Try to sleep	______	______
(5) Get nauseated and sometimes vomit	______	______
(6) Cry and bang or hold head	______	______
j. Is there a change in behavior before the onset of the headache? (an aura)	______	______
(1) How long before the headache	______________	
(2) What is the nature of the change	______________	
(3) Can you tell a headache is imminent?	______	______
(4) Can the child describe the aura?	______	______
k. How long does it take the child to get back to normal after the headache?	______________	
l. Headaches not relieved by nonprescription pain medicine	______________	
m. Headaches not relieved by prescription pain medicine	______________	
n. Headaches occurring in the middle of the night or upon awakening	______________	

CHAPTER 2

The Neurologic Examination of the Preterm and Full-term Neonate and of the Infant

Patricia H. Ellison and Donna Kathryn Daily

Outline

Does the neurologic examination of infants still contribute to the diagnosis and treatment of neurologic disorders? Can it be used as a measure of improvement from either systemic disease or neurologic injury? Does it have other attributes, such as reassurance to the parents and clinicians, or to identify the need for early intervention services? Has imaging technology changed the need for clinical examination?

The considerable diversity that exists in the numbers and types of items recorded by physicians as part of the neonatal neurologic examination makes it difficult to answer these questions. Generally, a report is modest, with notes often consisting of brief phrases such as "alert, moves all extremities." The most detailed examinations are often those of the physical or occupational therapist or those of a developmental pediatrician or pediatric neurologist, if consulted. The neurologic abnormality may be first noted after a clinical event, such as a seizure, an abnormal imaging study indicating cerebral hemorrhage, or after the observation of significant lack of response following birth or failure to suck well.

Single-item abnormalities, such as a facial palsy or brachial plexus injury, appear to be noted fairly soon, if not in the delivery room, then in the initial newborn examination. Other neurologic abnormalities, such as decreased alertness or even fairly diffuse hypotonia, may not be identified in the current brief newborn hospitalization, thus placing an increased obligation on physicians providing primary care or specialty services.

Who should do the neurologic examination?

It is obvious in reading charts that neurologic examinations are being done by clinicians and therapists with varying levels and types of training. The documentation of the neurologic examination as performed by other healthcare professionals, such as nurses or rehabilitation therapists, can complement that of the treating physician.

What should be part of the neurologic examination?

The traditional newborn and infant neurologic examination can be divided into four main areas: general description, cranial nerves, special situations such as altered mental status and spinal lesions, and data from the Premie-Neuro, NeoNeuro & Up, and Infanib scoring sheets described later. The traditional examination is described in more detail in the Appendix of this chapter. In addition, some other basic information needs to be gathered. Maternal, fetal, and perinatal history may be helpful, as well as the current medical history of the infant. A general physical examination may provide information to support the neurologic examination. Growth patterns are particularly important. Serial head circumferences seem so basic that this measurement would not need to be mentioned in a learned chapter. Yet circumferences have been missing in charts under review from the initial newborn evaluation; serial evaluations have been missing in newborns already identified with brain abnormality and in infants with a chief complaint that could refer to the brain.

The emphasis of this chapter is on scored assessment instruments. Fortunately, a number of clinicians have keenly observed newborns and infants and have created a large pool of items that could be used for neurologic examinations. The French angles are an excellent example, forming a part of the measure of gestational age by assessment when both physical and neurologic items are combined (Amiel-Tison 1976). The progressions are described from extreme immaturity to full term. Reversed progressions occur from full term to approximately 9–10 months in infancy. The scarf sign, heel-to-ear, popliteal angle, and leg abduction look similar in the preterm neonate who has a gestational age of 28 weeks and in the 9- to 10-month-old infant. Significant deviations are indicative of hypotonia or hypertonia.

Most of these clinicians have described and recommended a far larger number of items than can be done due to limitations of time for the clinician or tolerance of the sick newborn. Our first consideration has been to find some method of limiting the number of items. Second, the examination needs to be reliable, using scientific definitions for clinical measurement. In short, the examination method should have a mathematical cohesiveness of reliability, should be highly correlated when used from one time of examination to another, and should be highly correlated when used from one examiner to another. To this end, we have developed instruments of measurement for the neurologic examination of three age groups: the Premie-Neuro for gestational ages 23–37 weeks (Daily and Ellison 2005); the NeoNeuro & Up for the gestational ages 38 weeks to age 4 months (Sheridan-Pereira and Ellison 1991); and the Infanib for infants, ages 4–18 months (Ellison and Horn 1985a; Ellison 1994). The details of the methodology have been described previously (Ellison 1990). These three examinations assess aspects at the different ages, each of which has a number of items sufficient to assure validity (Table 2.1).

Scored assessment instruments

The Premie-Neuro scoring sheet

The Premie-Neuro is a neurologic examination of preterm infants between the ages of 23 and 37 weeks of gestational age. It consists of 24 items divided into three factors (Neurological, Movement, Responsiveness), each with eight items. Only the first 16 items are scored if the infant is very immature or on the ventilator because these checks can be done with minimal disturbance of the infant. The items in Factor 1 (Neurological) address reflexive behavior, progression of muscle tone, and movement type. The items in Factor 2 (Movement) document rate per minute of behaviors and limb movement. Last, the items in Factor 3 (Responsiveness) address head and trunk control as well as alertness and responsiveness. The examination should be scheduled .5 to 1 hour before a feeding. Asymmetry of findings should be noted for scoring. The examination consists of techniques commonly used for more mature infants but criteria for describing the very immature infant's responses differ (see photographs in NeoNeuro examination).

1. *Arm Recoil.* With the infant in supine position, take both hands and extend them alongside the trunk, hold 3 seconds and release. Note the amount of flexion at the elbow that is observed within 5 seconds.

   (a) >180° (b) 100–180° (c) 60–100° (d) <60°.

2. *Arm Traction.* With the infant in supine position, grasp the wrist slowly and pull arms to vertical.

Table 2.1 Scored neurologic assessments of the newborn and infant—comparative characteristics

	Premie-Neuro	NeoNeuro & Up	Infanib
Age group to be tested	23–37 weeks gestational age or post menstrual age	38 weeks gestation or post menstrual age to 16 weeks of age	4–18 months of age
Diagnostic category for total score	Abnormal, questionable, normal	Severely abnormal, moderately abnormal, mildly abnormal, normal	Abnormal, transient, normal
Factors (elements which comprise the total score)	Neurologic, movement, responsiveness	Hypertonus, primitive reflexes, limb tone, neck support, reflexes and tremor, alertness, fussiness	Spasticity, vestibular function, head and trunk, French angles, legs
Number of items	16 (<28 weeks/on respirator) 24 (≥28 weeks/off respirator)	32	20
Behavioral measures	2 items	8 items	0 items

Score the amount of elbow flexion and resistance that is noted at the moment the infant is initially lifted off the surface.

(a) >180° (b) 160–180° (c) 120–160° (d) 100–120° (e) <100°.

3. *Palmar Grasp*. With the infant in supine position, insert index finger into hand and gently press palmar surface. Grade according to strength of finger flexion.

   (a) absent (b) weak flexion (c) medium flexion (d) strong flexion spread to forearm (e) very strong–lifts off bed.

4. *Plantar Grasp*. With the infant in supine position, give pressure to the ball of the infant's foot. Grade according to strength of toe flexion.

   (a) absent (b) weak (c) medium (d) strong (e) very strong.

5. *Scarf Sign*. Hold the infant's arm near the elbow and move the arm across the infant's chest until resistance is met. Observe the angle formed by the upper arm and a line parallel to the trunk.

   (a) >85° (b) 60–85° (c) 45–60° (d) 15–45° (e) 0–15°.

6. *Popliteal Angle*. With both hips abducted, approximate knees and thighs to abdomen; extend legs by gentle pressure with index finger behind each ankle at the same time until resistance is met. When scoring this test, measure the angle of extension such that 180° equals a fully extended knee.

   (a) >180° (b) 150–180° (c) 130–150° (d) 110–130° (e) 90–110° (f) <90°.

7. *Heel-to-ear*. With the infant's feet held together, grasp both thighs and flex hips with knees extended until resistance is met. Measure the angle between the infant's trunk and legs.

   (a) <10° (b) 10–40° (c) 40–60° (d) 60–90° (e) 90–100° (f) >100°.

8. *Movement Type*. Observe predominant type of movement: sluggish, uncoordinated, jerky, athetoid, stretching, smooth, alternating, both spontaneous and elicited seen throughout the examination.

   (a) mostly sluggish (b) mostly stretching or smooth (c) smooth alternating (d) markedly asymmetrical (e) mostly tremulous.

9. *Tremors*. Record the number of episodes of tremors (trembling, shaking) observed in any part of the body, including face, and extremities.
10. *Thrashing*. Record episodes of overshooting, flailing movements, which could involve head and trunk, whole body, or single extremity.
11. *Facial Grimace*. Record number of facial movements (frowns, grimaces, quizzical) seen during the examination.
12. *Startle*. Observe the infant for a sudden flexor response of the arms in response to a loud noise, bright light, or if one is elicited spontaneously.
13. *Yawn*. Record the number of yawns observed during the examination.
14. *Color Change*. Observe the infant for any noticeable color change that is observed during the examination, including mottling, duskiness, pallor, or increased redness anywhere on the body.
15. *Arm Movements*. Record the number of spontaneous arm movements observed during the examination.
16. *Leg Movements*. Record the number of spontaneous leg movements observed during the examination.
17. *Arm Flexion*. With the infant in the supine position, grasp both wrists and by applying gently traction, elevate the shoulders about 45°. Note the flexion response at the elbows. (Done simultaneously with No. 18).

    (a) >170° (b) 140–170° (c) 110–140° (d) 70–110° (e) <70°.

18. *Head Lag*. Grasp both wrists and by applying gentle traction, elevate the shoulders about 45°. Observe the amount of head lag.
19. *Held Sit*. Hold the infant in an upright position with examiner's hands used to support the infant's shoulders. Observe the length of time the head is held in an upright position.

    (a) head stays forward or backward (b) head up <3 seconds (c) head up 3–10 seconds (d) head up >10 seconds.

20. *Posterior Neck*. Place the infant in supported sitting. Allow head to fall forward as you hold the shoulders, wait 15 seconds. Grade according to ability to lift head and maintain it upright.

    (a) no attempt to raise head (b) tries but cannot raise head (c) head upright by 30 seconds, drops head (d) head upright by 30 seconds, maintained (e) examiner cannot extend head.

21. *Anterior Neck*. Place the infant in supported sitting. Allow head to drop backward as you hold the shoulders, wait 15 seconds. Grade according to ability to lift head and maintain it upright.

    (a) no attempt to raise head (b) tries but cannot raise head (c) head upright by 30 seconds, drops head (d) head upright by 30 seconds, maintained (e) examiner cannot flex head.

22. *Alert.* Estimate the amount of time the infant is in the quiet, alert state, i.e. alert, with a bright look, minimal motor activity, and regular respirations.

    (a) 0–4 sec. (b) 5–10 sec. (c) 11–30 sec. (d) 31–60 sec. (e) > 60 sec.

23. *Ventral Suspension.* Place one hand under infant's abdomen in prone position and suspend horizontally. Observe curvature of back, flexion of limbs, and relationship of head to trunk.
24. *Responsiveness.* Note the infant's awareness level throughout the examination, a subjective and qualitative assessment of the infant's response to movement, touching, handling, noise, hunger, etc.

    (a) not very responsive (b) average (c) very responsive.

Using the Premie-Neuro scoring sheet

The Premie-Neuro scoring sheet lists the test items and their descriptions on the left side of the examination sheet. Each item should be evaluated and the appropriate description letter circled at that time. On the right-hand side of the page is the scoring for gestational ages 23–37 weeks. When scoring items 1–7, record a score for both the right and left extremities. When an asymmetry is present, score the lower value if there is a one-letter difference. When the asymmetry is greater than or equal to two levels, score the letter indicated in the central column and its corresponding value for the postmenstrual age. Enter the points that correspond to the letter circled in the scoring columns at the far right. For items 9–16, determine rate based on number of observations divided by total time taken to complete the examination. Each column is summed to yield a factor score. Factor scores are then summed to yield a total score. Scoring ranges for three categories (normal, questionable, and abnormal) are indicated for neonates of less than 28 weeks/on a respirator and more than 28 weeks/off a respirator. The scoring sheet and manual are available from the authors.

NeoNeuro & Up scoring sheet

Items 1–4. These four questions are asked of the main caretaker by the examiner. They make a nice introduction to the baby and immediately give the examiner helpful information about apathy/irritability.

1. *Caretaker must awaken infant to feed:*

   (a) rarely (b) sometimes (c) often.

2. *Number of feedings between 6 pm and 6 am:*

   (a) none (b) 1 (c) 2 (d) 3 (e) 4 (f) 5 (g) 6 or more.

3. *Ease of caring for:*

   (a) too easy (b) easy (c) not so easy (d) difficult.

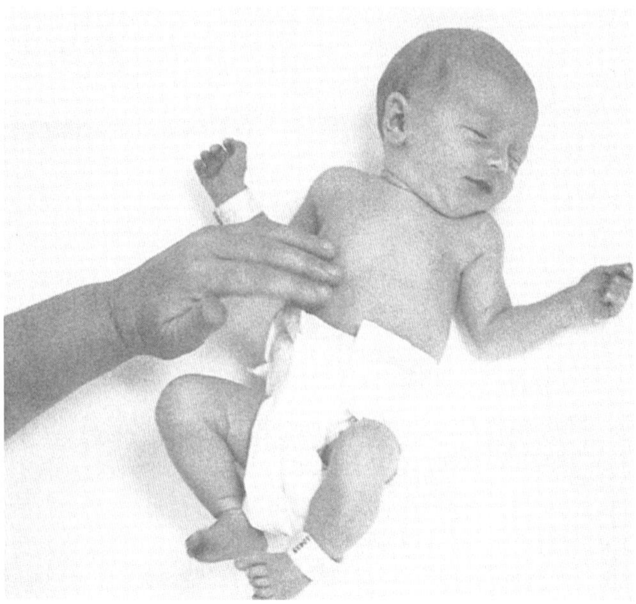

Figure 2.1 Normal posture of full-term infant.

4. *Cries how long before consoled?*

   (a) 1–3 min (b) 4–7 min (c) 8–12 min (d) 13–18 min (e) 19–24 min (f) 25 min or more.

5. *Posture.* Observe the predominant posture at rest. Make separate note of extension, semiflexion, flexion, or strong flexion for arms and for legs. Also note recurrent asymmetry. The normal position for a full-term neonate is one of semiflexion or flexion of both arms and legs (Figure 2.1).
6. *Abnormal Posturing.* Observe throughout the examination for decorticate, decerebrate, or opisthotonic posturing. In Figure 2.2A, there is flexion of the arms and extension of the legs (decorticate). There is also some neck retraction. In Figure 2.2B, there is extension of the arms and extension of the legs (decerebrate). In Figure 2.2C, the neonate assumes an opisthotonic posture. Note also extension of the arms and the clenched hands.
7. *Hands Open/Closed.* Observe whether the hands are clenched, clenched with stress, closed, sometimes closed, open. In Figure 2.3A, the hands of a normal newborn are shown. In Figure 2.3B, the hands are persistently clenched. Note also the opisthotonic posturing.
8. *Palmar Grasp.* Place a finger across the palm from the little finger side of the hand. Observe the degree of flexion of the fingers and arm. The normal degree of flexion for a newborn is shown in Figure 2.4.
9. *Plantar Grasp.* Press a thumb or finger against the balls of the feet and observe the degree of plantar flexion of the toes. The normal degree of flexion for a newborn is shown in Figure 2.5.

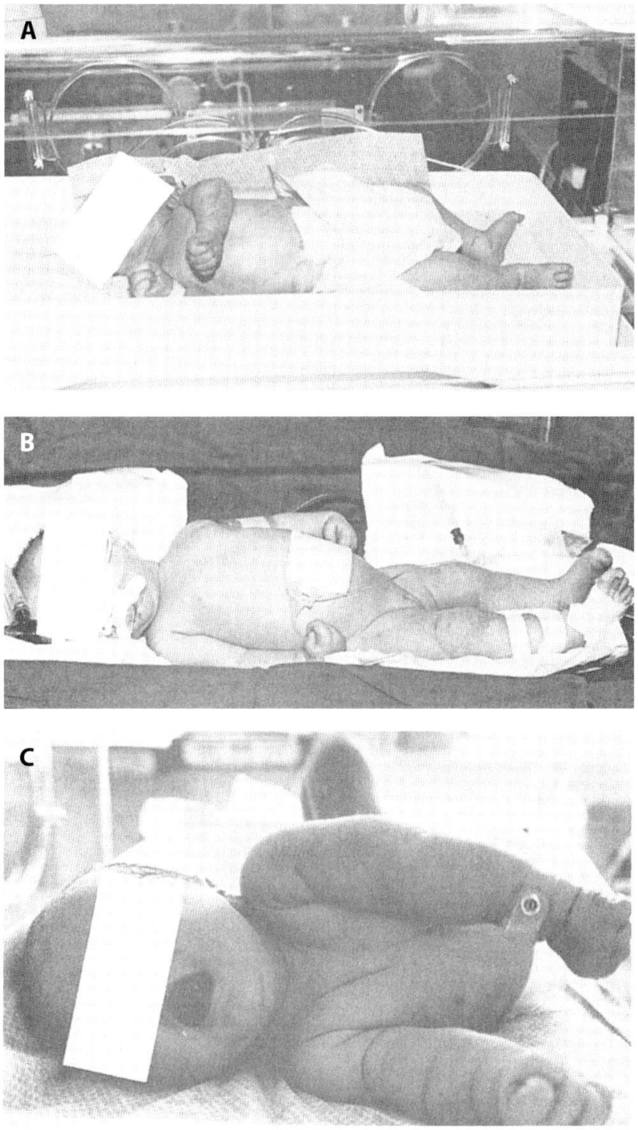

Figure 2.2 (A) Decorticate posturing. (B) Decerebrate posturing. (C) Opisthotonic posturing.

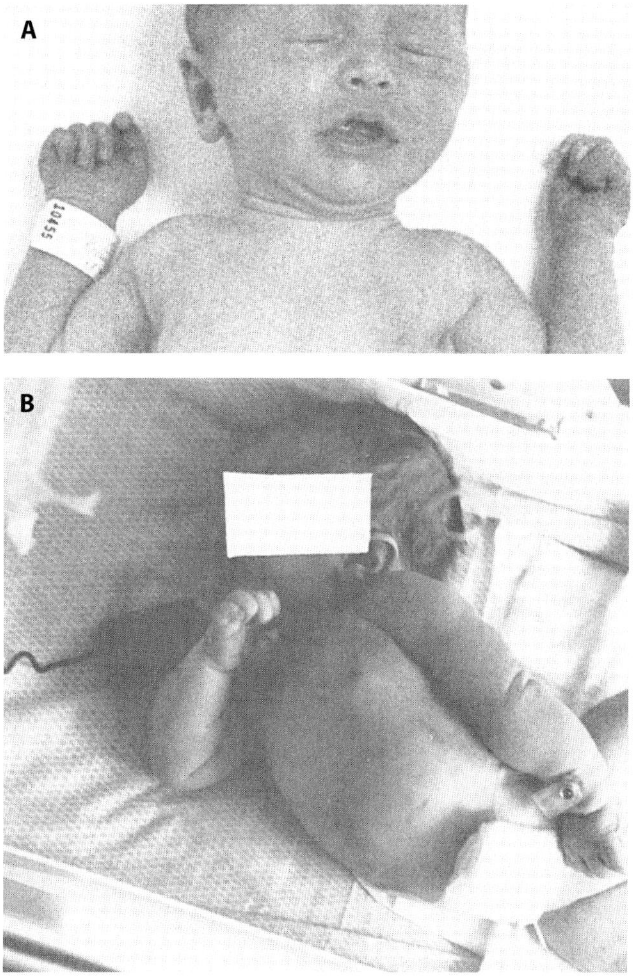

Figure 2.3 (A) Hand position of normal newborn. (B) Hands clenched in abnormal pattern.

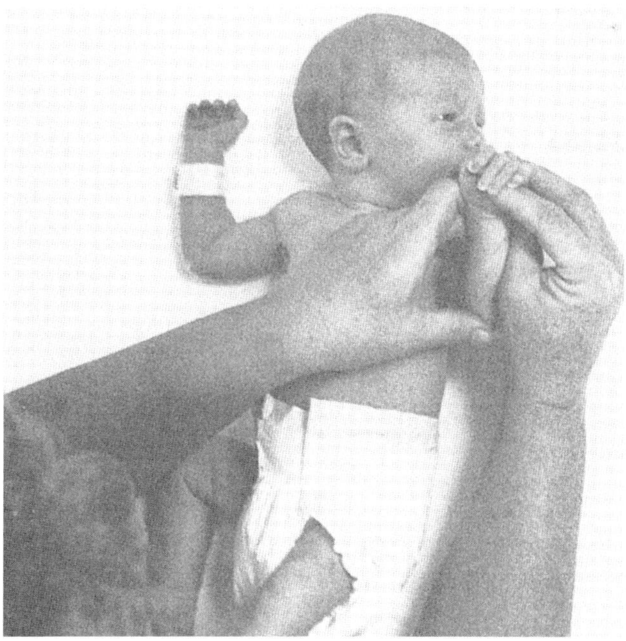

Figure 2.4 Palmar grasp.

10. *Asymmetric Tonic Neck Reflex*. Turn the head slowly to one side, and hold it. Observe for a fencing position: extension of the arm near the face and flexion of the opposite arm. Repeat on the other side. Observe whether this response is absent or present. If present, observe for ability of the infant to overcome the position and for persistence of the position. The position for a normal newborn is shown in Figure 2.6.
11. *Scarf Sign*. Grasp the upper arm near the elbow and move the arm across the chest. Observe the angle formed by the upper arm and a line parallel to the body. In Figure 2.7A, the angle is shown for a normal neonate. In Figure 2.7B, the infant demonstrates the excessive excursion of hypotonia or of prematurity.

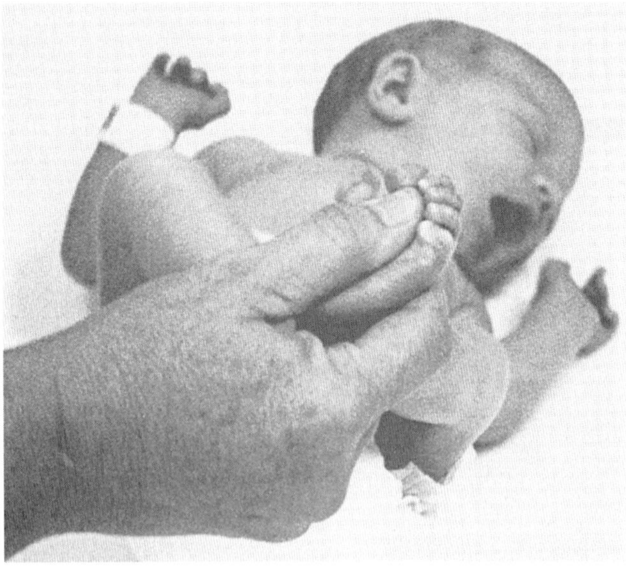

Figure 2.5 Plantar grasp.

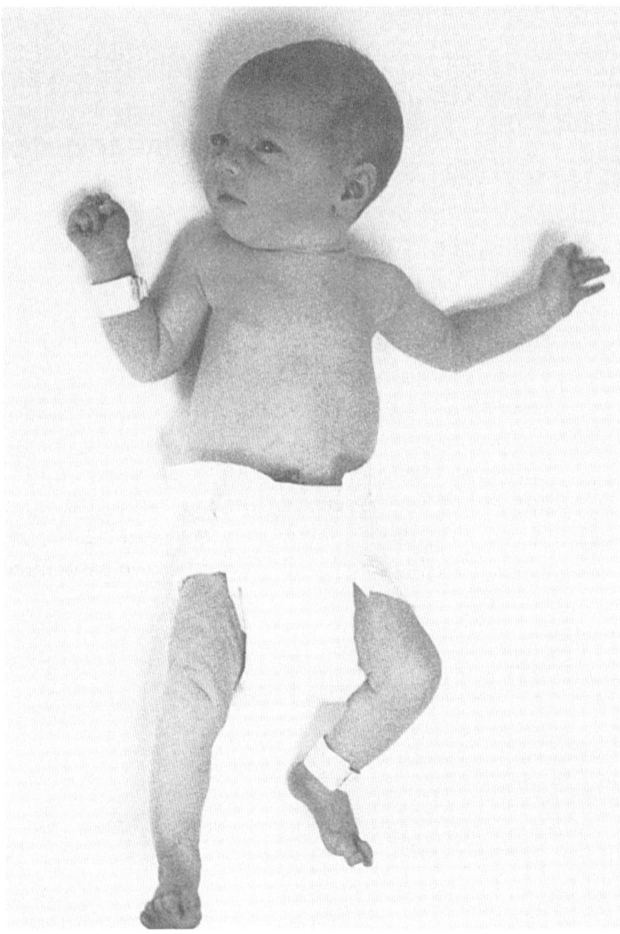

Figure 2.6 Asymmetric tonic neck reflex.

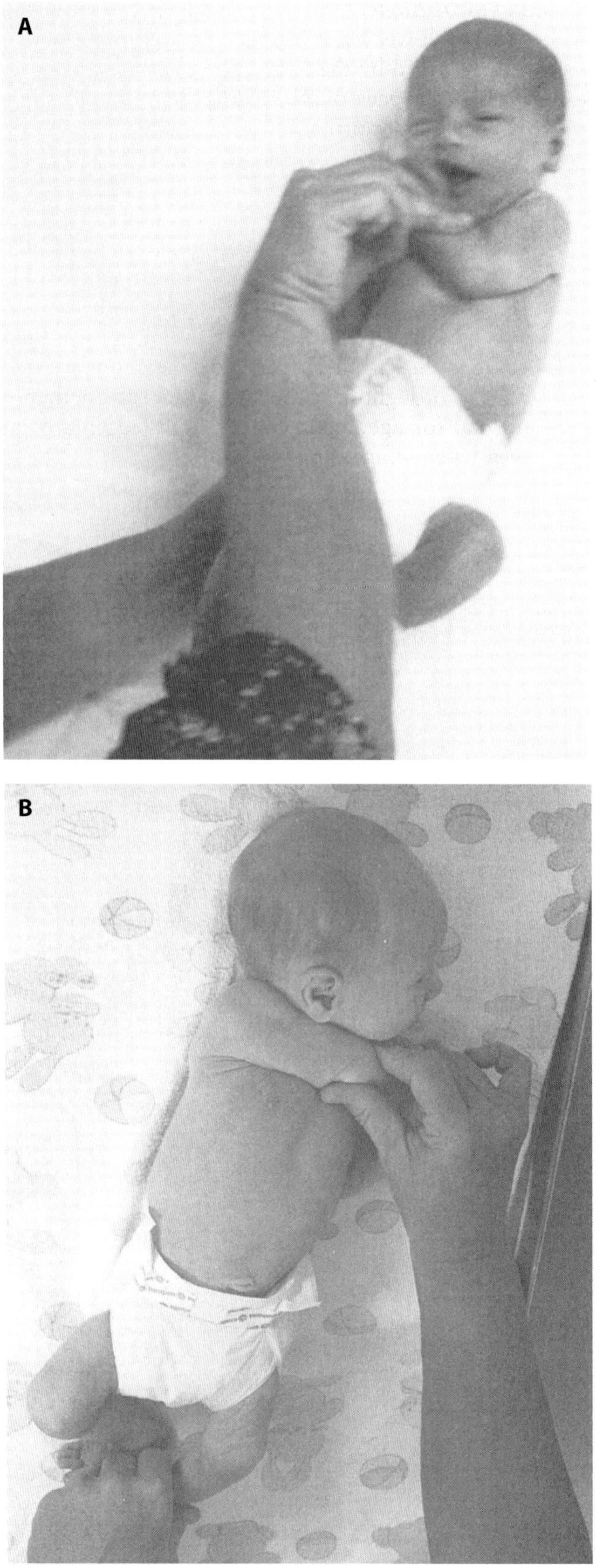

Figure 2.7 (A) Scarf sign of normal full term newborn. (B) Excessive excursion of arm in hypotonia.

12. *Popliteal Angle.* Grasp the legs near the knee. Extend the lower leg by gentle pressure. Observe the angle formed by the neonate's upper leg and lower leg with the back of the knee as the fulcrum. In Figure 2.8A, the normal popliteal angle is shown. In Figure 2.8B, the excessively wide angle of hypotonia or prematurity is demonstrated.
13. *Heel to Ear.* Grasp the legs near the ankles. Draw the feet as close to the head as they will go, keeping the buttocks on the table. Observe the angle between the infant's trunk and legs with the hips as the fulcrum. In Figure 2.9A, the normal newborn angle is shown. In Figure 2.9B, the neonate's toes may be brought near the nose more readily than is normal for age, again indicating hypotonia or as seen when infant is premature.

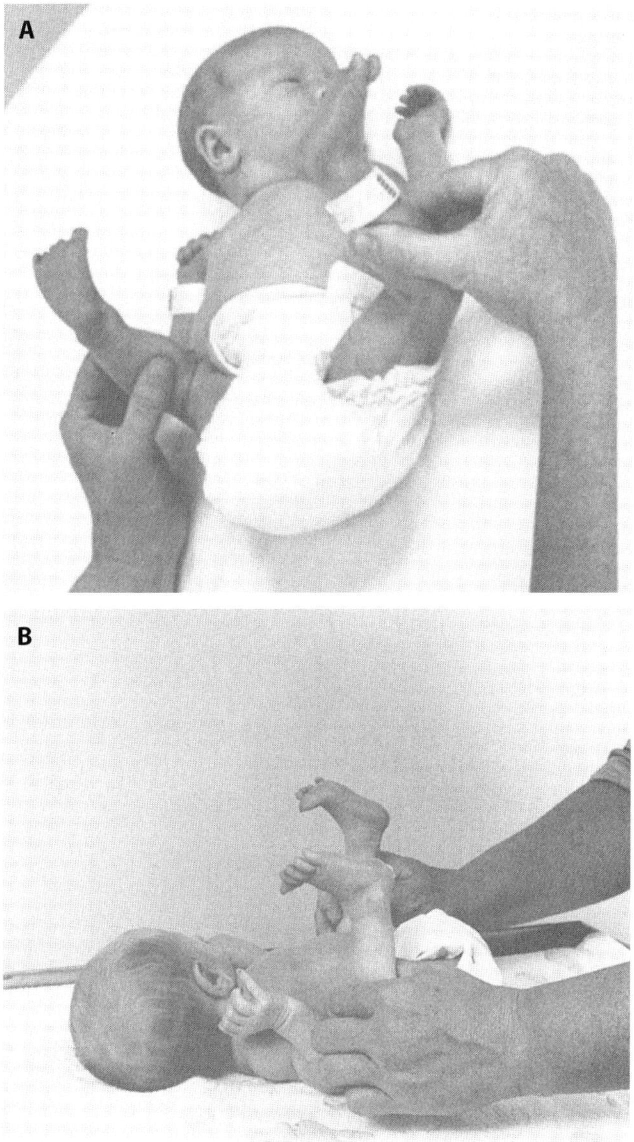

Figure 2.8 (A) Normal popliteal angle. (B) Excessive angle in hypotonia.

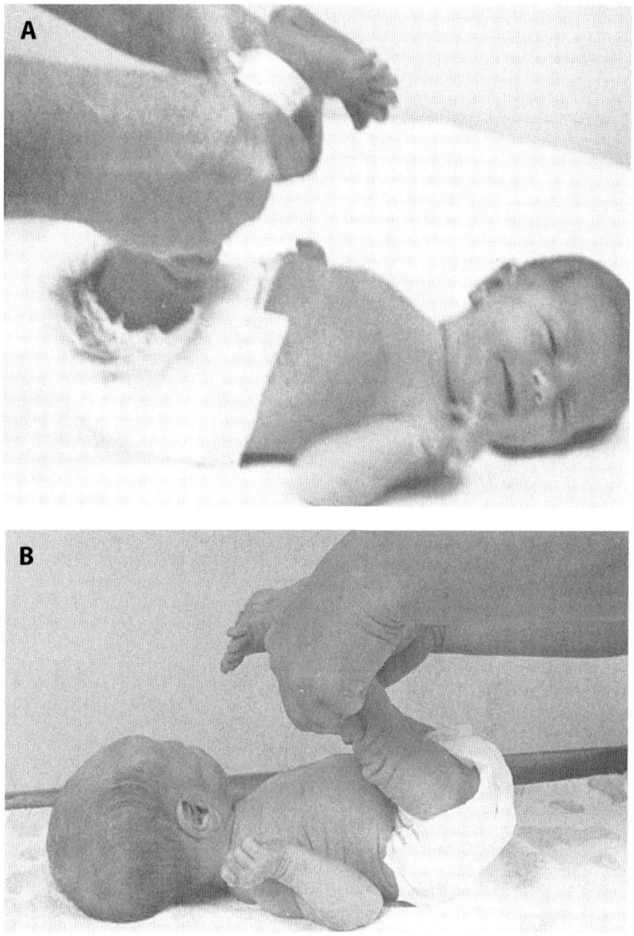

Figure 2.9 (A) Normal heel-to-ear. (B) Excessive heel-to-ear.

14. *Knee Reflex.* Relax the leg by slight flexion at the knee. Tap the patellar area with a finger or with a small reflex hammer.
15. *Ankle Clonus.* Rapidly press the distal side of the foot while maintaining the leg slightly flexed. Observe for a response of quick, jerking movements of the foot.
16. *Pull to Sit.* Use traction on both wrists to pull the infant slowly to the sitting position. Score the head lag and arm flexion separately. In Figure 2.10, the delayed head lag and lack of arm flexion associated with hypotonia are demonstrated.
17. *Pull to Sit.* Use traction on both wrists to pull the infant slowly to the sitting position. Score the head lag and arm flexion separately. In Figure 2.10, the delayed head lag and lack of arm flexion associated with hypotonia are demonstrated.
18. *Held Sit.* Hold the infant in an upright position with the examiner's hands used to support the infant's shoulders. Observe the length of time the head is held in an upright position. See item 19 for support at the shoulders; note that in 19, the head has been allowed to fall forward.

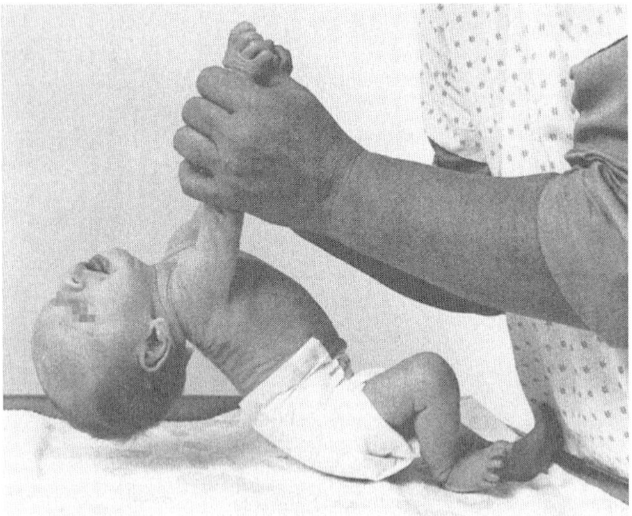

Figure 2.10 Excessive head lag.

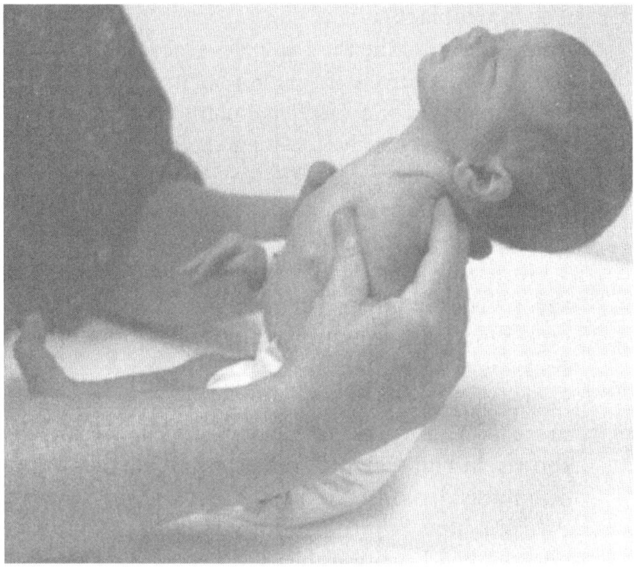

Figure 2.12 Held sit, anterior neck.

19. *Posterior Neck*. Support the infant at the shoulders, as in item 18. Allow the head to fall forward, and wait 30 seconds. Note attempts to raise the head and ability to maintain the head in an upright position. See Figure 2.11.
20. *Anterior Neck*. Support the infant at the shoulders, as in item 19. Allow the head to fall backward, and wait 30 seconds. Note attempts to raise the head and maintain the head in an upright position. See Figure 2.12.
21. *Auditory* (to rattle or to mother's voice). Support the infant's head in midline position, permitting head to rotate. The infant may be placed supine on the table. The mother's voice is a powerful stimulus for young infants. Ask her to call the infant's name from a meter away, to either side. Grade the response.

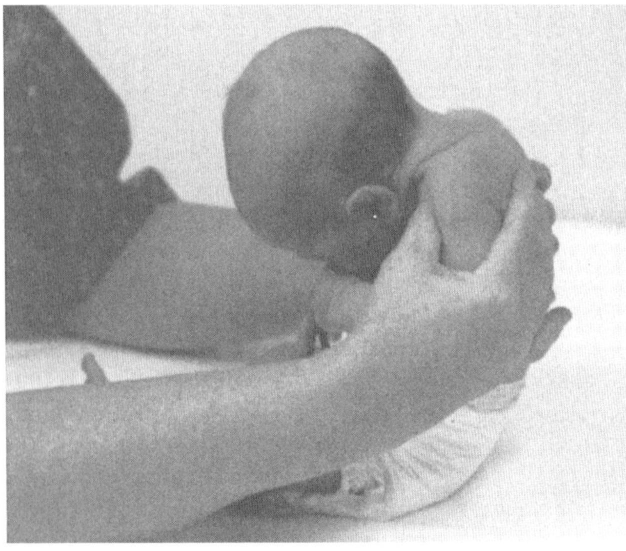

Figure 2.11 Held sit, posterior neck.

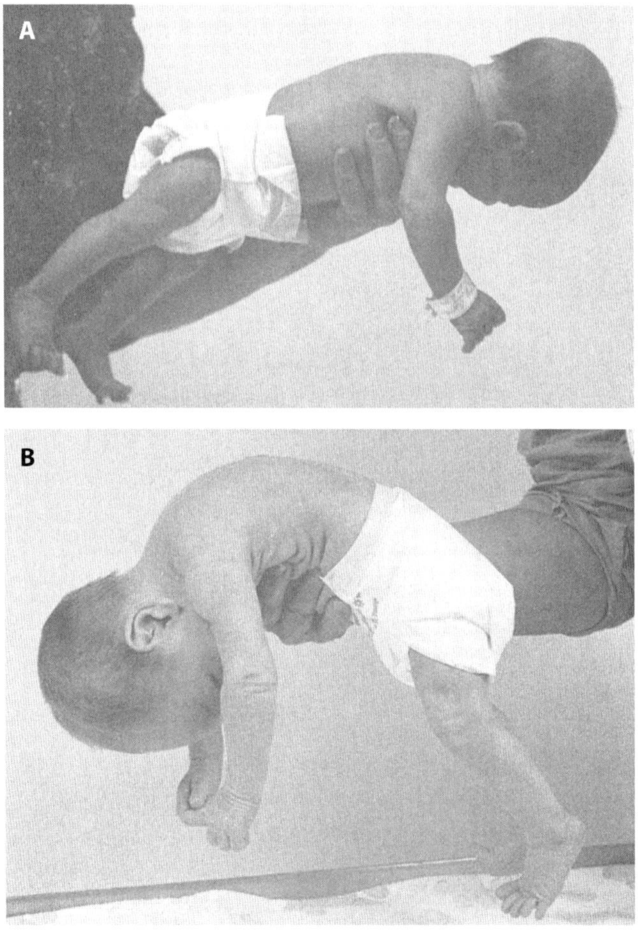

Figure 2.13 (A) Normal neonatal ventral suspension. (B) Hypotonic ventral suspension.

22. *Visual* (to black-and-white bull's eye). Support the infant's head in the midline supine position. Present the bull's-eye in the midline about 12 inches from the face. Move it laterally in either direction, then vertically, and finally in an arc.
23. *Alert*. The examiner talks or makes noises to the infant to obtain his or her attention and counts the seconds before the gaze is averted.
24. *Ventral Suspension*. Place one hand under the infant's abdomen in the prone position and suspend the infant horizontally. Observe the curvature of the back, the position of the head in relation to the trunk, and the flexion of the arms and legs. In Figure 2.13A, normal neonatal ventral suspension is shown. In Figure 2.13B, the drooping quality of hypotonia is demonstrated.
25. *All Fours and Prone*. Place infant in prone position; observe head turning, head and arms positioning. Talk to the infant to encourage the best performance. The normal infant in Figure 2.14A at age 2 months holds her head up 90°; she extends on the left arm and rests on the right arm. In Figure 2.14B, this 2-month-old infant, who is otherwise normal, has difficulty holding up his head. Note: This is seen frequently now because infants are positioned to sleep on their backs or sides. As an isolated finding, it does not indicate neurologic abnormality.

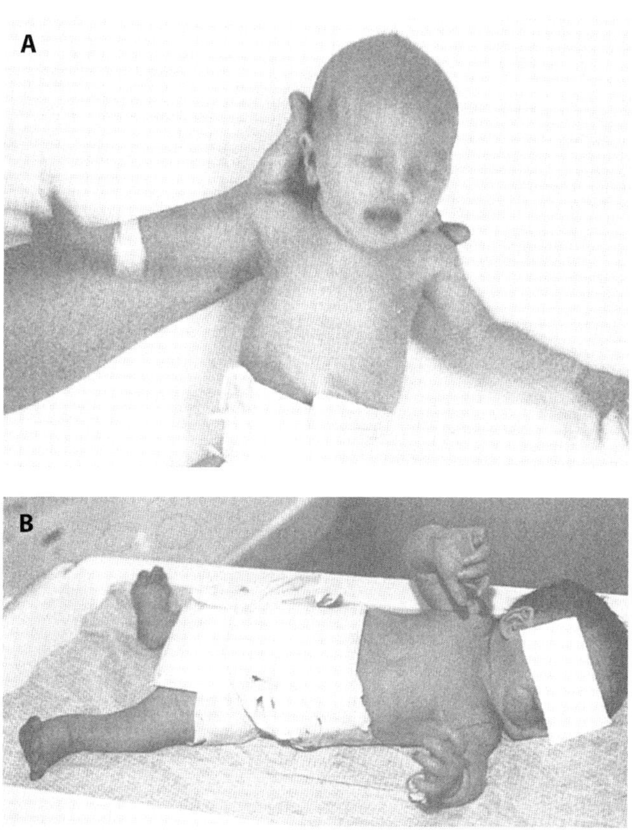

Figure 2.15 (A) Normal Moro response. (B) Exaggerated Moro response.

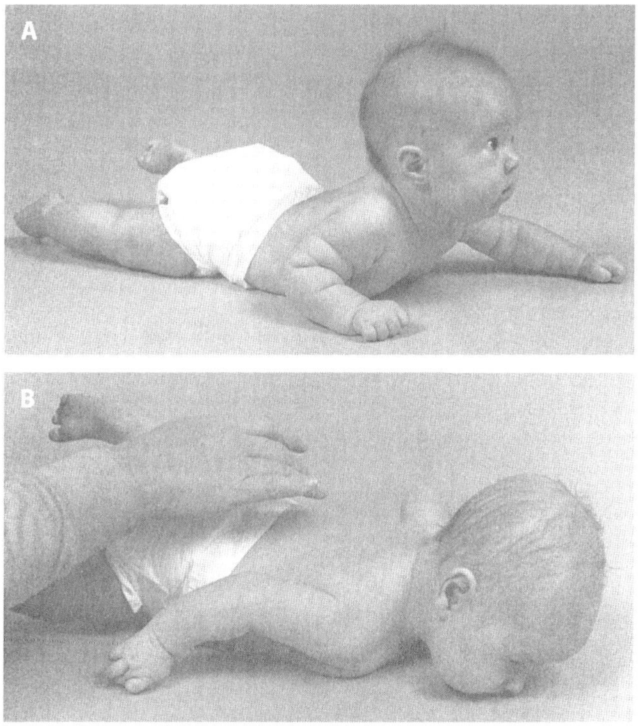

Figure 2.14 (A) Normal prone posture at 2 months. (B) Inability to hold head up at 2 months.

26. *Moro Reflex*. Support the neonate's head with one hand and the back in the midline with the other hand. Suddenly, drop the neonate 4–8 inches and observe the response of the hands and arms. In Figure 2.15A, the neonate demonstrates a normal response. In Figure 2.15B, the neonate has a spontaneous exaggerated Moro reflex.
27. *Suck*. Place index finger in the mouth with finger pad toward the palate. Assess strength and rhythm of suck.
28. *Tremor*. Observe the frequency of tremor throughout the examination. Observe also the state of the neonate at the time of tremor.
29. *Responsiveness*. The examiner talks or makes noises to the infant in an attempt to elicit a response.
30. *Vocalization*. The examiner talks or makes noises to the infant, then pauses, awaiting response from the infant.
31. *Attends to Examiner*. The examiner assesses the amount of stimulation needed to attract the infant's attention.
32. *Attends during Exam*. The examiner notes the attentiveness of the infant to the examiner throughout the examination.

Using the NeoNeuro & Up scoring sheet

The NeoNeuro & Up scoring sheet has two facing pages. The left side of each page is used for the description of items. Items are listed in an order logical from a clinical viewpoint. Each should be evaluated and circled at the time of examination.

To the right of the description for each item lies the scoring for 38 weeks to age 4 months corrected age for prematurity, if applicable. The points for each item are then entered in the scoring columns, far right. Each column is summed to yield a factor score. Factor scores are then summed to yield a total score. Two time periods are given: 0 through 48 hours, 48 hours to 4 months.

Scoring ranges for four categories of normality and abnormality are indicated for each of the two time periods. The categories are normal, mildly abnormal, moderately abnormal, and severely abnormal.

Much thought has been given to further description of early infancy. Our data indicated that a variety of types of abnormal newborns appeared in the moderately and severely abnormal ranges. These types are more numerous than the three types described by Prechtl and Dijkstra (1960): hemisyndrome, apathetic, and hyperexcitable. There were two basic types of mildly abnormal newborns with extension of these characteristics into early infancy: (a) irritability or apathy (irritability was more frequent) and (b) less-than-normal head control, some hypotonia of arms (scarf sign), some delay in held sit, posterior neck, anterior neck. Because this is frequent, the author has lightened these requirements from previous work. This should increase the predictive validity of the assessment method.

Infanib scoring sheet

1. *Hands Open/Closed.* Observe the infant's hands for constant return to a clenched hand or a tightly closed hand often noted with any of the stress maneuvers. These may be induced by the examiner, as in the tonic labyrinthine supine maneuver, or induced spontaneously by the infant, as with even a slight turning of the head. At age 5 months, the normal infant in Figure 2.16A holds his hands open. At age 2 months, the infant with transient neuromotor abnormalities in Figure 2.16B holds his hands clenched with even the slightest stimulation. At age 3.5 months, the abnormal infant in Figure 2.16C also clenches his hands with any stimulation, either examiner- or self-induced.
2. *Scarf Sign.* Hold the infant's arm near the elbow and move the arm across the infant's chest until resistance is met, as indicated in Figure 2.17C. (In the other figures, the maneuver is performed less well technically but the angle is seen more clearly.) Observe the angle between a vertical line dropped from the insertion of the arm and the upper arm.

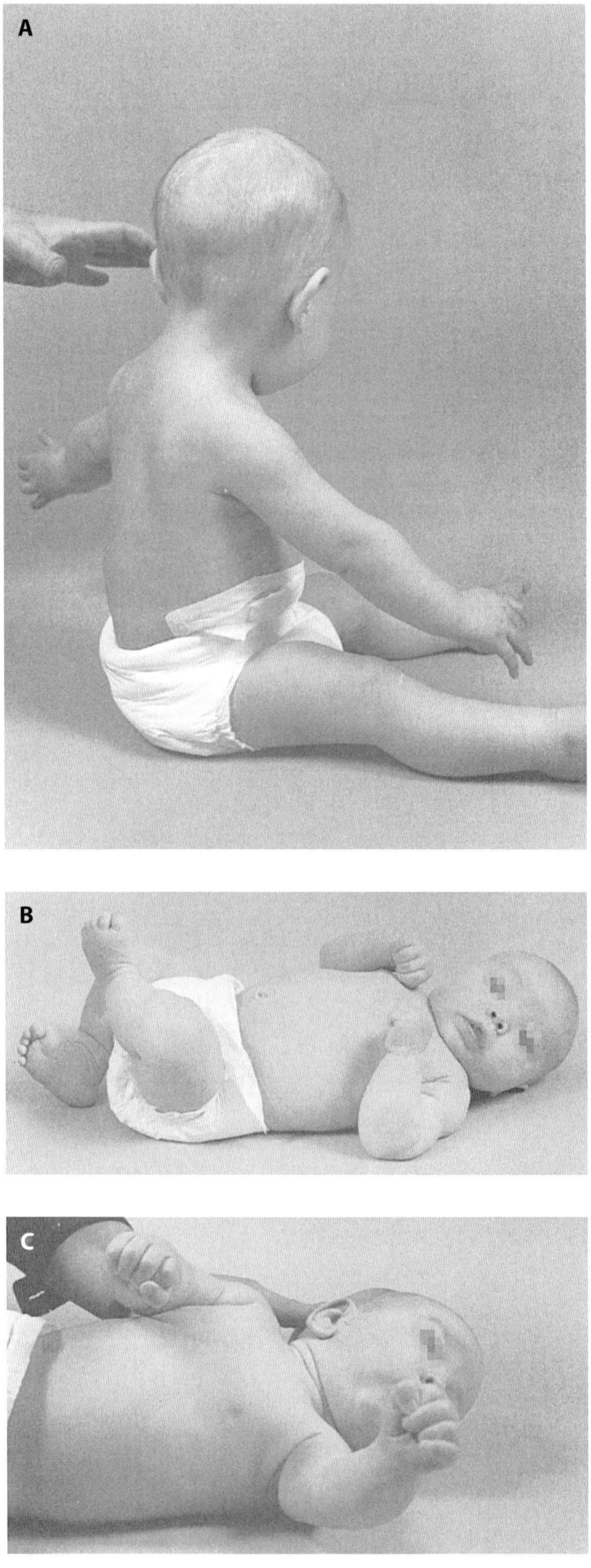

Figure 2.16 Hands open/closed. (B) Hands slightly clenched. (C) Hands clenched, abnormal.

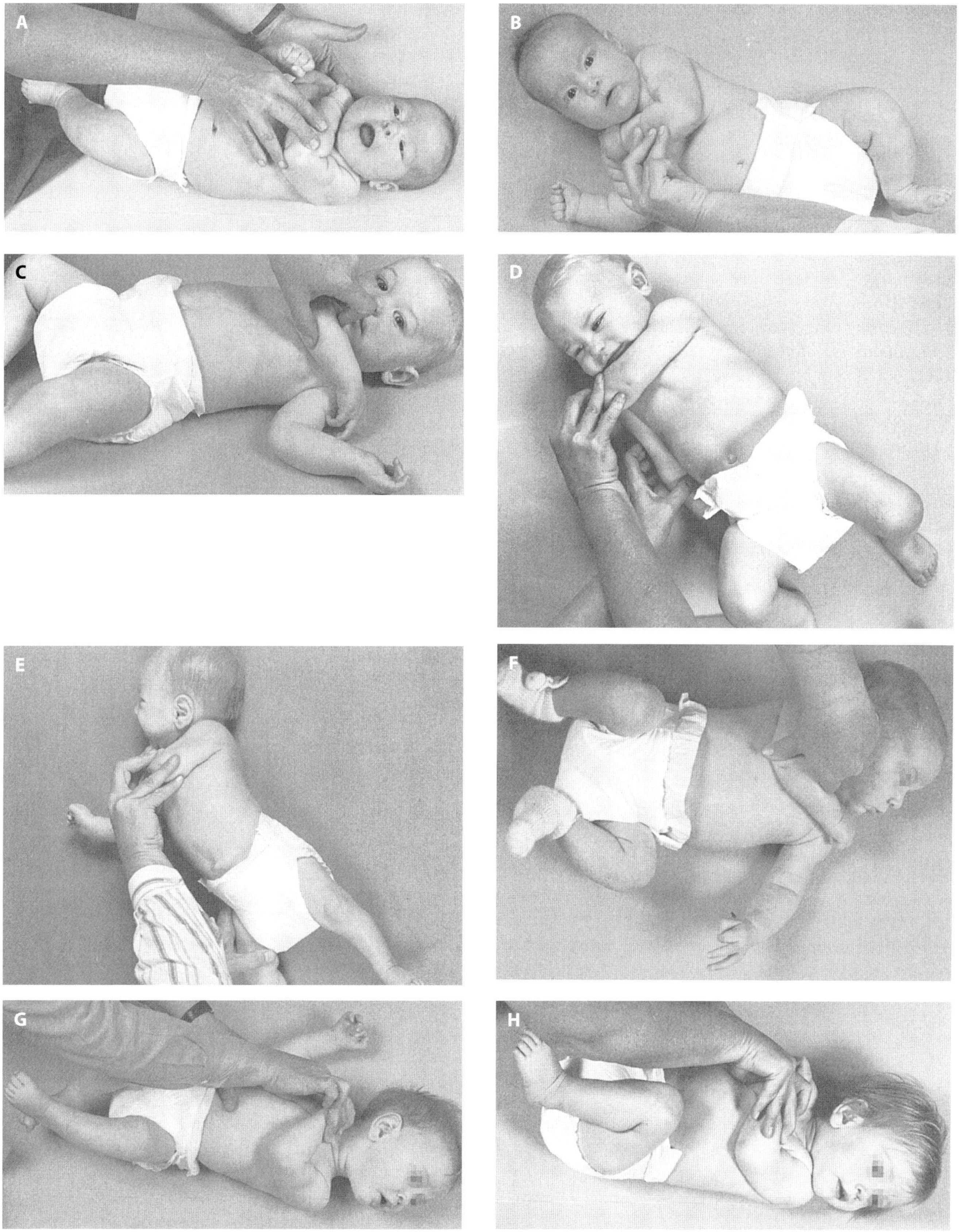

Figure 2.17 (A) Scarf sign, 0–3 months. (B) Scarf sign, 4–6 months. (C) Scarf sign, 7–9 months. (D) Scarf sign, 10–12 months. (E) Abnormal scarf sign, 0–3 months. (F) Abnormal scarf sign, 4–6 months. (G) Abnormal scarf sign, 7–9 months. (H) Abnormal scarf sign, 10–12 months.

A scarf sign with larger excursion than normal is an excellent indicator of hypotonia of the upper body, a very common finding in infants with other indicators of neurologic abnormality. Early hypertonia is uncommon. Progression from hypotonia to hypertonia in the upper body occurs in those infants with spastic quadriparesis and dyskinesia.

In the first series, the normal progression is shown from Figure 2.17A, 0–3 months; to Figure 2.17B, 4–6 months; to Figure 2.17C, 7–9 months; and Figure 2.17D, 10–12 months. Note the increasing ease with which the shoulder (and trapezius muscle) extends and the arm is moved across the chest. In the second series (Figures 2.17E–2.17H), the progression is reversed. Initially (0–3 months), the arm is extended too easily, indicating hypotonia. At each subsequent step (4–6, 7–9, and 10–12 months), the shoulder extends less easily, indicating a progression from hypotonia to hypertonia.

3. *Heel-to-ear*. Grasp the legs at the knees with legs extended and control the position of the buttocks. The buttocks should remain on or near the examining table (specifically this is not a measure of the flexibility of the spine; it is a measure of the flexibility of the hips). Measure the angle between the infant's trunk and legs.

   This is one of the best early indicators of hypertonia of the lower body. Infants with spastic diplegia or spastic quadriparesis and dyskinesia generally show change first in the flexibility of the hips or knees (see item 4). This later translates into the developmental milestone of an infant's ability to play with its feet.

   In the first series (Figures 2.18A–D), the normal infant shows the normal progression from 0–3, to 4–6, to 7–9, to 10–12 months. In the second series (Figures 2.18E–H), the abnormal infant fails to decrease the heel-to-ear angle after 0–3 months. He

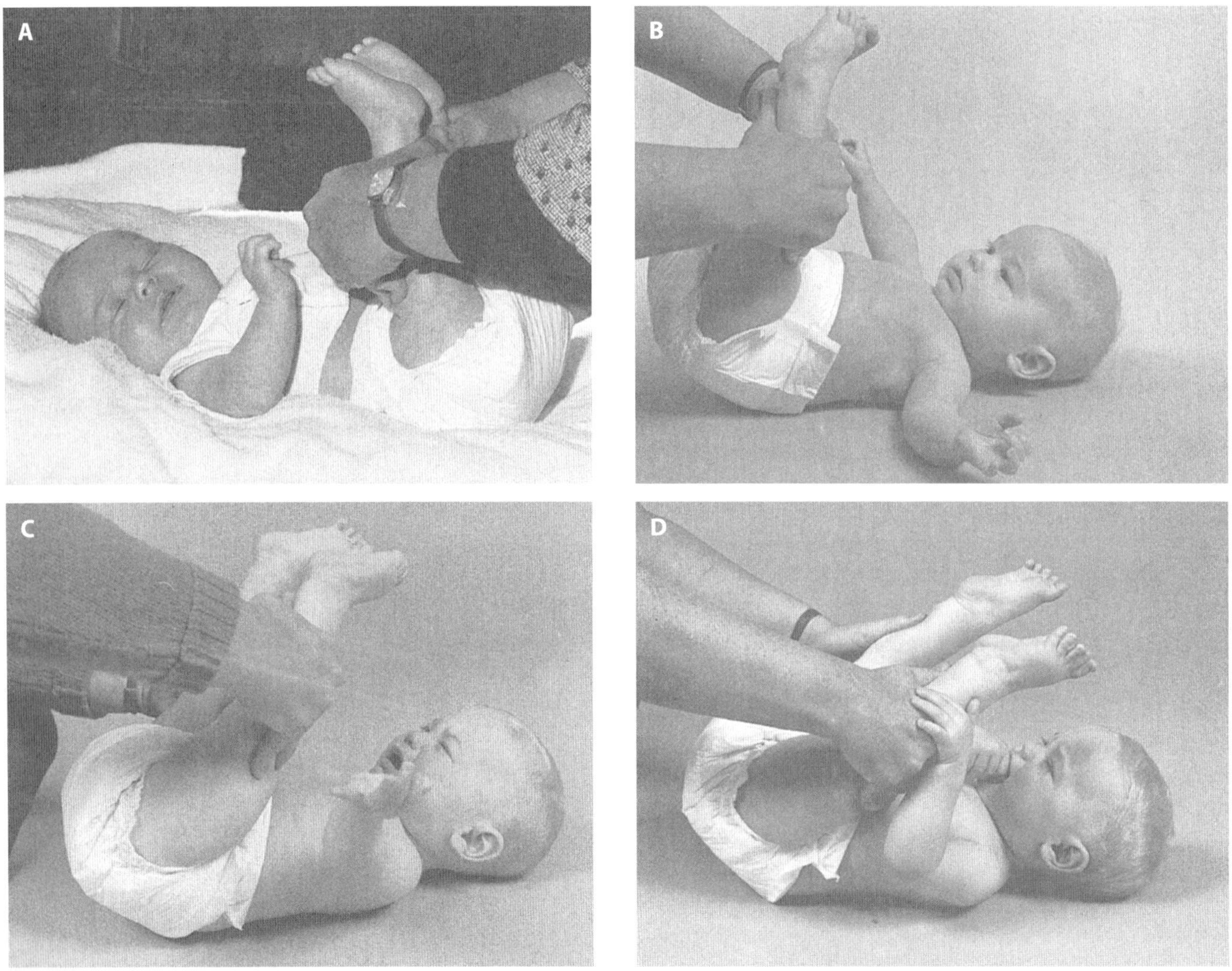

Figure 2.18 (A) Heel-to-ear, 0–3 months. (B) Heel-to-ear, 4–6 months. (C) Heel-to-ear, 7–9 months. (D) Heel-to-ear, 10–12 months.

departs increasingly from the normal progression (4–6 months, 7–9 months, 10–12 months). He also assumes an asymmetric tonic neck posture and keeps his hands closed (Figure 2.18F).

4. *Popliteal Angle*. Hold the legs near the knee, flex the leg at the hip, and abduct the legs, extending the lower leg until resistance is met. With the back of the knee as the fulcrum, measure the angle between the upper and lower parts of the leg. As indicated in item 3, popliteal angle is another excellent indicator of hypertonia in the lower body. Failure of the angle to increase throughout early and middle infancy often indicates spastic quadriparesis and dyskinesia, spastic diplegia, and asymmetrically, spastic hemiparesis.

   In the first series (Figures 2.19A–D), the infant shows the normal progression from 0–3, to 4–6, to 7–9, to 10–12 months. In the second series (Figures 2.19E–H), the popliteal angle is initially hypotonic, but then becomes hypertonic.

5. *Leg Abduction*. Hold the legs at the knee such that they are extended; abduct the legs. With the crotch as a fulcrum, measure the angle between the legs. This item is generally less sensitive than heel-to-ear or popliteal angle as an early indicator of hypertonia. It is an excellent indicator of hypotonia, but there are many other excellent indicators of hypotonia.

   In the first series, the normal infant demonstrates the normal progression from 0–3 (Figure 2.20A), to 4–6 (Figure 2.20B), to 7–9 (Figure 2.20C), to 10–12 (Figure 2.20D). In the second series, the abnormal infant has no increase in the angle at 4–6 months (Figure 2.20E) or at any other age range (Figures 2.20F–H).

6. *Dorsiflexion of the Foot*. Flex the foot, pushing it against the leg until resistance is met. With the ankle as a fulcrum, measure the angle between the foot and the leg.

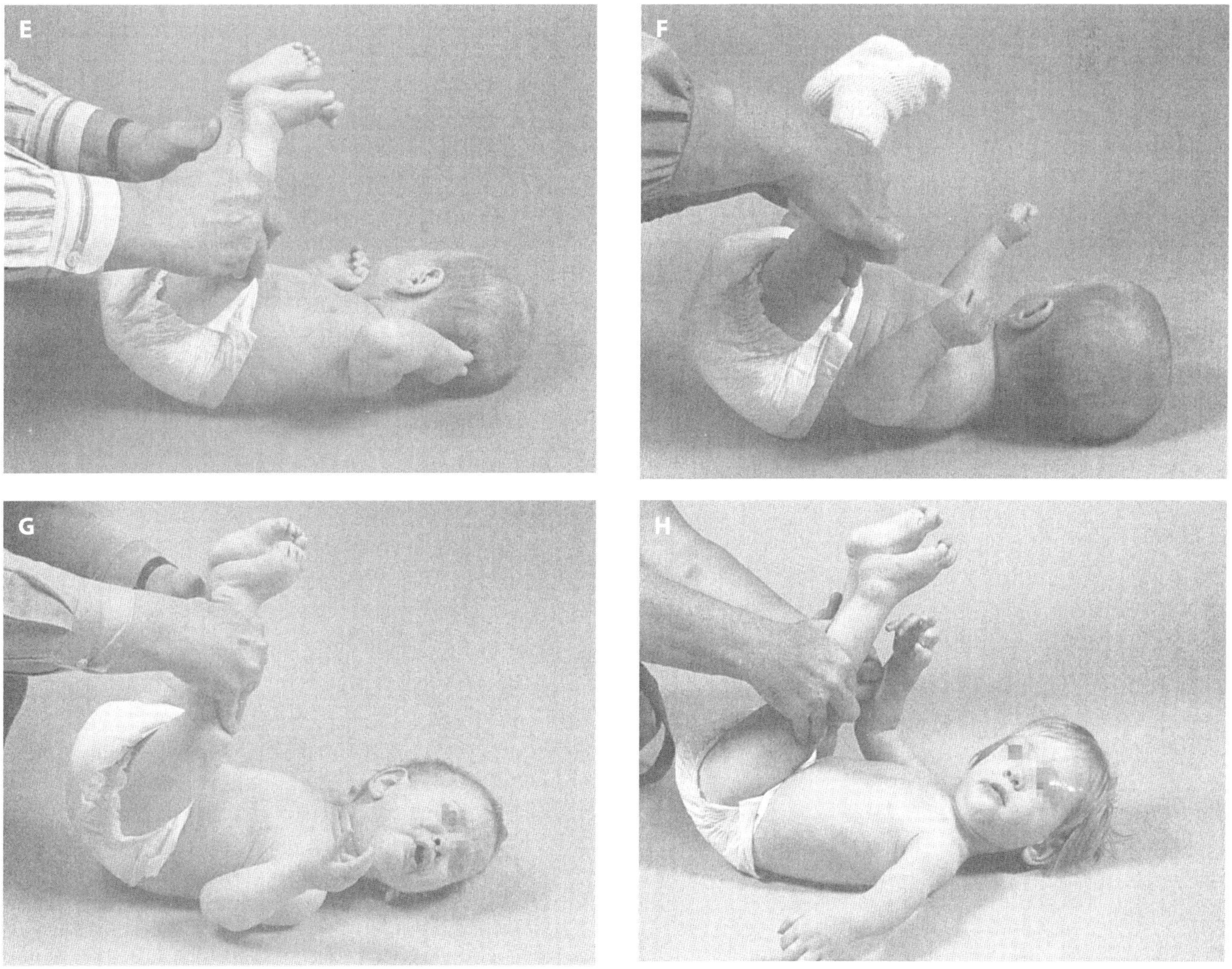

Figure 2.18 (E) Abnormal heel-to-ear, 0–3 months. (F) Abnormal heel-to-ear, 4–6 months. (G) Abnormal heel-to-ear, 7–9 months. (H) Abnormal heel-to-ear, 10–12 months.

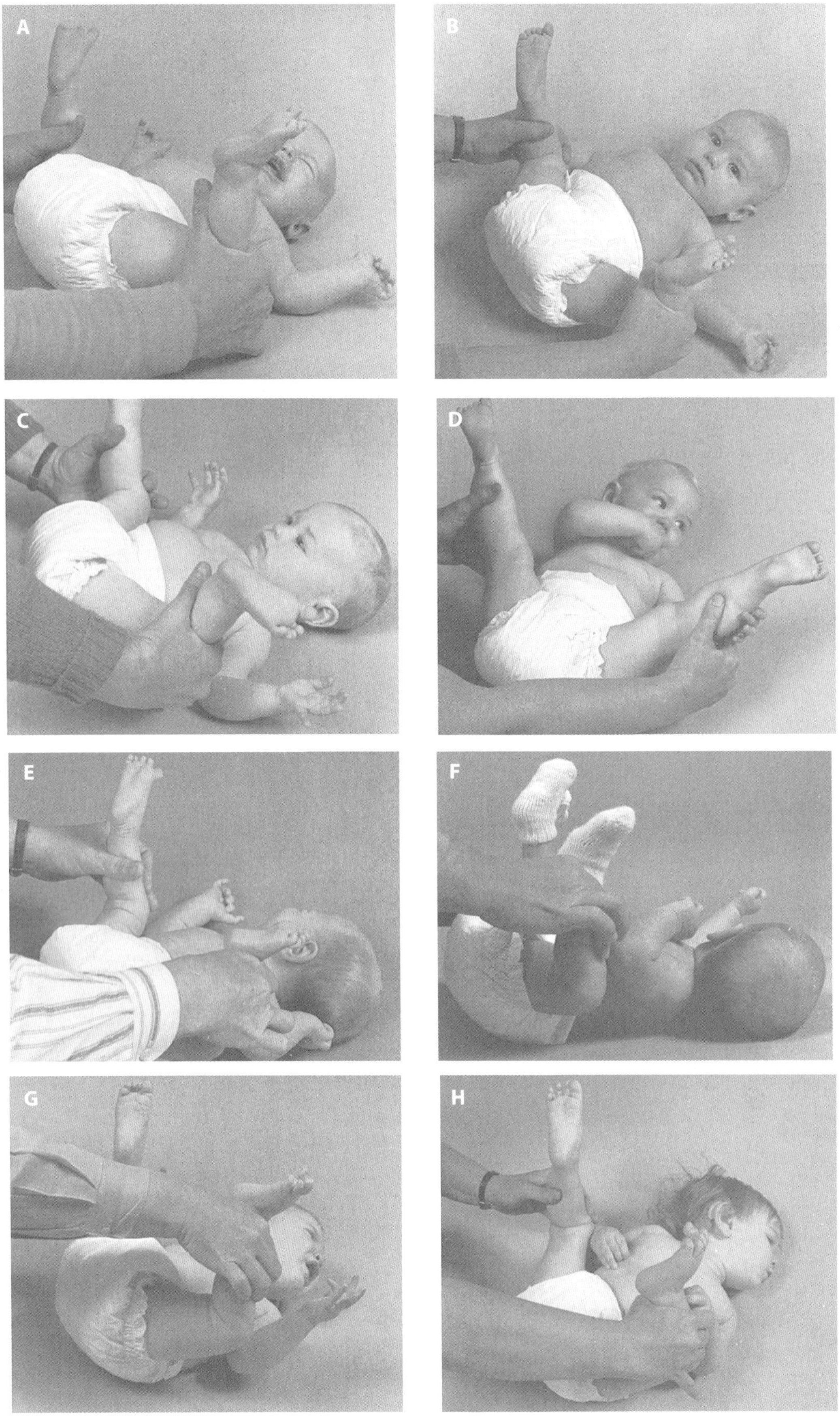

Figure 2.19 (A) Popliteal angle, 0–3 months. (B) Popliteal angle, 4–6 months. (C) Popliteal angle, 7–9 months. (D) Popliteal angle, 10–12 months. (E) Abnormal popliteal angle, 0–3 months. (F) Abnormal popliteal angle, 4–6 months. (G) Abnormal popliteal angle, 7–9 months. (H) Abnormal popliteal angle, 10–12 months.

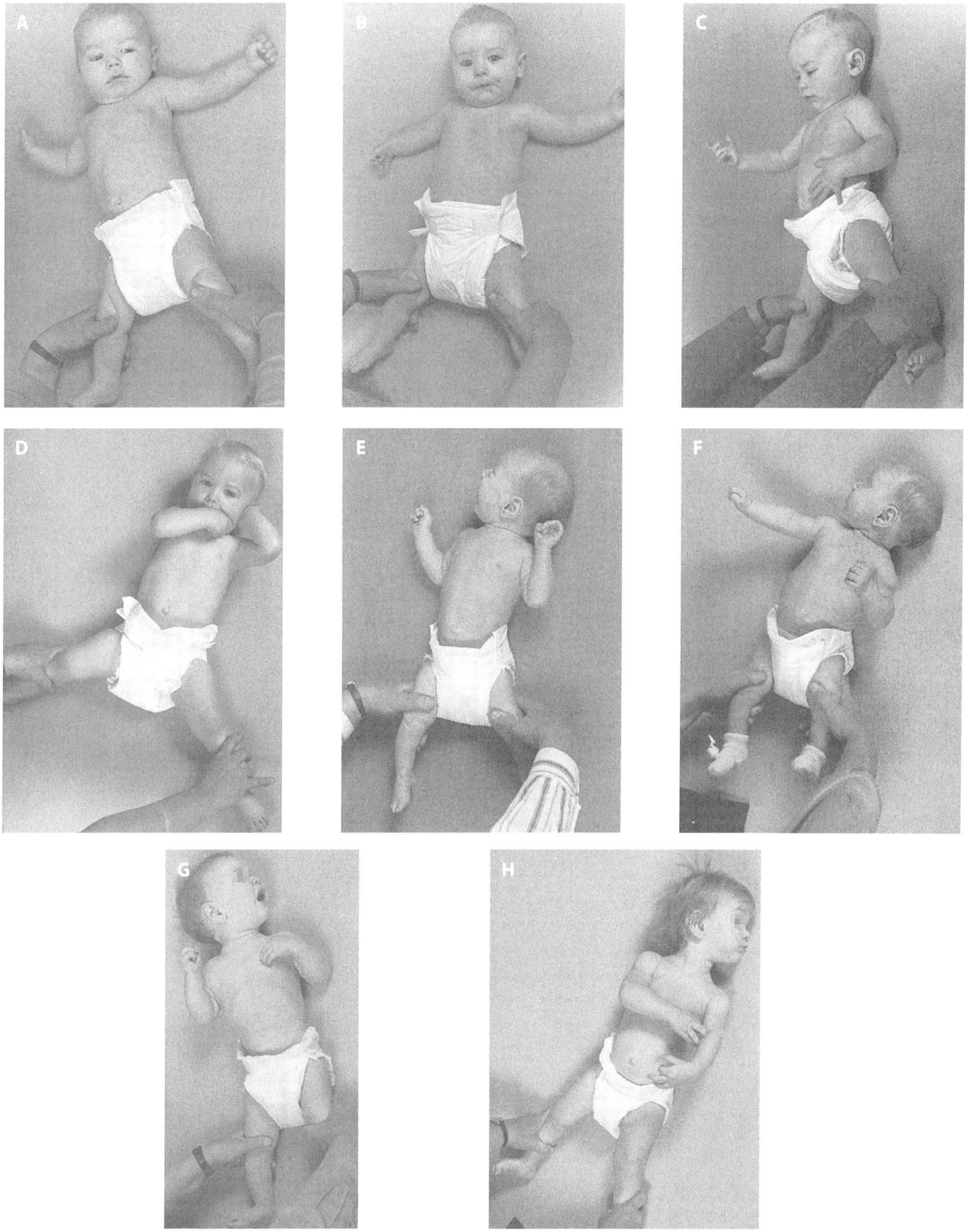

Figure 2.20 (A) Leg abduction, 0–3 months. (B) Leg abduction, 4–6 months. (C) Leg abduction, 7–9 months. (D) Leg abduction, 10–12 months. (E) Abnormal leg abduction, 0–3 months. (F) Abnormal leg abduction, 4–6 months. (G) Abnormal leg abduction, 7–9 months. (H) Abnormal leg abduction, 10–12 months.

The feet are generally the last to show hypertonia, except in situations of very early severe hypertonicity, in which they may be in an extended position that is very difficult to change. More frequently, the feet are hypotonic until middle or late infancy, even in infants with spastic quadriparesis and dyskinesia.

At age 2 months, the normal infant (Figure 2.21A) has a normal angle of dorsiflexion of the foot. At 4 months, the abnormal infant (Figure 2.21B) has an increased angle of dorsiflexion of the foot.

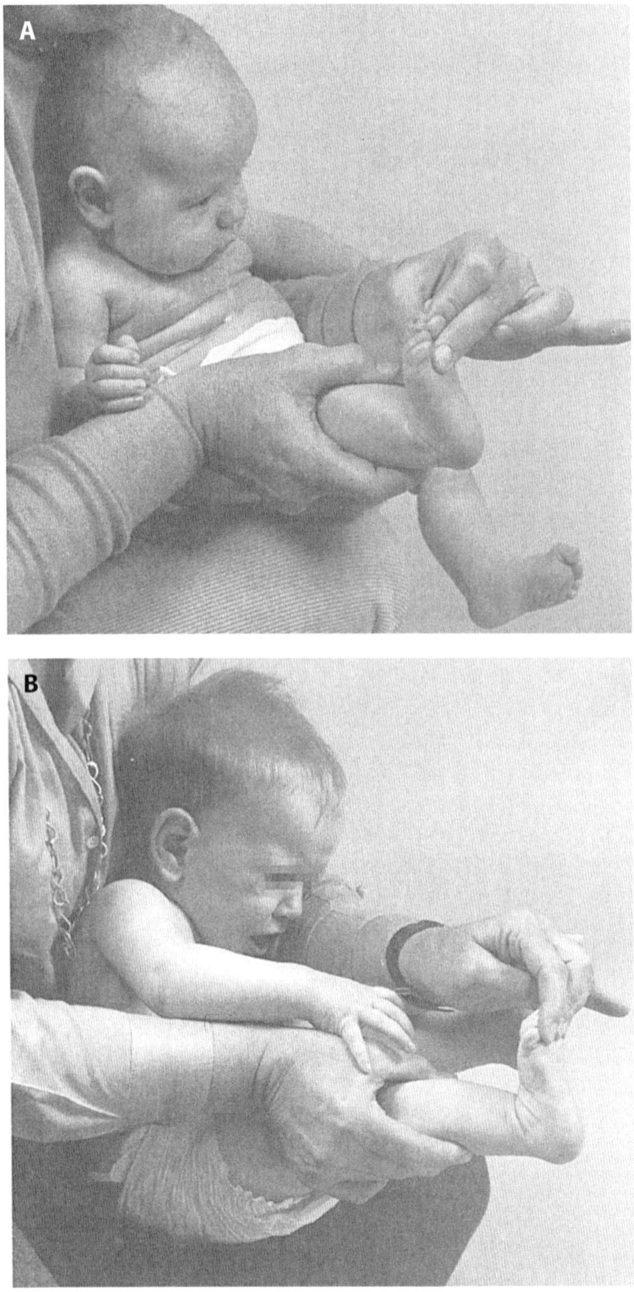

Figure 2.21 (A) Dorsiflexion of foot, 2 months. (B) Abnormal dorsiflexion of foot, 4 months.

7. *Foot Grasp*. Place the thumb or finger firmly in the footpad and observe for curling of the infant's toes toward the bottom of the foot.

   Foot grasp is a primitive reflex; specifically it is an item that is normal in the neonate but disappears over the course of infancy. For many of the primitive reflexes, the range of time that is considered normal for disappearance is long. It can also be exaggerated in its manifestation in early infancy; these exaggerations are abnormal. After the age at which the item should no longer be present, it can be graded to represent levels of normality and abnormality (no grasp, barely grasps, grasp).

   At 1 month of age, the normal infant (Figure 2.22A) has a prominent but not exaggerated foot grasp. At 3 months, the abnormal infant (Figure 2.22B) has an exaggerated foot grasp.

8. *Tonic Labyrinthine Supine*. Stimulate the intrascapular area with the hand. Observation is made of shoulder retraction and extension or flexion of arms, legs, or trunk. This item is also a primitive reflex.

   At 1 month of age, the normal infant (Figure 2.23A) demonstrates little response to this maneu-

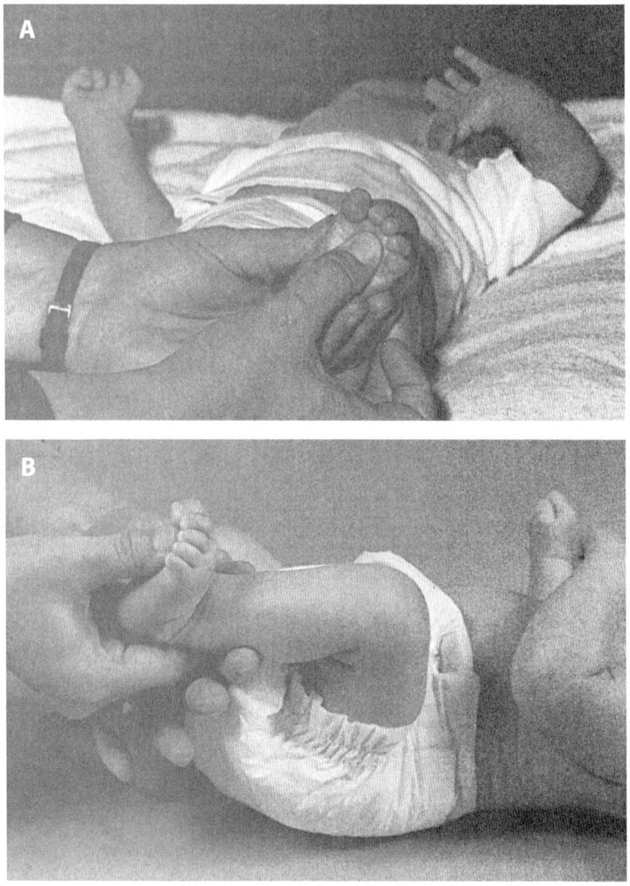

Figure 2.22 (A) Foot grasp. (B) Exaggerated foot grasp.

ver. The infant in Figure 2.23B has a dramatic response, with extension of both arms and legs; this response was graded as abnormal. The abnormal infant (Figure 2.23C) has flexion of both arms and legs at 2 months; this response was also graded as abnormal.

9. *Asymmetric Tonic Neck Reflex*. Turn the infant's head from side to side, observing the assumption of

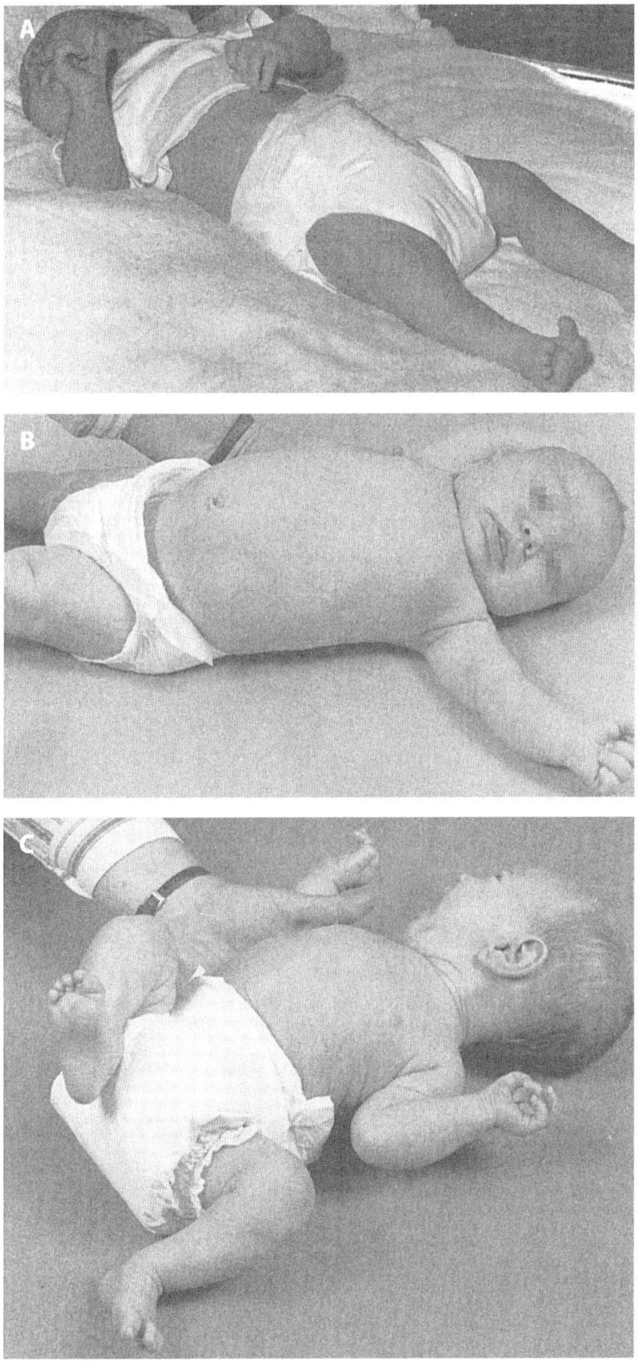

Figure 2.23 (A) Tonic labyrinthine supine, 1 month. (B) Abnormal tonic labyrinthine supine. (C) Abnormal tonic labyrinthine supine.

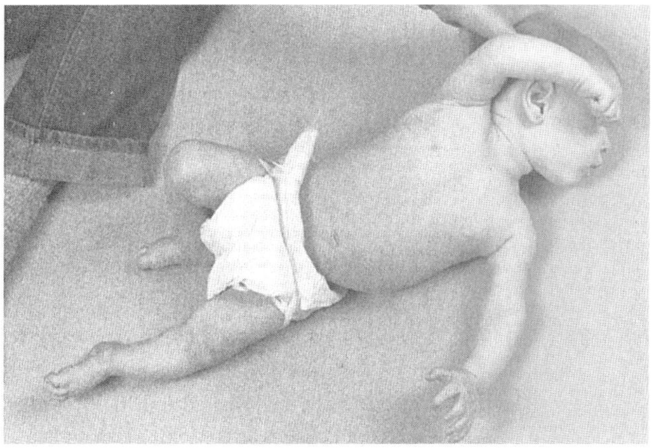

Figure 2.24 Abnormal tonic neck reflex, 5 months.

a fencing position, the extension of the arm faced, the flexion of the arm behind the head, and the extension of the leg faced. Also note the persistence of the posture: whether the infant assumes the posture and then moves out of it, in contrast to persisting in the posture. Persistence is abnormal at any age and is the manifestation of exaggeration of the reflex.

At age 1 month, the normal infant (Figure 2.6 NeoNeuro exam) manifests an asymmetric tonic neck reflex, which he then overcomes. The abnormal infant (Figure 2.24) at 5 months has a strong, persistent asymmetric tonic neck reflex. It may be noted than an infant with neurologic abnormality goes into an asymmetric tonic neck reflex with many neurologic maneuvers, as well as spontaneously and repetitively when he is supine.

10. *Pull to Sitting*. Grasp the infant's hands and pull the infant to a sitting position. As seen in the figures, a small sandbag may be used as a weight to maintain the position of the buttocks. Observe first the position of the head: extended, straight up, or flexed. Second, observe the position of the arms: extended or flexed. If there is a discrepancy in the two observations, the scoring is based on the position of the head.

The most common abnormal finding is that of delay in head control or hypotonia of the neck and upper trunk. Hypertonia is noted much less frequently. The manifestation is precocious head control with extension of the head. This is demonstrated by the infant in Figure 2.25A at age 2 months. His head control is "superior" to that expected for his age, an indication of the hypertonicity of his neck muscles. The normal infant (Figure 2.25B) at 2 months has normal head control. The abnormal infant (Figure 2.25C) at 7 months persists in poor head control, which he has had since his neonatal neurologic examination.

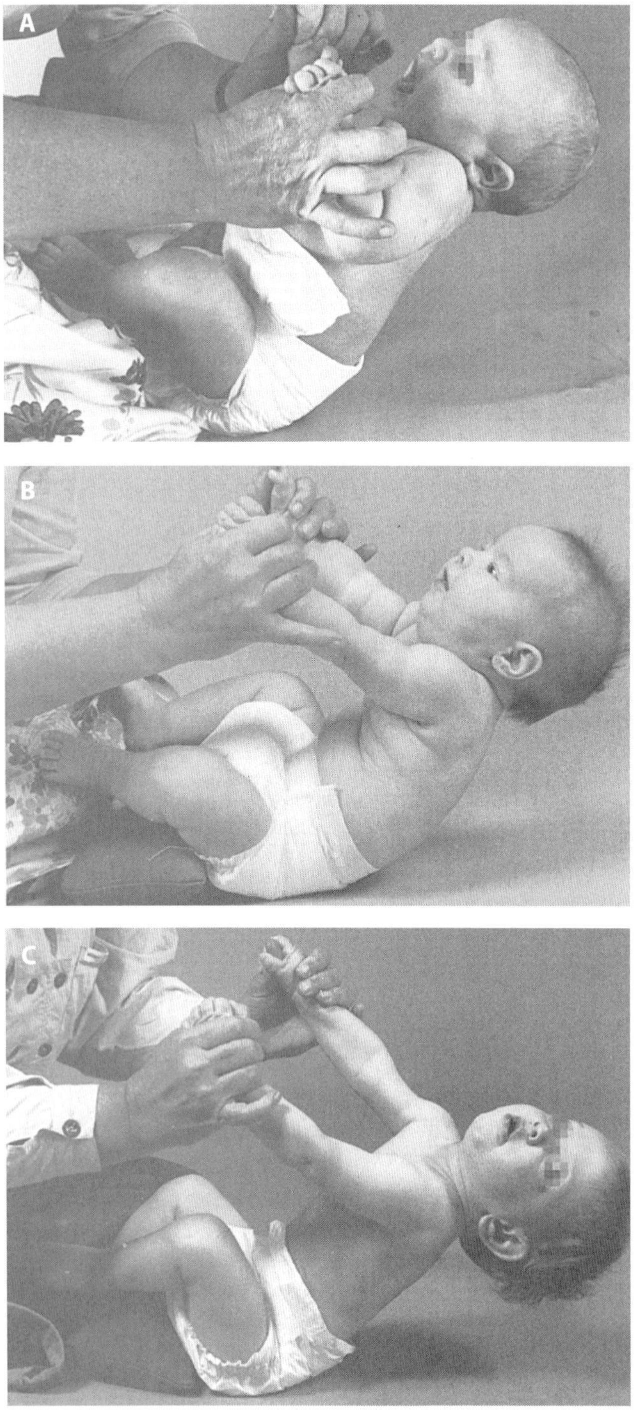

Figure 2.25 (A) Abnormal pull to sit, 2 months. (B) Pull to sit, 2 months. (C) Abnormal pull to sit, 7 months.

11. *Body Derotative*. Hold the infant by the lower legs, then rotate the legs to initiate rolling from supine to prone. Observe the infant's continuation of the maneuver. An infant with neurologic impairment may not be able to accomplish this or may do so slowly or awkwardly. To check for noncompliance, ask the parent if spontaneous rolling from supine to prone occurs at home. Full credit is given for a reported supine-to-prone roll.

    At age 4 months, the normal (Figure 2.26A) infant readily raises the upper arm and participates in the maneuver. The abnormal infant (Figure 2.26B) flexes his arms, extends his trunk and head, and cannot complete the maneuver.
12. *Body Rotative*. The infant spontaneously rolls from supine to prone, then pulls to standing position. In normal infants, the maneuver is often accomplished spontaneously in the course of the examination. The normal infant's ease is seen in Figures 2.27A and 2.27B. The abnormal infant (Figure 2.27C) accomplishes the maneuver, but he is slower and has a log-rolling style: his upper and lower body are rolled as a unit.
13. *All Fours*. Move the infant to the prone position. The rating of this item is based on observation of head position, arm position, and leg position. The major component is head position. The examiner is seeking optimal performance; encouragement of the infant is not only permitted but preferable.

    The normal infant (Figure 2.28) at age 5 months holds his head up 90° and extends his arms. An abnormal infant does not lift his head at all, even with much encouragement.
14. *Tonic Labyrinthine Prone*. Move the infant to the prone position. Flex the infant's head, and observe

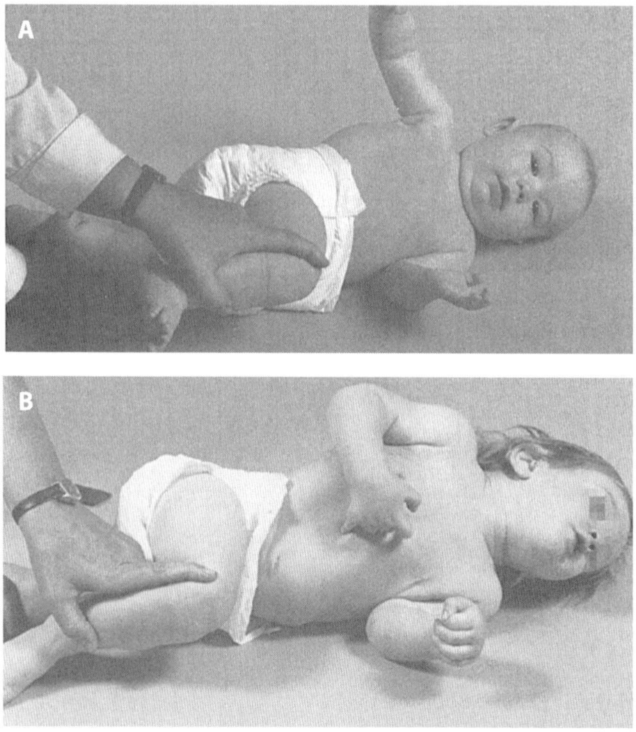

Figure 2.26 (A) Body derotative, 4 months. (B) Abnormal body derotative.

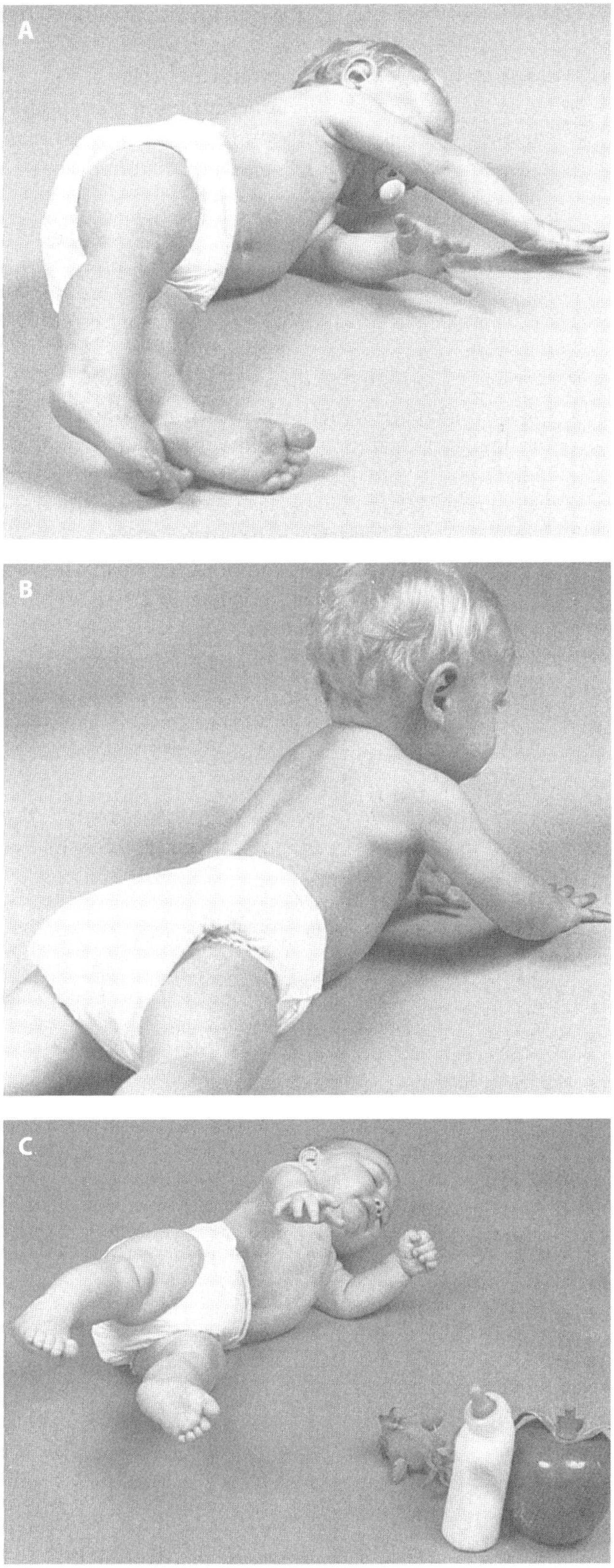

Figure 2.27 (A) Body rotative. (B) Body rotative. (C) Abnormal body rotative.

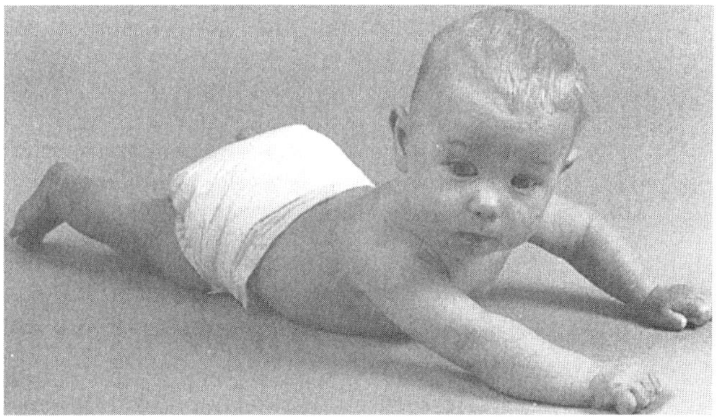

Figure 2.28 All fours, 5 months.

shoulder retraction and flexion of arms, hips, or legs under the trunk. The infant's body may be stabilized by placement of the examiner's hand under the abdomen. This is another primitive reflex, thus exaggeration is an abnormal response in early infancy. At 7 months, the abnormal infant has a prompt and vigorous response to head flexion (Figure 2.29).

15. *Sitting*. The examiner holds or places the infant in a sitting position and notes the point at which bending occurs (L3, L5). It may not be possible to get the infant into a sitting position if there is repetitive extensor posturing. Other items (such as tonic labyrinthine prone, tonic labyrinthine supine, and asymmetric tonic neck reflex) should also be abnormal with extensor posturing of this degree. More frequently, abnormality is manifested by poor trunk control with a delay in the progression of sitting positions.

    At age 4 months, the normal infant (Figure 2.30A) bends forward from L3. At the same age, the abnormal infant (Figure 2.30B) bends forward from L5 and holds his head in an extended position. This precocious sitting position is abnormal, indicating

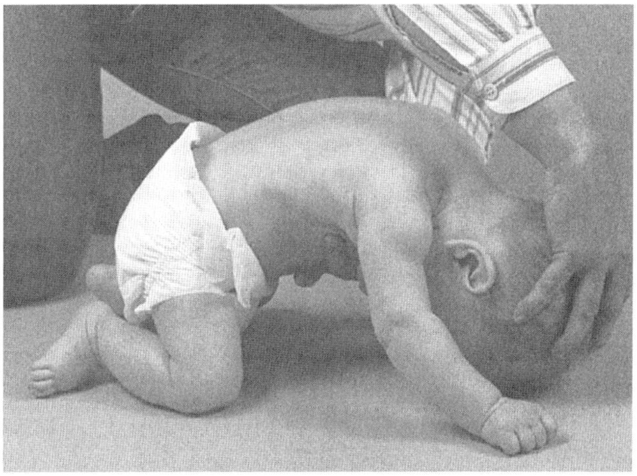

Figure 2.29 Abnormal tonic labyrinthine prone

excessive extension. At age 6 months, the abnormal infant (Figure 2.30C) bends forward from L3, indicating a delay in trunk control.

16. *Sideways Parachute*. Hold the infant in a sitting position, then tip the infant gently but firmly to each side and observe for the extension of the infant's hand to "prevent" falling or provide support. The

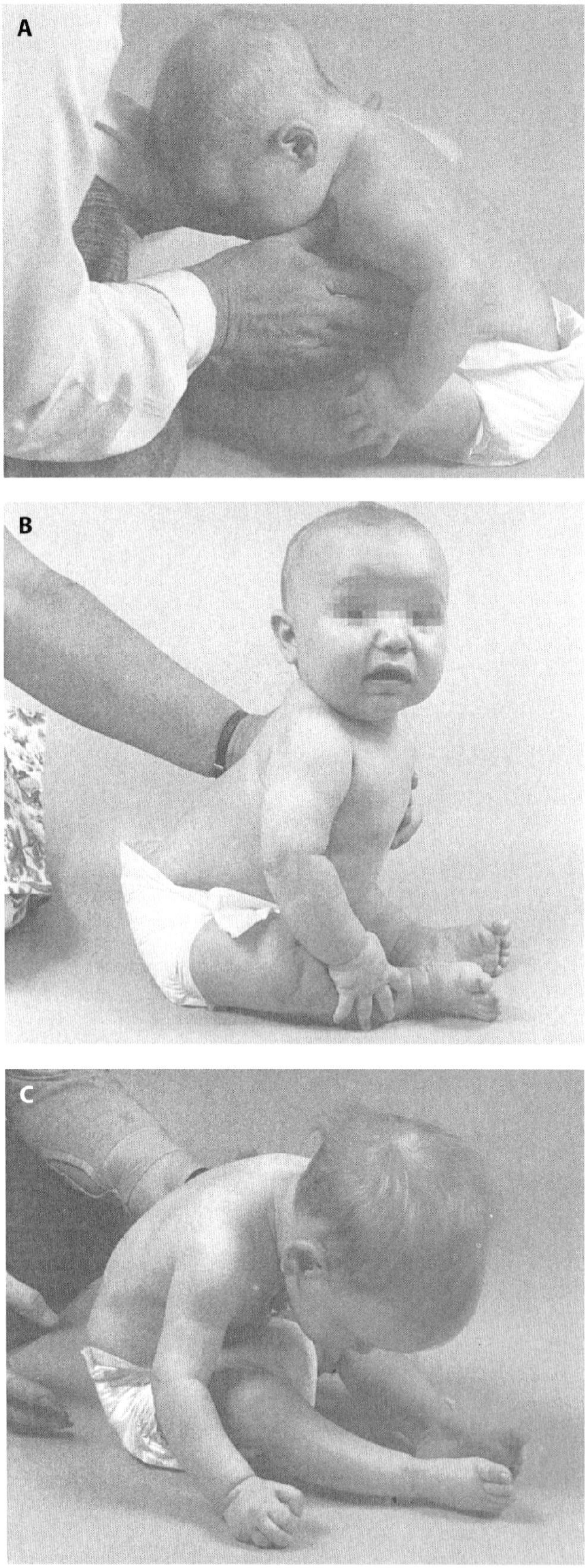

Figure 2.30 (A) Sitting, 4 months. (B) Abnormal sitting, 4 months. (C) Abnormal sitting, 6 months.

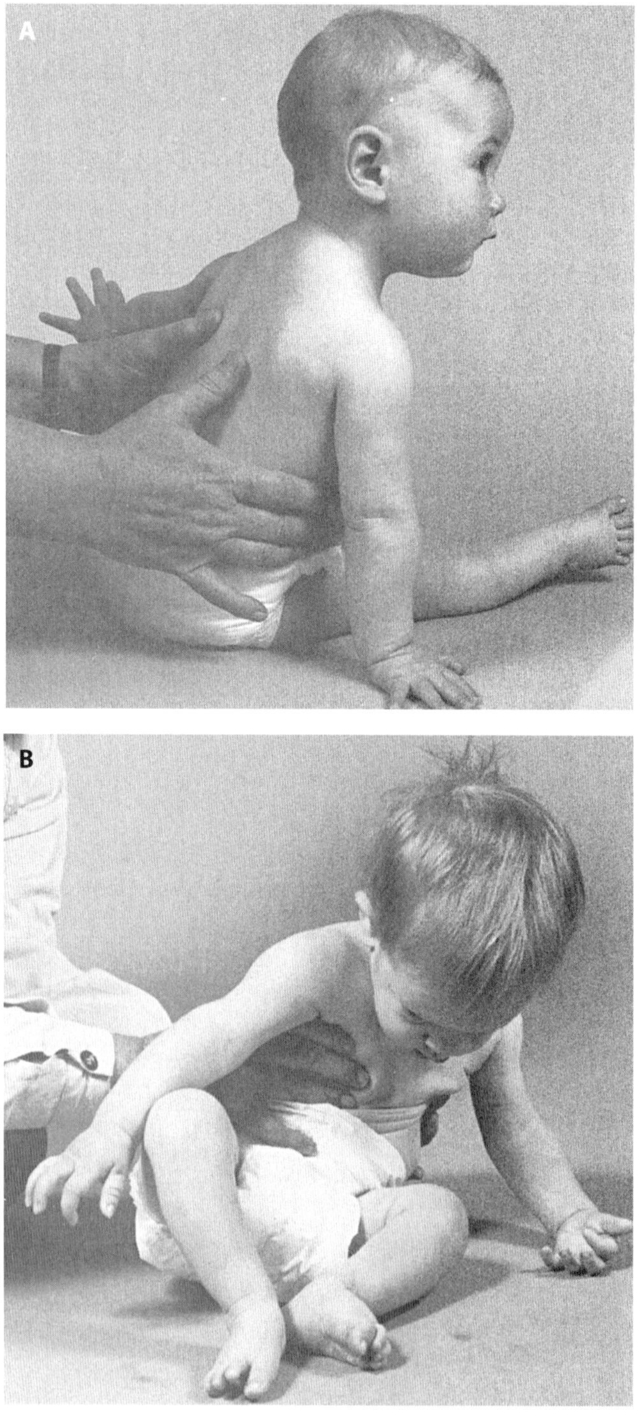

Figure 2.31 (A) Sideways parachute, 8 months. (B) Abnormal sideways parachute.

parachute items, including sideways, forward, and backward parachutes, probably provide a measure of the maturation of vestibular function. Sideways and forward parachute maneuvers are also useful in the identification of hemiparesis. A hemiparetic infant demonstrates less thrust with the impaired arm.

At 8 months of age, the normal infant (Figure 2.31A) readily thrusts his arm and head out in support. At the same age, the abnormal infant (Figure 2.31B) makes no effort to support himself with his arm and hand.

17. *Backward Parachute*. Gently but firmly thrust the infant backward, holding the infant at the trunk so that he or she will not lose balance and fall. Observe the posturing of the infant's arms. Some infants may turn to one side, appearing to use one arm more than the other. Because of this, the backward parachute maneuver is less useful in distinguishing asymmetry.

At 9 months of age, the normal infant (Figure 2.32A) thrusts both arms toward the back. The abnormal infant (Figure 2.32B) makes no effort to do so.

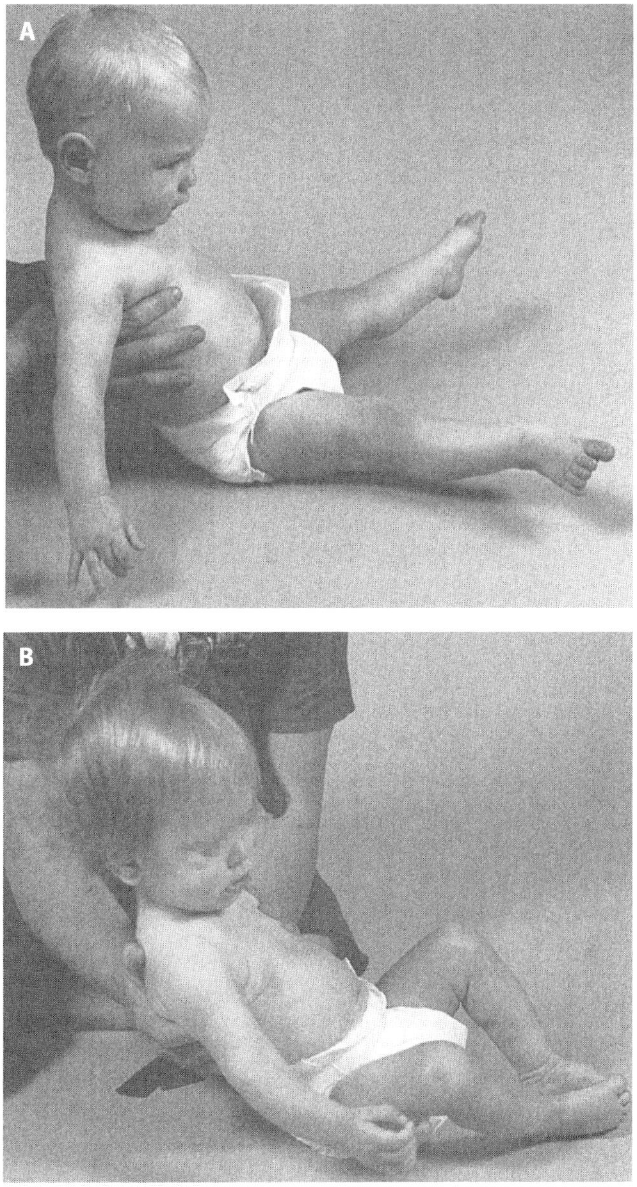

Figure 2.32 (A) Backwards parachute, 9 months. (B) Abnormal backwards parachute.

18. *Standing (Weight-bearing)*. Place the infant in a standing position, and observe the position of the infant's body. Most newborns assume a standing position because of primitive reflexes. This tendency is lost variably but is almost always gone by age 2 months. Then the infant makes no attempt to weight-bear, or is at best unable to weight-bear.

Early weight-bearing, at approximately 2–5 months, should be associated with buckling at the knee. Specifically, the infant stands with legs straight, then bends or flexes the knees briefly and resumes a more straight-legged stance. Persistent standing without buckling often indicates hypertonia. Thus, it is scored as abnormal. Unequal weight-bearing is less clear-cut; the infant may shift weight from one leg to another or stand such that the weight appears to be borne by one leg more than the other.

At 10 months, the normal infant (Figure 2.33A) is sufficiently relaxed in a standing position

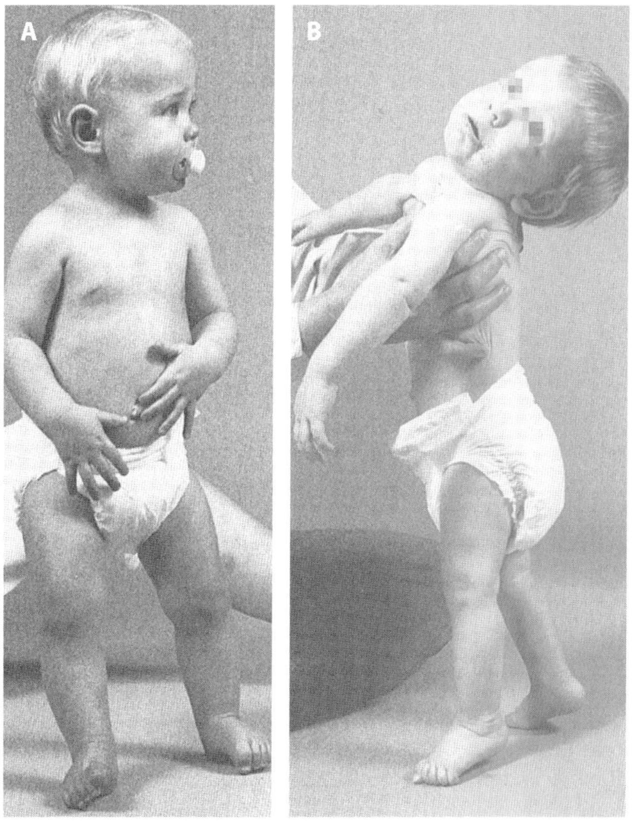

Figure 2.33 (A) Standing, 10 months. (B) Abnormal standing.

that he appears casual and at ease. The abnormal infant (Figure 2.33B) cannot maintain his trunk well and exhibits extensor posturing in a standing position (feet extended and head thrust back).

19. *Positive Support Reaction.* Observe the position of the infant's feet as the infant is placed in a standing position. The item is described and scored here a bit differently from usual, in order to focus attention on the feet. The item belongs with other items that describe the legs and feet: dorsiflexion of the foot, foot grasp, and weight-bearing. The abnormal infant fails to drop the heel flat to the floor (Figure 2.34).

20. *Suspended Position: Forward Parachute.* Hold the infant at the trunk, and propel the infant forward toward a surface, such as a table, thrusting the infant's head downward. Observe the infant's thrusting of arms forward for protection or support. As noted in item 16, this item is also an excellent indicator of asymmetry as manifested by unilateral arm thrust.

    At age 7 months, the normal infant (Figure 2.35A) thrusts his arms and hands forward. At the same age, the abnormal infant (Figure 2.35B) makes no effort to do this.

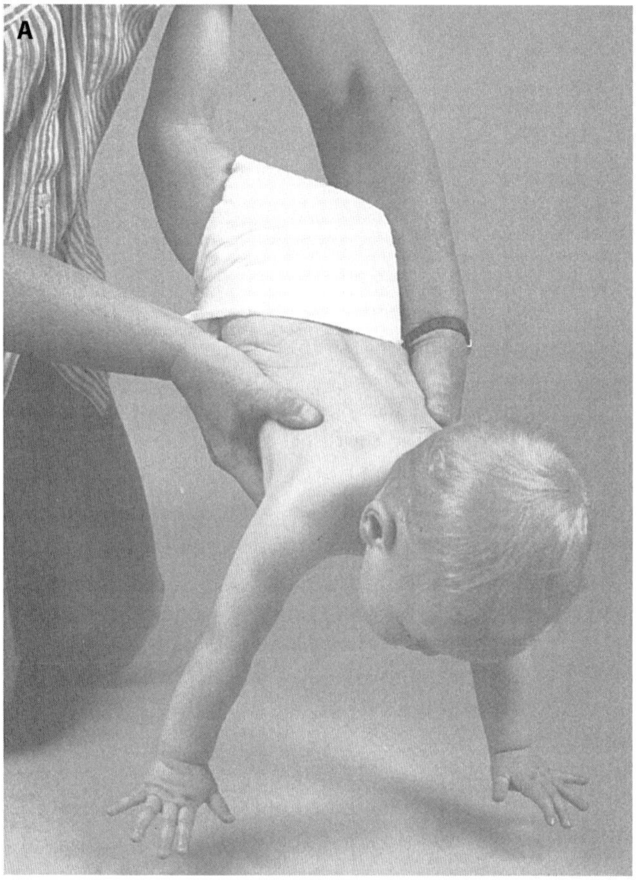

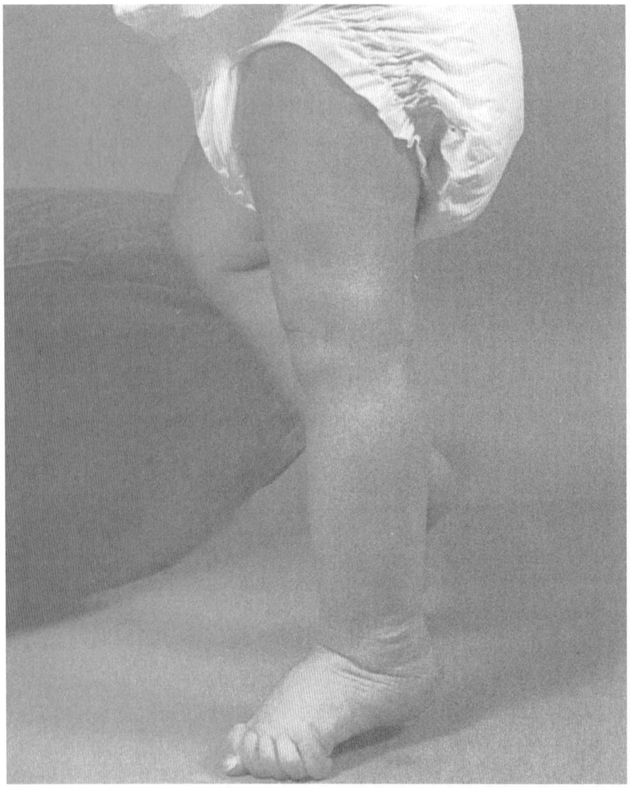

Figure 2.34 Abnormal positive support reaction.

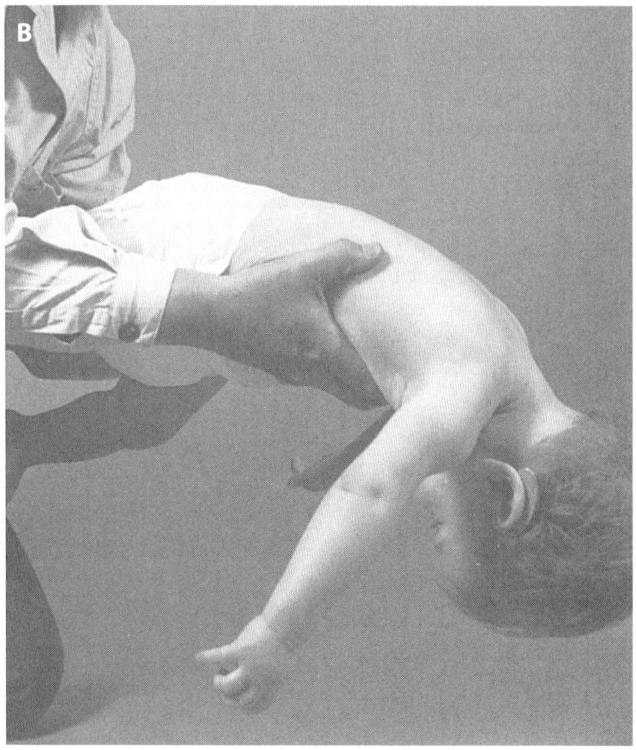

Figure 2.35 (A) Forward parachute, 7 months. (B) Abnormal forward parachute, 7 months.

Using the Infanib Scoring Sheet

The items on the Infanib are listed in a logical order, progressing from supine to prone to sitting to standing to suspension (Ellison 1994). The age at which the item appears is listed at the far left. For each item, the examiner circles the description that most closely approximates the infant being examined. An item is not scored unless it is appropriate for the infant's corrected gestational age (thus, 0 points are given for items above the infant's corrected gestational age). The age at which a major change occurs appears in the second column at the left.

The examiner uses the second page of the scoring sheet to ascertain the score per item. The age of the infant (or age corrected for degree of prematurity) is indicated at the top. Each item is scored by its relation to the infant's age. In general, items that are normal are scored 5, items that are mildly abnormal are scored 3, and items that are markedly abnormal are scored 1. For items that progress with age, a delay of one stage is scored 3 and a delay of two stages is scored 1. For the French angles items, the deviation may be in either direction, permitting a description of hypotonia (delay) or hypertonia (precocious). As noted previously, hands closed and open, foot grasp, tonic labyrinthine supine, asymmetric tonic neck reflex, and tonic labyrinthine prone are scored in the early months as abnormal only if the response is exaggerated. Early acquisition of a skill may be abnormal. For example, infants between 2.5 and 5 months who do not buckle at the knee within 60 seconds receive a score of 1 (abnormal). Similarly, young infants who bring their heads forward too well on pull to sit are scored as abnormal. All asymmetric positions are also given a score of 1. This approach assists in a diagnosis of hemiparesis.

The scores for each item should be placed in the allotted spaces on the first page of the scoring sheet. Each column is summed to obtain a factor score. This helps the examiner think about the items in groups. The factor scores are then summed to obtain a total score.

The degree of normality and abnormality based on the total score is ascertained from the chart on the second page of the scoring sheet for the three age divisions: less than 4 months (it is preferable to use the NeoNeuro & Up for ages less than 4 months), 4–8 months, and 8 months or more. For those infants whose scores fall in the range of abnormal, a category of abnormality is selected by the examiner.

In most of our work with infants, we have used a limited choice of categories for designation of neurologic abnormality: spastic quadriparesis/dyskinesia, spastic hemiparesis, spastic diplegia, and moderate to severe hypotonia. The mild hypotonias are included in transient neuromotor abnormalities. These categories evolved with experience and in working with other clinicians. When more categories of abnormality were used, clinicians often disagreed. Thus, the slightly broader categories were used when the research required that each category be graded for purposes of data analysis or for description of the progression of the category through infancy (Ellison et al. 1983). The types of abnormality and their outcome have been discussed in detail in other work (Ellison 1984a, 1984). Any examiner who evaluates and scores an infant should have knowledge of these progressions before discussing the infant with the parents.

What is the prognosis for neurologic abnormality?

Premature Newborns

Clinical researchers have varied in their approaches to the identification of those premature infants at risk for later neurologic dysfunction. Some have shown that the progression to a normal neurologic examination at 40 weeks post menstrual age establishes strong indication of neurologic normality and, in the past, this has been more reliable than electrophysiological or imaging studies.

Newer imaging techniques have been introduced to study newborn brains and improve prediction of outcome. Evidence of severely abnormal ultrasound findings, grade 4 intracranial hemorrhage, periventricular leukomalacia at term, or ventriculomegaly at term, have been useful in defining subsequent neurologic injury (Ment et al. 2003). However, sensitivity and positive predictive value have not been as powerful as hoped, especially in the more common case of noncystic white matter injury (Inder et al. 2003). Abnormal MRI findings at term-equivalent in preterm infants may also be useful in stratifying infants at risk, although gray matter abnormalities were less strongly associated with adverse neurodevelopmental outcome (Woodward et al. 2006). Combined methods of assessment may be the most useful in predicting cerebral palsy, although cognitive delays in preterm infants without overt neurologic injury may prove the most challenging to detect early.

We have used statistical techniques of path coefficients to tease out the contributions of various neonatal illnesses to later neurologic dysfunction (Ellison and Foster 1992).

Neonates

Full-term newborns who are normal neurologically are, in general, normal at follow-up. This was noted in the studies of Prechtl, in which 8% of the normal neonates had neurologic aberrations at 2–4 years (Prechtl and Dijkstra 1960), and others (Amiel-Tison 1976; Amiel-Tison and Grenier 1986). Abnormal neonates, on the other hand, are much more difficult to classify in regard to prediction:

citing Prechtl, 68% of the abnormal neonates had neurologic aberrations at 2–4 years. (Prechtl's "neurologic abnormality of the neonate" and "neurologic aberrations at 2–4 years" are both broad-spectrum categories.)

In our experience, neonatal factor scores, or elements of the neurologic examination, may have very low relationships with each other. Even with total scores in the severely abnormal range, certain factor scores were normal for some neonates. Neonates who scored in the moderately or severely abnormal categories had different combinations of low factor scores. Neonates with mildly abnormal total scores had lower scores for irritability or the head-on-neck support factors. Clinicians should be able to determine through further research which combinations tend to improve and which do not. We should also be able to determine which combinations respond to which intervention therapies. In short, the use of the subscores should help us in untangling some of the unsolved problems. This process may also be aided by newer electrophysiologic techniques. Amplitude-integrated electroencephalograph (EEG) has recently been found useful in predicting outcome in term infants with hypoxic–ischemic encephalopathy and again even more powerful when combined with the infant neurologic examination (Spitzmiller et al. 2007).

Infants

Considerable information is already available about the progression of neurologic normality and abnormality from infancy through the early school years. Again, infants who are normal tend to remain so, unless there is an intervening event such as meningitis, seizures, or head injury.

Infants who are abnormal often look worse or score worse during the course of infancy. Many of them will improve in their neurologic function between infancy and early school years; they may even "outgrow" cerebral palsy. In the National Collaborative Perinatal Project, 16% of infants with a diagnosis of moderate or severe quadriplegia did not carry a diagnosis of cerebral palsy at age 7 years; 72% of infants with mild spastic diplegia outgrew their cerebral palsy, and 50% of infants with moderate to severe spastic diplegia outgrew it. Only 48% of infants with mild hemiparesis and 13% of those with moderate to severe hemiparesis outgrew it by age 7 years (Nelson and Ellenberg 1982). This also speaks to the importance of not labeling a child with cerebral palsy until the motor pattern is obvious, although early intervention can be initiated in the meantime.

Hypotonia, the most common category of abnormality for infants initially treated in the neonatal intensive care unit, tends to improve. We prefer to consider mild hypotonia as part of transient neuromotor abnormalities. In a series of 999 infants from the neonatal intensive care unit, 21% demonstrated transient neuromotor abnormalities in infancy (Ellison and Browning 1982). Of these minor abnormalities, 79% had disappeared by 15 months. Infants with moderate to severe hypotonia also tend to outgrow it, more quickly if their other developmental skills (adaptive and personal-social) are normal.

Key Clinical Questions

- What are the early signs of cerebral palsy?
  The constellation of delayed head control, hypotonia of arms, and limited popliteal angle or heel-to-ear angle is an excellent indicator.
- What is the clinical significance of increased tone in the preterm infant?
  Increased tone without abnormality of posture or movement may be transient in the preterm infant.
- Will early spasticity in infants change over time?
  Quadriparesis may increase over time; diplegia may decrease or appear less so; and monoparesis generally changes either by disappearing or progressing to hemiplegia or diplegia.

Pearls and Perils

- Use of the reflex hammer is less reliable than evaluation of tone and posture.
- Young (0–3 months) hypotonic infants may become spastic.
- Older (6–12 months) hypotonic infants tend to become less hypotonic.
- Always obtain serial head circumference measurements.
- Do not name a neurologic condition on the basis of one or two signs; most conditions comprise a constellation of signs. Some exceptions include facial nerve palsy or brachial plexus injury.
- Address parental anxiety, as their concerns are usually well founded.

Transient neuromotor abnormalities

Much of the neurologic abnormality noted in the neonatal intensive care may disappear at varying ages in infancy depending on the assessment items used by the examiner. What remains is a reasonable marker that "something" happened to the brain. In the National Collaborative Perinatal Project, children who were given a label of "suspected" cerebral palsy at 1 year and who did not have cerebral palsy at age 7 years had a significantly increased frequency of mental retardation, refractive errors, hyperactivity, and immature behavior (Nelson and Ellenberg 1982). Drillien found significantly lower scores in reading and spelling achievement, speech, and motor tasks in those children from a sample of 261 low-birth-weight infants who had transient neurologic abnormalities (Drillien and Thomson 1980). In our work, these children had an increased frequency of combinations of problems at age 7 years: cognitive deficits, motor dysfunction, learning disabilities, and behavioral problems (Ellison, et al. 1985). In all of these studies, the majority of children with transient neurologic abnormalities were normal at preschool or early school years.

Appendix: Neonatal and infant neurologic examination

The examination has been divided into four subsections: I, General description; II, Cranial nerves; III, Special situations: altered mental status and spinal lesions; and IV, Data from Premie-Neuro, NeoNeuro & Up, and Infanib scoring sheets described earlier.

I. General description

Most experienced examiners are continually assessing the baby from the initial encounter, constantly forming and reforming a "gestalt" of the neurologic condition.

Head

The size of the head is recorded, preferably at every evaluation. The initial newborn head circumference may be misleading because of molding during the birth process. Severe molding with marked overlap of the sutures should be noted and recorded. Such a neonate may be mistakenly labeled as microcephalic. We prefer a definition of microcephaly as greater than two standard deviations below the mean (approximately the 2nd percentile). Even two standard deviations is not highly predictive of mental retardation. Three standard deviations below the mean (the 0.6 percentile) is the better predictor of brain dysfunction.

A decrease of percentiles to the second percentile in the first 6 months or later may indicate severe damage to the brain through a process such as hypoxia–ischemia. Excessively rapid growth may indicate hydrocephalus, subdural hematoma effusion, tumor, or rapid brain growth.

The shape of the skull is noted, with particular attention to unusual configurations. Most of the craniosynostoses can be diagnosed by inspection, although 3-D imaging techniques are now used as well.

Infants who sleep or constantly rest their heads in the same position often get unusual head shapes, labeled positional plagiocephaly. Frequently overlooked is the rather remarkable skull configuration secondary to trauma and secondary fibrosis of the sternocleidomastoid muscle (torticollis).

The size of the anterior and posterior fontanels is noted and recorded, as is any bulging, fullness, or tension. The size of the anterior fontanels for those infants with either larger or smaller head circumference should be recorded.

For newborns, the size and location of any caput are recorded, either cephalohematoma (restricted to one section of the skull) or caput succedaneum (crossing a suture line).

The definition of a head circumference that is abnormal should be straightforward. Any head circumference two standard deviations from the mean is abnormal (macrocephaly = 98th percentile or above; microcephaly = 2nd percentile or below). In addition, inappropriately enlarging heads need attention. Both accelerations and decelerations of growth should trigger concern. Obtain an imaging study with any measurement at the 98th percentile or above. In infants less than 6 months of age, an ultrasound will define the size of the ventricles. In most hospitals, computed tomography (CT) is readily available, quick, and much more infant-friendly than in the past. Magnetic resonance imaging (MRI), however, will more precisely define brain matter.

Eyes

Conjugate deviation and repetitive nystagmus are especially good indicators of seizures. Wandering eye movements and sustained nystagmus may indicate any of several abnormalities: coma, malformation, or decreased visual acuity. Other noteworthy findings may include abnormal pupil shape, various malformations of the anterior eye (e.g., coloboma), "setting sun" sign, and conjunctival hemorrhage. Special attention must be directed to acquired signs such as nystagmus (otherwise lesions such as optic glioma, hypothalamic tumors, or metabolic disorders will be missed).

The most common eye abnormality of infancy is strabismus. Strabismus per se does not equal brain dysfunction, but infants with a history of brain insults have an increased frequency of strabismus and are at increased risk of amblyopia.

Skin

Every inch of the skin is inspected for café-au-lait spots, depigmented spots, hemangiomas, and nevi. Particularly in babies with seizures, look for neurophakomatosis. Inspect every baby for ecchymoses. The size and location of all lesions must be recorded. For all ages, trauma is an important cause; other important causes include bleeding disorders and infectious causes.

Dysmorphologic features

If the physician cannot recognize basic dysmorphologic features, diagnoses of various syndromes may be delayed. Pay attention to distance between the eyes, ear shape and placement, hair whorls, hair texture, hair line, coarseness of facial features, shortness or webbing of neck, distance between nipples, presence of a gibbus formation, pectus excavatum, dermatoglyphics, number and placement of digits, webbing of fingers or toes, contracture of joints, and malformations of the limbs. Search the findings through one of the texts of dysmorphology or computer programs. Order appropriate diagnostic tests. The expertise of a dysmorphologist may be needed for genetic counseling or for further diagnostic evaluation.

Organomegaly

The size of the organs is usually assessed quickly and may give an important clue to a neurologic diagnosis (for example, hepatomegaly may suggest glycogen storage disease).

Seizures

Attention to seizures is of key importance in the neonatal period. In infancy, obvious seizures receive immediate attention by physicians. More subtle seizures—particularly the frequent, brief extension or flexion of infantile spasms—may be delayed in both diagnosis and treatment.

Apnea

The absence or presence and approximate frequency of apnea are noted.

Brachial plexus injury

This injury is usually noted in the hospital nursery. The injury is easily distinguished from hemiparesis. Brachial plexus injuries are associated with depressed reflexes and hypotonia of the arm. Hemiparesis can be associated with facial weakness and increased tone and reflexes in both arm and leg. The timing is also different: brachial plexus injury is identified early; hemiparetic lesions tend to be identified later in the first year.

Hand preference

Asymmetry of hand fisting, especially excessive clenching versus open position, is an important indicator of hemiparesis from the neonatal period through infancy. Development of handedness at less than 1 year is another indicator of hemiparesis.

II. Cranial nerves

With an alert, conscious neonate or infant, the following examinations should be carried out.

Vision and hearing

Funduscopic examination. In the neonate, look for cataracts, retinal hemorrhages, chorioretinitis, and anomalies such as optic nerve hypoplasia. For infants who are normal developmentally, the most one usually sees is a glimpse of the outline of the passing fundi. For at-risk or neurologically abnormal infants, a more thorough examination is needed to find a "cherry-red spot," a phakoma, or chorioretinitis. Extra patience will often yield evidence for more obscure diagnoses.

Visual acuity. Ordinarily, visual acuity is not tested. However, one must test whether the neonate or infant sees. (The use of a black-and-white bull's-eye is strongly recommended for testing, especially in neonates and young infants.) Testing of cranial nerves III, IV, and VI helps assess vision in infants. For infants who do not respond, further testing is often necessary to separate decreased visual function from limited cognitive processing.

Assessment of a visual field cut, as in a hemiparetic infant, can be performed by having the child sit on the caregiver's lap. The infant's attention is first attracted by a small toy; then the examiner brings another object from behind the head and observes the infant's head turning to that object. A dangling stethoscope or tape measure works well.

Often the determination of progressive loss of visual acuity is even more difficult. The caregiver may offer clues; for example, the observation that the baby used to pick up small items (such as cereal) and no longer does.

Cranial nerves III, IV, and VI. Although a human face or red yarn ball has been recommended as a stimulus for the neonate, a black-and-white bull's-eye is preferred. By 1 month of age, most neonates should track well if care is taken to test them while they are in an alert state. The bull's-eye can also be used to check the infant's ability to focus while the examiner covers one of the infant's eyes for the cover test, then removes the cover to observe for eye movement as a test for strabismus.

Cranial nerve VIII. For infants, hearing can be tested by the response to the crinkling of paper at either ear, unobserved by the infant. Another person may speak in a low voice and call the infant's name. Or the examiner may ring a bell, again unobserved by the infant. Any neonate or infant for whom there is evidence of poor response to sound deserves further evaluation, including behavioral audiometry or measurement of brainstem auditory evoked responses or both. As with vision, either decreased hearing or decreased mental function may contribute to decreased function.

Facial

Cranial nerve V. Response to tactile or painful stimuli on the face may be used to assess the function of this nerve.

Cranial nerve VII. Facial movement is generally best observed through spontaneous facial expression. The examiner may choose to test further for facial asymmetry by flicking the bottom of the foot to stimulate a cry, if the infant has not already done so spontaneously.

Bulbar function

Cranial nerves IX, X, and XI. Testing of the gag reflex is readily done with a wooden tongue blade. The infant's ability to swallow is best evaluated by report of the caregiver or nurse.

Cranial nerve XII. Fasciculations of the tongue have been observed but may be difficult to distinguish from normal movements. Unusual tongue movements such as tongue thrusting and a large, obtrusive tongue should be noted.

III. Special situations

Altered mental status

Special attention should be directed to the cranial nerves in all neonates or infants with altered mental states. This strategy can aid in localizing the site or sites of central nervous system injury. The degree of alteration should be noted.

Pupillary responses to light. Constricted pupils generally indicate brainstem dysfunction. Conversely, the dilated, poorly responsive pupil or pupils may indicate increased intracranial pressure owing to third-nerve compression.

Corneal reflexes. The examiner holds the lids apart and uses a small wisp of cotton to touch the cornea and elicit the reflex. Absence indicates brainstem dysfunction.

Doll's eyes (oculocephalic) reflex. The so-called doll's eyes reflex is the most readily elicited response indicating brainstem dysfunction. The baby's head is turned from side to side. Failure of the eyes to move so as to maintain midposition indicates brainstem dysfunction. Note that this is true only when unresponsive or comatose. Older infants, when alert, will focus or fix their gaze voluntarily.

Gag reflex. In the comatose baby, the gag reflex, when absent, also reflects brainstem dysfunction.

Spontaneous respirations. Clinicians have long used the presence and vigor of spontaneous respirations as an indicator of brainstem dysfunction.

Spinal cord

For the neonate or infant with suspected or obvious spinal cord lesion, such as myelomeningocele, further testing is mandatory.

Sensation to touch or pinprick. When a sensory level is sought, pinprick testing is most effective. This should be done with care, as the skin of the neonate, and even of the infant, may be readily marred by pinprick. Several examiners may wish to watch a single examination rather than each performing separate trials. The testing should be done under optimal circumstances. The baby should be quiet Testing should begin distally and proceed proximally.

Sweating. The level of a cord lesion may also be detected by the observance of abnormal sweating, but this method is less precise for localization.

Stream of urination. Observation of the stream is preferable. Percussion of the bladder outline may help confirm suspicions of a neurogenic bladder. Further information about infants may be gained from questioning the mother about the stream and the length of periods for which the diaper is dry. Constant dribbling also often indicates a neurogenic bladder.

Anal wink. Testing for anal wink is done with a pin. In general, this is reserved for infants about whom there is concern about a cord lesion.

Colon function. Decreased colon innervation generally results in constipation such that the bowel becomes distended and filled with feces. Then there may be recurrent diarrhea-like stools. The combination of a history of constipation and palpation of the abdomen for firm lumps of stool generally yields the correct interpretation. Many infants with abnormal neurologic function, particularly those with poor spontaneous movements, have constipation or less-frequent stools. They do not necessarily have poor innervation of the colon. As in most neurologic diagnoses, the constellation of findings yields the correct localization of the lesion.

IV. Scored Assessment Instruments

See Premie-Neuro, NeoNeuro, and Infanib discussed earlier. Contact donna.daily@vanderbilt.edu for scoring sheets.

Annotated bibliography

Amiel-Tison C, Grenier A. *Neurological assessment during the first year of life*. New York: Oxford University Press, 1986.
An explanation of the French angles, plus additional items that two very experienced examiners have incorporated into their examinations over the years. For those with less experience, the assimilation of the many items for an overall "picture" of the infant may be less clear.

Ellison P. The infant neurological examination. In: M Wolraich, DK Routh, eds. *Advances in developmental and behavioral pediatrics*. London: Jessica Kingsley Publishers, 1990; Volume 9: 75–138.
Details the reasoning for more reliable, mathematically coherent neurologic assessments of infants.

Ellison P. *The Infanib: A reliable method for the neuromotor assessment of infants*. Tucson: Therapy Skill Builders, 1994.
Manual providing a large number of photographs about the neurologic examination of infants.

CHAPTER 3

The Neurologic Examination of the Young Child

Ruth D. Nass

Outline

- The seated examination
- The sensory examination
- The standing examination
- The prone or supine examination
- Seated assessment of the head
- Office measures
- Evaluation

The goal of this chapter is to review the neurologic and developmental/psychometric assessment of the toddler and preschool child. The reader is provided with a prototypic examination and the rationale behind it. Because no toddler or preschooler will cooperate for the entire examination, Table 3.1 provides a basic examination that, if completed, will provide sufficient information for most purposes.

Touwen and Prechtl's 1970 monograph *The Neurological Examination of the Child with Minor Central Nervous System Dysfunction* remains a classic. Some general suggestions about the approach to the examination of the younger child deserve mention at the outset. As children generally dislike being undressed for examination, this should be done in stages and as necessary. Remove shoes and socks immediately, so that movements of the feet and legs can be monitored throughout. At some point, the child must be completely undressed to look for skin markings diagnostic of a neurocutaneous syndrome. A Wood's lamp examination for less visible ash leaf spots should be considered, especially in an autistic child. Inspection of the head, as well as that of the hands and feet, should include assessment for the minor physical anomalies (Table 3.2). High anomaly scores in preschoolers may correlate with conduct problems and hyperactivity at school age (Waldrup et al. 1968). Head circumference should also be measured, since there is an increased frequency of macro- and microcephaly in children with developmental disabilities. Macrocephaly should be pursued for potentially treatable causes like hydrocephalus and for genetic causes like fragile X chromosome disorder. Special attention should be paid to the motor function of the child with macrocephaly, since these children are at increased risk for both gross and fine motor dysfunction (Lewis et al. 1989; Nevo et al. 2002).

Touwen and Prechtl (1970) are very specific about the order of the neurologic examination in the preschool child. While the history is being taken from the parent(s), the child can be observed as she plays with toys. The seated examination is performed first (with a young child often sitting in the parent's lap), followed in order by those parts of the examination that are performed in the standing position, those dealing with locomotion, any part of the examination requiring a prone or supine position, and finally the examination of the head (Table 3.1).

The seated examination

Spontaneous motility

Spontaneous gross and fine motility is assessed over a 3-minute period while taking the history from the parents. Both the quantity and quality of movements are assessed, each on a scale of 0–3. Speed, smoothness, and adequacy are the qualitative parameters. High scores in the quantity domain suggest attentional difficulties. Note, however, that the diagnosis of attention deficit hyperactivity disorder (ADHD) is based on parent and teacher assessments of behavior, not office behavior.

Table 3.1 Soft-sign examination in the preschool child

Sitting assessment

1. Spontaneous motility (3-minute observation)
2. Muscle power, tone, and mass
3. Reflexes
4. Sensory examination: finger localization, double simultaneous stimulation, graphesthesia, stereoagnosis

Standing assessment

1. Posture
2. Spontaneous motility (2-minute observation)
3. Posture with arms extended palms up and palms down
4. Assessment for involuntary movements (Prechtl sign)
5. Mouth opening/finger spreading phenomenon
6. Diadochokinesis and associated movements
7. Finger-to-nose test
8. Fingertip touching test
9. Finger opposition test
10. Standing with eyes closed

Assessment of gait and station

1. Gait
2. Walking a straight line
3. Walking on tiptoes
4. Walking on heels
5. One-foot stand
6. Hopping on one foot
7. Catch a ball
8. Trunk

Prone or supine assessment

1. Examine spine
2. Knee-heel test
3. Sitting up without the use of the hands

Sitting assessment of the head

1. Musculature of face
2. Eyes
3. Ears
4. Mouth

Table 3.2 Anomalies seen with attention deficit hyperactivity disorder (ADHD)

Head

1. Electric hair
2. Very fine hair that will not comb down
3. Fine hair that is soon awry after combing
4. Two or more whorls

Eyes

1. Epicanthus (where upper and lower lids join nose point of union)
   Deeply covered
   Partly covered
2. Hypertelorism: approximate distance between tear ducts:
   Greater than or equal to 1½ inches
   Between 1¼ and 1½ inches

Ears

1. Low-seated ears
2. Bottom of ears in line with
   Mouth (or lower)
   Area between mouth and nose
3. Adherent lobes
4. Lower edges of ears extend
   Upward and back toward crown of head
   Straight back toward rear of neck
5. Malformed ears
6. Asymmetric ears
7. Soft and pliable ears

Mouth

1. High palate
2. Roof of mouth
   Definitely steepled
   Flat and narrow at the top
3. Furrowed tongue (one with deep ridges)
4. Smooth or rough spots on tongue

Hands

1. Fifth finger
   Markedly curved inward toward other fingers
   Slightly curved inward toward other fingers
2. Single transverse palmar crease
3. Index finger longer than middle finger

Feet

1. Third toe
   Definitely longer than second toe
   Appears equal in length to second toe
2. Partial syndactyly of two middle toes
3. Gap between first and second toe (greater than or equal to ¼ in)

Muscle power

Muscle power, tone, and mass are assessed in the same fashion as in the older child. Often functional assessment of the legs during gait maneuvers proves more useful than standard push-pull testing.

Assessment of reflexes

Reflex assessment is standard. Younger children sometimes show spread, for example, to the adductors when the knee is tapped, which is not necessarily pathologic. Touwen and Prechtl suggest that the plantar reflex be elicited by stroking with a sharp object or a thumbnail from toe to heel. The reverse technique prevents eliciting a grasp reflex as one approaches the toes.

The sensory examination

Although the sensory examination is difficult to perform in the young child, it is vital in providing information about the early development of sensory functions.

Finger localization

Many 3-year-olds (the percentages indicated in parentheses) and almost all 4- and 5-year-olds can oppose the thumb to the finger touched by the examiner (85%), find the fingers touched by the examiner with the contralateral hand (75%), oppose the thumb to the finger pointed to by the examiner (70%), find the fingers pointed to by the examiner with the contralateral hand (65%), and oppose the thumb to the finger indicated by the examiner while the subject's view is obstructed (50%) (Lefford et al. 1974). Finger imitation skills can be assessed in the 4- to 6-year-old (Levine & Schneider 1985). Sitting opposite the child, the examiner opposes his thumb to another finger on the same hand, holding that position for 5–8 seconds while the child imitates. Mirror movements and dyskinesias (opposition movements that are slow to release) should be noted. Children who require excessive visual input of their own hand movements may have true finger agnosia. Most 4- to 6-year-olds will perform correctly on three to four trials. Most 5-year-olds can even oppose the thumb to the proximal, distal, or middle phalanx of each finger when it is touched by the examiner out of the child's view (uncrossed localization) (Galin et al. 1977). However, most children are unable to perform a crossed localization task, that is, touch the homologous spot on the opposite hand with the opposite thumb, until age 8 or 9. Difficulty with crossed localization is also seen in disconnection syndromes caused by surgical section of the corpus callosum. The young child may indeed look functionally acallosal in some respects. The more classic finger agnosia tasks of "How many fingers were touched, one or two?" and "How many between?" are too difficult for the preschooler. They are performed by only 30% and 15%, respectively, of 5-year-olds, 45% and 30% of 6-year-olds, and 85% and 65% of almost-7-year-olds (Kinsbourne & Warrington 1963).

Finger localization skill in kindergarten predicts reading and arithmetic achievement at the end of the first grade (Lindgren 1978). Normal somatosensory system maturation may play a role in optimizing academic achievement. Furthermore, children with finger localization problems may try to compensate by adopting an awkward pencil grip with resultant dysgraphia (Levine 1985). It is interesting that finger localization difficulties in the preschooler can cause dysgraphia and predict later arithmetic skill, because finger agnosia, dysgraphia, and dyscalculia are three of the four deficits (right–left disorientation the other) seen in Gerstmann syndrome, which occurs in 2% of school-age children (Suresh & Sebastian 2000).

Double simultaneous stimulation

Extinction to face on double simultaneous stimulation of hand and face is common in the child until about age 10 years, presumably because the face is more elaborately represented and because the facial sensory pathways mature earlier than those of the hand. In the preschool child, there is also a right–left distinction, with the testable child (sometimes as young as 2 years old) being more likely to extinguish the stimulus presented to the left hand, when right and left are touched simultaneously (Kinsbourne & Hicks 1978). Asymmetric lateralization of attention may be a phase of normal development (Roeltgen et al. 1986).

Graphesthesia

In the preschool child, a matching format test in which the child picks out from drawings of a circle, line, square, and cross, the shape that has been made on her preferred hand can be used (Levine & Schneider 1985). Three of four correct is the norm for the 4- to 6-year-old.

Stereoagnosis

Using duplicate shaped pieces of wood, stereoagnosis can be tested in the preschooler (Levine & Schneider 1985). One by one, the forms are placed in the child's fisted hand and she is asked to pick visually the matching form. Most 4- to 6-year-olds will identify three of the four.

The standing examination

Posture

The posture of the preschooler differs from that of the older child. The 2-year-old has a rather broad-based stance and often postures the arms even when just standing in place. The 3-year-old has a slightly broad-based stance. The 5-year-old holds her body straight, and the base is narrow.

Spontaneous motility

Spontaneous motility is assessed in the standing position for 2 minutes, while the child is "standing around waiting for things to happen." Many preschoolers move around during a 2-minute observation period.

Posture with extended arms

Posture is checked in both the palms-up and the palms-down position for 20 seconds. The 2-year-old's arms drift

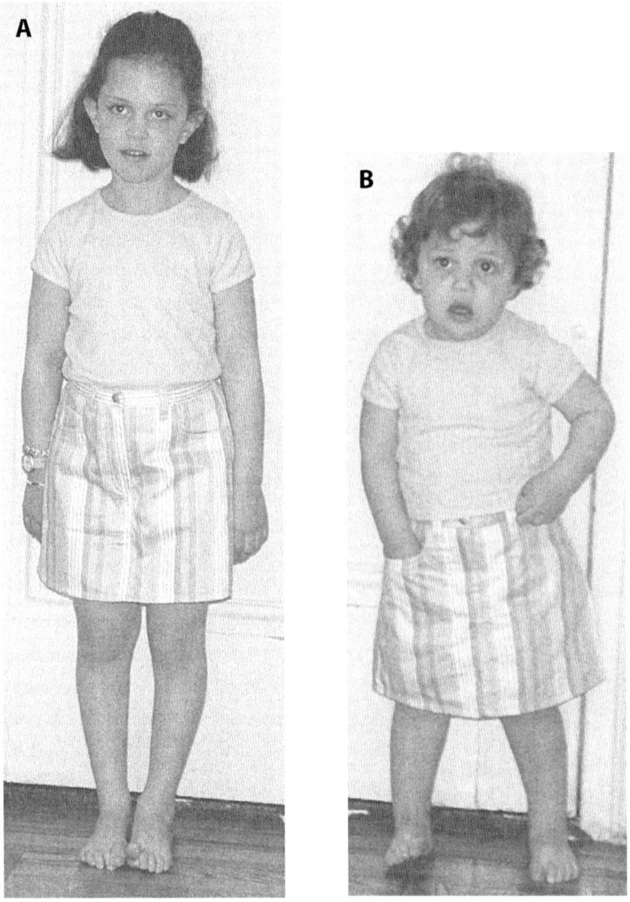

Figure 3.1 (A) The 5-year-old holds her body straight and her base is narrow. Note the spontaneous striatal toe here, presumably reflecting a relatively immature basal ganglia. Photo by Nora Gross. (B) The 2-year-old has a rather broad-based stance and often postures the arms even when just standing in place. The feet are not always flat on the ground.

up and down, as well as flexing at the elbows. The 3-year-old preschooler's arms tend to drift in the direction of the palms and to be laterally displaced on both tasks by 30–60 degrees. The older preschooler's arm doesn't drift up or down, but the child clearly has to concentrate to maintain a straight arm position. Spooning of the wrist and hands is often present through age 5 years.

Assessment for involuntary movements

Assessment for involuntary movements, including the Prechtl sign, is only accurate if the child can maintain a quiet standing position for 2 minutes (i.e., passes the initial motility test). Thus, a reliable result is unlikely in the child under 4 years. To assess for choreiform movements, the child stands with feet together and with the fingers of the pronated outstretched hands apart for 20 seconds. Under 6 years, the eyes are open, over 6, the eyes are closed. The Prechtl sign is probably very common.

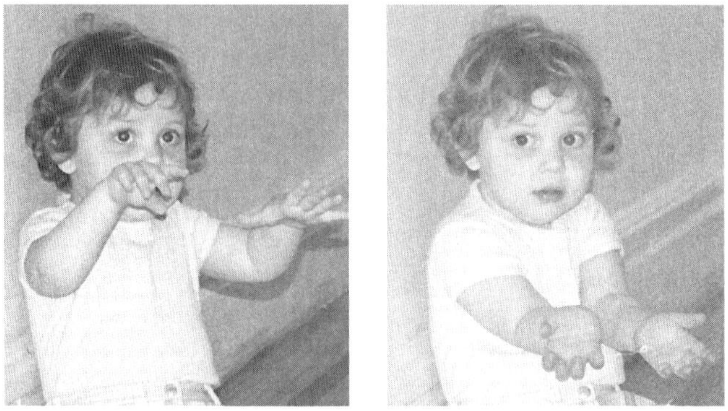

Figure 3.2 The 2-year-old's arms drift up and down, as well as flexing at the elbows. The hands take on cupped and capped positions. Photo by Nora Gross.

Overflow movements

Examination for overflow movements is an important part of the soft sign assessment. *Overflow movements*, *associated movements*, and *synkinesis* are defined as movements occurring in parts of the body other than the part attempting the task; they may be symmetric (mirror) or asymmetric. Overflow is common in young children and disappears around age 10 (Connolly & Stratton 1968), reflecting maturational changes in the motor system.

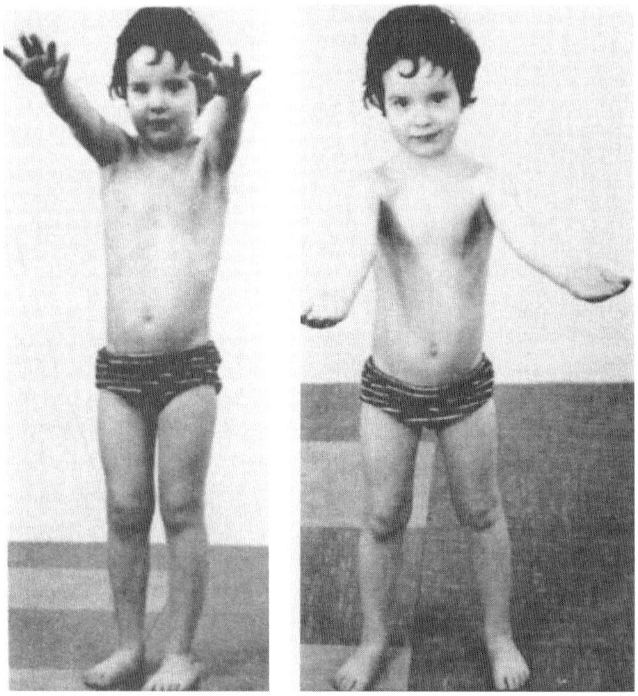

Figure 3.3 The 3-year-old preschooler's arms tend to drift in the direction of the palms and to be laterally displaced on both tasks by 30–60 degrees. Reproduced with permission from Touwen BC, Prechtl HFR. *The neurological examination of the child with minor central nervous system dysfunction*. London: Spastics International, 1970.

For example, the crossed pyramid motor system, mediating rapid independent finger movements, matures later than the less specific medial motor system, which provides proximal limb and ipsilateral motor innervation. The uncrossed motor pathways may function tonically during childhood, resulting in mirror movements. With maturation, these noncrossing pathways come under the inhibitory control of the contralateral hemisphere via the corpus callosum (Dennis 1976; Nass 1985). Myelination of the corpus callosum is largely completed at about the same time that mirror movements disappear around the age of 10 years (Yakovlev & LeCours 1967).

Touwen and Prechtl (1970) suggest three tasks for assessing overflow and mirror movements: mouth opening/finger spreading, diadochokinesis, and the finger opposition test. The first task requires the child to open her mouth, close her eyes, and stick out her tongue while the extended arms, with hands and wrists relaxed, are supported by the examiner. The response of spreading the fingers is marked in the preschooler and muted by age 7–8 years. The second and third tasks are standard parts of the neurologic assessment of cerebellar and motor function, respectively. On the diadochokinesis task, the preschooler will often mirror in the opposite limb. Associated movements are scored as follows: 0, none; 1, barely visible or slight elbow flexion; 2, mirror movements without elbow flexion; 3, mirror movements with elbow flexion. On Denckla's (1973, 1974) time-for-20 version of this task, about 20% of 5-year-olds evidence mirroring (Wolff et al. 1983). The finger opposition test has been described by Touwen and Prechtl as five sequences to and fro of thumb to 2, 3, 4, 5, 4, 3, 2, 3, 4, 5, and so on, and by Denckla (1973, 1974; Rudel et al. 1984) as time to do 20 movements; that is, five sequences of thumb to 2, 3, 4, 5, 2, 3, 4, 5, and so on. Although excellent for bringing out associated movements (65–90% of 5-year-olds show mirroring; Wolff et al. 1983), these tests are often too difficult for children under 5 years. Denckla's time-for-20 finger tapping task, thumb-to-index finger, can be performed by many children 3 years old and is, at least for the younger child, a good task for uncovering the overflow (30–45% of 5-year-olds show mirroring; Wolff et al. 1983), as well as looking at fine motor function. A number of other tasks have also been used to assess for associated movements, including clip pinching, finger spreading, and finger lifting (Wolff et al. 1983). Of these, only index finger lifting (passed by about 50% of 5-year-olds) would be a useful preschool measure. Interestingly, there is little difference between dominant- and nondominant-hand performance for clip pinching and finger spreading at any age. Thus, an asymmetry here might be a useful marker of a hemisyndrome, unlike a number of other gross and fine motor skills, for which dominance effects are common until age 7 years.

Cerebellar function

Tests of cerebellar function that Touwen and Prechtl (1970) perform in the standing position include diadochokinesis, the finger/nose test (the preschooler requires visual guidance and needs to hold her arm against the body for stabilization), the fingertip touching test, and standing with eyes closed for 15 seconds. Obvious asymmetries of function are suggestive of ipsilateral cerebellar disease. On the diadochokinesis task, the regularity of the movements and the presence of elbow movements are scored (Touwen & Prechtl 1970). It is the exception rather than the rule for the preschooler to perform this task with precision. Pronounced deviation of the elbow during rapid alternating movements, rather than maintaining the action at the wrist, suggests overuse of proximal musculature around the shoulder. In most children, right arm performance is better than left (Njiokikjien et al. 1986). However, Denckla (1974) found little asymmetry on a time-for-20 pronation/supination task.

Assessment of gait and station

The standing examination is followed by an evaluation of gait (Touwen & Prechtl 1970). Children under 6 years generally show little arching of the foot when walking and little arm swing. The 2- to 4-year-old should have minimal gait asymmetry. The 2-year-old may have a lunging gait. The normal gait width after age 3 is 11–20 cm. Narrowing may result from hypertonia of the leg adductors and widening from hypotonia or sensory or cerebellar disease. Children under 7 years may have difficulty

Pearls and Perils

- A position-oriented neurologic examination may be more useful in the preschooler than the classic systems-oriented examination.
- A Babinski reflex elicited from toe to heel avoids a false-negative result from the masking of a true Babinski sign by the grasp reflex, which is often still apparent in the toddler.
- Assessment for overflow movements can provide an index of neural maturation even in the preschooler, given the correct elicitation procedures. Excess overflow may be a marker of later learning disabilities.
- Gait and heel-and-toe walking are excellent sources of information about the neurologic status of the preschooler.
- Preschoolers often show dominance effects in both gross and fine motor skills. Beware of overcalling a left hemisyndrome.

with prolonged tandem walking. Difficulty with very simple line walking at age 4 is a risk factor for both hyperactivity and the neurologic soft sign syndromes at age 7 (Nichols & Chen 1981).

Children over 3 years should be able to walk on tiptoes. Any movements in upper extremities and face not present during the standard gait examination are counted as associated movements. Diminishing degrees of extension of arms, ventriflexion of the hands, and lip and tongue movements are seen through age 7 years. Clenching of the fists is counted as an associated movement only if the arms are also extended. About 25% of 5-year-olds evidence overflow (Wolff et al. 1983). Heel walking can also be performed by children over 3 years. Again, any movements not seen during the normal walk are considered associated movements. They occur in about 50–80% of 5-year-olds (Wolff et al. 1983). Associated movements noted during heel walking persist longer, sometimes until 10 years, than do associated movements noted with toe walking. Arms are extended and wrists are dorsiflexed. Poor performance may also reflect hypotonia, paresis, or both. Paresis of the peroneal muscles may occur without other muscles being impaired to the same degree (Touwen & Prechtl 1970). Such children will walk on the outer side of the foot rather than the heels. Even children with mild spastic diplegia have trouble heel walking.

The ability to stand on one leg develops suddenly and matures rapidly. At 3 years, only a few children can stand on one leg for more than a few seconds. The one-foot stand can be sustained for 10 seconds by a 4-year-old given a couple of false starts (Levine & Schneider 1985). By 5 years, most children can sustain the one-foot stand for about 10 seconds. There may be a marked difference between the performance on the dominant and the non-dominant leg between ages 4 and 5 years, a finding that does not usually indicate a hemiparesis. Hopping on one foot also develops suddenly and matures rapidly. At 3 years, only a few children are able to hop at all, and then only on the dominant foot. At age 4 years, five to eight hops are normal, and at age 5 years, nine to 12. Prior to the age of 7 years, one leg is generally better than the other, although, as with the one-foot stand, the better leg may not be the one preferred for athletics. When the asymmetry is marked, the possibility of a hemiparesis must be considered. Among a group of 150 5-year-olds, 28% hopped more than 13 times on their left leg and 39% hopped more than 13 times on their right leg (Touwen & Prechtl 1970). In the National Collaborative Perinatal Project Study failure at age 4 on a hopping task was a risk factor for both hyperactivity and the neurologic soft sign syndromes at age 7 years (Nichols & Chen 1981).

Ability to catch a ball can be assessed in the preschooler. The average 4- to 6-year-old will catch a 2-inch ball in three to four of five tries (Levine & Schneider 1985). Associated movements of the face should be noted since they are not present in most preschoolers. In the National Collaborative Perinatal Project Study failure at age 4 years on a ball catch task was a risk factor for the neurologic soft sign syndromes at age 7 years (Nichols & Chen 1981).

In general, motor system maturation often correlates with overall functioning at school age and beyond (Blondis et al. 1993; Gillberg 1989; Kadesjo & Gillberg 1999). In one study of children at the time of school entry, four motor tests (standing on one foot, Fog test, design copying, and diadochokinesis) combined with a brief structured clinical observation and a structured parent interview identified 80% of children with disorders of attention, motor, and perception (DAMP)—and all those with severe DAMP—as well as a small number of false positives (Landgren et al. 2000).

The prone or supine examination

Touwen and Prechtl (1970) begin this phase of the assessment by inspecting the spine. This is followed by inspecting the posture of the feet, legs, and hip joints. A 5-year-old can perform a sit up without using the hands only by lifting the legs off the table, whereas by age 7 years the legs stay in contact with the table, another marker of diminishing overflow.

Seated assessment of the head

Musculature of the face

Assessment of the head begins with inspection of the musculature of the face for asymmetry at rest, during voluntary movement, and during an emotional response. Peripheral lesions of the seventh nerve affect both the upper and lower face. After early injuries, improvement is often accompanied by synkinesias like crocodile tears. Bilateral facial nerve palsies are often the most prominent finding in the Mobius sequence, which consists, in addition, of gaze palsies, esotropia, and sometimes abnormalities of cranial nerves IX–XII. Generally, children present with feeding problems, lack of facial expression, and articulation difficulties (Smith 2006; Stromland et al. 2002). Central upper motor neuron seventh nerve deficits involve primarily the lower face, as the upper face is bilaterally innervated. The subcortically mediated emotional smile is relatively spared by supranuclear pathology, whereas with peripheral palsies the emotional smile is equally as impaired as the voluntary smile. Congenital absence of the depressor muscle of the mouth should not be confused with a facial palsy. In this disorder, the abnormal side of the mouth is not pulled down when the child cries and the resting face is relatively normal. The side that appears to droop during crying is really the normal side. The diagnosis is important, as the incidence of associated abnormalities, particularly cardiac, is high (Nelson & Eng 1972).

Eyes and ears

The examination of the eyes includes an assessment for strabismus. About 5% of normal children and about 50% of children with brain damage have strabismus. Strabismus is classified in several ways. Heterophoria is a latent condition that is brought out only in certain circumstances like fatigue and testing. A heterotropia is constantly present and may be either exo- (outward) or eso- (inward) in the horizontal direction or hyper- or hypo- in the vertical direction. Strabismus may be alternating, with the fixating eye switching back and forth, or it may be monocular. In monocular strabismus, the involved eye is at risk for a disuse amblyopia, since the immature nervous system can suppress fixation in order to prevent diplopia. Paralytic or noncomitant strabismus is due to paresis of one or more extraocular muscles. It is worst on gaze into the field of the affected muscle, and diplopia may be a symptom. Acquired paralytic strabismus raises concern for intracranial pathology. The one exception is the benign sixth-nerve palsy, which is sometimes seen in children in a parainfectious setting. This is, however, a diagnosis of exclusion. (Imaging should be performed to rule out intracranial pathology). Congenital paralytic strabismus is usually caused by developmental defects of the extraocular system or birth trauma. Nonparalytic or comitant strabismus is the more common type. Extraocular muscles function normally, and the defect is equal in all directions of gaze. Sometimes nonparalytic strabismus is due to underlying ocular or visual pathology; mostly it is idiopathic. Pseudostrabismus must be differentiated from true strabismus. The former is a reflection of certain anatomic variations like prominent epicanthal folds, a broad and flat nasal bridge, and hypertelorism. Two simple tests can be used to identify strabismus. In the Hirschberg test, the symmetry of the corneal reflex is documented. In the cover/uncover and cross/cover tests the eyes are observed for refixation movements. With the child fixing on a distant target, alternately covering the two eyes elicits no movement. With esotropia, the deviating eye will move outward as the fixating eye is occluded; with exotropia the deviating eye will move inward as the fixating eye is occluded. With a phoria, the occluded eye tends to deviate, because binocular vision is temporarily disrupted, and refixation will be seen at the moment of uncovering.

Extraocular motility is then assessed. Congenital anomalies of the oculomotor system are often not brought to the attention of the physician until the preschool years. Distinguishing between congenital and acquired oculomotor problems has obvious therapeutic implications; old photographs are often very useful for this purpose. The Duane retraction syndrome is of three types, all involving retraction of the globe and narrowing of the lid fissure on attempted adduction: (a) palsy of abduction with retraction on adduction, (b) palsy of adduction with retraction and intact abduction, and (c) palsy of adduction and abduction with retraction on attempted adduction. Occasionally, the Duane retraction syndrome is mistaken for an acquired sixth-nerve palsy; however, diplopia is rare with congenital palsies (Glaser 2000). In Brown tendon sheath syndrome, upgaze in the adducted position is restricted even during forced duction owing to the absence of the inferior oblique and thickening of the superior oblique tendon sheath. The deficit may be intermittent and even disappear during adulthood (Glaser 2000). A double elevator palsy has also been reported, involving both inferior oblique and superior rectus muscles. A homolateral ptosis is present, but there is no diplopia and the pupil is spared. Preservation of the Bell phenomenon suggests that this is a supranuclear problem (Glaser 2000). The Marcus Gunn jaw-winking phenomenon is a congenital trigeminal oculomotor synkinesis involving jaw and lid that is due to anomalous innervation. Generally the disorder presents in infancy as a (usually left) unilateral ptosis that jerks rhythmically upward during nursing. The jaw-winking phenomenon is an exaggeration of a normally existing reflex. The phenomenon often disappears over time. Congenital fourth-nerve palsies are not uncommon and are often uncovered after minor head trauma. Review of old photographs will reveal the compensatory head tilt—head away from, chin toward the side of the paretic superior oblique muscle. Examination of extraocular motility is concluded by assessment of the child's ability to converge. Accommodative esotropia tends to appear most commonly in the preschool years. This disorder is a reflection of excessive accommodation with overconvergence.

The pupils should then be examined. Anisocoria, which may actually have been congenital, is sometimes not noted until the toddler years. In general, anisocoria in which the difference is maintained in different illuminations is not pathologic; however, anisocoria that increases or diminishes when the light changes should be considered pathologic. If the pupillary difference is more pronounced in bright light, it is the larger pupil that is abnormal; if the anisocoria is worse in dim light, it is the smaller pupil that is abnormal. In Horner syndrome, seen for example with a brachial plexus palsy, anisocoria is more marked in dim light (which puts demands on the abnormal dilator mechanism) than in bright light (which puts demands on the intact constrictor mechanism) (Glaser 2000). If Horner syndrome occurs before age 2, the iris is often hypopigmented.

The examination of the pupils is followed by an assessment of acuity and of the visual fields. Acuity can be measured in the toddler using a finger-mimicking game with alternating eye occlusion. The acuity is recorded as finger counting at X feet (20 feet equals 20/200, 40 feet equals 20/100) and is limited only by the distance that the examiner can stand from the child (Glaser 2000). Visual fields can be measured in the preschooler by finger mimicking of one, two, or five fingers flashed by the examiner. When fixation is a problem, the face may be turned so that the abducted eye can be moved no further toward the right or left (Glaser 2000).

Auditory acuity is then assessed with a ticking watch. The tongue and pharyngeal arches are inspected (cranial nerves IX–XII). Finally, the funduscopic examination is performed.

Mental status

Much information about the child's cognitive functioning can be gleaned from observation during the neurologic examination. Attentional difficulties for example, are seen as an inability to stick with such tasks as motor stance or heel or toe walking. An impression about the child's general language skills can be gleaned from her contribution to the history and ability to follow verbal requests during the examination. However, a formal assessment of higher cortical function should nonetheless be attempted. The assessment of higher cortical function in the preschooler is limited not only by the availability of appropriate measures, but by the cooperation of the child and the patience of the examiner. However, it is generally possible for the neurologist to get an impression of the child's functioning in the office and to obtain supporting and elaborating data from a psychometrician, neuropsychologist, and/or speech and language pathologist. In this chapter, useful office measures for assessing the preschooler will be discussed.

Office measures

Historic

Although historic data are potentially biased by the parent/historian, the advantages in the preschool-age group are temporal proximity and the cooperative nature of the informant. The Anser system, developed by Levine (1996), includes parent and teacher questionnaires for the 3- to 5-year-old. Although it is biased toward behavioral issues, a useful medical and developmental history can also be obtained using the parent questionnaire. The Denver Developmental Screening Test (DDST-II, Frankenburg & Dodds 2002) is a classic tool for assessing development in the personal–social, fine motor, language, and gross motor domains. By and large, except for the personal–social domain, assessment beyond 2 years requires the cooperation of the child. However, a prescreening developmental questionnaire filled out by the parent identifies over 80% of non-normal DDSTs (Frankenburg et al. 1987). An abnormal DDST predicts school problems at the end of the first grade with 84% accuracy (Sturner et al. 1985). However, the DDST is not as sensitive to speech and language problems as some specific language inventories (Glascoe et al. 1992) (discussed later). The Early Screening Inventory (Meisels et al. 1997) for 3- to 6-year-old children and their parents and the Developmental Assessment of Young Children (Voress & Maddox 2003) are both new instruments that can be used in the office to perform a general developmental screen.

Language

Table 3.3 lists pertinent questions to ask the parents of preschoolers suspected of experiencing language delay (Schwartz & Murphy 1975). Tables 3.4 and 3.5 list anticipated 50th-percentile receptive and expressive language milestones from ages 1–5 years. Assessment of language functioning using these milestones provides a general idea of language level. Additional information can

Table 3.3 Pertinent questions to ask parents of preschool children with suspected language disorders

Key questions	Likely parent responses
1. How old was your child when he began to speak his first words?	24 months or older
2. How old was your child when she began to put words into sentences?	36 months or older
3. Does your child have difficulty learning new vocabulary words?	Yes
4. Does your child omit words from sentences (e.g., do his sentences sound telegraphic)?	Yes
5. Does your child speak in short or incomplete sentences?	Yes
6. Does your child have trouble with verbs such as *is, am, are, was,* and *were*?	Yes
7. Does your child have difficulty following directions?	Yes
8. Does your child seem to have difficulty in understanding you if you use long sentences?	Yes
9. Does your child respond appropriately to questions?	No
10. Does your child ask questions beginning with *who, what, where,* and *why*?	No
11. Does your child use present and past tense verbs correctly?	No
12. Does it seem that your child has made little or no progress in speech and language in the last 6–12 months?	Yes
13. Does your child omit sounds from her words?	Yes
14. Do you feel your child's speech is more difficult to understand than it should be in view of his age?	Yes
15. Does it seem as though your child uses t, d, k, or g in place of most other consonants when she speaks?	Yes

Table 3.4 Receptive language skills

Years	Expected abilities of a child at this age
1	Understands "Where is mother?"
1½	Points to one body part
1½	Follows two-step commands two times out of three (*me spoon/mom ball, me ball/mom spoon, mom ball/cup me*)
2	Knows six body parts
2–2½	Understands concept of "one"
2½	Points to spoon, ball, cup by use
3	Recognizes day and night
3½	Knows three out of four prepositions (*on, under, in front, behind*)
4	Recognizes colors
4–4½	Understands concept of "three"
4½–5	Identifies right and left on self

be gleaned from observations of communicative language use (pragmatics). Considering language in terms of its subcomponents of phonology, syntax, and semantics, and evaluating prosody and pragmatics may provide the skilled clinician with enough information to make a subtype diagnosis from among the developmental language disorders (see Chapter 23). Achenbach & Rescorla (2000) have recently developed and validated a brief screening checklist language inventory for 2-year-olds, which can be used to document the presence of an at least 50-word vocabulary and at least some two-word phrases. Coplan's (1987) Early Language Milestone Scale is useful through age 3 years. The clinical adaptive test/clinical linguistic auditory milestone scales (CAT/CLAMS), which can be administered in the office from ages 1–36 months, are both sensitive and specific to mental retardation and correlate well with Bayley scale scores of mental development (Capute & Accardo 2005; Hoon et al. 1993). To obtain a measure of receptive vocabulary skills that correlates with overall language status, the Peabody Picture Vocabulary Test (Dunn & Dunn 2005) can be administered from 2.5 years on by secretary, nurse, or physician. The Pediatric Extended Examination at Three (PEET) and Pediatric Examination of Educational Readiness (PEER) (Levine & Schneider 1985; Blackman et al. 1986) have language subtests—including spatial directions, complex sentences, categories, temporal directions, word span, and rote language skills (e.g., counting, days)—that can be used in isolation or in conjunction with the whole examination for the 3- to 6-year-old. The Preschool Language Scale (Zimmerman et al. 2006) provides a more specific and extensive assessment of language, but also takes longer to administer.

Table 3.5 Expressive language skills

Years	Expected abilities of a child at this age
1	Knows two to four single words
1½	Uses two-word sentences
2	Refers to self by name
2–2½	Uses plurals, *I*
2–2½	Converses in sentences
2½–3	Gives full name
3–3½	Comprehends *cold, tired, hungry*
3–3½	Can draw opposite analogies two times out of three (*fire/ice; mother/father; horse/mouse*)
4	Comprehends senses
4½–5	Defines words correctly six times out of nine (ball, lake, desk, house, banana, curtain, ceiling, hedge, pavement)

Visual-spatial and motor

Tables 3.6 and 3.7 list anticipated 50th-percentile gross and fine motor milestones from ages 1–5. Attention should be paid to crayon-holding posture. Egan (1990) describes several early grasps: (a) supinate (pencil grasped at the distal end and often held vertically; present from 18 months but virtually gone by 36 months); (b) pronate (pencil is grasped in the middle of its length with flexed fingers and thumb gone at 42 months); and (c) tripod (pencil held near to the point with thumb, index, and middle fingers functioning together). This grasp is used by 50% of children from 36 months onward. Eighty percent of children have a tripod grasp at 48 months. The preschooler uses a rigid tripod, with the thumb opposed to index finger supported by middle finger, but without flexion extension of the interphalangeal joints, which becomes a dynamic tripod at age 6–7 years.

The Developmental Test of Visual Motor Integration (Beery & Buktenica 2003) can be administered in the office starting at age 2 years. The PEET and PEER (Levine & Schneider 1985; Blackman et al. 1986) have visuomotor subtests including visual matching, copying figures,

Table 3.6 Motor milestones

Years	Expected abilities of a child at this age
1½	Walks up steps, throws overhand
2	Tricycles
2½	Balances on one leg for 1 second
3	Toe and heel walks
3½	Balances for 5 seconds
4	Hops, tandems
5	Hops 10 times
6	Tandems well

Table 3.7 Visuospatial and visuomotor milestones

Years	Typical abilities of a child at this age
1	Scribbles
2	Copies vertical line
2½	Copies circle
3½	Copies +, draws circle, Humpty-Dumpty
4½	Draws square, oblique lines, 6-part person
5–6	Draws triangle, 10-part person
6–7	Draws diamond

and drawing from memory that can be used in isolation or in conjunction with the whole examination for ages 3–6 years. Having a child draw a person is a simple way to monitor development. Egan (1990) suggests that there are three main stages of development in drawing the human figure by the preschooler: (a) "Humpty-Dumpty" has a head and arms and legs are on the head; (b) intermediate man, who has a head, no body, legs on head and arms at the right level on the legs (it is not clear that all children necessarily go through this intermediate stage, although some 25% do so); and (c) mature man, with head, body, and limbs on body. Developmental delay should be suspected if a child of 42 months is not yet drawing at least a "Humpty-Dumpty" man, or a child of 54 months is still drawing a "Humpty-Dumpty" man. The Draw a Person Test (Goodenough & Harris 1963) can be used to generate a developmental quotient, as well as a projective about the child's emotional status (Jolles 1996). Drawings are scored for the presence of 73 details. Raw scores are converted into standard scores distributed similarly to IQ scores. The number of body part details expected increases with age. Two parts are expected at age 3.5, six parts at 4.5, and ten parts at 5½.

Attention

Attentional deficits can be a problem in the preschool years (see Chapter 22) and are best assessed by observation and by history. Connors' questionnaire (2008) can be used, as can Levine's Anser questionnaires (1996), the Child Behavior Checklist (Achenbach & Rescorla 2002), the Preschool Behavior Questionnaire (Behar 1977), and the Early Childhood Inventory (Gadow & Sprafkin 2002).

Dominance

Finally, dominance should be assessed by demonstration: show me which hand you use for writing. A dominance battery (eye, hand, foot) filled out by the parents is a useful way of assessing for mixed dominance. In general, it is atypical for the eventual right-hander to declare strongly prior to age 1 year or to have failed to declare by age 5 years (Annett 1985). Left-handers tend to be more ambidextrous, so they declare later. Pathological left-handedness (a genetic right-hander who, perhaps because of perinatal injury to the left hemisphere, becomes a manifest left-hander) should be considered when the child is clearly left-handed before age 1. The increased frequency of left-handers among preterms may reflect this (Ross et al. 1987). Relatively little information is available about the right- versus left-hand skill of right-handers during the preschool years. Annett (1985) found a stable right-hand advantage on her peg-moving task from ages 3.5 to 15 years. A right-hand advantage on finger tapping and sequencing tasks paralleling the right-hand advantage to age 7 years found by Denckla (1973, 1974) is present in preschoolers. Although left-handers are in general less strongly left-handed than right-handers are right-handed, the left hand of the young left-hander is the equal in terms of dexterous performance to the right hand of the young right-hander (Rudel et al. 1984).

Consider Consultation When...

- The examination shows unilateral soft signs.
- Testing shows a domain-specific deficit.
- Testing shows a learning disability, but there is no family history.

Evaluation

Practice parameters have recently been put forward by several different groups with suggested workups of the young child with developmental delay (Committee on Children with Disabilities 2001; Filipek et al. 2000; Shevell et al. 2003).

Annotated bibliography

Annett M. *Left, right, hand and brain: The right shift theory.* Hillsdale NJ: Erlbaum Associates, 1985.

Comprehensive book on all aspects of dominance.

Blackman J, Levine M, Markowitz M. *Pediatric extended examination at three* (PEET). Cambridge, MA: Educators Publishing Service, 1986.

Egan D. Developmental examination of infants and preschool children. *Clinics in Developmental Medicine #12.* Philadelphia: J.B. Lippincott, 1990.

These are comprehensive references on the neurologic examination of the preschool and early elementary school-age child.

Frankenburg W, Dodds J. *Denver Developmental Screening Test II (DDST-II)*; 1990. Denver, CO: Available by calling (303) 355–4729.

Frankenburg WK, Fandal AW, Thornton SM. Revision of Denver Prescreening Developmental Questionnaire. *J Pediatr* 1987;110:653–658.
This remains the classic, easy-to-administer developmental screen.

Glaser JS. *Neuro-ophthalmology*. New York: Harper & Row, 2000.
A readable and, for its size, amazingly comprehensive Neuro-ophthalmology text.

Kinsbourne M, Warrington EK. The development of finger differentiation. *J Exp Psychol* 1963;15:13–137.
These articles provide a theoretic approach to the development of sensory skills and the understanding of body schema.

Nichols P, Chen T. Minimal brain dysfunction. Hillsdale, NJ: Lawrence Erlbaum, 1981.
Presents the preschool neurologic examination from the National Perinatal Collaborative Project and examines its predictive value.

Lefford A, Birch HG, Green G. The perceptual and cognitive basis for finger localization and selective finger movement in preschool children. *Child Dev* 1974;45:335–343.

Levine, M, Schneider E. *The pediatric examination of educational readiness* (PEER). Cambridge, MA: Educators Publishing Service, 1985.

Levine MD. *The Anser system*. Cambridge, MA: Educators Publishing Service, 1996.
This system, devised by a developmental pediatrician, provides parent and teacher history forms for the preschooler.

Nass R. Mirror movement asymmetries in congenital hemiparesis. *Neurology* 1985;35:1059–1062.
Provides a good review of the theoretic basis for overflow in the child.

Touwen BCL, Prechtl, HFR. *The neurological examination of the child with minor central nervous system dysfunction*. London: Spastics International, 1970.

Wolff P, Gunnoe C, Cohen C. Associated movements as a measure of developmental age. *Dev Med Child Neurol* 1983;25: 417–429.
Provides a good practical review of the extent of mirroring in the preschooler on common motor tasks.

CHAPTER 4

The Neurologic Examination of the School-age and Adolescent Child

Ruthmary K. Deuel and Amy C. Rauchway

Outline

- Items of the general physical examination
- The neurologic examination

Virtually all items used in the neurologic examination of the adult may also be employed in the neurologic examination of the school-age child and adolescent. The items to be included must be chosen with care, commensurate with the information that is required from the examination.

Certain domains must always be evaluated in any neurologic examination. Thus, every neurologic examination should include an evaluation of the patient's mental status, cranial nerves, motor system, deep tendon reflexes, and responses to sensory stimulation. Depending on the presenting complaint and the general purposes of the examination, each of these domains may then be evaluated in greater or lesser detail. To aid in examination of developmentally delayed or anomalous children, specific variations of the neurologic examination may prove useful.

Rapport with the child is a major factor in ensuring an efficient neurologic examination. The examiner should bear in mind that the child's best effort on each item is more informative than grudging or partial performance. In general, a cheerful, positive attitude toward the child and a stubborn insistence on repeated efforts if the first response to a command is insufficient are rewarded by a better examination. Just as developmental norms are important for the neurologic examination at younger ages, they are important in the school-age child, particularly on the mental status and motor performance items. To obtain as much information as possible with the least amount of effort, it is good to use certain items in the neurologic examination to define more than one factor. For instance, response to commands and negative or positive reinforcement on the part of the examiner give considerable information about the child's compliance. Hand preference and fine motor performance are other aspects that are readily evaluated concomitantly with the ongoing examination. If the child is instructed to use "your fastest hand first" or "your strongest hand first" on unimanual motor items, a measure of hand preference will be obtained (Deuel & Moran 1980). The historic information gathered concerning the child's conduct should be supplemented by the physician's direct observations during the examination.

In the sections that follow, the individual items of the neurologic examination will not all be discussed in detail. An excellent standard text on the general subject is DeJong's *The Neurologic Examination* (Campbell 2005). The chapter by Dodge and Volpe in Farmer's textbook *Pediatric Neurology* (1983) remains a detailed overview of the more specialized pediatric neurologic examination. A newer, very well referenced chapter is in the seventh edition of Menkes, Sarnat, and Maria, *Child Neurology* (2006). The goal of conducting a neurologic examination in a school-age child is to arrive at the correct diagnosis. If one appropriately applies the formal examination to test hypotheses constructed from the chief complaint and history, and also observes the child's spontaneous actions and interactions, at the end of 30 or so minutes, sufficient information should be available to make a positive diagnosis of localized or lateralized nervous system abnormalities. Mental retardation, specific learning disabilities, as well as attention deficit disorder, developmental language disorder, or developmental apraxia are equally identifiable. In addition, psychiatric disorders such as childhood depression, anxiety, and conduct disorder may be positively identified by a versatile and thorough neurologic examination. For a standardized examination protocol, see David's *Child and Adolescent Neurology, Second Edition* (Deuel & Rauchway 2005, chap. 4).

Items of the general physical examination

For a complete neurologic assessment, aspects of the general physical examination are pertinent and should always be evaluated. The number of the general examination items actually conducted is of course dependent on the question that the examination is attempting to resolve. In infants and children, height, weight, and head circumference should always be accurately measured and plotted according to the percentile for chronologic age. For school-age children, the Nellhaus Composite International and Interracial Graph for head circumference is most accurate (Nellhaus 1968). More recent head circumference growth charts published by the Centers for Disease Control and Prevention (Kuczmarski et al. 2000) are for children up to age 3 years. For countries other than the United States, some nation-specific guidelines apply (Wright et al. 2002). Blood pressure and pulse rate are also part of the standard neurologic examination, as is evaluation of the head, eyes, ears, nose, throat, skin, skeleton, and thoracic and abdominal organs.

In observing the hair, texture and thickness are important. The skull should be palpated for bone defects and for unusual shape or contour, such as is seen in plagiocephaly or hydrocephalus. The facies should be described if any irregularities at all are observed. External examination of the eyes is important, including the anatomic structure of the lids, cornea, sclerae, conjunctivae, and iridies. Interpupillary distance should be recorded. Hypertelorism or hypotelorism is an important stigma of some chromosomal disorders (Pryor 1969). Excessive conjunctival vasculature is a subtle but important indicator of ataxia-telangiectasia (Taylor et al. 1975). The external examination of the ears likewise may yield information regarding branchial cleft and other less common anomalies. The otoscopic examination is best carried out after first testing for tympanic movement. A full examination of the mouth, lips, palate, and tongue structures is valuable. In general, facial and other dysmorphisms may be an indicator of specific acquired or genetic conditions. A detailed catalogue with developmental norms is the *Handbook of Physical Measurements* (Hall et al. 2007). An oral examination pertinent to speech mechanisms and articulation should be carried out in any child with speech or language delay (Spriesterbach et al. 1978). Dentition may give a clue to skeletal abnormalities. In certain syndromes, abnormal dentition is the rule (Beumer et al. 1973). Evaluation of the thyroid gland should be carried out by palpation and auscultation of the gland. The thorax should be examined, the heart and lungs auscultated, and pulses in the neck examined with auscultation of the head and neck after it is ascertained that the cardiac rhythm is regular and there are no intrinsic cardiac auscultatory findings. The radial, carotid, and femoral pulses also should be palpated. It is important to palpate the abdomen for enlarged organs. The genitalia should also be examined with a view to Tanner staging (Tanner 1962). This is particularly important in suspected sex chromosome aneuploidies (Waber 1979; Pennington et al. 1980; Ratcliffe 1982; Scriver et al. 2000). The spinal column should be examined with the patient prone, standing, and bending over to evaluate scoliosis and lordosis. The sacral region should be particularly carefully observed for dimples or bony defects, particularly if any lower extremity difficulties have been noted. Skin changes overlying the spine, such as hemangioma or hair tufts, are of importance because they may herald underlying bony and neural tube defects. Shagreen patches of tuberous sclerosis are also found in this location (Berg 1985). The extremities should be carefully evaluated for structural abnormalities that may yield the clue to various heritable syndromes, such as homocystinuria, the mucopolysaccharidoses, and pseudohypoparathyroidism (Schimke 1965; Grossman & Dorst 1973; Scriver 2000).

During all phases of the history and examination, it is convenient to note whether the patient remains attentive to the examination, cooperative with commands, and responsive to positive and negative reinforcement. Because the physical examination is primary, we have called this latter group of assessments *concomitant observations*. Extra boxes for noting these observations are pro-

Key Clinical Questions

A 9-year-old girl is brought by her family because of the sudden onset, yesterday, of a "twisted" smile and an inability to close her right eye, without history of antecedent infection, trauma, or toxic exposure. On examination, you find no general physical abnormalities, and on thorough neurological examination only mild decrease in right seventh nerve functions, including taste discrimination, eye closure, lacrimation, and facial expression. You find no hyper- or hypoacusis.

What is the most likely cause of the isolated seventh-nerve paralysis you have defined? What should be done to protect the eye?

Most likely the child has idiopathic facial palsy (IFP; Bell palsy). Use of an eye lubricant and a "pirate patch" are needed for corneal protection. Certain factors, such as severity of paralysis (if severe, minimal excitability of the facial nerve allows an estimate of residual nerve function if done soon after onset) or endemic Lyme disease, should influence the intensity of your pursuit of underlying and treatment-demanding etiologies.

vided on the preschool and school-age pediatric and neurologic examination scoring form in David's *Child and Adolescent Neurology, Second Edition* (Deuel & Rauchway, 2005, chap. 4). It is usually easy to find at least two or three opportunities to use positive reinforcement. For example, when the child opens his mouth, one can say, "That's good" or when she relaxes her abdominal muscles, one can respond with, "You're doing a good job at that. Would you keep it up?" Of course there are usually also opportunities for negative reinforcement, for example, "Don't breathe so fast" or "Don't put your shirt on yet." It is likewise valuable to consider the quality and quantity of the subject's distractibility. Observe the results of external interruptions (for example, comments from parents, knocks at the door) to determine if they distract the child from following instructions for the formal examination. Does the child become distracted without any obvious external stimuli? Finally, as a concomitant observation, is the child impulsive, interrupting the examination with sudden self-initiated actions or talk? Structured conscious rating of these responses is valuable and necessary to the evaluation of the cognitive, attentional, and motivational abilities of the child. It is thus an integral part of the mental status examination. Although further testing may certainly be required to refine behavioral and cognitive observations, the directed pediatric and neurologic examination combination should suffice for initial detection and categorization of pervasive developmental, cognitive, attentional, motivational, and conduct disorders, as well as more specific entities such as cerebral palsy, fragile X, and childhood migraine.

Children with deviant communication styles are usually sent to a physician for at least one diagnostic evaluation. Such children, however, present a major challenge to any physician's examining expertise. Careful initial consideration of the child's interactions with parents and objects in the room before paying overt attention to the child should direct the physician's approach to the hands-on examination. For example, nonverbal cues may be the operative ones for this particular child. To break the ice, the child may be handed a fascinating toy appropriate to his or her estimated cognitive level. Then, very obviously, attention is directed back to the adult historian while the child's reaction to the move, and interaction with the toy are covertly monitored. Does the child make some kind of attempt to retrieve the examiner's attention? If so, some valuable information has been gained about social abilities and communication style that is not available through quantitative testing. Is the child interacting appropriately with the toy? Is the child also attending to the examiner's interactions with the historian? Of course, carrying on an interview with a historian and at the same time observing the child may tax the physician's own attentional capacities, but it will be rewarded by observational material that is informative in and of itself, as well as affording a chance to plan strategy for completion of the funduscopic examination and other items of the basic neurologic examination.

The neurologic examination

The neurologic examination is actually a series of functional tests aimed at determining whether different segments and subsystems within the nervous system are normal. Some of the functions assessed will vary, depending on the chief complaint of the patient. Thus, the "standard" neurologic examination is designed to answer pertinent questions regarding sensory, motor, and higher cortical functions.

The subject of the examination cannot be passive during most tests but must comply and attempt to carry out commands. For example, any detailed sensory examination is impossible without good patient compliance. In children, the order of the neurologic examination items should be dictated by common sense and the need to maintain good compliance. It is more important to assess all the necessary items than to follow some set rule for their presentation. At the beginning of the examination of the school-age child, it is often useful to introduce yourself by asking some of the conversational items in the mental status examination. For example, an assessment of orientation is often a good opener. This allows an evaluation

Key Clinical Questions

A 14-year-old high school freshman reports excellent health and school grades since you last saw him 3 years ago, but gradually increasing difficulty in walking. General physical examination is normal, with no change in growth parameters. On neurological examination, the mental status, cranial nerves, and complete sensory examination are also normal, as is the upper extremity motor examination. Power in all muscles of both legs is excellent, but gait testing reveals slow progression with intoeing and no heel-strike. Reflexes at the knees and ankles are 4+, and there is ankle clonus bilaterally, with bilateral upgoing toes.

What descriptive diagnosis will you give the condition? What causes will you investigate? Irrespective of cause, what therapies could be helpful to ambulation?

On the basis of your examination findings of spasticity in both lower extremities, the child has a progressive spastic paraparesis. There are multiple etiologies, most common of which is familial spastic paraplegia (FSP). Physical therapy is most helpful in prolonging ambulation in this slowly progressive degenerative disease.

Key Clinical Questions

A 6-year-old boy is brought by his newly adopting parents because of his problems with kindergarten schoolwork. Birth, family, and developmental history are sketchy, but recent health has been fine. His pediatric examination shows macrocephaly, a long face, large protuberant ears, frequent inattention to commands, distractibility, and poor articulatory skills. On neurologic examination, he is eager and interactive, but cannot explain where he is, cannot draw a triangle nor print his name. Otherwise he has only mild diffuse hypotonia. *Given the history limitations, are you able to consider any diagnoses at this point? What further evaluations will you recommend?*

The combined examination findings, namely large ears, long face, big head, moderate cognitive and language problems, attention difficulties, and mild hypotonia are in themselves suggestive of fragile X or other genetic syndromes. Given the unknown history (injury, abuse?) and large head (acquired?), a brain imaging study may be helpful. Psychometric, and speech and language evaluations should be planned, and possibly a stimulant trial.

of the child's knowledge of where he or she is, who the doctor is, the day of the week, and, for older children, the date and year. Other items that can be used are the names of the child's school and school teacher. For middle and junior high school-age children, the address and zip code of the child's school is a good item, as is the question about presidents of the United States.

Handedness may also be identified conversationally by inquiring about several everyday activities (Bryden 1977) (and later checking the responses with performance during pantomime on command and use of actual objects; Provins & Cunliffe 1972), such as "What hand do you use when you cut with a pair of scissors?" "What hand do you use when you eat with a fork?" The patient should be asked to identify his right hand and then given a three-part command using left and right items (for example, "Close your eyes and put your left thumb on your right ear").

If the chief complaint is failure or poor performance in school, the mental status examination should definitely include grade- and age-appropriate testing of school skills: letter identification or reading, copying shapes, and writing spontaneously, as well as to dictation and copying. The writing should be evaluated for speed and the output for legibility. The child should be asked to count or work arithmetic problems, including word problems, as grade-appropriate. He should be asked to draw a picture of a person.

Some of these tasks may be incorporated into an informal assessment of attention and memory: Hand the child a clean sheet of unlined paper and a sharpened pencil with an eraser. Seat the child comfortably at a good writing surface. Tell the child to (a) write her full name, (b) draw a picture of a person, and (c) write a sample. The sample should be of the child's own composition, and the examiner should specify a grade-appropriate task (the alphabet, a word, a few words, a sentence, paragraph, or short essay on the subject of the child's choice). Have the child repeat the commands. When they have been repeated correctly, ask the child to carry out the tasks and (d) inform you when they are complete. This constitutes a complex, developmentally appropriate four-part command that assesses attention and memory.

Then, out of the corner of the eye, while ostensibly discussing historic information with the parent, the examiner should observe several facets of the patient's performance: (a) how the hands are used, (b) how attentive the child is to the task, and (c) how rapidly or painstakingly the task is accomplished. To present a distractor, the examiner may ask the parent a question about a subject that is emotionally charged for the child. Several types of information may be derived from this exercise. First, if the child successfully follows the complex four-part command without interrupting the adult conversation, one has an estimate of her memory span, attention focus span, and compliance. If, in addition to completing the assigned task, she has been monitoring the adult conversation, and interjecting comments about it, the examiner can be assured the child has adequate capacity (to be distinguished from actual everyday performance) to refocus attention on a task after having shifted attention to distractors. Second, the examiner can judge the age-appropriateness of the writing and drawing samples and note any major discrepancies in this factor between the two types of graphic production. The picture the child produces may be scored using the Goodenough criteria (Taylor 1959; Robertson & Shilkofski 2005). The spontaneous writing sample may be judged for grade-appropriate configuration, spelling, and punctuation. Such screening allows the physician direct observational insight that may then be supplemented by formal individual psychometric and school achievement tests performed at a school or other facility.

The direct, first-hand testing of school skills by the neurologic examiner affords that examiner an opportunity to detect uneven development of different cognitive abilities. This portion of the examination should thus help evaluate the validity of any formal cognitive testing that may have been performed. More importantly, it may point up areas where more detailed and quantitative testing should be requested. Without direct examination of the cognitive aspects of the child's development, the neurologic examination will not be helpful in solving diagnostic dilemmas concerning attention, and specific learning and language disorders. This is particularly relevant to the child with a pervasive attention or conduct disorder secondary to an underlying cognitive deficit. It is much less important in the evaluation of other common problems, such as seizures or neuropathy, in which case these added cognitive elements of the examination may be minimized.

Examination of the cranial nerves includes evaluation of the important special senses, vision, and hearing. It is usually unnecessary to test smell. However, if there is a question of frontal lobe or anterior fossa pathology, this examination should be performed. The use of commercially available tests allows one to present familiar fruit smells (orange and banana are most easily recognized by school-children) to each nostril. Confrontation visual fields are usually easily undertaken with one eye covered with a 3 × 5 index card in the child 10 years old and older. The optimal object is a small white-headed pin. The tester should sight on the subject's pupil and use her own visual field as a measure of the subject's visual field, placing the pin equidistant between the tester and the subject. With this technique, the blind spot that confirms accurate field mapping can usually be found in the alert cooperative school child (Traquiar 1949; Thompson 1979). In younger or less able children, fingers may be presented spontaneously to both fields or to one for at least a gross estimate of field integrity. In any child who will fixate, optokinetic nystagmus can be used to estimate responses to visual stimuli (Campbell 2005). Optokinetic testing should definitely be performed when there is a question of cortical blindness in a child of any age (Brindley 1969). Visual acuity can be tested using a standard Snellen chart at 6 meters, in first graders or older children.[1] Visual acuity testing should be performed with and without glasses. Eye position should be noted without glasses. A cover test—consisting of having the patient fixate with both eyes forward, then covering one eye and seeing if the position of the remaining uncovered eye changes—may be used if there is a question concerning extraocular muscle abnormality (Cogan 1956). Versions of the eyes in conjugate following should also be tested. Pupillary symmetry and reactions to direct stimulation with light, and to light in the opposite eye, should be noted, as should nystagmus. Spontaneous and reactive nystagmus may have various connotations, depending on the type and direction of the movements (Cogan 1956).

Funduscopy should be carried out so that both disks, both maculae, and the peripheral retina of each eye can be visualized. If, for any reason, a satisfactory view of the fundi cannot be obtained, and this appears necessary for diagnosis, referral to a pediatric ophthalmologist is recommended. Jaw movements should be assessed. The symmetry of both the upper and the lower face should be evaluated. To test hearing crudely, finger rustling or whispering in the right and left ear with the other ear occluded is a reasonable test of conversation level. Deafness is still often undetected (Coplen 1987); losses in selected frequencies particularly may go unnoticed as a cause of "inattention," as are central auditory processing deficits. Taste is sometimes tested, and children older than age 4 usually readily respond to salt/sugar taste in the anterior two-thirds for the seventh nerve or the posterior third for the ninth nerve of the tongue. Palate elevation must be tested, both voluntarily and as part of the gag reflex. The sternocleidomastoid muscle is tested by having the child turn the face away from the side of the muscle tested. Tilting the chin up toward the ear will make the contracting

[1] In first graders or older children, a Rosenbaum pack vision or screener may be used.

Pearls and Perils

Neurologic Examination of the School-Age Child

- There is no such thing as the standard neurologic examination. Rather, an infinite variety of neurologic examinations exists, the items of which depend heavily on the individual performing them and the hypotheses being tested. Even with a standard protocol, as in the Collaborative Perinatal Project, different neurologic examiners will ascertain somewhat different incidences of disorders (Nichols & Chen 1981).
- Mild degrees of hemiparesis may be markedly accentuated by the Fog maneuver, which may elicit marked asymmetries of the upper extremities and assumption of a hemiparetic posture by the arm on the affected side (see items N93 and N94).
- Aneuploidies and their associated physical features are often accompanied by distinctive neuropsychologic profiles called *behavioral phenotypes* (Cassidy 2002). An example is Turner syndrome, with abnormal spatial understanding and motor skills, but normal verbal skills (Money 1993).
- Williams syndrome and its associated physical features are also accompanied by a distinctive neuropsychologic profile, including a fluent receptive language disorder and clumsiness (Bellugi 2000).
- The nondominant hand is often more accurate in stereognostic discrimination than the dominant one (Witelson 1978).
- Most standardized psychometric tests—for example, the WISC-IV (Wechsler 2003), Stanford-Binet, Fifth Edition (Roid 2003), and Slosson (SIT-R3) (Slosson et al. 2002)—are somewhat dependent on verbal instructions. Even though they have become more sophisticated, they may still underestimate certain learning disabilities.

sternocleidomastoid more prominent for palpation. Shrugging of the shoulders also allows testing of the eleventh nerve. Tongue protrusion and lateral movements are evaluated to test the twelfth nerve. Repeated syllables such as PA-TA-KA (Spriesterbach et al. 1978) allow for evaluation of orobuccal agility. Obviously, it may be necessary to carry out further, more refined and quantitative tests of visual and auditory sensation, such as the measurement of visual evoked potentials or brainstem auditory evoked potentials (BAEP). It is well to bear in mind that measurement of BAEP to clicks (composed of multiple frequencies) is not designed for testing hearing thresholds.

Introducing the motor examination with gait testing allows the youngster a chance to stretch. Running should be tested with at least a 6-meter leeway; a hall is useful for this test. Children 6 years old or older should be able to skip or able to learn from a demonstration.[2] Tandem walking should be tested to evaluate lower extremity coordination. The Fog maneuver may be used, which requires the child to walk on the insides or the outside of the soles (Fog & Fog 1963). This is useful in determining whether there are adventitious movements in the face and hands during this "stress" gait. Toe and heel gait are also helpful to test active strength in the lower extremity muscle groups. The pronator drift test should be performed with the child standing, arms extended, palms up. The child should be asked to hold the posture for 20 seconds. To evaluate for chorea, the child should stand unsupported for 20 seconds with eyes closed, arms extended, and hands pronated with wrists extended and fingers abducted and extended (Barlow 1974). Resistive strength testing of the upper and lower extremities may be carried out in standard fashion in children 6 years old and older. For screening purposes, shoulder girdle, distal extremity, and hip girdle strength should be tested. Stair climbing or stepping up to the seat of a chair, guided by safety concerns, is an excellent test for hip girdle strength. If a musculoskeletal or neuromuscular disorder is suspected, more thorough testing of each muscle group should be carried out, with grading of muscle strength from 0 to 5. Of course, evaluation of sitting posture should be made during this portion of the examination.

Cerebellar coordination of the upper extremities is best tested with the finger-to-nose test. The elbow should come to full extension and the wrist to full pronation before the child's finger is allowed to touch the examiner's finger. It is best to require three positions—center, 30 degrees to the left, and 30 degrees to the right—with each hand, and to require two trials in each position for each hand. To evaluate coordination more proximally in the upper extremities, several tests are used. With all of them, observation of body parts not involved in the demanded action may yield information about synkinesis, particularly mirror movements. Resting tremor, intention tremor, titubation of the trunk or head, and other involuntary adventitious movements may also become apparent. To test wrist turning, alternating taps of the palm, and the dorsum of the hand on the knee should be done as rapidly as possible, or the child may be given an object, such as a reflex hammer, to turn back and forth in a regular rhythmic fashion. The child may also be asked to pretend to screw a light bulb into a ceiling fixture. Movements are normally performed in a rhythmic, alternating fashion. With cerebellar disorders, however, they frequently assume an extremely erratic, nonrepetitive pattern. The heel–shin knee–ankle maneuver further tests coordination of the lower extremities.

To assess isolated finger movements as a measure of pyramidal tract function, a finger-tapping task is often used, and has the advantage of standardization as to rate expected at different ages and for both genders (Denckla 1974). During such unimanual distal movements, it is valuable to have the other hand held in the air without support. One may then note whether associated mirror movements occur when the hand that is designated to be active is in fact carrying out the required action. Associated movements mirroring a variety of actions may occur in the hand not voluntarily engaged. Thus it is well to observe for them during the entire examination. Foot tapping can be done in the time-for-20 format described by Denckla (1974) and compared with standards. Hopping in place on either foot should be possible for any child older than 5 years of age.

Testing for developmental apraxia and clumsiness, a source of school and home failure that cannot be determined from paper-and-pencil tests, is very important in any child with school or attention difficulties. The tapping test just discussed is excellent to define clumsiness and accompanying adventitious movements but does not suffice to demonstrate apraxia. Apraxia (or dyspraxia) may be defined as the inability to carry out age-appropriate voluntary motor sequences in the absence of a primary motor or sensory deficit (David 1981). It is only determined by direct testing during the neurologic examination. Copying hand postures (using for instance the Luria Fist Test), pantomiming acts (pouring milk into a glass), and using actual objects (putting a flashlight together and turning it on) are the three types of performance that should be covered in any complete examination for apraxia (Damasio et al. 1985). A standard manual apraxia battery is incorporated in the neurologic protocol in David's *Child and Adolescent Neurology, Second Edition* in Chapter 18.

Upper extremity reflexes should be tested with the arms relaxed and in a symmetric position. Relaxation can

[2] Skipping requires a step on one foot, next a hop, landing on the first foot, then a step on the second foot, followed by a hop, landing on the second foot. If a child has no prior experience with skipping, he or she should be able to learn from one demonstration trial.

somctimes be accomplished by asking complex questions of the patient as the respective tendons are tapped or by reinforcement maneuvers. The Hoffman sign, otherwise called the "Babinski of the upper extremity," should be attempted with a flick of the nail of the middle fingernail. Examination of reflexes in the lower extremities may be performed with the patient sitting and the legs in a symmetric dependent position, which is also advantageous for eliciting clonus. However, the deep tendon reflexes and clonus may also be checked in the supine position.

Sensation may be tested in 6- to 12-year-old children in the same manner as in adults. For a screening examination, light touch and position sense or light touch and vibration sense may be adequate. If there is any question of a spinal lesion, then examination of responses to thermal and pinprick stimuli becomes mandatory. Even in school-age children, it is wise to introduce the pin carefully before starting the examination, in which the entire dermatomal distribution should be tested, including the lower sacral segments. Stereognosis can be readily evaluated in this age group by using small common objects such as clips, safety pins, keys, and coins. Graphesthesia (writing on the skin) may be evaluated. Normative data for graphesthesia of a relatively psychometric quality is given in the Halsted-Reitan battery (Reitan 1969), although the testing routine they recommend is lengthy. Bilateral, simultaneous somatosensory stimulation with fingers on the face, the hands, and the legs should be part of every screening examination. Finally, autonomic responses, vasomotor responses, and sweating should be noted.

In conclusion, the neurologic examination is a versatile diagnostic instrument. Using it, one should detect localizing and lateralizing signs of nervous system abnormalities, and determine reliably the maturational level of cognitive, emotional, and motor capacities, as well as physical growth and development. Supplemented by a careful comprehensive history, the examination frequently yields all the basic information necessary to make a full diagnosis, not only of neurologic disease but also of neuropsychiatric and developmental disorders of higher cerebral function. Standardized tests are usually helpful to analyze age appropriate specific hearing and visual loss problems found on the neurologic evaluation; to evaluate nerve and muscle functions further; or to quantitatively characterize developmental language disorders, dyslexia, dysgraphia, and dyscalculia.

Annotated bibliography

Deuel RK, Rauchway AC. Preschool and school-age pediatric and neurologic examination scoring form. In: David RB, ed., *Child and adolescent neurology*, 2nd ed. Oxford: Blackwell, 2005; 74–80.

Dodge PR, Volpe JJ. Neurologic history and examination. In: Farmer TW, ed. *Pediatric neurology*, 3rd ed. Philadelphia: Harper & Row, 1983; 1–41.

A very succinctly written and well-illustrated chapter. In addition, it explains how to take a good history and provides excellent advice on how to engage the patient's interest and cooperation, issues as pertinent today as 20 years ago. The chapter contains good detail concerning examination of the cranial nerves and gives various "tricks of the trade" for eliciting valid sensory responses from immature subjects.

Roid G, Miller L. *Leiter International Performance Scale–Revised*. Wood Dale, IL: Stoelting Company, 1996.

This test requires a highly trained psychometrician. It was specifically designed to be a nonverbal test of IQ. As such, the language medium is almost irrelevant (although the gestural idioms of the culture from which the tested child comes are important). Thus it is a much better reflection of cognitive ability in most language-disabled children. However, the child with severe visual-spatial disabilities will not do well on the LIPS-R.

Slosson R, Nicholson CL, Hibpshman TL. *Slosson intelligence test revised 3rd ed. (SIT-R3) for children and adults*. East Aurora, NY: Slosson Educational Publications, Inc., 2002.

The Slosson is a quick-screening IQ test that, with proper precautions against testing artifacts, can be very useful to the neurologic examiner. However, the Slosson, like all screening tests, particularly if it provides an abnormal estimate, should be checked by more reliable (and complex, requiring a person fully trained in their administration) tests of intelligence.

Spriesterbach D, Morris HL, Darley FL. Examination of the speech mechanisms. In: Darley FL, Spriesterbach D, eds., *Diagnostic methods in speech pathology*, 2nd ed. New York: Harper & Row, 1978; 215–231.

This chapter describes methods of examining speech mechanisms that are practical and often not covered by the medical school physical examination course. Examination of the speech mechanism is highly important in any school-age child suspected of having a language disorder but is often omitted for lack of familiarity with the proper method.

Taylor, EM. Psychological appraisal of children with cerebral defects. Cambridge, MA: Harvard University Press, 1959.

Wechsler D. *Wechsler intelligence scale for children*, 4th ed. (WISC-IV). San Antonio, TX: Psychological Corporation, 2003.

The W1SC-IV is an individually administered, well-standardized test that breaks down cognitive function into indices including Verbal Comprehension and Perceptual Reasoning. Although these indices (and the individual subtests that compose them) are highly useful, it is important to bear in mind that the WISC-IV and the fifth edition of the Stanford-Binet (SB5), despite their sophistication, may underestimate the ability of a child with a language disorder. Thus, a child with a language disorder should be sent for testing with the neurologist's suspicion clearly outlined.

CHAPTER 5

The Electroencephalogram

Warren T. Blume

Outline

- The normal electroencephalogram
- Maturation milestones
- Electroencephalography and epilepsy
- Certain central nervous system disorders

The normal electroencephalogram

To read the electroencephalogram (EEG) of a child or adolescent properly, one must be aware of several aspects that distinguish it from that of an adult. Many of its features are age dependent, and a brief review of these follows. Maturational and state factors create a wider variety of waveforms than is usually found among adults; such multiple waveforms may become superimposed to create sharply contoured waves that can be mistaken for spikes. Infants and young children often fall asleep during the recording, and the consequent EEG changes are more marked than those found in older age groups. These factors of maturation and state create wider fluctuations of EEG readings among normal children, a factor that commonly leads to overinterpretation of the recording. Finally, interhemispheric asymmetries of normal features occur commonly in youth, including alpha activity, mu rhythm, and the so-called "posterior slow of youth."

The sometimes bewildering array of components can be simplified by asking five questions for each state of alertness in determining whether a recording is normal:

1. In what state of alertness is the child?
2. Is the background activity appropriate for age?
3. Are any asymmetries present, beyond those normally accepted for certain waveforms, which cannot be ascribed to artifact?
4. Are any definite spikes present?
5. Is there any focal or diffuse excessive delta activity?

Maturation milestones

Wakefulness

The first discernible background frequency is 3–4 Hz, which appears at age 3 months. This frequency increases to about 5 Hz at age 5 months, to 6–7 Hz at 12 months, and to 7–8 Hz at 2 years and, by 6 years, stabilizes at about a 9-Hz rhythm (Figure 5.1). The mean frequency at 15 years is about 10 Hz. Alpha amplitude varies from 30 to 100 μV in the first year of life; it may increase to a maximum at 6–9 years and then decline. Gentle passive eye closure by the technologist may elicit background frequencies not otherwise apparent. An asymmetry of alpha is commonly seen in pediatric EEGs; it is usually higher to the right, but a higher left-sided amplitude is not clearly an abnormality. Asymmetries of amplitude are more accepted than asymmetries of frequency, and a left-to-right frequency difference exceeding 1 Hz usually indicates an abnormality on the slower side.

The rhythmic background activity in youth is commonly interrupted by 250- to 500-msec posterior waves occurring singly or repeating at 2–4 Hz. Their amplitude is equal to or slightly greater than that of the background rhythms (Figure 5.2). The combination of such waveforms with alpha creates sharply contoured, spike-like deflections in the occipital regions, which are not as sharp as occipital spikes. Such posterior slow activity blocks with eye opening and generally waxes and wanes with alpha. The quantity and amplitude of such activity gradually increases in the first decade of life, reaching an apex in early adolescence. As with the background activity, the abundance of such posterior slow of youth can be considerably greater in the right hemisphere as compared to

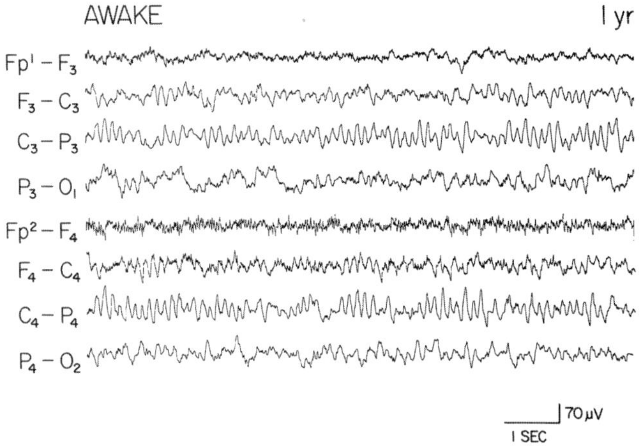

Figure 5.1 Rich mixture of waveforms in alert infant. This tracing is dominated by 7- to 8-Hz central-parietal activity, but 1- to 2-Hz diffuse activity is also evident. The slightly greater quantity of delta on one side (left) is insignificant at this age. None of the apiculate waves is a spike. Normal recording.

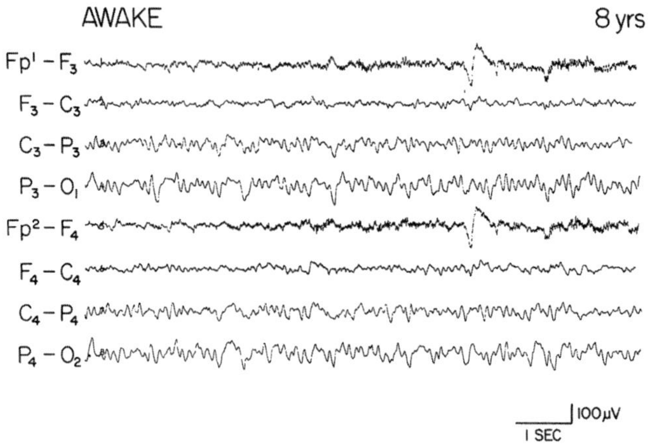

Figure 5.2 Electropositive occipital waves of 200–250 msec separate the sharply contoured alpha to constitute the "posterior slow of youth," which can normally be abundant, as in this example.

the left. Such activity can be rhythmic at about 3–4 Hz and may appear in prolonged runs. In addition to an intermittent and rhythmic form, a halving of the alpha-frequency occurs on occasion in children, usually with drowsiness. All such potentials occur only with the eyes closed.

In contrast, lambda waves may be particularly prominent as primarily electropositive, sharply contoured waves seen over the occipital head regions with the eyes open and particularly during scanning eye movements. Asymmetry of lambda waves is not an abnormality.

Theta (4–7 Hz) activity is present in varying amounts in the EEGs of children. Its quantity relative to other waveforms increases considerably in the first years of life, reaches a peak at age 5–6 years, and then declines somewhat thereafter. Therefore, with the eyes closed or open, theta is the dominant diffuse activity in recordings in the 2- to 5-year age group. With eyes closed, its quantity equals that of alpha activity at age 5–6 years, after which alpha becomes the more prominent. As with adults, theta activity tends to predominate over the left hemisphere at most ages. It would be very difficult to interpret a pediatric recording as containing excess theta activity, given its normal predominance.

Delta (1–3 Hz) and theta are approximately equal in quantity during the first year of life. Although the absolute quantity of delta increases during the first year and continues to do so to the fifth year, proportionally, it declines in relation to theta. However, low-voltage delta persists into adolescence in steadily declining quantities. Delta is never normally accentuated in drowsiness.

Persistent background activity develops earlier in the central (rolandic) head regions than in any other area. A 6- to 7-Hz rhythm may appear before 3 months of age and its frequency gradually increases to 8–10 Hz after 3 months. In the 1- to 5-year-old age group, the most prominent awake activity with eyes open resides in the central region (Figure 5.1). Asymmetries of such activity appear commonly and usually shift back and forth between hemispheres. A persistent central-rhythm asymmetry usually suggests an abnormality on the lower side unless some defect in the skull is present. As such central rhythms combine with other rhythms, a sharply contoured appearance may result; this factor should be taken into account when identifying any central morphology as a spike.

The main purpose of hyperventilation in children's recordings is to elicit spike-wave discharges if they are not present during the resting recording. Regional spikes or

Pearls and Perils

The Normal Electroencephalogram

- Maturation criteria must be considered when reading a child's EEG.
- The modifications of the EEG with drowsiness are considerably greater for children than for adults, and such modifications vary with age.
- When assessing the frequency of background activity, make sure the child is not drowsy, as this will slow the rate.
- The rich mixture of normal activity in children's EEGs creates sharply contoured waves. Only those apiculate waves that contrast clearly with ongoing activity can be identified as spikes.
- A wide variety of normal findings exists in children's EEGs. Therefore, great caution should be exerted before stating that a mild abnormality exists.

excess slow waves are less commonly revealed in children than in adults. The accentuation of 2- to 3-Hz waves with hyperventilation is usually more marked in children than in adults, particularly around ages 10–12 years. Their location is often initially posterior in the early phases of hyperventilation, before becoming anterior.

Drowsiness

Because the EEG signs of drowsiness commonly appear before the child appears drowsy, the associated slowing of background rhythms may be misinterpreted as abnormal. Sinusoidal theta is the most common drowsy pattern in children from ages 3 months to about 5 years. Its frequency is 3–5 Hz in the first year of life, increasing gradually to 4–6 Hz by age 4 years. Its amplitude declines thereafter. From ages 6–16 years, rhythmic 5- to 7-Hz waves, maximum anteriorly, can accompany drowsiness.

Prominent generalized bisynchronous bursts of 2- to 5-Hz rhythmic activity occasionally attaining 350 µV or more can be seen over the frontal and central regions in drowsiness from age 14 months to about 10 years (Figure 5.3). They are most common at ages 3–5 years. Such bursts are commonly mistaken for abnormalities. If sharply contoured background waves are intermingled, the composite can be falsely identified as spike waves.

Beta activity at 20–25 Hz becomes more prominent in drowsiness and light sleep and may be distributed diffusely with a maximum anteriorly. Alpha activity classically disappears in moderate drowsiness, but the aforementioned phenomena may appear before alpha wanes. In some children, the transition from wakefulness to sleep resembles an adult pattern, without the previously mentioned features.

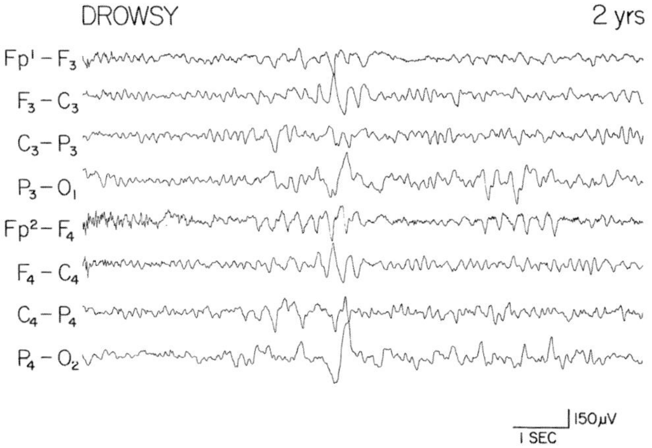

Figure 5.3 Bursts of theta and delta in drowsiness, a normal phenomenon of childhood.

Sleep

Rudimentary vertex (V) waves appear in light sleep as early as 3–4 months of age and become well developed by age 5 months. They achieve maximum expression as high-voltage, sharply contoured monophasic or diphasic electronegative or electropositive waves at age 3–4 years, and may be mistaken for rolandic spikes (Figure 5.4). On bipolar montages, their amplitude may appear asymmetrical, but such asymmetries should shift from side to side. When in doubt, use a referential montage to assess the symmetries of such V waves.

Spindles appear first at age 3–4 months and are almost invariably present during ages 3–9 months if adequate quantity and different levels of sleep are attained. Occasionally, a child of this age may descend too rapidly to very deep sleep and omit the spindle phase. Spindles may shift in prominence from side to side, but the overall quantity should be approximately equal in the two hemispheres. Spindles are often at a maximum in the central and parietal regions in youth. After infancy, almost all recorded sleep is non-REM. Therefore, the features previously discussed describe this phase.

Delta activity (1–3 Hz) is invariably present in non-REM sleep. In children, it should be accentuated posteriorly, a feature best illustrated by a bipolar anteroposterior montage or an ipsilateral ear reference. Such posterior activity may be sharply contoured.

Arousal

In infants younger than 2 months of age, arousal consists of a decrease in the voltage of ongoing activity. At age 3 months, a diphasic slow wave may occur in response to an afferent stimulus. This phenomenon, initially resembling a V wave, becomes better developed by 5 months, when it merges with a series of delta waves. If further arousal occurs, 4- to 8-Hz rhythmic theta lasting 1–5 seconds or more may appear in children age 7 months to 4 years. With continuing arousal, this theta is followed

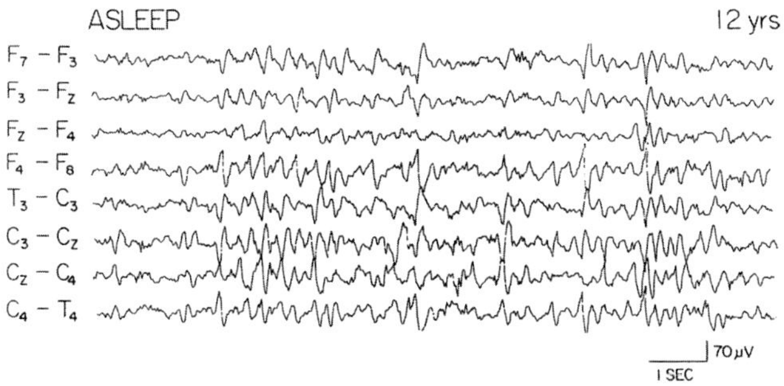

Figure 5.4 Very apiculate V waves of varying morphology may appear in sequences, particularly in youth. Note their central-frontal (Cz-Fz) maxima.

(paradoxically) by 1- to 3-Hz diffuse delta; this appears first at age 2–3 months, is maximally expressed at ages 12–18 months, and declines after age 5 years.

Electroencephalography and epilepsy

With access to a vast array of laboratory tests, the physician can easily forget that epilepsy is, and always will be, a clinical diagnosis based on a differential diagnosis based on a painstaking history and physical examination. In many instances, these two effective, safe, and relatively inexpensive diagnostic procedures leave no unsolved questions. At other times, they will focus the attention on several questions to be addressed by the EEG, thus maximizing its clinical value: Is there a seizure disorder? Is it focal or generalized? If it is focal, is it unifocal (where?) or multifocal? How severe is the seizure disorder?

To answer such questions with confidence, a recording of high technical quality is required. It must be interpreted by a physician knowledgeable in pediatric electroencephalography.

Interictal electroencephalography

It is unusual for a patient to have an epileptic seizure in front of the physician, and a clinical seizure occurs only rarely in routine EEG, with the occasional exception of absence attacks with 3-second spike waves. Therefore, interictal abnormalities, particularly spikes, are in practice the chief correlate of the epileptic condition that can help answer the questions posed earlier.

A reasonable correlation between epileptiform activity in the resting EEG and seizure disorders exists in children. Of 242 children with spike foci, 82% were found to have epilepsy (Trojaborg 1968), whereas in another study, epileptiform activity was found in only 1.9% of the 743 normal children (Eeg-Olofsson et al. 1971). Spikes occur in about 30% of children after a first seizure (Shinnar et al. 1994). Such discharges appear on an initial EEG in 50% (Carpay et al. 1997) to 76% (Yoshinaga et al. 2001) of children and adolescents with epilepsy. This incidence range likely reflects varying proportions of syndromes included in their studies. The Carpay study found that two EEGs will disclose spikes in approximately 66% of cases if sleep is included. Ninety-two percent of the Yoshinaga study patients demonstrated spikes at some point over three EEGs. Younger children will more likely have spikes, but spike specificity for epilepsy at this age may be lower (Pedley et al. 2003). However, two cautionary notes should be added. The first concerns the normal sharply contoured waves that appear ubiquitously in the recordings of children. In addition, several types of epileptiform phenomena, which can properly be called spikes, do not correlate with epileptic conditions (see Klass and Westmoreland 1985, for a review). These include small sharp spikes, 14-second and 6-second positive spikes, wicket spikes, 6-second spike-waves, and rhythmic midtemporal discharges. Definitions and descriptions of these phenomena are found in that article and in most EEG textbooks and atlases.

Generalized epileptiform abnormalities

Generalized spike-waves

The most classic of all EEG–clinical correlations is that observed between bilaterally synchronous spike-wave complex and absence attacks. Usually, both the spike and the wave component emerge abruptly and distinctively from the background activity. However, occasionally, the spike discharge is obscure, leaving only a burst of rhythmic 3- to 4-Hz bilaterally synchronous waves. Such "generalized" phenomena may be confined to the anterior head regions, to the posterior head regions, to one hemisphere, or even to a region of one hemisphere. When the phenomena are topologically confined, differentiation from focal spikes may be difficult. Descriptions of these phenomena appear in Weir (1965), Blume and Kaibara (1999), and Lemieux and Blume (1986).

About 97% of patients with bilaterally synchronous spike waves on the resting EEG or with hyperventilation have a generalized seizure disorder (Blume & Kaibara 1999). About 60% of these patients have absence attacks. The incidence of generalized tonic–clonic (grand mal) attacks varies considerably according to age at recording. A smaller number of patients with 3-second spike waves, usually in the younger age groups, have myoclonic seizures.

Because impairment of awareness, as studied by reaction times, is most profound between 0.5 and 1.5 seconds after onset of spike-waves (Browne et al. 1974), some have considered that even a single spike-wave represents an absence attack. Although this may be true theoretically, an absence attack is unlikely to be clinically detectable unless sequential spike-waves last more than 5 seconds (Niedermeyer 1987).

Pearls and Perils

Electroencephalograms (EEGs) and Epilepsy

- Slow spike waves are characteristically more abundant than 3-Hz spike waves.
- Rolandic spikes are characteristically abundant, even though seizures are rare.
- Distinction between sharply contoured mu rhythm and rolandic spikes can occasionally be most difficult. When in doubt, consider the phenomenon mu.

Hyperventilation is the most effective means to elicit bisynchronous spike-waves when they are not present in the resting recording. Hyperventilation was found to be more effective than a 6-hour recording in predicting clinical seizure frequency (Adams & Lueders 1981). Photic stimulation may also elicit spike waves, but these may appear in clinically normal subjects who do not have a history of spontaneously appearing seizures.

Continuous spike waves of sleep (electrical status epilepticus of sleep) is a condition in which sequential bilaterally synchronous spike waves are very abundant in non-REM sleep and therefore represent reiterative absence (Patry et al. 1971; Tassinari et al. 1984). In this disorder, atypical absences with atonic components are among the seizure disorders present in wakefulness, as varying quantities of 3-Hz spike-wave discharges occur during the awake recording as well. Behavioral and mental deterioration, including a reduction in speech, occurs. Therefore, the syndrome shares clinical and electrographic properties with the Landau-Kleffner syndrome.

Bilaterally synchronous myoclonic seizures are usually associated with bilateral spike waves or polyspike waves. These may appear in an otherwise normal EEG, with slow spike waves in the Lennox-Gastaut syndrome, or with excess delta in degenerative central nervous system (CNS) disorders and metabolic encephalopathies. Although spike-waves accompany the myoclonus, the specific timing between the spike and the myoclonic jerk varies (Gastaut et al. 1974).

The EEG may be normal in patients with generalized tonic–clonic (grand mal) seizure disorders such as juvenile myoclonic epilepsy. In other cases, it may show diffuse bursts of theta or may contain sporadic 4- to 5-Hz spike-wave or polyspike-waves. Asymmetric or focal spike waves, or both, may appear commonly, but these can be considered fragments or regional expressions of essentially bilaterally synchronous phenomena (Aliberti et al. 1994; Lancman et al. 1994; Blume & Kaibara 1999). During a rarely recorded generalized tonic–clonic (GTC) attack, 20- to 40-Hz diffuse waves, slowing to about 10 Hz, appear during the tonic phase, followed by bilaterally synchronous and diffuse polyspike waves during the clonic phase. Unfortunately, muscle artifact rapidly obscures the tracing during GTC. Postictally, diffuse delta and theta predominate, with a return toward a normal recording within several minutes. No regional postictal abnormalities should occur if the attack was a primary generalized GTC. In those patients with secondarily generalized GTC, the attack itself may predominate in one hemisphere, and its postictal effects would reflect the side or area of most intense involvement.

Slow spike waves

Gibbs and associates (1939) first distinguished slow spike waves from 3-Hz spike-waves; the former repeats at 1.5–2 Hz. The epileptiform component may be either a spike or a sharp wave. These bilaterally synchronous discharges occupy a considerably greater quantity of the awake resting recording than do 3-Hz spike-waves (Figure 5.5). No clinical alteration may be discerned in such patients at the onset of a burst of slow spike-waves, in contradistinction to 3-Hz spike-wave discharges in which a closer correlation between the EEG and clinical findings occurs. As compared to 3-Hz spike waves, which appear principally in the 5- to 14-year-age group, the maximum incidence of slow spike waves occurs in children 1–5 years old (Blume et al. 1973). In earlier years, this pattern may be intermixed with hypsarrhythmia; in later years, it may merge with 3-Hz spike waves. The nonparoxysmal portion of the recording is abnormally slow, in contrast to the traditionally normal findings with 3-Hz spike waves. Hyperventilation less commonly elicits slow spike waves, and photic stimulation is not effective. Sinusoidal-like waves at 10–20 Hz may appear diffusely in such recordings (fast rhythmic waves [FRW] known also as epileptic recruiting rhythm [ERR]), accompanied either by tonic seizures or absence attacks (Fig. 5.8).

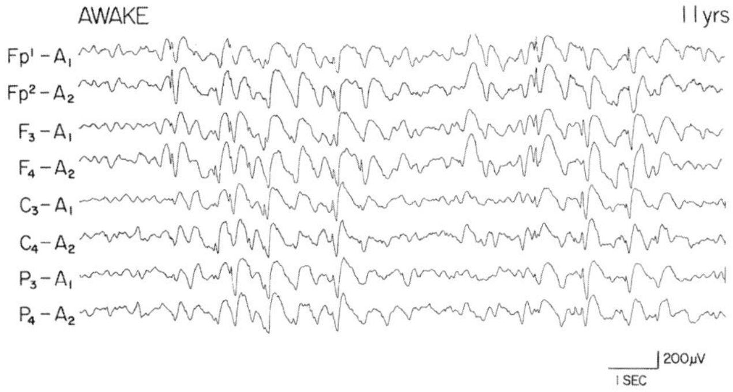

Figure 5.5 Abundant bisynchronous 1.5- to 2.5-Hz spike waves are "slow spike waves" (SSW) seen with the Lennox-Gastaut syndrome or during absence status epilepticus. The unilateral (*right*) accentuation of some SSW occurs commonly and shifts from side to side. This is not secondary bisynchrony.

As with 3-Hz spike waves, about 98% of patients with spikes of varying waves have seizures. Tonic seizures are the most common, followed by atypical absence and myoclonic attacks. Intelligence varies inversely with age of seizure onset. Intractable generalized seizures and bilaterally synchronous slow spike waves and ERR on the EEG constitute the Lennox-Gastaut syndrome (Genton et al. 2000).

Hypsarrhythmia

High-voltage 1- to 3-Hz waves with multifocal asynchronous spikes and sharp waves of varying morphology and amplitude constitute the pattern known as *hypsarrhythmia* (Figure 5.6). "Chaotic" is an appropriate description of the waveforms in their full expression.

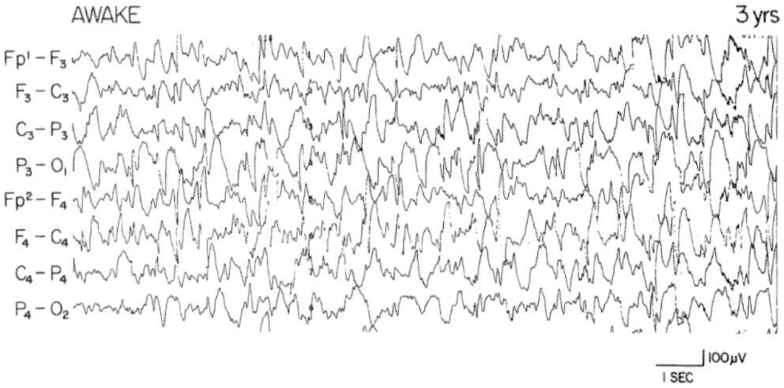

Figure 5.6 High-voltage diffuse delta with abundant multifocal spikes comprise the hypsarrythmia pattern. These phenomena are at least moderately persistent in wakefulness, but may appear in bursts during sleep.

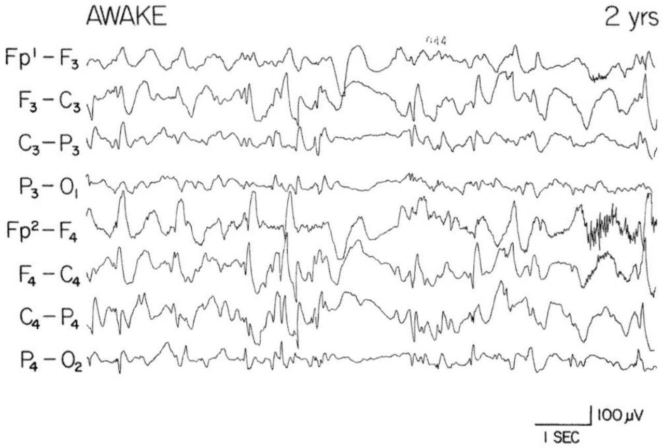

Figure 5.7 An electrodecremental event. Sudden regional or diffuse (*center*) attenuation may interrupt the hypsarrhythmia or slow spike-wave pattern. Although no clinical change was evident on this occasion, such change may be associated with epileptic spasms. Note chaotic hypsarrhythmia and bisynchronous slow spike-wave patterns here.

Virtually continuous during wakefulness when fully present, hypsarrhythmia may become discontinuous in moderate and deep sleep, and this effect of state should be considered whenever sequential EEGs are compared.

Hrachovy and coworkers (1984) described dramatic changes in the character of hypsarrhythmia over the course of recordings from all their 67 patients. In addition to the description already given, epochs of increased interhemispheric synchronization were found that may be the forerunners of slow spike waves. Hypsarrhythmia may predominate in one hemisphere or even be associated with consistently focal spike discharge. Epochs of attenuation may interrupt the hypsarrhythmic pattern. Finally, asynchronous high-voltage activity with minimal epileptiform potentials can appear. The appearance of such varying EEG features depends on the duration of the recording, the clinical state of the patient, and the presence of structural abnormalities. For example, a large cystic defect in one hemisphere could impair the expression of hypsarrhythmia on that side, creating the asymmetric form. Attenuation is most common in deep non-REM sleep, as already mentioned.

Despite the abundance of spikes and abnormal slow waves, the hypsarrhythmic pattern is considered an interictal phenomenon although one could consider the patient as being in an atypical absence during its presence. The most common clinical correlate of hypsarrhythmia is epileptic spasms. During these spasms, the hypsarrhythmic pattern is abruptly and diffusely replaced by a single high-voltage wave with or without an accompanying spike. Immediately following this, a diffuse or regional attenuation of electrical activity occurs, occasionally accompanied by low-voltage, high-frequency activity. Such phenomena are termed *electrodecremental events* (EDEs) (Figure 5.7).

The hypsarrhythmic pattern is not always present when infantile spasms first occur, but it ultimately appears. Therefore, the hypsarrhythmic pattern is helpful in differential diagnosis of epileptic and nonepileptic spasmodic conditions in infancy. Hypsarrhythmia is an age-related phenomenon, being confined usually to children aged 3 months to 5 years, approximately paralleling the time course of epileptic spasms. In younger patients, with the Ohtahara syndrome, a burst suppression pattern is characteristic (Ohtahara et al. 1976). In children of older ages, it may be replaced by slow spike waves, focal or multifocal epileptiform abnormalities, or nonepileptiform abnormalities.

No aspect of the hypsarrhythmic pattern has been found to correlate reliably with the ultimate evolution of mental development. Etiology and clinical course are more likely to be of value in this respect: Haga et al. (1995) found that those with focal ictal semiology had a poorer outcome.

Electroencephalographic changes during generalized seizures

In some instances, an electrographic seizure is manifested simply as sequential interictal potentials, such as a series of 3-Hz spike-wave discharges with absence attacks. Given the usual abundance of 3-Hz spike-waves discharges, at times it is difficult to determine whether the patient is having an atypical absence attack. Rhythmic waves of 10–20 Hz appearing diffusely may have absence or tonic seizures as the clinical correlate (Blume & Kaibara 1999) (Figure 5.8). Generalized myoclonic seizures have high-voltage, diffuse, bilaterally synchronous spike waves as the clinical correlate, even though the precise timing relationship between the EEG spike and the myoclonic jerk varies among patients and even in the same patient over time. GTC seizures combine many of these aforementioned EEG features: very-low-voltage

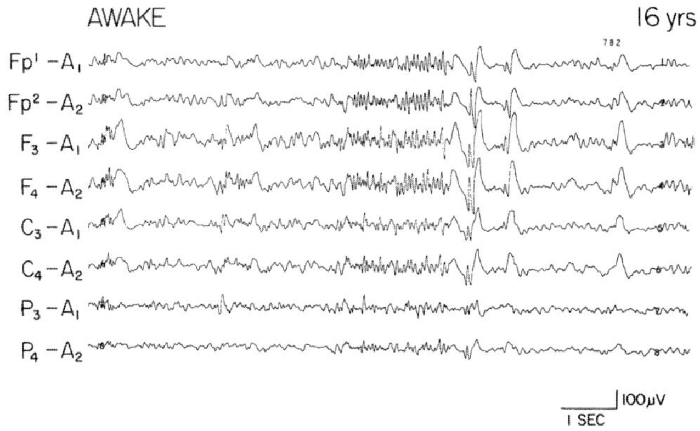

Figure 5.8 Fast rhythmic waves (epileptic recruiting rhythm) appear bilaterally in a 2-second burst (*center*), followed by bisynchronous slow spike waves. Such fast waves may be associated with either absence or tonic seizures, but this burst ended before any clinical change could be discerned. The short (0.05) time constant of this segment abbreviated the slow waves of the slow spike waves.

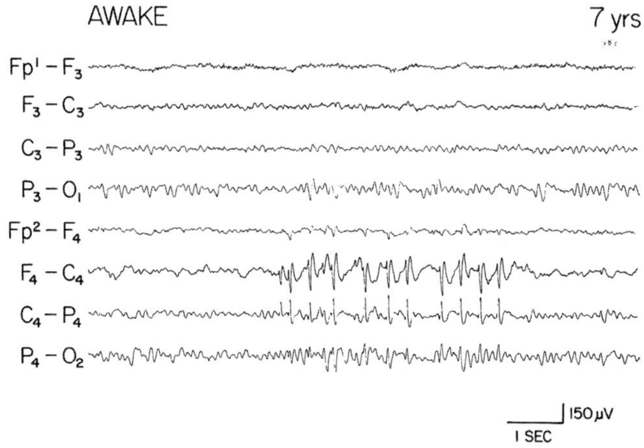

Figure 5.9 Right rolandic spikes. Their abundance is usually considerable, *not* in keeping with the infrequent associated seizures.

high-frequency waves, 10- to 20-Hz rhythmic waves, or both appear during the tonic phase. These waves are then interrupted by 300- to 400-msec bilaterally synchronous slow waves to constitute polyspike-wave discharges during the clonic phase. The ictal phase of epileptic spasms and hypsarrhythmia has been described. See Gastaut and Broughton (1974) for a full discussion of these ictal EEG–clinical relationships.

Focal epileptiform potentials

Rolandic spikes

Confined to children and adolescents, rolandic spikes are frequent, stereotyped, and distinct discharges that have as their most prominent component a downward deflection on anterior-posterior bipolar montages (Figure 5.9). This prominent downward deflection reflects the dipolarity of its field distribution, which can be proven by referential montages with simultaneous anterior positivity and posterior negativity (Blume 1982). Although the negative component of the field is usually over the central-parietal regions, with extension to the midtemporal areas, a sagittal or even parietal-occipital location may be seen, all identified by the characteristic morphology and abundance. Such spikes may be virtually limited to one hemisphere in a recording but can be seen independently bilaterally and even synchronously bilaterally, in which case they resemble spike waves. Rolandic spikes appear more abundantly in sleep; in some patients they occur exclusively in sleep. Beydoun and colleagues (1992) noted generalized spike waves in 15% of patients with rolandic spikes and other foci in 10%. The clinical course of patients with these features did not differ from those with rolandic spikes alone. Distinction of these spikes from rhythm may be difficult. Mu is more confined to central regions (C3,4); rolandic spike quantity would increase in non-REM sleep when the mu rhythm disappears.

When such spikes are abundant, they may be accompanied by slow waves in the same region. With this exception, the remainder of the EEG should be normal. Rolandic spikes do not usually represent a structural lesion. However, when a persistent attenuation of background activity or focal delta appears, particularly if independent of spikes, then a structural lesion might be present.

The associated seizure disorder is benign epilepsy of childhood with rolandic spikes (BECRs), which occurs most commonly during non-REM sleep as GTC with occasional unilateral predominance. During the daytime, partial sensory–motor attacks appearing principally in the face or arm may occur. Intellect and neurologic examinations are normal. Both the seizure tendency and the spikes tend to disappear by mid adolescence, but the quantity of spikes bears no relationship to the quantity of epileptic seizures. About 50–70% of patients with rolandic spikes have seizures (Niedermeyer 1987). Therefore, it is possible to find this pattern by chance in an EEG performed in the course of looking for another condition. For example, this author has seen this pattern in patients with definite syncope. If a patient has a seizure disorder the characteristics of which are not those of BECRs, then additional electrographic abnormalities must be sought for correlation. Conversely, if a patient with a seizure disorder implicating the rolandic region does not have classic rolandic spikes, then an epileptogenic lesion should be sought if a second EEG including sleep fails to disclose such discharges.

Occipital spikes

Occipital spikes are well-defined electronegative spikes that appear unilaterally or bilaterally in synchronous or independent fashion over the occipital lobes and may spread to the posterior temporal or parietal regions. They are more abundant with the eyes closed and therefore can be distinguished from lambda waves which, in contrast, are normal electropositive potentials that occur when scanning a complex field.

Eeg-Olofsson and associates (1971) found occipital spikes in less than 1% of the normal children they studied. Occipital spikes are the most common focal discharges in children younger than 4 years of age, and they appear most commonly at that time. Smith and Kellaway (1964) found epilepsy in only 54% of their studied children with occipital spikes. However, Maher and colleagues' 1995 study of occipital spikes in a referral center laboratory found 29 of 31 children to have seizure disorders.

There are several types of occipital spikes and several conditions in which they appear. Discharges resembling rolandic spikes may appear in the occipital region and may be associated with a benign partial epilepsy of childhood consisting of visual, hemisensory-motor, autonomic, oculoversive and limbic-like seizures (Gastaut 1992; Panayiotopoulos 1999). Not all children with occipital spikes that attenuate with eye opening have easily controlled seizures, and therefore gradations between benign and more therapy-resistant syndromes occur (Cooper & Lee 1991). Very brief occipital spikes may appear in congenitally blind children without any occipital lesion or seizure disorder (Lairy et al. 1964). Syndromes encompassing migraine, occipital and other seizure disorders, and occipital spikes have been described (Andermann 1987). Occipital spikes associated with other focal occipital EEG abnormalities occur in children with epileptogenic lesions in this area including arteriovenous malformations, tumors, and cortical developmental abnormalities. Gobbi and coworkers (1991) described patients with occipital spikes, epilepsy, and calcifications in association with celiac disease. The seizures gradually become intractable. Finally, patients with a progressive myoclonus epilepsy, such as Lafora body disease, may have occipital spikes and light-sensitive seizures (Tassinari et al. 1978).

Photic stimulation may elicit occipital spikes in patients with both regional (Jones & Blume, unpublished results) and generalized encephalopathies, such as neuronal ceroid lipofuscinosis (Pampiglione & Harden 1977).

Anterior temporal spikes

Although anterior temporal spikes are thought to be more common among adults, they do appear in childhood and have similar clinical correlates. This is not surprising, because temporal lobe seizures may begin as early as 3–4 years of age. Montages that distinguish these discharges from the temporal extension of rolandic spikes are necessary; rolandic spikes extend principally to the midtemporal or posterior temporal region and are less prominent anteriorly and inferiorly. Eeg-Olofsson and colleagues (1971) found temporal spikes in less than 1% of their series of normal children.

The etiology of such spikes includes any anterior temporal chronic lesion including mesial temporal sclerosis (MTS), malformative lesions with or without MTS, and tumors (Falconer & Taylor 1968; Blume et al. 1982; Pringle et al. 1993; Aicardi 1994).

Periodic epileptiform phenomena

Periodic lateralized epileptiform discharges (unilateral, PLEDs; bilateral, BIPLEDs) appear in children. More precisely, PLEDs are repetitive regional discharges, as they seldom repeat with metronomic regularity (Gross et al. 1999). These discharges usually reflect acute conditions with metabolic/electrolytic derangements complicated by seizures. Two-thirds of patients in a study by Chen and coworkers (2003) had CNS infections, particularly herpes simplex encephalitis. All 15 patients of Garg and colleagues (1995) had seizures, of whom eight had status epilepticus; only one of seven survivors was seizure-free.

Periodic discharges may also accompany the hemispheric epileptiform and nonepileptiform abnormalities of Rasmussen encephalitis.

Periodic high-voltage broad spikes occur in subacute sclerosing panencephalitis (SSPE). These 100–1,000 μV complexes appear as 1- to 3-Hz waves with intermingled spikes that may occur at 2- to 20-second intervals and may be distributed diffusely or regionally. These waves correlate irregularly with brief axial or proximal limb myotonic phenomena.

Electroencephalographic changes during focal seizures

Focal seizures are characterized by the regional appearance of sequential waves that differ from background, the morphology of which evolves over the course of the seizure (Blume et al. 1984). Such waves may resemble single or multiple sine wave sequences or a series of spikes or sharp waves (Figure 5.10).

Activation procedures

Any method that may elicit an EEG abnormality that has not occurred in a routine recording falls under the broad category of an activation procedure.

Hyperventilation

From age 4 years, children can cooperate with hyperventilation; their enthusiasm for the procedure is usually greater than among adults. Consequently and for reasons of brain immaturity, the effect of hyperventilation is more prominent in children than among adolescents and adults. Rhythmic theta and delta activity appears initially posteriorly and then diffusely. It may not remit when the technologist asks the patient to stop hyperventilating because

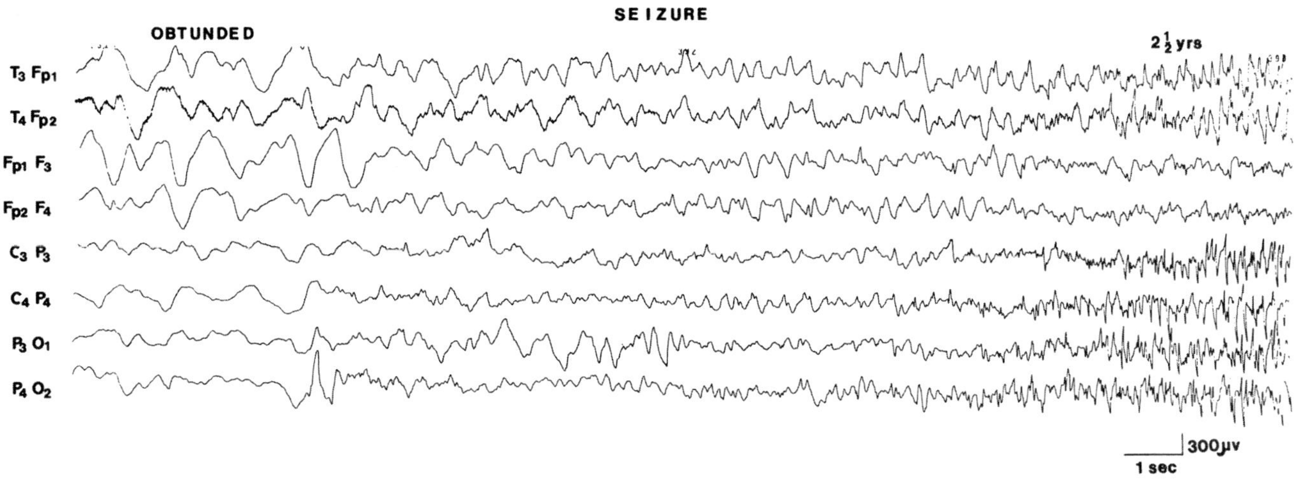

Figure 5.10 From an excessively slow, delta-dominated background, a seizure gradually begins—first as theta (*center*), then as sequential polyspikes (*right*). Note left-right alternating montage.

some patients may continue to do so. Hypoglycemia may augment the response. Therefore the quantity of this response and its persistence are not criteria of abnormality.

Photic stimulation

Four types of results occur with photic stimulation: (1) "driving," that is, response of varying morphology that is time-locked to the flash rate; (2) frontal myoclonic potentials, also time-locked, reflecting myoclonus of periocular and scalp musculature; (3) photoparoxysmal response, described later; and (4) no apparent effect. Full discussions of these phenomena can be found in EEG textbooks and atlases.

The most clinically significant phenomenon with photic stimulation is the photoparoxysmal response, a bilaterally synchronous polyspike or polyspike-wave discharge that is not time-locked to the flash rate and that may continue beyond the cessation of the flash stimulus (Reilly & Peters 1973) (Figure 5.11). This response is most readily elicited with flash rates of about 14–18 per second, particularly on eye closure. It appears in about 3% of all patients referred for EEG and of those with focal seizure disorders, and in about 20–50% of patients with GTC, myoclonic, or absence attacks (Takahashi 1987). As the photoparoxysmal response may be seen in normal individuals and in patients with metabolic or drug withdrawal conditions, a diagnosis of a seizure disorder cannot conclusively be made on this basis. Moreover, relatives of patients with primary generalized seizures may demonstrate a photoparoxysmal response without necessarily having a seizure disorder. On the other hand, such polyspike waves may confirm questionable spike-wave discharges on the resting recording. A photoparoxysmal response in a child with febrile convulsions suggests that these may be the first manifestations of a myoclonic epilepsy of childhood (Dalla Bernardina et al. 1982; Dravet et al. 1985). The photoparoxysmal response suggests that seizures of patients with primary generalized seizures may be precipitated by light flashes. Spike-wave discharges to photic stimulation are uncommon in children younger than 5 years of age, and the incidence in children aged 5–15 years is relatively stable.

Ambulatory electroencephalography

To record sporadic, usually unpredictable clinical events in the patient's habitual environment is the goal of ambulatory monitoring (AM), which provides long-term recording without continuous technical supervision.

Although the currently most reliable method uses collodion-applied disk electrodes to achieve stable long-term

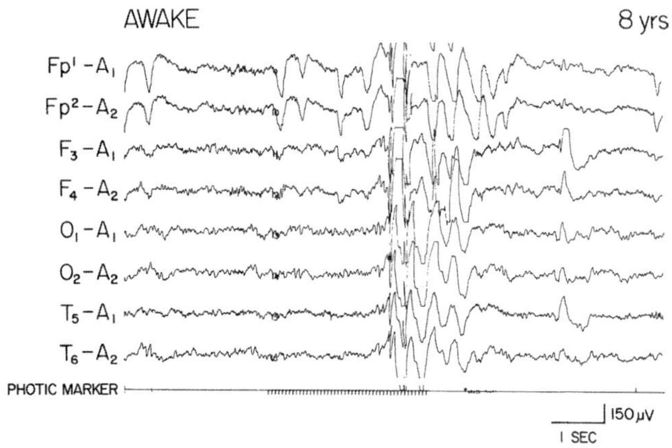

Figure 5.11 The photoparoxysmal response, consisting of spike waves that have a repetition rate that is wholly independent of the flash rate and that outlast termination of the photic stimulation. Such spike waves correlate better with a generalized seizure disorder than do spike waves that are time-locked to the stimulus and do not outlast the flash.

recordings (Ebersole et al. 2003), Young and coworkers (2003) have developed a small subdermal needle electrode even less susceptible to artifact.

Ebersole's group (Leroy & Ebersole 1983) devised montages to emphasize the anterior temporal and frontal regions, as most epileptiform discharges arise in these areas. With careful adherence to conservative standards of montage design and electrode application, about 80% of focal epileptiform abnormalities could be accurately identified and localized and 100% of seizures detected by ambulatory monitoring as compared to inpatient telemetry. Both systems were superior to routine EEG in this respect (Leroy & Ebersole 1983; Bridgers & Ebersole 1985), although routine EEG is probably superior for nonepileptiform abnormalities.

Ambulatory EEG may help distinguish epileptic seizures from nonepileptic events such as pseudoseizures, syncope, or sleep attacks. It could assist in determining seizure quantity, particularly absence. Classification of known seizures, for example, temporal lobe from absence, may be accomplished. Technical limitations must be acknowledged, particularly when localization of seizure onset is paramount. Epileptiform activity could arise from areas not covered by the limited montages, and the design of such montages should be flexible. Patient selection and technical factors may affect yield. Thus, while Saravanan and colleagues (2001) obtained clarification of management in only 31%, Olson (2001) obtained useful information in 84% of 167 children.

Outpatient video-electroencephalography

In instances in which the clinical description and standard EEG fail to identify the nature of some events, combining video-recording and EEG in a 2- to 3-hour session has been diagnostically helpful in 50–90% (Al-Qudah 1999; Carmant et al. 1996; Chen et al. 1995; Kramer et al. 1995; Valente et al. 2003). Distinction of epileptic seizures from other intermittent episodes, reclassification of known epileptic seizures, and management changes have been realized in these studies.

Certain central nervous system disorders

Febrile seizures

Three mechanisms may predispose a child to seizures with a fever. The classic febrile seizure represents a genetically determined susceptibility to generalized seizures occurring only with fever. A second group of patients have seizures with fever because of a cerebral lesion occurring either before or during the febrile episode. A third group consists of children who have a chronic generalized epileptic condition that first becomes evident as seizures during a febrile episode.

Complex febrile seizures are those that last more than 15 minutes, are unilateral or focal, or are repeated within a single febrile episode. Such attacks tend to occur in patients whose neurologic development before the febrile attack was already abnormal and are usually associated with a higher risk of later epilepsy. Conversely, a single, brief, generalized febrile seizure may have a relatively favorable prognosis. However, in practice, classifying each episode into either the simple or the complex category may be clinically difficult, as may be the determination of prognosis. Therefore, EEG may help categorize the mechanism of the febrile seizure if its nature is clinically ambiguous.

EEGs obtained less than a week after a febrile seizure may show various quantities of delta activity, appearing either diffusely or posteriorly, with the quantity depending on the duration of the febrile seizure and the interval between its termination and the EEG recording. Such bilateral delta activity would fail to reveal the febrile seizure mechanism. A postictal EEG with regionally accentuated delta or focal spikes would suggest that the seizure with a fever represented the second category outlined previously, that is, a seizure secondary to a previous or current regional CNS abnormality.

EEG could be valuable in the emergent situation for any patient who fails to regain consciousness within a reasonable time after the apparent end of a febrile seizure, to exclude the possibility of continuing seizure activity.

Generalized spike-waves on a routine EEG in a patient with febrile seizures does not increase the incidence of nonfebrile generalized seizures later in life. For example, about 20% of the patients of Frantzen and colleagues (1968) had sporadic generalized spike waves that were not predictive of the recurrence of febrile seizures or the later development of nonfebrile seizures. Such spike waves appear more commonly after age 4 years. On the other hand, abundant spike waves suggest that the febrile seizure is the first manifestation of a generalized nonfebrile seizure disorder, particularly if a photoparoxys-

Pearls and Perils

Central Nervous System Conditions with Epilepsy

- The patient with a simple febrile seizure does not necessarily need an electroencephalogram (EEG).
- Sporadic spike-wave discharges in a patient with febrile seizures do not necessarily indicate that epilepsy will supervene.

mal response is readily elicited (Dalla Bernardina et al. 1982; Dravet et al. 1985).

An EEG is not mandatory in most patients with a simple febrile seizure. Clinical judgment would be required as to whether an EEG could help unravel the mechanism of a more complex attack.

Hemiconvulsion-hemiplegia-epilepsy

The hemiconvulsion-hemiplegia-epilepsy (HH&E) syndrome described by Gastaut and coworkers (1960) consists of a unilateral or predominantly unilateral prolonged motor seizure, a postictal hemiplegia that may or may not persist, and a focal epileptic seizure disorder, either as seizures from the temporal lobe of the implicated hemisphere or focal motor and possible secondarily generalized seizures. Because the young child is often febrile at the onset of the status epilepticus, a distinction from predominantly unilateral febrile seizures is clinically and nosologically impossible. Postictally, high-voltage 1- to 2-Hz delta activity may be seen bilaterally, with emphasis on the implicated hemisphere, and this EEG abnormality may persist in less prominent form for several years. Multifocal spikes chronically appear independently in either hemisphere but principally over the clinically implicated hemisphere. Secondarily generalized spike waves are also a feature.

Continuous spike-waves during slow sleep (CSWS)

Synonymous with electrical status epilepticus during sleep (ESES) (Patry et al. 1971; Tassinari et al. 1982; 2000), the EEG features of this rare syndrome consist of abundant (~85% of slow-wave sleep) bisynchronous spike waves and slow spike waves with occasional regional expression, usually best expressed over the frontal-central regions (Pedley et al. 2003). Spike waves and slow spike waves also appear in wakefulness, but less abundantly. These phenomena appear principally at 4–7 years of age, but the associated generalized and focal seizure disorder may begin 1–2 years earlier. The CSWS phenomenon persists for 1–6 years; it gradually resolves along with the associated seizure disorder, leaving cognitive, behavioral, and motor deficits in some.

Acquired epileptic aphasia (Landau-Kleffner syndrome)

The Landau-Kleffner syndrome is closely associated with the CSWS syndrome (Dulac 2001; Veggiotti et al. 1999). Abundant spikes or spike-wave complexes appear bilaterally with predominance over the temporal, parietal, and occipital regions in acquired epileptic aphasia, with the emphasis shifting from side to side. Background activity is normal (Hirsch et al. 1990). Sleep onset and non-REM sleep may augment spike quantity, but they may persist in REM sleep (Roger et al. 1993). Such EEG abnormalities become less prominent in adolescents, in rough parallel with the decline in the seizure disorder for most patients. This syndrome and electrographic status epilepticus of sleep may be variants of the same disorder.

Malformations of cortical development

Several EEG phenomena may be associated with cerebral malformations, including a paucity of EEG activity either focally or diffusely, monorhythmic theta, or diffuse or focal delta activity. Encephalopathy caused by perinatal insults such as infection or trauma may have similar constellations of abnormalities, depending on the severity. In patients with relatively restricted abnormalities, such as porencephaly, most cerebral activity may be normal except in the implicated area, where paucity of activity, excessive slowing, or spike discharges may appear. Agenesis of the corpus callosum may be associated with a normal EEG or with hypsarrhythmia in infants with Aicardi syndrome.

Patients with focal cortical malformations who have epilepsy may show multifocal spikes that extend beyond the lobe of the malformation (Palmini et al. 1991), but these are usually principally seen in the region of the malformation. Such epileptiform discharges may be very abundant and may appear in repetitive sequences, paralleling the very frequent seizures with which these patients are afflicted (Gambardella et al. 1996; Raymond et al. 1995).

Trauma

The magnitude of EEG changes following trauma is considerably greater in children than in adults with the same neurologic status. A mild head injury in a child may produce prominent EEG changes that do not necessarily connote irreversible brain injury. Posteriorly accentuated excess activity is the most prominent single abnormality in the acute phase. The frequency of this delta activity is lower in the younger age groups. Such delta declines rapidly after the second week postinjury (Silverman 1962).

Because a head injury involves both direct and contrecoup effects, it is possible that the EEG would reveal dysfunction that is not clinically apparent. For example, the author has seen hemispheric arrhythmic delta activity ipsilateral to trauma-produced hemiplegia.

In addition to direct cerebral injury, other mechanisms may pertain. Carotid artery injury in neck trauma may produce a dissection-related stroke. Hypoxia from a chest injury would give diffuse abnormalities. Fat embolism from long bone fractures may rarely occur.

When assessing the effects of head injury on EEG, the presence of preexisting EEG abnormalities must always be considered; for example, 3-Hz bilaterally synchronous

> **Pearls and Perils**
>
> **Acute Conditions**
>
> - Electroencephalography (EEG) can help monitor the effectiveness of anticonvulsant medication in acutely ill patients whose epileptic seizures may have subtle or bizarre manifestations.
> - Sequential EEGs are often of greater prognostic value than a single EEG in assessing the prognosis of a comatose child.
> - EEG can be helpful in assessing whether coma is irreversible, but its value is considerably less than that of clinical data in this respect.

spike-waves and slow spike-wave changes characterize the result of trauma.

Epileptiform abnormalities are a not uncommon late consequence of trauma. To ensure the relative or complete absence of these abnormalities, one or more recordings, including one taken during sleep, may be required.

Encephalitis

In encephalitis, normal background rhythms are replaced by theta and excess delta activity. These slow waves are usually diffuse but may have regional accentuation. Although the abnormalities correlate reasonably well with the neurologic state of the patient, both the severity of the encephalitis and any associated systemic disease with metabolic derangements may contribute. Electrolytic derangements alter the EEG more prominently in children than in adults.

Epileptic seizures may complicate encephalitis, and their clinical manifestations may be unusual or subtle. The EEG, particularly if adequate recording time is allowed, can detect electrographic seizures or at least abundant epileptiform activity. In this manner, it may also monitor the effectiveness of anticonvulsant therapy.

Periodic broad spikes are particularly characteristic of herpes simplex encephalitis; such phenomena may be diffuse, temporal-frontal, unilateral, or bilateral in a shifting manner.

In the past, EEG was useful in localizing focal or multifocal abscesses, but advances in neuroimaging have largely supplanted this role in developed countries.

Meningitis

If meningitis has a minimal encephalitic component, the associated EEG changes could be slight. Moreover, they may also represent any metabolic or electrolytic derangements attendant on the acute condition. Once again, focal delta activity should alert the clinician to the possibility of abscess or cerebral vein thrombosis as a complication.

Coma

Because the clinical examination of a patient with a subnormal level of consciousness, particularly coma, is primarily confined to assessment of brainstem function, the EEG provides a valuable adjunct by recording cortically originating activity.

Several phenomena can be seen in comatose conditions. The most common is diffuse persistent excess delta and theta activity. Lack of attenuation or other alteration of this activity by afferent stimuli indicates deep coma. The occurrence of triphasic waves in association with a depressed level of consciousness indicates a metabolically induced comatose condition (Bickford & Butt 1955; Sundaram & Blume 1987). Periodic lateralizing epileptiform discharges may be seen in patients with overriding regional abnormalities (Chatrian et al. 1964).

When recurrent seizures complicate the situation, the effectiveness of anticonvulsant treatment can be monitored by assessing the abundance of clinical and subclinical electrographic seizures and the quantity of spikes (Figure 5.10).

Burst suppression activity may appear in deep coma: Bursts or brief runs of intermixed theta, delta, and spikes are separated by equal or longer periods of relative or complete inactivity, either diffusely or regionally. In other situations, diffuse, nonreactive sinusoidal patterns in the theta or alpha range have been described by several authors (see Bauer 1987, for review).

The prognosis of any of these patterns depends on the etiology of the comatose condition, its duration, and the direction of which sequential EEG recordings are headed. Thus, if anesthetics or other CNS depressants have been used, the value of EEG patterns in prognosis is virtually nil. Metabolic and toxic states usually have a better prognosis than structural or anoxic encephalopathies for a given EEG picture. Within this context, prognostically favorable signs are EEG reactivity to exogenous stimuli, spontaneous variability, and normal sleep potentials. The following suggest an unfavorable outcome: lack of reactivity to deep painful afferent stimuli, the burst suppression pattern, monorhythmic alpha or theta frequencies, a very-low-voltage EEG, or electrocerebral inactivity.

Pampiglione and Harden (1968) carried out EEGs within the first 12 hours of cardiac arrest in children aged 1 day to 10 years. Those children whose EEGs contained at least some normal features appropriate to age, either on the initial recording or within a few hours, recovered well. Patients with continuous delta that failed to resolve over several hours and those with burst suppression or electrocerebral inactivity died.

The electroencephalogram in determination of irreversible coma

Bobele and colleagues (1993) found clinical examination to more reliably predict outcome or death in newborns and infants than either EEG or radionuclide cerebral perfusion scans.

With respect to the EEG, even apparent electrocerebral inactivity cannot be equated with total cessation of cortical function. A limiting factor is machine noise, from which cerebrally originating potentials of less than 2 μV cannot be distinguished. Neuronal discharges from the thalamus have been recorded when no EEG activity is apparent (Carbonell et al. 1963; Jonkman 1969; Visser 1969). Ashwal and Schneider (1979) showed the presence of EEG activity in patients up to 30 months of age who fulfilled other criteria for brain death; none of these five patients survived.

Instead of requiring physicians to use EEG in the determination of irreversible coma, it could be suggested as an ancillary test in situations during which full evaluation of brainstem function is not possible from a practical standpoint. This would occur when trauma to structures reflecting brainstem function had occurred. Even in this circumstance, EEG data would not necessarily assume primary importance but would be considered along with other data in arriving at a clinical decision of irreversible coma.

If one accepts the concept of irreversible coma instead of brain death, demonstration of complete cortical electrical inactivity may not be required. Reactivity of any pattern to afferent stimuli would assume paramount importance. Technical requirements can be found in many publications, particularly in the work of Bauer (1987).

Reye syndrome

Aoki and Lombroso (1973) demonstrated a close relationship between clinical staging of neurologic impairment and EEG. Although the prognosis at each stage has likely improved since their original publication because of improvements in management, the close clinical–EEG relationship may be useful in monitoring patients who have been pharmacologically paralyzed as part of management.

As with any comatose condition, unfavorable EEG prognostic signs would include lack of reactivity to afferent stimuli, very-low-voltage activity, electrocerebral inactivity, and the burst suppression pattern.

Cerebral palsy

Among patients with cerebral palsy, those with hemiplegia have the highest incidence of EEG changes (90%), followed by quadriplegics (85%) (Gibbs & Gibbs 1964). Because the pathology is more deeply seated among patients with paraplegia and athetosis, EEG abnormalities are less common.

Asymmetries of awake and sleep potentials may appear among patients with hemiplegia, the side of lower voltage corresponding to the clinically implicated hemisphere. Such abnormalities would be less common for patients with athetosis or diplegia.

Multiple independent spike foci are probably the most common single EEG abnormality. Usually these spike foci are more common over the implicated hemisphere, but if both hemispheres are extensively damaged, the spikes may be better expressed over the relatively healthy side.

Syncope

Sequential EEG events occur in fortuitously recorded syncope: loss of alpha, a brief period of low-voltage beta, then rapidly augmenting diffuse theta, then delta activity followed by transient electrocerebral inactivity, then progressive recovery. Nonetheless, diagnosis of syncope does not depend on demonstration of this sequence, as was thought in the past.

The danger of performing an EEG in patients with syncope is that some irrelevant abnormality or anomaly might be disclosed. Therefore, the purpose of the recording should be thoroughly communicated to the patient and parents before the fact. When myoclonic or tonic movements are a prominent or prolonged feature of the syncopal attack (brief myoclonies are common), the clinician may be justified in wondering if a generalized epileptic condition is so represented. However, this is a rarity and an EEG is unnecessary in almost all cases of syncope.

As syncope may reflect cardiac arrhythmias, scrutiny of the electrocardiac (ECG) monitor recorded during the EEG is prudent although this single ECG lead would not be a sufficient cardiac examination in itself.

Headache

Although a high percentage of nonspecific abnormalities may be seen in children and adults with migraine or other forms of headache, the value of such abnormalities

Pearls and Perils

Chronic Conditions

- History and neurologic examination are better than an electroencephalogram (EEG) in diagnosing syncope and determining the cause of headache.

in differential diagnosis has never been adequately established. Thus, an EEG would be of less value than clinical judgment in evaluating the cause of headache.

Progressive disorders

The EEG does not play a major role in the differential diagnosis of most degenerative diseases encountered; of greater significance are age, symptoms, neurologic examination, family history, and the course of the disease. However, EEG changes are often prominent and, therefore their unexpected presence may signal the existence of a degenerative disorder.

Slowing then disappearance of normal background rhythms combined with excessive delta or theta activity is a common finding whether gray or white matter is primarily involved. Spike discharges are more common in primarily gray matter disorders, whereas activity is relatively more prominent in white matter disorders; however, these distinctions are not absolute (Gloor et al. 1968).

At younger ages, patients with neuronal ceroid lipofuscinosis may respond to low-frequency flash stimulation with large occipital spikes (Pampiglione & Harden 1973). Early-onset degenerative conditions such as globoid leukodystrophy or phenylketonuria may be represented by the hypsarrhythmic pattern.

High-voltage posteriorly situated delta activity during wakefulness may represent adrenoleukodystrophy in any patient in whom more likely causes of this EEG phenomenon, such as recent seizures or trauma, are not present.

The electroretinogram (ERG) may help in the differentiation of some degenerative conditions. For example, in GM_2 gangliosidosis (Tay-Sachs disease), the ERG remains normal, whereas it may become abolished with neuronal ceroid lipofuscinosis.

Electroencephalography in progressive myoclonus epilepsies

Slowing of background activity and frequent generalized spike-waves and slow spike-waves characterize this group of disorders. In mitochondrial encephalopathy with ragged red fibers (MERRF), focal abnormalities and photosensitivity may appear. Normal physiologic sleep patterns may be abolished. In ceroid lipofuscinosis, low-frequency flashes may elicit high-voltage posterior polyphasic spikes. Visual evoked potentials are also large in this disorder. In Lafora disease, focal occipital paroxysms may be seen in the same recording that demonstrates generalized polyspike waves. In Unverricht-Lundborg disease, photic stimuli may elicit polyspike-wave discharges in about 90% of patients, particularly in the early phases of the disease (Genton & Roger 1993).

Epilepsy and brain tumors

The classic EEG sign of brain tumor is persistent regional delta activity with spike discharges in the same region if the tumor is slowly growing. Thus we found persistent EEG delta activity in 10 of 16 patients whose tumors presented as chronic uncontrolled partial seizure disorders (Blume et al. 1982). However, multiple independent spike discharges occurred in a majority of epileptic patients with

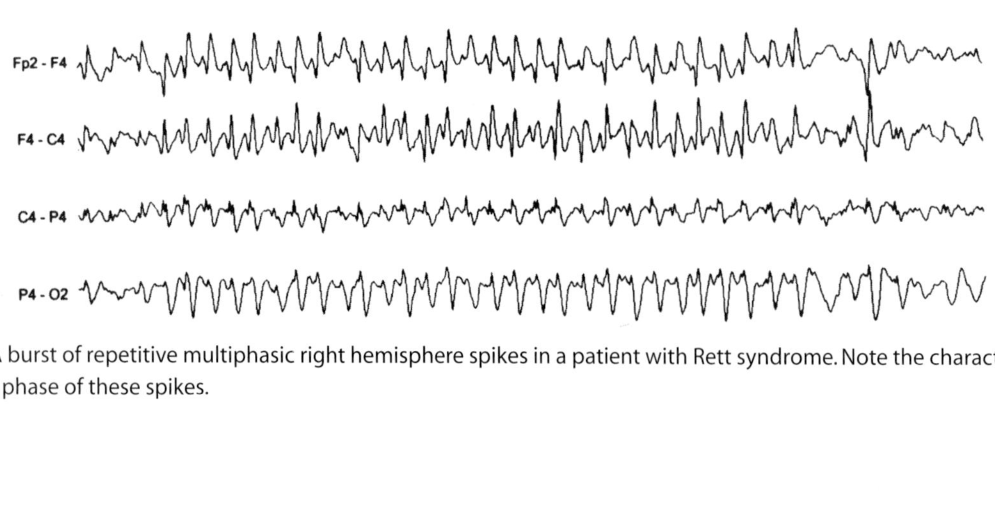

Figure 5.12 A burst of repetitive multiphasic right hemisphere spikes in a patient with Rett syndrome. Note the characteristic brevity of at least one phase of these spikes.

tumors; 4 of the 16 with tumor had generalized spike-wave discharges. Thus, the type and distribution of epileptiform discharges does not distinguish patients with tumors, but persistent focal delta activity over several recordings may suggest its presence. Of course, improved neuroimaging has lessened the EEG's value in tumor detection.

Angelman syndrome

Characteristic EEG features are bursts of high-voltage, rhythmic, anterior-predominant delta activity that may appear in one or more forms: (a) hypsarrhythmic, with multifocal spikes; (b) rhythmic delta bursts only; (c) superimposed spikes creating a slow spike-wave or notched appearance; and (d) triphasic morphology (Valente et al. 2003). Although one or more of these appeared in 96% of their patients, Hou and colleagues (1997) indicate that clinical features become obvious before characteristic EEG features appear. Similar delta bursts may appear posteriorly and may be precipitated by eye closure (Rubin et al. 1997).

Rett syndrome

Reflecting the severe epilepsy that afflicts most girls with Rett syndrome, epileptiform activity is prominent in the EEGs. Slow spike waves are a major feature, and these waves usually achieve maximum expression posteriorly, as compared to the usual anterior field distribution of slow spike waves in the Lennox-Gastaut syndrome (Niedermeyer & Naidu 1987). Multifocal spikes may also appear. Needle-like central spikes, occasionally evoked by stimulation of the contralateral fingernails, are characteristic (Nordli et al. 2003) (Figure 5.12). Trauner and Haas (1985) also found disorganized and slow background activity during wakefulness and quasiperiodic bursts of high-amplitude delta or theta with interspersed epochs of attenuation lasting 3–4 seconds. These features develop particularly between ages 2–10 years, when seizures and neurologic signs appear (Nordli et al. 2003). Although EEGs of Angelman and Rett syndromes differ substantially (Nordli et al. 2003), features of each have been found in the same patient (Laan & Vein 2003).

Annotated bibliography

Blume WT, Kaibara M. *Atlas of pediatric electroencephalography*. New York: Lipincott-Raven, 1999.
A more complete series of illustrations can be found in this atlas.

Niedermeyer E, Lopes da Silva F. *Electroencephalography: Basic principles, clinical applications and related fields*, 5th ed. Philadelphia: Lippincott Williams & Wilkins, 2005.
This textbook covers the topic of the EEG in greater detail.

CHAPTER 6

Electrodiagnostic Evaluation of Pediatric Neuromuscular Disease

Laurie Gutmann and Jack E. Riggs

Outline

- Challenges of pediatric electromyography
- Abnormalities in pediatric electromyography
- Examples of questions to be addressed by pediatric EMG
- Concluding remarks

This section on electrodiagnostic studies in the evaluation of pediatric neuromuscular disease will review the special challenges encountered and the types of electromyographic (EMG) abnormalities that the physician can reasonably expect to detect in this age group. No attempt has been made to describe the actual performance of pediatric EMG. Since specific neuromuscular disorders are reviewed elsewhere in this text, we will not review the specific electrodiagnostic abnormalities associated with each of these disorders. This chapter will review the specific questions that are commonly addressed by EMG in the evaluation of pediatric neuromuscular disease.

Challenges of pediatric electromyography

Pediatric EMG presents an array of special challenges to both the physician ordering the study and the physician performing the study. These challenges create potential pitfalls that can greatly affect the interpretation of the EMG study. Recognizing these differences when performing an electrodiagnostic evaluation of a pediatric patient as compared to an adult are extremely important for accurate performance and interpretation of the study.

Limited capacity to cooperate

The limited capacity of infants and young children to cooperate during an EMG has several practical implications. Foremost, before ordering an EMG on a young child or infant, the physician should be able to explicitly ask the electromyographer a specific question that is to be addressed by the EMG study. If the electromyographer does not have a specific question to address, he will not know how to prioritize the examination. Since young children may not be able to cooperate with the examination or may be sedated for it, the study is often performed in a nonstandard sequence. The electromyographer may need to alter the examination in such a way as to obtain information as the opportunity arises. The examination may have to be curtailed without doing all that was initially planned.

If the physician ordering the EMG does not have a specific question for the electromyographer, everyone involved would be better served by referring the patient first to a physician with experience in pediatric neuromuscular disease. Similarly, if the electromyographer does not have experience in performing EMGs on young children or infants, it is best to refer the patient to an electromyographer with such experience. Much time can be wasted and ill feelings can evolve when parents suspect that physicians and electromyographers are not sure what they are looking for or how to interpret what they have done, particularly when it has involved repeatedly sticking needles into and delivering electrical shocks to their children. Parents may not allow these studies to be repeated elsewhere, thereby hindering the diagnostic process.

Conscious sedation is sometimes utilized by our EMG laboratory, depending on the age of the child. With or without conscious sedation, the child may be able to cooperate for only a limited time during the examination, again emphasizing the need for a specific question and plan for the study. We encourage the presence of parents in the laboratory. Every attempt to reduce the anxiety of both is made through explanation of the question(s) the procedure may help to answer.

Large body surface area to body mass

The relatively large body surface area to body mass of a small child means that children are more prone to cooling. Abnormal temperature of the patient during nerve conduction studies and EMG can alter the results of the test, giving either a false-positive or a false-negative result. Although the importance of maintaining normal body temperature when screening for defects of neuromuscular junction transmission is widely acknowledged, the patient's temperature is also important when obtaining standard nerve conduction studies and needle EMG. A false-positive diagnosis of a mild demyelinating generalized peripheral neuropathy can occur if the patient is too cool, with distal latencies mildly prolonged and nerve conduction velocities mildly slowed. These alterations are partially due to alteration of the sodium/potassium (Na^+/K^+) pump activity and Na^+ channel open time.

On the other hand, conduction block in demyelinating disease improves with cooling. Sodium channel open time is prolonged with cooling, allowing for depolarization of the nerve in demyelinated areas. Warming can actually enhance the abnormalities in focal compressive lesions such as carpal tunnel syndrome by shortening Na^+ channel open time, improving the accuracy of the test. However, warming will not make a normal study look abnormal.

On needle EMG, fibrillation and fasciculation potentials are reduced with focal cooling and may even disappear in early disease. This effect could result in a normal appearing study in a patient with early axonal loss or early motor neuron disease.

At the neuromuscular junction, cooling will enhance neuromuscular transmission, resulting in a less prominent decrement with repetitive stimulation, despite a defect of the neuromuscular junction. The alterations from cooling are complex, having to do with a combination of calcium (Ca^{2+}) influx and prolonged half-life, reduced acetylcholinesterase activity, and vesicle and acetylcholine binding. However, warming or cooling will not give you an abnormal result in a patient without disease. The safety margin in a normal neuromuscular junction is high enough to compensate for temperature effects.

In our EMG laboratory, blankets are utilized to warm young children or infants if their extremity skin temperature is low. While utilization of heat lamps might be faster, we do not use them on young children or infants who cannot reliably notify laboratory personnel if they become too hot.

Pearls and Perils

Nerve Conduction Techniques

- Nerve conduction techniques can help differentiate among the many similarly presenting disorders of the motor unit by outlining the types of nerve fibers involved, the pattern of involvement, and the type and degree of the physiologic insult.
- The referring physician plays a critical role in the successful completion of the examination by appropriately preparing the parent and child, as well as by developing a differential diagnosis and set of specific questions from which the electromyographer plans the examination.
- Infants under 12 months of age will frequently sleep through nerve conduction studies if the examination is timed to take advantage of a natural sleep period and the stimuli are well spaced.
- Children who have had a negative experience with painful medical or dental procedures benefit from special preparation for their examination, with consideration being given to use of guided imagery or self-hypnosis and use of analgesic medication or conscious sedation.
- The presence of a parent or familiar adult frequently improves the quality of the study by maximizing patient relaxation and cooperation.
- Normal values depend on the technique used and change dramatically between preterm infants and toddlers. Slower maturational changes occur between toddler age and adulthood. If adequate normative data do not exist for the technique being used, the sensitivity of the test greatly diminishes.
- Inaccurate results can be caused by imprecise distance measurements, excessive shock artifact, or cool extremity temperatures.

Absolute small dimensions

Since nerve conduction velocities are calculated using measured distances on the child's extremities, any measurement inaccuracies will be magnified as the size of the patient decreases. For example, an inaccuracy of 5 mm is relatively greater if the interelectrode distance is 50 mm than if it is 300 mm. Studies of children, especially infants, require accurate measurements for calculations of conduction velocities to avoid a false-positive finding. In addition, until age 2 years, children have slower conduction and may have smaller amplitudes. Tables are available for the expected range of normal values in young children and infants.

Pearls and Perils

Needle Electromyography (EMG)

- Standard needle EMG can reliably differentiate neurogenic processes from other motor problems in infants and children.
- Needle EMG can provide important information about the pathophysiology of the disease process, for example, the presence or absence of ongoing reinnervation.
- Many myopathic processes—carrier states or subclinical phases of muscular dystrophies as well as congenital, structurally distinct myopathies—can produce motor unit potentials with characteristics and recruitment patterns that are too difficult to differentiate from normal values for age.
- Muscles that are going to be biopsied should not be studied by needle EMG within several weeks before biopsy because the muscle trauma incurred can produce changes that are difficult to differentiate from disease states.
- Serum muscle enzymes should be drawn before needle EMG, because the repeated needle insertions involved in most studies can produce a transient elevation of muscle enzymes that may confound the diagnostic effort.

The effect of limb length must also be taken into account for parameters such as F-wave latency and H-reflex. Calculations are available to correct for limb length.

Intensive care unit settings

As in adults, electrophysiologic testing is prone to electrical interference and artifacts, particularly in the intensive care unit setting. Needle EMG can be difficult to interpret, and sensory nerve action potentials may be obscured, due to their small amplitudes. It is important to be aware of these limitations and to make the referring physician aware of them as well.

Abnormalities in pediatric electromyography

The motor unit includes the motor neuron, peripheral nerve (motor axon), neuromuscular junction, and the muscle fiber. Nerve conduction studies (NCS) and EMG are an integral part of the neurologist's diagnostic armamentarium. It is important to remember that NCS and EMG results alone are not pathognomonic of any specific disease and do not give a definitive diagnosis. However, in conjunction with a good history and physical examination, these studies often clinch a diagnosis.

Abnormalities of the motor neuron

Fibrillation potentials are the most frequent EMG abnormality seen that indicates the presence of a possible underlying motor neuron disorder. In the floppy infant syndrome, the implications of fibrillation potentials are so grave that care must be exercised in calling this abnormality. One must be certain not to confuse the fibrillations seen with motor neuron disease with the fibrillations seen, for example, with myofiber necrosis in muscular dystrophy (Figure 6.1). The motor units may have some polyphasia but they may not be large, as seen in adult motor neuron disease. Increased size and polyphasic motor units are evidence of denervation with reinnervation.

Abnormalities of peripheral nerve

Nerve conductions studies are a reliable method of detecting the presence of peripheral nerve disease in a child, after correcting for age-related maturational effects. Peripheral nerve disease may be diffuse or focal. NCS in combination with the needle EMG can help to distinguish whether the problem is demyelinating, axonal, or conduction block, as well as generalized, focal, or multifocal. NCS look at the latency (ms), amplitude (mV or μV), and conduction velocity (m/s) of a response to an electrical stimulus over the nerve.

Before age 2 or 3 years, normal values are much reduced. Premature infants have even slower velocities and prolonged latencies. Gestational age is more important for determining these values than is age from birth. Normal reference values for infants and young children are available in most electrophysiology texts.

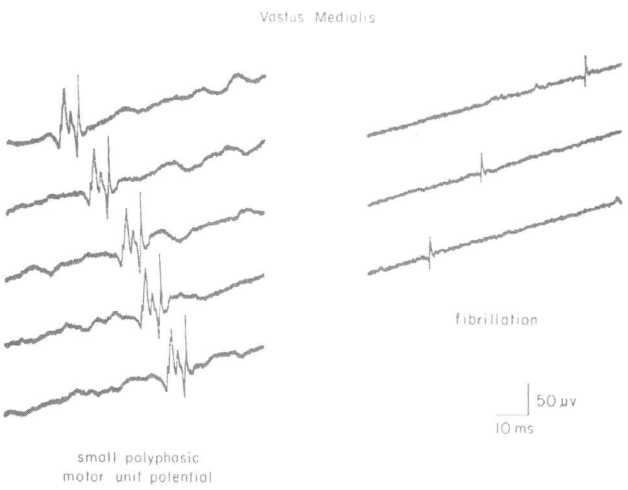

Figure 6.1 Duchenne muscular dystrophy with small motor unit action potentials (MUAPs) and fibrillation potentials.

Abnormalities of the neuromuscular junction

Repetitive nerve stimulation is useful in the evaluation of infantile botulism, as well as in the evaluation of the congenital myasthenic syndromes, although the latter are extremely rare. To ensure accurate findings on repetitive stimulation, it is important that the patient be warmed to enhance the neuromuscular junction defect (see above) and, if they are old enough, understand what is expected of them. Movement artifact can give a seemingly abnormal response. If the repetitive responses amplitudes go up and down, the patient is either moving or the limb is not being stabilized during the testing. If there is amplitude decrement from a defect of the neuromuscular junction, the decrement should stabilize after the fourth response.

For infants and children who cannot voluntarily exercise for the testing, either due to severe weakness or poor cooperation, it may be necessary to use 50-Hz stimulation (Figure 6.2). Although 50 Hz is more uncomfortable than slower rates of stimulation, it is especially important to use if there is suspicion for a presynaptic defect of the neuromuscular junction, such as botulism. Most other times, 2–3 Hz of repetitive stimulation is adequate, especially when used before and after exercise.

If there is concern about a postsynaptic defect of the neuromuscular junction, prolonged 50-Hz stimulation may give a false-positive result in an infant, especially a premature infant. The immaturity of the neuromuscular junction results in a poor safety factor and a decremental response that can be seen in healthy infants with a high rate of stimulation. Slower rates of stimulation (2–3 Hz), with some mild sedation to reduce movement artifact, would be preferred in this situation.

Although single-fiber EMG (SFEMG) gives useful information in patients with defects of the neuromuscular junction, a significant amount of cooperation and concentration from the patient is required. SFEMG requires patience from both the examiner and the patient. Most children cannot participate in SFEMG before the age of 8 years.

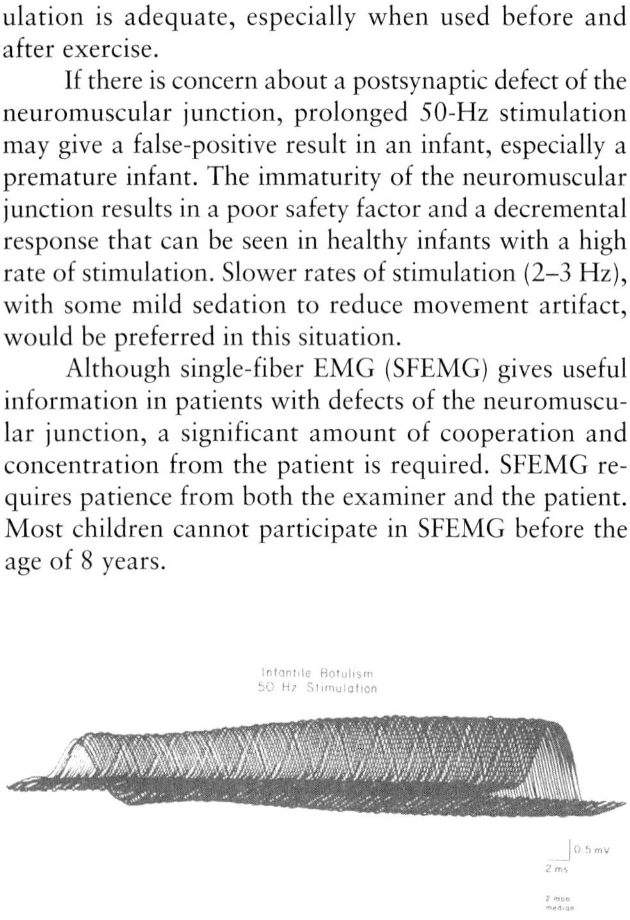

Figure 6.2 6.2 50-Hz stimulation in a 2-month-old child with botulism.

Abnormalities of muscle

EMG may be limited in the evaluation of congenital myopathies. Mild degrees of polyphasia are can be difficult to assess in infants or young children. Fibrillation potentials associated with myofiber necrosis or myositis are often readily apparent, especially if associated with the early recruitment of many small motor unit potentials. The presence of fibrillation potentials may make it difficult to rule out a neuropathic process, as noted above.

Loss of insertional activity during needle examination may occur with fibrotic replacement of muscle in some myopathic processes.

Myotonic discharges, with their characteristic waxing and waning sound, may be an unexpected finding. The discharges are seen with needle insertion in a muscle at rest. In infants, the myotonic discharges may be absent or less sustained and quieter than in adults. Sometimes they can be confused with end-plate noise.

Examples of questions to be addressed by pediatric EMG

Floppy infant: Myopathy, neuropathy, or central weakness?

Muscle weakness is a frequent reason pediatric patients are referred to our EMG laboratory. In this situation, trying to differentiate between a central nervous system (CNS) versus a peripheral cause for the weakness may be the primary question. Weakness from either cause may have similar clinical presentations. Newborns or infants who have respiratory difficulties or feeding difficulties with no CNS etiology may have spinal muscular atrophy, a myopathy (such as myotonic dystrophy or other congenital myopathies), or infantile botulism. For myotonic dystrophy, the parents should be studied for myotonic discharges, with the mother most likely being the disease carrier when a newborn presents as above. The myotonic discharges may not be present in the newborn, but will typically be found in the mother.

For other congenital myopathies, abnormal motor unit action potentials on needle EMG may be seen. Small amplitudes in motor NCS may be seen in motor neuron disease, motor neuropathies, botulism, or significant myopathies. Remember that fibrillation potentials may occur in some myopathic disorders, as well as in neuropathic disorders (Figure 6.3).

H-reflexes are long-latency responses that are present in the ulnar nerve in infants, disappearing by about 1 year of age. Their presence in this nerve is due to lack of CNS myelination. Reoccurrence or persistence at a later age would be indicative of CNS demyelination or continued lack of myelination.

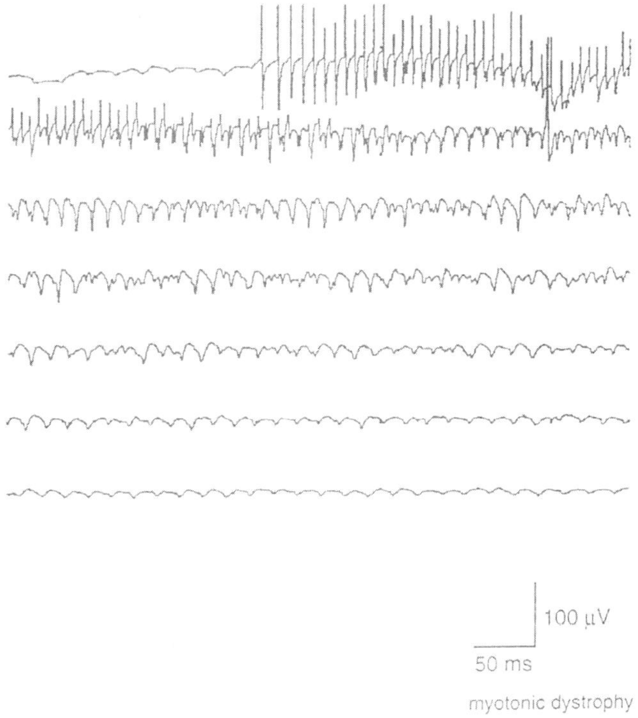

Figure 6.3 Myotonic discharge in a 7-year-old child with myotonic dystrophy.

Is a neuropathy present?

Loss of sensation, with or without associated weakness, may occur with neuropathies, both acquired and hereditary. Ascending numbness may be from a CNS (spinal cord) lesion or an acquired neuropathy, such as acute inflammatory demyelinating polyneuropathy. Hereditary neuropathies are more common than toxic/metabolic neuropathies. We frequently do NCS on parents of children with abnormal nerve conduction studies and EMG findings consistent with a polyneuropathy.

The combination of both central and peripheral nervous system involvement causing weakness is uncommon in adults. In children, this combination is usually a hereditary demyelinating disorder, such as metachromatic leukodystrophy or Krabbe disease.

The time course of the illness is an important clue in differentiating between an acquired and a hereditary neuropathy. For demyelinating neuropathies, the presence of temporal dispersion and/or conduction block of the compound muscle action potential (CMAP) usually indicates an acquired disease. This is more noticeable with proximal stimulation of nerves. The latencies and conduction velocities will be prolonged in both hereditary and acquired neuropathies, so the numbers may be very similar. However, the pictures of the CMAPs show the spread (dispersion) of the conduction velocities in all the axons, based on the uneven demyelination throughout the nerve. Hereditary neuropathies have a more even distribution of demyelination.

When should the EMG be performed?

With infants and children, the electromyographer may only get one opportunity or very limited opportunities to do the test, with parents and/or patient refusing a repeat study. In a mononeuropathy or plexopathy, if the question involves prognosis, waiting 3–4 weeks after the onset of the symptoms would be appropriate. However, if the question is that of postpartum brachial plexopathy, an early EMG may help answer the question of whether the plexopathy occurred in utero or in the perinatal period. Fibrillation potentials take 7–10 days to develop. Their presence soon after delivery would indicate a prenatal onset.

If the EMG is being performed for prognosis, the presence of motor unit action potentials, either large/rapidly firing or small, nascent units, in a plegic muscle are encouraging. Lack of motor unit action potentials and continued presence of fibrillation potentials would be discouraging. Parents and patients should be warned that repeat study may be necessary for continued assessment of prognosis in the latter case.

Concluding remarks

Electrodiagnosis is an important part of the diagnostic evaluation of children with neuromuscular disease. With the increased use of DNA testing, pediatric EMGs are not done as frequently, making it more important that the electromyographer is familiar with doing EMGs in children. The key component in successful electrodiagnostic studies in pediatric cases remains being aware of the limitations of what information can be obtained and knowing what question you must have answered.

Annotated bibliography

Gutmann L. Pearls and pitfalls in the use of electromyography and nerve conduction studies. *Semin Neurol* 2003;23:77–82.
An introduction for many of the technical issues introduced in this chapter, along with appropriate additional references.

Jones HR, Harmon RL, Harper CM, Bolton CF. An approach to pediatric electromyography. In: Jones HR, Bolton CF, Harper CM, eds. *Pediatric clinical electromyography.* Philadelphia: Lippincott-Raven, 1996; 1–36.
A nice technical summary of the issues covered in this chapter as well as normal values for infants and young children, along with appropriate additional references.

CHAPTER 7

Clinical Evaluation with Evoked Responses

John F. Kerrigan

Outline

- Basic principles
- Electroretinography
- Visual evoked responses
- Brainstem auditory evoked responses
- Somatosensory evoked potentials
- Concluding remarks

Evoked potentials (EPs) are a noninvasive tool for evaluating the functional integrity of peripheral and central sensory pathways. As such, they complement the neurologic examination and other diagnostic studies. The relative clinical utility of EPs has been diminished somewhat in the current era of imaging technology. In contrast, the pace of new developments in clinical neurophysiology over the past one or two decades has been more modest. Nevertheless, EPs remain important, providing information regarding the functional integrity of neurologic pathways, the localization of deficits within these pathways, and changes in function over time that may not be accessible by physical examination or other techniques.

EPs may be expected to provide clinically useful information in the following situations: (a) evaluating the integrity of sensory (or motor) pathways in those patients unable to cooperate with conventional methods of neurologic examination; this may apply to patients who lack behavioral maturity and voluntary cooperation, or who are otherwise impaired; (b) providing specific diagnostic clues in selected patients that may complement other diagnostic or imaging studies; (c) providing evidence for or against possible sites of pathologic localization that may elude other studies; and (d) providing a means of functionally evaluating sensory pathways during surgical interventions or other procedures that place these anatomic pathways at risk in a sedated or anesthetized patient.

In contemporary practice, the most common clinical applications for EPs in children are screening of high-risk neonates and infants to identify possible hearing loss, and intraoperative monitoring. However, all EP modalities are important in selected clinical circumstances. This chapter seeks to provide an overview of EP modalities in the context of evaluation and management of infants, children, and adolescents with neurologic concerns or established neurologic disease. The study of evoked responses is appropriate for neurologists and neurosurgeons, as well as for a host of practitioners in other disciplines that deal with sick or impaired children, including audiologists, ophthalmologists, and anesthesiologists. These techniques also shed light on the maturation of sensory function in the developing newborn and infant.

Basic principles

This chapter provides the interested clinician with a basic understanding of the indications, diagnostic potential, and pitfalls of each of the various EP modalities, while abbreviating technical aspects of study performance. Several excellent texts are available to the reader with more advanced interests (Chiappa 1997; Levin & Luders 2000; Aminoff 2005).

Electrical activity of the brain is continuously present as "resting" or baseline activity, with distinct features that allow identification of waking, sleeping, or encephalopathic states. However, the nervous system will also demonstrate evidence of responsiveness (activation) that is time-locked to external events or stimulation, typically conducted by sensory pathways. EP studies attempt to record and quantify evidence of this neural activation, serving as a functional assessment of the sensory pathway in question. Most of the electrical potentials elicited by these sensory stimuli possess very-low-amplitude features, and consequently repeated stimulation and digital averaging of a large number of individual stimulation events is required to separate the evoked signal from the background neurophysiologic "noise" of ongoing activity. (The exception to this rule is familiar to all electroencephalographers, as the occipital response to photic stimulation may be visually detectable with just a single stimulus.) Typically two trials (two sets of repeated stimulation) are performed and visually compared to confirm reproducibility of the findings.

Evoked potential teaching tends to imply that each waveform can be attributed to a single specific structure within the sensory conduction pathway. The reality is more nuanced. Peripheral nerve responses, such as the Erb peak with median nerve stimulation, result from the passage of an axonal volley through the local nerve or plexus. However, central nervous system (CNS) responses usually defy such easy attribution, as the individual waveforms consist of a composite of responses from multiple structures, potentially including both near-field and far-field responses. Fortunately, in most cases, the *predominant* feature of an identified waveform can be assigned to activation of a particular structure. This is usually validated with the study of patients with well-localized, discrete lesions. We will identify the "primary" generator of the principal waveforms for each EP modality, which serves to provide localizing information for focal sensory conduction deficits.

The technical features of each EP modality are unique. Details regarding the stimulation system (including such features as simulation intensity, duration, and repetition rate), and the recording system (relating to features such as electrode placement, sweep speed, gain, and bandpass) are discussed in the comprehensive references noted above. In comparison to other diagnostic studies, EPs possess relatively poor signal-to-noise ratios, particularly in children, and waveform changes resulting from a physiologic abnormality must be differentiated from artifact. The expertise of the clinical neurophysiologist, interpreting a study after its performance, cannot make up for technical problems occurring at the time the study was performed. Oversight of the technical performance of these studies is of paramount importance.

Electroretinography

Anatomic considerations

Functional integrity of certain cellular elements within the retina can be assessed with electroretinography (ERG). A light flash delivers photic energy to the retina and evokes predictable changes in photosensitive cells and, secondarily, in their supporting cellular network. The a-wave identified in normal individuals is due to activation of the photoreceptor layer. The b-wave is generated by activity of supporting glial elements (Müller cells) and probably other cells within the bipolar layer (inner nuclear layer) of the retina (Figure 7.1A and 7.1B)

Testing of cone cell responses (mediating high-resolution, color, light-adapted vision) can be preferentially performed with bright-white flash stimulation in the light-

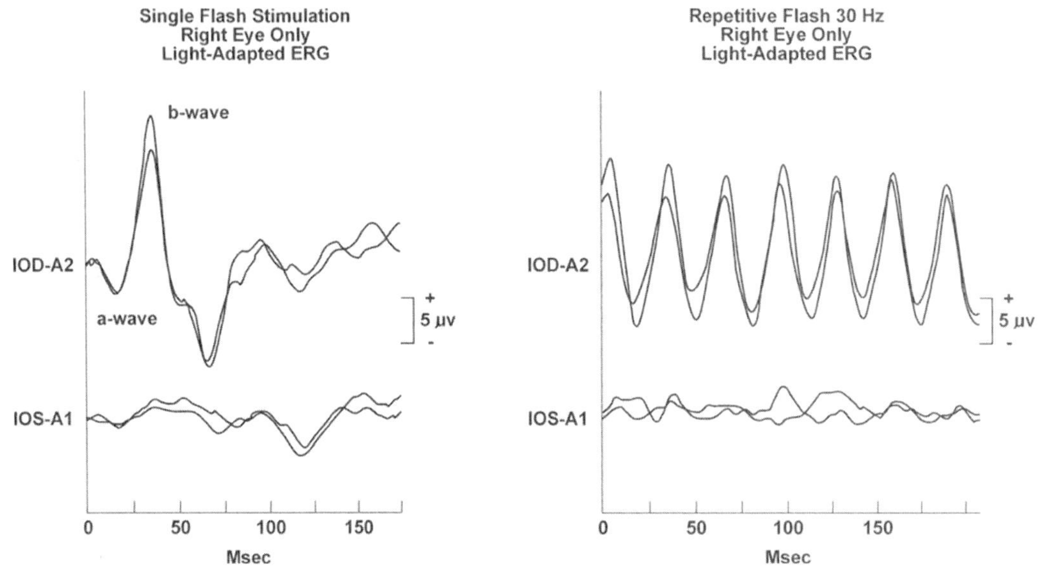

Figure 7.1 (A) The principal electroretinography waveforms, with monocular stimulation of the right eye, identifying a-wave and b-wave responses. This response was obtained to bright full-field flash in a light-adapted state. (B) The "frequency following" response to repetitive flash stimulation of the right eye. IOD = right eye electrode, IOS = left eye electrode, A2 = right ear electrode, A1 = left ear electrode.

adapted state, whereas rod responses (mediating lower-resolution, dark-adapted vision) can be preferentially tested by a lower-intensity blue-flash stimulation under dark-adapted conditions. Flash stimulation is diffused over the entire retina, and consequently ERG tends to be a study that is more sensitive for diffuse retinal disease processes, and is relatively less sensitive for macular degenerations (even when utilizing the light-adapted, cone-predominant stimulation conditions). Focal ERG techniques (for regional evaluation of the retina) have been developed, but are technically demanding.

Key Clinical Questions

ERG studies are helpful for...

- Evaluation of children with unexplained visual loss and/or nystagmus.
- Differentiating pigmentary retinopathy from normal variants of retinal pigmentation.
- Confirming visual dysfunction in the retina prior to pathologic changes in the funduscopic examination.

VER studies are helpful for...

- Children with unexplained visual loss and/or nystagmus (often performed with ERG).
- Localizing a visual conduction deficit to the optic nerve or chiasm.
- Following visual function in young patient with known optic nerve glioma.
- Usually not helpful for evaluating children with cortical visual impairment.

BAER studies are helpful for...

- Children with suspected hearing loss who are younger or otherwise unable to cooperate.
- High-risk newborns with prematurity, intrauterine growth retardation, hyperbilirubinemia, possible intrauterine infection, meningitis or sepsis, exposure to ototoxic medications such as aminoglycosides, presence of a syndrome associated with hearing impairment, or family history of deafness.
- Infants or young children recovering from meningitis.

SSEP studies are helpful for...

- Children with suspected multifocal or demyelinating diseases processes.
- Evaluating patients with possible posterior column dysfunction, particularly if imaging studies are unrevealing.
- Evaluating prognosis in children (but not newborns) with acute coma, due to known hypoxic–ischemic injury or severe cerebral trauma. Absent SSEP waveforms bilaterally at the scalp electrodes correlates with a poor outcome.

Pearls and Perils

Electroretinogram (ERG)

- Most ERG techniques use flash, and do not require cooperation for visual fixation on a target.
- The ERG is more sensitive to diffuse retinal diseases than to diseases affecting the macula (maculopathies).
- ERG abnormalities usually precede funduscopic findings in Leber's congenital amaurosis and neuronal ceroid lipofuscinosis.

Developmental changes

The a-wave and b-wave responses are present at birth in term newborns, but typically show lower-amplitude features and slightly longer latencies. Mature a-wave and b-wave latencies are usually seen by 6 months of age, and fully mature ERG responses (considering both light-adapted and dark-adapted conditions) are typically obtained by age 1 year (Flores-Guevara 1996).

Clinical aspects

ERG studies, often together with visual evoked responses (VER), can be helpful in evaluating children with visual loss and/or nystagmus, either due to disease processes that affect the eye alone, or in conjunction with other features of neurologic disease. These studies should be obtained *after* ophthalmologic examination, including funduscopy, to exclude the presence of conditions that affect the preretinal structures of the eye, such as corneal opacification and cataracts. However, it is also important to recognize that abnormalities of the ERG may be present in disorders of retinal function, including certain neurodegenerative conditions, prior to observable changes in the retina by direct funduscopic examination (Harden 1989).

Retinal disorders

A large number of primary diseases of the retina, without other neurologic symptoms, occur in children. The single most common genetic cause of childhood blindness is *Leber congenital amaurosis*, an autosomal recessive retinal dystrophy that affects both cones and rods. This disorder is genetically diverse, mapping to a number of different loci. Some of the specific gene mutations have been identified. These children present in infancy with visual inattention and nystagmus. Initially, the funduscopic examination is normal. However, ERG responses at this time are markedly abnormal, if not entirely absent, and, accordingly, assist with the diagnosis of this disorder.

Pigmentary retinal degenerations, including retinitis pigmentosa (RP), also show abnormal ERG results. RP typically presents with night blindness and progressive restriction of the visual fields. It is largely due to degeneration of rods, with relative sparing of the cones, and thus, central vision. At the point in time during the clinical course at which pathologic pigmentary changes are seen, the ERG, particularly for dark-adapted (rod-optimized) conditions, should always be abnormal (Baker 1995). Consequently, the ERG can be of great practical usefulness in distinguishing pathologic versus nonpathologic pigmentary features.

Leber congenital amaurosis and RP represent two of the more common retinopathies in which ERG can help with the diagnosis. There are a large number of other "pure" retinal diseases, both progressive and nonprogressive, and a partial list is provided in Table 7.1.

Table 7.1 Disorders associated with electroretinographic abnormalities

"Pure" Retinopathies (Modified from Kriss 1992)
- Static
  - Congenital stationary night blindness
  - Color blindness, complete and incomplete subtypes
  - Albinism
- Progressive
  - Leber congenital amaurosis
  - Retinitis pigmentosa
  - Cone dystrophies
  - Cone–rod dystrophies
  - X-linked juvenile retinoschisis

Neuro-ophthalmologic Disorders (Modified from Baker 1995)
- Nonprogressive Syndromes
  - Usher syndrome (multiple subtypes)
  - Laurence-Moon syndrome
  - Bardet-Biedl syndrome
  - Joubert syndrome (some subtypes)
- Degenerative Diseases
  - Neuronal ceroid lipofuscinosis (infantile and juvenile subtypes)
  - Gangliosidoses
    - GM2 Type I (Tay-Sachs disease)
    - GM2 Type II (Sandhoff disease)
  - Mucopolysaccharidoses
    - MPS Type 1H (Hurler syndrome)
    - MPS Type 1S (Scheie syndrome)
    - MPS Type 2 (Hunter syndrome)
    - MPS Type 3 (Sanfilippo syndrome)
    - MPS Type 7 (Sly syndrome)
  - Mucolipidoses
    - Type IV
  - Peroxisomal Disorders
    - Zellweger syndrome
    - Neonatal adrenoleukodystrophy
    - Hyperpipecolic acidemia
    - Infantile Refsum disease
  - Abetalipoproteinemia

Neuro-ophthalmologic disorders

Perhaps more commonly, the child neurologist is asked to evaluate children in whom neurologic symptoms, in addition to visual disturbance, are present. Most children with brain disorders and visual inattention will be determined to have cortical visual impairment (the preferred term to "cortical blindness," since most of these children have some partial retention of visual function). Although usually unnecessary, an intact ERG can help make the case that visual disturbance originates posterior to the retina.

Several nonprogressive syndromes can include retinopathy, and an abnormal ERG may assist with the diagnosis. Usher syndrome, combining sensorineural hearing impairment and visual loss secondary to a pigmentary retinopathy, has several clinical subtypes. Linkage studies have shown that it is genetically diverse, but usually autosomal recessive. Abnormalities of the ERG may predate the changes on funduscopy, and therefore can help to establish the diagnosis in a child with congenital deafness. Bardet-Biedl syndrome, and the phenotypically similar Laurence-Moon syndrome, combines pigmentary degeneration (and an abnormal ERG) with retardation and hypogonadism. Some subtypes of Joubert syndrome include retinopathy and visual loss.

Abnormal suppression and eventually complete loss of ERG responses is seen in several neurodegenerative diseases that affect children. The infantile and juvenile subtypes of neuronal ceroid lipofuscinosis (NCL) show early abnormalities of the ERG, even before clinical visual disturbance may be evident. Although counterintuitive, the ERG response can be completely absent in the presence of preserved flash VER. The late infantile form of NCL (Jansky-Bielschowsky) actually shows VER waveforms with *high*-amplitude features ("giant VERs"), despite suppressed or absent ERGs. Roughly 70% of the late infantile cases will show pathogenic mutations of the *CLN2* gene. ERGs are also abnormal in GM2 gangliosidosis (although not the Type III subtype) and some forms of mucopolysaccharidoses, mucolipidoses, and peroxisomal diseases. Some of these disorders combine corneal opacification and retinal degeneration, making interpretation of the ERG more problematic (Baker 1995). Conversely, ERG abnormalities are generally not seen with leukodystrophies. See Table 7.1 for a more detailed list of those disorders associated with ERG abnormalities.

Visual evoked responses

Anatomic considerations

Assessment of the visual pathways posterior to the retina is performed using the VER. The latency and amplitude

Pearls and Perils

Visual Evoked Responses (VER)

- Pattern-reversal testing is the most useful, but requires a cooperative patient for visual fixation, often not possible in children.
- Flash VER can be obtained simultaneously with the ERG.
- Asymmetrical responses over the occipital region may falsely lateralize to the side opposite of the abnormality (due to tangential projection of the electrical field). Confirmation with structural imaging is recommended.
- ERG and VER abnormalities must *always* be correlated with ophthalmoscopic examination. Ocular problems such as corneal opacification and cataracts should be excluded.

of the waveform response from the occipital cortex provides information about visual conduction through these anterior visual pathways (optic nerves, chiasm, tracts, and radiations), as well as the functional integrity of the visual cortex itself. The major waveform response (the P100) appears to be generated by postsynaptic potentials in the pyramidal cells of layer IV of occipital cortex, primarily from the macular area of representation (Ducati 1988). As the name implies, this peak occurs roughly 100 msec following stimulation with a pattern-reversal checkerboard. Negative potentials precede and follow the major positive peak (N85 and N135, respectively). These negative peaks have lower-amplitude features and can be more difficult to identify (Figure 7.2).

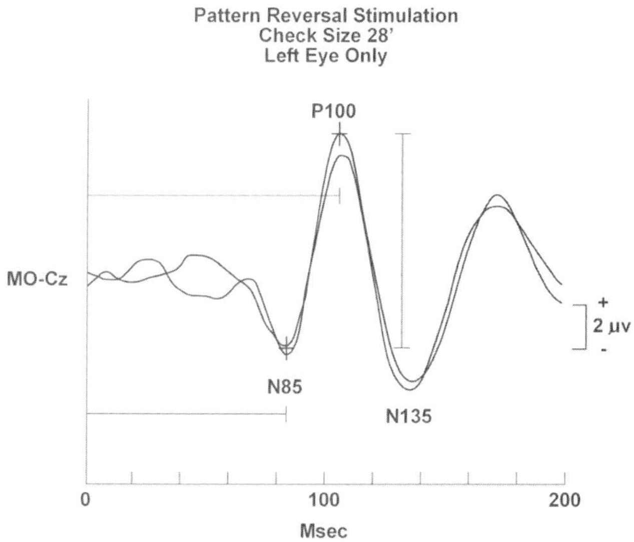

Figure 7.2 Normal visual evoked responses waveform, showing major positive peak (P100) and smaller negative peaks preceding and following (N85 and N135). Measurements relating to peak latency and amplitude (trough of N85 to peak of P100) are shown. A scalp positive electrical field shows an up-going deflection. Some laboratories use a reversed polarity convention, however, with the P100 showing a downward deflection. MO, midline occipital electrode; Cz, vertex electrode.

Although localization of the abnormality is relatively imprecise with VER, the presence of an asymmetrical response to monocular stimulation suggests a conduction defect in anterior (optic nerve or chiasm) pathways. In the absence of ocular pathology or retinal abnormality demonstrated by ophthalmologic examination or ERG, this type of pattern strongly suggests an optic nerve disturbance. Conversely, an asymmetric field to the VER over the occipital region to monocular stimulation of *both* eyes suggests a unilateral or asymmetrical post-chiasmal visual conduction defect or unilateral dysfunction of visual cortex. It is important to be aware that in some patients the field potential of the occipital (visual) cortex to VER stimulation may actually project its maximum to the contralateral side of the head, potentially resulting in false localization. Correlation with structural imaging would be recommended. The visual pathways are shown in Figure 7.3.

Developmental changes

A great deal of individual variation occurs with regard to the latency and amplitude of flash VER. These are usually judged to be normal based upon the presence or absence of a consistent and symmetric response to monocular stimulation (Baker 1995). The pattern-reversal VER shows higher amplitude responses with a tighter and more highly validated range of normal latency values. However, as noted earlier, pattern reversal study may not be possible in young or inattentive children.

Flash responses can be recorded as a long-latency, surface-negative wave in preterm infants as young as 24 weeks postconceptual age. A major surface-positive waveform can be seen at 32 weeks, is consistently identifiable by 37 weeks postconceptual age, and is very well-defined by term. The latency of this surface-positive peak decreases rapidly until 5–6 months of age, when it approximates adult values.

For high-risk newborns screened at 40 weeks postconceptual age with flash VER, an intact response is strongly associated with normal visual function at 1 year of age, whereas an abnormal response is associated with abnormal visual function at 1 year in approximately 50% of cases. Consequently, an abnormal VER during the newborn period should identify the child as "at risk" and requiring follow-up, but does not necessarily imply an abnormal outcome (Kurtzberg 1982).

Clinical aspects

VER results can be influenced by ocular pathology, such as opacifying lesions of the cornea, lens, or vitreous, and

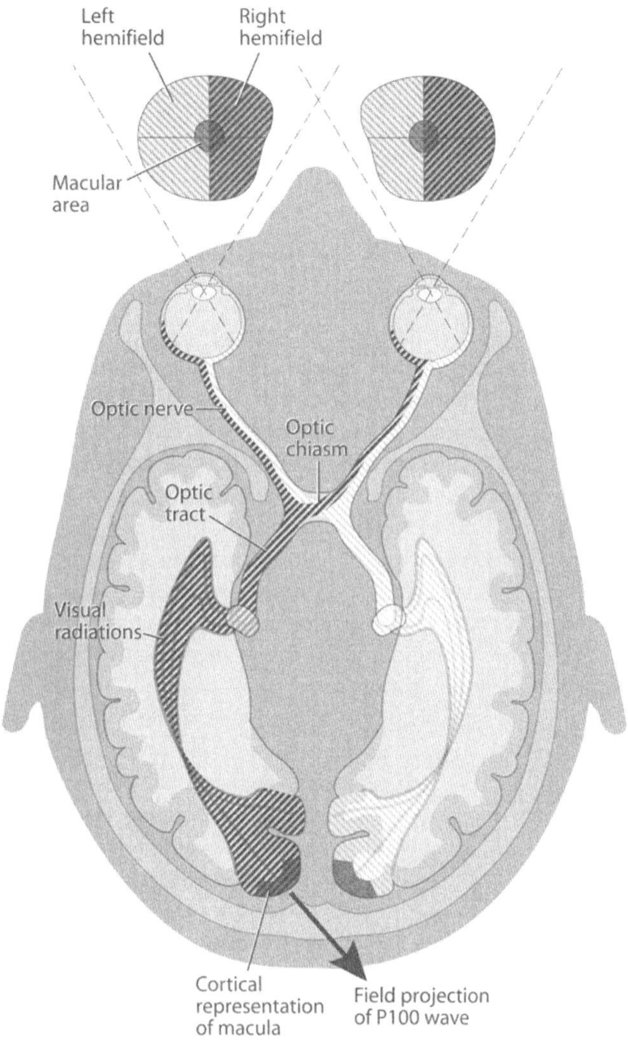

Figure 7.3 Anatomy of the visual pathways, with ipsilateral projection of fibers from the temporal fields of the retina, and crossed projection of the nasal fields through the optic chiasm. The region of representation in the calcarine cortex for the macula is relatively enlarged in comparison to other areas of the retinal surface and is located at the posterior occipital pole (*heavy black line*). The tangential field of the occipital visual evoked responses is also represented.

therefore should always be preceded by funduscopic examination.

Attempts to demonstrate a tight correlation between visual acuity and findings on VER testing for young or uncooperative children have been made, but thus far these techniques are technically demanding and unsatisfactory for practical use. Even so, the VER remains the best proxy for functional assessment of the visual system in these patients.

VER studies are most useful in detecting conduction defects in the anterior optic pathways (optic nerve and chiasm). Pattern-reversal VERs are highly sensitive to signal conduction changes of the optic nerve, particularly if the pathologic process is unilateral or asymmetric. VERs can detect optic nerve lesions in the absence of obvious changes on MR imaging, such as with optic neuritis resulting from acute disseminated encephalomyelitis (ADEM), neuromyelitis optica (Devic disease), or the uncommon pediatric case of multiple sclerosis. VER can confirm or supplement the clinical examination in patients with optic nerve hypoplasia or atrophy. For patients with known structural abnormalities, such as a glioma of the optic nerve or chiasm, the VER can offer a powerful noninvasive method for serial studies, looking for progressive changes that may mandate a change in therapy.

VERs for diseases that affect the posterior optic pathways (posterior to the optic chiasm) are less useful. VERs have proven to have limited value in evaluating patients with cortical blindness (cortical visual impairment), as patients with intact responses may still demonstrate disabling visual impairment when old enough for behavioral testing of visual function. Conversely, patients with absent VERs may still demonstrate useful (although usually not normal) vision.

Brainstem auditory evoked responses

Clinical indications

Peripheral and central auditory conduction pathways can be evaluated with brainstem auditory evoked responses (BAER). BAERs are used to evaluate two related functions. First, they can evaluate hearing in infants and children who are unable to cooperate for conventional auditory threshold testing. Secondly, they can assess the functional integrity of brainstem conduction in an effort to localize pathology to the brainstem or to a specific location within it. A normal BAER study is shown in Figure 7.4.

Pearls and Perils

Brainstem Auditory Evoked Responses (BAER)

- BAER (or another suitable auditory screening modality) should *always* be performed in high-risk newborns before hospital discharge.
- Alternative technologies for screening include otoacoustic emission (OAE) or automated auditory brainstem response (A-ABR).
- BAER abnormalities in children should *always* be correlated with physical examination of the external auditory canal and tympanic membrane to exclude obstructing problems or middle ear disease.

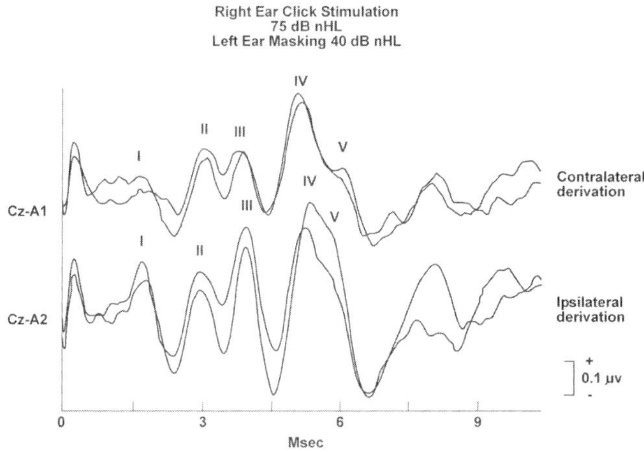

Figure 7.4 Normal brainstem auditory evoked response (BAER). Waves I, III, and V are of the greatest clinical significance. A2, R ear electrode; A1, L ear electrode; Cz, vertex electrode.

Anatomic considerations

Auditory stimulation usually consists of clicks, delivered at the selected intensity via insert-type earphones. The responses are recorded by electrodes placed at the vertex and bilaterally on the earlobes or mastoid regions. Sound intensities up to 95 or 100 dBnHL can be used.

The most commonly used and validated modality, the short-latency BAER, demonstrates auditory signal transmission through peripheral and brainstem structures that occur during the first 10 msec after click stimulation (Figure 7.4). Waves I, III, and V are the most consistent and easily identified. Lesion studies and microelectrode recordings in humans and animal models have established that wave I originates from the peripheral (most lateral) aspect of the VIIIth (auditory) cranial nerve, wave III from the lower pons (superior olivary nucleus and possibly cochlear nucleus), and wave V from the lower midbrain (inferior colliculus). Auditory pathways through the brainstem have bilateral representation, but lesions ipsilateral to the stimulus are more likely to attenuate or abolish BAER waveforms.

By making use of these relationships, the BAER may help to localize a neurologic deficit. As an example, a tumor in the cerebellopontine angle will tend to increase the ipsilateral wave I–III interpeak latency, or may abolish completely all waves subsequent to wave I (to ipsilateral stimulation). However, magnetic resonance imaging (MRI) has largely superseded the clinical utility of BAER studies in localizing neurologic lesions. Mid-latency and long-latency BAER studies are recorded by some laboratories, but are highly variable and of limited clinical usefulness.

Audiologic assessment

For patients who are too young or unable to cooperate with traditional behavioral-response audiology, the BAER provides a tool for assessing hearing. The sound intensity threshold at which wave V appears (generally the most robust and easily identified of the BAER waveforms) provides a clue as to the hearing threshold. A threshold of 15–20 dBnHL is considered normal. This threshold is affected by either conductive or sensorineural disturbances, so correlation with the otologic examination is required for abnormal results. Additionally, BAER waveform latencies decrease as the intensity of the sound stimulus increases. The detailed measurement of wave V latency against sound stimulation intensity yields a latency–intensity curve, the characteristics of which may help differentiate conductive versus sensorineural hearing loss (Figure 7.5).

BAER studies are very commonly used to screen for hearing impairment in high-risk newborns. Factors that would include a newborn in this high-risk category include premature birth, low birth weight, possible intrauterine infection, hyperbilirubinemia, meningitis or sepsis, exposure to aminoglycoside or other ototoxic medications, the presence of a congenital syndrome associated with hearing impairment, or family history of deafness. The presence of other neurologic problems, including neonatal seizures, hypoxic–ischemic encephalopathy, or intracerebral hemorrhage, also calls for audiologic screening. Alternative studies, more easily performed but still sensitive to the conductive or sensorineural (cochlear) deficits that are common in newborns, such as the otoacoustic emission (OAE), are also performed at some institutions. Automated auditory brainstem response studies (A-ABR) are a new technology

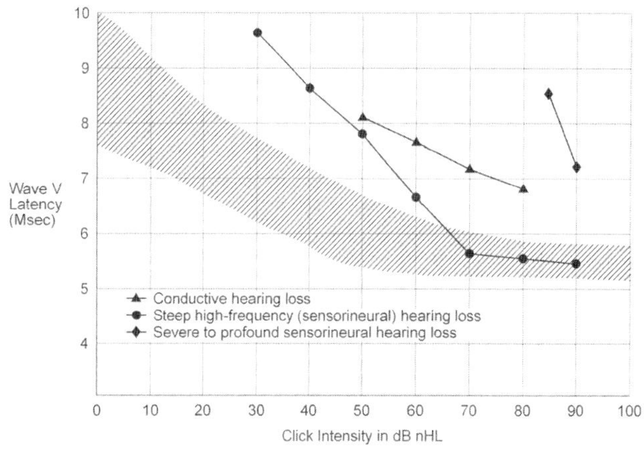

Figure 7.5 Latency-intensity graph, with normal range and idealized representations of sensorineural and conductive hearing loss. *Stippled area* shows range of normal for children; *arrow line* represents mild–moderate sensorineural hearing loss (example: history of hypoxic-ischemic injury at birth); *circle line* shows conductive hearing loss (example: chronic middle ear effusion); *diamond line* demonstrates profound sensorineural hearing loss (example: history of bacterial meningitis).

now used at a large number of institutions for screening purposes.

Developmental changes

BAER waveforms can be elicited in preterm newborns, with wave V appearing as early as 27 weeks postconceptual age. A progressive decrease in waveform latency occurs, and an increase in waveform amplitude during maturation, so that normal adult values are approximated at 1–2 years of age.

Clinical aspects

Newborn screening is by far the most important and common use of the BAER modality in clinical use. Older but still uncooperative patients with some of the problems identified above as neonatal risk factors may also be studied in this way, such as infants and young children recovering from bacterial meningitis.

The latency of wave I may be delayed by conductive problems, such as an occluded external ear canal, or middle ear infection or effusion. However, in the absence of neurologic disease, subsequent waveforms and interpeak latencies should be normal.

BAER studies are known to be abnormal in a number of different clinical conditions and therefore may complement the clinical examination and other areas of testing in selected circumstances. BAER studies are sensitive to brainstem dysfunction but are nonspecific as to the underlying cause. Many of the neurodegenerative diseases, particularly the leukodystrophies, result in BAER abnormality. For some, most importantly Pelizaeus-Merzbacher (PM) disease, the BAER may be markedly abnormal early in the course of the illness and therefore helpful with the initial diagnostic evaluation. (Definitive diagnosis for most PM cases is made by determining a mutation in the *PLP* gene, coding for proteolipid protein.) The degree of abnormality typically increases with disease progression, and therefore BAER findings may offer an objective way of following the clinical course of these diseases and, potentially, the response to therapeutic interventions. BAER studies do not appear to be helpful with respect to identifying children or family members at risk for sudden infant death syndrome (SIDS).

Somatosensory evoked potentials (SSEPs) appear to be more specific than BAERs with regard to predicting poor outcome from hypoxic–ischemic injury in children (see below).

> **Pearls and Perils**
>
> **Somatosensory Evoked Potentials (SSEP)**
>
> - SSEPs provide information about both peripheral and central sensory conduction pathways. If a peripheral disturbance is suggested, results should be correlated with electromyograph (EMG) and nerve conduction studies.
> - Peripheral nerves mature more quickly than central sensory pathways.
> - Most of the signal for SSEPs travels through the posterior columns of the spinal cord. Accordingly, SSEPs are relatively insensitive to diseases that may affect the anterior portions of the cord exclusively.

Somatosensory evoked potentials

Clinical indications

SSEPs allow for noninvasive and objective assessment of the peripheral, spinal, and cerebral somatosensory pathways. As with other evoked potential modalities, SSEPs complement the clinical examination and other diagnostic studies in selected circumstances. SSEPs can demonstrate the presence or absence of conduction deficits in the somatosensory pathways and, in the process, can contribute to the localization of neurologic lesions.

Technical features and anatomic considerations

Peripheral nerves are stimulated with very brief but repetitive application of alternating electrical current to the overlying skin. The peripheral nerves utilized in common clinical practice are mixed sensory and motor nerves. Sensory conduction activated by electrical stimulation is mediated almost exclusively by large, myelinated nerve fibers. Activation of motor nerve fibers also results in orthodromic conduction to innervated muscles, resulting in a visible twitch, which acts as an easily observed clinical confirmation of successful electrical activation. Antidromic (proximal) conduction through motor nerves also contributes to the recordable waveforms generated by peripheral structures such as brachial plexus at the Erb point or other peripheral recording points.

Waveforms recorded from central (spinal or cerebral) electrode locations result from activity in sensory conduction pathways only. Common recording locations are the posterior cervical spinous process of C7, and the contralateral scalp for upper extremity (median or ulnar) stimulation. For lower extremity stimulation (posterior tibial or peroneal), a lumbar recording electrode, commonly at the L1 level, is also used.

The physiologic generator of the peripheral waveforms, such as the Erb point response, is the collective volley of action potentials traveling through the subjacent nerve structures. The central waveforms are more complex. Spinal responses are generated both by the volley of ascending action potentials in the posterior columns, as well as by postsynaptic activity in the dorsal gray matter of the cord. It is important to be aware that SSEP signals are conducted primarily through the posterior columns. Therefore SSEP studies are typically not sensitive to pathology that may affect the anterior portions of the spinal cord.

The scalp response, recorded by electrodes placed over the cortical sensory representation areas for either upper or lower extremities, consists of postsynaptic activity in the sensory nuclei of the thalamus, projected to the scalp as a far-field surface-negative wave. This is followed shortly thereafter by a largely surface-negative near-field wave generated by activation of sensory cortex in the parietal lobe, followed by an equally prominent surface-positive peak. These findings are illustrated in Figure 7.6A and B.

Developmental changes

Myelination, and therefore conduction velocity, matures more quickly in the peripheral nerves in comparison to the central sensory conduction pathways. Peripheral nerve conduction velocities reach adult values around 3–4 years of age, whereas interpeak latencies that reflect central conduction velocities appear to reach adult values around 6–8 years of age.

Because of this relative immaturity, SSEP waveform components, most commonly the cortical peaks, may not be present in all normal newborns. In one study, 33% of term newborns failed to demonstrate a cortical SSEP re-

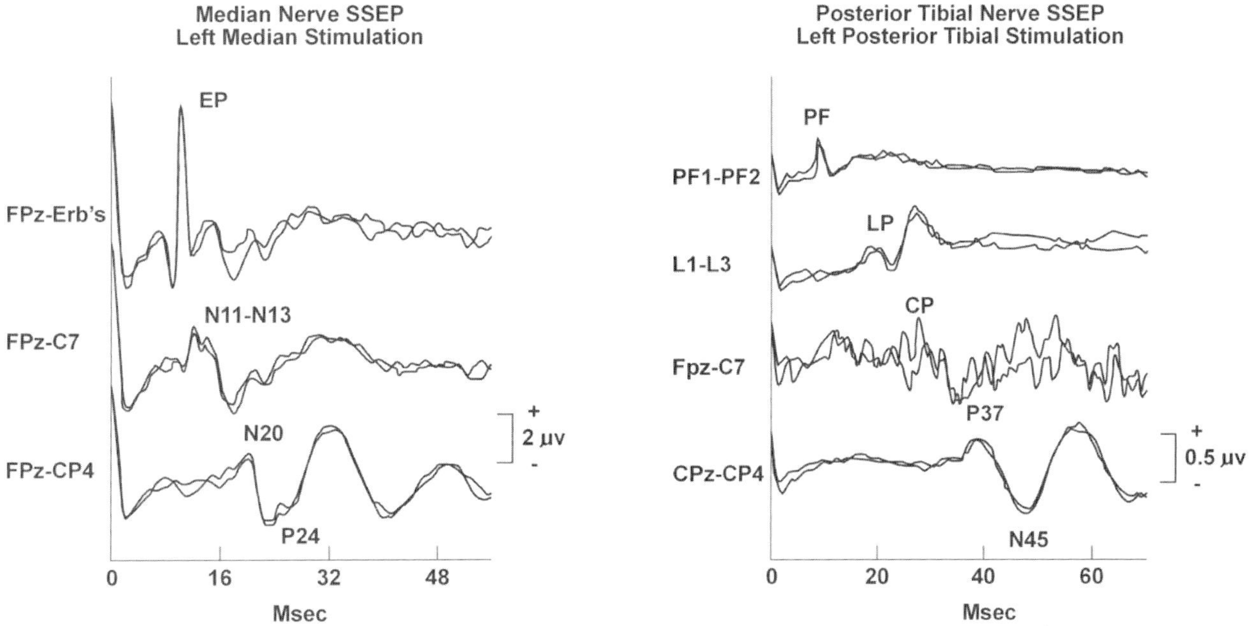

Figure 7.6 (A) Representative somatosensory evoked potentials (SSEP) waveforms in a normal 14-year-old boy. Median nerve stimulation results are shown in three channels. The top channel shows the peak at the Erb point, representing the volley of action potentials traveling through the brachial plexus. The second channel down shows the cervical peak, with bifid features. The first negative potential (N11 in this derivation) represents the volley of action potentials traveling through the underlying posterior columns, whereas the second of the two peaks (N13) is due to postsynaptic activity in dorsal gray matter of the cord. The bottom channel demonstrates the response at the contralateral scalp. CP4 is the "active" electrode over the arm/hand area, and the polarity convention reveals an initial up-going, scalp-negative peak (N20), followed by a down-going, scalp-positive peak (P24). The N20 is due to thalamic activation, projected out to the scalp electrodes, whereas the subsequent P24 is generated in parietal sensory cortex. (B) SSEPs study of lower extremity in same normal 14-year-old boy. Responses to stimulation of posterior tibial nerve at the ankle are shown in four channels. The top channel shows the ascending volley of action potentials recorded at the popliteal fossa (PF). The second channel demonstrates the lumber peak (LP), recorded with a pair of electrodes at L1 and L3. Like the cervical peak with median nerve stimulation, this waveform is a combination of the ascending volley in posterior columns, as well as postsynaptic activity in dorsal gray matter of cord at the level of entry. The ascending volley traveling through cervical cord from the lower extremities is shown in the third channel. This waveform is difficult to record and may be absent in normals. The bottom channel shows the response at the scalp. CPz is now the "active" electrode, as it is closer to the sensory cortex for leg near the sagittal midline. The surface-negative peak due to thalamic activation is not well seen, and the major up-going, scalp-positive potential is due to activation of the primary sensory cortex (analogous to the P24 to median nerve stimulation). The polarity conventions used in our laboratory account for the P24 going downward in Figure 7.6A and the P37 going upward in Figure 7.6B. However, both are surface-positive potentials generated by activation of somatotopic cortex.

sponse, with all subjects demonstrating this peak at 2 months of age (Willis 1984). This highlights the need to avoid overinterpretation of abnormal SSEP studies in the newborn.

Clinical aspects

SSEPs can help localize single lesions within the nervous system, although their anatomic specificity is poor. As an example, a lesion can be localized to the thoracic spinal cord (involving the posterior columns) with normal median nerve SSEP results, along with abnormal posterior tibial SSEPs that show normal peripheral nerve and lumbar peaks, but delayed or abolished cervical and cortical peaks. From time to time an SSEP study can supplement the clinical examination and other studies. However, as discussed in the introduction to this chapter, the evolution of MRI has largely eclipsed the role of EP studies in localizing solitary lesions (tumor, hemorrhage, stroke, etc.).

SSEPs continue to be useful in demonstrating the involvement of sensory pathways in multifocal neurologic disorders. The classic example is the role of SSEPs to help establish multiple lesions in "space and time" that are the hallmark feature of multiple sclerosis (MS). Although the lesions within cerebral white matter are usually clearly seen on MRI, demyelinating lesions affecting the optic nerves or the spinal cord may not be seen. Accordingly, EP studies (most notably VER and SSEP modalities) are clinically useful for those relatively uncommon cases of MS presenting in children or adolescents. They are equally useful for establishing the multifocal nature of monophasic, acquired disorders with demyelination, such as ADEM, seen more commonly in children.

Not unexpectedly, most of the leukodystrophies have been reported to show abnormalities of SSEPs, including adrenoleukodystrophy, metachromatic leukodystrophy (MLD), Krabbe disease, Pelizaeus-Merzbacher disease, and others. SSEPs may help to demonstrate peripheral as well as central sensory conduction disturbances in diseases where these coexist, such as MLD, Krabbe disease, and Friedreich ataxia.

Similar to electroencephalography (EEG), the role of evoked potential studies in modern pediatric neurology practice is to noninvasively assess neurophysiologic function, rather than to provide neuroanatomic localization. A clinically important example of this role is the evaluation of children with coma, specifically with respect to making predictions of outcome. The absence of scalp responses to SSEP study is highly correlated with poor outcome (death, vegetative state, or severe disability) in children with coma due to hypoxic–ischemic injury or cerebral trauma (DeMeirleir 1987, and multiple others).

Consider Consultation When...

- Ophthalmologic consultation is needed in all patients with visual complaints or abnormal ERG or VER results, to exclude ocular disease and to provide a full examination of the retina.
- An audiologist is needed to evaluate children with hearing complaints or abnormal BAER findings. An ear, nose and throat specialist should see patients with suspected middle ear disease, or abnormalities of the cochlea or vestibular structures.
- Further study with electromyography and nerve conduction studies is being considered for patients with SSEP findings that suggest a peripheral nerve disease process.

Concluding remarks

Although the role of evoked potential studies has been reduced significantly in our current era of imaging and molecular diagnostics, they continue to provide an important tool for the *functional* assessment of selected patients, particularly those who are too young or otherwise uncooperative for other means of testing. Newborn screening for hearing impairment and intraoperative monitoring are the most common use for these modalities in current clinical practice.

Acknowledgments

I wish to thank Dana L. Day, AuD., CCCA for her assistance with the preparation of this chapter. I would also like to acknowledge the technologists in the EEG and Evoked Potential Laboratory at the Barrow Neurological Institute for their expertise and support.

Annotated bibliography

Aminoff MJ, ed. *Electrodiagnosis in clinical neurology*, 5th ed. London: Churchill Livingstone, 2005.

Baker RS, Schmeisser ET, Epstein AD. Visual system electrodiagnosis in neurological disease of childhood. *Pediatr Neurol* 1995;12:99–110.

An excellent review of the technical features of ERG and VER studies in children, as well as the ophthalmologic and neurologic disease states in pediatric patients that make them useful.

Chiappa KH, ed. *Evoked potentials in clinical medicine*, 3rd ed. Philadelphia: Lippincott-Raven, 1997.

The best and most scholarly textbook resource for the field of evoked potentials in either adults or children. Each evoked potential modality has a separate chapter addressing issues in children.

DeMeirleir LJ, Taylor MJ. Prognostic utility of SEPs in comatose children. *Pediatr Neurol* 1987;3:78–82.

This study, along with multiple others (see SSEP chapter in Chiappa's textbook, above) demonstrates that bilateral absence of scalp SSEP waveforms in children with acute coma (most hypoxic–ischemic or traumatic) is associated with death or a poor functional outcome.

Ducati A, Fava E, Motti EDF. Neuronal generators of the visual evoked potentials: Intracerebral recording in awake humans. *EEG Clin Neurol* 1988;71:89–99.

Flores-Guevara R, Renault F, Ostre C, Richard P. Maturation of the electroretinogram in children: Stability of the amplitude ratio a/b. *Electroencephalogr Clin Neurophysiol* 1996;100:422–427.

Harden A, Adams GGW, Taylor DSI. The electroretinogram. *Arch Dis Child* 1989;64:1080–1087.

Kriss A, Jeffrey B, Taylor D. The electroretinogram in infants and children. *J Clin Neurophysiol* 1992;9:373–393.

An excellent ERG review, based upon the large experience at the Hospital for Sick Children, Great Ormond Street, London.

Kurtzberg D. Event-related potentials in the evaluation of high-risk infants. *Ann N Y Acad Sci* 1982;388:557–571.

Levin KH, Luders HO, eds. *Comprehensive clinical neurophysiology*. Philadelphia: W.B. Saunders, 2000.

As the title states, a comprehensive textbook on clinical neurophysiology, including electromyography (EMG), electroencephalography (EEG), and evoked potentials. An excellent single-text resource.

Willis J, Seales D, Frazier E. Short latency somatosensory evoked potentials in infants. *Electroencephalogr Clin Neurophysiol* 1984;59:366–373.

CHAPTER 8

Neuroimaging Techniques

Russell J. Butterfield, Gary Hedlund, and James F. Bale, Jr.

Outline

- Pediatric neuroimaging
- Clinical applications
- Disorders of children and adolescents

The past three decades have brought remarkable advances in the ability to image the nervous system of the young child. All of the imaging tools used to diagnose pediatric central nervous system (CNS) disease, including sonography; computed tomography (CT); magnetic resonance imaging (MRI); nuclear medicine brain imaging, including single-photon emission computed tomography (SPECT) and positron emission tomography (PET); magnetoencephalography (MEG); and conventional angiography, have shown robust development. The purpose of this chapter is to emphasize the practical applications, strengths, and weaknesses of currently available imaging techniques.

The first section provides a technical summary of the available imaging modalities and presents a conceptual framework by which clinicians can make relevant decisions regarding the choice of modalities. The remainder of the chapter focuses on common neurologic conditions, including the complications of the neonatal period, infections (congenital or acquired), cranial cerebral trauma, headaches, stroke, neurocutaneous disorders, and seizures. By collaborating with radiologists, clinicians can make safe and cost-effective decisions regarding the optimum utilization of these new and sensitive techniques.

Pediatric neuroimaging

Patient preparation and sedation

The success of a pediatric neuroimaging study begins with consultation between the clinician and the neuroradiologist. The exchange of relevant clinical information allows selection of the best imaging tool to answer the clinical question at hand. The imaging process continues with further preparation of the patient, including sedation when necessary. The majority of cranial-spinal ultrasound and CT/CTAs are accomplished without sedation or with a short-acting agent (midazolam and/or ketamine). When scheduling patients for longer imaging examinations, such as MRI, sedation with an agent such as pentobarbital for patients younger than 8 years of age is typically necessary. Anesthesia-directed sedation is considered for our pediatric patients over 37 kg in weight, and in children with autism, severe developmental delay, or movement disorders. Patients of any age with airway obstruction, achondroplasia, cardiovascular disease, pulmonary compromise, or other complex medical conditions require an anesthesiology consultation. Pediatric patients undergoing cerebral angiography may be studied with either conscious sedation or general anesthesia depending upon patient age, level of patient cooperation, and anticipated length of examination.

Ultrasonography

With the evolution of high-resolution variable-megahertz probes, robust Doppler, and harmonic imaging, ultrasound image quality has expanded the applications of pediatric neurosonography. The portability of the ultrasound unit allows this technology to come to the bedside. The most frequent neurologic indication for sonography is the evaluation of the neonatal brain for intracranial hemorrhage (Figure 8.1). The anterior and posterior fontanels and transmastoid foramen provide acoustic windows for the investigation of anatomic regions susceptible to hemorrhage.

Other important neonatal applications of cranial sonography include the evaluation of periventricular leukomalacia (PVL), cerebral edema, congenital brain malformations, hydrocephalus, and destructive lesions. The robust color and pulse Doppler capabilities of current ultrasound equipment allow interrogation of central intracranial arteries and veins. In infants and children, transcranial Doppler (TCD) has been useful in the evaluation of vasculopathy, such as sickle cell disease. Spinal sonography is an efficient screening tool to evaluate the dorsal lumbosacral spine in newborns and infants up to 6 months of age with sacral dimples to detect occult spinal dysraphism and cord tethering.

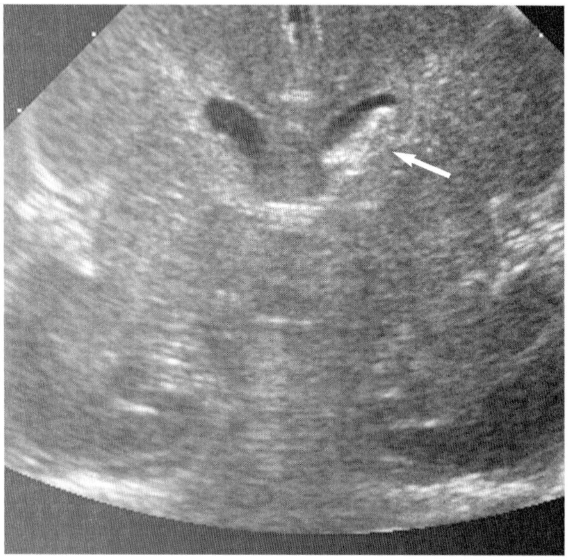

Figure 8.1 Neonatal cranial ultrasound. Coronal ultrasound in a very-low-birth-weight (VLBW) preterm newborn shows a smooth appearance of the cerebral hemispheres, consistent with prematurity and a left grade I germinal matrix hemorrhage (*arrow*).

Computed tomography

The use of CT scanning technology has increased dramatically in recent years, prompting concerns about the long-term effects of radiation exposure. CT-related radiation in children is a particular concern as they are more radiosensitive and have a longer expected lifespan. As many as 4 million children undergo CT scans annually in the United States, contributing to an estimated one additional cancer per 10,000 scans. Continued improvements in technology, attention to size and weight of the patient, and careful consideration of appropriateness of the test by physicians will help to minimize the risk of radiation exposure from this technology.

Conventional CT remains an important tool for the assessment of acute head injury, detection of intracranial hemorrhage, calcification, acute neurologic decline, status

Pearls and Perils

Sonography

- The cranial fontanels are reliable acoustic windows up to 8–10 months of age.
- The major limitations of cranial sonography are the "blind spots" of the peripheral cerebral hemispheres.
- Periventricular leukomalacia is underestimated with cranial ultrasound. The gold standard for infants at risk is magnetic resonance imaging (MRI).
- Spinal sonography for occult spinal dysraphism is most useful for patients less than 3 months of age, but diagnostic studies can be performed up to 6 months. Beyond this age MRI is advised due to increasing acoustic impedance of the posterior neural arch elements.
- In the evaluation of complex lumbosacral skin lesions (skin-covered mass, verrucous hemangioma, dermal sinus, hypertrichosis, or a combination of the above) MRI is recommended.

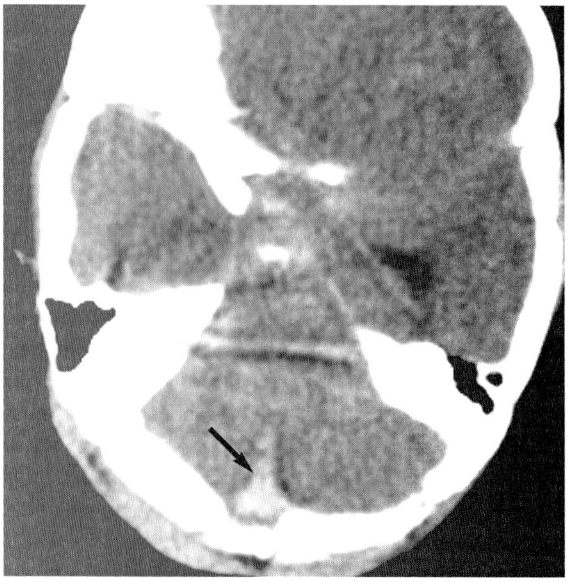

Figure 8.2 Subarachnoid hemorrhage secondary to spinal vascular malformation. Axial noncontrast computed tomography (NCCT) demonstrates hemorrhage filling the cisterna magna (*arrow*).

Pearls and Perils

Computed Tomography (CT)

- Requires exposure to ionizing radiation.
- Scan times are brief, rarely requiring sedation.
- Remains the method of choice for detecting acute hemorrhage and parenchymal calcifications.
- Lower anatomic resolution compared to magnetic resonance imaging (MRI) for the evaluation of temporal lobes, posterior fossa, and the cranial–cortical interface due to beam-hardening artifact.
- Underestimates acute ischemia.
- CT angiography (CTA) is becoming a viable option to magnet resonance angiography (MRA) and catheter angiography in many clinical settings.
- Remains a helpful adjunct in the evaluation of sinonasal diseases and their relationship to intracranial structures.

epilepticus, cranial facial malformations, investigation of lesions of the temporal bone and skull base, nasal obstruction in the newborn without evidence of intranasal mass, and the follow-up of patients with intracranial shunts (Figure 8.2).

Contrast enhanced CT contributes to the diagnostic evaluation of patients with cranial tumefactions, meningoencephalitis, suspected arteriovenous malformations, intracranial venous thrombosis, and complicated sinonasal infections (Figure 8.3).

CT angiography is a less invasive alternative to conventional catheter angiography. Indications for CTA in the pediatric population include detection of intracranial aneurysms (screening patients at high risk and detection of low-profile "blister" aneurysms), evaluating CNS and visceral vasculature in the work-up of suspected vasculitis, particularly in the patient weighing less than 10 kg (where the risk of femoral artery injury is highest), penetrating neck injuries, and the evaluation of nonocclusive arterial dissection (Figure 8.4). CTA used in the acute assessment of the unstable patient with cerebral hematoma secondary to ruptured arteriovenous malformation or aneurysm may provide valuable preoperative information to the neurosurgeon regarding the relationship of the malformation to the clot bed. Patients who are not good candidates for MR angiography (MRA; those with pacemakers and surgical clips juxtaposed to vessels of interest) can often be successfully studied using CTA. The spatial resolution of CTA exceeds MRA when studying the neck vasculature due to artifact in MRA studies introduced by motion from swallowing and respiration. CT venography presents an option to magnetic resonance venography (MRV) in the evaluation of dural venous sinuses.

Perfusion CT affords a quantitative measurement of regional cerebral blood flow. Sequential acquisition of CT sections occurs during IV contrast administration. Using the central volume principle, regional cerebral blood volume, blood mean transit time, and regional cerebral blood flow can be computed. Some centers are gaining experience with perfusion CT in the assessment of acute stroke. This technology may find a role with respect to inclusion criteria for thrombolysis protocols. Perfusion CT may also be utilized following cerebral synangiosis to evaluate for improved regional cerebral perfusion.

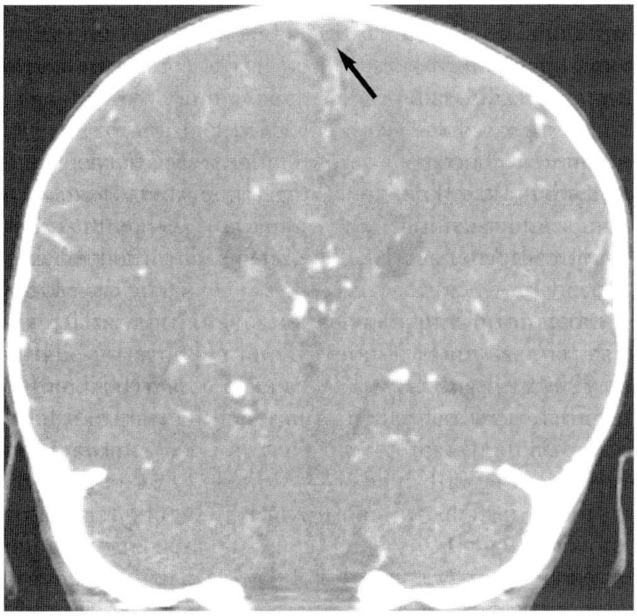

Figure 8.3 Venous sinus thrombosis of the superior sagittal sinus (*arrow*).

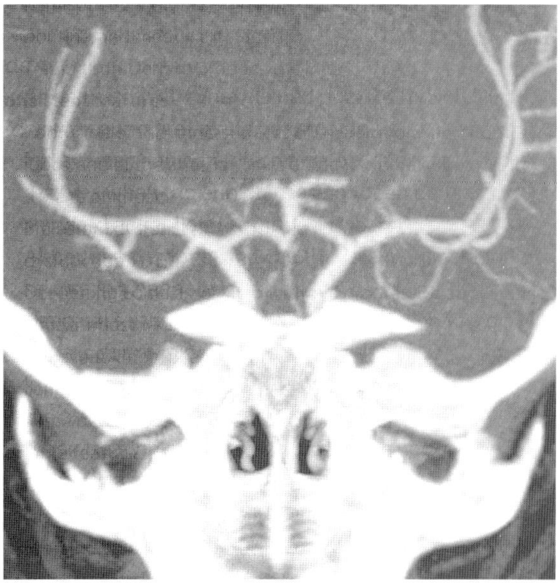

Figure 8.4 Normal circle of Willis computed tomography angiography (CTA).

Magnetic resonance imaging

The development of biologically safe high-field-strength MR systems, more powerful MR gradients, novel coil development, reengineered image processing, and robust scan sequences has led to faster scan times and the capability to overlay functional MR information upon high-resolution anatomic imaging. The ability to create multimodal MR acquisitions within practical scanning times has led to the rapid accumulation of clinically useful information.

Conventional magnetic resonance imaging (MRI) is a clinically useful modality that represents the backbone for investigation of diseases of the pediatric CNS. Evaluation of cerebral malformations, assessment of traumatic injury, characterization of neoplastic and inflammatory disorders, and the diagnosis of early neurodegenerative disease are a few of the practical clinical applications of MRI (Figure 8.5). An important consideration in the evaluation of pediatric MRI is the myelination pattern, as this reflects ongoing motor and cognitive development (Table 8.1). In this respect, attention to the patient's gestational age is critical in the first 18–24 months. Contrast administration becomes a helpful adjunct in the evaluation of neoplasms, demyelinating disease, suspected meningoencephalitis and its complications, and vascular malformations.

The signal intensity in a *diffusion weighted MR image* (d-MRI) is a function of the random translational motion of water molecules (Brownian motion). Conditions that produce cell membrane depolarization such as acute ischemic stroke will result in cytotoxic edema, dis-

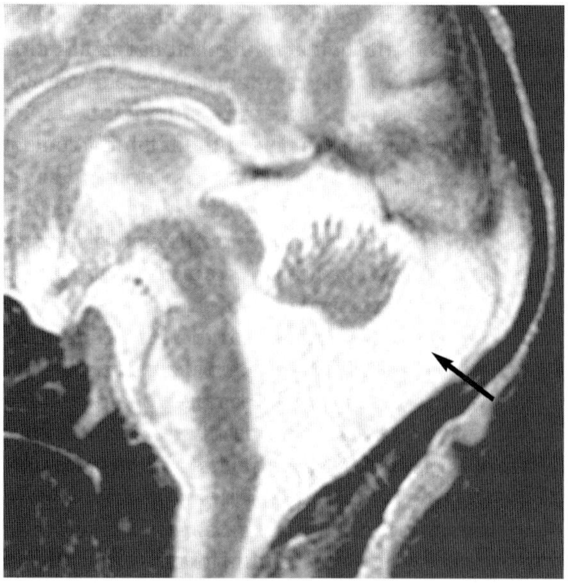

Figure 8.5 Dandy-Walker complex. Sagittal fast spin-echo T2 (FSE T2) image demonstrates upward rotation of the hypogenetic vermis (*arrow*). Note the prominent retrocerebellar cerebrospinal fluid collection.

Pearls and Perils

Magnetic Resonance Imaging (MRI)

- With increases in MRI field strength, anatomic resolution continues to improve.
- The peripheral cerebral cortex, temporal lobes, cerebellum, and brainstem are exquisitely visualized without the osseous artifact that is typical with computed tomography (CT).
- Contrast agents (gadolinium) can enhance evaluation of the blood–brain barrier, the central nervous system reticulo-endothelial system and the extracellular spaces.
- Sensitivity is greater than CT for detecting structural lesions, developmental malformations, demyelinating foci, and disruptions of the blood–brain barrier.
- Magnetic resonance spectroscopy may aid in distinguishing tumefactions (neoplasm versus tumefactive demyelination), inflammatory/infectious conditions, toxic/metabolic insults, and ischemia.
- MRI is insensitive to intracranial calcification.
- Sedation or video goggle distraction is required in almost all children younger than 8 years of age.
- MRI and all advanced MR techniques such as MR angiography (MRA) and venography (MRV) are susceptible to motion (swallowing, respiration, and vascular pulsation). Thus, we currently prefer CTA to MRA when evaluating cervical vasculature.
- MRV may overestimate the degree of venous sinus narrowing.

Table 8.1 Myelination by age

Region	T1	T2
Internal capsule		
Posterior limb posterior portion	36 wk gestation	40 wk gestation
Posterior limb anterior portion	First month	4–7 mo
Anterior limb	2–3 mo	7–11 mo
Corpus callosum		
Splenium	3–4 mo	4–6 mo
Genu	4–6 mo	5–8 mo
White matter		
Occipital	3–5 mo (4–7 mo subcortical)	9–14 mo (11–15 mo subcortical)
Frontal	3–6 mo (7–18mo subcortical)	11–18 mo (14–30 mo subcortical)
Centrum semiovale	2–4 mo	7–11 mo

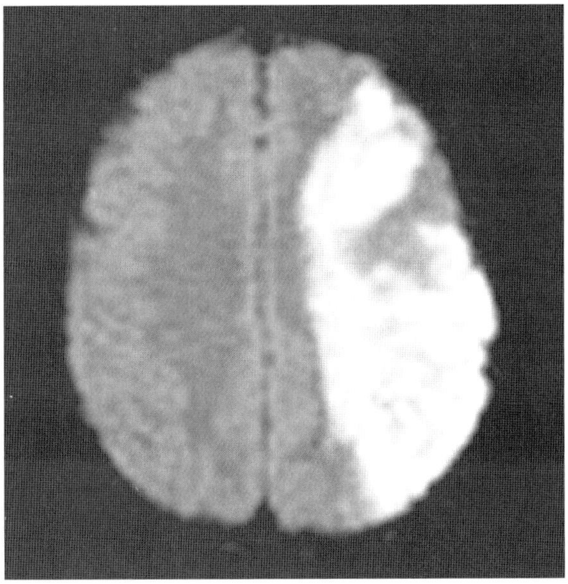

Figure 8.6 Thromboembolic stroke secondary to carotid dissection. Diffusion-weighted image shows a large left middle cerebral artery territory infarction.

rupting normal diffusion patterns in the brain, which are detected in d-MRI scans (Figure 8.6). In cytotoxic edema, the apparent diffusion coefficient (ADC) of water in ischemic tissue is reduced relative to that of normal brain water and allows the ischemic territory to be visualized as a hyperintense region on trace diffusion images and a hypointense region on the ADC map. Diffusion abnormalities can be detected within minutes of infarction, and begin to normalize in 7–10 days. Other causes of restricted diffusion include necrotizing infection (herpes encephalitis), mitochondrial cytopathies, toxic substances such as intermediary metabolites and organic acids, highly cellular tumors, empyema, abscess, and acute demyelination.

Diffusion tensor imaging (DTI) and fiber tracking (tractography) exploit the concepts of water molecule motion properties in all directions (isotropy) and in prescribed paths (anisotropy). These techniques are helpful in the evaluation of a structural lesion and its relationship to white matter tracts. Additionally, further investigation of developmental malformations, such as agenesis of the corpus callosum and holoprosencephaly, may be further understood by assessing the structural neural pathways with DTI. DTI and fiber tracking will play a future role in the investigation of cognitive abnormalities and developmental delay, as well.

Noninvasive MRI vascular imaging (MRA, MRV) techniques provide valuable alternatives to catheter angiography and venography in the evaluation of intracranial vascular disease. The MRA signal is generated from protons in flowing blood. Flow direction, volume, and velocity of flow affect the signal and thus the apparent size of the vessel being studied. The MRA techniques most commonly utilized in the setting of pediatric neuroradiology are time-of-flight (TOF) MRA and phase-contrast angiography (PCA). Time-of-flight techniques take advantage of the differences in signal amplitude between stationary tissue and flowing blood, whereas phase-contrast angiography exploits the differences in signal phase between flowing and stationary spins (protons). Physiologic and anatomic factors influence the image quality and signal from vascular imaging studies. Relevant factors include direction and velocity of blood flow relative to the imaging plane, geometry of the vessel being studied, and complex flow patterns. The T1 relaxation of stationary tissue as in parenchymal hemorrhage may create a pitfall to TOF MRA image interpretation. In the setting of parenchymal bleed, PCA is preferred.

Clinical applications of MRA include the investigation of developmental vascular anomalies or anatomic variations, such as embryonic basilar to carotid connections, evaluation of unusual vessel turns that may mimic an aneurysm or varix, relationship of tumors to vessels (displacement versus encasement), vessel occlusion, dissection, and suspected arteriovenous malformations (Figures 8.7 and 8.8). Emphasizing venous flow (MRV) is helpful in children with intracranial venous thrombosis or pseudotumor cerebri and in the preoperative evaluation of tumors and encephaloceles juxtaposed to venous sinuses.

Magnetic resonance spectroscopy (MRS) is a clinically useful MRI technique that allows the evaluation of brain metabolism in vivo. The primary identifiable metabolites include N-acetyl aspartate, choline, creatine,

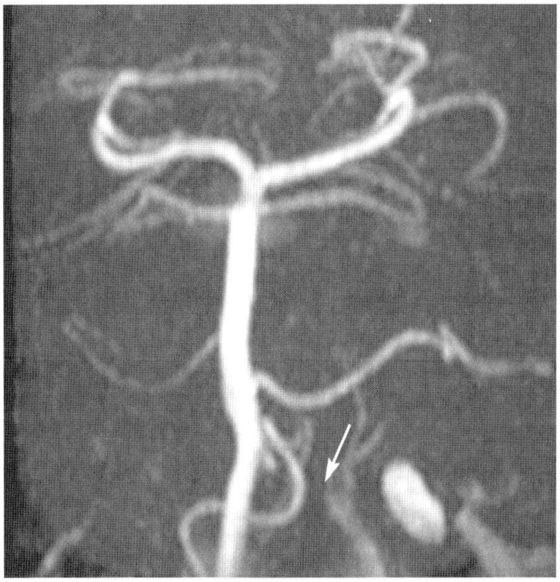

Figure 8.7 Vertebral artery dissection. Time-of-flight magnetic resonance angiography shows occlusion of the left vertebral artery (*arrow*).

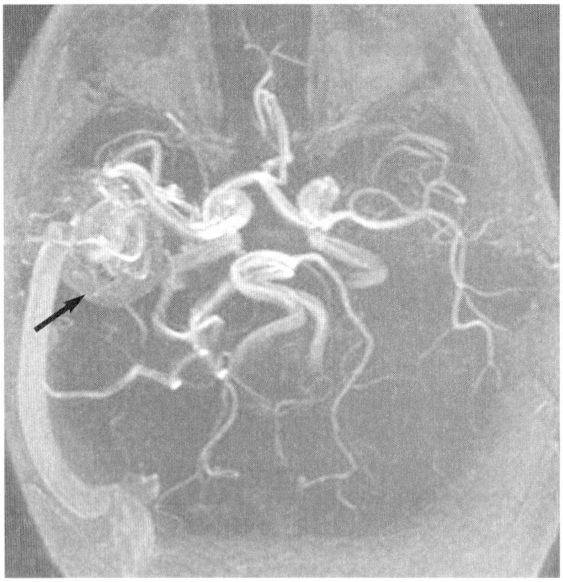

Figure 8.8 Arteriovenous malformation (AVM). Magnetic resonance angiography shows prominent flow signal within a peripheral right meddle cranial fossa AVM (*arrow*).

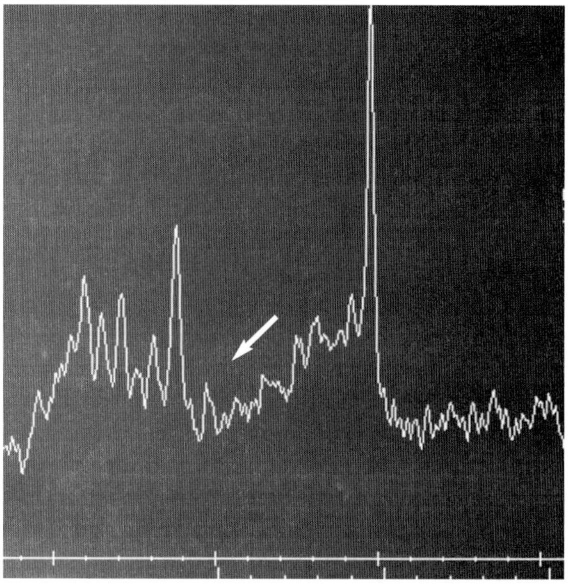

Figure 8.9 Magnetic resonance spectroscopy (MRS). There is absence of the creatine peak (*arrow*) in a patient with guanidinoacetate methyltransferase (GAMT) deficiency.

lactate, myoinositol, and lipid (Table 8.2). MRS is useful in the evaluation of pediatric brain tumors, metabolic disorders, epilepsy, chronic infection (HIV), demyelinating disease, hypoxic ischemic encephalopathy, head trauma, developmental delay, and hypotonia (e.g., creatine deficiency) (Figure 8.9). Technical limitations include the presence of dental braces, intracranial hemorrhage, and patient motion, all of which create susceptibility artifacts.

Cortical activation/functional MRI (fMRI) utilizes changes in the ratio of oxygenated and deoxygenated hemoglobin as an indirect measure of cerebral blood flow and neuronal activity. Scans are performed during activities designed to stimulate a particular area of the brain. Functional MRI is useful for noninvasively mapping eloquent regions of the brain during presurgical planning for structural lesions including neoplasms and epileptic foci. Functional MRI paradigms may activate the motor and visual cortex, interrogate language, and query memory. In many centers fMRI has replaced Wada testing.

Table 8.2 Magnetic resonance spectroscopy

Metabolite	Peak (ppm)	Composition	Utility
NAA[1]	2.02	Neuron-specific	Depressed in disorders causing decline in number and/or function of neurons
Choline	3.2	Phosphatidyl- and other cholines	Elevation reflects increased membrane turnover (gliosis, neoplasm), or membrane breakdown (demyelination)
Creatine	3.0, 3.9	Combination of creatine and phosphocreatine	Reflects energy stores. Commonly used as internal reference. Decreased in pilocytic astrocytoma, SIADH, and hyponatremia
Lactate	Doublet at 1.3	Lactic acid	Not present in normal spectra. Presence reflects anaerobic metabolism. Can be seen in hypoxia, stroke, seizure, or in mitochondrial cytopathies.
mI[2]	3.56	Glial marker	Component of membrane phospholipids, may be elevated in myelin breakdown, low-grade neoplasms, hyperosmolar states, and renal failure.
Glx[3]	2.1–2.5	Neurotransmitters	Elevated in early hypoxic ischemic injury, acute demyelination, and hepatic encephalopathy.
Lipid	0.9–2.0		Elevated in necrosis, high-grade tumor, myelin breakdown, and some inborn errors of metabolism

[1]N-acetyl aspartate; [2]Myoinositol; [3]Glutamate, glutamine, γ-aminobutyric acid

Pearls and Perils

Nuclear Medicine Brain Imaging

- The choice of ictal or interictal studies is somewhat dependent upon institutional logistics.
- The availability of image integration software allows a fusion of single-photon emission computed tomography (SPECT) and positron emission tomography (PET) data with computed tomography (CT) and magnetic resonance imaging (MRI) images.

Nuclear medicine brain imaging

In contrast to structural imaging modalities such as CT or MRI, nuclear medicine techniques derive images that reflect brain metabolism and neural chemistry. These techniques rely on the assumption that cerebral metabolism and blood flow are linked. The most developed techniques are single-photon emission computed tomography (SPECT) and positron-emission tomography (PET). For either SPECT or PET, knowledge of the type of lesion suspected and its clinical localization is useful to the neuroradiologist and allows more accurate image interpretation. SPECT may offer the most widely available and applicable measure of neural behavior and offers spatial resolution similar to PET imaging. A SPECT tracer such as technetium^{99m} hexamethylpropyleneamine (Tc-HMPAO) is extracted by brain tissue on the first arterial pass after intravenous injection and is retained in the brain for several hours. In the evaluation of seizure, the tracer is delivered ictally, and imaging can be performed within several hours. The seizure focus shows increased ictal uptake (Figure 8.10) and decreased interictal uptake. The currently used PET radiopharmaceuticals include 18FFDG, 11Cflumazenil (for temporal lobe epilepsy), and $^{11C}\alpha$-methyltryptofane (identifies epileptogenic tubers in tuberous sclerosis).

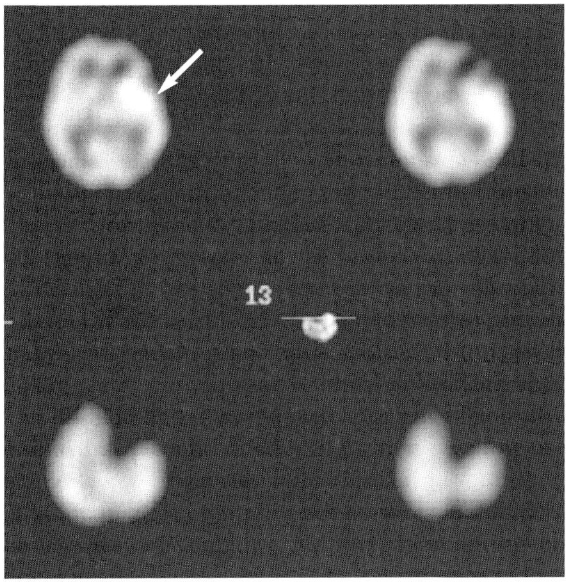

Figure 8.10 Single-proton emission computed tomography (SPECT) nuclear medicine brain imaging. Axial ictal Tc-HMPAO SPECT image demonstrating increased radiotracer uptake adjacent to a region of brain injury (*arrow*).

Catheter angiography

In many clinical situations MRA, MRV, and CTA have supplanted catheter angiography (CA). However, several important indications for CA remain. These include the initial characterization and follow-up of arteriovenous malformations or nonocclusive arterial dissections, preoperative evaluation of suspected meningothelial tumors, petrosal venous sampling in patients with Cushing syndrome, and therapeutic applications, such as embolization of tumors, clot removal in the setting of venous thrombosis, and coil occlusion of congenital vascular abnormalities, such as vein of Galen malformations. In addition, the development of spiral (3D) angiographic techniques has diminished the contrast requirement and shortened examination time, which is critically important in the pediatric population (Figure 8.11).

Clinical applications

Disorders of the neonate

Full-term and premature infants commonly experience neurologic complications, including intracranial hemorrhage, seizures, posthemorrhagic hydrocephalus, stroke, and infection. The choice of neuroimaging modalities depends greatly upon the suspicions of the clinician and the stability of the infant for transport to the imaging suite. Although

Pearls and Perils

Catheter Angiography

- Risks of femoral artery occlusion rise with catheter angiography in patients weighing less than 10 kg.
- General anesthesia is necessary in many pediatric patients requiring cerebral angiography.
- 3D and spiral catheter angiographic techniques reduce requirements for contrast and shorten examination time.
- Flow characteristics and associated stenoses within arteriovenous malformations are best evaluated with a catheter angiography.

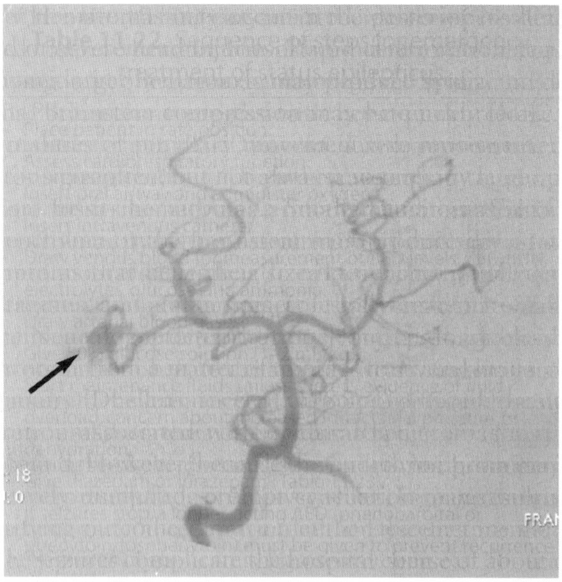

Figure 8.11 Three-dimensional catheter angiography. In this patient with hereditary hemorrhagic telangiectasia (HHT), a right paratentorial arteriovenous fistula (*arrow*) is fed by the right posterior temporal artery.

cranial ultrasound, by virtue of its portability, has great utility in the unstable newborn infant, rapid-acquisition CT and MRI can supplant ultrasound in certain disorders.

Intracranial hemorrhage

Premature infants experience intracranial hemorrhage as a complication of germinal matrix hemorrhage and intraventricular hemorrhage (IVH). The likelihood of IVH corresponds inversely with gestational age and reflects the integrity of the immature germinal matrix vasculature and alterations of cerebral blood flow that accompany prematurity. Approximately 20% of very-low-birth-weight (VLBW) infants experience IVH, whereas the prevalence of IVH among infants older than 36 weeks is negligible. The severity of IVH is designated by grades I–IV (Table 8.3); infants with grades III and IV have increased risks of adverse outcomes, including developmental delay, seizures, and cerebral palsy (Figure 8.1).

Infants with germinal matrix hemorrhage and severe IVH are at increased risk for posthemorrhagic hydrocephalus. Hydrocephalus in these patients reflects arachnoiditis and/or ventricular outlet obstruction and affects 25–35% of VLBW infants with IVH. Posthemorrhagic hydrocephalus usually appears gradually during the first several weeks after birth and may be difficult to distinguish from passive ventriculomegaly during the early stages of evolution.

In contrast to premature infants, term infants experience intracranial hemorrhage as a consequence of hypoxic ischemic encephalopathy, clotting disorders, or

Table 8.3 Germinal matrix and intraventricular hemorrhage

Grade I	Germinal matrix hemorrhage without intraventricular extension
Grade II	Germinal matrix hemorrhage with intraventricular extension filling <50% of the ventricular space
Grade III	Germinal matrix hemorrhage with intraventricular extension filling >50% of the ventricular space and causing ventricular dilation.
Grade IV	Germinal matrix hemorrhage with periventricular hemorrhagic infarction

stroke. Term infants who sustain intracranial hemorrhagic with intraventricular extension are also at risk of posthemorrhagic hydrocephalus. Cystic encephalomalacia, passive ventriculomegaly, or focal cerebral atrophy commonly develops in premature or term infants with stroke.

Cranial ultrasound remains an important screening tool for IVH in the VLBW neonate. We perform the first cranial ultrasound between 7 and 10 days of life. Serial sonograms track the evolution of intracranial hemorrhage and complications, such as hydrocephalus. Periventricular leukomalacia (PVL) is manifest by early periventricular regions of hyperechogenicity, followed by the development of periventricular cysts and passive ventricular dilation (Figure 8.12). Unfortunately, a significant number of neonates with PVL will have a normal initial and follow-up cranial sonogram. The subtle evolution of unexplained ventricular dilation suggests underlying PVL.

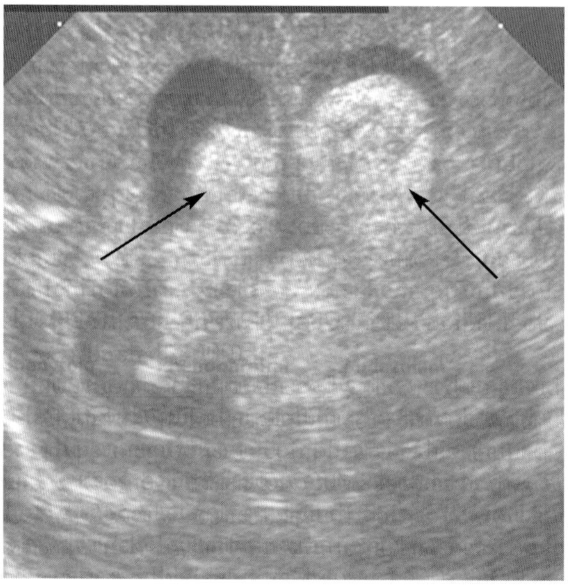

Figure 8.12 Neonatal intracranial hemorrhage. Coronal cranial sonogram demonstrates intraventricular clot and ventricular dilation (*arrows*).

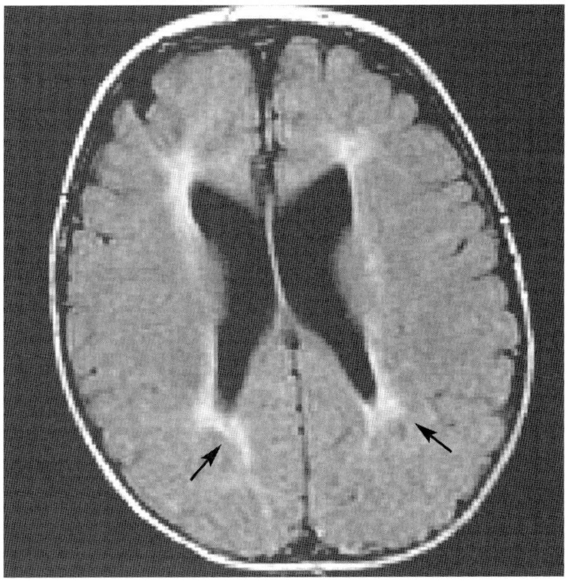

Figure 8.13 Periventricular leukomalacia (PVL). Axial FLAIR magnetic resonance imaging shows periventricular gliosis (*arrows*) and passive ventricular dilation.

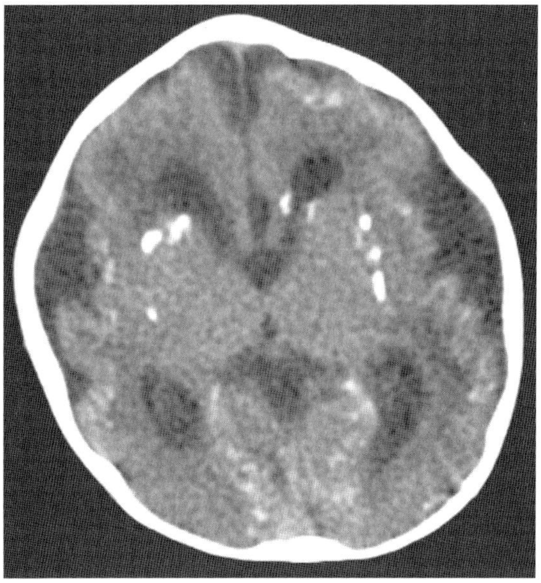

Figure 8.14 CT of an infant with congenital cytomegalovirus infection shows multiple periventricular and intraparenchymal calcifications.

It has become our practice to study VLBW neonates (<1,200 g) with MRI near the time of discharge. This remains the gold standard for detecting PVL (Figure 8.13).

Infection

Many different microorganisms, including bacteria, viruses, fungi, and protozoa, can infect the neonate as the result of intrauterine or postnatal acquisition. Congenital infections, historically designated as TORCH (*To*xoplasma gondii, *r*ubella, *c*ytomegalovirus, and *h*erpes) infections can produce intracranial calcifications, hydrocephalus, and cortical dysplasia (Table 8.4, Figure 8.14). Infections during the neonatal period, such as late-onset neonatal meningitis or herpes encephalitis, can produce hydrocephalus, stroke-like lesions, and cystic encephalomalacia.

Table 8.4 Congenital infections and their associated imaging abnormalities

Agent	Imaging features
Toxoplasma gondii	Hydrocephalus, scattered intracranial calcifications
Rubella	Microcephaly, periventricular calcifications
Cytomegalovirus	Microcephaly, periventricular calcifications, cortical dysplasia, cerebellar hypoplasia, porencephaly, schizencephaly, lissencephaly
Herpes simplex virus (congenital)	Cystic encephalomalacia, calcifications of the thalamus and basal ganglia
Lymphocytic choriomeningitis virus	Hydrocephalus, periventricular calcifications, cortical dysplasia
Varicella zoster virus (congenital)	Calcifications of the thalamus and basal ganglia, hydranencephaly, porencephaly

In the neonate suspected of having a congenital infection, cranial sonography may show regions of periventricular germinolysis (cysts) and scattered parenchymal foci of echogenicity (calcification). Additionally, sonography may show branching linear foci of hyperechogenicity within the thalami and basal ganglia indicative of mineralizing vasculopathy, which has been associated with a congenital infection, sepsis, and certain trisomies. Unfortunately, the peripheral cortex and regions of the posterior fossa are not completely characterized with sonography. MRI remains the most sensitive tool to evaluate the extent of injury with congenital infection, detecting demyelination, germinolytic periventricular changes, encephalomalacia, ventriculomegaly, and associated cortical malformations (Figure 8.15). Nonenhanced CT of the brain often is used as an adjunct to MRI, given its greater sensitivity to detect calcification.

Hypoxic ischemic encephalopathy

Hypoxic ischemic encephalopathy (HIE), or neonatal encephalopathy, represents a common neurologic complication in both term and preterm infants. Coma, seizures, and stroke can be acute manifestations of HIE. Infants who survive HIE, like infants with IVH, have increased risks of epilepsy, cerebral palsy, and developmental delays. Cerebral palsy typically reflects PVL, a lesion that

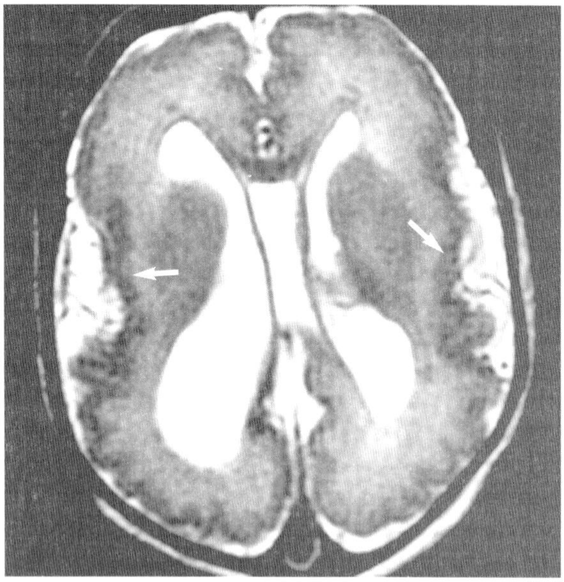

Figure 8.15 Cytomegalovirus (CMV). Axial T2 magnetic resonance imaging shows bilateral perisylvian polymicrogyria (*arrows*).

commonly affects premature infants and can be a sequela of HIE or indicate a predisposing thrombophilic disorder such as factor V Leiden mutation.

In the acute and subacute setting, MRI supplemented with diffusion-weighted imaging and MR spectroscopy are standard imaging techniques used to detect HIE, characterize extent of abnormality, and, when possible, to prognosticate outcome (Figure 8.16). Timing for the MRI scan in infants with suspected HIE is optimal at 4–5 days post-event, as diffusion-weighted changes are maximal at this time. In the late subacute and chronic setting following hypoxic–ischemic injury, MRI remains a powerful tool to detect and characterize encephalomalacia, ventriculomegaly, cortical necrosis, gliosis, and extra-axial fluid accumulations such as subdural hemorrhages (Figure 8.17).

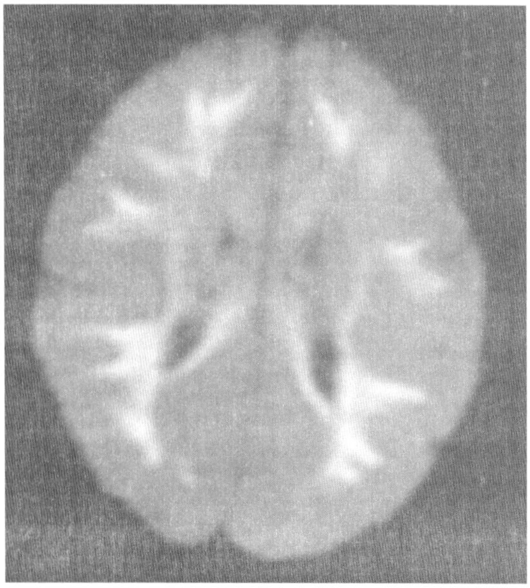

Figure 8.16 Axial diffusion-weighted MRI showing extensive white matter injury in an infant with HIE.

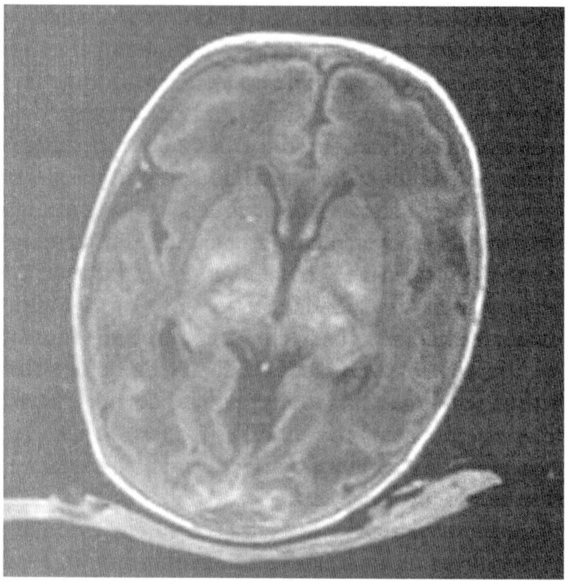

Figure 8.17 Hypoxic–ischemic encephalography in the preterm newborn. Axial T1-weighted magnetic resonance imaging shows basal ganglia and thalamic T1 shortening, indicating profound preterm hypoxic–ischemic insult.

CNS malformations, including lissencephaly, schizencephaly, Chiari malformation, and cortical dysplasia

Infants with severe CNS malformations, such as lissencephaly, holoprosencephaly, schizencephaly, or diffuse cortical dysplasias, frequently become symptomatic in the neonatal period because of seizures, abnormalities of muscle tone, or dysmorphic features. Microcephaly or macrocephaly may also provide the initial clinical clue regarding a cerebral malformation. Chiari malformation, when recognized in the neonatal period, accompanies a meningomyelocele (Chiari type II) or occipital encephalocele (Chiari type III). Occasionally, Chiari type I is identified as an incidental finding during cranial imaging for other reasons.

Imaging the CNS of pediatric patients with disorders of cleavage, neuronal migration, and cortical organization is best accomplished with MRI (Figure 8.18). With the advent of multichannel head coil technology and the ability to image at higher clinical field strengths, the sensitivity in detecting subtle cortical malformations has improved. The use of diffusion tensor imaging and tractography has already brought insights into the organiza-

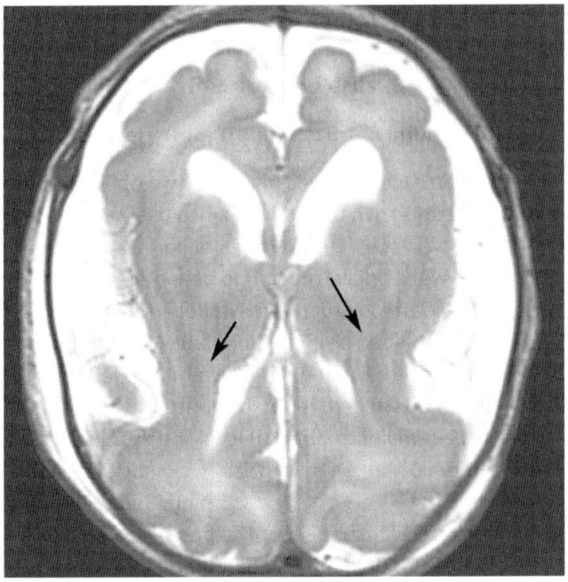

Figure 8.18 Pachygyria. Axial T2-weighted magnetic resonance imaging shows hourglass configuration of the brain, smooth cortex, and subcortical band heterotopia (*arrows*). Findings are consistent with incomplete lissencephaly-subcortical band heterotopia spectrum.

tion of the cortical spinal tracts in patients with holoprosencephaly.

Disorders of children and adolescents

Seizures and epilepsy

Each year thousands of children have their first unprovoked seizure, and many more children have seizures provoked by fever, illness, or trauma. Seizures have many distinct etiologies, ranging from life-threatening CNS infections to benign, inherited conditions, such as rolandic (centrotemporal) epilepsy. Epilepsy, affecting 0.5–1% of the pediatric population, can be symptomatic (reflecting remote or acute CNS pathology), idiopathic (indicating a genetic etiology), or cryptogenic (indicating an unknown etiology).

Practice parameters have examined in detail the role of neuroimaging in children with seizures. Children with uncomplicated febrile seizures do not routinely require neuroimaging. By contrast, imaging should be considered strongly in children with fever-provoked seizures and complicating factors such as focal onset, prolonged seizures or postictal state, or signs suggesting meningitis or encephalitis. Indications for emergent neuroimaging include cranial trauma, status epilepticus, focal seizure, focal postictal deficits, or prolonged postictal states. When urgent cranial imaging is indicated, nonenhanced cranial CT remains a front-line imaging tool, given its availability and short scan times. Traumatic extra-axial hemorrhages, parenchymal hematomas, and tumors are quickly detected.

Neuroimaging studies in children with unprovoked seizures frequently reveal abnormalities, but the majority of these abnormalities do not affect urgent treatment decisions. Young children (<1 year of age) or children with unexplained cognitive or motor delays require nonurgent imaging. When nonurgent imaging is considered in children with seizures or epilepsy, MRI is the study of choice. MRI accurately detects cortical dysplasia, heterotopias, atrophy (including mesial temporal sclerosis), arteriovenous malformations, and other developmental or acquired disorders that can be associated with seizures or epilepsy (Figures 8.19 and 8.20). Contrast administration in patients with seizures becomes important in CT and MRI to characterize suspected meningoencephalitis, cerebral tumefactions, extra-axial fluid collections, venous thrombosis, and suspected vascular malformations. In patients with partial complex seizures and normal MRI examinations, ictal SPECT, interictal PET, or MEG may be employed to add additional useful information (Figure 8.10).

Global developmental delay

Neuroimaging has a major role in the evaluation of children with developmental delay, especially when children have dysmorphic features or abnormal neurologic findings. Imaging studies yield useful information in approximately one-third of children with global developmental delays. However, in many cases of global developmental delay, such as the autistic spectrum disorder, Rett syndrome, and fragile-X, imaging studies (including MRI and MRS) are normal.

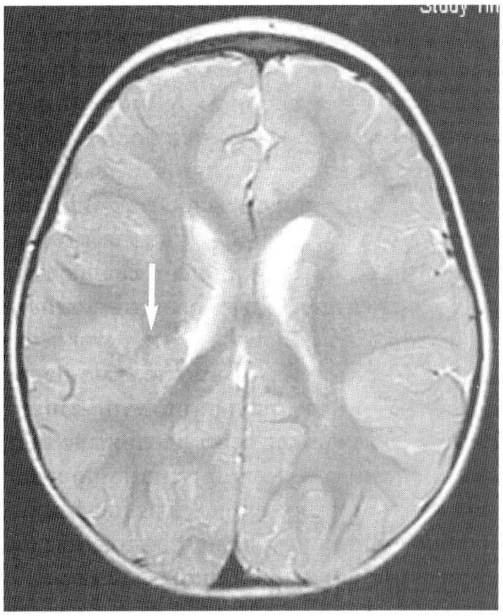

Figure 8.19 Axial T2 MRI demonstrating right parietal-temporal heterotopia (*arrow*).

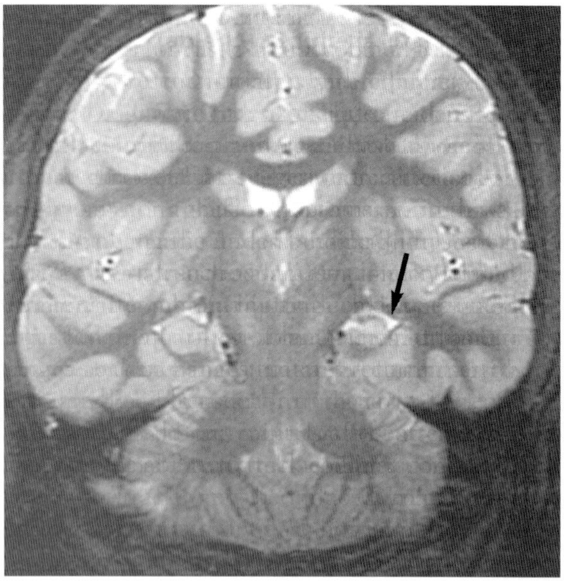

Figure 8.20 Mesial temporal sclerosis (MTS). Coronal fast spin echo T2 magnetic resonance imaging demonstrates atrophy of the left hippocampus (*arrow*).

Although CT can have utility in infants or children with microcephaly and suspected intrauterine infections, MRI should be obtained in children with global developmental delay, especially when accompanied by clinical features compatible with cerebral palsy. MRI may reveal abnormalities of white matter; severe developmental cortical anomalies, such as lissencephaly, porencephaly, or schizencephaly; or less obvious abnormalities such as heterotopias, polymicrogyria, and cortical dysplasia. Periventricular leukomalacia, manifesting as white matter volume loss, passive ventriculomegaly, and T2 signal prolongation, especially evident on fluid attenuated inversion recovery (FLAIR) images, is commonly identified in children with global delays and cerebral palsy. Because of its relatively high yield, MRI is recommended as part of the diagnostic evaluation of children with global developmental delay.

Metabolic and neurodegenerative disorders

Neuroimaging has a useful role in evaluating children with suspected metabolic or neurodegenerative disorders, and certain findings, as summarized in Table 8.5, may

Table 8.5 Imaging features of selected metabolic and degenerative disorders of the central nervous system

Disorder	Imaging features
Disorders of organic acid metabolism	
Glutaric acidemia	Extra-axial fluid collections, especially of the middle fossae and sylvian sulci; basal ganglia T2 prolongation and diffusion restriction
Propionic acidemia	T2 prolongation in putamen and caudate nuclei
Methylmalonic acidemia	T2 prolongation within globi pallidi
Mevalonic acidemia	Progressive cerebellar atrophy
Mitochondrial disorders	
MELAS	Multifocal areas of T2 prolongation; elevated lactate peak in basal ganglia
Leigh disease	T2 prolongation and lactate elevation of caudate nuclei and putamina
Leukodystrophies	
Metachromatic leukodystrophy	T2 prolongation in frontal and occipital white matter
Adrenoleukodystrophy	T2 prolongation prominent in peritrigonal white matter; gadolinium enhancement of the leading margin of demyelination
Vanishing white matter disease	Diffuse, near complete T2 prolongation of cerebral and cerebellar white matter; ± cysts
Pelizaeus-Merzbacher disease	Profound delay in white matter maturation
Alexander disease	T2 prolongation of frontal white matter; macrocephaly
Miscellaneous	
Hallervorden-Spatz disease	Iron deposition in the globi pallidi leading to "eye of the tiger" sign
Guanidinoacetate methyltransferase	Absent creatine peak on MRS; deficiency (creatine deficiency) T2 prolongation and diffusion restriction within globi pallidi
Wilson disease	Signal alteration of basal ganglia, thalami, brainstem; MRS shows decrease in NAA[1]/Cr[2], increased ml[3]/Cr[2], and increased iron/copper deposition
Huntington disease	T2 prolongation of caudate, globus pallidi; caudate and cortical atrophy
Subacute sclerosing panencephalitis	Focal periventricular demyelination, progressive cortical atrophy; reduced NAA peak and elevated myoinositol peak (MRS)

[1]NAA, N-acetyl aspartate; [2]Cr, creatine; [3] ml, myoinositol

lead to specific genetic and metabolic diagnoses. Children with suspected neurodegenerative disorders should undergo complete MRI studies as a routine part of their diagnostic evaluations; MR spectroscopy should be obtained when available, especially in children with suspected mitochondrial disorders.

Headaches

Like seizures and epilepsy, headaches can reflect many distinct disorders affecting the CNS of children and adolescents. Migraine, one of the most common causes of headaches in the pediatric population, consists of intermittent headaches that fulfill several clinical and historical criteria. Most importantly, children with migraine typically have family histories of the disorder. Imaging is not routinely indicated with children with migraine, normal neurologic examinations, and compatible family histories. Imaging should be considered strongly in children or adolescents with headaches of longer than 6 months' duration and features suggesting a space-occupying lesion, such as early morning headaches that awaken the patient from sleep, unexplained vomiting, absence of a family history of migraine, or abnormalities on neurologic examination.

When benign intracranial hypertension is suspected, children or adolescents require MRI, to exclude intracranial mass lesions, and MRV, to exclude sinovenous occlusion. Children with headaches and seizures also require CNS imaging, usually MRI. CNS imaging is always considered urgent whenever a CNS tumor is considered to be the cause of a child's headache or in the presence of abnormal neurologic findings on examination.

Intracranial infections

Children with suspected bacterial meningitis, papilledema, obtundation, seizures, or focal neurologic signs require cranial imaging prior to lumbar puncture. CT without contrast provides sufficient information regarding ventricular morphology and cerebral parenchyma to guide clinical management. Lumbar puncture should be deferred and empiric antimicrobial treatment provided to children with substantial hydrocephalus, mass lesions, cerebral edema, or compressed basal cisterns. Subsequent neuroimaging features in children with bacterial meningitis can include subdural effusions, cerebritis, abscess, communicating hydrocephalus, sinovenous thrombosis, or stroke (Figure 8.21).

Children or adolescents with viral meningitis do not typically have imaging abnormalities. By contrast, pediatric patients with viral encephalitis often have imaging findings that provide important clues to the etiology. Thus, neuroimaging studies, usually MRI, should be obtained in all patients with suspected viral encephalitis. Patients with herpes simplex virus type I (HSV-1) encephalitis display T2 prolongation and gadolinium enhancement of the mesial temporal lobe and insular cortex (Figure 8.22). Children or adolescents with encephalitis due to Epstein-Barr virus or Japanese encephalitis virus often have abnormalities of the basal ganglia or white matter. Patients with acute disseminated encephalomyelitis, a disorder that accounts for approximately 10–15% of encephalitis cases, have multifocal areas of T2 prolongation in the subcortical white matter, corpus callosum, cerebellum, brainstem, thalami, or basal ganglia.

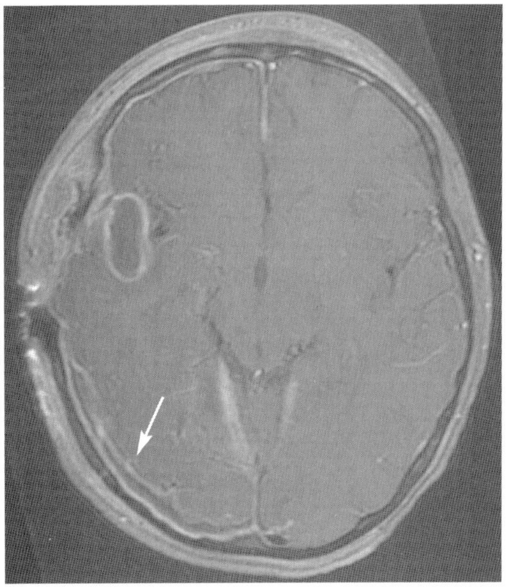

Figure 8.21 T1 enhanced MRI showing subdural empyema (*arrow*) and a ring-enhancing abscess.

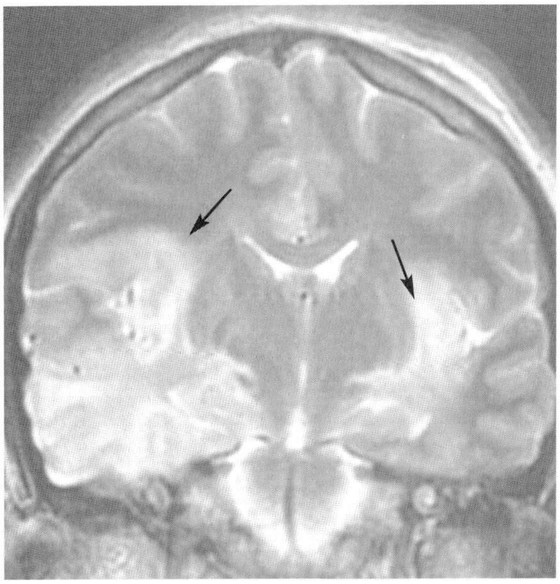

Figure 8.22 Coronal T2 MRI showing bilateral asymmetric insular and temporal lobe edema in child with herpes simplex type 1 encephalitis (*arrows*).

Stroke

Stroke, either ischemic or hemorrhagic, occurs in approximately 3–6 per 100,000 children annually. Multiple conditions predispose to stroke, including trauma, congenital or acquired heart disease, thrombophilic disorders, infection, inflammatory disorders, and vascular anomalies. Many children and adolescents with stroke lack identifiable predisposing factors despite extensive evaluation.

Patients with acute, focal neurologic deficits require urgent neuroimaging. Noncontrast CT is the modality of choice initially, to exclude lesions that require acute neurosurgical intervention such as hemorrhage or intracranial mass. If the CT is normal or detects a nonsurgical lesion, the evaluation should proceed to MRI, including DWI and ADC maps, and as deemed necessary, MRA. If the MRI confirms ischemic stroke, the MRA is normal, and no systemic reason has been identified, many centers consider CA to detect subtle vascular lesions, such as vasculitis or arterial dissection, since identifying such abnormalities influences clinical management. CT angiography through the circle of Willis may be useful when Moyamoya syndrome is suspected.

The precise sequence and timing of the neuroimaging evaluation should be tailored to the patient's condition and the potential for neurosurgical or medical intervention. Although the administration of thrombolytic agents has become the standard of care for adults with stroke, the role of thrombolytic agents or other medical interventions in pediatric stroke are not yet known.

Craniocerebral and spinal trauma

Children with acute head injury require emergent CT to exclude lesions, such as an epidural or subdural hematoma, that require urgent neurosurgical evacuation. Associated spinal injury should not be overlooked in unconscious or obtunded patients, and the imaging evaluation of the injured child or adolescent should also include plain radiography of the spine. When cervical spine injury is suspected, radiographs should be obtained in the neutral position and cautiously in flexion and extension with neurosurgical assistance, as required. Depending upon these findings, thin section CT through the region(s) of interest may be necessary.

MRI displays greater sensitivity than CT for focal cerebral edema and shearing injuries to subcortical white matter; gradient echo MRI can be used to detect small intraparenchymal hemorrhages. MRI also readily detects posttraumatic lesions of the spinal cord. Findings include focal regions of cord swelling secondary to edema or intramedullary areas of T2 prolongation; perispinal hemorrhage, ligamentous tears, or disruption of tissue planes. MRI during the convalescent stages of craniocerebral or spinal trauma can assist clinicians in making more accurate prognostications.

Neuroimaging with CT and MRI plays an essential role in evaluating infants and young children with suspected nonaccidental trauma (NAT). Detecting subdural hemorrhage and fluid accumulations of different ages strongly supports recurrent events as might occur with NAT. Identifying acute intrafalcine subdural hematomas and frontal lobe parenchymal lacerations also supports NAT as the likely mechanism for the child's injury. When the trauma is severe, follow-up imaging can show cystic encephalomalacia, chronic subdural hematoma, or stroke secondary to vascular injury.

Neoplasia

Children or adolescents with suspected intracranial tumors require urgent imaging evaluation, usually starting with CT. In general, MRI has superior sensitivity to CT, especially when imaging the posterior fossa, a common location for CNS tumors in childhood. However, CT can more readily detect intratumor calcifications, particularly when small. MRI should be obtained with and without enhancement, because these modalities provide useful correlates to tumor histopathology. When primitive neuroectodermal tumors or other tumors that frequently disseminate throughout the neuroaxis are suspected, spinal MRI should be obtained, as well.

Children and adolescents who undergo irradiation or chemotherapy for leukemia are at risk for post-therapy CNS injury. Because cranial irradiation under the age of 3 years commonly produces intracranial calcifications of the white matter and basal ganglia, cranial irradiation of young children is avoided whenever possible. Radiation-related CNS effects can present acutely or chronically and be associated with atrophy or cystic degeneration. Methotrexate-related demyelination commonly presents with headache, focal deficits, and altered mental status. MRI usually detects focal areas of T2 prolongation in the white matter.

Neurocutaneous disorders

Neurocutaneous disorders, including tuberous sclerosis, neurofibromatosis (NF) types I and II, and Sturge-Weber syndrome, cause considerable neurologic disability among children and adolescents. Neuroimaging has a major role in identifying these disorders and monitoring children and adults for their associated complications. In addition, neuroimaging represents an essential component of the diagnostic evaluation of children with less common neurocutaneous disorders, such as incontinentia pigmenti, Bannayan-Riley-Ruvalcaba syndrome, von Hippel-Lindau disease, and the epidermal nevus syndrome. Table 8.6 summarizes the characteristic neuroimaging features of these disorders.

Table 8.6 Imaging features of neurocutaneous disorders

Disorder	Imaging feature (CT or MRI)
Neurofibromatosis type I	T2 prolongation in basal ganglia, brainstem, and cerebellum (MRI); optic pathway tumor (MRI); nerve root neurofibroma (MRI); intracranial tumors (CT or MRI)
Neurofibromatosis type II	Acoustic nerve schwannoma (CT or MRI), meningioma (CT or MRI), spinal cord ependymoma (MRI)
Tuberous sclerosis	Periventricular calcifications (CT), periventricular glial nodules (CT or MRI), cortical and subcortical tubers (MRI), radial and glial bands within white matter (MRI), hydrocephalus (CT or MRI) giant cell astrocytoma (CT or MRI)
Sturge-Weber syndrome	Dural and parenchymal calcifications (CT), cortical atrophy (CT or MRI), accelerated myelination (early) and demyelination (late) (MRI)
von Hippel-Lindau syndrome	Vascular lesions of brain, cerebellum, and spinal cord (MRI with contrast) endolymphatic sac tumors (MRI)
Incontinentia pigmenti	Hemiatrophy (CT or MRI), heterotopia (MRI)
Epidermal nevus syndrome	Hemimegalencephaly (MRI), cortical dysplasia (MRI)
Bannayan-Riley-Ruvalcaba syndrome	Heterotopia (MRI)

Patients with suspected NF type I require MRI at the time of diagnosis to establish the extent of their intracranial disease. Optic nerve pathway gliomas are a common finding and can be monitored by annual ophthalmologic examinations and periodic MRIs. Some authors have suggested that MRIs be obtained annually in patients with known optic nerve gliomas to guide therapeutic interventions. Because patients with NF type I are at risk of other intracranial lesions, brain MRIs should be considered when new symptoms, such as headache, seizures, or unexplained focal deficits occur. Spinal MRI is necessary in patients with NF type 1 and back pain, long track signs, or bladder dysfunction as nerve root neurofibromas are a common complication.

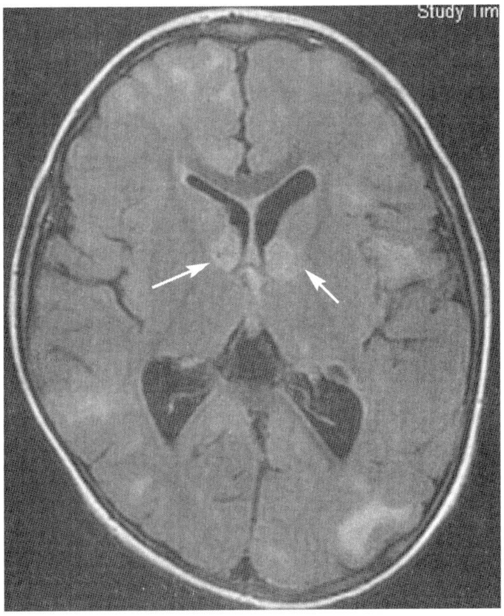

Figure 8.23 Axial FLAIR MRI showing cortical and subcortical tumors in a child with tuberous sclerosis. Bilateral masses near the formina of Monro (*arrows*) are indicative of subependymal giant cell tumors, a common feature in tuberous sclerosis.

Young children with tuberous sclerosis (TS) complex often undergo CT when being evaluated for the new onset of seizures, especially infantile spasms. Characteristic CT features of TS complex include periventricular calcifications and glial nodules; the demonstration of symmetric bilateral calcific glial lesions near the foramina of Monro can be considered diagnostic of TS. These lesions can evolve to giant cell astrocytomas, obstruct cerebrospinal fluid pathways, and cause progressive hydrocephalus (Figure 8.23). Some authors suggest imaging studies be obtained annually to monitor such patients for tumors and hydrocephalus. Because MRI detects TS-associated cortical tubers more readily than CT, MRI should be considered at the time of diagnosis to establish the extent of intracranial disease and periodically thereafter based on the presence of new clinical symptoms and signs.

Annotated bibliography

Ball WS, ed. *Pediatric neuroradiology*. Philadelphia: Lippincott-Raven, 1997.

A comprehensive, clinically oriented pediatric neuroradiology textbook.

Barkovich AJ. Magnetic resonance techniques in assessment of myelin and myelination. *J Inherit Metab Dis* 2005;28:311–343.

Thorough review of physiology and development of normal and abnormal myelination patterns in children.

Barkovich AJ, ed. *Pediatric neuroradiology*. Salt Lake City UT: Amirsys, 2007.

An excellent resource for pediatric neuroimaging with excellent sections on developmental anatomy.

Brody AS, Frush DP, Huda W, et al. Radiation risk to children from computed tomography. *Pediatrics* 2007;120:677–682.
Excellent review of issues related to radiation exposure in children.

Castillo M, ed. New techniques in MR neuroimaging. *Magn Reson Imaging Clin N Am* 1998;6(1).
A comprehensive review of state-of-the-art MRI techniques.

Hedlund GL. Neuroradiology of the central nervous system in childhood. In: Bodensteiner JB, Bale JF, eds. *Neurologic clinics: Pediatric neurology*, Part I. Philadelphia: WB Saunders, 2002; 965–981.
A current review of pediatric neuroimaging techniques.

Hirtz D, Ashwal S, Berg A, et al. Practice parameter: Evaluating a first nonfebrile seizure in children. *Neurology* 2002;55: 616–623.
A thoughtful, well-organized assessment of the child with seizure.

Shevell M, Ashwal S, Donley B, et al. Practice parameter: Evaluation of the child with global developmental delay. *Neurology* 2003;60:367–380.
A practical guide to evaluating the child with developmental delay.

SECTION 2

GENERAL PEDIATRIC NEUROLOGIC DISEASES AND DISORDERS

David E. Mandelbaum

CHAPTER 9

Toxic and Metabolic Encephalopathies

Michael Flink and Doris A. Trauner

Outline

Definitions and general features

Encephalopathy refers to a generalized disturbance in neuronal or glial metabolism that results in alteration of consciousness, cognition, or behavior.

Acute encephalopathy refers to a condition in which a sudden alteration in brain function is induced by an alteration in normal metabolic homeostasis or exposure to a toxic substance. Typically, the individual was functioning at a normal level prior to the onset of the encephalopathy, and a sudden observable change occurs over a few hours. A subacute change in consciousness or cognitive function evolves over several days.

Chronic encephalopathy evolves insidiously over days, weeks, or even months. Chronic or recurrent exposure to toxins, drugs, or metabolic derangements leads to progressive deterioration in cognitive function. The initial changes may be so subtle as to be missed for some time.

General symptoms of acute encephalopathy may include indifference, confusion, disorientation, other behavioral changes such as hyperactivity, irritability, or aggression, hallucinations, seizures, and alterations in the level of consciousness ranging from mild (lethargy) to severe (coma). The neurologic examination of the encephalopathic child typically demonstrates evidence of diffuse dysfunction, including generalized hyperreflexia, positive Babinski signs, and preservation of cranial nerve function until late in the course. Focal findings are uncommon with metabolic or toxic encephalopathies (Table 9.1).

Chronic encephalopathies may have very subtle neurologic changes over time. Symptoms often appear to be static or very slowly progressive. Some children may be misdiagnosed as having cerebral palsy, developmental delay, or attention deficit disorder. The neurologic examination provides some information, but is nonspecific. Reflexes may be normal or increased, although occasionally they can be diminished, such as with certain mitochondrial disorders and with arsenic poisoning. Muscle tone may be normal or decreased, depending on the etiology of the disorder. Hyperactivity and behavioral symptoms are prominent features of some chronic encephalopathies. In assessing any child with developmental delay, hyperactivity, or behavior problems, it is very important to ask the parent or caretaker about loss of previously acquired skills by the child. Even subtle impairments in skills previously acquired may indicate the presence of a chronic encephalopathy and suggest that further studies are required.

Neuroimaging procedures such as computed tomography (CT) or magnetic resonance imaging (MRI), in acute encephalopathies generally demonstrate either no structural change or evidence of diffuse cerebral edema. Such procedures are helpful in ruling out structural lesions such as tumors, bleeds, or cerebral infarcts. Electroencephalography (EEG) reveals diffuse slowing of background electrical activity. Multifocal or generalized epileptiform abnormalities may also be seen on EEG. The

Table 9.1 Features of metabolic encephalopathy

Discriminating features
- Generalized or multifocal brain dysfunction
- Nonlocalizing findings on neurologic examination
- Laboratory evidence of metabolic derangement or organ dysfunction

Consistent features
- Altered mental status
- Diffuse slowing of background activity on EEG

Variable features
- Hyperreflexia, clonus
- Generalized or focal seizures
- Epileptiform discharges on EEG

EEG rarely has focal abnormalities, although shifting asymmetries may occur.

Hypoxic ischemic encephalopathy

One of the most common causes of acute neurologic deterioration in infants and young children is hypoxic–ischemic encephalopathy (HIE). Acute hypoxia may result from severe respiratory distress (e.g., asthma, pneumonia), near-drowning, asphyxia, or respiratory arrest. Chronic hypoxia may be caused by cyanotic congenital heart disease or severe chronic pulmonary disease. Lack of sufficient oxygen to the brain adversely affects all cellular elements and all areas of the brain, although certain brain regions are particularly sensitive to the detrimental effects of hypoxia (e.g., hippocampus). Inadequate blood flow to the brain (ischemia) may also cause widespread damage, but the most severe insult occurs at the border zones or watershed areas of blood supply from major arteries such as anterior and middle cerebral arteries. In the case of ischemic brain damage, multiple infarcts of brain tissue may occur, resulting in a multifocal distribution of deficits.

Symptoms and signs of HIE are rapid in onset and progression. Agitation, followed quickly by depression in the level of consciousness, follows an acute hypoxic–ischemic insult. Cortical depression with obtundation and coma are followed by decorticate or decerebrate posturing, and in the young child in particular, opisthotonic posturing may persist for long periods. Generalized or multifocal seizures may be seen at any time during the course of the encephalopathy. The brain damage progresses in a rostral-caudal direction, so that brainstem dysfunction with involvement of cranial nerves develops late in the course of the encephalopathy, and respiratory arrest occurs as a result of involvement of the medulla.

After a hypoxic insult, the patient may appear to be improving in the first 24 hours, only to deteriorate over the next 48–72 hours as a result of severe cerebral edema. This second phase is often fatal, with tonsillar herniation causing cardiorespiratory arrest.

Recovery from a severe hypoxic or ischemic event is gradual, and return of function follows a caudal-rostral progression. Recovery is often incomplete, with permanent neurologic dysfunction, including seizure disorder, spastic quadriplegia, microcephaly, and mental retardation.

The EEG in HIE typically demonstrates diffuse slowing in the θ or δ range, at times with multifocal epileptiform discharges and even electrographic seizures. A burst-suppression pattern may be seen in severe cases.

A history of respiratory compromise (e.g., near-drowning) or an event that caused reduced cerebral blood flow (e.g., strangulation, severe hypotensive episode) suggests the probability of HIE. Arterial blood gas determinations minutes and possibly up to 1–2 hours after the event typically show a respiratory acidosis and increased CO_2 concentrations. This is followed by a metabolic acidosis. Intensive supportive therapy is required, including maintenance of adequate oxygenation and systemic arterial pressure, as well as careful fluid and electrolyte balance. Anticonvulsant therapy, such as intravenous fosphenytoin or benzodiazepines, may be necessary to control seizures. Intracranial pressure (ICP) monitoring and control of ICP may be necessary in severe cases. Treatment of elevated ICP may include controlled hyperventilation, neuromuscular paralysis, elevation of the head of the bed, and osmotic diuretics. If the child is paralyzed or heavily sedated, continuous EEG monitoring is useful in detecting electrographic seizure activity.

Pearls and Perils

Metabolic Encephalopathy

- Cerebral edema and increased intracranial pressure (ICP) are major complications of most metabolic encephalopathies, and a frequent cause of death.
- Pupillary light reflexes are preserved until late in the course of acute metabolic encephalopathies and can be helpful in differentiating metabolic from structural causes of coma.
- It is uncommon for children with metabolic encephalopathies to have focal abnormalities on neurologic examination; however, focal findings do not rule out a metabolic etiology.
- The electroencephalograph (EEG) in metabolic encephalopathy usually shows diffuse slowing of background activity; generalized or multifocal epileptiform activity is also common.

Disorders of fluid and electrolyte balance

Water and electrolytes are constantly moving across capillary and cell membranes, maintaining equilibrium. Fluid and electrolyte homeostasis is regulated by the interactions of the kidney, skin, lungs, adrenal glands, and brain. A malfunction in any one of these organs can cause disturbances in fluid or electrolyte balance. Persistent or severe diarrhea or vomiting, particularly when coupled with poor fluid intake, results in excessive depletion of body water, or dehydration. Other causes of dehydration include excessive sweating, polyuria, diabetes mellitus, and diabetes insipidus. Infants and young children are particularly prone to the detrimental effects of dehydration. Dehydration is often accompanied by electrolyte imbalances. Excessive loss of water over salt results in hypertonic dehydration; excessive loss of salt results in a hypotonic state. Both of these conditions can be detrimental to the developing brain. With hypertonic dehydration, cell shrinkage occurs, and venous thromboses may develop. Rapid correction of a hypertonic state may result in cerebral edema. In the hypotonic state, excess water moves into brain cells, and cerebral edema with intracellular swelling may develop.

The clinical signs of dehydration depend on the rapidity of the fluid and electrolyte changes, as well as the degree of hypo- or hypernatremia. Lethargy and confusion occur in the presence of acute isotonic dehydration. If the condition persists, systemic hypotension may develop and lead to cerebral ischemia and coma. In addition to mental status changes, hypotonic dehydration may be accompanied by seizures. Acute hypertonic states present with irritability, increased muscle tone, hyperreflexia, seizures, and mental status changes. Overly rapid rehydration and reduction in serum sodium in this condition may result in intraparenchymal brain hemorrhages with worsening coma, multifocal abnormalities on examination, and seizures.

A history of vomiting and/or diarrhea, and poor fluid intake, combined with evidence of poor skin turgor, dried mucus membranes, sunken eyes, and lack of tear production, make the diagnosis of dehydration readily apparent. However, these findings may be less apparent in the presence of hypertonic dehydration, because extracellular fluid volume is relatively preserved.

Intravenous fluid replacement is the mainstay of treatment. Initial rapid replacement of fluid and electrolytes is required to establish or maintain adequate cardiovascular and renal function and organ perfusion. After that, slower replacement of fluids and electrolytes is needed to more fully replace what was lost and to maintain adequate fluid volume.

Specific parameters of fluid and electrolyte replacement must be determined on a case-by-case basis, using age, neurologic and cardiovascular status, degree of electrolyte imbalance, and other factors in the decision-making. Monitoring of serum electrolytes and renal function is necessary to determine the course of therapy.

If severe acidosis is present, bicarbonate solutions may be useful. With hypernatremic dehydration, hypotonic solutions may be used for fluid replacement, but it is important to lower serum sodium levels gradually over about 72 hours, to minimize the potential complications that occur with rapid correction. The primary concern is development of cerebral edema, with the potential for worsening encephalopathy and even herniation, as fluid shifts back into the dehydrated neurons. Seizures usually respond to correction of the dehydration and electrolyte imbalance and generally do not require anticonvulsant medication after the initial acute illness.

Outcome is generally favorable unless severe cerebral edema or intraparenchymal hemorrhages have occurred.

> **Pearls and Perils**
>
> **Disorders of Fluid, Electrolyte, and Glycemic Balance**
>
> - When seizures occur as a consequence of electrolyte imbalance or hypoglycemia, treatment of the metabolic derangement generally results in seizure remission.
> - Infants of diabetic mothers, premature infants, and those who are small for gestational age are most at risk for hypocalcemia, hypomagnesemia, and hypoglycemia in the neonatal period.
> - Most myopathies are not associated with altered mental status, whereas metabolic causes of muscle weakness often have concomitant changes in alertness or cognition.
> - Severe dehydration, hyperglycemia, and hypernatremia may cause tearing of superficial cortical veins and bleeding or cerebral thromboses, leading to focal neurologic deficits.
> - Prolonged or recurrent episodes of symptomatic hypoglycemia may lead to irreversible brain damage.

Disorders of calcium homeostasis

Regulation of calcium homeostasis is the function of parathyroid hormone, vitamin D, and thyrocalcitonin; renal function and movement of calcium into and out of bone tissue also alter calcium concentration. Calcium has a number of important functions in the nervous system, including membrane stabilization and modulation of the excitable threshold of the cell. Thus, either hypo- or hypercalcemia may cause neurologic symptoms.

Hypocalcemia occurs in the premature neonate, in infants of diabetic mothers, and in small-for-gestational-age infants. In older children, hypocalcemia may be seen with vitamin D deficiency, hypoparathyroidism, pseudohypoparathyroidism, renal failure, acute pancreatitis, malabsorption syndromes, magnesium deficiency, as a complication of treatment with certain medications (e.g., phenytoin), and following infusion of large concentrations of citrate during blood transfusions.

Jitteriness, clonus, increased extensor tone, and hyperreflexia are the common findings on neurologic examination of the hypocalcemic newborn. Seizures, either generalized or focal, may be the presenting symptom in some infants. In older children, muscle cramps, paresthesias, carpopedal spasms, and laryngospasm are typical manifestations of hypocalcemia. Lethargy, hyperreflexia, and focal or generalized seizures may also be found in older children. Positive Chvostek and Trousseau signs can be elicited in children with low calcium levels. Chvostek sign is elicited by tapping the lateral aspect of the face over the facial nerve. A positive response is a brief contraction of the facial muscles on the side percussed. Trousseau sign is elicited by applying pressure to the upper arm. Carpal pedal spasm is induced in the presence of low calcium levels.

Diagnosis is made by obtaining a serum calcium concentration below 7 mg/dL. If serum albumin is low, it is important to check ionized calcium, which may be within the normal range even if total calcium concentrations are low. The Q-T interval may be prolonged on electrocardiography (EKG). The EEG often shows diffuse slowing of background activity; multifocal epileptiform discharges may also be seen.

Treatment consists of intravenous infusion of calcium salt solutions. Seizures and other neurologic manifestations typically disappear with this treatment. Long-term anticonvulsant medication is usually not necessary.

Hypercalcemia is found in conditions such as vitamin D or A toxicity, thyrotoxicosis, hyperparathyroidism, bony metastases, prolonged immobilization, hypophosphatasia, sarcoidosis, and Williams syndrome. High calcium levels adversely affect the nervous system by blocking synaptic transmission.

Infants with hypercalcemia have failure to thrive, weakness, and hypotonia. In older children, symptoms are nonspecific and include headache, constipation, anorexia, vomiting, irritability, lethargy, and weakness. Chronic hypercalcemia can predispose to renal stones and renal failure.

Since weakness and hypotonia are common features of hypercalcemia, this condition should be considered in any child who appears to have a neuromuscular disorder. Serum calcium concentrations make the diagnosis.

Treatment consists of administration of a chelating agent to bind excess calcium. Infants with hypercalcemia usually respond to lowering the vitamin D and calcium intake in the diet. If hyperparathyroidism is the cause, surgical removal of the parathyroid may be necessary.

Disorders of magnesium homeostasis

Normal magnesium concentrations in the blood are 1.5–2.5 mg/dL. Levels under 1.0 mg/dL or over 4 mg/dL may produce symptoms. The diagnosis is based on serum calcium, phosphorus, and magnesium levels.

Hypermagnesemia is rare in healthy children. The usual cause is an overdose of magnesium-containing medications, although elevated magnesium levels may be found in association with uremia and adrenocortical insufficiency. Symptoms of hypermagnesemia include muscle weakness, hypotonia, and loss of reflexes. In extreme cases, alterations in consciousness may occur, as well as respiratory depression, hypotension, and flaccid paralysis. Symptoms of hypermagnesemia may resemble myasthenia gravis, infantile botulism, or toxin ingestions. For elevated magnesium levels, intravenous hydration, administration of calcium gluconate and, at times, diuretics, are the usual treatments.

Hypomagnesemia is seen in newborn infants of diabetic mothers, in infants who are small for gestational age, and after exchange transfusions. Hypocalcemia is usually present as well, but correction of the calcium level alone does not reverse the symptoms. In older children, prolonged vomiting or diarrhea, excessive use of diuretics, rickets, diabetic ketoacidosis, malabsorption syndromes, and hypoparathyroidism may result in hypomagnesemia. Hypomagnesemia produces symptoms that are similar to those of hypocalcemia, including tetany, irritability, increased muscle tone, and hyperreflexia. Treatment consists of intravenous infusion of magnesium sulfate.

Disorders of glucose homeostasis

Glucose is the primary energy substrate for the brain. Hypoglycemia produces seizures and altered mental status within 30–45 minutes after a severe drop in serum glucose concentration. If not treated rapidly, irreversible brain damage can result as early as 90 minutes following onset of severe hypoglycemia. Focal as well as generalized neurologic abnormalities can be seen with hypoglycemic encephalopathy.

Hyperglycemia produces a hyperosmolar state with subsequent intracellular dehydration. CNS manifestations of this condition include seizures, hallucinations, tremor, lethargy, and coma. Treatment consists of cautious hydration and exogenous insulin administration. Rapid rehydration may result in sudden fluid shifts that can lead to cerebral edema and worsening neurologic dysfunction.

Nutritional disorders

Vitamins are necessary cofactors for many enzymatic reactions in the brain. Neurologic dysfunction can occur in the face of vitamin deficiency states and in some cases in the presence of excess vitamin concentrations. In some cases, a dependency state exists in which the individual requires higher than usual levels of certain vitamins for the body to carry out normal enzymatic reactions. Vitamin deficiencies generally result from nutritional deprivation, malabsorption states, chronic infections, or malignancies.

Vitamin A deficiency

Deficiency of vitamin A may lead to night-blindness, facial nerve palsy, and reduced sense of smell. Excess vitamin A ingestion in infants and children may cause seizures and cognitive slowing. Either a deficiency or an excess of vitamin A may cause pseudotumor cerebri, the symptoms and signs of which include headache, visual impairment, and papilledema.

Vitamin D deficiency

Vitamin D deficiency produces signs and symptoms associated with hypocalcemia. Excess vitamin D may cause pseudotumor cerebri.

Pearls and Perils

Nutritional Disorders

- The most common causes of vitamin deficiencies are malabsorption syndromes and inadequate nutrition.
- Deficiencies of the B-complex vitamins may result in cognitive delay or regression.
- Excessive intake of the fat-soluble vitamins A or D may cause pseudotumor cerebri with increased intracranial pressure (ICP).
- Vitamin E deficiency causes a neurologic syndrome of ataxia and gait disturbance.
- Early recognition and treatment are key factors in reversing the neurologic abnormalities caused by vitamin deficiencies.

Key Clinical Questions

- *What major features differentiate metabolic encephalopathy from intracranial hemorrhage or closed head injury?* Typically, an absence of focal findings is present in metabolic encephalopathy, although focal findings can occur (see Pearls & Perils), generalized slowing on the EEG, brain MRI either normal, or diffuse cerebral edema.
- *How long is it necessary to treat a child who has hypoglycemic seizures with anticonvulsant therapy?* In most cases, anticonvulsant medications can be discontinued once the acute metabolic problem has resolved.

Vitamin B deficiencies

Most of the B vitamins are cofactors for mitochondrial electron transport chain enzymes. Deficiencies in any of these are uncommon, but can lead to impaired energy production and serious neurologic complications.

Vitamin B_1 (thiamine) deficiency interferes with cellular metabolism and may cause cerebral lactic acidosis. Thiamine deficiency is responsible for beriberi, a condition in which a mixed sensory and motor neuropathy occurs, with weakness, absence of tendon reflexes, sensory loss, and ataxia. In severe cases, altered mental status and increased ICP may occur. In adults, thiamine deficiency can also cause Wernicke encephalopathy, but this condition is very rare in children. Symptoms include ophthalmoplegia, ataxia, and altered mental status (e.g., inattentiveness, lethargy, or dementia). Permanent neurologic impairment may result from prolonged thiamine deficiency.

Vitamin B_2 (riboflavin) deficiency causes a chronic encephalopathy with mental retardation and slowing of the EEG.

Vitamin B_3 (niacin) deficiency is the cause of pellagra, consisting of dermatitis, diarrhea, and dementia.

Vitamin B_6 (pyridoxine) deficiency can be caused by certain drugs (e.g., isoniazid), as well as by malnutrition and malabsorption. Symptoms of pyridoxine deficiency include seizures and irritability. Infants with pyridoxine dependency syndrome present with intractable epilepsy, markedly abnormal EEGs, and developmental regression. Early treatment with large daily doses of pyridoxine may reverse or at least ameliorate these problems.

Vitamin B_{12} (cobalamin) is necessary for the synthesis of DNA during cell division. It also plays a role in the maintenance of myelin. Deficiency states are usually caused by malabsorption. Weakness, fatigue, and apathy may be the only CNS manifestations of cobalamin deficiency. Decreased reflexes, loss of balance, and sensory loss in the lower extremities (subacute combined degeneration) may be found in adults with chronic B_{12} deficiency.

Vitamin E deficiency

Vitamin E deficiency can occur in cystic fibrosis, chronic cholestasis, abetalipoproteinemia, and as a familial condition of isolated vitamin E deficiency. These conditions may result in a chronic encephalopathy that consists of cognitive slowing, progressive ataxia, muscle weakness, impaired position and vibratory sensations, and inability to walk. Measurement of serum vitamin E levels may not accurately reflect the degree of the deficiency state. The presence of any underlying condition that predisposes to vitamin E deficiency should raise suspicion of this condition in a child presenting with the typical clinical features. Administration of high daily doses of vitamin E will ameliorate the symptoms of this condition, especially if treated relatively early in the course.

Pearls and Perils

Encephalopathies Associated with Systemic Diseases

- Bleeding tendencies are increased in patients with hepatic injury and may lead to additional neurologic complications. Correction of clotting disorders in patients with hepatic encephalopathy is difficult and may require exchange transfusion or plasmapheresis.
- Systemic disorders, such as liver and kidney disease, can cause chronic, slowly progressive encephalopathy that may be difficult to recognize in the early stages.
- Asymptomatic peripheral neuropathy is found in many children with chronic uremia.
- Children with chronic liver or renal disease may decompensate and develop encephalopathic symptoms in the presence of acute infection or electrolyte imbalance, even when organ function has been fairly stable.

Encephalopathies associated with systemic disease

Hepatic encephalopathy

Liver failure, regardless of etiology, is associated with multiple metabolic disturbances, including hyperammonemia, hyperbilirubinemia, and disturbances in carbohydrate and fatty acid metabolism. Both acute and chronic forms of hepatic encephalopathy (HE) may occur, depending in part on the rapidity and severity of the liver disease.

In acute HE, agitation, disorientation, and lethargy are the early symptoms. Asterixis can be demonstrated during the early stages. Asterixis is a loss of postural tone in the outstretched wrists that produces a flapping movement of the hands. Obtundation and coma may follow in severe cases. The EEG in HE demonstrates diffuse slowing, and a pattern of triphasic waves may appear, although this is much less common in children than adults.

Treatment of HE involves multiple approaches, including intensive supportive care, correction of bleeding abnormalities, and reduction in ammonia levels using neomycin orally and/or rectally, or oral lactulose. Fulminant hepatic failure may require liver transplantation.

Cerebral edema complicates liver failure and treatment should include measures to reduce ICP, including osmotic diuretics, controlled hyperventilation, and elevation of the head.

Chronic HE occurs with liver damage that is prolonged and sufficient to cause metabolic derangements. Symptoms and signs include cognitive impairments, at times with frank dementia, and movement disorders such as choreoathetosis or dystonia. Some evidence suggests that liver transplant may improve cognitive function in these patients.

Inflammatory bowel disease (IBD)

Both ulcerative colitis and Crohn disease are associated with a number of complications, including a hypercoagulable state in which the patient is prone to develop thromboses. The etiology of this coagulopathy is unknown. Elevated levels of factor VIII have been found in some patients with this condition, whereas thrombocytosis has also been reported in association with thromboembolic events in IBD. Arterial and venous cerebral thromboses have been reported in children with these disorders. Acute arterial thrombosis typically presents with a stroke-like picture of hemiplegia, aphasia, or other focal signs. Venous sinus thromboses cause acute alterations in mental status, with lethargy, headache, vomiting, seizures, and possibly coma. This complication can be fatal, although many patients survive with few or no sequelae. Treatment with steroids and anticoagulation may be warranted, but treatment must depend on the clinical severity as well as other factors including evidence of hemorrhagic infarct or other bleeding diathesis that might contraindicate the use of anticoagulation therapy.

Celiac disease

Celiac disease is a fairly common gastrointestinal disorder associated with gluten intolerance and malabsorption syndrome. Children with this condition have a history of chronic diarrhea, at times associated with short stature. Performing a small-intestine biopsy and demonstrating villous atrophy and crypt hyperplasia makes the diagnosis. Circulating antigliadin, antireticulin, and antiendomysial antibodies are also diagnostic of this condition. There is some controversy as to whether IgA antibodies are required to make the diagnosis as opposed to IgG only. Institution of a gluten-free diet and replacement of vitamins and other cofactors that were reduced because of malabsorption leads to a reduction or resolution of clinical symptoms.

Neurologic complications of untreated celiac disease include a chronic encephalopathy in which there is cognitive decline, with psychomotor delay or retardation, or dementia with loss of previously acquired cognitive function. Behavioral disorders, depression, ataxia, and seizures have all been reported in association with celiac disease. Dietary control generally improves the neurologic condition.

Renal failure

Renal failure results in a number of metabolic derangements, including uremia, hypocalcemia, acidosis, and other abnormalities. Hypertension is also a complication of renal disease. The encephalopathy associated with renal failure may be caused by the metabolic derangements or by severe hypertension.

Acute uremic encephalopathy develops in the presence of sudden marked elevations of blood urea. Symptoms include lethargy, restlessness, agitation, and slurred speech. Muscle weakness with fasciculations may also be present, as well as tremors and other movement disorders. Progressive impairment in mental status may culminate in coma, with focal or generalized seizures, diffuse hyperreflexia, and rigidity.

Chronic renal failure is associated with a slowly progressive encephalopathy consisting of cognitive slowing (at times quite severe) and seizure disorders.

Diagnosis of uremic encephalopathy includes elevations of blood urea nitrogen, typically >90 mg/dl, as well as elevations in serum creatinine. Diffuse slowing is seen on the EEG, at times with triphasic slow waves.

Treatment of the acute encephalopathy consists of dialysis to reduce the uremia. Long-term anticonvulsant therapy may be required, as seizures may persist beyond the acute stage. Chronic uremic encephalopathy is poorly responsive to dialysis and tends to have a slowly progressive course despite treatment.

Hypertensive encephalopathy begins abruptly, in association with a sudden and severe rise in systemic arterial blood pressure, and typically presents with a sudden marked alteration in consciousness (usually coma) with generalized or focal seizures. Rapid control of systemic arterial pressure is necessary to treat hypertensive encephalopathy. Seizures may not recur once the acute episode is over. However, there may be long-term sequelae from hypertensive encephalopathy as a consequence of cerebral edema and petechial hemorrhages into the brain during the acute stages.

Pearls and Perils

Thyroid Dysfunction

- Thyroid dysfunction should be considered in a child with unexplained muscle weakness and hypertrophy.
- Children with thyroid dysfunction may have symptoms reminiscent of attention deficit disorder.

Thyroid dysfunction

Both hypo- and hyperthyroid states cause chronic encephalopathies with impairment in cognitive function and behavior. Hypothyroidism that begins after infancy produces a slow deterioration in cognitive function, with worsening school performance, inattentiveness, slurred speech, and general slowing. These children are occasionally misdiagnosed as having attention deficit disorder. Treatment with daily L-thyroxine replacement may reduce or reverse the neurologic problems, but often some residual CNS dysfunction will remain despite adequate treatment.

Hyperthyroid conditions typically manifest neurologically as hyperactivity, restlessness, poor concentration, and occasionally mania or psychosis. Often, a fine tremor can be observed in the outstretched hands. Treatment with agents that suppress thyroid function usually reverses the encephalopathic symptoms.

Steroid-responsive encephalopathy associated with Hashimoto encephalopathy

Although steroid-responsive encephalopathy associated with Hashimoto encephalopathy (SREHT) is rare and etiologically a somewhat controversial diagnosis, it deserves mention. Hashimoto thyroiditis is an autoimmune disorder and the most common cause of acquired hypothyroidism. At time of diagnosis most patients are hypothyroid or euthyroid and less commonly hyperthyroid and may present with the above-mentioned symptoms depending on the thyroid state. In rare instances, some patients with Hashimoto thyroiditis can present with confusion, hallucinations, seizures, and/or focal neurologic deficits. These symptoms reflect SREHT when associated with elevated thyroid antibody titers, clinical symptoms respond to corticosteroid treatment, and other etiologies have been excluded. Although elevated thyroid antibodies are part of SREHT, titers do not correlate with the extent of encephalopathy. The onset of SREHT can be acute, subacute, or more slowly progressive. To date, no clear guidelines on treatment exist, as controlled trials are lacking. However, most treatment strategies include use of high-dose intravenous steroids followed by prednisone for several months. Many of the clinical symptoms will resolve, but can eventually relapse.

Toxic encephalopathies

Heavy metals

Lead exposure continues to be a common occurrence. Although lead paint is no longer used in homes, older buildings still may have some residual lead paint undercoats. Infants and toddlers can ingest chipped paint. Lead is also found in some china, pottery, and glassware products. Drinking water can be contaminated by lead pipes or by waste from industrial plants. Burned storage batteries emit fumes containing lead. Low-income, inner-city children are at highest risk for lead exposure, and African American children have a higher incidence of lead exposure than do other ethnic groups.

Acute lead intoxication causes a severe encephalopathy consisting of vomiting, ataxia, and seizures, followed by coma with increased ICP. Diffuse hyperreflexia and increased tone are found on examination, with few focal features. Seizures may accompany the acute encephalopathy.

Chronic lead intoxication has been associated with more subtle effects on the CNS. Behavior problems, hyperactivity, learning disabilities, and at times frank mental retardation have been attributed to chronic high levels of lead in the blood.

Diagnosis is made by blood lead-level determinations. Elevated free erythrocyte porphyrin levels and low hemoglobin are also found.

Pearls and Perils

Toxic Encephalopathies

- All children are at risk for lead exposure from many sources in the environment.
- Low levels of lead exposure over a long period of time have been associated with subtle cognitive and behavioral deficits.
- A serum salicylate level should be obtained in acute encephalopathy of unknown cause in young children, especially when hyperventilation and acidosis are present.
- Acetaminophen toxicity can cause acute hepatic failure and encephalopathy.

Treatment consists of chelation therapy, but the lead level at which chelation is warranted remains an area of controversy. In acute encephalopathic conditions, supportive care and treatment of elevated ICP are necessary. Anticonvulsant therapy may also be required. Toxic encephalopathies associated with other metals are outlined in Table 9.2.

Insecticides

Organophosphates and carbamates are common components of insecticides used worldwide. Exposure can occur via skin absorption, inhalation, or ingestion from in-home containers of insecticide agents or treated outdoor areas. These agents act by inhibiting cholinesterases, the enzymes involved in the degradation of acetylcholine. Thus, activity of acetylcholine is prolonged, leading to overexcitation of the cholinergic nervous system. Toxicity can affect both the peripheral (PNS) and central nervous systems (CNS) and can occur within 12 hours of exposure. In children, CNS symptoms such as altered level of consciousness, confusion, restlessness, anxiety, seizures, or ataxia more commonly occur before PNS symptoms are exhibited. However, when affected, PNS symptoms can include muscle fasciculations, weakness, miosis, diaphoresis, increased pulmonary secretions, bronchospasms, pulmonary edema, cardiac arrhythmias, excessive salivation, and diarrhea.

Treatment initially involves patient stabilization by securing an airway and cardiovascular evaluation and management if needed. Skin and clothing decontamination of the child is necessary to avoid exposure of the agent to others. In cases of ingestion, activated charcoal should be used. Anticholinergic agents such as atropine should be immediately introduced. Use of the cholinesterase reactivator, pralidoxime remains controversial; in fact, some studies have not only shown lack of efficacy, but possible harm as well. Thus, the role of pralidoxime in organophosphate toxicity is not clear.

Immunosuppressive agents

Immunosuppressive agents have contributed significantly to transplant survival and quality of life. Many of these agents, including cyclosporin, tacrolimus, and methotrexate (MTX) can cause encephalopathy, usually, but not exclusively at toxic serum levels. Acute cyclosporine toxicity is characterized by tremulousness and restlessness, as well as an acute confusional state, at times with psychosis. Speech problems and myoclonus have also been reported in this condition. Tacrolimus has been reported to cause similar adverse symptoms. Both cyclosporin and tacrolimus have also been associated with posterior reversible leukoencephalopathy syndrome (PRES), which usually manifests as headache, seizures, vision changes,

Table 9.2 Heavy metal toxicity

Heavy metal	Exposure source	Central nervous system symptoms	Diagnosis	Treatment
Thallium	Insecticides Rodenticides	Headaches Ataxia Seizures Somnolence Cranial nerve palsies	Urine thallium level	Bithizone KCl and charcoal hemodialysis
Arsenic	Insecticides Herbicides	Headaches Irritability Seizures Sensory neuropathy	Urine and hair arsenic levels	British antilewisite penicillamine
Mercury	Fungicides	Ataxia Movement disorders Tremor	Red blood cell mercury level	Chelation (?)
Manganese	Industrial exposure Impaired elimination of dietary Mn (from liver disease)	Mild cognitive impairment Tremor Parkinsonian symptoms	Blood manganese levels	Withdrawal of source of excess Mn

and/or altered consciousness. In cyclosporin and tacrolimus-induced PRES, the onset of symptoms usually occurs 7–30 days after exposure. Although in PRES white matter changes (edema) in the parieto-occipital regions are typically observed via imaging studies, the gray matter and other areas of the brain may be involved as well. In contrast to the name, this syndrome is not always reversible. However, most cases will resolve with either removal or lowering the dose of the offending agent. Other factors, such as hypertension or renal insufficiency may increase the risk for developing immunosuppressive agent–induced PRES. Controlling these other predisposing factors may lessen the need for complete cessation of the immunosuppressive agent.

Route of administration and dosage of these agents are also important. Methotrexate, given either intrathecally or as a high-dose intravenous agent can also acutely cause neurologic deficits, including headache, alterations in levels of consciousness, vision changes, and seizures. Alternatively, MTX can cause a subclinical leukoencephalopathy that can slowly progress to permanent cognitive changes, seizures, focal neurologic deficits, and possibly coma. This type of MTX-induced neurotoxicity can occur many months after treatment and is often associated with other adjunctive therapies, including radiation or cytosine arabinoside. Case reports have suggested that dextromethorphan may be beneficial in the treatment of MTX encephalopathy.

In addition, corticosteroids, often used in treatment of cancer, rheumatologic disorders, multiple sclerosis exacerbations, or vasogenic brain edema, can adversely affect the CNS. Given in high doses, particularly intravenously, agitation, hallucinations, or even psychosis can occur.

Drug intoxication

Iatrogenic and accidental drug ingestion or overdose can often have deleterious effects on the CNS either directly or indirectly by producing numerous metabolic derangements. A careful history regarding potential medication exposures and clinical manifestations can help elucidate the etiologic cause of the encephalopathy. For example, narcotic ingestion, which can lead to alterations in the level of consciousness, will also produce respiratory depression and miotic pupils. Along these lines, anticholinergic drugs, such as atropine, antihistamines, or tricyclic antidepressants can produce predictable symptoms: confusion, agitation, psychosis, mydriasis, dry skin and mucus membranes, tachycardia, hypoactive bowel sounds, and urinary retention.

In general, the mainstay of treatment in drug intoxication involves removal of the offending agent and supportive care, but more specific therapies and treatments vary depending on the drug involved.

The number of drugs that can cause a diffuse encephalopathy is quite vast and beyond the scope of this text, however, some are worth mentioning.

Psychiatric medications

The medications used to treat psychiatric illness in children have been quite beneficial, but can have adverse effects on the CNS at therapeutic or supratherapeutic doses, or when administered in conjunction with other drugs. Treatment of depression with selective serotonin reuptake inhibitors (SSRI) can, rarely, lead to serotonin syndrome. This condition usually occurs acutely upon initial administration, change in dosing, or overdose of a SSRI. In addition, serotonin syndrome can occur with use of many other drugs in a similar manner to SSRI or when used in conjunction via a mechanism that affects SSRI metabolism or concomitantly increases total serotonin levels; the list is quite extensive, but includes dextromethorphan, meperidine, metoclopramide, tricyclic antidepressants, buspirone, venlafaxine, Demerol, fentanyl, tramadol, and linezolid.

The serotonin syndrome consists of altered mental status, autonomic instability, and neuromuscular abnormalities. However, not all findings may be observed. In fact, clinical presentation may be mild, presenting as only mydriasis, hyperactive bowel sounds, diaphoresis, and/or tachycardia and only later progressing to myoclonus, hyperreflexia, agitation, motor restlessness, hypertension, and hyperthermia. If left untreated, this condition can rapidly progress to altered mental status, severe hypertension, hypertonicity, and rigidity greatest in the lower extremities and then abruptly become life-threatening. Thus, it is important to recognize this syndrome during the early manifestations.

Treatment includes immediate discontinuation of the offending agent, supportive care, including control of cardiac and respiratory abnormalities, administration of antipyretics for hyperthermia, and benzodiazepine use to control agitation. In more severe cases, 5-HT_{2a} antagonists, such as cyproheptadine have shown some benefit and, when core body temperatures are significantly increased, further sedation, intubation, and neuromuscular paralysis with nondepolarizing medications should be performed.

Consider Consultation When...

- An infant or child develops a sudden change in mental status that is not explained by fluid or electrolyte imbalance or hypoglycemia.
- A previously typically developing child begins to have difficulty with school performance, motor functions, or behavior.
- A previously healthy child complains of headache or has persistent vomiting and lethargy without clear gastrointestinal cause.
- Findings on neurologic examination demonstrate hyperreflexia, positive Babinski signs, and/or papilledema.

Neuroleptic malignant syndrome (NMS), a somewhat similar condition to serotonin syndrome, can also occur during the management of childhood psychiatric conditions, but is associated with neuroleptic and atypical antipsychotic medications. Classically, NMS consists of muscle rigidity, autonomic instability, including hyperpyrexia, and altered mental status. In contrast to serotonin syndrome, clinical manifestations in NMS occur after subacute to chronic treatment. Furthermore, extrapyramidal rigidity is present equally in all extremities, pupil size is unchanged, reflexes are not increased, and myoclonus does not occur.

Treatment of NMS also involves cessation of the offending agent and supportive care, including hydration, antipyretics, dantrolene, and use of dopamine agonists such as bromocriptine.

Salicylism

Although warnings on medications that contain salicylates have significantly reduced the administration of these drugs to children, accidental ingestion is still a concern in children, particularly those under the age of 5 years. Salicylate compounds are found in many over-the-counter medications. Salicylate overdose produces a number of metabolic derangements that lead to CNS compromise. These include metabolic acidosis, respiratory alkalosis, hypoglycemia, and lactic acidosis. Acute poisoning can also cause hepatocellular damage with additional metabolic problems, including hyperammonemia.

Signs and symptoms of acute salicylate intoxication include vomiting, dizziness, hyperventilation, delirium, and coma. Increased ICP with cerebral edema is a common complication, as is excessive bleeding.

Diagnosis is suspected from the history and the laboratory findings of mixed metabolic acidosis and respiratory alkalosis, hypoglycemia, and elevated salicylate levels in the blood.

Treatment includes intensive cardiorespiratory support, correction of the metabolic derangements, treatment of elevated ICP, and administration of vitamin K to attempt to reduce the potential for bleeding.

Annotated bibliography

Frank Y, Pavlakis SG. Toxic and metabolic encephalopathies. In: David RB, ed. *Child and adolescent neurology*. St. Louis: Mosby, 1997.

A concise chapter summarizing the same topic.

Trauner DA. Toxic and metabolic encephalopathies. In: David RB, ed. *Pediatric neurology for the clinician*. Norwalk, CT: Appleton & Lange, 1992; 153–168.

A very good short chapter summarizing the topic in the previous edition of this book.

Trauner DA, Neurologic manifestations of gastrointestinal and liver disease. In: Berg B, ed. *Principles of child neurology*. New York: McGraw-Hill, 1996.

Trauner DA. Cognitive and behavioral manifestations of metabolic and endocrine diseases. In: Frank Y, ed. *Pediatric behavioral neurology*. Boca Raton FL: CRC Press, 1996.

Each of these references provides additional information on this topic.

CHAPTER 10

Traumatic Encephalopathies

H. Terry Hutchison and Paul C. Lebby

Outline

- Severe, acute traumatic brain injury
- Mild traumatic brain injury
- Deterioration following acute brain injury
- Recovery from traumatic brain injury

Each year in the United States, approximately 564,000 children between the ages of 0 and 19 years are seen in emergency departments with traumatic brain injury (TBI). About 79,300 are hospitalized and 781 die from their injuries. The death rate in 15–19-year-olds is 5.4 times greater than for 0–14-year-olds. Much of this difference is accounted for by motor vehicle accidents (Langlois et al. 2006). Most children with moderate to severe head injury suffer some disability lasting months or years.

Traumatic brain injuries range from very mild, with minor cognitive compromise for only a few minutes, to severe with profound permanent compromise to all brain functions. Mild brain injuries generally cause mostly transient disruption of functioning at the cortical level. Moderate injuries cause damage to the cortex and often deeper structures of the diencephalon and mesencephalon. Severe TBIs often cause damage to all levels of the brain, from the cortex to the subcortical structures of the diencephalon, midbrain, and brainstem (Lebby & Asbell 2007).

Severe, acute traumatic brain injury

Immediate loss of consciousness is a hallmark of severe brain injury that involves both hemispheres or the brainstem. These injuries invariably involve shearing of axons, referred to as *diffuse axonal injury* (DAI) located in the cerebral white matter or, less frequently, within the corpus callosum, brainstem, or cerebellum. Persistent deep coma, often with gradual recovery, is a consistent feature of those patients whose brains at autopsy show DAI (Jennett & Teasdale 1981).

Pathology

Several mechanisms of injury occur simultaneously in severe TBI (Marshall 2000). Direct contusion of the gray matter of the brain may occur at the site of impact or opposite the point of impact (contrecoup) as a result of the brain being thrust against the inside of the cranium. More commonly, the brain is contused on the undersurface of the temporal and frontal lobes, and on the anterior poles of the temporal lobes, whatever the site of impact. This pattern results from the brain striking against the bony prominences at the base of the cranial vault. This pattern accounts for the almost universal signs and symptoms of frontal and anterior temporal lobe dysfunction seen in TBI (Baddeley & Wilson 1988; Garth et al. 1997; Hanten et al. 2002; Levin 1982; Schwartz et al. 2003). Shearing forces are major contributors to the pathogenesis of the contusions (Adams et al. 1989). Rotational acceleration exaggerates these forces. A cascade of biochemical changes triggered by the mechanical disruption contributes to the pathogenesis of the injury.

Primary brainstem lesions in the absence of hemispheric DAI are rare. They often involve the reticular activating system, and may include hemorrhage, necrosis, and axonal injury. They often occur by centroaxial injury with downward shift of the brain, and are exaggerated by rotational forces or by flexion–extension of the cervical spine (Besenski 2002).

Contusions may be extensive without loss of consciousness, although they may become more significant subsequent to the genesis of events such as hemorrhage and swelling. Laceration of the brain occurs with penetrating trauma, and may or may not include more extensive contusion or shearing forces depending on the velocity of the projectile. For example, gunshot wounds may result in direct injuries along the trajectory of the bullet as well as more diffuse injury owing to the shock wave produced by a high-speed projectile.

Intracerebral hematoma account for a major portion of focal symptoms. Encephalomalacia (loss of brain substance due to necrosis) almost always can be detected in the area of the hematoma. Penetrating trauma produces similar focal injuries. Compared to diffuse brain injury, *focal injuries* are more frequently associated with posttraumatic epilepsy.

Diffuse axonal injury is characterized by predominantly white matter injury owing to shearing forces in brain trauma. Electron microscopy very early after fatal injury shows disruption of axon filaments. Later, axon retraction balls and myelin blebs may be seen in the light microscope. The histopathologic classification of DAI includes three grades based on the extent of brain involvement. Grade 1 involves DAI in the white matter of the cerebral hemispheres, the corpus callosum, the brainstem, and sometimes the cerebellum. Grade 2 includes focal lesions in the corpus callosum. Grade 3 includes focal lesions in the dorsolateral quadrants of the rostral brainstem.

Animal studies have suggested that injuries of increasing severity involve first the cerebral hemispheres, then the diencephalon. Only the most severe injuries involve dysfunction of the mesencephalon directly. Direct brainstem contusion, without concomitant injury to the cerebral hemispheres, is rarely seen pathologically. However, several lines of evidence suggest that transient functional changes in the reticular activating system, without gross structural changes in the brainstem, may be involved in the initial loss of consciousness in TBI.

Some measure of anoxia or ischemia accompanies most severe TBIs. Hypoventilation and hypotension, and unequal distribution of blood flow, are present to some degree with most head injuries. Multiple trauma increases the risk of anoxic (hypoxic)–ischemic injury. Anoxia affects the gray matter preferentially; the amygdala, hippocampus, and basal ganglia are quite sensitive to such injury, although the cerebral cortex and cerebellum are also prone to anoxic–ischemic injury. More severe anoxic–ischemic injury affects the gray matter globally, usually with severe sequelae (Kriel et al. 1994). Diffuse white matter destruction is typical following very severe anoxic-ischemic injuries, with often poor outcome.

Secondary brain damage occurring after the initial injury may be due to anoxic–ischemic events or transtentorial herniation. Herniation, in turn, may be due to diffuse brain swelling or expanding intracranial masses. These secondary brain injuries may be more significant than the primary injury and are discussed in more detail later in this chapter.

Pearls and Perils

Acute Diffuse Traumatic Brain Injury

- Worsening vital signs (blood pressure may be increased) owing to brain injury almost always occur after a decrease in the level of consciousness. Therefore, deteriorating mental status and level of consciousness is the most sensitive indicator of neurologic deterioration. The Glasgow Coma Scale (GCS) is widely used to monitor level of consciousness.
- People with GCS scores of less than 8 account for 30% of all head injury admissions, but more than 95% of deaths.
- Maintenance of airway, breathing, and circulation are of the highest priority for the treatment of brain-injured children.
- Some severe or fatal brain injuries occur without external evidence of trauma.
- The presence of retinal hemorrhages in an infant suggests child abuse.
- Secondary brain damage may be preventable. The major causes of secondary brain damage are anoxic–ischemic injury and transtentorial herniation.
- In an individual child, it is not possible to predict outcome reliably from the length or severity of coma.
- Severe focal brain injuries and cervical spinal cord injury may be overlooked in comatose children because of the lack of responsiveness and motor signs associated with coma.
- The tendency to ascribe warning signs of other injury to brain dysfunction should be avoided.
- Hypotension rarely occurs as a result of acute brain injury. Hypertension is the usual response. Fever over 102°F rarely is due to brain dysfunction.
- A long-bone series should be done in cases of child abuse.
- The most common conditions resulting from inadequate treatment include hypoxia, hypotension, sepsis, and seizures.
- Comatose children with traumatic brain injury usually require intubation, intravenous lines, and transfer to an appropriate intensive care unit.

Signs and symptoms

Loss of consciousness is characteristic of severe diffuse TBI. The extent and duration of the loss of consciousness correlate with outcome. However, in an individual child, it is not possible to predict outcome reliably from length of coma. A few children present an alarming but short-lived picture of deep coma with unreactive pupils, followed by rapid recovery. Others may have a brief loss of consciousness followed by deterioration and a poor outcome.

With the exception of primary brainstem injuries or medication-induced coma, the severity of loss of consciousness (or of coma) correlates with the severity of injury. Deeper levels of unconsciousness imply more severe injury. Posner and colleagues (2007) have defined stages of consciousness corresponding to dysfunction of progressively more caudal structures in the brain. Recovery from loss of consciousness follows the reverse order of caudal-rostral progression.

The diencephalic stage is the first of these stages. At this level, consciousness is altered, but not necessarily lost. Some children are agitated or combative. Others are somnolent, but may become agitated transiently with stimulation. Appropriate motor responses to noxious stimulation are present. Except for babies in the newborn period, children can usually move their limbs toward the source of noxious stimulation. Children of all ages withdraw from pain. Oculocephalic and pupillary reflexes are intact.

The second, or late diencephalic, stage is marked by loss of consciousness and flexor (decorticate) posturing. Posturing occurs in response to stimulation, discomfort, or sometimes at rest. Oculocephalic and pupillary reflexes remain intact. Hypoventilation may occur and respirations are irregular.

The third stage correlates with dysfunction of the midbrain and upper pons. Responsiveness is deeply impaired. Extensor rigidity (decerebrate posturing) is the maximum motor response. Oculocephalic and pupillary reflexes are impaired because the brainstem nuclei controlling these reflexes are located in the damaged midbrain. Respiration is usually irregular, with hyper- or hypoventilation.

The fourth stage corresponds to dysfunction of the lower pons and upper medulla. The limbs are motionless and flaccid except possibly for leg flexion to stimulation above the neck. Spontaneous breathing is present, but hypoventilation is the rule.

Periods of apnea commonly occur in more severely head-injured children. This, in part, accounts for the high incidence of anoxic damage complicating TBI. Anoxic injury carries a worse prognosis than purely traumatic injury producing the same level of coma.

Sometimes symptoms do not fit a pattern of rostral-caudal progression. For example, a child may exhibit extensor rigidity with the eyes open and with conjugate eye movements. This suggests patchy compromise, and is often due to anoxic–ischemic injury to the brainstem, or to DAI, cortical contusions, or damage to subcortical gray matter. Careful examination may reveal other focal neurologic deficits even in a comatose patient. Such deficits are more likely to occur with more severe injury, but are easily overlooked because of the motor signs and lack of responsiveness associated with coma. These signs are important because they may suggest severe focal brain injuries that are not reflected in the level of consciousness.

Diagnostic studies

Computed tomography (CT) has greatly aided the diagnosis and management of TBI. This technique allows direct visualization of the brain and is particularly sensitive to the presence of intracranial bleeding. Although diffuse axonal shear injuries are often not evident on CT, the presence of petechial hemorrhages (small spots of blood) is a good sign that DAIs are also present. All imaging modalities underestimate the true extent of DAI. Skull fractures also may be seen on CT. Other body areas, including the cervical spine, should also be examined radiographically, and a long-bone series should be obtained in cases of suspected child abuse.

Magnetic resonance imaging (MRI) is superior to CT in resolution, but the problems of gaining access to a patient in a strong magnetic field, the longer times needed to acquire each image, and image degradation due to even small movements preclude its routine use in acute head trauma. Currently, however, there is no appreciable difference between CT and MRI in the diagnosis of clinically significant acute intracranial injury and bleeding that requires neurosurgical intervention (Coombs 1999). CT offers substantial advantages because of ease of obtaining the study and lower cost. It is important to keep in mind that the CT findings after brain injury may evolve over hours to days. Therefore repeat CT should be considered in view of changing neurologic condition (Adelson et al. 2003; Giza et al. 2007). MRI is particularly useful in the diagnosis of acute spinal cord injuries. It is also quite helpful in the evaluation of the patient who has not improved as rapidly as expected.

Seizures may complicate the management of severely injured children (Adelson et al. 2003). Often, these children are sedated and given neuromuscular paralyzing agents. This may mask the physical signs of seizures, but does not ameliorate their deleterious effects. The electroencephalograph (EEG) is helpful in identifying seizures in these children. Continuous EEG, compressed EEG spectral array monitoring, and evoked potential monitoring are of great interest, but their usefulness in the management of individual patients is still being studied. EEG is of limited value for prognosis of the acutely injured child. If brain death is suspected, a formal protocol should be followed for the determination of death by neurologic criteria (Ashwal 1997). EEG, by itself, is not a reliable determinant of death in children.

Although these diagnostic studies are useful, their utility is limited by their poor sensitivity to milder injuries, or those involving diffuse axonal shearing, which often does not show well on brain scans but can present as diffuse slowing on EEG. In these cases, the functioning of the child on bedside examination can be the most accurate measure of brain injury, with more subtle cognitive limitations only presenting on more sensitive neuropsychological assessment.

Treatment

The importance of adequate management of severe traumatically brain-injured children cannot be overemphasized (Mazzola & Adelson 2002). Maintenance of airway, breathing, and circulation are the principles of basic life support and are of first priority.

The taking of a history and examination for other injuries are essential. Life-threatening injuries of the chest, abdomen, spine, and limbs are easily overlooked in children with impaired consciousness. This is particularly true of abdominal injuries, in which tenderness, guarding, and rigidity may be absent despite severe bleeding or peritonitis. Stabilization of the neck and subsequent imaging studies of the spine, the chest, and, if indicated, the limbs are the next important steps. A history is often difficult to obtain but may be important. The details of the injury, information regarding the onset of symptoms, prodromal illness or the ingestion of poisons, and the use of drugs or alcohol must be sought. Scalp injuries or other signs of trauma are important in the assessment of brain injury. But some severe or fatal TBIs occur with no external evidence of trauma. Retinal hemorrhages accompany severe deceleration or shaking injuries, but also occur with asphyxia. Marked retinal and preretinal hemorrhages in young children, without a history of severe head trauma, strongly suggest child abuse (Johnson et al. 1993; Bechtel et al. 2004).

Severe brain injury rarely occurs in infants who fall from a height less than that of an adult (Chadwick et al. 1991). DAI has been reported in young infants who suffer TBI, and in most infants who die from abuse. Gliding contusions (tears at the junction of gray and white matter) are more prominent in infants under 6 months of age compared to the callosal damage in older infants. Roughly half of abused children who die lack external evidence of trauma. It has been argued that simple shaking does not produce sufficient force to cause DAI (Alexander et al. 1990) whereas impact of the head against a cushioned surface generates forces up to 300 times gravity, more than enough to cause DAI (Prange et al. 2003). Thus the term *shaken-impact syndrome* has been coined to suggest the role of forceful impact against a cushioned surface producing severe brain injury, but without external marks (Bruce 1992). An older term, coined by C. Henry Kempe, the "battered child syndrome," is perhaps more descriptive. Additional autopsy findings include acute subdural hematoma, usually posterior and along the falx. Subarachnoid hemorrhage is frequent. Severe

Table 10.1 Glasgow Coma Scale

Response	Value	Explanation
Eye opening		
Spontaneous	4	Eyes are open without stimulation
To speech	3	Eyes open to speech or sound. This does not imply obeying commands
To pain	2	Eyes open only to noxious stimuli
None	1	Do not score if eyes are swollen shut
Motor response		
Obeys commands	6	Follows commands like "stick out your tongue"
Localizes pain	5	Limb moves toward source of pain
Withdrawal	4	Normal response with abduction of the shoulder (this is the maximum response babies can generate)
Flexion	3	"Decorticate" posturing with adduction of the shoulder, elbows flexed, legs extended, rigid
Extension	2	"Decerebrate" posturing with elbows and legs extended, rigid
No response	1	Tone is flaccid
Verbal response		
Oriented	5	Knows time, place, person
Confused	4	Conversational speech but confused
Inappropriate	3	Words but no coherent speech—often swearing and combativeness
Incomprehensible	2	No recognizable words—moans and groans or crying in babies (this is the maximum response babies can generate)
No response	1	Makes no sounds—score of 1 is given for intubated patients

The maximum score generated with maximum stimulation is added in each section. Maximum possible is 15 (10 in babies). Remember that words are a perfectly adequate form of communication and that a description of what happens in each area is more useful than numbers alone. From Teasdale G, Jennett B. The Glasgow Coma Scale. *Lancet* 1974;2:81.

brain swelling usually occurs, often with ischemic neuronal damage and tentorial herniation. The swelling may be quite asymmetric, affecting one hemisphere more than the other, even lacking any other evidence of focal injury. Occasionally, children who die of abuse show evidence of asphyxia, with traumatic damage absent or confined to the cervicomedullary junction.

Assessment of the level of consciousness should be carried out accurately. The Glasgow Coma Scale (GCS) is widely used for this purpose and is described in Table 10.1. One great advantage of this scale is that it may be applied quickly, repeatedly, and accurately by professionals with all levels of training. The scale records responses in terms of eye opening, movements, and vocalization. This information can be transmitted quickly and unambiguously to others involved in the care of the patient. It is not necessary to use, or remember, the numbers of the scale; words are sufficient and communicate more information.

According to the GCS, a child is in coma who fails to open his eyes, to speak, and to obey commands. Coma in babies is less well characterized but may be defined as existing in those babies with abnormal motor responses who fail to open their eyes or to cry. All children whose GCS is 7 or below are in coma by these definitions. Furthermore, many children with a GCS score of 8 will also be in coma. This is of great predictive importance. Patients with GCS scores of greater than 8 account for 70% of all head injury admissions but less than 5% of deaths. Those who die most often have severe injury to other organs, although brain swelling, and, less often, expanding intracranial hematomas contribute to their mortality. Conversely, those with GCS scores of less than 8 account for only 30% of admissions but more than 95% of deaths. A similar dichotomy exists for other causes of acute brain injury, including drowning and metabolic encephalopathy.

Once the initial assessment and stabilization have been accomplished, ongoing careful observation and management are essential to prevent secondary brain injury and to treat injuries not involving the brain directly. This is often best accomplished in an intensive care unit. This further management will be discussed in the following section.

Clear and compassionate communication with the families of acutely injured children is an essential part of medical management (Jurkovich et al. 2000). A wealth of printed material is available that is designed to answer some of their questions (Hutchison & Hutchison 1983; Lebby & Asbell, 2007). When discussing a child's injury with parents, it is critical that the clinician understand the inherent difficulty in predicting outcome. Two children with seemingly identical injuries, in respect to etiology, severity, symptom presentation, and the like may have vastly different outcomes, with one recovering to functional levels and the other remaining significantly compromised. Due to the numerous factors influencing recovery of function following a brain injury, prognosis becomes an educated guess. Accordingly, when discussing prognosis with parents of a brain-injured child, often it is better to be vague, giving both a best-case scenario and a worst-case scenario, but without removing hope. As time passes, prognosis become easier and more accurate, as most recovery of brain functioning takes place in the first year. Honesty is the best approach, but with the caveat that one cannot easily predict outcome of an individual patient (Table 10.2).

Mild traumatic brain injury

At the opposite end of the spectrum from those with severe TBI are those children who have suffered no loss, or no more than a brief loss of consciousness, and who have no focal neurologic deficits. These children are said to have suffered a minor or mild head injury. The term *concussion* is also used to describe these children, although to be specific, this is actually a term relating to the neurologic and cognitive effects of a mild brain injury. Confusion and amnesia are the hallmarks of concussion and can last from minutes to days or even months depending on

Table 10.2 Severe acute traumatic brain injury (TBI)

Discriminating features

- Loss of consciousness in all severe TBI, except purely focal injuries.
- Deepening coma following a rostral-caudal progression from hemispheric dysfunction through diencephalic, midbrain, pontine, and medullary stages.
- Trauma sufficient to produce the injury.

Consistent features

- Contusion of the undersurfaces of the temporal and frontal lobes, and of the anterior poles of the temporal lobes, whatever the site of impact.
- Brainstem dysfunction associated invariably with hemispheric dysfunction.
- Deepening coma associated with the progressive appearance of flexor posturing, extensor posturing, and finally flaccidity.
- Hypoventilation, or apnea, accompanying deeper levels of coma.
- Some degree of anoxic–ischemic brain injury.

Variable features

- Contusion of the brain on the side opposite the point of impact (contrecoup lesions).
- In an individual child, the depth of coma is only roughly correlated with the severity of injury. Focal traumatic injury and anoxia account for some of this variability.

Pearls and Perils

Mild Traumatic Brain Injury (MTBI)

- Children who have experienced loss of consciousness, vomiting, or seizures have been found to have a prevalence of intracranial injury ranging from 2% to 5%. A few percent of children are quite disabled by such seemingly trivial injuries, and the organic deficits may persist for months.
- Confusion and amnesia are the hallmarks of MTBI. However, normal people also sometimes endorse these symptoms.
- Rarely, children who initially appear to have suffered a mild head injury show marked deterioration.
- Most symptoms of MTBI resolve entirely within 2–3 months. Depending on the situation, up to a third of children with MTBI continue to have some complaint at 3 months. Headache is the most frequent complaint.
- When evaluating a child with mild traumatic brain injury, it is important to consider the child's condition before the injury.

the severity. The confusional episode and amnesia may occur immediately after the blow or occur several minutes later. Some children with such an injury have persistent, subtle, but disabling symptoms of brain dysfunction lasting hours to months. Rarely, children who initially appear to have suffered a mild head injury show marked deterioration owing to brain swelling or, less often, to an expanding intracranial hematoma.

Signs and symptoms

The evaluation and management of injured children may be influenced by the local practice customs, settings where children are evaluated, the type and extent of financial coverage, and the availability of technology and medical staffing.

Mild TBI (MTBI) is defined using a variety of criteria (Barth & Macciocchi 1993; Coombs 1999; Kay et al. 1993). Lebby and Asbell (2007) identified the following criteria for MTBI:

- Alteration of mental status, which may or may not include a brief loss of consciousness no longer than 20–30 minutes.
- Glasgow Coma Score of 13–15.
- No evidence of physical injury on brain imaging.
- Less than an hour of posttraumatic amnesia.
- Less than 2 days of hospitalization relating to the brain injury.

The physical signs of MTBI include nausea, vomiting, dizziness, headache, blurred vision, sleep disturbance, fatigue, and lethargy.

Cognitive and behavioral symptoms of MTBI initially include deficits in executive functioning, memory, thinking, attention and concentration, behavioral and mood lability, and lethargy. In a few patients, these symptoms persist longer than 2–3 months.

Lately, much interest has been given to the issue of sports-related brain injuries. The American Academy of Neurology (AAN) (Greenberg 1997) has developed a practice parameter for the management of concussion in sports. Brain injury may occur in any sport. At least 60,000 American high school football players suffer concussion every year (Daniel et al. 1999). Several approaches to sideline evaluation of the injured athlete have been pro-

Table 10.3 Summary of guidelines for evaluation of injured athletes

Grade 1: Mild concussion with confusion.

This includes athletes who have had no loss of consciousness observed by team mates, coaches or spectators. Confusion lasting less than 15–30 minutes is the hallmark sign of mild concussion. These players sometimes are referred to as having been "dinged." They may be able to function unnoticed during the course of the athletic contest. This is a common condition that occurs at least once in most American football games. After 20–30 minutes, if the athlete is absolutely symptom-free and has no headache dizziness or confusion, then she may return to play. Most of the published guidelines include a sideline mental status examination, so that more subtle confusion and lack of coordination is not overlooked.

Moderate concussion with amnesia.

No observed loss of consciousness occurs, or loss of consciousness occurs but is less than 5 minutes in duration. Loss of memory of the events surrounding the blow is present. The athlete may have retrograde amnesia for some of the events preceding the injury and anterograde amnesia for some events that have occurred after the injury. This anterograde or posttraumatic amnesia must not exceed 30 minutes. Evaluation of such memory deficits is included in the sideline mental status examination. The athlete is removed from play and not permitted to return the same day. If she still is symptomatic the following day, then urgent medical evaluation is indicated.

Severe concussion.

Athletes who have loss of consciousness longer than 5 minutes or posttraumatic amnesia longer than 24 hours should be transported to a medical facility equipped to handle traumatic brain injury (TBI). Care should be exercised to protect the cervical spine and the airway. Consideration should be given to prohibiting play for the remainder of the season.

Adapted from Bailes JE, Hudson V. Classification of sport-related head trauma: A spectrum of mild to severe injury. *J Athl Train* 2001;36:236–243.

posed to provide a rapid and reliable evaluation of the risks of further injury and the athlete's ability to return to play (Cantu 2001; Greenberg 1997). Bailes and Hudson (2001), Table 10.3, nicely summarize no fewer than eight guidelines for return to play, including the AAN practice parameter. Very rarely, athletes suffer diffuse cerebral swelling following a seemingly minor injury. Cantu (2001) and others argue that this syndrome is related to a "second impact" or the result of a second concussion on a brain that has not yet recovered from the first. McCrory (2001) argues that little evidence supports a "second-impact" rather than just "diffuse cerebral swelling."

Diagnostic studies

Estimates of the likelihood of intracranial injury in children with no loss of consciousness are varied. Simon et al. (2001) report that 35 (16%) of 215 children seen at a Level 1 trauma center, but with normal neurologic examination and without history of loss of consciousness, had signs of intracranial injury on CT scan. On neuropsychological assessment, most children with a MTBI recover most, if not all cognitive abilities by 6 months. Compromised executive functioning can sometimes persist for more than a year.

Treatment

In spite of the publication of the AAP/AAFP practice parameter (Coombs 1999), Blostein and Jones (2003) found no standard practice for defining, evaluating, or managing MTBI at Level 1 trauma centers. It is clear that detailed physical and mental status examinations are essential to appropriately assess a child's need for further treatment and observation. When no loss of consciousness occurs, then observation by a competent caregiver may be safe (Coombs 1999). More worrisome signs may appear, and then the child should return immediately for repeat examination, including CT of the head.

Deterioration following acute brain injury

Immediate loss of consciousness is the rule is most cases of severe TBI. There are some exceptions to this rule. About 4% of adults with severe diffuse brain injury have a lucid interval during which they are able to talk before lapsing into deeper coma. Up to a third of children may have some lucid interval (Bruce 1992). Most children with secondary deterioration have a benign course with a spontaneous and full recovery. A few children may go on to more prolonged and deeper coma, or even death.

Neurologic deterioration following acute TBI often warns of life-threatening complications. Many of these complications are treatable and most are preventable. The most sensitive indicator of neurologic deterioration is a progressive decrease in mental status and ultimately the level of consciousness. Brain damage secondary to events occurring after the initial injury is often more severe than the primary traumatic damage. Two mechanisms underlie these secondary injuries (Marshall 2000). First, there is a high risk of ongoing anoxic–ischemic injury in severely injured children. Other metabolic derangements,

Pearls and Perils

Deterioration Following Acute Brain Injury

- Fever of any source aggravates brain swelling.
- Nutrition is critically important in head-injured children. Orogastric feeding or parenteral nutrition should begin early.
- The Cushing reflex associated with intracranial hypertension involves arterial hypertension and bradycardia. Arterial hypertension and tachycardia are also often seen together, but this combination of symptoms is due to catecholamine release rather than intracranial hypertension.
- Lumbar puncture is relatively contraindicated in the presence of diffuse brain swelling because of the risk of herniation.
- Paralyzing drugs mask the clinical signs of seizures, but the brain hypoxia and acidosis caused by seizures may continue.
- Early posttraumatic seizures occur more often, and late seizures less often, in children than in adults.
- The outcome in patients with intracranial hematomas has more to do with the underlying brain injury than with the presence of blood.
- Most children with gradually deteriorating mental status and consciousness do not have an intracerebral hematoma.
- Computed tomography (CT) (or magnetic resonance imaging [MRI]) scanning is an essential part of the diagnosis of intracerebral hematoma.
- Prompt drainage (within 4 hours) may yield dramatic improvement with subdural hematoma.
- Prompt drainage of epidural hematoma may be life-saving.
- The appearance of a third-nerve palsy is often more useful as a sign of impending herniation than as an early sign of an intracranial hematoma.
- Life-threatening intracranial hematoma may follow mild head trauma.
- New bleeding may occur for a week or more after head trauma.
- Brain edema associated with a hematoma may be more dangerous to the child than the bleeding.

such as electrolyte imbalance, hypoglycemia, and hyperosmolar states, are also common. The effects of alterations involving excess excitatory amino acids, free radicals, cytokines, apoptosis, calpain proteolysis, and axonal stretch are under active investigation (Adelson et al. 2003; Giza et al., 2007; Marshall 2000). The second major process, increased volume within the cranial vault due to diffuse brain swelling and/or an expanding intracranial hemorrhage, may lead to herniation of the brain through the tentorium, compression of the brainstem as it is pushed caudally, or to global ischemic injury through lack of blood perfusion to brain tissue. Infection and fever may aggravate diffuse swelling.

Seizures occur in more than one in five patients during the first week after moderate to severe brain injury (early posttraumatic seizures) and may be associated with a worse outcome (Vespa et al. 1999). Seizures may be even more problematic in victims of child abuse (Barlow et al. 2000; Gilles & Nelson 1998).

In recovering patients, seizures may cause a temporary loss of consciousness with a period of postictal depression. Status epilepticus may lead to prolonged worsening, and to hypoxic–ischemic injury and more severe brain edema (Jennett & Teasdale 1981; Vespa et al. 1999). Seizures may be more important as a cause of secondary deterioration in children than in adults. Late-onset posttraumatic epilepsy adversely affects the outcome of brain injury (Asikainen et al. 1999; Jennett & Teasdale 1981). Prophylactic anticonvulsants may reduce the incidence of early posttraumatic seizures, but do not affect outcome (Adelson et al. 2003).

Subacute diffuse brain swelling is more likely to cause secondary neurologic deterioration in children than in adults (Bruce 1992). In young children, this swelling is sometimes so dramatic that it has been called the syndrome of "malignant brain edema." This condition is often treatable with good outcome if herniation and brain ischemia are prevented. On the other hand, diffuse brain swelling may cause death owing to increased intracranial pressure (ICP) or transtentorial herniation. The pressure in the head may become so high that it exceeds the arterial pressure generated by the heart, making it incapable of perfusing the brain. This results in diffuse ischemic death of brain tissue. Once blood flow to the whole brain, or to portions of the brain, has ceased entirely for more than a period of minutes to hours, reperfusion and recovery do not occur (see Ashwal 1997 for discussion of the relationship between absent cerebral blood flow and brain death).

Intracranial hematomas occur in a minority of children with deteriorating neurologic signs (Aoki & Masuzawa 1984; Dhellemmes et al. 1985; Oertel et al. 2002; Stein et al. 1993). Focal deficits, such as hemiparesis or eye deviation, may warn of bleeding in the head. This is especially so when these signs appear gradually after an injury. Similarly, a gradual deterioration of mental status and ultimately consciousness may warn of bleeding, causing increasing ICP or pressure on the brainstem. Seizures commonly are associated with hematomas, and at times may contribute to clinical deterioration. If the child survives the initial deterioration, the outcome often has more to do with the underlying brain injury than with the presence of intracranial blood.

Pathology

Traumatic brain injury often disrupts the blood–brain barrier. Tight junctions between the endothelial cells of brain capillaries form this barrier and prevent passage of larger molecules out of the capillaries. The capillary barrier is susceptible to traumatic damage, thus permitting a transudate to fill the extracellular spaces in the brain. This vascular compromise, termed *vasogenic edema*, involves biochemical mediators and is not due to direct mechanical disruption of the vessels. It affects the white matter preferentially. Cytotoxic edema, on the other hand, affects all parts of the brain and involves swelling of the neuronal and glial cells without an increase in extracellular fluid. Anoxic–ischemic injury, and injury resulting from most metabolic causes, is the major contributor to cytotoxic edema. Hyperemia also increases the volume of the brain and is the major contributor to brain swelling in children during the first 24 hours or so following injury (Bruce 1992). The cerebrospinal fluid may be trapped within the ventricles or it may fail to be absorbed into the venous system.

Intracranial hematomas may arise from bleeding in the epidural space, in the subdural space, in the ventricles, or within the parenchyma of the brain. The clinical and pathologic findings and the mechanisms of injury differ among these sites of bleeding.

Epidural hematomas (Dhellemmes et al. 1985) often are associated with a fracture of the skull and the subsequent rupture of an artery lying next to the skull. The middle meningeal artery often is injured, leading to a temporal fossa clot. However, epidural hematomas may also occur in the posterior fossa. The bleeding may be brisk, accounting for rapid neurologic deterioration (over minutes), especially if the main branches of the middle meningeal artery are involved. Damage to smaller branches of the artery can result in less rapid (over several hours) deterioration of neurologic functioning. The clot of blood often forms a lens-shaped mass as it dissects the dura away from the skull. This mass then deforms the underlying brain, which may herniate if the bleeding continues. Except for this mass effect and the pressure it exerts, the underlying brain may be relatively uninjured.

Subdural hematomas (Aoki & Masuzawa 1984), on the other hand, more often are associated with underlying brain injury. They appear to result from tearing of the veins bridging the subdural space. The bleeding is venous and therefore often slower and under less pressure than epidural arterial bleeding. Strong shearing forces appear to mediate the formation of subdural hematomas. These shearing forces are particularly disruptive to cortical nerve fibers. Microscopic evidence of axonal disruption (DAI) (Hoskote et al. 2002; Tomita et al. 1997) frequently is found in the brain underlying a subdural hematoma. This underlying brain may become quite edematous. As has been discussed earlier, such shearing does not occur in trivial injuries.

Intracerebral blood often is associated with focal contusions or lacerations of the brain. Contusions alone, although they may be extensive, rarely are large enough to account for loss of consciousness. However, they frequently are accompanied by focal or diffuse brain edema and axonal injury, which accentuates their clinical importance. Petechial hemorrhages, and small hemorrhages in the hemispheres, corpus callosum, or brainstem, suggest DAI. Persistent evidence on MRI of contusion or DAI suggests a worse prognosis.

Collections of blood occasionally are found within the ventricular system, usually when subdural, epidural, or intraparenchymal hematomas are also present. Intraventricular hemorrhage often is correlated with more severe injury and with a worse outcome.

Occasionally, intraparenchymal bleeding is delayed by hours or days following the injury (Givner et al. 2002; Oertel et al. 2002). The mechanism of this curious circumstance is unknown but may be related to local or diffuse clotting abnormalities induced by the trauma. Evidence of intravascular fibrinolysis is frequently obtained. The tendency to form delayed hematomas may be related to the severity of the underlying brain injury.

Signs and symptoms

Brain swelling causes clinically significant signs and symptoms by two mechanisms: increased ICP and transtentorial herniation. The GCS score reflects the sequential rostral-caudal progression of symptoms caused by downward herniation of the brain and brainstem (Jennett & Teasdale 1981), resulting in compromise of the diencephalon, midbrain, pons, and medulla. Brain swelling can also exert pressure on the third cranial nerves, resulting in dilated and unresponsive pupils bilaterally for diffuse swelling and unilaterally when swelling is restricted to one hemisphere.

Inadequate ventilation with hypoxia and hypercarbia is the most common condition aggravating brain swelling and leading to neurologic compromise following head trauma. Hypoventilation, with its attendant deleterious effects, sometimes occurs in association with acute brain injury before medical assistance arrives. Primary pulmonary complications cause hypoventilation and may include pneumonia or pneumonitis from aspiration of gastric contents, or of water as in drowning. Intubation, or sometimes tracheostomy, may be necessary to maintain an open airway. Almost every seriously head-injured child has difficulty swallowing and handling secretions, a problem that may lead to airway obstruction or pneumonia. Infection and fever from any source may aggravate brain swelling.

Rigid posturing also may interfere with ventilation and require management with neuromuscular paralysis. Pulmonary edema caused by injudicious fluid management is a preventable complication. On the other hand, hypotension owing to inadequate fluid administration may further damage the brain and other organs. Good hemodynamic balance is essential (Marshall 2000).

The hallmark of clinically significant intracranial bleeding is gradual neurologic deterioration with the appearance of focal neurologic signs, deterioration of mental status, and a decreasing level of consciousness. Seizures frequently are associated with hematomas and may suggest their presence. Although these signs and symptoms are consistent with an expanding hematoma, only a minority of children with these symptoms has clinically significant intracranial bleeding (Stein et al. 1993). More often, these symptoms are the result of progressive brain swelling. Similarly, not all intracranial hematomas are symptomatic. Furthermore, the symptoms of the various kinds of intracranial bleeding often overlap. Thus, the clinical evaluation of intracranial hematomas is not entirely reliable.

Hemiparesis is sometimes associated with intracranial hematoma. This condition may be difficult to evaluate in a comatose child, but careful observation of spontaneous movements and movements in response to stimulation may reveal the deficit. Reflex asymmetry or the *Babinski sign* is sometimes helpful. Conjugate eye deviation or a gaze preference sometimes correlates with a hemispheric hematoma. As a rule, the eyes look toward the side of the lesion. In a small percentage of cases, this sign may be "false-localizing" and the eyes look toward the side opposite the lesion (Tijssen 1994).

Unilateral pupil dilation with ptosis and failure of adduction of the affected eye suggests third-nerve palsy. When this sign appears after an injury, it suggests an expanding intracranial mass and incipient uncal herniation. In a majority of cases, the affected eye is on the same side as the mass. Unfortunately, this clinical sign occurs late and is more important as a herald of impending uncal herniation than as an early sign of intracranial bleeding.

Retinal and preretinal hemorrhages may be associated with traumatic hematomas, especially when they involve acceleration–deceleration injury. Extensive retinal and preretinal hemorrhages and retinal tears, without a history of trauma adequate to explain the injury, strongly suggest nonaccidental injury (Bechtel et al. 2004).

Hematomas may occur in the posterior fossa after mild or severe head injuries. Rapid deterioration accompanying larger hematomas may produce apnea and deep coma. Brainstem compression may be quickly fatal. Abnormalities of pupillary movement, eye movement, and motor signs often, but not always, accompany larger posterior fossa hematomas. Small hematomas in the parenchyma of the brainstem may produce devastating symptoms that belie their size. Headache, papilledema, nystagmus, and ataxia suggest less severe hematomas.

Neurologic deterioration from epidural bleeding may occur from a matter of minutes to several hours after the injury (Dhellemmes et al. 1985). Untreated, the deterioration associated with epidural hematomas may be profound. However, because the underlying brain may be relatively uninjured, prompt evacuation may result in a gratifying outcome.

Seizures complicate the hospital course of about one in five children with TBI. Roughly 50% of children with penetrating injury or intracranial hematoma have seizures (Jennett & Teasdale 1981; Vespa et al. 1999). In about 60% of cases, seizures occur within the first 24 hours after injury. Seizures further aggravate the effects of brain injury by increasing brain metabolism and producing acidosis. Hypoxia, systemic acidosis, increased ICP, and fever may accompany the muscle contractions of seizures. These movements may worsen other injuries. Furthermore, seizures may not be detected clinically in patients being treated with paralytic agents, and may not be prevented by prophylactic administration of phenytoin. Recently, continuous EEG recording has been shown to be useful for detection of seizures under these conditions (Vespa et al. 1999). Paralyzing the child does not reverse the central effects of seizures. Local brain tissue hypoxia and acidosis may continue to damage the brain even though paralyzing drugs mask the clinical signs of seizures.

Late posttraumatic epilepsy (seizures occurring more than 1 week after the injury) is more likely to occur in the presence of penetrating brain injury or hematoma, or if early seizures have occurred. Early posttraumatic seizures occur more often, and late seizures less often, in children than in adults (Adelson et al. 2003; Asikainen et al. 1999; Jennett & Teasdale 1981).

Electrolyte abnormalities are common following severe head trauma. Inattention to electrolyte balance may add to the problems caused by diabetes insipidus or inappropriate antidiuretic hormone secretion. These latter abnormalities may occur at different times in the same patient. Poor temperature regulation accompanies severe brain injury. However, as already noted, hypothermia rather than fever is the rule.

A hypermetabolic state occurs in many children with traumatic or metabolic brain injury. Increased catecholamine secretion into the peripheral circulation, triggered by the injured brain, causes arterial hypertension and tachycardia. Direct cardiac injury and cerebral perfusion disturbances may result when this condition is severe. Although the arterial blood pressure is high, the ICP also may be high and the cerebral blood flow compromised. Excessive catecholamine release is to be distinguished from the Cushing reflex that comprises *arterial hypertension and bradycardia*, in response to increased ICP. The hypermetabolic state caused by excess catecholamine secretion may be treated with β-adrenergic blockade. As the arterial blood pressure is reduced, the ICP often follows, without further compromise of the cerebral perfusion pressure (for a more complete discussion, see Marshall 2000).

Nutrition is compromised by the need for fluid restriction and the relative inability to provide oral feedings. Hypermetabolism complicates this nutritional deficiency. Some children lose 20% of their body weight in the first 2 weeks in the hospital. This condition can be alleviated partly by early institution of nasogastric feedings or parenteral hyperalimentation.

Penetrating head trauma is a special problem because of the risks of infection and the need for surgical intervention to debride the wound. If the penetration is

Consider Consultation When...

- A decreasing level of consciousness is detected by history, on examination, or on the Glasgow Coma Scale.
- Focal neurologic signs or hemiparesis is noted on neurologic examination.
- Pupillary and eye movement abnormalities are detected. A gradually developing third-nerve palsy is most worrisome.
- A child has any prolonged seizures (more than about 1 minute) or if seizures occur after the first 24 hours, especially after the first week.
- Fever or other symptoms suggest a complicating systemic illness.
- A persistent hypermetabolic state is present, with arterial hypertension and tachycardia. Even more worrisome is arterial hypertension and bradycardia.
- Electrolyte abnormalities suggest diabetes insipidus or the syndrome of inappropriate antidiuretic hormone secretion.
- Imaging studies suggest collections of free blood in the epidural space, in the subdural space, in the ventricles, or within the brain parenchyma.
- Imaging studies present a picture of small ventricles and lucent brain with blurring of the gray-white borders.
- Radiographs show a fracture of the skull that might be associated with rupture of an artery lying near the skull.

by a low-velocity object, the signs and symptoms are those of purely focal brain injury, with any swelling being restricted to the damaged tissue. Unless there is involvement of both hemispheres, or of the brainstem, there is no, or only brief, loss of consciousness, with the sequelae being related to the injured portion of the brain.

Diagnostic studies

CT provides a rapid, reliable, and noninvasive means of diagnosing and following intracranial bleeding (Adelson et al. 2003; Stein et al. 1993; Tomita et al. 1997). MRI may detect some hematomas not seen on CT. However, the small increase in yield rarely justifies the extra time required and risk of placing an acutely ill patient in a device with which monitoring is difficult and all magnetic materials must be removed from the room.

CT is the major diagnostic tool for the evaluation of brain swelling (Givner et al. 2002; Oertel et al. 2002), but it is limited because it cannot measure ICP. Thus, clinically significant swelling may accompany a normal CT, and marked swelling on CT may accompany normal ICP. CT in acute head injury often shows small ventricles and reduced size of the perimesencephalic cistern, which is immediately posterior to the mesencephalic structures of the superior and inferior colliculi (quadrigeminal plate). The parenchyma may be lucent with blurring of the border between the gray matter and the white matter appearing as reduced gray–white differentiation. In children, these changes may be difficult to distinguish from normal. Acute or incipient herniation of the brainstem may be suspected if obliteration of the perimesencephalic cistern is present. The lateral recesses of this cistern separate the midbrain from the unci of the temporal lobes. Although CT is most often used, MRI also is sometimes useful in detecting early edema.

Treatment

Intubation and hyperventilation are the most rapid and effective ways of treating progressive brain and brainstem compromise caused by increased ICP. This procedure is not without risk because hyperventilation sometimes exacerbates cerebral ischemia (van den Brink et al. 2000). Injudicious use of hyperventilation will not consistently cause a reduction of ICP and may cause loss of autoregulation and reduced cerebral blood flow (see Marshall 2000 for a more complete discussion). Hypothermia has also been used to control brain swelling and subsequent injury.

For severe brain injury, it is standard practice to paralyze the patient to prevent "fighting" the ventilator and to reduce intrathoracic pressure that is transmitted to the brain. Hyperosmolar agents, such as mannitol or sodium, may be helpful to reduce brain water. However, early in the course, brain swelling may result from hyperemia with little increase in brain water. Therefore these agents may worsen the problem initially by increasing blood volume and also may contribute to hyperosmolar damage and electrolyte imbalance. Their use should be limited to an intensive care unit, and to medical and nursing personnel who are familiar with their effects (Marshall 2000; van den Brink et al. 2000).

Monitoring of ICP is a standard of care in the management of brain swelling (Adelson et al. 2004; Giza et al. 2007; Marshall 2000). Ventricular catheterization is the most invasive of the monitoring procedures. Furthermore, the catheter cannot always successfully be placed because of small ventricular size owing to brain swelling. On the other hand, ventricular catheterization allows for the most direct measurement of ICP and permits some reduction of intracranial hypertension by venting cerebrospinal fluid. A fiberoptic pressure monitor in the subarachnoid space threaded through a screw in the skull provides reliable readings and is less invasive than the ventricular catheter.

Little evidence suggests that intracranial hypertension per se causes secondary brain injury. Rather, the increased pressure is transmitted to the intracranial vascular tree and may compromise cerebral blood flow. The maintenance of brain cellular oxygenation is of fundamental importance, and is the subject of current research. Brain tissue hypoxia occurs frequently during the treatment of severely brain-injured patients and is significantly related to poor outcome (Marshall 2000; van den Brink et al. 2000).

Prompt evacuation of larger extra-axial hematomas is often lifesaving. In spite of the underlying brain injury associated with subdural hematomas, evacuation within 4 hours greatly improves survival. With large epidural hematomas, survival is dramatically better with prompt drainage. Thus, the early diagnosis of intracranial hematomas is essential. CT scans should be obtained initially in all children with severe TBIs, and should be done whenever evidence of neurologic deterioration appears (Givner et al. 2002; Oertel et al. 2002; Stein et al. 1993).

Smaller clots that do not produce clinically significant mass effects need not be evacuated acutely. Debridement of contused and lacerated brain may be necessary because of increasing ICP and local mass effect. Delayed intraparenchymal hematomas usually do not require drainage. Furthermore, the location of these hematomas within the brain parenchyma and the coagulopathy associated with them makes surgical removal more difficult.

The brain edema associated especially with subdural and intracerebral hematomas may pose important therapeutic problems. Craniectomy and removal of portions of the damaged brain may be of benefit in the treatment of expanding masses aggravated by focal brain edema. The amelioration of the effects of brain edema by bilateral craniectomy, barbiturate coma, glucocorticoids, and hypothermia are subjects of ongoing study (Marshall 2000; van den Brink et al. 2000).

Children who are comatose (GCS of 8 or less) or whose deteriorating level of consciousness suggests they may become comatose should be treated in an appropriate intensive care unit. The presence of other injuries or systemic illness increases the risk of deterioration and complicates the management of brain injury.

The most important feature of an appropriate intensive care unit is a multidisciplinary team that is familiar and comfortable with the management of acutely brain-injured children. Round-the-clock availability of neurosurgical care committed to the management of TBI is also important. CT capability must be immediately available.

Transport to an appropriate facility should involve initial stabilization, which usually includes intubation. Many units now have transport teams to ensure against secondary brain damage in transit. Some features of deterioration following TBI are shown in Table 10.4.

Table 10.4 Deterioration following acute brain injury

Discriminating features

- Subacute decreasing level of consciousness is the most sensitive indicator of progressive brain and brainstem compromise.
- Increased brain volume is due to greater quantities of extracellular fluid (vasogenic edema), intracellular fluid (cytotoxic edema), or blood (hyperemia).
- Collections of free blood in the epidural space, in the subdural space, in the ventricles, or within the brain parenchyma.

Consistent features

- Increased intracranial pressure.
- Computed tomography (CT) picture of small ventricles and lucent brain with blurring of the gray-white borders.
- Focal neurologic signs.
- Hemiparesis with a supratentorial hematoma.
- Pupillary and eye movement abnormalities and motor signs suggest a posterior fossa hematoma.
- Seizures.
- Gradually developing third-nerve palsy suggests an intracerebral hematoma and may herald impending uncal herniation.

Variable features

- Obliteration of the perimesencephalic cisterns may be seen in incipient or actual herniation.
- Seizures worsen brain swelling, but are more likely to occur if some focal injury to the brain is present.
- Electrolyte abnormalities may be due to diabetes insipidus or to the syndrome of inappropriate antidiuretic hormone secretion.
- A hypermetabolic state with arterial hypertension and tachycardia.
- Epidural hematomas often are associated with fracture of the skull and rupture of an artery lying near the skull.
- Subdural hematomas often are associated with marked underlying brain injury owing to the shearing forces involved in the formation of the hematoma.
- Intracerebral bleeding often complicates focal contusion and lacerations and may be delayed by hours or days following the injury.
- Retinal and preretinal hemorrhages may accompany intracerebral hematomas especially those involving acceleration/deceleration injuries.
- Retinal and preretinal hemorrhages suggest nonaccidental trauma.

Recovery from traumatic brain injury

Recovery from a TBI in childhood is variable. Those children with the worst injuries die or remain in a coma or persistent minimally conscious or vegetative state. Surviving children show transient or permanent neurologic deficits. Less obvious lasting deficits often become evident as difficulties in school or as findings on more detailed neuropsychological evaluation. The rate and extent of recovery from TBI follows a characteristic course when one looks at many patients (Catroppa & Anderson 2002; Ewing-Cobbs et al. 2003; Jaffe et al. 1995; Levin 1982; Levin et al. 1997). No two children have identical deficits involving motor, cognition, or behavioral functioning. The pattern of recovery similarly is variable. Yet the similarities in the patterns of impairment and recovery tend to outweigh the individual differences. Early in the course, it is hardly possible to reliably predict the outcome of any particular patient. For those children who have not recovered fully within the first year after injury, the rate of recovery slows. Those children with greater severity of injury improve less over the 2 years following the injury than do children with less severe injuries (Jaffe et al. 1995). It is clear, however, that in a population of brain-injured children, significant recovery continues for several years following a TBI (Ewing-Cobbs et al. 2003; Jaffe et al. 1995; Johnson et al. 2003). Traumatic brain injury differs from severe anoxic–ischemic injury (Kriel et al. 1994) in that good recovery from prolonged coma is the rule and not the exception. More than half of children who have been in coma for 3 months eventually walk, talk, and go to school (Brink et al. 1980). Among former students who had suffered TBI, 62% had returned to school by 6 months after injury (Ruff et al. 1993). Recovery from coma lasting longer than 3–6 months is unusual.

At first glance, the prognosis for recovery from TBI in children might seem better than that for adults. This is true for older children and adolescents. In contrast, the immature brains of young children are particularly vulnerable to diffuse damage, and they are more likely to show residual neuropsychological deficits. Because injury takes place during sensitive developmental periods, some deficits may not present until several years later in a child's life, when the functions were expected to mature

Pearls and Perils

Recovery from Traumatic Brain Injury (TBI)

- A few children will have an alarming but transient picture of deep coma with unreactive pupils, but with rapid and complete recovery.
- An extended period of mutism lasting a few days to several months, followed by complete resolution, occurs in about 3% of adult brain-injured patients. The frequency of occurrence in brain-injured children is unknown, but certainly higher than in adults.
- Gaze palsies and visual tracking problems usually are transient, but may persist for more than 6 months in a third of brain-injured patients.
- The brains of young children appear to be more vulnerable to lasting damage than do those of older children and adolescents.
- It is not possible to predict reliably, for most individual children, the rate and extent of recovery.
- Children with severe cognitive disability owing to TBI do not necessarily score in the abnormal range on standardized intelligence tests.
- The normal emergence of continuing developmental skills may limit the recognition of residual deficits of TBI until the deficient skill would be expected to appear.

naturally. Later deficits frequently include difficulties with executive functions such as foresight, hindsight, planning, organization, and the conceptualization of abstract concepts (Ewing-Cobbs et al. 2003; Hanten et al. 2002; Johnson et al. 2003; Lebby & Asbell 2007; Levin et al. 2002).

Injuries in primary cortical areas that produce specific deficits such as visual field scotomas or anopias, motor paralysis, and tactile deficits typically show rapid and mostly compete recovery. However, recovery from problems persisting for more than a few months is likely to be incomplete.

Lesions in the posterior cortical association areas of the parietal lobe involve more complex functions such as constructional abilities, visual–motor coordination, higher order language and visual processing, and one's ability to allocate attention appropriately. These problems show more gradual improvement that continues beyond the first year after injury (Ewing-Cobbs et al. 2003; Lebby & Asbell 2007).

Patterns of behavior involving the prefrontal and anterior temporal cortical areas or those that are symptomatic of more diffuse injury portend prolonged impairment (Schwartz et al. 2003). Even if a brain-injured child returns to fully independent and functional living, subtle deficits that reflect the child's injury may be apparent to the experienced eye. Problems in memory, organization, speed of thinking, attention and concentration, affective control and irritability, motivation, judgment, and socialization are the hallmarks of TBI (Hutchison 1992).

Signs and symptoms

The relationships of brain injury to observed deficits have been discussed in great detail (Heilman & Valenstein 2003; Kolb & Wilshaw 1996; Lebby & Asbell 2007; Levin 1982; Lezak 1995). Receptive deficits following TBI may include signs and symptoms related to primary cortical sensory areas. Visual field deficits are common after severe hemispheric injury. Tactile sensory deficits are subserved by redundant systems, and therefore pain and touch are rarely lost completely. The residual sensory deficits are easily overlooked in children. Discriminatory touch including stereognosis is more susceptible to injury, but may be quite difficult to test in children. The vestibular system is easily damaged, leading to dizziness and eye movement problems (Jennett & Teasdale 1981). Hearing loss or loss of smell can also result from a brain injury.

More complex receptive deficits involving the perception of language from auditory or visual material suggest damage to the posterior association cortex. Deficits in visual–spatial perception may be more subtle, but still quite debilitating. Constructional deficits and poor drawing or writing skills suggest disruption of the integration of sensory information with motor functions.

Spastic paralysis results from injury anywhere along the length of the pyramidal tracts. More subtle limitations involving motor efficiency suggest disruption of secondary and tertiary motor cortices. Abnormalities of tone and posture, inaccuracy and poor coordination of movements, and movement disorders such as tremor, ataxia, choreoathetosis, dystonia, and ballism, suggest injury to the extrapyramidal motor system. Slow, irregular, robot-like movements and gait are characteristic of children with severe brain injury and may persist in spite of otherwise excellent functional recovery. These deficits interfere with normal psychosocial development and preclude recreational activities requiring grace of movement. It is important to remember that extrapyramidal abnormalities may be quite delayed in their manifestation, a year or more after injury (Krauss & Jankovic 2002).

Focal motor and sensory signs may reflect circumscribed injury anywhere in the brain or brainstem. The localization of these lesions benefits from the rich heritage of the study of vascular lesions in neurology. Brainstem signs, particularly gaze palsies and visual tracking problems owing to frontal lobe dysfunction, usually are transient but may persist for more than 6 months in a third of brain-injured patients (Jennett & Teasdale 1981). Unilateral frontal lobe damage close to the eye-gaze center can result in a period of eye deviation to one side or the other, making it important to interact with the child from the side that allows for easier visual contact. Rarely, transient blindness is present initially, with complete resolution over time.

Problems in the planning and execution of complex coordinated movements suggest more anterior cortical injury. Some motor aphasic symptoms are in this category. Deficits involving the understanding and use of complex linguistic material, such as sarcasm, innuendo, and humor is common after a brain injury. Such deficits undoubtedly account for peculiarities of language and limitations involving verbal exchanges that are recurrent attributes of brain-injured children.

More global brain injuries affect attention, concentration, and the ability to track complex concepts and reasoning. Executive functioning deficits result in slow and inefficient cognitive processing and deficient ability to multitask, track, or efficiently switch between multiple components of a task. Children with executive dysfunction may have difficulty processing complex material or functioning in a classroom when required to simultaneously listen to the teacher, take notes, and keep track of textbook material. School and social functioning are impaired even when primary cognitive skills such as reading and computation are intact. Impulsivity, distractibility, and motor hyperactivity are frequent attributes of brain-injured children, as are states of apathy and inactivity. These deficits are particularly difficult to rehabilitate, in part because they lead to poor participation in a therapy regimen. Children who are fastidious in other ways may become erratic and careless in dress and hygiene. Children with impaired ability to start and stop activities, or to shift activities, may appear rigid and apparently uncooperative. Explosive behavior, catastrophic anxiety, and intractable indifference are exasperating to parents, teachers, and peers. These problems may hamper goal-directed behavior in children who otherwise have shown excellent cognitive recovery.

The opportunity for the development of secondary emotional and behavioral problems is obvious. Preinjury family and child functioning play major roles in outcome (Rivara et al. 1994; Schwartz et al. 2003; Yeates et al. 1997). The family's ability to cope with the child's injury also is important, and family environment has been shown to influence postinjury progress (Rivara et al. 1994; Taylor et al. 2002). Unfortunately, the preconceptions of parents and siblings, as well as of teachers and peers (Hawley et al. 2004), may have forceful negative impact on the brain-injured child. There is no substitute for an appropriately supportive and structured home and school environment in the rehabilitation of the child with TBI.

Memory is a highly complex brain function that depends on several structures and processes. Thus, it is not surprising that memory difficulties are virtually universal in TBI (Catroppa & Anderson 2002; Levin et al. 2002). Memory consolidation, subserved by the limbic system and thalamus, is often impaired after TBI because the hippocampus, in particular, is exquisitely susceptible to anoxia and also to direct mechanical contusion of the temporal poles (Catroppa & Anderson 2002; Levin 1982).

Immediate memory recovers quickly in patients who regain consciousness. Thus, they can grasp and remember the events around them for some seconds. However, recovery of the next process, short-term memory, is more likely to be prolonged. Conscious children with short-term memory deficits are unable to lay down any lasting new memories and may remain confused and disoriented even though they can recognize faces, speak, and converse on a perfunctory level. After further recovery, children have little or no memory of this period of dis-

Consider Consultation When...

- A child remains in coma for more than a day or so following brain injury, and when a team approach to rehabilitation seems essential because several overlapping areas of expertise are needed.
- It is anticipated that a structured and supportive environment is essential for a child (and family) with impaired executive functions and whose performance deteriorates with extraneous stimulation.
- Memory is lost of the events of the accident and immediately afterward.
- Motor deficits persist including spasticity, disorders of tone and posture, movement disorders, ataxia, and deficits in the planning and execution of complex coordinated movements.
- Language problems persist including comprehension, visual perceptual, naming, expressive difficulties, and nonaphasic speech disturbances.
- Hearing loss is present.
- A child demonstrates the hallmarks of traumatic brain injury that include impairments in:
  - Memory
  - Organization
  - Speed of thinking
  - Attention and concentration
  - Affective control and irritability
  - Motivation
  - Judgment
  - Socialization
- School performance remains below that expected from standardized testing given in a one-on-one setting.
- During the normal emergence of developmental skills, deficiencies become apparent that were not previously noted

orientation following their injury, a phenomenon called *posttraumatic amnesia*. In addition to the extent of recovery, the length of posttraumatic amnesia is commonly used as a measure of the severity of injury (Levin 1982). The hippocampus plays an important role in short-term memory. It is quite sensitive to anoxia and also may be injured directly by contusion of the temporal poles.

Confabulations are more prominent in children with posttraumatic amnesia who also have a frontally based *dysexecutive syndrome* (Baddeley & Wilson 1988; Fischer et al. 1995), or diencephalic injury (Lebby & Asbell 2007).

Retrograde amnesia (loss of memory for events preceding the trauma) commonly occurs with any degree of TBI. An injury sufficient to produce posttraumatic amnesia also disrupts those memories that, at the time of the accident, had not yet been consolidated into long-term memory. This period rarely exceeds 30 minutes before the injury. In another phenomenon, called *shrinking retrograde amnesia*, memories of events several months before the accident are lost, but gradually return. Their loss reflects abnormalities in memory retrieval. Older and often-rehearsed memories are the most easily retrieved, but these represent only a small part of the stored experiences of a normal child (Levin 1982).

Deficits in speech and language are present in about a third of brain-injured adults and children at 6 months post injury (Levin 1982). Naming errors and word-finding difficulties routinely persist in brain-injured children. These deficits contribute to the use of inappropriate words, paraphasias (production of unintended syllables, words, or phrases), verbal approximations, and circumlocution, in which the child uses inefficient means to communicate verbally. Dysnomia following brain injury is related to disruption of the language association areas of the posterior temporal cortex (Kolb & Wilshaw 1996). Aphasias are complex and involve a spectrum of deficits from subtle word-finding problems and agrammatism (disrupted sentence structure), to more severe deficits involving impaired comprehension and expression of the most basic language functions. In a minority of children, these problems may continue to improve for years after a severe head injury (Chapman et al. 2001). Nonaphasic speech disturbances—including dysarthria, mutism, echolalia, palilalia, stuttering, difficulty with intonation and prosody, and nonaphasic misnaming—also occur in brain-injured children. Mutism lasting a few days to several months, followed by complete resolution, occurs in about 3% of adult brain-injured patients. The frequency of occurrence in brain-injured children is unknown, but certainly higher than in adults (Dayer et al. 1998; Levin 1982). The prognosis for recovery of speech and language generally is better in children than in adults.

Younger children with focal left-brain injuries may show excellent recovery of language with time. This is apparently because bihemispheric language potential is present, particularly in younger children. This recovery of language is in contrast to the greater susceptibility of the immature brain to the effects of diffuse injury.

Diagnostic studies

Neuropsychological testing is useful for assessing the functional consequences of brain injury (Lebby & Asbell 2007; Levin 1982; Lezak 1995). Prediction of the course of recovery from brain injury is hampered by the relative paucity of studies in children and by the variability from case to case. Furthermore, deficits from brain injury are superimposed on normally emerging and continuing developmental skills. Many skills that one would like to measure have not yet appeared in younger children (Ewing-Cobbs et al. 2003). Thus different test instruments, each with age-adjusted norms, must be used. However, care should be taken when using normative values with a heterogeneous TBI population, as they can be misleading (Jaffe et al. 1993). Even so, discovery of motor, cognitive, and behavior deficits resulting from brain injury may not be possible for years after the injury (Blosser & DePompei 1994). By then, the myriad factors influencing normal development and adjustment to disability confound the test results. Normal school performance and normal performance on intellectual tests does not guarantee a good long-term outcome (Chapman et al. 2001; Hawley et al. 2004; Koskiniemi et al. 1995). With continuing difficulties involving social functioning and executive skills (Slomine et al. 2002), navigating a post school environment can be a daunting task for a survivor of childhood TBI.

Detailed assessment of a head-injured child is a complex process that includes formal and informal evaluation and also the integration of the child's premorbid functioning and personal-social history. Because of the child's limitations in arousal and attention, and in motor and language skills, informal assessment of a child's abilities during therapy sessions, play activities, and other less structured times can be very helpful in evaluating functioning. The major purpose of an assessment is to guide rational therapy in an inpatient or outpatient rehabilitation setting, or in school (Hawley et al. 2004). No simple test battery reliably identifies all the areas of residual injury. Many head-injured children are severely debilitated by their injuries and yet score within the normal range of standardized intellectual tests. This paradox is particularly true in ordinary school evaluations, when only simple reading, word recognition, and computational skills are tested (Chapman et al. 2001; Hawley et al. 2004; Jaffe et al. 1993). When the test situation is highly structured within a one-on-one setting, and with minimal if any distractions, subtle but disabling difficulties experienced by these children may go unnoticed. The caution that, "absence of evidence is not evidence of absence" should be well considered when assessing TBI children. Thus the organic deficits preventing the child's success in the classroom are ascribed to "behavioral problems," and the child may be denied appropriate special education services. Recently, tests of selective learning, and of working memory and prospective memory, show promise of sensitivity to some of the higher cognitive functions that so limit the participation of brain-injured children in school and community (Hanten et al. 2002; Levin et al. 2002). Tests of executive functioning have also shown promise in clarifying subtle deficits that significantly impact school functioning, but do not show up on basic tests of cognition. Interestingly, although skills involved with executive functioning are not generally considered important in younger children, a younger age at injury has been shown to place children at greater risk of impairment on measures of executive functioning (Garth et al. 1997; Levin et al. 1997; Slomine et al. 2002). In contrast, because many children perform inconsistently in the classroom due to variations in attention, fatigue, and executive functioning, any poor performance may be attributed to behavior or effort, and not due to brain-related limitations (Hawley et al. 2004). Furthermore, the standard categories of special education—"learning disabled," "emotionally disabled," "mildly mentally retarded," and so on—do not address the patterns of deficits seen in traumatically brain-injured children, in whom variability of functioning is the rule, not the exception. Thus, knowledge of the special patterns of recovery, special needs and problems, and use of more sophisticated neuropsychological testing are of great importance to the brain-injured child, especially at the time of return to school (Hawley et al. 2004).

In the acute period following a TBI, the child's abilities may change daily. Thus, the team involved in his treatment is advised to assess the child's deficits regularly. The team may be directed by a child neurologist, neuropsychologist, or pediatrician and includes therapists from several disciplines. Individuals involved in assessments should be trained and skilled in working with hard-to-test children, as formal testing techniques may not be applicable to a particular patient due to motor and language processing limitations, or by the executive dysfunctions described earlier. The Lebby-Asbell Neurocognitive Status Examination for Children (LANSE-C) and the Lebby-Asbell Neurocognitive Status Examination for Adolescents (LANSE-A) are useful in efficiently assessing multiple areas of neurologic and cognitive functioning in acutely brain injured patients who cannot tolerate longer examination.

Measures of functional ability, such as the FRESNO (Roberts et al. 1999), are sensitive to daily or weekly changes in performance in the areas of mobility, self-care, language, cognition, and socialization. The FRESNO has proven to be useful in the acute rehabilitation setting and after discharge.

Rehabilitation

The more severely brain-injured child requires acute inpatient rehabilitation, which should begin even while the child is in coma. A team approach to rehabilitation is essential because several overlapping areas of expertise are needed to address a child with multiple problems (Esselman & Dillman-Long 2002). Furthermore, a structured and supportive environment is essential for children with impaired executive functions and whose performance deteriorates with extraneous stimulation. The family is an essential part of the rehabilitation team, and appropriate social and family interactions are fostered by the team approach (Esselman & Dillman-Long 2002). The rehabilitation nurse typically spends the most time with the child and acts as liaison between the team and the family. The speech and language pathologist assesses and treats language problems and deficits in cognitive functioning, including learning style as it relates to academic skills. The occupational therapist is concerned with the functional use of limbs, motor planning, and visual–spatial or perceptual skills related to activities of daily living. A feeding team is assembled for children who are not able to take adequate nutrition by mouth. The physical therapist is concerned with tone and posture, seating and positioning, and ambulation. The psychologist addresses problems in the control of emotions, behavior, and family issues. Formal neuropsychological testing is done when appropriate to assist other team members in understanding neurocognitive limitations and how they impact therapy. In addition, the neuropsychologist is important in educating the family about the functional effects of the brain injury, and how that may influence transition to home or to an educational environment. The child life specialist acts as an advocate for the child as a whole person, integrating play and recreation into the child's therapeutic regimen. Patient education and play activities are designed to reduce stress and to foster the integration of the child with family and community. The schoolteacher involves the child in educational activities and begins the reintegration of the child into an appropriate school upon discharge. The social worker is involved in maintaining and supporting the family, and in coordinating community resources for the child's benefit. The discharge planner or case manager provides a smooth and timely transition to home and community, and secures needed equipment and funding to continue the child's rehabilitation outside the hospital.

Some children benefit from a post acute rehabilitation setting, which may involve residential care. These are children who have recovered some measure of independent mobility and cognition and need additional intensive help in achieving successful reintegration in home and community.

Less severely injured children do not require a full team approach to rehabilitation. But an awareness of the problems unique to traumatic brain-injured children is essential to assess and treat them adequately.

School is the major occupational activity of children beyond 5 or 6 years of age. Reintegration into an appropriate school situation is essential for children with injuries of all degrees. When children require assistance in school, the federal law encompassed by the Individuals with Disabilities Education Act (IDEA) mandates that schools provide special education services and/or accommodations to students who qualify because of special needs that result from a brain injury. Importantly, children with brain injury typically require different services than do children with impairments that are developmental in origin. One major difference is that, characteristically, brain injury leads to inconsistencies in cognitive functioning, with some retained old learning. Thus, it is difficult to understand why a child can do well in some areas and yet have so much difficulty with other skills (Chapman et al. 2001; Hawley et al. 2004). Too often this results in the attribution of "not trying" or "lazy" to the child. Brain-injured children with limitations involving attention and problem-solving strategies have difficulty utilizing trial-and-error techniques to solve problems. Therefore, mentoring and small-group tutoring is much more helpful as the child learns by repeated successes, and techniques of problem-solving and organization of work can be taught directly. Children who have poor understanding or awareness of cognitive problems, and who fail to understand the need for external assistance, should be monitored and not just asked whether they need assistance (Hawley et al. 2004).

Brain-injured children with reduced cognitive processing speed and deficits in sustained attention have difficulty completing assignments in the expected time. Motor limitations that impact writing and drawing skills exacerbate these cognitive problems. Provision of additional time for assignments and tests becomes necessary to facilitate functioning for these children within a school environment.

Within school and at home, it is important to accentuate the positive in a child with brain injury. Decreased confidence and self-esteem follows from overemphasis on the remediation of deficits, especially within an educational environment. It also is important for family members, friends, and teachers to normalize their interactions with the child and not treat the child differently. Treating the child as disabled or damaged becomes a self-fulfilling prophecy (Hawley et al. 2004; Yeates et al. 1997).

The protection and safety of the brain-injured child require caution upon re-entering the community following discharge from the hospital. The child's intellectual ability is likely to be overestimated because physical impairments typically improve faster than cognitive impairments. Thus, following recovery from physical injuries, the child may appear to be functioning normally in spite of subtle deficits in thinking ability. One must anticipate that the brain-injured child will not exercise the same degree of concern for the safety of himself or others as would be expected in another child of the same age. In addition, the child may be impulsive owing to reduced ability to self-monitor and regulate his actions. Impaired or diminished judgment may result in the child inadvertently doing things that are dangerous, or the child failing to recognize when he is in a dangerous situation. This imposes upon those who care for a child with a TBI the duty to exercise a high degree of vigilance and caution, and to provide more stringent structure and boundaries for safety.

Annotated bibliography

Adams JH, Doyle D, Ford I, et al. Diffuse axonal injury in head injury: Definition, diagnosis and grading. *Histopathology* 1989;15:49–59.
Defines the pathological entity of DAI.

Adelson PD, Bratton SL, Carney NA, et al. Guidelines for the acute medical management of severe traumatic brain injury in infants, children, and adolescents. *Pediatr Crit Care Med* 2003;4;S1–S75.
Extensive evidence-based review of current standards for the treatment of TBI in children.

Alexander R, Sato Y, Smith W, Bennett T. Incidence of impact trauma with cranial injuries ascribed to shaking. *Am J Dis Child* 1990;144:724–726.
Argues that shaking, rather than impact, is the major cause of acute brain injury in abused children.

Aoki N, Masuzawa H. Infantile acute subdural hematoma: Clinical analysis of 26 cases. *J Neurosurg* 1984;61:273–280.
Discusses infantile subdural hematomas associated with minor trauma. Mechanism of injury is discussed with particular reference to the battered child syndrome.

Ashwal S. Brain death in the newborn. *Clin Perinatol* 1997;24:859–882.
Includes thorough discussion of the relationship of absent blood flow to brain death particularly in the newborn, but also in older children.

Asikainen I, Kaste M, Sarna S, et al. Early and late post-traumatic seizures in traumatic brain injury rehabilitation patients: Brain injury factors causing late seizures and influence of seizures on long-term outcome. *Epilepsia* 1999;40:584–589.
Young children are more prone to early seizures, and adolescents and adults, to late seizures. Late-onset posttraumatic epilepsy adversely affects the outcome of brain injury.

Baddeley A, Wilson B. Frontal amnesia and the dysexecutive syndrome. *Brain Cogn* 1988;7:212–230.
Study of an amnestic patient with bilateral frontal damage and dysexecutive syndrome, who presented with poor autobiographical memory and substantial confabulations. Sug-

gests that the deficits result from of a classic amnestic syndrome with additional problems associated with a frontal dysexecutive syndrome.

Bailes JE, Hudson V. Classification of sport-related head trauma: A spectrum of mild to severe injury. *J Athl Train* 2001;36:236–243.
Discusses the pathophysiology of concussion, including diffuse brain injury and intracranial hemorrhages. Summarizes the various classifications proposed for management of sport-related concussions.

Barlow KM, Spowart JJ, Minns RA. Early posttraumatic seizures in non-accidental head injury: relation to outcome. *Dev Med Child Neurol* 2000;42:591–594.
Out of 44 children with TBI owing to nonaccidental trauma, 32 developed early posttraumatic seizures. The outcome in those with seizures was significantly worse than those without.

Barth JT, Macciocchi SN, eds. Mild traumatic brain injury. *J Head Trauma Rehabil* 1993;8:1–87.
This issue is devoted to mild TBI, including definition, mechanisms, and treatment.

Bechtel K, Stoessel K, Leventhal JM, et al. Characteristics that distinguish accidental from abusive injury in hospitalized young children with head trauma. *Pediatrics* 2004;114:165–168.
Describes the clinical features that distinguish accidental from abusive head injury in hospitalized children younger than 24 months. During hospitalization, children had CT scans of the brain, serial neurologic examinations, dilated ophthalmoscopic eye examinations, and evaluation by a social worker, and, in some cases, a child abuse specialist.

Besenski N. Traumatic injuries: Imaging of head injuries. *Eur Radiol* 2002;12:1237–1252.
Excellent discussion of the pathologic mechanisms underlying imaging findings, including DAI, focal injuries, hematomas, gliding injuries, secondary edema, and late effects of trauma.

Blosser JL, DePompei R. *Pediatric traumatic brain injury. Proactive Intervention, Neurogenic Communication Disorders Series.* San Diego: Singular Publishing Group, 1994; 27–31.
Focuses on the reintegration of children with brain injuries into community and educational systems. Written at a level that will be helpful to professionals, family members, and anyone else who wants to learn more about how to face the challenges intertwined with brain injury in young people.

Blostein P, Jones SJ. Identification and evaluation of patients with mild traumatic brain injury: Results of a national survey of level I trauma centers. *J Trauma* 2003;55:450–453.
Currently, no standard practice defines, evaluates, or manages MTBI at Level 1 trauma centers. The incidence of symptoms of postconcussive syndrome is 32% at 1 month and 17% at 2 months.

Brink JD, Imbus C, Woo-Sam J. Physical recovery after severe closed head trauma in children and adolescents. *J Pediatr* 1980;97:721–727.
Classic paper describing the recovery of brain-injured patients from coma. When coma lasts less than 3 months, a majority of children recover some mobility and are able to go to school.

Bruce DA. Neurosurgical aspects of child abuse. In: Ludwig S, Kornberg AE, eds. *Child abuse*, 2nd ed. New York: Churchill Livingstone, 1992.
Thorough discussion of pathophysiology, with discussion of surgical treatment and outcome, of TBI in children, especially as related to nonaccidental injury. The role of impact injury is discussed.

Cantu RC. Post-traumatic retrograde and anterograde amnesia: Pathophysiology and implications in grading and safe return to play. *J Athl Train* 2001;36:244–248.
An evidence-based discussion of the risks of returning to play after an athlete has suffered a concussion or repeated concussions. Presents guidelines for returning to play.

Catroppa C, Anderson V. Recovery in memory function in the first year following TBI in children. *Brain Injury* 2002;16:369–384.
Memory difficulties are present during the acute 6–12 months following childhood TBI. Appropriate strategies and interventions for brain-injured children are discussed.

Chadwick DL, Chin S, Salerno C, et al. Deaths from falls in children: How far is fatal? *J Trauma* 1991;30:1353–1355.
Review of the mortality of falls from various heights. Argues that children rarely die from falls of 4 feet or less.

Chapman SB, McKinnon L, Levin HS, et al. Longitudinal outcome of verbal discourse in children with traumatic brain injury: Three-year follow-up. *J Head Trauma Rehabil* 2001;16: 441–455.
Severe TBI can have a pernicious effect on discourse abilities in children years after injury compared with children with mild/moderate injuries. Discourse measures must be sufficiently challenging when used to assess older children and children with milder forms of TBI.

Coombs JB, chairperson. The management of minor closed head injury in children. *Pediatrics* 1999;104:1407–1415.
This AAP/AAFP practice parameter is intended for previously neurologically healthy children between 2 and 20 years of age with isolated minor closed head injury; defined as children who have normal mental status at the initial examination, who have no abnormal or focal findings, and who have no physical evidence of skull fracture. It includes children who may have experienced loss of consciousness of less than 1 minute in duration, who may have had a seizure immediately after injury, or who may have had physical symptoms such as vomiting, headache, and lethargy.

Daniel JC, Olesniewicz MH, Reeves DL, et al. Repeated measures of cognitive processing efficiency in adolescent athletes: Implications for monitoring recovery from concussion. *Neuropsychiatry Neuropsychol Behav Neurol* 1999;12:167–169.
Discusses that "return to baseline" cognitive function as the criterion for recovery from concussion may be insufficient in adolescents.

Dayer A, Roulet E, Maeder P, Deonna T. Post-traumatic mutism in children: Clinical characteristics, pattern of recovery and clinicopathological correlations. *Eur J Paediatr Neurol* 1998; 2:109–116.
Seven of 14 children in this study went through a period of total absence of verbal production lasting from 5 to 94 days, followed by the recovery of nonverbal communication skills and emotional vocalization.

Dhellemmes P, Lejeune JP, Christianens JL, Combelles G. Traumatic extradural hematomas in infancy and childhood: Experience with 144 cases. *J Neurosurg* 1985;62:861–864.
Discusses the incidence and clinical course of extradural (epidural) hematomas in children.

Esselman PC, Dillman-Long J. Morbidity and management conference: An approach to quality improvement in brain injury rehabilitation. *J Head Trauma Rehabil* 2002;17:257–262.
Rehabilitation medicine has a long history of working as a coordinated multidisciplinary team caring for complex patients with chronic conditions and is in a position to be a leader in quality improvement activities.

Ewing-Cobbs L, Barnes MA, Fletcher JM et al. Early brain injury in children: Development and reorganization of cognitive function. *Dev Neuropsychol* 2003;24:669–704.
Development and recovery after brain injury reflects both restoration and reorganization of cognitive functions.

Fischer RS, Alexander MP, D'Esposito M, Otto R. Neuropsychological and neuroanatomical correlates of confabulation. *J Clin Exp Neuropsychol* 1995;17:20–28.
A common profile from nine confabulatory patients suggests that spontaneous confabulations require extensive, simultaneous disruption of medial basal forebrain and frontal cognitive systems, resulting in profound executive and memory deficits.

Garth J, Anderson V, Wrennall J. Executive functions following moderate to severe frontal lobe injury: Impact of injury and age at injury. *Pediatr Rehabil* 1997;1:99–108.
Twenty-two children with moderate to severe frontal lobe injuries (FLI) were examined on several tasks of executive functioning and on intelligence to determine the impact of FLI on the development of executive functioning through childhood.

Gilles EE, Nelson MD, Jr. Cerebral complications of nonaccidental head injury in childhood. *Pediatr Neurol* 1998; 19:119–128.

Givner A, Gurney J, O'Connor D, et al. Reimaging in pediatric neurotrauma: Factors associated with progression of intracranial injury. *J Pediatr Surg* 2002;37:381–385.
Children with more severe injury are more likely to show progressive lesions of edema and hematomas, especially if intracranial injury is present on the initial CT scan. Of 14 children, 11 (79%) had early posttraumatic seizures. Cerebral infarction developed in all survivors.

Giza CC, Mink RB, Madikins A. Pediatric traumatic brain injury: Not just little adults. *Curr Opin Crit Care* 2007;13: 143–152.
Recent updates in evidence-based treatment of TBI in children.

Greenberg MK, chairperson. Practice parameter: The management of concussion in sports (summary statement). *Neurology* 1997;48:581–585.
Grades concussion on the basis of loss of consciousness and mental status abnormalities. This AAN practice parameter contains detailed criteria for return to play after each grade of concussion.

Hanten G, Zhang L, Levin HS. Selective learning in children after traumatic brain injury: A preliminary study. *Neuropsychol Dev Cog Sect C Child Neurospychol* 2002;8:107–120.
Selective learning is the ability to select important items to learn from among other items of lesser importance. Traumatically brain-injured children are disproportionately compromised in selective learning compared to simple word recall.

Hawley CA, Ward AB, Magnay AR, Mychalkiw W. Return to school after brain injury. *Arch Dis Child* 2004;89:136–142.
One-third of teachers were unaware of the TBI. Two-thirds of children with TBI had difficulties with school work, one-half had attention/concentration problems, and 26 (39%) had memory problems. Compared to other pupils in the class, one-third of children with TBI were performing below average.

Heilman KM, Valenstein E. *Clinical neuropsychology*, 4th ed. New York: Oxford, 2003.
Focuses on the clinical presentation of the major neurobehavioral syndromes. Includes clinical descriptions, neuropsychological mechanisms that might account for the disorders, brain pathology associated with the conditions, and possible aspects of therapy and management.

Hoskote A, Richards P, Anslow P, McShane T. Subdural haematoma and non-accidental head injury in children. *Childs Nerv Syst* 2002;18:311–317.
Subdural hemorrhage in nonaccidental injury tends to present before 4 months of age. The patients are more seriously ill and have other findings, such as fractures and retinal hemorrhages.

Hutchison HT. Traumatic encephalopathies. In: David RB, ed. *Pediatric neurology for the clinician*. Norwalk CT: Appleton & Lange, 1992; 180.
The first edition of this chapter defines the hallmarks of TBI.

Hutchison R, Hutchison HT. *Head injury: A booklet for families*. Houston: Texas Head Injury Foundation, 1983.
A compendium of answers to questions frequently asked by families of acutely head-injured persons. The booklet explains some of the equipment and terminology of the intensive care unit.

Jaffe KM, Fay GC, Polissar NL et al. Severity of pediatric traumatic brain injury and neurobehavioral recovery at one year: A cohort study. *Arch Phys Med Rehabil* 1993;74:587–595.
Children between the ages of 6 and 15 who suffered mild, moderate, or severe TBI were followed for 1 year after injury. Neurobehavioral outcomes were statistically evaluated on three levels: a case score, case-control scores, and case/difference scores minus control/difference scores. Results showed that the use of population normative values to evaluate impairment was misleading. Although the mean scores of all severity groups fell within the normal range of standardized tests, the means for the moderately and severely injured were substantially below those of their matched controls on many tests.

Jaffe KM, Polissar NL, Fay GC, Liao S. Recovery trends over three years following pediatric traumatic brain injury. *Arch Phys Med Rehabil* 1995;76:17–26.
This cohort study shows chronic neurobehavioral deficits across all 3 years for moderately and severely injured children. They show a strong improvement rate during the first year, but a negligible rate of change during the following 2 years postinjury in most domains. Domains investigated include intelligence, real-world functioning, behavior, and academic achievement. Mildly injured children, however, exhibit negligible deficits or change in performance over time.

Jennett B, Teasdale G. *Management of head injuries*. Philadelphia: FA Davis, 1981; 19–75, 211–252.
A clear presentation of the pathophysiology of diffuse brain swelling and its management. This book also discusses posttraumatic epilepsy.

Johnson DL, Braun D, Friendly D. Accidental head trauma and retinal hemorrhage. *Neurosurgery* 1993;33:231–235.
Retinal hemorrhage is associated with extraordinary force and rarely occurs in accidental head injury.

Johnson DA, Rose FD, Brooks BM, Eyeres S. Age and recovery from brain injury: Legal opinions, clinical beliefs and experimental evidence. *Pediatr Rehabil* 2003;6:103–109.
Despite scientific evidence to the contrary, many medical practitioners maintain that children recover from brain injury better than adults.

Jurkovich GJ Pierce B, Pananen L, Rivara FP. Giving bad news: The family perspective. *J Trauma* 2000;48:865–870.
Of the characteristics of persons giving bad news, families value attitude, clarity, privacy, and ability to answer questions most.

Kay T, et al. Definition of mild traumatic brain injury. *J Head Trauma Rehabil* 1993;8:86–87.
A standard definition often used to define mild TBI. This definition includes all but the most severe athletic injuries.

Kolb B, Whishaw I. *Fundamentals of human neuropsychology*, 4th ed. New York: WH Freeman, 1996; 387–416.
An examination of neuropsychology from the perspective of cognitive neuroscience, human and nonhuman studies, and recent advances in the technology of brain study. This work covers general topics related to neuropsychology, in addition to specific topics related to clinical brain disorders.

Koskiniemi M, Kyykka T, Nybo T, Jarho L. Long-term outcome after severe brain injury in preschoolers is worse than expected. *Arch Pediatr Adolesc Med* 1995;149:249–254.
This study followed 39 preschoolers with severe TBI into adulthood. Outcome measures of ability to work and living independently indicated the overall outcome is worse than originally thought.

Krauss JK, Jankovic J. Head injury and posttraumatic movement disorders. *Neurosurgery* 2002;50:927–940.
Movement disorders after severe head injury have been reported in 13–66% of patients, and may be delayed in appearance. Although movement disorders after mild or moderate head injury are frequently transient and, in general, do not result in additional disability, kinetic tremors and dystonia may be a source of marked disability in survivors of severe head injury.

Kriel RL, Krach LE, Luxenberg MG, et al. Outcome of severe anoxic/ischemic brain injury in children. *Pediatr Neurol* 1994;10:207–212.
Cognitive and motor outcomes were correlated with the severity of injury as indicated by the duration of unconsciousness. All children who regained language skills or the ability to walk were unconscious less than 60 days.

Langlois JA, Rutland-Brown W, Thomas KE. *Traumatic brain injury in the United States: Emergency department visits, hospitalizations, and deaths.* Atlanta: Centers for Disease Control and Prevention, National Center for Injury Prevention and Control, 2006; 17.
Current statistics on the incidence of TBI at all ages.

Lebby PC, Asbell SJ. *The source for traumatic brain injury: Children and adolescents.* Chicago IL: Linguisystems, 2007.
This book provides a comprehensive discussion of TBI in children and adolescents from neuroanatomy and neurodevelopment, to brain injury and pathology, to recovery and family/school issues. Two tests of neurocognitive functioning, one for children and one for adolescents, are also provided with the text.

Levin HS et al. *Neurobehavioral consequences of closed head injury*. New York: Oxford, 1982; 189–207.
A classic treatise on outcome issues, including assessment, pathophysiology, and rehabilitation. Chapter 10, in particular, is devoted to children.

Levin HS, Song J, Scheibel RS et al. Concept formation and problem solving following closed head injury in children. *J Int Neuropsychol Soc* 1997;3:598–607.
Three measures of executive functioning were used in 151 head-injured children, and 89 controls, from 5 to 18 years of age. Fifty-seven of the patients were included in a longitudinal study (3 months and 36 months). The three measures of executive functioning were evaluated in relation to age, severity of injury, and time post injury. All three EF measures depicted changes in performance over 3 years.

Levin HS, Hanten G, Chang CC, et al. Working memory after traumatic brain injury in children. *Ann Neurol* 2002;52:82–88.
Traumatic brain injury results in preferentially impaired working memory and diminished inhibition in children.

Lezak MD. *Neuropsychological assessment*, 3rd ed. New York: Oxford, 1995.
Discusses the brain–behavior relationships underlying neuropsychologic assessment. This book also contains a detailed compendium of testing instruments.

Marshall LF. Head injury: Recent past, present, and future. *Neurosurgery* 2000;47:546–562.
A particularly cogent and articulate discussion of neurobiology and its application in the treatment of severe TBI.

Mazzola CA, Adelson PD. Critical care management of head trauma in children. *Crit Care Med* 2002;30:S393-S401.
Summarizes current treatment and outcome of children with TBI.

McCrory P. Does second impact syndrome exist? *Clin J Sport Med* 2001;11:144–149.
Suggests that the very rare condition of delayed catastrophic deterioration following some athletic injuries is related to diffuse cerebral swelling and is not due to the effects of repeated concussion.

Oertel M, Kelly DF, McArthur D, et al. Progressive hemorrhage after head trauma: predictors and consequences of the evolving injury. *J Neurosurg* 2002;96:109–116.
CT scans within 2 hours of severe head injury do not reveal the full extent of the hemorrhagic injury. Progressive hemorrhage is apparent in nearly 50% of these patients within the next 6 hours, particularly parenchymal lesions in the frontal and temporal lobes. These patients have a greater degree of ICP elevations and account for almost 25% of those who require craniotomy for hematoma removal.

Posner JB, Saper CB, Schiff ND, Plum F. *Plum and Posner's diagnosis of stupor and coma*, 4th ed. New York: Oxford, 2007.
Classic text that still contains very detailed and understandable descriptions of the causes and manifestations of coma.

Prange MT, Coats B, Duhaime AD, Margulies SS. Anthropomorphic simulation of falls, shakes, and inflicted impacts in infants. *J Neurosurg* 2003;99:143–150.

Inflicted impacts against hard surfaces are more likely to be associated with brain injuries than falls from a height of less than 1.5 m, or from shaking alone.

Rivara JB, Jaffe KM, Pollissar NL, et al. Family functioning and children's academic performance and behavior problems in the year following traumatic brain injury. *Arch Phys Med Rehabil* 1994;75:369–379.
Poor academic and cognitive outcomes at 1 year were associated with injury severity and, to a lesser degree, poor preinjury family and child functioning. In contrast, most of the variation in behavioral outcomes was explained by preinjury child or family factors.

Roberts SD, Wells RD, Brown IS, et al. The FRESNO: A pediatric functional outcome measurement system. *J Rehabil Outcomes Meas* 1999;3:11–99.
The FRESNO is useful for the concurrent measurement of performance of brain-injured children during rehabilitation, and after discharge.

Ruff RM, Marshall LF, Crouch J et al. Predictors of outcome following severe head trauma: Follow-up data from the Traumatic Coma Data Bank. *Brain Inj* 1993;7:101–111.
Among former students who had suffered TBI, 62% had returned to school by 6 months after injury. Age, length of coma, speed for both attending and motor movements, spatial integration, and intact vocabulary were all significantly related to returning to work or school.

Schwartz L, Taylor HG, Drotar D, et al. Long-term behavior problems following pediatric traumatic brain injury: Prevalence, predictors, and correlates. *J Pediatr Psychol* 2003;28: 251–263.
The risks of long-term posttraumatic behavior problems are multifactorial, and correlates include child dysfunction and family sequelae.

Simon B, Latourneau P, Vitorino E, McCall J. Pediatric minor head trauma: Indications for computed tomographic scanning revisited. *J Trauma* 2001;51:231–237.
Fourteen percent of children treated at a Level 1 trauma center had CT evidence of intracranial injury despite normal neurologic examination and lack of loss of consciousness. A liberal policy of CT scanning is advocated for children with mild TBI.

Slomine BS, Gerring JP, Grados MA, et al. Performance on measures of executive function following pediatric traumatic brain injury. *Brain Inj* 2002;16:759–772.
This study followed 68 children with moderate to severe TBI between the ages of 7 and 15 in an attempt to investigate the relationships between age at injury, neuroanatomic lesion location, and executive function (EF) in a pediatric population. Results supported the vulnerability theory for the pediatric population. Younger age at injury places children at greater risk of impairment on measures of EF. Performance on measures of EF depends on brain variables other than frontal lobes, including extrafrontal cortical brain areas and total number of lesions. The relationship between extrafrontal brain regions and EF suggests that domain-specific cognitive content (i.e., language or visuospatial analysis), mediated by the parietal or temporal lobes, may disrupt underlying cognitive processes necessary for successful performance on measures of EF. In addition, the association between total number of lesions and EF may be related to disconnections and disruption of frontal/subcortical systems.

Stein SC, Spettell C, Young G, Ross SE. Delayed and progressive brain injury in closed-head trauma: Radiological demonstration. *Neurosurgery* 1993;32:25–31.
The severity of the initial brain trauma contributes significantly to neurologic outcome. The presence of delayed cerebral injury makes the outcome dramatically worse. Only 20% of patients (mostly adults) in this series with radiologic worsening had subdural or epidural hematomas.

Taylor HG, Yeates KO, Wade SL, et al. A prospective study of short- and long-term outcomes after traumatic brain injury in children: Behavior and achievement. *Neuropsychology* 2002;16:15–27.
Behavioral and academic sequelae for moderate to severe TBI pediatric patients were evaluated, taking into account family environment and how that influences recovery. Mixed model analyses revealed persistent neuropsychological sequelae of TBI that generally did not vary as a function of time postinjury. Some recovery occurred during the first year post injury, but recovery reached a plateau after that time, and deficits were still apparent at the extended follow-up. Further recovery was uncommon after the first year post injury. The findings suggest that pediatric TBI has long-term effects on behavior and achievement but that post injury progress is influenced by the family environment.

Tijssen CC. Contralateral conjugate eye deviation in acute supratentorial lesions. *Stroke* 1994;25:1516–1519.
In 5 of 133 patients with conjugate eye deviation caused by an acute supratentorial lesion, the eye deviation proved to be a "false-localizing" sign with the gaze deviated to the side opposite the lesion.

Tomita H, Tone O, Ito U. Hemispheric cerebral atrophy after traumatic extra-axial hematoma in adults. *Neurol Med Chir* 1997;37:819–824.
Acute swelling and subsequent atrophy are more prominent in the hemisphere underlying an acute hematoma.

van den Brink VA, van Santbrink H, Steyerberg EW, et al. Brain oxygen tension in severe head injury. *Neurosurgery* 2000;46: 868–876.
Discusses the measurement of brain tissue oxygenation and the role of this measure in intensive care, and in predicting outcome, in victims of severe brain injury.

Vespa PM, Nuwer MR, Nenov V et al. Increased incidence and impact of nonconvulsive and convulsive seizures after traumatic brain injury as detected by continuous electroencephalographic monitoring. *J Neurosurg* 1999;91:750–760.
Seizures occur in more than one in five patients during the first week after moderate to severe brain injury and may play a role in the pathobiologic conditions associated with brain injury.

Violence in America: A public health crisis—the role of firearms. *J Trauma* 1995;38:163–168.
A review of the alarming increase of the role of firearms in childhood trauma.

Yeates K, Taylor HG, Drotar D, et al. Pre-injury family environment as a determinant of recovery from traumatic brain injuries in school-aged children. *J Int Neuropsychol Soc* 1997;3:617–630.

A prospective study emphasizing environmental factors as determinants of brain injury recovery in children aged 6–12 years. Outcomes were assessed at 6- and 12-month follow-ups. Measures of preinjury family environment consistently predicted both the level of cognitive and behavioral functioning at 12 months post injury, and the rate of intraindividual change during the 12-month period, even after taking into account group membership (Severe TBI, Moderate TBI, Orthopedic injury), and injury severity.

CHAPTER 11

The Epilepsies

Carl E. Stafstrom

Outline

- Epidemiology
- Classification of seizures and epilepsies
- Pathophysiology and genetics
- Evaluation of the child with seizures
- Differential diagnosis
- Epilepsy syndromes in children
- Prognosis of childhood epilepsy
- Nonepileptic disorders that may mimic epilepsy
- Treatment of the child with seizures and epilepsy
- Withdrawing antiepileptic drugs
- Pharmacology of antiepileptic drugs
- Other epilepsy therapies
- Concluding remarks

Epidemiology

This chapter reviews the diagnosis and treatment of epilepsy in childhood. Several excellent resources also discuss childhood epilepsy in detail (Arzimanoglou et al. 2004a; Guerrini 2006; Raspall–Chaure et al. 2008).

A seizure is a paroxysmal alteration of neurologic function caused by the abnormal discharge of neurons in the brain. Epileptic seizure is sometimes used to distinguish a seizure caused by abnormal neuronal firing from a paroxysmal nonepileptic event such as a pseudoseizure or syncope. Epilepsy is a chronic condition of recurrent, unprovoked seizures. Epilepsy is not a single disease but rather a sign of underlying brain dysfunction. Seizures provoked by a reversible insult (e.g., fever, hypoglycemia) do not fall under the definition of epilepsy because they are a short-lived, secondary condition rather than a chronic state. An epilepsy syndrome refers to a group of clinical characteristics that consistently occur together, with similar seizure type, age of onset, electroencephalographic (EEG) findings, precipitating factors, inheritance pattern, natural history, prognosis, and response to antiepileptic drugs (AEDs) (Benbadis 2001). The nonspecific term "seizure disorder" should be avoided.

Epilepsy is a common disorder, with an incidence of approximately 50 new cases per year per 100,000 population (Hauser 1995; Shinnar & Pellock 2002). Approximately 1–2% of the population suffers from epilepsy. The highest incidence occurs in childhood, with a second peak of increased incidence in the elderly. Approximately 75% of epilepsy begins during childhood (Hauser 1995).

Classification of seizures and epilepsies

The International League Against Epilepsy (ILAE) has developed separate classifications of seizures and epilepsies (epilepsy syndromes). The International Classification of Epileptic Seizures (ICES, Table 11.1; Commission 1981) is based on three factors: (1) clinical seizure manifestations, (2) ictal EEG patterns, and (3) interictal EEG patterns. In this classification scheme, seizures are subdivided into two broad categories: partial (focal) or generalized. Using clinical criteria, partial seizures begin focally in the brain and present with focal clinical signs, whereas generalized seizures begin simultaneously in both hemispheres, and do not have a focal onset (Figure 11.1). Seizures are then further classified by their interictal and ictal EEG features, if available. Based on a reliable history and interictal EEG, the physician can often classify the seizure, after which an appropriate diagnostic evaluation and treatment plan can be formulated.

Although the ICES describes the seizure itself, it does not consider the many epilepsy syndromes that occur in

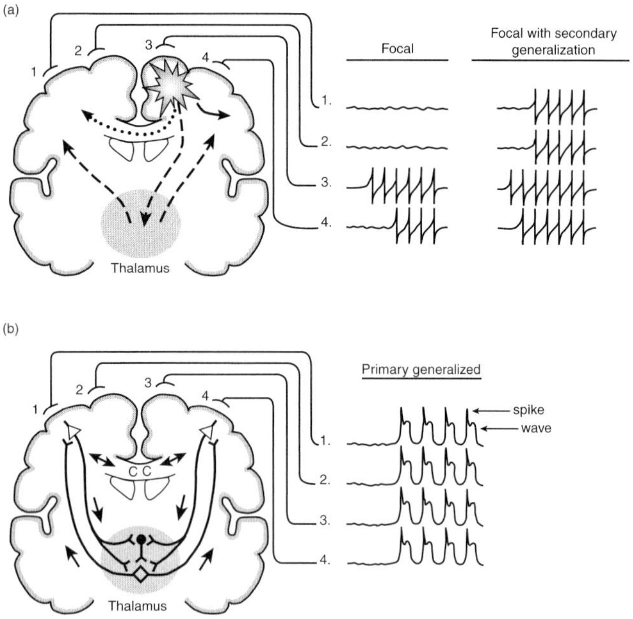

Figure 11.1 Coronal brain sections depicting seizure types and potential routes of seizure spread. (A) Focal area of hyperexcitability (*star*) and spread to nearby neocortex (*solid arrow*), via corpus callosum or other commissures to the contralateral cerebral hemisphere (*dotted arrow*), or via subcortical pathways (e.g., thalamus, brainstem; *downward dashed arrow*) resulting in secondary generalization (*upward dashed arrows*). Accompanying electroencephalographs (EEGs) show brain electrical activity under numbered electrodes. Focal epileptiform activity (*spikes*) is maximal at electrode 3 and is also seen nearby at electrode 4 (*left traces*). If a seizure secondarily generalizes, spike activity may be seen synchronously at all electrodes, after a delay (*far right traces*). (B) A primary generalized seizure begins simultaneously in both hemispheres. The characteristic bilateral synchronous "spike-wave" pattern on EEG is generated by interactions between cortex and thalamus, with rapid spread via corpus callosum (CC) contributing to the rapid bilateral synchrony. One type of thalamic neuron (*filled circle*) is a GABAergic inhibitory cell with intrinsic oscillatory properties; it is able to fire in bursts of action potentials due to a specific type of calcium channel, allowing these cells to modulate ongoing excitatory corticothalamic activity. Cortical neurons send impulses to both inhibitory thalamic neurons (*filled circle*) and excitatory thalamic neurons (*diamond*), setting up oscillations of excitatory and inhibitory activity, which gives rise to the rhythmic spike waves on EEG.

children. Therefore, the International Classification of Epilepsies and Epilepsy Syndromes was developed (Commission 1989). Two broad categories are used to shape the major classes of epilepsies and epileptic syndromes (Table 11.2). The first category separates generalized epilepsy syndromes (generalized epilepsies) from those with partial or focal onset (localization-related partial epilepsies). The other category separates epilepsies of known etiology (symptomatic or secondary epilepsies) from those that are idiopathic (primary) or cryptogenic (cause unknown).

The classifications of seizures and epilepsies just described may not fully account for modern genetic and clinical data, particularly in children (Nordli 2002). A new classification system is being developed that takes into account ictal phenomenology, seizure type, syndrome diagnosis (if present), etiology, and degree of functional impairment (Table 11.3) (Engel 2001, 2006). Classification schemes will evolve to reflect growing knowledge about epilepsy genetics and pathophysiology.

Pathophysiology and genetics

The developing brain is prone to seizures for a variety of reasons (Stafstrom 1998; Ben-Ari & Holmes 2006). A seizure may result when there is distortion of the usual balance between excitation and inhibition in the brain (Table 11.4). This balance can be disrupted by genetic or acquired factors. Genetic pathologies leading to epilepsy can occur anywhere from the circuit level (e.g., abnormal synaptic connections in cortical dysplasia), to the receptor level (e.g., abnormal γ-aminobutyric acid [GABA] receptor subunits in Angelman syndrome), to abnormal ionic channel function (e.g., potassium channel mutations in benign familial neonatal convulsions). Similarly, acquired cerebral insults can alter circuit function (e.g., structural alterations of hippocampal circuitry following prolonged febrile seizures or head trauma). In the developing brain, excitatory synaptic function develops prior to inhibitory synaptic function, favoring seizure generation. In addition, early in life GABA can act as an excitatory neurotransmitter rather than an inhibitory one, due to a reversed chloride ion gradient and immature pattern of chloride transport by membrane pumps (Staley 2006). These observations partly explain why the very young brain is especially susceptible to seizures. Fortunately, seizures seem to cause less structural damage in the developing brain compared to the adult brain.

There has been an explosion of information about the genetic basis of epilepsy syndromes (Noebels 2003; Scheffer & Berkovic 2003), some of which is summarized in Table 11.5. Both monogenic and polygenic mutations can lead to epilepsy. Mutations in proteins governing a wide variety of physiologic functions can lead to a state of hyperexcitability that underlies epilepsy. As these syndromes become better elucidated, there is hope that syndrome-specific therapeutic interventions can be designed.

Evaluation of the child with seizures

The history and neurologic examination are the cornerstones of neurologic diagnosis; laboratory studies are properly used to augment or confirm the diagnosis. Historical features include the clinical context in which the

Table 11.1 International classification of epileptic seizures

Partial (focal) seizures
Simple partial
Motor signs
Somatosensory or special sensory symptoms
Autonomic symptoms or signs
Psychic symptoms
Complex partial
Simple partial onset followed by impaired consciousness
Consciousness impaired at onset
Partial seizures with secondary generalization (tonic, clonic, or tonic–clonic)
Simple partial seizures evolving to generalized seizures
Complex partial seizures evolving to generalized seizures
Simple partial seizures evolving to complex partial seizures evolving to generalized seizures
Generalized seizures (convulsive or nonconvulsive)
Absence
Typical
Atypical
Myoclonic
Clonic
Tonic
Tonic–clonic
Atonic
Unclassified epileptic seizures

From Commission 1981.

Table 11.2 International classification of epilepsies and epilepsy syndromes

Localization-related (focal, partial) epilepsies
Idiopathic
Benign childhood epilepsy with centrotemporal spikes (rolandic epilepsy)
Childhood epilepsy with occipital paroxysms
Primary reading epilepsy
Symptomatic or cryptogenic (presumed to be symptomatic but cause is unknown)
Temporal lobe epilepsy
Frontal lobe epilepsy
Occipital lobe epilepsy
Parietal lobe epilepsy
Chronic progressive epilepsia partialis continua
Generalized epilepsies
Idiopathic (with age-related onset, listed in order of age)
Benign neonatal convulsions
Benign familial neonatal convulsions
Benign myoclonic epilepsy in infancy
Childhood absence epilepsy
Juvenile absence epilepsy
Juvenile myoclonic epilepsy
Epilepsy with generalized tonic–clonic seizures on awakening
Symptomatic
Nonspecific etiology
Early myoclonic encephalopathy
Early infantile epileptic encephalopathy with suppression burst
Other symptomatic generalized epilepsies
Cryptogenic
West syndrome (infantile spasms)
Lennox-Gastaut syndrome
Epilepsy with myoclonic-astatic seizures (Doose syndrome)
Epilepsy with myoclonic absences
Specific syndromes (disease states in which seizures are present as a predominant feature)
Indeterminate epilepsies
Generalized and focal features
Neonatal seizures
Severe myoclonic epilepsy of infancy (Dravet syndrome)
Epilepsy with continuous spike waves during slow wave sleep
Acquired epileptic aphasia (Landau-Kleffner syndrome)
Other indeterminate epilepsies without unequivocal generalized or focal features
Special syndromes
Situation-related seizures
Febrile seizures
Isolated seizures or status epilepticus
Seizures caused by an acute or toxic event, such as alcohol or drugs, eclampsia, or hyperglycemia

From Commission 1989.

seizure occurred, features of the seizure itself, seizure duration, and postictal signs. It is imperative to determine whether an epileptic syndrome is present, to guide the nature and extent of the evaluation, treatment, and prognosis. If uncertainty exists about the diagnosis, it is more prudent to wait for another attack than to embark on an extensive workup and initiate AEDs.

Diagnostic studies

Electroencephalography

An EEG is a recording of the electrical activity of the brain. It can detect abnormal electrical activity such as focal spikes or waves (consistent with partial epilepsy) or diffuse, bilateral spike waves (consistent with generalized epilepsy). A routine EEG should be obtained on any child with suspected epilepsy, preferably during wakefulness and sleep and with photic stimulation and hyperventilation. Prolonged video-EEG monitoring can increase the diagnostic yield or differentiate an epileptic seizure from a nonepileptic event.

Table 11.3 Proposed new diagnostic scheme for persons with epileptic seizures or epilepsy

Axis	Comments	Example
1. Ictal phenomenology	Detailed description of the ictal event	Right lower facial clonus and dysarthric speech
2. Seizure type	Specify localization within the brain and precipitating stimuli for reflex seizures when appropriate	Focal motor with elementary clonic motor signs (simple partial)
3. Syndrome	Syndrome diagnosis is not possible in every patient	Benign childhood epilepsy with centrotemporal spikes (rolandic epilepsy)
4. Etiology	When possible, list specific pathology or genetic defect	Idiopathic (genetic basis assumed)
5. Impairment	Specific impairments of function associated with the epilepsy	a. Anxiety associated with stigma of epilepsy b. Fatigue associated with anticonvulsant medication

Table 11.6 summarizes typical EEG findings in various seizure types and syndromes. The EEG can be normal in a child with epilepsy, especially with partial-onset seizures. The diagnosis of epilepsy is based on clinical information, and the EEG should be regarded as confirmatory, not diagnostic. Although we ordinarily "treat the child, not the EEG," certain exceptions exist in which electrographic abnormalities themselves are pathognomonic of an epilepsy syndrome, including 3-Hz spike-waves in absence epilepsy, continuous spike-wave discharges during slow wave sleep, and hypsarrhythmia in infantile spasms.

Neuroimaging

Computed tomography (CT) and magnetic resonance imaging (MRI) scans are important adjuncts to the clinical examination and EEG, in the evaluation of a child with seizures (Kuzniecky & Knowlton 2002). Neuroimaging techniques are especially sensitive for CNS structural lesions. MRI is more likely to show an abnormality in a child with partial seizures, abnormal neurologic findings, or focal discharges on the EEG. A child with focal neurologic findings on examination generally requires neuroimaging.

MRI is more sensitive than CT and therefore is the preferred modality to detect cortical malformation, dysgenesis, or hippocampal sclerosis (Porter et al. 2002; Guerrini & Filippi 2005). Quantitative, computer-assisted volume analysis of the temporal lobes may allow detection of asymmetries that are not readily apparent on visual analysis of the scan. CT is valuable in the acute setting to detect hemorrhage, calcification, tumor, or other lesions that requires immediate attention.

Several new imaging techniques can aid in the assessment of epilepsy. Structural information (MRI) can be correlated directly with functional activity (EEG). MR spectroscopy measures the concentrations of a variety of neurochemicals in different brain regions and can sometimes help to localize a seizure focus. Positron emission tomography (PET) images the brain's regional utilization of glucose, with asymmetries suggesting areas of interictal or ictal abnormality (Henry & Heertum 2003). Single-photon emission computed tomography (SPECT) compares local blood flow discrepancies, information that is most useful when recorded during a seizure.

Table 11.4 Some factors predisposing the developing brain to hyperexcitability and seizures

- Early development of excitatory sodium and calcium channels
- Earlier development of excitatory synapses and neurotransmitters
- Delayed development of inhibitory synapses and neurotransmitters
- Exuberant axonal branching pattern early in life (more excitatory synapses)
- Depolarizing action of γ-aminobutyric acid (GABA) early in development
- Delayed ability of glia to clear extracellular potassium ions

Table 11.5 Epilepsy genetics in selected syndromes

Syndrome	Chromosome(s)	Genes
Autosomal dominant nocturnal frontal lobe epilepsy (ADNFLE)	20q13, 1p21	Acetylcholine receptors
Benign familial neonatal convulsions (BFNC)	20q13, 8q24	Potassium channels
Generalized epilepsy with febrile seizures plus (GEFS+)	19q13, 2q24, 5q34	Sodium channels; $GABA_A$ receptors
Severe myoclonic epilepsy of infancy (SMEI)	2q24, 5q31	Sodium channels
Juvenile myoclonic epilepsy	5q34, 2q22–23	$GABA_A$ receptors; calcium channels
Childhood absence epilepsy	5q34 19p	$GABA_A$ receptors; calcium channels

GABA, γ-aminobutyric acid

Table 11.6 Characteristic electroencephalographic (EEG) features in various seizure types

Seizure type	Interictal EEG abnormalities
Partial seizures	
Simple partial	Variable; spikes over involved area of cortex; may be normal
Complex partial	Variable; frontal/temporal lobe spikes; may be normal
Generalized seizures	
Absence	Generalized spike-wave, often activated by sleep, hyperventilation, or photic stimulation
Generalized tonic–clonic	Variable; often normal
Myoclonic	Usually abnormal; generalized spike-wave, multiple spike-waves
Tonic/atonic	Usually abnormal; generalized abnormalities, spikes, multiple spike-waves
Infantile spasms	Hypsarhythmia (interictal); electrodecrement (ictal)

Magnetoencephalography (MEG) assesses the brain's dynamic electromagnetic fields and localizes areas of abnormal function (Otsubo & Snead 2001). These new techniques are used primarily in epilepsy centers for presurgical evaluations.

Metabolic evaluation

The type of seizure and epilepsy syndrome dictates the extent of the metabolic workup (DeVivo 2002; Hylund & Arnold 1999; Rice & Hsu 2005). In metabolic disorders, seizures typically accompany other abnormal findings such as developmental delay. In neonatal seizures, a metabolic evaluation is mandatory (see later Neonatal Seizures section). Table 11.7 lists some recommended studies for children with a variety of seizure types and epilepsy syndromes.

Differential diagnosis

Seizure types

Partial seizures

As discussed earlier (under Classification of Seizures and Epilepsies), seizures are classified according to their onset as partial or generalized. Partial (focal) seizures are those in which the first clinical and EEG changes indicate activation of neurons limited to part of one cerebral hemisphere. Partial seizures are further classified as to whether or not consciousness is impaired during the attack. When consciousness is not impaired, the seizure is termed simple partial (Table 11.8). When consciousness is impaired—that is, the child is unable to respond normally to environmental stimuli—the seizure is classified as complex partial (Table 11.9). The clinical manifestations of partial seizures are determined by the cortical area involved. For example, a simple partial seizure arising from the occipital lobe presents with visual phenomena; from the precentral gyrus, with motor activity; and from the postcentral gyrus, with sensory symptoms. Seizures arising from the temporal lobe are usually associated with an altered state of consciousness and are therefore classified as complex partial. Partial

Table 11.7 Tests to consider in the evaluation of a child with seizures

Seizure type/syndrome	Test	Comments
Simple partial	MRI	Rule out structural lesion
Complex partial	MRI	Rule out structural lesion
Generalized tonic–clonic	MRI	Rule out structural lesion
Absence	None required	
Infantile spasms and other refractory epilepsies and epileptic encephalopathies	Skin examination (Wood's lamp)	Hypopigmented lesions (tuberous sclerosis)
	MRI	Rule out congenital malformation, neuronal migration disorder
	Serum/urine amino/organic acids; serum biotinidase	Metabolic screening tests
	Serum ammonia	Screen for urea cycle defects
	Lactate/pyruvate	Screen for mitochondrial disorder
	Pyridoxine infusion	Rule out vitamin B_6-dependent seizures
	Ophthalmologic examination	Chorioretinitis may indicate congenital infection Chorioretinal lacunes may indicate Aicardi syndrome
	Lumbar puncture	Rule out neurotransmitter disorder, chronic infection

MRI, magnetic resonance imaging

Table 11.8 Simple partial seizures

Discriminating features
- No impairment of consciousness

Consistent features
- Seizures are usually brief and stereotyped
- Symptoms and signs are referable to a particular brain region

Variable features
- Motor symptoms
- Somatosensory symptoms
- Psychic symptoms
- Autonomic symptoms
- Postictal symptoms
- Association with structural brain lesion
- Interictal EEG abnormalities
- Responsiveness to AEDs

Table 11.9 Complex partial seizures

Discriminating features
- Consciousness is impaired

Consistent features
- May begin with an aura
- Clinical features are stereotyped from seizure to seizure
- Gradual onset and termination

Variable features
- Automatisms
- Affective and psychic symptoms
- Somatosensory symptoms
- Aura
- Postictal impairment
- Duration
- Association with structural brain lesions
- Interictal electroencephalographic findings
- Responds to antiepileptic drugs

seizures can secondarily generalize; that is, spread from the focus to both sides of the brain.

Generalized seizures

Generalized seizures begin in both cerebral hemispheres simultaneously, with alteration of responsiveness and sometimes other clinical signs. Several types of generalized seizure exist. Absence seizures (formerly called petit mal) involve sudden staring with unresponsiveness, and often eye blinking or head nodding. Note that "absence" refers to both a seizure type and an epilepsy syndrome (see later section on Childhood Absence Epilepsy).

Generalized tonic–clonic seizures (formerly called grand mal) consist of bilaterally symmetric convulsive movements of all limbs, with impairment of consciousness. Some children have prodromal symptoms, such as headache, insomnia, irritability, or a change in mood hours or even days before a seizure. Prodromal symptoms are distinguished from an aura, which generally precedes the GTC by seconds or minutes. The aura is actually a partial seizure, whereas a prodrome is not considered a seizure. An aura is useful in identifying a secondarily generalized seizure. Auras vary considerably from patient to patient and may encompass any of the manifestations of simple partial seizures including focal motor, sensory, autonomic, or psychic symptoms. Occasionally, a seizure is clonic or tonic without the other component.

Atonic seizures consist of sudden loss of tone in the axial musculature, causing the individual to fall or slump to the ground. Atonic seizures are often associated with other seizure types in the same person, and are often seen

Pearls and Perils

Simple Partial Seizures

- Simple partial seizures are usually short, lasting less than a minute.
- Structural brain lesions must be considered in children with simple partial seizures.
- The lack of an EEG abnormality during a seizure does not rule out the possibility of a simple partial seizure.
- The choice of AEDs for treatment of simple partial seizures is the same as that for complex partial seizures.

Pearls and Perils

Complex Partial Seizures

- The child with epileptic staring spells, especially if they occur less than once per day, is more likely to have complex partial seizures than absence seizures.
- Children with complex partial seizures who do not respond to trials of two antiepileptic drugs (AEDs) are unlikely to achieve complete seizure control, and the possibility of surgery should be considered.
- Violent behavior is rarely caused by an epileptic seizure. Although patients may become agitated during a seizure or in the postictal period, especially if they are restrained, directed violence is extremely uncommon.
- Seizures rarely cause abdominal pain. Abdominal epilepsy, a very rare disorder, is usually partial complex in type and is associated with impairment of consciousness.

Pearls and Perils

Generalized Tonic–Clonic Seizures

- Most generalized tonic–clonic seizures are secondarily generalized; that is, the seizures have a focal onset and then become generalized.
- Seizures in a given child are typically stereotyped. In patients who experience different symptoms with different spells, pseudoseizures should be considered.

in epilepsies such as Lennox-Gastaut syndrome. A child with atonic seizures usually has significant neurologic impairment and may need to wear a protective helmet due to the high risk of head injury.

Myoclonic seizures consist of sudden, brief ("lightning-like") movements that are not associated with any obvious disturbance of consciousness (Table 11.10). These brief involuntary muscle contractions may affect one or several muscles; therefore, myoclonic seizures can be generalized or partial. Myoclonus can be associated with a lesion at any level of the neuraxis, including cortex, cerebellum, brainstem, or spinal cord (Table 11.11). Myoclonic seizures have numerous causes. Myoclonic movements may be normal phenomena such as hypnagogic jerks or sleep starts. Conversely, myoclonus can be associated with virtually any severe insult to the brain, including toxic, metabolic, infectious, traumatic, or degenerative insults. Likewise, the pathophysiology of myoclonus varies; some myoclonus is nonepileptic and classified as a movement disorder, whereas other myoclonus has an epileptic basis.

Table 11.10 Myoclonic seizures

Discriminating features

- May be confused with atonic seizures. Electromyographic (EMG) monitoring demonstrates increased muscle activity during a myoclonic seizure and decreased muscle activity during an atonic seizure

Consistent features

- Very brief
- Sudden onset without aura or postictal impairment

Variable features

- Distribution of muscle groups involved
- Frequency
- Severity varies greatly; some myoclonic seizures are subtle and difficult to recognize, others may cause child to fall to the ground
- Association with structural brain lesions
- Response to VPA or clonazepam

Pearls and Perils

Myoclonic Seizures

- In children, epileptic myoclonus is most frequently seen as a component of absence epilepsy or juvenile myoclonic epilepsy.
- Not all myoclonus is epileptic in origin. Nonepileptic myoclonus can be seen in conditions varying from benign sleep states to devastating degenerative disorders.

Epilepsy syndromes in children

The following examples of childhood epilepsy syndromes were selected based on their importance or frequency, and are categorized according to the 1989 ILAE classification scheme.

Generalized epilepsy syndromes

Idiopathic generalized epilepsy syndromes

Benign familial neonatal convulsions. In benign familial neonatal convulsions (BFNC), seizures begin in the first week of life (Chahine & Mikati 2006; Singh et al 1998). The seizure type is focal clonic or focal tonic (although it is currently classified as a generalized epilepsy), often accompanied by apnea. The seizures occur in sleep and are usually brief, lasting 1–2 minutes, but may occur as many as 30 times per day. They usually stop after a few days or weeks. Ictal EEG recordings show initial generalized voltage attenuation followed by bilateral spikes and sharp waves. Except for seizures, the infants are normal, and evaluation fails to detect an etiology of the seizures. The key to the diagnosis is a positive family history of newborn or infantile seizures with benign outcome. However, even with a positive family history, other more ominous causes of seizures should be ruled out before concluding that the seizures are inherited.

Infants can be treated with phenobarbital until seizures remit. The prognosis of BFNC is good, although 10–15% of affected infants continue to have seizures beyond the neonatal period, even into adulthood.

BFNC has been linked to two chromosomal loci. The identified genes (*KCNQ2* on chromosome 20q and *KCNQ3* on chromosome 8q) encode voltage-gated potassium channel subunits that regulate the M-current, a muscarine-activated neuronal current that turns off a class of potassium channels. The M-current ordinarily stabilizes resting membrane potential, so its dysfunction in BFNC causes increased neuronal excitability and seizures. It is not known why seizures in BFNC affect neonates primarily, since the genetic defect is presumably present throughout life (Wong 2005).

Table 11.11 Classification of myoclonus

Nonepileptic myoclonus
Physiologic myoclonus
Sleep starts (hypnic jerks)
Benign awake myoclonus
Pathologic myoclonus
Hyperekplexia (startle disease)
Shuddering attacks
Periodic movements of sleep (sleep myoclonus)
Restless leg syndrome
Benign neonatal sleep myoclonus
Benign myoclonus of early infancy
Benign familial myoclonus
Segmental myoclonus
Brainstem
Opsoclonus
Palatal myoclonus
Spinal cord
Symptomatic epileptic myoclonus
Infections
Subacute sclerosing panencephalitis
Creutzfeldt-Jakob disease
Encephalitis
Congenital brain anomalies
Toxins
Systemic diseases (uremia, hepatic insufficiency)
Medications
Postanoxic
Component of inherited progressive neurologic disease
Progressive myoclonic epilepsy with Lafora bodies
Progressive myoclonic epilepsy without Lafora bodies
Ramsay-Hunt syndrome
Metabolic disorders
Neuronal ceroid lipofuscinosis
Gaucher disease
Sialidosis (cherry red-spot myoclonus)
Gangliosidosis (GM1, GM2)
Mitochondrial disorders
Myoclonic epilepsy with ragged red fibers (MERRF)
Mitochondrial encephalopathy, lactic acidosis, and stroke-like episodes (MELAS)
Primary epileptic myoclonus
Generalized epileptic myoclonus of early childhood
Juvenile myoclonic epilepsy
Focal cortical myoclonus
As a component of other epilepsies
Absence with myoclonic component
Eyelid myoclonus with absences
Component of generalized tonic–clonic seizures
Myoclonic–astatic absence (Doose syndrome)
Lennox-Gastaut syndrome

Generalized epilepsy with febrile seizures plus. Generalized epilepsy with febrile seizures plus (GEFS+) is a recently described disorder in which children have febrile seizures beyond the age at which febrile seizures usually stop (age 5 years) (Scheffer et al. 1997, 2005). In addition, these children may develop afebrile seizure types, including generalized tonic–clonic, absence, myoclonic, and atonic. Therefore, this syndrome is not the same as simple febrile seizures and represents a genetic predisposition to epilepsy. GEFS+ is transmitted in an autosomal dominant pattern with high penetrance. In different families, genetic defects have been identified in neuronal sodium channels and GABA receptors. In GEFS+, the outcome is variable: seizures resolve in some children, whereas in others, epilepsy persists. GEFS+ may be a spectrum of disorders with different phenotypes caused by sodium channel dysfunction. For example, the same sodium channel mutation (SCN1A) has been identified in GEFS+ and in severe myoclonic epilepsy of infancy (Dravet syndrome). Recent research has implicated SCN1A mutations in several cases of presumed vaccine encephalopathy (Berkovic et al. 2006).

Childhood absence epilepsy. Absence seizures can be part of several epilepsy syndromes, including childhood absence epilepsy (CAE), juvenile absence epilepsy, and juvenile myoclonic epilepsy (JME). CAE is characterized by typical absence seizures with an onset between 4 and 10 years of age. In CAE, absence seizures consist of staring, with altered alertness, sometimes with motor phenomena such as blinking or head nodding (Table 11.12). Because absence seizures are brief and nonconvulsive, they can be easily missed or misdiagnosed. Their recognition and treatment is important because frequent absence seizures can cause a decline in school performance or result in injury.

Clinical characteristics. The hallmark of a typical absence spell is the suppression of mental function, usually to the point of complete abolition of awareness, responsiveness, and memory. The seizures start abruptly and generally last from 5 to 15 seconds. Ongoing activity is suddenly interrupted, the facial expression changes, and the child stares off. When the seizure ends, the child immediately resumes her previous conversation or activity. There may be momentary confusion afterward, but no prolonged postictal state. Atypical absence seizures, usually seen in neurologically impaired children, involve an altered state of awareness or staring with an onset and cessation that is not as abrupt as a typical absence seizure. Atypical absences are often accompanied by automatisms, clonic movements, autonomic components, and changes in tone. Atypical absence seizures can last several minutes.

The frequency of absence seizures varies considerably, from a few per day to hundreds per day. Stress and fatigue can increase their frequency. Most children with typical absence seizures have a normal neurologic examination and intelligence, although school performance

Table 11.12 Absence seizures

Discriminating features
- Usually brief (<15 seconds)
- Ictal electroencephalograph (EEG) consists of 3-Hz generalized spike-waves

Consistent features
- Impairment of consciousness
- Abrupt onset and termination
- No aura or postictal period

Variable features
- Duration
- Automatisms
- Changes in body tone
- Responds to ethosuximide or valproate

may be impaired if seizures are frequent. GTC seizures later occur in 10–20% of patients with CAE.

Electroencephalography. The EEG background is normal. The ictal EEG pattern of an absence seizure consists of the sudden onset of generalized spike-wave complexes at a frequency of 3 Hz. For practical purposes, generalized spike-wave activity lasting longer than 1 second or so can be considered a seizure. Hyperventilation is a potent activator of absence seizures, and this simple test can be used in the clinic to diagnose absence seizures and assess treatment effectiveness. Failure to induce an absence attack with several trials of hyperventilation of 3- to 5-minutes duration in an untreated patient would make the diagnosis of absence seizures unlikely.

Unlike the usual 3 Hz spike-wave discharges of typical absence seizures, slower spike-wave discharges occurring at 1.5–2.5 Hz are more characteristic of atypical absence seizures. The interictal EEG is usually abnormal in children with atypical absences, many of whom have Lennox-Gastaut syndrome (see later section on Lennox Gastaut syndrome).

Etiology. The differential diagnosis of staring spells includes absence seizures, complex partial seizures, and inattention (Table 11.13). The pathophysiology of absence seizures involves altered function of thalamocortical circuits (Crunelli & Leresche 2002). CAE has a genetic basis, although a single gene mutation has not yet been found. Some families with CAE have been identified with GABA receptor loss-of-function mutations. EEG studies of families with CAE have shown age-related increased incidences of spike-wave abnormalities among asymptomatic siblings. Therefore, the EEG abnormality is a marker for genetic susceptibility to absence epilepsy, although the seizures will not manifest in everyone with the EEG trait. The EEG abnormality is the expression of an autosomal dominant gene with the unusual characteristic of having a very low penetrance at birth that rises to nearly complete penetrance during childhood before decreasing again.

Evaluation. In a child with typical absence seizures, a classic 3-Hz spike-wave ictal EEG, a normal interictal EEG, and a normal neurologic examination, no further diagnostic studies are necessary. If there is an abnormal developmental history, neurologic deficits, or focality on the EEG, a brain MRI scan is recommended. Because absence seizures are brief and subtle, their frequency is often underestimated. Each follow-up evaluation should include a trial of hyperventilation. Activation of a seizure by hyperventilation indicates that the seizures are not under optimal control, regardless of the history supplied by the parent or other observer.

Treatment. Ethosuximide and valproic acid (VPA) are equally effective in the treatment of absence seizures (Posner 2006). A child with CAE has a better than 70% chance of achieving seizure control on either drug. Ethosuximide is usually tried first, because of concerns about adverse reactions with VPA. VPA is the drug of choice in a child who has both absence and GTC seizures. The combination of ethosuximide and VPA sometimes works better than either drug alone, although signs of toxicity must be closely monitored. Lamotrigine is also effective in CAE.

Prognosis. The prognosis of CAE is good, with most children outgrowing the absence seizures during adolescence. However, at least 15% of children with CAE have persistent seizures or evolve into JME. A general guideline is to withdraw AEDs slowly after the child has been seizure free for 2 years and no longer has generalized spike-wave discharges on the EEG (including a hyperventilation trial). Spike-wave discharges on the routine EEG indicate a high recurrence risk if the medication is withdrawn.

Pearls and Perils

Absence Seizures

- A helpful test in the office to determine whether a child's absence seizures are well controlled is to have the child hyperventilate for 3 minutes (e.g., by blowing on a pinwheel). Failure to induce an absence attack indicates that the child's seizures are under satisfactory control.
- Most children who stare are not having a seizure. Staring as the sole manifestation of absence seizures is unusual; many children with absence seizures have other clinical changes during the seizure, such as eye blinking, facial clonus, or head nods.

Juvenile myoclonic epilepsy. Myoclonic seizures in children may occur as a component of an epilepsy syndrome

Table 11.13 Diagnosis of typical absence seizures and complex partial seizures

Clinical data	Absence seizures	Complex partial seizures
Frequency per day	Multiple	Rarely >1 or 2
Duration	Frequently less <10 seconds; rarely >30 seconds	Average duration >1 minute; rarely <10 seconds
Aura	Never	Frequently
Onset and termination	Abrupt	Gradual
Eye blinking	Common	Occasionally
Automatisms	Common	Frequently
Postictal impairment	None	Common
Seizures activated by:		
Hyperventilation	Very frequently	Occasionally
Photic stimulation	Frequently	Rarely
EEG:		
Ictal	Generalized spike-wave	Usually unilateral or bilateral temporal or frontal discharges
Interictal	Usually normal	Variable; may be spikes or sharp waves in frontal or temporal lobes

known as JME (Table 11.14) (Welty 2006). JME typically begins in adolescence, and 15% of JME cases evolve from CAE. The myoclonic seizures in JME involve jerks of the neck, shoulders, or arms, occurring singly or repetitively. The myoclonic jerks may cause the patient to drop objects, which may be attributed to nervousness or clumsiness. The myoclonic seizures most often occur shortly after awakening from sleep and are exacerbated by fatigue, sleep deprivation, and alcohol use.

GTC seizures also occur in as many as 90% of patients with JME, and the syndrome often presents with a GTC seizure. GTC seizures also occur soon after awakening. Sometimes a series of myoclonic seizures culminates in a GTC seizure. Up to 35% of patients with JME also have absence seizures.

The neurologic examination and intelligence are usually normal in JME. Multifactorial inheritance is presumed. Studies have linked the syndrome to chromosome 6p, a locus that appears to be dominantly inherited.

The interictal EEG in JME shows characteristic bursts of fast (3.5–6 Hz) spike-waves. This pattern contrasts with the 3-Hz spike waves seen in childhood absence epilepsy and the slow (1.5–2.5 Hz) spike-waves of Lennox-Gastaut syndrome. Photic stimulation may activate the epileptiform discharges in JME. If the diagnosis is suspected and the awake EEG is normal, a sleep-deprived EEG should be obtained.

VPA is the treatment of choice for JME, although other broad-spectrum AEDs (e.g., lamotrigine, topiramate) may be effective. The seizures in JME often respond quite promptly to VPA, but long-term treatment is required. Patients rarely tolerate drug withdrawal and seizures rarely remit spontaneously, hence treatment during childbearing years will likely be necessary; this will influence AED choice. JME is considered relatively benign because most patients continue to exhibit normal neurologic function. However, some myoclonic epilepsies are progressive (Conry 2002).

Cryptogenic or symptomatic generalized epilepsy syndromes

Infantile spasms. Infantile spasms (IS) is an epilepsy syndrome characterized by seizures known as epileptic spasms, an interictal EEG pattern called *hypsarhythmia*, and mental retardation (Fukuyama 2001) (Table 11.15). This triad is known as *West syndrome*. IS is an age-specific disorder beginning primarily in the first year of life, with a peak age of onset between 4 and 6 months. The underlying pathophysiology of this developmental epilepsy syndrome is unknown; IS may represent alteration of the developing brain's stress response or age-specific hyperexcitability due to immature neurotransmitter function (Brunson et al 2002; Frost & Hrachovy 2005).

Clinical characteristics. The epileptic spasms of IS vary considerably, and the diagnosis is often delayed due

Table 11.14 Juvenile myoclonic epilepsy

Discriminating features
- Bursts of generalized fast spike-wave discharges (4–6 Hz) on electroencephalograph (EEG)

Consistent features
- Myoclonic jerks, especially in the morning
- Onset in adolescence
- Normal examination and intelligence
- Responds to valproic acid

Variable features
- Photic sensitivity
- Generalized tonic–clonic seizures

to their subtle features. The duration of a spasm is intermediate between a myoclonic jerk (which is briefer) and a tonic seizure (which is more sustained). Some seizures are characterized by brief head nods, whereas others consist of forceful flexion or extension of the trunk and limbs. The epileptic spasms may be predominantly flexor, extensor, or mixed flexor-extensor. The seizures characteristically occur in a cluster of a few to tens of individual spasms. The number of clusters varies up to 50 or more per day. Spasms typically occur during sleep transitions, especially upon awakening.

Differential diagnosis. Several disorders may be confused with infantile spasms. IS is often misdiagnosed as colic or another nonepileptic phenomenon. In *benign myoclonus of early infancy*, infants have clusters of tonic or myoclonic movements, but unlike infants with IS, these children are normal neurologically and developmentally, have normal EEGs, and the movements stop by 18 months of age. *Benign neonatal sleep myoclonus* consists of erratic myoclonic jerks only when the child is asleep. The jerks are usually quicker than IS. The myoclonus occurs during non-REM sleep and stops upon awakening; neurologic function and EEG are normal and treatment is unnecessary.

Electroencephalography. The interictal EEG in children with IS is called hypsarhythmia, which consists of a disorganized, "chaotic" pattern of very-high-voltage slow waves and spikes in multiple cortical areas. Variants include hypsarhythmia that is more prominent over one hemisphere or the presence of a focus of spikes. The ictal EEG pattern is a generalized slow wave followed by background voltage attenuation in all channels (electrodecrement), usually accompanied by a clinical spasm.

Etiology. IS cases are conventionally classified into those in which there is no identified preceding neurologic disorder or etiology (cryptogenic) and those in which there is a preexisting pathologic event or disorder (symptomatic). With modern neuroimaging and other diagnostic modalities, the proportion of cryptogenic cases is decreasing: less than 20% of cases are currently considered cryptogenic.

Table 11.15 Infantile spasms

Discriminating features
- The clustering of infantile spasms differentiates them from tonic or myoclonic seizures
- Interictal electroencephalograph (EEG) pattern usually demonstrates hypsarhythmia or modified hypsarhythmia

Consistent features
- Begin in the first year of life
- Each spasm is brief (<5 seconds)
- Responds to treatment with adrenocorticotrophic hormone or vigabatrin

Variable features
- Clinical spasms may be flexor, extensor, or, most commonly, mixed flexor and extensor
- Responds to valproate, clonazepam, or topiramate
- Developmental stagnation or regression (more likely if symptomatic etiology)

Pearls and Perils

Infantile Spasms

- Drugs that work in infantile spasms usually do so within days of starting therapy.
- If the spasms have a focal onset, a surgical evaluation should be considered.

Several specific conditions are associated with IS. Common etiologies include hypoxic–ischemic encephalopathy, neonatal intracranial hemorrhage, meningitis or encephalitis, congenital infection, developmental anomaly of the CNS, and metabolic disease. *Tuberous sclerosis complex* (TSC) is associated with an especially high incidence of infantile spasms (up to 50% of TSC patients) (Holmes & Stafstrom 2007).

Evaluation. An infant who presents with IS requires a thorough developmental assessment, neurologic examination, and laboratory studies. The neurodevelopmental status at the time of diagnosis is an important indicator of prognosis. Every child with the possible diagnosis should have an EEG and neuroimaging. A normal EEG (including sleep) would suggest that the child has benign myoclonus of early infancy rather than IS, although in some affected children, hypsarhythmia develops after the onset of spasms. An MRI scan may uncover a brain anomaly such as cortical dysplasia.

In children in whom an etiology cannot be established definitively, an infusion of 50–100 mg pyridoxine intravenously during EEG monitoring may be useful. Infants with pyridoxine dependency should have an improvement in the seizures and EEG within minutes. Infants with frequent vomiting, lethargy, failure to thrive, peculiar odors, and unexplained neurologic findings should have urine amino and organic acid screening, serum ammonia and liver function tests. Because many children will be treated with adrenocorticotropic hormone (ACTH), analysis of electrolytes, calcium, phosphorous, glucose, and urine should be obtained. Examination of the spinal fluid (CSF), including CSF glycine, is indicated if there is concern about an active infection or a metabolic disorder.

Treatment. In the United States, ACTH and corticosteroids have been the primary drugs used to treat IS (Mackay et al. 2002, 2004). The anticonvulsant mechanism of ACTH is not known; it may work via the hypothalamic–pituitary axis or directly decrease neuronal membrane excitability (Brunson et al. 2002).

The effects of ACTH on long-term outcome are controversial. Several authors have found no developmental differences as a function of treatment. For infants with preexisting brain damage, it is unlikely that any form of therapy will greatly influence the long-range mental and motor outcome. An important question is whether treatment of cryptogenic IS in children who were normal before the onset of seizures alters outcome. Long-term studies on infants with cryptogenic IS who received either ACTH, oral steroids, or other AEDs, show that those who received ACTH had a lower incidence of seizures and better psychomotor development.

There is no consensus about the optimal ACTH dosage regimen or treatment duration. A commonly used protocol uses a starting dose of nonsynthetic ACTH gel 40 international units (IU) per day given intramuscularly. The response to ACTH can be dramatic, with cessation of seizures and EEG improvement within a few days. ACTH is given for 1 month following the cessation of seizures. At that time, a taper is begun, decreasing the dosage by 10 units per week. If the seizures do not completely resolve by 2 weeks, the dosage should be increased by 10 IU increments each week until the seizures cease or a daily dose of 80 IU is reached. If, at that point, the seizures persist, VPA, topiramate, or a benzodiazepine can be tried. If relapse occurs during the taper or after ACTH discontinuation, ACTH can be restarted at the dosage that originally stopped the spasms.

Adverse ACTH side effects include cushingoid obesity, growth retardation, acne, and irritability. Serious side effects include infection, hypertension, cardiomyopathy, osteoporosis, gastrointestinal bleeding, and electrolyte disturbances. Monitoring should include twice weekly blood pressure and stool guaiac checks and weekly serum electrolytes. If the child develops hypertension or hypokalemic alkalosis, a reduction in dosage is warranted. Some children require salt restriction or antihypertensives. Fever should be investigated promptly, as infections are more likely during steroid-induced immunosuppression. Tuberculosis testing and urine culture for cytomegalovirus (CMV) should be obtained prior to initiating ACTH therapy.

A recent exponential increase in the cost of ACTH gel has prompted physicians to reconsider other modes of therapy (Baram et al. 1996). One protocol consists of oral steroids (prednisolone) 40–60 mg daily with a tapering regimen over several weeks (Lux et al. 2005). Vigabatrin, a selective inhibitor of GABA-transaminase, exerts a favorable effect on IS, especially in children with TSC. Vigabatrin is not approved for use in the United States. There have been some reports of vigabatrin-induced visual field defects. Other therapies that have been reported to be beneficial in the treatment of IS are topiramate, benzodiazepines, VPA, and the ketogenic diet.

Infants whose spasms have a consistent focal onset may benefit from resective surgery. A structural lesion such as focal dysgenesis may correlate with the focal EEG and clinical features. Some infants with cryptogenic infantile spasms and normal MRI scans have deficits of cerebral metabolism (detected by PET). When this area of cortical hypometabolism is removed under the guidance of intraoperative corticography, the seizures may be reduced or eliminated (Shields 2006). This is also true in cases of tuberous sclerosis.

Prognosis. As an epileptic encephalopathy, the prognosis of IS is poor (Riikonen 2001). Many affected children have psychomotor retardation and persistent seizures. With age, the seizures often change from spasms to mixed seizures of the types seen in Lennox-Gastaut syndrome. About two-thirds of affected children are mentally retarded and have motor impairment. Because a large number of children have neurologic impairment before the onset of the spasms, it is not surprising that the outcome is so poor. Prognosis is directly related to etiology, with cryptogenic cases having a significantly better prognosis than symptomatic ones.

Lennox-Gastaut syndrome. Lennox-Gastaut syndrome (LGS) is a generalized epilepsy syndrome in which children have frequent, medically intractable seizures (up to hundreds per day) (Wheless & Constantinou 1997). LGS is characterized by a slow spike-wave EEG pattern (<3 Hz), mental retardation, and multiple seizure types (Table 11.16). Most children with LGS also have motor impairments.

Clinical characteristics. LGS begins between the ages of 1 and 6 years. Seizure types include tonic, GTC, atypical absence, atonic, or myoclonic. Tonic seizures consist of periods of sustained muscle contractions accompanied by altered consciousness. These are especially frequent during sleep. Atonic (astatic) seizures, or drop attacks, occur without warning. If standing, the child will lose tone and fall to the floor. Head or facial injuries often occur, and these children often need to wear a protective helmet. Head drops can occur singly or in a series of head nods. Consciousness is momentarily impaired, but the child regains alertness promptly.

Atypical absence seizures occur frequently in children with LGS. These have a gradual onset and cessation, and may involve clonic components, automatisms, autonomic changes, and myoclonic jerks. Atypical absences may be prolonged, during which the child has a dull, confused appearance with drooling and behavioral arrest. It is often difficult to tell when one seizure ends and the next one begins, because alertness and activity level do not improve between the absences. GTC seizures also occur in children with LGS, usually at night or during sleep transitions.

Electroencephalography. The characteristic EEG finding in LGS is generalized slow spike-wave discharges,

Table 11.16 Lennox-Gastaut syndrome

Discriminating features
- Tonic seizures during sleep

Consistent features
- Severe, mixed seizures
- Mental retardation
- Slow spike-wave discharges on electroencephalogram (EEG)

Variable features
- Types of seizures (usually tonic, myoclonic, atypical absence, generalized tonic–clonic)
- Frequency of seizures
- Symptomatic or idiopathic etiology

at a frequency of 1.5–2.5 Hz. These discharges occur in long runs during wakefulness and are even more frequent in sleep.

Etiology. Children with LGS are already neurologically or mentally handicapped. The etiology may uncertain (cryptogenic) or result from a definable etiology, such as hypoxic brain injury, cerebral dysgenesis, or a neurocutaneous disorder. The etiologies of LGS overlap those of IS. The majority of children with symptomatic LGS have a static encephalopathy, although children with a degenerative disorder such as neuronal ceroid lipofuscinosis can also present with LGS.

Evaluation. In the absence of an obvious medical condition, the child needs to be thoroughly evaluated, with the specific evaluation guided by the history and physical examination. In view of the devastating nature of the syndrome, every effort should be made to rule out a treatable disorder. Abnormalities on neuroimaging are common, especially cortical or subcortical atrophy or dysplasia.

Treatment. Children with LGS are notoriously refractory to AEDs (Conry 2004; Hancock & Cross 2003). Because the syndrome is heterogeneous, variability occurs in responsiveness to AEDs. Drug therapy should be individualized to address the types and frequency of seizures in each child. Children with LGS may benefit from VPA, clonazepam, lamotrigine, or topiramate, or some combination of these. Felbamate is reserved for particularly refractory cases and tends to be an activating rather than a sedating drug. Because of the intractable nature of the seizures, there is a tendency to place the children on numerous AEDs. This polypharmaceutical approach usually results in drug toxicity with somnolence, fatigue, nausea, ataxia, and rarely optimal seizure control.

Prognosis. Children with LGS have a poor neurologic prognosis. Over time, the atonic, myoclonic, and atypical absence seizures may decrease, but GTC seizures increase and partial seizures emerge. In addition to debilitating seizures, intellectual impairment hinders children with LGS from leading independent lives. Some children have a progressive deterioration in mental function despite vigorous attempts to control their seizures.

Pearls and Perils

Lennox-Gastaut Syndrome

- Complete seizure control in children with Lennox-Gastaut syndrome is unlikely. Avoid the temptation to place the patient on multiple antiepileptic drugs (AEDs). Usually one or two drugs work better than three or four.
- Daily seizure frequency varies considerably in patients with Lennox-Gastaut syndrome. Avoid changing AEDs too quickly.

Localization-related epilepsy syndromes

Idiopathic localization-related epilepsy syndromes

Rolandic epilepsy (benign childhood epilepsy with centrotemporal spikes). Rolandic epilepsy (RE) is a common, distinctive epilepsy syndrome of childhood characterized by seizures arising from the lower central sulcus of Rolando (Table 11.17) (Gobbi et al. 2006). The evaluation and prognosis of a child with RE differs considerably from other, less benign focal epilepsies.

Clinical characteristics. Seizures typically begin between the ages of 5 and 11 years and usually remit in early adolescence. Children have a normal neurologic examination and normal intellectual function. The classic presentation is a nocturnal seizure with clonic movements of the mouth and face, salivation, and garbled or arrested speech, but maintained consciousness. Motor phenomena during RE attacks are usually restricted to one side of the body, typically the face, but sometimes affect the arm or leg. This simple partial seizure may secondarily generalize. Little or no postictal state is present. Seizures of RE are distinguishable from partial complex seizures because they lack automatisms, auras, hallucinations, and affective symptoms.

Electroencephalography. The classic interictal EEG shows a normal background with superimposed high-amplitude spike-wave complexes, which occur singly or in brief runs over one or both midtemporal and central (rolandic) regions. Rolandic spikes are not diagnostic of epilepsy and may occur in children without a seizure history.

Genetics. RE has a strong familial occurrence (Neubauer 2002). The EEG trait, but not the clinical syndrome, is inherited as autosomal dominant, with age-dependency and incomplete penetrance. About half of first-degree relatives demonstrate the EEG abnormality between the ages of 5 and 15 years. Before 5 and after 15

Table 11.17 Rolandic epilepsy

Discriminating features
- Partial seizures with or without secondary generalization
- Unilateral or bilateral independent central-temporal spikes

Consistent features
- Begins before 13 years of age; not seen after second decade
- Nocturnal generalized tonic–clonic seizures or diurnal seizures, or both, with clinical signs referable to the lower rolandic region (speech arrest, facial clonus, and sometimes tonic–clonic activity of ipsilateral upper extremity)
- Normal neurologic examination
- Benign prognosis

Variable features
- Responds to carbamazepine and most other antiepileptic drugs (AEDs)
- Seizures may occur day, night, or both
- Electroencephalographic abnormality may be seen during wakefulness, sleep, or both

years of age, penetrance is low, with few patients exhibiting the EEG abnormality. Only about 12% of children who inherit the EEG abnormality develop seizures.

Evaluation. If the child has a clinical history and EEG characteristic of RE, plus a normal neurologic examination, further workup is not necessary. If the neurologic examination is abnormal or the EEG demonstrates any atypical features, a brain MRI is warranted.

Treatment and prognosis. Since the seizures of RE are benign and often infrequent, many clinicians do not treat the first or even the second seizure. Seizures are usually controlled with a single AED, such as carbamazepine (usually the first choice), phenytoin, or VPA. The efficacy of the newer AEDs in RE is not known. In Europe, sulthiame has proven effective in clinical trials.

Pearls and Perils

Rolandic Epilepsy (RE)

- Children with RE and a normal neurologic examination do not require neuroimaging. However, if seizures do not respond to antiepileptic drugs (AEDs), focal slowing develops on electroencephalogram (EEG), or the neurologic examination changes, a magnetic resonance imaging (MRI) scan should be obtained.
- RE has a strong genetic basis.
- Many children with RE have only one or two clinical seizures, and AED treatment may not be necessary in every case.

Treatment is recommended for 1–2 years before the AED is tapered. Resolution of the EEG abnormalities is a favorable sign. Children usually outgrow both seizures and EEG abnormalities around adolescence. Long-term prognosis is usually excellent, although caution is advised if atypical clinical or electrographic features are present.

Benign childhood epilepsy with occipital paroxysms. Benign childhood epilepsy with occipital paroxysms (BCEOP, Gastaut syndrome) resembles RE in that focal seizures occur in neurologically normal children who tend to outgrow their epilepsy before adulthood. The syndromes differ in the localization of the epileptiform discharges and the phenomenology of the seizures. In BCEOP, the peak age of seizure onset is between 5 and 9 years. The seizures consist of elementary visual phenomena such as hallucinations, illusions, blindness, or phosphenes, although any seizure type may occur. Progression to a hemiclonic seizure is common. A seizure is often followed by a migraine headache. Interictal occipital rhythmic spikes are maximal upon eye closure. A genetic etiology is assumed.

Panayiotopoulos syndrome is a variant of BCEOP, seen in slightly younger children (3–7 years old) (Panayiotopoulos 2002). Nocturnal seizures predominate, accompanied by eye deviation and vomiting, but description of visual phenomena may be minimal. This syndrome also remits by adolescence. Both BCEOP and Panayiotopoulos syndrome are commonly associated with migraine, and these disorders may share a similar pathogenetic mechanism (Andermann & Zifkin 1998).

Symptomatic localization-related epilepsy syndromes

Symptomatic localization-related epilepsy syndromes are those that arise in a particular region of brain due to an acquired or congenital lesion. Etiologies include tumors, gliosis (e.g., hippocampal sclerosis), cortical dysplasias, porencephalic cysts (resulting from perinatal infarction), and vascular malformations. Seizure features are related to the region of brain affected; usually, the seizures will begin as simple partial or complex partial and then generalize secondarily. The EEG may show focal spikes, sharp waves, or slowing, related to the area of brain involved.

These syndromes are sometimes divided into those originating in the neocortex or mesial temporal structures. In children, a neocortical localization is more common, whereas in adults, the mesial temporal lobe is a frequent epileptogenic site. Neocortical etiologies in children may include low-grade neoplasms and a wide spectrum of migrational abnormalities and developmental dysplasias. Epilepsy of temporal lobe origin can occur in children, often associated with hippocampal sclerosis, which can be caused by a prolonged seizure or other genetic or developmental lesions (Bourgeois 1998; Guerrini

2006). Research is in progress to determine if febrile seizures are a cause of hippocampal sclerosis.

Some important childhood localization-related epilepsy syndromes involve an entire hemisphere. *Rasmussen encephalitis* is a focal encephalitis that affects only one hemisphere and results in progressive hemiparesis, intractable epilepsy (partial seizures that may progress to epilepsia partialis continua), and cognitive decline. The etiology of Rasmussen encephalitis is unknown but it might have an autoimmune basis, with antibodies developing to certain glutamate receptor subunits (McNamara et al. 1999). The unilateral pathology may be due to focal breakdown of the blood–brain barrier. Neuroimaging shows progressive unilateral cortical atrophy. Another hemispheric syndrome, *Sturge-Weber syndrome* (encephalotrigeminal angiomatosis), consists of a hemispheric vascular malformation, leading to intractable epilepsy and hemiparesis. The degree of cerebral involvement is reflected by the degree of facial angiomatosis. Some authorities recommend early surgery (hemispherectomy) to afford a better prognosis in the hemispheric localization-related epilepsy syndromes.

Indeterminate epilepsy syndromes

Neonatal seizures. Neonatal seizures are classified as "indeterminate" because the typical seizure types in newborns do not conform to the ILAE scheme. Seizures may be the first and only sign of central nervous system (CNS) dysfunction in a newborn, so their recognition is critical. Despite advances in obstetrics and perinatal care, many infants with neonatal seizures have a poor neurologic outcome.

Clinical characteristics. Seizures in the neonatal period (first 30 days of life) differ considerably from those in older children and adults (Table 11.18) (Stafstrom 1995; Silverstein & Jensen 2007). Due to immature myelination and cortical organization, the neonatal brain is unable to sustain generalized epileptiform discharges, so GTC seizures rarely, if ever, occur in neonates, and absence seizures never do.

Neonatal seizures are classified clinically into four types, based on behavioral manifestations: subtle, generalized tonic, focal or multifocal clonic, and myoclonic. Subtle seizures may include repetitive oral-buccal-lingual movements such as sucking, pedaling movements of the legs or arms, eye deviation, nystagmus, or apnea. Subtle seizures are often associated with severe CNS insults. Neonatal tonic seizures resemble decerebrate or opisthotonic posturing with intermittent tonic extension of the arms and legs; they are usually associated with severe brain lesions and most often occur in preterm infants. Clonic seizures consist of rhythmic jerking of groups of muscles in a focal or multifocal pattern. In multifocal clonic seizures, movements may migrate from one part of the body to another. Focal seizures may be seen with localized brain malformations or insults, such as a perinatal stroke, as well as in disorders that diffusely affect the brain, such as asphyxia, metabolic derangement, or infection. Myoclonic seizures are similar to those seen in older children, with rapid isolated jerks, occurring either focally or bilaterally.

Simultaneous video-EEG monitoring can differentiate behaviors with an EEG correlate ("epileptic seizures") from behaviors that do not have associated EEG changes (Table 11.19) (Mizrahi & Kellaway 1987). Focal clonic seizures have the highest correlation with EEG ictal abnormalities. Many behaviors considered to be subtle seizures on clinical grounds (for example, chewing or pedaling movements) are not associated with EEG abnormalities,

Table 11.18 Neonatal seizures

Discriminating features
- Occurrence in first 30 days of life
- May be difficult to differentiate from nonepileptic behavior without the aid of electroencephalographic monitoring

Consistent features
- Stereotyped activity with clear onset and cessation

Variable features
- Clinical manifestations are variable; may consist of focal clonic, multifocal clonic, tonic, or myoclonic seizures, subtle manifestations, or autonomic dysfunction
- Associated with virtually any insult to the neonatal brain
- Responds to antiepileptic drugs (AEDs)

Pearls and Perils

Neonatal Seizures

- All neonates with unexplained seizures must have a lumbar puncture to rule out meningitis.
- Pyridoxine should be given to every neonate with seizures when the etiology has not been determined or standard antiepileptic drugs (AEDs) fail.
- Although rare, apnea may be the sole manifestation of a seizure in a neonate.
- Neonatal seizures may be over- or underdiagnosed. When there is doubt, it is better to withhold AED treatment.
- In neonatal seizures, the priority should be to determine the etiology rather than rushing to treat.
- When treating neonatal seizures with phenobarbital, it usually takes a full 15–20 mg/kg loading dose to reach a therapeutic level; giving two 10 mg/kg boluses separated in time often undertreats the seizures.
- It is prudent to have intubation equipment ready when treating neonates with seizures.

suggesting that these behaviors are not epileptic in nature. Subtle seizures may represent "brainstem release" phenomena or epileptic seizures originating from deep subcortical structures not recordable on surface EEG. In either case, subtle seizures often reflect severe CNS dysfunction. Apnea alone is rarely the sole manifestation of a neonatal seizure. Myoclonic and tonic events have a variable relationship to EEG abnormalities.

Neonatal jitteriness must be distinguished from neonatal seizures (Rosman et al. 1984). *Jitteriness* is an intermittent involuntary movement of the limbs that may mimic a seizure. The movements resemble a coarse tremor of the limbs and are not accompanied by eye deviation. The movements can be spontaneous or evoked by limb movement, and can be suppressed by passive flexion of an involved extremity. Jitteriness often appears in the context of other CNS excitation, such as irritability and excessive startle. It is often seen in infants of substance-abusing mothers and in hypoxic–ischemic encephalopathy. The etiologies of seizures and jitteriness overlap, but in jitteriness the EEG does not show epileptiform abnormalities.

Table 11.19 Classification of neonatal seizures

Seizures with a close association to electroencephalographic (EEG) seizure discharges
Focal clonic
Unifocal
Multifocal
Alternating
Migrating
Hemiconvulsive
Axial
Myoclonic
Focal tonic
Apnea
Seizures with an inconsistent or no relationship to EEG seizure discharges
Motor automatisms
Oral-buccal-lingual movements
Ocular signs
Progression movements
Pedaling
Stepping
Rotary arm movements
Generalized tonic
Extensor
Flexor
Mixed flexor/extensor
Myoclonic
Generalized
Focal
Fragmentary

From Mizrahi EM Kellaway P. Characterization and classification of neonatal seizures. *Neurology* 1987;37:1837–1844, with permission.

Electroencephalography. The neonatal EEG is usually not specific for a particular etiology, but it may provide clues about the severity and time course of a CNS insult. The EEG may support the clinical diagnosis of seizures in infants with atypical or minimal behavioral manifestations if the recording includes the episode in question. The EEG may also document seizure discharges that are not accompanied by overt clinical manifestations ("uncoupling" of electrographic and clinical seizures, or "electroclinical dissociation"). In infants who are paralyzed and dependent on respiratory support, the EEG may be the only objective means for assessing cerebral function and determining the presence of seizure activity. For prognostic purposes, EEG background patterns and sleep–wake cycles are especially important.

Etiology. Establishing the etiology of a neonatal seizure is critical because the cause determines the therapy and is highly correlated with outcome. Major causes of neonatal seizures are hypoxia–ischemia, hypocalcemia, hypoglycemia, hyponatremia, intracranial hemorrhage, infection, congenital malformations, genetic factors, inherited metabolic disorders, and drug withdrawal. Hypoxia–ischemia is the most common cause of neonatal seizures. Most asphyxia occurs before delivery (20% of cases), during delivery (35%), or a combination of antepartum and intrapartum (35%); only 10% of cases result from postnatal causes. Timing of the seizure is related to etiology. Seizures due to hypoxia–ischemia usually occur in the first day of life; those caused by metabolic derangements begin in the first few days; whereas those secondary to cortical malformations do not appear until several weeks of life or later.

Treatment. After ventilation and adequate glucose levels are ensured, initial goals are to establish the underlying cause and institute appropriate therapy. Metabolic derangements should be corrected and antibiotics given when appropriate. The decision to treat an infant with recurrent seizures is based on the seizure duration and frequency, associated autonomic dysfunction, etiology, and EEG abnormalities. If seizures are brief and not associated with autonomic instability, treatment may be deferred or a short-acting benzodiazepine used. Conversely, neonates with frequent seizures, especially if they interfere with ventilation, require prompt and vigorous treatment.

Phenobarbital is the primary drug used to treat neonatal seizures, despite its limited effectiveness (Sankar & Painter 2005). The initial loading dose is 20 mg/kg intravenously with a maintenance dosage of 5–6 mg/kg per day, given once or twice daily. Most infants require serum levels between 10 and 40 mg/dL to suppress seizures, but the dose is often pushed higher before resorting to polytherapy. Serum levels above 40 mg/dL may result in lethargy.

If phenobarbital is ineffective, a second drug is added (usually fosphenytoin). As in older children, phenytoin follows nonlinear kinetics in the newborn period. The drug is usually administered in two boluses of 10 mg/kg intravenously, which results in a blood level of 15–20 mg/dL. Phenytoin is poorly absorbed from the gastrointestinal tract of newborns and it is often difficult to maintain therapeutic levels using the oral route; 8 mg/kg per day or higher is sometimes required to obtain a therapeutic level. Commonly, phenobarbital or phenytoin will suppress clinical seizures but the baby continues to have electrographic seizures ("uncoupling") (Scher et al. 2003). In such cases, the physician must decide, in the context of the clinical situation, how far to push medications to suppress electrographic seizures. In infants with refractory seizures, a trial of pyridoxine (50–100 mg intravenously) should be administered with concurrent EEG monitoring (Gospe 2002).

Diazepam and lorazepam are commonly used to treat neonatal seizures. A diazepam dose of 0.2–0.5 mg/kg intravenously is recommended for the acute management of neonatal seizures. Due to its short distribution phase, diazepam is not an optimal maintenance AED.

There is little information about the efficacy of the newer AEDs in neonatal seizures. In general, AEDs should be weaned once seizures stop and medical abnormalities are corrected, preferably before the infant is discharged from the nursery.

Neonatal epilepsy syndromes. Most neonatal seizures are reactions of the brain to a neurologic insult. However, several neonatal epilepsy syndromes have been defined (Mizrahi 2001). The syndrome of benign familial neonatal convulsions was discussed earlier.

Early myoclonic encephalopathy (EME) is characterized by sporadic and erratic fragmentary myoclonus, usually in combination with other seizure types. The EEG shows burst suppression. A variety of etiologies has been associated with EME, including metabolic diseases, cerebral dysgenesis, and hypoxic–ischemic insults. The prognosis is very poor. Most infants die within a year or survive with severe neurologic sequelae. Another syndrome with myoclonic seizures, severe myoclonic epilepsy of infancy (SMEI, Dravet syndrome) was discussed earlier under Idiopathic Generalized Epilepsy Syndromes.

Ohtahara syndrome, or *early infantile epileptic encephalopathy (EIEE)*, begins in early infancy, with severe, frequent tonic seizures and burst suppression on the EEG. Affected infants have severe developmental deficits. EIEE may evolve into West syndrome. As with EME, a host of etiologies has been described in EIEE, but cerebral dysgenesis is the most common association.

Landau-Kleffner syndrome

Landau-Kleffner syndrome (LKS; acquired epileptic aphasia) is a rare epilepsy in which a child loses previously acquired language abilities and has seizures or epileptiform abnormalities on EEG (Table 11.20) (Ballaban-Gil & Tuchman 2000; Landau & Kleffner 1957; Nieuwenhuis & Nicolai 2006). In its pure form, LKS occurs in previously normal children with normal language development, who gradually lose the ability to understand spoken language and produce speech. Recently, some authors have expanded the syndrome to include behavioral and cognitive deterioration, including symptoms seen in autistic spectrum disorders. Regression of social and language skills is frequently seen in children with autism, with or without accompanying seizures, so the differentiation of autism and LKS can be difficult. In LKS, compared to autism, social skills are better preserved. The pathophysiology of LKS is unknown. Imaging studies are generally negative although recent PET studies have shown bitemporal abnormalities, supporting the hypothesis that language-related brain regions are dysfunctional in LKS.

EEG abnormalities in LKS may include generalized, focal, or multifocal spikes, spike-waves, or sharp waves. If focal, the discharges commonly involve one or both temporal or temporoparietal (perisylvian) regions. The hypothesis has arisen that the epileptiform discharges interfere with language production, although it is possible that both the language dysfunction and EEG abnormalities are independent consequences of the same underlying brain pathology. Successful treatment of the seizures or even the EEG discharges is not usually accompanied by language or behavioral improvement. The outcome is quite variable; some children recover completely, usually in adolescence, whereas others have persistent aphasia in adulthood.

Evaluation should include hearing assessment, an overnight EEG, and a MRI scan of brain. The seizures usually respond readily to AEDs, whereas the language impairment does not. Attempts to treat children with steroids or subpial resection have been controversial.

Table 11.20 Landau-Kleffner syndrome (LKS)

Discriminating features
- Loss of language following a period of normal language development

Consistent features
- Loss of receptive language ("word deafness") precedes loss of expressive language

Variable features
- Autistic behaviors; compared to autism, social skills are better preserved in LKS
- Electroencephalographic (EEG) findings
- Responds to antiepileptic drugs
- Age of language loss (usually age 5–7 years)

Electrical status epilepticus of sleep (ESES; Continuous spike-wave discharges during slow-wave sleep or CSWDS)

ESES is an electrographic diagnosis and CSWDS is considered the electroclinical syndrome (Tassinari et al. 2000). Children have normal language development prior to the onset of seizures, which are usually partial-complex in type, followed by language and cognitive or behavioral deterioration. The cognitive changes may range from inattention to psychosis. The EEG shows a fairly normal background during wakefulness and rapid eye movement (REM) sleep, but more than 85% of the slow-wave sleep (non-REM) record consists of generalized spike-wave discharges (although focal spikes or fragmentary generalized spike-wave can be seen during wakefulness). These discharges are often slow (1.5–2 Hz) and have a frontocentral predominance. The cognitive and behavioral deterioration is often less dramatic than in children with LKS, and ESES often remits during adolescence. Similar treatment options are used in ESES and LKS. Carbamazepine may worsen the syndrome. The outcome of ESES is quite variable; some children eventually regain normal language function.

Special syndromes (situation related)

Febrile seizures. Febrile seizures occur in children from about 6 months to 5 years of age and represent an age-dependent response of the developing brain to fever (Baram & Shinnar 2002; Dubé et al 2007). A genetic association exists, with febrile seizures occurring two to three times more frequently in affected families than in the general population. Overall, febrile seizures occur in 2–5% of children in the susceptible age range. Seizures with fever before or after those ages suggest a different cause.

Clinical characteristics. The two main types of febrile seizures are: (a) simple and (b) complex or complicated. (The term "complicated" is preferred, to avoid confusion with complex partial seizures). Simple febrile seizures are brief (<15 minutes), generalized, and do not recur within 24 hours of the first one. Simple febrile seizures usually occur in neurologically normal children. Complicated febrile seizures are either prolonged (>15 minutes), the seizures have focal components (e.g., the seizure begins on one side of the body or there is lateralized eye deviation), or another seizure occurs within 24 hours of the initial one. Simple and complicated febrile seizures differ in their prognosis and in the risk for development of epilepsy.

Differential diagnosis and evaluation. In a child presenting with fever and seizure, there are three possibilities: febrile seizure, seizure secondary to meningitis or intracranial infection, or underlying epilepsy unmasked by the fever. If the seizure was brief, the child promptly returns to baseline mental status, and a source of fever is identified (e.g., otitis media or gastroenteritis), a simple febrile seizure is the most likely cause and an extensive evaluation is not necessary. On the other hand, if a concern exists about persistent lethargy or diminished responsiveness, a lumbar puncture should be performed to rule out meningitis or encephalitis. In a complicated febrile seizure, especially if there is focality to the seizure, a neuroimaging study should be performed to rule out an intracranial injury, stroke, mass, or dysplasia. A head CT scan will rule out an acute bleed, but an MRI scan is preferred to evaluate for cortical malformations and dysplasia. In a simple febrile seizure, an EEG will usually be unrevealing, whereas in a complicated febrile seizure, an EEG is useful to evaluate for focal spikes or slowing.

Treatment. Simple febrile seizures do not require treatment, nor do most complicated febrile seizures. For a child with prolonged febrile seizures, diazepam can be administered rectally or midazolam intranasally for seizures lasting 5 minutes or more. For children with frequent febrile seizures, intermittent oral diazepam can be given for the duration of the fever only, at a dose of 0.3 mg/kg every 8 hours. Only in exceptional circumstances would prophylactic medication be prescribed, and usually only if there is concern about epilepsy rather than febrile seizures. Only phenobarbital and VPA have been shown to be effective in preventing febrile seizures; the newer AEDs have not been studied systematically.

Prognosis. A child who has had a single simple febrile seizure has about a 33% chance of another febrile seizure with a subsequent fever (50% chance if the first febrile seizure occurs at less than 12 months of age). If a child has had two simple febrile seizures, there is about a 50% chance of a third febrile seizure. The recurrence risk for additional febrile seizures is greatest if a child has had a first febrile seizure under 12 months of age or there is a family history of febrile seizures.

Concern is greatest not for recurrent febrile seizures, but rather for the development of afebrile seizures (i.e., epilepsy). A significant proportion of adults with temporal lobe epilepsy (due to mesial temporal sclerosis) had a prolonged febrile seizure as a child. After a simple febrile seizure, the risk for epilepsy later in life is only slightly higher than for the general population, about 2%. The risk of developing epilepsy after febrile seizures is greatest if the child has preexisting neurologic impairment such as developmental delay or cerebral palsy, if there is a family history of epilepsy, or if the febrile seizure was complicated in type. Depending on the specific complicated febrile seizure feature (prolonged, focal, recurrent), the risk for epilepsy varies from 6.5% to 9.3%; if all three features are present, the risk for epilepsy is as high as 49%.

Status epilepticus

Status epilepticus (SE) is defined as more than 30 minutes of continuous seizure activity, or multiple shorter seizures over the same time period without full recovery of consciousness between seizures (Table 11.21). There is unequivocal clinical and experimental evidence that SE can lead to brain damage and therefore must be stopped as quickly as possible.

Clinical features. Any seizure type can progress into SE (Mitchell 2002). SE is usually classified as convulsive or nonconvulsive. In convulsive SE, the seizure type is usually GTC, accompanied by significant autonomic manifestations including tachycardia, respiratory compromise, and hypersecretion. If the seizure continues, the patient may develop fever, hypotension, acidosis, and respiratory depression. Nonconvulsive status refers to SE with absence or partial seizures. Nonconvulsive SE can present as a continuous or fluctuating state of confusion and incomplete responsiveness. In addition, partial status may involve motor function (epilepsia partialis continua), sensation, or focal impairment of function (e.g., aphasia) not associated with altered consciousness.

Etiology. The etiologies of SE are as varied as those of epilepsy in general. Most SE is symptomatic. In children, fever, hypoxic–ischemic encephalopathy, and CNS infection account for the majority of cases of symptomatic SE. In patients already being treated for epilepsy, SE can be precipitated by abrupt withdrawal of anticonvulsant medications (particularly barbiturates and benzodiazepines), sleep deprivation, or intercurrent infection.

Treatment. In practical terms, any child seizing upon arrival at the emergency department or found seizing in the community should be treated for SE. Failure to treat SE quickly may result in neurologic sequelae or even death. A protocol for the treatment of SE is found in Table 11.22. Systemic abnormalities such as hyperpyrexia, hypoglycemia, hypotension, and hypoxia may occur during SE and exacerbate the cerebral damage. Therefore, it is critical to achieve systemic metabolic stability as well as stop the seizures. As the SE is being treated, the search for precipitating causes should proceed.

Initial therapy aims to provide basic life support, such as adequate cardiac output and cerebral perfusion and prevention of injury from excessive motor activity. Because cerebral hypoxia can be both a cause and consequence of status epilepticus, immediate needs are to assess cardiorespiratory function and insert an oral airway. Oxygen should be administered and endotracheal intubation may be necessary. Once the airway is secure, intravenous access should be obtained. Blood should then be sent for laboratory studies (Table 11.22), glucose given by bolus injection, and maintenance fluids started. Blood pressure must be monitored, especially during AED administration. Body temperature should be monitored continuously as it may rise quickly during SE and necessitate a cooling blanket or ice packs.

Once systemic conditions are addressed, AEDs should be given. Table 11.23 lists the doses and other data about the five most commonly used drugs in children with SE. Each drug is efficacious, and there is no proscribed order of administration. The usual protocol is to administer a fast-acting benzodiazepine (one or more times) to stop the SE, then load with a longer-acting agent such as fosphenytoin or phenobarbital. For SE refractory to these agents, more drastic measures may need to be undertaken, such as a midazolam drip or pentobarbital coma.

Refractory status epilepticus. When status epilepticus fails to respond to the medications described previously, more drastic treatment must be initiated. Until recently, the first step in stopping refractory status has been induction of coma using pentobarbital. The depth of coma can be assessed using EEG monitoring; the appearance of

Pearls and Perils

Status Epilepticus

- The water-soluble form of phenytoin (fosphenytoin) can be given intramuscularly to treat status epilepticus.
- Failure to give a sufficient dose of an antiepileptic drug (AED) is a common error in the treatment of status epilepticus.
- Although benzodiazepines are critical in the acute treatment of status epilepticus, the patient should also be loaded with a long-acting AED.
- Children who remain stuporous or comatose after a prolonged seizure should have an electroencephalogram (EEG) to determine whether the symptoms are due to nonconvulsive status.

Table 11.21 Status epilepticus

Discriminating features
- Diagnosis of convulsive status epilepticus is usually straightforward. Nonconvulsive status epilepticus may be mimicked by drug intoxication, psychosis, or migraine, and may require electroencephalogram (EEG) monitoring for diagnosis
- Defined as clinical or EEG seizure activity lasting 30 minutes or more, or intermittent seizures over a 30-minute period without full return of awareness between seizures. This definition may be too restrictive (see text)

Consistent features
- Convulsive status epilepticus is associated with hypoxia, hyperthermia, and other toxic and metabolic derangements

Variable features
- Clinical seizures may be convulsive (i.e., tonic, clonic, or tonic–clonic) or nonconvulsive (i.e., absence or partial complex)
- Etiologies are as broad as for any seizure
- Responds to antiepileptic drugs

Table 11.22 Sequence of steps for emergency treatment of status epilepticus

- Place patient in safe position.
- Assess cardiorespiratory function.
- Insert oral airway and administer oxygen.
- Insert intravenous catheter.
- Draw venous blood for measurement of AED levels, CBC, BUN, electrolytes, glucose, and ammonia.
- Draw arterial blood gases.
- Give 50% glucose solution (1–2 mL/kg).
- Start maintenance fluids unless there is evidence of fluid overload, concern about increased intracranial pressure, or dehydration.
- Give diazepam or lorazepam (Table 11.23).
- If seizures stop, a longer-acting AED (phenobarbital or phenytoin/fosphenytoin) must be given to prevent recurrence of status.
- If status continues, give phenobarbital or phenytoin/fosphenytoin (Table 11.23).
- If status continues, intubate child and admit to intensive care unit. Give propofol bolus then drip. Alternatively, use a midazolam bolus (0.15–0.3 mg/kg) and maintenance (Doses in Table 11.23).
- If status continues, consider general anesthesia.

AED, antiepileptic drug; BUN, blood urea nitrogen; CBC, complete blood count.

burst suppression on the EEG suggests that the brain's metabolic rate is slowed and that ongoing status epilepticus should be suppressed. However, distinguishing burst suppression from epileptic discharges can be difficult, and some authorities recommend pushing the medication until the EEG is completely flat, since any persistence of EEG activity predicted recurrence of status epilepticus when the infusion is stopped (Treiman 2001).

The child must be intubated and mechanically ventilated before pentobarbital coma is induced. Although it is often effective at stopping status, pentobarbital coma is associated with significant hypotension and myocardial depression. There are few guidelines as to the use of pentobarbital coma in children, such as the most efficacious duration of coma, optimal interburst interval, and best approach if seizures recur.

An alternative to pentobarbital coma is continuous infusion of the water-soluble benzodiazepine midazolam (Versed; see Table 11.23), which has a rapid onset of action and excellent effectiveness. In one large series of children, midazolam promptly stopped status (usually in <1 hour) and was associated with a very low morbidity (Rivera et al. 1993). In critical care units, the anesthetic agent propofol is becoming more widely used, especially for refractory status (Claassen et al. 2002). It has a rapid onset and minimal hemodynamic side effects. Some authorities recommend general anesthesia by inhalation of halothane or enflurane, but these agents must be administered in the controlled environment of an operating suite, which poses practical problems for a child in an intensive care unit. Future studies will clarify the role of these and other agents in the management of status in children.

Prognosis. The outcome of SE is improving with earlier and more effective medical management (Maytal et al. 1989; Sillanpää & Shinnar 2002). The SE-related mortality rate in children is less than 5%. Fewer than 10% of children with SE develop new neurologic deficits, and most of those patients have preexisting neurologic impairment. The consensus is that the etiology of SE, rather than the seizure itself, is the main determinant of neurologic outcome. Risk factors for neurologic sequelae from SE include age of onset under 6 years, a remote symptomatic cause, and partial seizures.

Prognosis of childhood epilepsy

It is difficult to ascribe an overall prognosis to childhood epilepsy, because the outcome is very dependent upon the epilepsy syndrome and several other factors, including preexisting neurologic impairment, duration of epilepsy, and ease with which seizures are controlled (Arzimanoglou et

Table 11.23 Properties of five antiepileptic drugs (AEDs) used for the intravenous treatment of status epilepticus

Property	Diazepam	Lorazepam	Fosphenytoin	Phenobarbital	Midazolam
Dose	0.2–0.4 mg/kg (maximum dose 20 mg)	0.05–0.1 mg/kg	15–20 mg/kg	15–20 mg/kg	Bolus: 0.15–0.3 mg/kg Drip: 0.75–10 μg/kg/min
Time to stop seizure	3–10 min	1–20 min	5–30 min	10–30 min	15 min
Half-life	50 hours	15 hours	10–15 hours	80–100 hours	1.7–4.0 hours
Duration of action	Minutes	Hours	12–24 hours	Days	30–80 min
Side effects	Hypotension Apnea Somnolence	Hypotension Apnea Somnolence	Cardiac arrhythmias Hypotension	Hypotension Apnea Somnolence	Hypotension Apnea Somnolence

al. 2004c; Sillanpää et al. 1998). Many childhood epilepsies remit over time (Berg et al. 2001).

It has been emphasized that in epilepsy, seizures are often just "the tip of the iceberg" (Bax 1999). Children with epilepsy often have significant psychological, social, and educational challenges that, in many cases, outweigh the burden of the seizures themselves (Austin & Caplan 2007). When discussing prognosis, seizure control (i.e., with AEDs) must be distinguished from seizure remission. Psychosocial adjustment and AED side effects play a prominent role in the self-image of a child with epilepsy.

Prognosis related to individual syndromes was discussed earlier. Generally, the idiopathic benign epilepsies of childhood (BCECTS, BEOP) have a favorable prognosis, with seizure resolution and continuance of normal neurologic function once the seizures remit in adolescence. Generalized epilepsy syndromes, such as childhood absence epilepsy and GEFS+, have an intermediate prognosis: seizures resolve in many cases but a significant proportion persists. Some epilepsy syndromes are considered "catastrophic" (Conry 2004). Catastrophic epilepsy syndromes include infantile spasms, Lennox-Gastaut syndrome, and Landau-Kleffner syndrome, in which seizures persist, become refractory to medical treatment, and are accompanied by severe cognitive impairment. It is an intriguing but unanswered question whether "seizures beget seizures"; that is, does the occurrence of a seizure increase the chance that a subsequent seizure will occur? Considerable experimental investigation is under way into determining whether epilepsy is a progressive disorder and whether this phenomenon is age-related (Holmes & Ben-Ari 1998; Pitkanen & Sutula 2002).

Finally, some children with epilepsy die unexpectedly, without an obvious cause determined either historically or by postmortem examination. Sudden unexplained death in epilepsy (SUDEP) has been seen in both adults and children (Breningstall 2001; Donner et al. 2001). Definitive risk factors have not been established, but children with severe, intractable generalized epilepsies may be at greater risk.

Nonepileptic disorders that may mimic epilepsy

Differentiating epileptic seizures from the wide variety of nonepileptic paroxysmal alterations of motor activity or behavior is a challenging task for the primary care physician and seasoned epilepsy specialist alike (Bleasel & Kotogal 1995; Obeid & Mikati 2007; Prensky 2001). Many nonepileptic disorders may mimic epilepsy by history or clinical presentation (Table 11.24). Here, a few of the more common disorders are described. From a therapeutic viewpoint, it is important to distinguish epileptic from nonepileptic behaviors, because some nonepileptic phenomena respond to medications other than AEDs and others require no specific treatment other than reassurance or avoidance of circumstances that precipitate the spell.

Benign paroxysmal vertigo

Benign paroxysmal vertigo (BPV) manifests as sudden, brief overwhelming sensations of vertigo that cause a child to stagger, lose balance, and sometimes fall. The child appears distressed and frightened and might become pale, diaphoretic, and nauseated. Nevertheless, consciousness is maintained. An episode may last from a few minutes to several hours, and episodes may occur once every few months to several times per week. BPV is thought to be a migraine variant; there is often a family history of migraine. The disorder usually affects preschool-age children and usually resolves by 7 years of age, although most affected children go on to develop more typical migraine symptoms later in life. As opposed to other causes of vertigo, in BPV there is no accompanying tinnitus, hearing impairment, or other brainstem dysfunction, although nystagmus can be present. Diagnosis is aided by a normal EEG and neurologic examination. The lack of rhythmic movements or alteration of consciousness further differentiates BPV from epilepsy. The attacks

Table 11.24 Some nonepileptic disorders that may mimic epilepsy

- Apnea
- Benign paroxysmal vertigo
- Breath-holding spells (cyanotic and pallid)
- Cardiac arrhythmias (e.g., prolonged QT syndrome)
- Cataplexy
- Daydreaming
- Episodic dyscontrol (rage attacks)
- Gastroesophageal reflux
- Hyperekplexia (startle disease)
- Hyperventilation
- Jitteriness
- Migraine
- Narcolepsy
- Night terrors
- Pediatric autoimmune neuropsychiatric disorder after streptococcus (PANDAS)
- Paroxysmal choreoathetosis
- Pseudoseizures (psychogenic seizures)
- Sandifer syndrome
- Shuddering attacks
- Spasmus nutans
- Syncope
- Tics, Tourette syndrome

typically fail to respond to anticonvulsant or antimigraine medications, and the only treatment is to reassure the parents of the benign nature of the spells.

Breath-holding spells

Despite their name, breath-holding spells (BHSs) are involuntary reflex responses with a benign prognosis. They are age-related and are typically outgrown by school age. Two types of BHSs occur: cyanotic (often called *cyanotic infantile syncope*) and pallid (often called *pallid infantile syncope* or *reflex anoxic seizures*). Features of each type are listed in Table 11.25. Their nomenclature, pathophysiology, and differentiation can be complex (Arzimanoglou et al. 2004b; Stephenson 1990).

Cyanotic BHSs, the more common type, are precipitated by upset, anger, or frustration. The hallmark is crying, during which the child will stop breathing (usually in expiration), become cyanotic, then lose consciousness. At that point, the child may become rigid, limp, or even shake, raising the concern about a seizure. The unconsciousness lasts from seconds to a minute. The pathogenesis of cyanotic BHS is complex, probably involving an interaction between hyperventilation, Valsalva maneuver, expiratory apnea, and intrinsic pulmonary mechanics (Breningstall 1996; Stephenson 1990).

Pallid BHSs are similar to cyanotic BHSs in some respects but are more likely to be provoked by fright or a mild unpleasant stimulus (such as a mild head bump or even stubbing a toe). There will be a gasp but little or no cry, followed by loss of consciousness, pallor, diaphoresis, and limpness. Pallid BHSs result from vasovagally mediated cardiac inhibition, causing diminished cerebral blood flow. During an attack, the pulse slows significantly. Such spells are very frightening to an observer, who may initiate cardiopulmonary resuscitation, thinking the child has died.

Neither type of BHS is associated with an increased predisposition to epilepsy, although seizure activity can occur during a cyanotic or pallid BHS. These so-called "seizures" manifest as tonic stiffening of the extremities, sometimes followed by brief clonic jerking. Such seizures are not epileptic in nature, however, and merely represent a response of the brain to acute, mild hypoxia. These seizures terminate spontaneously and do not require anticonvulsant treatment. Notably, in a BHS, cyanosis occurs before the seizure, whereas in an epileptic seizure, cyanosis usually occurs during or after the seizure.

Evaluation with an EEG is usually not needed. An electrocardiogram can rule out the possibility of prolonged QT syndrome, which can mimic epilepsy. In addition, anemia can worsen BHS and should be excluded; some authors have recommended iron therapy even in the absence of anemia (Daoud et al. 1997). Management of BHS consists mainly of reassurance that the spells will be outgrown, usually by school age, and will not lead to future epilepsy or brain damage. Children with the pallid type may develop syncope later in life. Parents of children with BHS may be reluctant to discipline their child in an age-appropriate manner for fear of provoking an attack. Counseling the parents about limit-setting is indicated. Medical therapy is advised only in exceptional circumstances. A child followed by the author had pallid BHS and leukemia; he was treated with a small dose of atropine before his frequent blood draws, which predictably precipitated attacks. Based on reports of efficacy of piracetam (not available in United States) for BHS, studies are in progress to assess the efficacy of levetiracetam in their treatment.

Syncope (fainting)

Syncope, seen commonly in older children and adolescents, can often be differentiated from an epileptic seizure by history. Attacks may be preceded by warning (presyncopal) signs such as lightheadedness, blurring of vision, pallor, nausea, or diaphoresis. These warning signs are followed by a

Table 11.25 Clinical differentiation of cyanotic and pallid breath-holding spells (BHS)

Clinical data	Cyanotic BHS	Pallid BHS
Onset of spells	0–18 months	12–24 months
Remission	Most by 4–6 years	Most by 4–6 mo
Percent of total*	60	20
Precipitant	Anger, frustration, fright	Sudden unpleasant stimulus, e.g. minor injury
Sequence of events	Cry → apnea, cyanosis → loss of consciousness and tone (or rigidity) → ± brief tonic–clonic seizure	Gasp or weak cry → pallor → loss of consciousness and tone → ± brief tonic–clonic seizure
Duration of unconsciousness	Usually less than 1 minute	May be longer than 1 minute
Mechanism	Multifactorial (see text)	Vasovagal
Therapy	Reassurance	Reassurance; rarely, atropine

*The remaining 20% consists of mixed types or indeterminate spells.

gradual loss of consciousness and a slow slump to the ground, as opposed to the more violent fall seen with a myoclonic or atonic seizure. Late in the syncopal spell, there may be a brief tonic or clonic seizure secondary to cerebral hypoperfusion and hypoxia; these are not epileptic seizures. Consciousness is regained rapidly, compared with a more prolonged epileptic postictal state. A child may be tired after syncope but is not ordinarily confused for more than a few seconds. Seizure is further differentiated from syncope in that a seizure is not associated with cold, clammy skin.

Syncope is caused by transiently diminished cerebral blood flow, due to an irregular heart rate (an arrhythmia causing decreased cardiac output), decreased venous return (orthostasis or Valsalva), a vasovagal mechanism (fright, pain, emotional upset), or, rarely, cough- or micturition-induced reflex syncope. Vasovagal attacks often occur in a hot, crowded environment. Orthostasis is most commonly precipitated by rising from a sitting or recumbent position.

A child who has an arrhythmia or who faints from any position other than standing requires a cardiac evaluation, including an electrocardiogram, echocardiogram, Holter monitor, and perhaps a tilt-table test. Orthostatic blood pressures should be documented; upon standing, a drop in pulse of more than 20 points or systolic blood pressure of more than 15 points is abnormal.

The hallmark of treatment is prevention. The child should avoid precipitating factors as much as possible. During a syncopal event, the observer should allow the child to lie horizontally or with the head at a lower level than the body; lifting or raising the head can delay return of consciousness by prolonging the duration of cerebral hypoperfusion.

Pseudoseizures

Pseudoseizures, also referred to as *psychogenic seizures* or simply *nonepileptic seizures* (to avoid a presumption of etiology or any pejorative connotation), are paroxysmal changes in motor activity or behavior that resemble epileptic seizures clinically but have no EEG correlate (Bhatia & Sapra 2005). The diagnosis of pseudoseizure should be considered in any child with seizures refractory to anticonvulsants or with consistently normal EEGs (awake, asleep, and with activation procedures). A history of strong emotional overlay or psychiatric disturbance in the child or family may suggest pseudoseizures. Clinically, it may be very difficult to differentiate between epileptic seizures and pseudoseizures (Table 11.26), and simultaneous video-EEG monitoring can be helpful. A single routine EEG is not usually useful, because even if a spell is captured, it is likely to be obscured by muscle artifact. Diagnosis relies on prolonged monitoring and careful correlation of clinical and electrographic findings. To complicate the diagnostic evaluation, pseudoseizures and epileptic seizures often coexist in the same child.

> **Pearls and Perils**
>
> **Pseudoseizures**
>
> - In most cases, prolonged video-electroencephalogram (EEG) monitoring is necessary to diagnose pseudoseizures.
> - Epileptic seizures and pseudoseizures often coexist in the same patient.
> - Urinary incontinence is an unsatisfactory discriminating feature, because it occurs in up to 20% of patients with nonepileptic seizures.
> - Some frontal lobe epileptic seizures present with ictal manifestations similar to classic pseudoseizures (e.g., bilateral motor activity with preserved consciousness, pelvic thrusting).
> - Pseudoseizures are real in the sense that they are the symptom of real (psychiatric) disease. Therapy is aimed at uncovering the underlying psychological etiology and teaching the child effective new coping skills. In evaluating pseudoseizures, always rule out physical and sexual abuse.

Pseudoseizures are no less serious and disabling than epileptic seizures, in that they reflect major underlying psychopathology that necessitates proper diagnosis and treatment. As with many psychosomatic illnesses, pseudoseizures can arise because of unresolved psychological conflicts and anxiety that are converted into a physical symptom. In children with pseudoseizures, one must always be suspicious of physical or sexual abuse. As noted earlier, many children with pseudoseizures have epilepsy. Others may have witnessed a real seizure, either first-hand or in the media.

Pseudoseizures present with a variety of clinical forms. Many resemble generalized tonic–clonic seizures, although the two sides of the body are more likely to be jerking out of phase with each other. Pseudoseizures can also simulate complex partial, atonic, myoclonic, and even absence seizures. Sometimes the behavioral manifestations of the spell are a clue to its nonepileptic nature. For example, GTC activity in the setting of preserved consciousness favors a nonepileptic event. However, it is becoming increasingly apparent that some behaviors previously thought to be pseudoseizures are, in fact, epileptic events generated by brain areas distant from scalp EEG electrodes. For example, seizures arising from the frontal lobe may give rise to behavioral ictal manifestations that were formerly thought to be characteristic of pseudoseizures. Seizures originating in the supplementary area (SMA) of the frontal lobe involve bilateral motor activity with preserved consciousness. Compared with pseudoseizures, SMA seizures are briefer, more stereotyped, frequently occur during sleep, and initially

Table 11.26 Criteria useful for differentiation of epileptic seizures from pseudoseizures

Clinical data	Pseudoseizures	Generalized tonic–clonic seizures
Changes in seizure frequency with medication change	Rare	Usual
Increased seizures with stress	Frequent	Occasional
Combativeness	Common	Rare
Vulgar language	Frequent	Rare
Self-injury	Rare	Common
Incontinence	Rare	Common
Tongue biting	Rare	Common
Nocturnal occurrence	Rare	Common
Stereotype of attacks	Often variable	Little variation
Postictal confusion, lethargy or sleepiness	Rare	Frequent
Electroencephalogram		
Interictal	Often normal	Frequently abnormal
During attack	Normal	Always abnormal

manifest with arm abduction (fencer's pose). Seizures originating in the orbitofrontal region are now recognized to include nonspecific screaming, affective changes such as intense fear, bilateral nonrhythmic leg or arm movements, and even sexual automatisms such as pelvic thrusting. Such behaviors were previously considered to be the sine qua non of pseudoseizures. These observations underscore the difficulty of differentiating between epileptic seizures and pseudoseizures on clinical grounds.

A child with pseudoseizures must be approached with a great deal of sensitivity. It is usually best to avoid confronting the child directly. The diagnostic suspicion should be discussed with the family in a supportive fashion. Therapy must involve both the child and family and might include psychotherapy (occasionally requiring inpatient management), stress management strategies, relaxation techniques, or biofeedback. Management is best instituted with the assistance of a psychiatrist experienced in this field. The family members must be counseled to reduce secondary gain engendered by the child's behavior. They should be assured that the symptom (pseudoseizure) is real but does not involve epileptic neuronal discharges, and that therapy is designed to address the underlying cause of the symptom. Pseudoseizures are a learned behavior, and the main therapeutic goal is to teach the child alternative coping skills, so that anxiety or psychological stress does not need to manifest in such a maladaptive fashion.

The psychopathology that causes a child to manifest pseudoseizures is varied and complex; it may simply be a reaction to death or illness in a family member or it may indicate subconscious repression of a serious insult such as physical or sexual abuse. Several methods have been described to induce or terminate a pseudoseizure, but interpretation of such procedures is difficult and produces many false-positive results. Therefore, provocative methods should be used with extreme caution if at all, ideally with concurrent EEG monitoring. Serum levels of prolactin, cortisol, and other substances have been reported to correlate with an epileptic seizure, thereby providing a way to differentiate epileptic seizures from pseudoseizures. In practice, interpretation of such levels is fraught with difficulty, and these are not routinely recommended in children for the diagnosis of pseudoseizures.

The outcome of pseudoseizures in children varies but may be more auspicious than in adults. In one study, 81% of children and adolescents were free of pseudoseizures 3 years after diagnosis, compared with only 40% of adults with pseudoseizures (Wyllie et al. 1991). Another group reported that all children with pseudoseizures resumed regular school attendance after treatment (Gudmundsson et al. 2001).

Episodic dyscontrol (rage attacks)

Rage attacks are episodes of aggression that are out of proportion to the precipitating event and social context (Gordon 1999). They are common in school-aged children and adolescents, especially boys. Children often come to neurologic attention when the primary caregiver or psychiatrist becomes concerned that a child's temper tantrum is out of character with his usual personality. The attacks may appear suddenly and explosively and consist of uncontrolled behaviors such as hitting, kicking, biting, spitting, and throwing objects around the room. After an attack, the child may be completely or partially amnestic for the event or show signs of remorse. Some fatigue may follow an episode, but not usually the prolonged postictal confusional state that follows an epileptic seizure. Guidelines to differentiate rage attacks from epileptic seizures are provided in Table 11.27. Some children with

Pearls and Perils

Episodic Dyscontrol

- Rage attacks are usually provoked, although the provocative stimulus may seem minor or trivial to the parent or other observer.
- In a rage attack, the violence is not random but goal-directed; violence during an epileptic seizure is usually very brief and not directed at a specific target.
- In rage attacks, the behavioral manifestations are varied and change with time. In an epileptic seizure, rhythmic or nonpurposeful behaviors are seen throughout the event.
- Rage attacks last minutes to hours, whereas seizures usually last seconds to minutes.
- The response to antiepileptic drugs (AEDs) does not discriminate between the two conditions. A positive response may reflect a placebo effect, and some AEDs (especially carbamazepine and valproate) have antidepressant, calming actions independent of their antiepileptic mechanism.

complex partial seizures exhibit episodic dyscontrol interictally. Rage attacks often occur in children who are mildly impaired neurologically, including those with such conditions as autism, attention deficit disorder, or following traumatic injury to the temporal or frontal lobe. Children who experience rage attacks sometimes respond to propanolol, carbamazepine, or selective serotonin reuptake inhibitors.

Spasmus nutans

Spasmus nutans is a condition usually seen in infants between 6 and 12 months of age. The child presents with a triad of symptoms including nystagmus, torticollis, and most commonly, horizontal but at times vertical head movements. The congenital nystagmus can be pendular and mistaken for the nystagmus seen as a consequence of impaired vision. Impaired vision and lesions of the optic tract should be excluded before this diagnosis is made. The condition is often self-limited and disappears by 3–4 years of age.

Sandifer syndrome

Sandifer syndrome is an episodic movement disorder that may mimic tonic seizures. It is associated with tilting or lateral flexion of the head and associated extension of the neck; limbs are rarely involved. Spells usually occur with feeding, and are due to gastroesophageal reflux with or without an associated hiatal hernia.

Night terrors

Night terrors (*pavor nocturnas*) are a common parasomnia that are often confused with seizures. Night terrors occur in children from about 18 months to 8 years of age, with a peak around 4–5 years of age. They occur in the early stages of sleep (non-REM, stages 3 and 4). The child will awaken with inconsolable, frantic screaming, sweating and other signs of sympathetic activation, and flailing of all extremities in a nonrhythmic fashion for several minutes, then fall back to sleep without memory of the episode in the morning. There is often a family history of night terrors. The diagnosis is a clinical one; video-EEG recording is rarely needed. The main differential diagnosis is nightmares (which occur out of REM sleep) and nocturnal epileptic seizures, such as frontal lobe seizures. The only treatment is reassurance.

Table 11.27 Differentiation of rage attacks from partial complex seizures

Clinical data	Complex partial seizures	Rage attacks
Duration	Seconds to minutes	Minutes
Stereotype of attacks	Variable but usually have consistent patterns	Patterns widely diverse
Aura	Frequent	Rare
Violence	Unusual, rarely directed	Frequent, may be directed
Precipitating event	None	Usual
Amnesia for event	Partial to total	None to total
Postictal confusion, lethargy, sleepiness	Common	Occasionally
Responds to antiepileptic drugs	Usually	Occasionally
Electroencephalogram		
Ictal	Variable, temporal or frontal lobe spikes	Normal or nonspecific abnormalities
Interictal	Unilateral or bilateral temporal or frontal discharges	No change

Treatment of the child with seizures and epilepsy

Initiating treatment

The decision to treat a child with antiepileptic therapy should consider both benefits and risks. The potential benefits of treatment (prevention of further seizures and development of epilepsy) must be weighed against potential adverse effects (cognitive/behavioral changes, toxicity, cost, stigma, etc.) (Hirtz et al. 2003). All AEDs have side effects, both dose-related and idiosyncratic. These include systemic effects such as bone marrow suppression, rashes, and alterations of bone density (Samaniego & Sheth 2007), as well as CNS-related side effects, such as drowsiness and mental slowing. The decision of whether or not to begin AEDs is related strongly to the syndrome diagnosis. For example, multiple absence seizures affecting attention span and school performance would warrant treatment. A single nocturnal seizure with an interictal EEG showing classic rolandic spikes may not require treatment.

On the other hand, the approach to a first unprovoked (nonsyndromic) seizure is more controversial, and is based on recurrence rates by 2 years of 37–54% (Hirtz et al. 2003; Shinnar et al. 2000; Stroink et al. 1998). Therefore, roughly half of children with a first unprovoked seizure will have another seizure in the ensuing 2 years (the period of greatest recurrence risk). Children with prior neurologic impairment are at the greatest risk for recurrence. Therapy does not seem to change the recurrence rate, and the EEG is a good predictor of recurrence.

Many factors need to be considered when deciding whether to start AED therapy, and each child must be evaluated individually. However, in view of the risk of adverse effects encountered with AEDs, in most children it appears reasonable to wait for a second seizure before subjecting the child to years of drug therapy.

Withdrawing antiepileptic drugs

Deciding when to withdraw AEDs from a child who is doing well can be as difficult as deciding when to start a drug, and again, considerations are based on age-specific risks and benefits (O'Dell & Shinnar 2001). Psychosocial as well as medical factors must be considered. If the child is tolerating the medication well, there is a tendency to leave well enough alone and continue with the drug. However, AEDs are expensive, often require laboratory monitoring, and may be associated with cognitive impairment. Therefore, the clinician should consider tapering and discontinuing AEDs in children who remain seizure-free for 2 years or sometimes sooner. A history of focal seizures is the main risk factor for seizure recurrence after AED taper in children who are well-controlled for more than 2 years, especially if the EEG remains abnormal (Hawash & Rosman 2003). As discussed earlier, syndrome classification can guide the decision to withdraw AEDs. For example, children with absence epilepsy or benign rolandic epilepsy have a high likelihood of outgrowing their seizures, whereas those with juvenile myoclonic epilepsy are less likely to remit.

Pharmacology of antiepileptic drugs

The primary mode of treatment in children with epilepsy is pharmacologic, although epilepsy surgery, vagus nerve stimulation, and ketogenic diet therapy are useful in selected cases. The medical treatment of epilepsy has changed decisively in the past decade, with regard to both the introduction of new AEDs and improved formulations and methods of administration. For children, it is fortunate that multiple formulations of AEDs are available (e.g., chewable tablets, sprinkles, suspension), as well as extended-release preparations and options to deliver the AED by different routes (sublingual, intravenous, intramuscular, rectal) (Wheless & Venkataraman 1999). These options decrease poor compliance, which is an important cause of breakthrough seizures and a source of ongoing family stress.

The goal in the pharmacologic treatment of epilepsy is to reduce or eliminate seizures while minimizing the adverse effects of treatment. Drug treatment is only one component of the overall management strategy—psychological, educational, and social complications of epilepsy and its treatment must also be considered. Failure to address these quality-of-life issues will result in treatment program failure, regardless of whether seizures are controlled.

Although there is no single drug of choice in the treatment of epilepsy, clinical trials have demonstrated that some drugs are more effective in certain seizure types and syndromes. Some AEDs, such as ethosuximide, are highly effective in controlling only one type of seizure (absence), whereas others, such as VPA, are useful in a broad spectrum of seizure types. Table 11.28 lists the AEDs found to be most useful in some seizure types. Table 11.29 provides analogous information for selected epilepsy syndromes. Treatment choices are reviewed further in the discussion of individual seizure types and epilepsy syndromes.

Medical treatment should always begin with a single AED. Monotherapy controls approximately 60% of newly diagnosed epilepsy (Camfield et al. 1997; Kwan & Brodie 2000). Even in patients with multiple seizure types, a single drug is started and increased to high therapeutic serum levels or until toxicity ensues. If, at that time, seizures are not controlled, a second drug can be initiated while the first one is either continued or tapered. The physician should avoid the temptation of adding a second

Table 11.28 Antiepileptic drugs of choice in the treatment of childhood seizures

Seizure type	Antiepileptic drugs: First choice	Second choice
Partial seizures		
Simple partial	Carbamazepine	Lamotrigine
	Phenytoin	Topiramate
	Valproic acid	Tiagabine
	Oxcarbazepine	Levetiracetam
		Zonisamide
		Gabapentin
		Phenobarbital
		Primidone
		Benzodiazepines
Complex partial	Carbamazepine	Lamotrigine
	Phenytoin	Topiramate
	Valproic acid	Tiagabine
	Oxcarbazepine	Levetiracetam
		Zonisamide
		Gabapentin
		Phenobarbital
		Primidone
		Benzodiazepines
Generalized seizures		
Absence	Ethosuximide	Lamotrigine
	Valproic acid	Acetazolamide
	Clonazepam	
Generalized tonic–clonic	Carbamazepine	Lamotrigine
	Phenytoin	Topiramate
	Valproic acid	Tiagabine
	Oxcarbazepine	Gabapentin
		Phenobarbital
		Primidone
		Benzodiazepines
Myoclonic	Valproic acid	Lamotrigine
	Clonazepam	
	Levetiracetam	
Clonic	Valproic acid	Lamotrigine
		Phenobarbital
Tonic	Valproic acid	Carbamazepine
		Phenytoin
		Lamotrigine
		Phenobarbital
Atonic	Valproic acid	Lamotrigine
		Clonazepam

Table 11.29 Antiepileptic drugs (AEDs) of choice in the treatment of selected childhood epilepsy syndromes

Seizure type	Antiepileptic drugs: First choice	Second choice
Infantile spasms	Adrenocortico-trophic hormone	Topiramate
		Lamotrigine
	Vigabatrin	Valproic acid
	Pyridoxine (vitamin B_6)	
Lennox-Gastaut syndrome	Valproic acid	Lamotrigine
		Topiramate
		Felbamate*
Childhood absence epilepsy	Ethosuximide	Lamotrigine
	Valproic acid	Clonazepam
Juvenile absence epilepsy	Valproic acid	Lamotrigine
Benign rolandic epilepsy	Carbamazepine	Gabapentin
	Phenytoin	Lamotrigine
	Valproic acid	Topiramate

*Consider in children refractory to several AEDs (see text).

AED too soon. If more than one AED is used simultaneously, one can never be sure which one is controlling seizures or causing toxicity. Addition of a second AED will control only another 10% of patients, and the side effects of multiple medications are cumulative. "Rational polytherapy," the use of more than one AED, is sometimes effective, especially if the AEDs are chosen to have complementary mechanisms of action.

Therapeutic ranges, the plasma concentrations for which optimal seizure control is likely to occur without side effects, have been established for most AEDs. However, these levels should be obtained judiciously. Individual patients may have complete control with levels below the therapeutic range, whereas others may tolerate and require levels above the usual therapeutic range. Conversely, some children develop intolerable side effects at serum levels within the quoted therapeutic range. Signs of clinical toxicity are particularly common in patients receiving multiple AEDs, even when the level of each individual drug is within the therapeutic range. Despite these caveats, clinical responses and toxicity correlate much better with serum levels than with dosage.

Physicians should be familiar with the basic principles of AED pharmacokinetics. In most instances, AEDs are administered orally on a long-term basis. Following initiation of therapy, the drug accumulates in the body until such a time as the rate of elimination equals the rate of administration. Over this period, body and plasma concentrations increase exponentially until they reach a steady state or plateau. *Steady state*, the balance between accumulation and elimination of the AED, results in a stable level below which the concentration in the serum will not fall. The time to reach a steady state is approximately five half-lives.

In the steady state, the range of fluctuation of plasma concentrations remains relatively constant. The minimum concentration (trough) occurs before a dose, whereas the maximum level is primarily dependent on the absorption rate. Because bioavailability varies considerably among the AEDs, it is usually preferable to obtain routine levels at trough, immediately before the next dose. AEDs with a long half-life, such as phenobarbital, have small daily fluctuations, and the timing of serum sampling is not as critical. However, when using a drug with a short serum half-life, such as carbamazepine or VPA, the serum level varies significantly depending on when the blood is sampled. If toxicity is the main concern, a peak level 1 to several hours after a dose would be most informative. Transient toxic effects of carbamazepine, such as diplopia, lethargy, and nausea, subside when the serum level decreases. Fluctuation between minimum and maximum AED levels are more pronounced in children who are on polytherapy. If a patient complains about side effects at the time of peak serum concentration, the frequency of administration may be increased without changing the total daily dose. For example, if a child is taking carbamazepine 300 mg twice daily and experiences diplopia 2 hours after taking a dose, a trial of 200 mg three times a day may be helpful.

A common error is to obtain a serum AED level before a steady state is reached; the serum level will be spuriously lower than the eventual steady-state level. Due to numerous drug interactions, it is important to obtain serum levels of all AEDs if the child is on polytherapy. Measurement of AED levels is expensive and levels should only be obtained when the information is clinically useful.

A summary of some important properties of the AEDs is found in Table 11.30. For further details of AED mechanisms, pharmacokinetics, dosing recommendations, and adverse effects, the reader is referred to several comprehensive resources (Hadjiloizou & Bourgeois 2007; Jarrar & Buchhalter 2003; LaRoche 2007; Levy et al. 2002).

Traditional antiepileptic drugs

Carbamazepine

Carbamazepine (Tegretol, Carbatrol), introduced in 1962, is effective against partial seizures, secondarily generalized seizures, and generalized tonic–clonic seizures. It has no cosmetic side effects, and does not usually significantly alter mood, behavior, or cognition. Carbamazepine acts by blocking active neuronal sodium channels.

Carbamazepine has linear pharmacokinetics, with the serum level directly proportional to the dosage. *Autoinduction*, a phenomenon whereby hepatic degradation increases over time, occurs during the first month of therapy. A trough serum level should be checked several weeks after beginning therapy, and periodically thereafter. The serum level tends to stabilize after a few months of treatment. Carbamazepine has a relatively short half-life, and although three daily doses are optimal, this regimen is often not practical for families. Longer-acting twice-daily dose formulations are now available (Carbatrol, Tegretol-XR). Carbamazepine increases the rate of metabolism of other AEDs but may increase phenytoin levels. Some common drugs, particularly erythromycin, decrease carbamazepine clearance and inadvertent coadministration can result in carbamazepine toxicity.

Carbamazepine has been associated with both dose-related and idiosyncratic reactions. The dose-related side effects are common but not life-threatening, whereas the idiosyncratic reactions are rare but serious. Common dose-related side effects include drowsiness, ataxia, nausea, diplopia, headache, irritability, and dizziness. These symptoms usually occur at peak serum concentrations and can often be alleviated by increasing dose frequency without changing total daily dose.

Idiosyncratic reactions of most concern involve the bone marrow. Most cases of carbamazepine hematopoietic toxicity occurred in patients on other AEDs. Estimated prevalences of hematologic toxicity are 0.002% for aplastic anemia, 10% for transient leukopenia, 2% for persistent leukopenia, 2% for thrombocytopenia, and less than 5% for anemia. Pancreatitis has also been reported with carbamazepine. Rash occurs in about 5% of children. As with phenytoin, rashes from carbamazepine can be mild or serious (e.g., Stevens-Johnson syndrome). The serious cutaneous reactions tend to occur in the first few months of treatment, and usually in patients with hypersensitivity to other medications. Carbamazepine may exacerbate some seizure types, most commonly atypical absences (Guerrini et al. 1998).

It is recommended that a complete blood count (CBC) and liver transaminases be obtained before therapy is initiated, at 2–4 weeks, at 2 months, and then every 6 months. These guidelines are reasonable unless there is clinical evidence of hepatic or hematologic dysfunction. Mild leukopenia does not usually require drug discontinuation. It is recommended that the daily dose of carbamazepine be reduced if the absolute neutrophil count falls below 900 mm^3. Families should be advised to contact their physician for such signs as easy bruising or petechiae.

Ethosuximide

Ethosuximide (Zarontin) is an excellent first-line AED for the treatment of absence seizures. It is rarely used for other seizure types. Ethosuximide works by blocking calcium channels in those thalamic neurons that project to neocortex, interrupting the thalamocortical feedback loop that underlies the generalized spike-wave discharges of absence seizures. Mild side effects occur in approximately one-third of children upon initiation of therapy, and include nausea, anorexia, dizziness, headaches, and

Table 11.30 Summary of commonly used antiepileptic drugs (AEDs)

AED (trade names)	Starting dosage	Typical maintenance dosage	Half-life (hours)	Therapeutic range (mg/L)	Common side effects	Serious idiosyncratic side effects
Phenobarbital	<1 year: 4–6 mg/kg/day >1 year: 3–4 mg/kg/day Teenagers, adults: 3 mg/kg/day	Same as starting dosage	40–70	15–40	Irritability Hyperactivity Lethargy	Rash Hepatic failure Agranulocytosis Stevens-Johnson syndrome
Primidone (Mysoline)	1–2 mg/kg	10–25 mg/kg/day once a day at bedtime	5–8	5–12	Irritability Hyperactivity Lethargy Nausea	Rash Agranulocytosis
Phenytoin (Dilantin)	5 mg/kg/day (may need higher dose in children <5 years)	Same as starting dosage	5–34	10–20	Lethargy Dizziness Ataxia Gingival hyperplasia Hirsutism	Rash Hepatic failure Lymphadenopathy Pancreatitis Agranulocytosis Stevens-Johnson syndrome
Carbamazepine (Tegretol, Tegretol XR, Carbatrol)	5–10 mg/kg/day	10–30 mg/kg/day	8–25	6–12	Diplopia Lethargy Blurred vision Ataxia	Rash Hepatic failure Pancreatitis Leukopenia Aplastic anemia Hyponatremia
Valproic acid (Depakote, Depakene, Depacon)	15 mg/kg/day	15–60 mg/kg/day	4–14	50–100	Lethargy Weight gain (or rarely, weight loss) Hair loss Tremor	Rash Hepatic failure Pancreatitis Thrombocytopenia Anemia Agranulocytosis Stevens-Johnson syndrome Polycystic ovary syndrome
Ethosuximide (Zarontin)	10 mg/kg/day	15–40 mg/kg/day	25–40	40–100	Gastric distress Hiccups Lethargy	Rash Leukopenia Pancytopenia Systemic lupus erythematosus
Gabapentin (Neurontin)	10 mg/kg/day; increase in 5 mg/kg increments	20–100 mg/kg/day; optimal dose not established	5–8	2–12 Usefulness not established	Lethargy Dizziness Ataxia Agitation Weight gain Headache	Rash

(continued on next page)

Table 11.30 Summary of commonly used antiepileptic drugs (AEDs) (continued)

AED (trade names)	Starting dosage	Typical maintenance dosage	Half-life (hours)	Therapeutic range (mg/L)	Common side effects	Serious idiosyncratic side effects
Lamotrigine (Lamictal)	Add-on therapy: If on valproate: Weeks 1–2: 0.2 mg/kg/day Weeks 3–4: 0.5 mg/kg/day If on other AEDs: Weeks 1–2: 2 mg/kg/day Weeks 3–4: 5 mg/kg/day	Add-on therapy: If on valproate: 1–5 mg/kg/day If on other AEDs: 5–15 mg/kg/day	On monotherapy: 25 On valproate: 30–70 On other AEDs: 15	4–20	Lethargy Dizziness Ataxia Headache	Rash Stevens-Johnson syndrome
Topiramate (Topamax)	0.5–1 mg/kg/day	5–9 mg/kg/day	12–24	4–10	Somnolence Dizziness Ataxia Headache Nausea Fatigue Weight loss Acidosis	Rash Glaucoma
Tiagabine (Gabatril)	0.1 mg/kg/day	0.6–1 mg/kg/day	3–9	0.1–0.3	Somnolence Dizziness Ataxia Nausea	Rash
Zonisamide (Zonegran)	1–2 mg/kg/day	4–8 mg/kg/day	30	20–40	Somnolence Dizziness Ataxia	Rash
Levetiracetam (Keppra)	10 mg/kg/day	40–60 mg/kg/day	6–8	5–40	Somnolence Dizziness Ataxia	Rash
Oxcarbazepine (Trileptal)	8–10 mg/kg/day	20–45 mg/kg/day	9 (of active metabolite, 10-monohydroxy-carbazepine)	4–12 (MHD* 12–30)	Somnolence Dizziness Ataxia Headache Nausea	Rash Hyponatremia
Felbamate (Felbatol)	15 mg/kg/day	15–45 mg/kg/day	16	30–80	Insomnia Nausea	Aplastic anemia Hepatic failure
Pregabalin (Lyrica)	3.5–5 mg/kg/day	15–20 mg/kg/day	5–7	Unknown	Somnolence Blurred vision Weight gain	None reported

*MHD (10-monohydroxy-carbazepine) is the active metabolite of oxcarbazepine.

drowsiness. Serious side effects are very rare and include leukopenia and pancytopenia. It is recommended that periodic CBCs be obtained.

Phenobarbital

Phenobarbital, available since 1912, is the oldest AED still used. It is relatively safe, inexpensive, and effective in several seizure types. Side effects such as hyperactivity (especially in toddlers and preschoolers) and concerns about adverse effects on cognition and behavior limit its use. It acts by enhancing GABAergic inhibition, by prolonging the time that chloride channels are open in response to GABA.

Phenobarbital is a broad-spectrum AED with proven efficacy in generalized tonic–clonic, simple partial, and complex partial seizures. It is not effective against absence and myoclonic seizures. Phenobarbital prevents recurrences of febrile seizures and is one of the primary drugs used to treat status epilepticus. Phenobarbital remains the drug of first choice for neonatal seizures (see below), due to its long half-life, although its effectiveness in neonatal seizures is modest. As an inducer of liver enzymes, phenobarbital can accelerate the metabolism of other AEDs, theophylline, cyclosporine, warfarin, and other drugs.

Phenobarbital causes few serious side effects. Rashes are common, but discontinuation of the drug is not required unless the rash is severe or persistent. The major side effects of phenobarbital are lethargy, learning difficulties, and behavioral changes such as hyperactivity, mood lability, irritability, and sleep disturbance. In both children and adults, phenobarbital can affect cognitive abilities such as memory and perceptual-motor function.

Primidone

Primidone (Mysoline), a congener of phenobarbital, is useful in the treatment of generalized tonic–clonic and partial seizures. It differs from many AEDs in that both the parent compound and metabolites have anticonvulsant properties. Primidone is metabolized through oxidation to phenobarbital and splitting of the ring to form phenylethylmalonamide (PEMA). Primidone, phenobarbital, and PEMA all have anticonvulsant actions, and primidone sometimes controls seizures that do not respond to phenobarbital. The side effects and drug interaction profile of primidone are similar to phenobarbital.

Phenytoin and fosphenytoin

Phenytoin (Dilantin) is an inexpensive, broad-spectrum AED that is effective against generalized tonic–clonic, partial, and tonic seizures. Although there are numerous side effects, some of which can be serious, it is generally considered to be safe. Its primary mechanism of action is use-dependent block of neuronal sodium channels.

Phenytoin is metabolized in the liver, but its metabolism differs from that of other AEDs because its biotransformation follows zero-order kinetics. Enzymes responsible for degradation of phenytoin become saturated within the serum therapeutic range, after which the metabolic rate is no longer dependent on substrate load but proceeds at a constant pace (zero-order or nonlinear kinetics). Once hepatic enzyme saturation occurs, small increases in dosage result in a large increase in serum level and subsequent clinical toxicity. After the child has a level in the lower therapeutic range, further increases in dose should be small, generally no more than 25 mg/day once the serum level is above 10 µg/mL. Monitoring serum levels is important. Since phenytoin is highly protein bound, it is useful to obtain free and total phenytoin levels in conditions of hypoproteinemia. Phenytoin is an inducer of

Pearls and Perils

Pharmacology of Antiepileptic Drugs (AEDs)

- Published therapeutic levels of AEDs should be used only as a guide. It is likely that each patient has his own therapeutic level.
- Blood levels are most useful when there is a change in seizure control or toxic side effect; routine levels are often not necessary.
- The most common reason for a subtherapeutic AED level is noncompliance.
- Owing to their erratic bioavailability, the generic preparations of several AEDs (including carbamazepine, valproate, and phenytoin) can sometimes result in erratic serum levels. Before switching drugs or adding a second AED, it may be worth trying the name-brand formulation.
- Blood levels obtained before the steady state is reached (five half-lives) are useful only in emergency situations. Otherwise, wait at least five half-lives after starting a new drug or changing the dosage before obtaining a level.
- The use of a single AED usually results in higher serum levels, less toxicity, and better seizure control than when polytherapy is employed.
- When using drugs with short half-lives, the timing of the level is important (best to get trough levels). In drugs with longer half-lives, timing of levels is less critical.
- When using AEDs that are highly protein bound (e.g., phenytoin or valproate), free or unbound levels can sometimes be more informative.
- The physician should pay close attention to parental observations about behavioral changes with AEDs.
- In some children with intractable seizures, a realistic goal might be to allow the child to function well at home and school even though occasional seizures occur. Cognitive side effects of AEDs can be equally or more detrimental than seizures.

hepatic enzymes, and it has complicated interactions with AEDs and other drugs (Levy et al. 2002).

Because intramuscularly injected phenytoin crystallizes and is subsequently absorbed slowly and erratically, the drug should not be given by this route. Fosphenytoin (Cerebyx), a phosphate-ester prodrug of phenytoin, is a water-soluble form of phenytoin that can be given intravenously or as an intramuscular injection. Fosphenytoin is now a standard AED for treating status epilepticus.

Phenytoin has both dose-dependent and idiosyncratic adverse effects. Monitoring serum levels can eliminate many of dose-related side effects including lethargy, dizziness, ataxia, tremors, and nystagmus. A correlation exists between serum levels and signs of toxicity, with nystagmus appearing around 20 g/mL, ataxia at 30 g/mL, and drowsiness at levels greater than 40 g/mL.

The most serious idiosyncratic reaction is a skin rash. The clinical spectrum of rash ranges from a common morbilliform rash occurring 1–14 days after the beginning of therapy, to the rare, severe toxic epidermal necrolysis, exfoliative dermatitis, and Stevens-Johnson syndrome. Although a morbilliform rash may be benign and self-limited, it is recommended that phenytoin be discontinued with any type of skin reaction because it may be an early indication of a hypersensitivity reaction. In the case of a mild rash, therapy may be resumed after the rash clears. If the rash recurs upon reinstitution of therapy, further phenytoin usage is contraindicated. Hepatic dysfunction is a rare but serious complication that usually occurs during the first 6 weeks of therapy. Lymphadenopathy is a rare complication of phenytoin treatment, requiring that the drug be discontinued.

Cosmetic side effects of chronic phenytoin use include gingival hyperplasia, hirsutism, coarsening of facial features, and acne. These cosmetic side effects reverse when phenytoin is discontinued. Chronic phenytoin use has been associated with cerebellar atrophy. With toxic serum levels, phenytoin has been associated with impairments in attention, memory, speed of information processing, and fatigue.

Valproic acid

Valproic acid (VPA, sodium valproate, Depakene, Depakote, Depacon) is one of the most commonly used AEDs for treating childhood epilepsy. VPA is a broad-spectrum AED effective for typical and atypical absence, partial, generalized tonic–clonic, and myoclonic seizures. Its mechanism of action is complex, likely involving enhanced GABAergic inhibition as well as block of sodium and calcium channels.

VPA is rapidly absorbed after parenteral administration. It is eliminated by the liver. Enzyme-inducing AEDs, such as carbamazepine and phenytoin, reduce VPA levels.

Mild side effects are common, including transient nausea, which usually dissipates over time and can be lessened by taking the drug with food or using the enteric-coated preparation. Sedation is also common upon VPA initiation, especially in children taking multiple AEDs. Hand tremors are related to serum level and are rarely severe enough to cause motor dysfunction; if so, lowering the dose or initiating propanolol may be helpful. Weight gain can be significant, especially in adolescent females. Mild hair loss is sometimes seen.

The teratogenic effects of VPA are well known. Use of VPA by pregnant mothers correlates with an increased incidence of neural tube defects (NTDs) in the fetus. There is a 1–2% risk of NTDs in newborns whose mothers take VPA in the first trimester (Bourgeois 2001). It is unclear whether this increased risk of NTDs is reduced by supplemental folic acid during the pregnancy. Certainly, all women on AEDs, VPA included, should be on supplemental folic acid and probably at doses higher than the standard dosing for pregnant women, although the exact dose remains an area of controversy. Recent concern has also arisen about an association between VPA and polycystic ovary syndrome (PCOS). Studies of children born to mothers with epilepsy have shown a lower mean verbal IQ in those exposed to VPA versus other medication (Adab et al. 2004).

Pancreatitis is a rare but serious side effect of VPA. Symptoms include abdominal pain, vomiting, and elevated serum amylase levels. Thrombocytopenia or platelet dysfunction have been reported with VPA. Except in children undergoing surgery, these findings usually have little clinical importance. Red blood cell aplasia, neutropenia, and bone marrow suppression have also been reported.

Stupor and coma have occurred at therapeutic serum VPA levels, both when used alone or in polytherapy. In some cases, these symptoms are due to hyperammonemia, but VPA-induced hyperammonemia is usually asymptomatic. It may occur in association with other evidence of hepatic dysfunction or with normal liver function tests. Elevated ammonia levels may be associated with increased seizure frequency, lethargy, stupor, and coma. However, elevated ammonia levels also occur without clinical impairment. Although a poor correlation exists between clinical symptoms and serum ammonia levels, reductions of VPA dosage in symptomatic patients may result in clinical improvement.

The most serious side effect associated with VPA is liver toxicity (Perucca 2002). This toxicity is of two types: a common, transient, dose-dependent asymptomatic rise in liver transaminases (ALT and AST), and a rare, idiosyncratic, non–dose-related symptomatic hepatitis that may be fatal. The first type usually occurs within the first 3 months of treatment and is seen in up to 30% of patients. Usually, the ALT and AST fall when the VPA dose is reduced; at other times the elevated enzymes recede spontaneously despite continuation of treatment. Concern is not usually warranted until transaminase levels exceed three times normal values.

Fatal liver toxicity due to VPA has been well documented (Bryant & Dreifuss 1996) and is heralded by jaundice, anorexia, lethargy, and clinical hepatitis. It usually occurs within the first few months of VPA treatment. The risk is highest in children under the age of 2 years on multiple AEDs. The most recent survey, covering the years 1987–1993, cites only one hepatic fatality among more than 600,000 patients on VPA monotherapy over the age of 10 years. Under age 10, the risk on monotherapy is about one in 16,000. Among patients who received VPA as part of polytherapy, the fatality rate was much higher. Under the age of 2 years, there was a 1 in 618 fatality rate, which declined to 1 in 8,307 in the 3- to 10-year-old group; further declines in the fatality rate were observed in older patients. Considering all groups, of more than 1 million patients receiving VPA during 1987–1993, 29 developed fatal hepatotoxicity (1 in 34,691). Although routine laboratory studies are warranted, parents must be warned that the onset of hepatic dysfunction can be rapid and fulminating, and that normal laboratory determinations do not guarantee safety.

All patients on VPA require close monitoring of liver function and hematologic parameters. Baseline CBC platelet count, AST, and ALT should be obtained before VPA is started. Repeat studies should then be performed within the first month and then every 3–6 months, depending on the child's age, concurrent medications, and clinical status. In patients on polytherapy, it is important to obtain levels of all AEDs, because drug interactions with VPA are common. These studies should be repeated immediately if there is any clinical indication of liver disease. An amylase level may be informative if the child has abdominal pain. The cause of easy bruising or bleeding should be pursued with a CBC, platelet count, and clotting studies. In children with lethargy or other mental status changes, serum ammonia should be checked. In children under 2 years of age on VPA, as well as any child with carnitine deficiency, carnitine supplementation is often recommended (50–100 mg/kg/day in divided doses) (DeVivo et al. 1998; Tein 2002). However, there are no conclusive data that coadministration of carnitine reduces the risk of hepatic dysfunction in children on VPA.

Newer antiepileptic drugs

Felbamate

Felbamate (Felbatol), released in the United States in 1993, is approved as monotherapy and adjunctive therapy of partial seizures with or without secondary generalization in adults 14 years of age and older, and as adjunctive therapy for partial and generalized seizures associated with Lennox-Gastaut syndrome in children 2–14 years of age. Unfortunately, in its first year of use, felbamate was linked to 34 cases of aplastic anemia and 18 cases of fatal hepatic failure. No child under 13 years old developed aplastic anemia, but some children under 5 years old did develop liver failure (Pellock et al. 2006). There have been no reported fatalities since then. Currently, felbamate is reserved for patients with severe refractory epilepsy, and only after the attendant risks have been explained fully. The adverse events were especially unfortunate because felbamate was the first AED shown to successfully treat seizures in children with Lennox-Gastaut syndrome. In addition, many of these children were more alert and interactive on the drug.

In children, the most common side effects of felbamate are weight loss, nausea, dizziness, anorexia, and insomnia. All of these side effects are more common with polytherapy. Close monitoring of CBCs and liver function is necessary.

Gabapentin

Gabapentin (Neurontin) was released in the United States in 1994. It is structurally related to the inhibitory neurotransmitter GABA, although its exact mechanism of action is uncertain. In patients 12 years of age or older, gabapentin is somewhat effective for the adjunctive treatment of partial seizures with or without secondarily generalization. In pediatric studies, adjunctive gabapentin had better efficacy than placebo in children with partial seizures (Appleton et al. 1999; McLean & Gidal 2003). Gabapentin is useful for neuropathic pain.

Adverse effects of gabapentin are uncommon and include somnolence, fatigue, dizziness, nausea, and weight gain. Most of these side effects are mild and transient. A major advantage of gabapentin is that it is relatively free of interactions with other drugs. Unlike other AEDs, gabapentin is not metabolized by the liver, does not induce hepatic enzymes, and is not protein bound. It is almost completely eliminated by renal excretion of the parent compound. Gabapentin does not affect the levels of other AEDs. The dose can be escalated and tapered quickly. Despite these advantages, it does not seem to be as effective in controlling seizures as most of the older and newer AEDs.

Lamotrigine

Lamotrigine (Lamictal) was released in 1994. It is approved for the treatment of partial and secondarily generalized seizures in adults, and in children and adults as add-on treatment of generalized seizures in Lennox-Gastaut syndrome (Messenheimer 2002).

Adverse effects may include diplopia, drowsiness, ataxia, and headache. Rashes have been a significant problem in children and adults. Although in some patients the rash is mild and transient, in others the severity of the rash has necessitated its discontinuation. Rash is particularly troublesome when lamotrigine is added to VPA; the rash may be avoided if lamotrigine is added very slowly. Carbamazepine and phenytoin increase the metabolism of lamotrigine, whereas VPA inhibits its metabolism. Smaller doses of lamotrigine are required when VPA is used concurrently, but not when carbamazepine and phenytoin are used with lamotrigine.

Levetiracetam

Levetiracetam (Keppra) is approved for the adjunctive therapy of adults with partial seizures with or without generalization. Its mechanism of action is unknown, but it is probably different from the mechanism of other AEDs. Because very little levetiracetam is protein bound, drug interactions are not common. Since levetiracetam has not been approved for children, dosing recommendations have not been determined. However, a number of open-label studies are providing some guidance on the dosing range and spectrum of activity of this drug in children. Levetiracetam holds promise as a drug with unique characteristics among AEDs.

Side effects include fatigue, lethargy, ataxia, and behavioral alterations, such as irritability, depression, and even psychosis. Such side effects usually appear within the first month of treatment and most are mild.

Oxcarbazepine

Oxcarbazepine (Trileptal) is approved for monotherapy or adjunctive therapy of partial seizures with or without secondary generalization in adults and children 4 years and older. Oxcarbazepine is a carbamazepine derivative that has a similar mechanism of action and a similar side-effect profile to carbamazepine. However, oxcarbazepine side effects (somnolence, fatigue, headache, dizziness, nausea) seem to be milder and the efficacy may be even better than that of carbamazepine (Glauser et al. 2000). There have been anecdotal reports that oxcarbazepine, like carbamazepine, may exacerbate generalized seizures (Mandelbaum et al. 2002). Oxcarbazepine is a weaker hepatic enzyme inducer than carbamazepine and does not exhibit autoinduction. Hyponatremia has been reported in patients using oxcarbazepine. Allergic rashes have been observed; there is approximately 30% cross-reactivity to patients allergic to carbamazepine. Recently, a warning has been added to the prescribing information regarding reports of serious dermatologic reactions, including Stevens-Johnson syndrome and toxic epidermal necrolysis.

Pregabalin

Pregabalin (Lyrica) was approved in 2005 as adjunctive therapy against partial seizures with or without secondary generalization in adults (Brodie 2004). Its efficacy in children is not yet established. Structurally related to gabapentin, this GABA analog has no effect at GABA receptors and might work by blocking calcium-dependent release of excitatory transmitters. Also similar to gabapentin, it is quite effective for neuropathic pain. Common side effects include weight gain, dizziness, somnolence, and constipation. It has little interaction with the metabolism of other drugs. Pregabalin has been reported to exacerbate myoclonic seizures.

Tiagabine

Tiagabine (Gabatril) is approved as adjunctive therapy for partial seizures in adolescents and adults, although it may exacerbate generalized seizures. Tiagabine works by preventing reuptake of synaptically released GABA back into the presynaptic terminal, thus prolonging the time that GABA is available for synaptic inhibition. Common side effects include mental slowing, dizziness, lethargy, and gastrointestinal symptoms such as nausea or pain. Drug interactions with tiagabine are not prominent, although caution should be exercised, especially when VPA is added, since it may worsen tiagabine side effects.

Topiramate

Topiramate (Topamax) has been approved for adjunctive therapy for partial seizures with or without generalization and generalized seizures in adults and children over 2 years of age. It is efficacious in Lennox-Gastaut syndrome and shows some promise for infantile spasms. The mechanism of action is complex, involving actions on sodium channels, calcium channels, and glutamate receptors of the non-N-methyl-D-aspartate (NMDA) type.

The most common side effects are mental slowing, dizziness, somnolence, ataxia, and headache. Patients often lose weight on topiramate, which has led to its proposed use as an appetite suppressant. Because topiramate is a weak carbonic anhydrase inhibitor 1–2% of patients develop renal stones. Acute glaucoma, presenting with severe ocular pain and myopia, may occur shortly after initiation of treatment.

Vigabatrin

Vigabatrin (Sabril) is a reversible inhibitor of GABA transaminase and may exert its anticonvulsant effect by decreasing the breakdown of GABA in the brain. Although it is not available in the United States at this time, vigabatrin merits mention because of its broad efficacy in refractory partial and secondarily generalized seizures, as well as in infantile spasms (particularly in children with tuberous sclerosis). Vigabatrin has relatively low toxicity but has caused psychosis in some patients. There are reports of visual field constriction due to vigabatrin (Iannetti et al. 2000). Otherwise, the drug appears to be well tolerated by children.

Zonisamide

Zonisamide (Zonegran) is a sulfonamide derivative approved in the United States for the adjunctive treatment of partial seizures in adults. However, experience worldwide has shown that it has a much broader spectrum of action and may also be useful in generalized seizures such as myoclonic, absence, and even Lennox-Gastaut syndrome and infantile spasms. The mechanism of action is unknown.

Zonisamide does not dramatically alter the metabolism of other AEDs. Patients may experience somnolence, ataxia, dizziness, fatigue, difficulty with concentration, mental slowing, or even a psychotic reaction, especially in the first few months of treatment. Renal stones occur in up to 4% of adult patients on zonisamide; data are not available for children. Severe idiosyncratic reactions are rare but have included Stevens-Johnson syndrome and aplastic anemia.

Other antiepileptic drugs

Many other medications may be useful in treating seizures in children. Clonazepam (Klonopin), a benzodiazepine, is effective in a variety of seizure types including absence, generalized tonic–clonic, and myoclonic. Clonazepam and other benzodiazepines are often used as adjunctive therapy in children with epilepsy. The development of tolerance requires progressive increases in dosage to achieve the same effect; unfortunately, side effects such as excessive drooling may then supervene. Acetazolamide (Diamox) is a carbonic anhydrase inhibitor with some anticonvulsant effect against generalized seizures, such as absence and generalized tonic–clonic. Methsuximide (Celontin), like ethosuximide, may be useful in absence and has also been shown to be effective in partial complex seizures.

Other epilepsy therapies

Ketogenic diet

The ketogenic diet (KD) was developed in 1920 to mimic the fasting state, which was known to be anticonvulsant. The KD is a specific dietary regimen that has proven efficacious in many children with medically refractory epilepsy. The diet, which must be monitored strictly by an experienced physician and dietician, is composed of a 4:1 ratio (by weight) of fats to carbohydrates and protein. Children consuming such a diet become ketotic, as assessed by increases in serum ketone bodies (acetoacetate and β-hydroxybutyrate). It is unknown how the ketotic state reduces seizures (Bough & Rho 2007; Hartman et al. 2007), but at some centers, up to half of children on the ketogenic diet experience a greater than 90% seizure reduction (Vining 1999; Kossoff 2004). Details of ketogenic diet formulation and administration, side effects, and sample diet plans, as well as answers to parents' frequently asked questions, are summarized in a useful handbook (Freeman et al. 2007).

Vagus nerve stimulation

The vagus nerve stimulator (VNS) is an implantable device that generates a programmed pattern of electrical stimulation to the vagus nerve. Afferent impulses travel to the brain along the vagus nerve and decrease seizures by an unknown mechanism, possibly by "desynchronizing" neuronal activity (Heck et al. 2002). The VNS was approved in the United States in 1997, and the technique is effective in diminishing seizure frequency in some patients. A major advantage is the patient's ability to activate the device when an aura is sensed, thereby averting the spread of the seizure. Disadvantages include the need for surgical implantation and its associated cost, although this must be weighed against the cost of AEDs and their attendant side effects. Minor side effects include a cough or hoarse voice during stimulations. Although the VNS is effective in some children, its place among antiepileptic therapies is still not fully defined (Sheth et al. 2005).

Epilepsy surgery

Some children with medically refractory seizures will benefit from epilepsy surgery. Epilepsy surgery has become an accepted therapeutic modality, with good outcome and

Key Clinical Questions

Epilepsy

- Was it an epileptic seizure?
  Differentiation of an epileptic seizure from a nonepileptic event is critical and is based largely on obtaining a careful history of the event. An electroencephalogram (EEG) may be helpful but can be normal in cases of epilepsy. A video-EEG also yields important information, but is most useful if spells are frequent. A home video recording of the event in question can also assist in the diagnosis.
- If so, what kind of seizure was it?
  The seizure semiology is important for classification and treatment choice.
- Does the seizure, in conjunction with other clinical information (e.g., age, EEG findings, family history, etiology) comprise an epilepsy syndrome?
  This information is crucial for discussion the treatment options and natural history of the epilepsy.
- What diagnostic workup is necessary and sufficient for a given patient?
  An efficient diagnostic evaluation should be tailored to the individual child, based on associated findings and potential for a treatable etiology.

Table 11.31 Summary of selected surgical procedures for children with medically intractable seizures

Procedure	Seizure types	Electroencephalogram	Risks	Benefits
Temporal lobectomy	Simple or complex partial ± secondary generalization	Interictal: Temporal or frontal spikes, sharp waves Ictal: Initially, focal temporal lobe discharges; later, spread	Visual field defect; cerebrovascular accident; third nerve palsy; memory/speech impairment	Seizure reduction or control
Nontemporal resection	Partial ± secondary generalization	Interictal: Focal spikes or sharp waves, occasionally generalized spike wave Ictal: Focal spikes, β activity or polyspike-wave	Dependent on surgical site; hemiparesis; visual field cut	Seizure reduction or control; improved development
Corpus callosotomy	Partial ± secondary generalization; tonic; atonic, drop attacks	Interictal: Multifocal spikes/sharp waves, generalized spike-wave, polyspike-wave Ictal: Rapid spikes, polyspike-wave	Disconnection syndrome; speech deficits; increase in frequency or intensity of partial seizures	Reduction in "drop" and generalized seizures; rarely do seizures totally remit
Hemispherectomy	Unilateral partial ± secondary generalization	Interictal: Lateralized discharges over involved hemisphere; may have bilateral spikes Ictal: Lateralized seizure onset over involved hemisphere	Hemiparesis; hemosiderosis; hydrocephalus	Seizure control; improved behavioral and cognitive status

low morbidity. The issues of patient selection, surgical options and workup, and prognosis are reviewed elsewhere (Cross 2002; Holmes 2002). Table 11.31 lists some of the more common epilepsy surgery techniques in children. Overall, the evidence suggests that earlier surgery is associated with a better neurodevelopmental outcome, since brain plasticity is greater at younger ages (Stafstrom et al. 2000).

Focal lesions, such as dysplasias or developmental tumors, can be resected with an excellent chance of seizure resolution. In adolescents with mesial hippocampal sclerosis (perhaps due to a prolonged febrile seizure or other insult early in life), temporal lobectomy has been shown to be very successful in affording seizure freedom. Corpus callosotomy is occasionally performed to reduce atonic seizures, although the success rate is modest. Hemispherectomy is most useful for children with Rasmussen encephalitis (see below), a focal encephalitis affecting the entire hemisphere (McNamara et al. 1999).

Concluding Remarks

From the plethora of treatment options just discussed, it is clear that the physician has many choices available to treat the child with epilepsy. Of course, if the seizures are due to a systemic derangement (e.g., hypocalcemia or hypoglycemia), the primary etiology can be corrected without AED therapy. Once the decision to treat with an AED is made, the choice of agent will depend on the child's age, lifestyle, syndrome, and concurrent medical conditions and treatments, as well as the side-effect profile of the AED and its cost, potential toxicity, kinetics, and drug interactions. Therefore, the decision is not always straightforward and must be tailored individually to the patient. Although the newer AEDs tend to have fewer idiosyncratic reactions, the full spectrum of drug interactions and side effects will not become clear until these newer AEDs have been used more extensively. For traditional AEDs, we have a better appreciation of the range of adverse reactions and side effects, but their efficacy is often not optimal. Finally, for refractory epilepsy, the complexities of multiple concurrent AEDs must be dealt with and consideration given to alternative epilepsy treatments such as the ketogenic diet, VNS, and epilepsy surgery. Treatment of the child with epilepsy is a truly challenging but rewarding endeavor.

Annotated bibliography

General resources

Arzimanoglou A. et al. *Aicardi's epilepsy in children*. Philadelphia: Lippincott Williams & Wilkins, 2004.
A recently updated edition of Aicardi's classic textbook on pediatric epilepsy. With more than 4,000 references, this

comprehensive guide covers all aspects of epilepsy diagnosis, common and rare syndromes, and a general approach to epilepsy management.

Guerrini R. Epilepsy in children. *Lancet* 2006;367:499–524.
A comprehensive overview of childhood epilepsy and its treatment.

Classification, pathophysiology, and genetics

Ben-Ari Y, Holmes GL. Effects of seizures on developmental process in the immature brain. *Lancet Neurol* 2006;5:1055–1063.
Reviews the mechanisms and consequences of seizures in the developing brain, reasons why the young brain is particularly seizure-prone, and animal models of developmental epilepsy.

Engel J Jr. A proposed diagnostic scheme for people with epileptic seizures and epilepsy: Report of the ILA task force on classification and terminology. *Epilepsia* 2001;42:796–803.
Presents the revised scheme for epilepsies and epilepsy syndromes.

Engel J Jr. (chair). Report of the ILAE classification core group. *Epilepsia* 2006;47:1558–1568.
Revision of 1981 and 1989 classifications of seizures and epilepsies.

Nordli DR Jr. Diagnostic difficulty in infants and children. *J Child Neurol* 2002;17(Suppl. 1):S28–S35.
Discusses difficulties in classification of seizures and epileptic syndromes in young children, compared to the ILAE scheme, as well as an orderly approach to epilepsy classification at very young ages.

Scheffer IE, Berkovic SF. The genetics of human epilepsy. *Trends Pharmacol Sci* 2003;24:428–433.
Excellent update by internationally recognized authorities who have made pivotal advances in the rapidly evolving field of epilepsy genetics.

Stafstrom CE. The pathophysiology of epileptic seizures: A primer for pediatricians. *Pediatr Rev* 1998;19:335–344.
Presents basic concepts of neurophysiology in a readable format.

Evaluation and treatment

Hirtz D, Berg A, Bettis D et al. Practice parameter: Treatment of the child with a first unprovoked seizure. *Neurology* 2003; 60:166–175.
Compiled by expert subcommittees of the American Academy of Neurology and the Child Neurology Society, this review presents detailed recommendations and rationale as to when to treat a first unprovoked seizure in a child.

Levy RH et al., eds. *Antiepileptic drugs*, 5th ed. Philadelphia: Lippincott, Williams & Wilkins, 2002.
This comprehensive book, now in its 5th edition, provides detailed information about all AEDs, old and new.

Raspall-Chaure M, Neville BG, Scott RC. The medical management of the epilepsies in children: Conceptual and practical considerations. *Lancet Neurol* 2008;7:57–69.
Discusses practical aspects of epilepsy diagnosis and treatment with emphasis on challenging situations.

Wheless JW, Clark DF, Carpenter D. Treatment of pediatric epilepsy: Expert opinion, 2005. *J Child Neurol* 2005; 20(Suppl 1):S1–S60.
Summary of recommendations of 41 pediatric epileptologists for treating variety of seizure types and epilepsy syndromes.

Epileptic seizures and epilepsy syndromes

Benbadis SR. Epileptic seizures and syndromes. *Neurol Clin* 2001;19:251–270.

Camfield P, Camfield C. Epileptic syndromes in childhood: Clinical features, outcomes, and treatment. *Epilepsia* 2002; 43(Suppl 3):27–32.
Both references discuss childhood epilepsy syndromes in detail, expanding upon the information presented in this chapter.

Absence epilepsy

Crunelli V, Leresche N. Childhood absence epilepsy: Genes, channels, neurons, and networks. *Nat Rev Neurosci* 2002;3: 371–382.
Describes the neuronal networks underlying absence epilepsy and provides a comprehensive catalog of animal mutants with absence seizures, which may shed some light on the pathophysiologic basis of this common epilepsy.

Posner E. Pharmacological treatment of childhood absence epilepsy. *Expert Rev Neurother* 2006;6:855–862.
Review of absence epilepsy treatments.

Infantile spasms

Brunson KL, Avishai-Eliner S, Baram TZ. ACTH treatment of infantile spasms: Mechanisms of its effects in modulation of neuronal excitability. *Int Rev Neurobiol* 2002;49:185–197.
The emerging understanding of the physiology of infantile spasms may relate to the intrinsic excitability of limbic neurons and its modulation by ACTH.

Frost JD Jr., Hrachovy RA. Pathogenesis of infantile spasms: A model based on developmental desynchronization. *J Clin Neurophysiol* 2005;22:25–36.
These authors, experts in the diagnosis and treatment of infantile spasms, present a plausible pathophysiologic schema of how infantile spasms might develop.

Fukuyama Y. West syndrome and other infantile epileptic encephalopathies. *Brain Dev* (special issue) 2002;23(7).
Contains articles on all aspects of infantile spasms, including epidemiology, diagnosis, EEG, and treatment.

Mackay MT, Weiss SK, Adams-Webber T, et al. Practice parameter: medical treatment of infantile spasms: Report of the American Academy of Neurology and the Child Neurology Society. *Neurology* 2004;62:1668–1681.
Current treatment modalities are critically reviewed.

Lennox-Gastaut syndrome

Conry JA. Pharmacologic treatment of the catastrophic epilepsies. *Epilepsia* 2004;45 (Suppl 5):12–16.

Wheless JW, Constantinou JEC. Lennox-Gastaut syndrome. *Pediatr Neurol* 1997;17:203–211.
These articles overview the diagnosis and treatment of this devastating epileptic encephalopathy, with helpful hints about patient management.

Neonatal seizures

Mizrahi EM, Kellaway P. Characterization and classification of neonatal seizures. *Neurology* 1987;37:1837–1844.
The authors used simultaneous video-EEG recording to develop a classification of neonatal seizures.

Silverstein FS, Jensen FE. Neonatal seizures. *Ann Neurol* 2007;62:112–120.
Overview of current thinking on neonatal seizure pathophysiology and treatment.

Volpe JJ. Neonatal seizures: Current concepts and classification. *Pediatrics* 1989;84:422–428.
Develops a classification of neonatal seizures using careful clinical observation.

Landau-Kleffner syndrome

Ballaban-Gil K, Tuchman R. Epilepsy and epileptiform EEG: Association with autism and language disorders. *Ment Retard Dev Disabil Res Rev* 2000;6:300–308.
Excellent overview of the role of epileptic discharges in language developmental disorders, including autism.

Landau WM, Kleffner FR. Syndrome of acquired aphasia with convulsive disorder in children. *Neurology* 1957;7:523–530.
Classic article that first described the pure syndrome of acquired epileptic aphasia.

Status epilepticus

Maytal J, Shinnar S, Mosche SL, Alvarez LA. Low morbidity and mortality of status epilepticus in children. *Pediatrics* 1989;83:323–331.
In this study of status epilepticus in children, the authors found low mortality and morbidity rates. The improvement in outcome likely relates to improved acute care in recent years.

Mitchell WG. Status epilepticus and acute serial seizures in children. *J Child Neurol* 2002;17 (Suppl 1):S36–S43.
Superb review of risk factors, consequences, and treatment of status epilepticus in children.

Nonepileptic disorders that may mimic epilepsy

Bleasel A, Kotogal P. Paroxysmal nonepileptic disorders in children and adolescents. *Semin Neurol* 1995;15:203–217.

Obeid M, Mikati MA. Expanding spectrum of paroxysmal events in children: Potential mimickers of epilepsy. *Pediatr Neurol* 2007;37:309–316.
Two articles that comprehensively review clinical events that mimic seizures.

Stephenson JBP. *Fits and faints*. Oxford: MacKeith Press, 1990.
Classic monograph that explores the pathophysiology and clinical manifestations of nonepileptic syncopal (hypoxic) seizures.

CHAPTER 12

Movement Disorders in Childhood

Kenneth J. Mack

Outline

Description of movements

Abnormal movements in children are typically classified as hemiballismus, chorea, athetosis, dystonia, tremors, tics, myoclonus, or ataxia. *Hemiballismus* is characterized by large-amplitude, wild, and irregular limb movements. This movement often occurs after an infarct of the subthalamic nucleus opposite the side of the movements. Often the movements will fade into chorea after a period of days (Hallett 1993).

The word *chorea* has been derived from the Greek word for "dance," and originally referred to the epidemic dancing manias of the Middle Ages (Hallett 1993). Choreic movements are single, quick, isolated muscle movements that result in uncoordinated jerks of the face, trunk, or extremities. Often choreic movements occur in combination with athetosis, in which case the term *choreoathetosis* is used.

Athetosis is characterized by slow, sinuous, writhing, and purposeless involuntary movements, which may flow into one another. The wrists are usually held in a flexed position, and the fingers, the shoulders, and much of the lower extremities are held in extension. Athetotic movements are exaggerated by voluntary activity and are not noted during sleep.

Dystonia refers to an abnormal maintenance of a posture, a result of sustained muscle contraction. This abnormal tone may last for seconds to minutes in an affected muscle group.

Tics are brief, involuntary contractions of a muscle or muscle group. This may include vocal tics such as throat clearing, or motor tics such as shoulder shrugging and facial grimacing. Tics are localized to the face and shoulder.

Tremors are involuntary, rhythmic, oscillatory movements caused by the alternate contractions of agonist and antagonist muscles. Typically, these movements oscillate around a single axis. Tremor may occur with action, maintenance of posture, or at rest.

Ataxia refers to a poor coordination of motor function. When a child with cerebellar disease is asked to touch her nose with the tip of an index finger, the movement is performed in an unsteady, halting manner. Ataxic movements may occur in the extremities (appendicular) and/or in the axial musculature (truncal).

Although multiple terms are used to describe abnormal movements, it may be more useful to think of these abnormal movements as flowing along a continuum, rather than as discrete entities. A dystonic child will exhibit an abnormal maintenance of posture in space. Dystonia may flow into the slow, writhing, snake-like movements of athetosis. Chorea is described as sudden jerk-like movements, but many of the disorders described in this chapter appear as a "chorea-athetosis" or "choreoathetosis." In the most severe form of jump-like movements, ballismus (or more typically, hemiballismus), the movements will be strong enough to knock a child off a chair. Many abnormal movements do not readily fit into a single descriptive category. Hence, it may be more informative to describe the actual movements than to attempt to label the movements.

Although these classifications are descriptively useful, some diseases are manifested by multiple movement abnormalities. For instance, patients with ataxia-telangiectasia may have both ataxic and choreiform movements. Wilson disease patients may exhibit tremor, dystonia, and/or rigidity. Similarly, patients with juvenile parkinsonism may have dystonia, tremor, bradykinesia, and rigidity.

Evaluation of the child

The history and physical examination will often be the most important factor in making the diagnosis. Historically, it is useful to determine whether the movements represent an acute or a slowly progressive process. Sudden onset of movements suggests some recent insult to the brain. Did the child recently have varicella (as in postinfectious varicella ataxia) or a streptococcal infection (as in Sydenham chorea)? Do certain activities trigger the movements, as in a paroxysmal movement disorder? Are there comorbid features, such as symptoms of attentional problems or obsessive-compulsive traits, as in tic disorders?

The past medical history and review of systems can be most helpful. A history of liver disease raises concern about Wilson disease; although neurological symptoms usually present later in life, they may present before liver abnormalities are identified. Huntington disease in childhood may first present as a difficult-to-control seizure disorder. A history of significant jaundice may suggest a bilirubin encephalopathy. Patients with ataxia-telangiectasia are subject to frequent sino-pulmonary infections.

A thorough family history is often crucial in making the diagnosis. Some movement disorders are inherited as a simple recessive or autosomal dominant trait. However, in other disorders, the genetics are more complex. Huntington disease shows anticipation in succeeding generations, so that newer generations may be symptomatic earlier and have a more severe course than their parents. The genetics of Tourette syndrome are poorly understood, although parents and siblings may show a subset of comorbid symptoms (attention deficit disorder, obsessive compulsive symptoms, or tics), and tics may be inherited as an autosomal dominant trait with variable penetrance.

A complete physical examination is often the most cost effective diagnostic study and the most significant segment of the evaluation of a child with a movement disorder. Some diseases have notable changes on the general examination, such as the bulbar conjunctival telangiectasias in ataxia-telangiectasia. The mental status examination will be of note in several disorders. Because of the behavioral, cognitive, and personality alterations that may occur in Huntington or Wilson disease, patients may be misdiagnosed with a psychiatric disorder. Patients with Sydenham chorea often display an emotional lability. In the opsoclonus-myoclonus syndrome, severe random chaotic eye movements will be noted. Ataxia is noted by observing the incoordination of the eye movements (nystagmus), trunk (titubation), and extremities (decomposition of movements during finger-to-nose testing). Many choreoathetotic movement disorders have an associated hypotonia. In choreoathetotic disorders, it is helpful to have the patient try to rest his hands on his legs. Often the patient is unable to maintain this position, eliciting the movements. Alternatively, the patient can stand with his hands outstretched and eyes closed, in which case quick jerking movements of the fingers may be noted. Reflexes are diminished or absent in several disorders, such as ataxia-telangiectasia. In the choreas, reflexes are often described as being "hung up." This has the appearance of a prolonged contraction in a muscle whose tendon has been tapped with a reflex hammer. Gait is a critical part of the examination. Parkinson patients will show a slow, shuffling gait. Hereditary dystonic disorders often show tonic posturing of the feet, often brought out by walking.

During the examination, it is more useful to see the abnormal movements than to rely on the patient's or another individual's labeling of these movements. When the movements are complex, it is often useful to describe the dyskinesia, rather than trying to force the movement into a descriptive category. The accessibility of video recorders has made photographic documentation of the severity, duration, and frequency of the movements more readily available for later study. This is particularly useful for movements that are not readily observed in the office, and parents can often bring in a videotape of a movement disorder that occurs infrequently.

Ancillary testing

The history and physical examination should direct which ancillary tests are ordered. Not every patient with a movement disorder needs all or any of the following tests.

It is useful to ask if a structural abnormality predisposes the child to the movement disorder. This is particularly true in an acute-onset disorder, in the choreoathetoses, or in the dystonias. Magnetic resonance imaging (MRI) is the most helpful test, and characteristic MRI abnormalities have been noted in Huntington (caudate atrophy), Sydenham (increased T2 signal in the basal ganglia), and neurodegeneration with brain iron accumulation (NBIA; "eye-of-the-tiger" MRI abnormality secondary to iron deposition in the basal ganglia). The MRI findings in kernicterus (bilateral globus pallidus lesions with or without lesions in the subthalamic nuclei) can distinguish it from hypoxic–ischemic encephalopathy.

The electroencephalograph (EEG) can sometimes be abnormal, although EEG abnormalities in these disorders tend to be nonspecific and therefore of limited use in making an etiologic diagnosis. The EEG is of most benefit when trying to differentiate abnormal movements from seizure activity. Video-EEG documentation of the abnormal movements is often helpful.

Blood tests can help confirm a diagnosis. Antistreptolysin O (ASO) titers for Sydenham, ceruloplasmin for Wilson, IgA levels for ataxia-telangiectasia, and thyroid studies to rule out thyroid abnormalities are easily performed. Specific genetic testing is now available for many movement disorders. The website GeneTests (http://genetests.org/) is particularly helpful in delineating the most up-to-date information on test availability for specific conditions. In certain conditions, such as Huntington disease, counseling must be done before the test is performed. In some of the intermittent ataxia syndromes, measurement of serum amino acids, short-chain fatty acids, and urine organic acids may detect some forms of metabolic causes.

Surface electromyograph (EMG) recording may help better characterize the specific movement disorder (Canavese et al. 2008). This is particularly true of tremors and myoclonic movements, whereas dystonic movements may be difficult to distinguish from voluntary movements.

Functional anatomy of the extrapyramidal system

The extrapyramidal system plays an important role in the control and execution of motor movements. It consists of the basal ganglia, thalamus, subthalamic nuclei, substantia nigra, red nuclei, and brainstem reticular formation. The basal ganglia are composed of the corpus striatum and the amygdaloid nuclear complex. The amygdala is not involved in movement and is not usually considered as part of the extrapyramidal system. The term *corpus striatum* refers to caudate, putamen, and globus pallidus. *Neostriatum*, or just *striatum*, refers to the caudate and putamen; *palladium* refers to globus pallidus. *Lenticular nucleus*, a descriptive term, refers to the combination of the putamen and globus pallidus. The neostriatum and palladium are phylogenetically, cytologically, and functionally distinct. The neostriatum receives fibers from the cerebral cortex, the intralaminar nuclei of the thalamus nuclei, the substantia nigra, and the globus pallidus, and it sends fibers to the substantia nigra and globus pallidus.

The extrapyramidal system can be thought of as a complex series of interconnected feedback loops that ultimately, through modulation of the direct corticospinal pyramidal pathways, influence movement. One example is a loop that connects cerebral cortex to striatum to globus pallidus to thalamus and back to cerebral cortex; another loops from striatum to substantia nigra and back again to striatum.

Striatal neurons discharge prior to the onset of movement, suggesting that the basal ganglia participate in the initiation of movement. The extrapyramidal system also participates in control of ongoing movement, posture, and automatic and skilled volitional movement.

A functional equilibrium exists between the acetylcholine and the dopamine systems of the extrapyramidal system. A reduction of dopamine in the striatum and substantia nigra in Parkinson disease, and this is associated with akinesia or bradykinesia. Therefore parkinsonian symptoms respond favorably to dopaminergic or to anticholinergic drugs. An excess in dopaminergic tone can produce chorea and other hyperkinesias. Similarly, the chorea of Huntington disease is exacerbated by L-dopa (a dopamine agonist) and treated with cholinergic agonists (trihexyphenidyl) or dopamine receptor blockers (haloperidol).

To understand the anatomy of these abnormal movements, one may think of two classes of movement disorders, *hyperkinetic* and *hypokinetic*. The hyperkinetic disorders (e.g., tics, chorea, athetosis, and ballismus) are characterized by an excess of movement, with uncontrollable and relatively rapid motor acts intruding into the normal flow of motor activity (Albin et al. 1989, for review). In addition to shared anatomy, some of these movements will share a common pharmacology. These abnormal movements tend to be exacerbated by dopamine agonists (e.g., methylphenidate) and attenuated by dopamine antagonists (e.g., haloperidol).

Choreoathetosis is seen in a variety of neurological diseases. Because of the association of Huntington disease with abnormalities in the striatum (i.e., the caudate and putamen), choreoathetosis has been assumed to be caused by a striatal lesion. However, traumatic, ischemic, or ablative lesions of the striatum in humans infrequently produce choreoathetosis. In Huntington disease, the degeneration of γ-aminobutyric acid (GABA) and cholinergic striatal neurons with relatively preserved dopaminergic function is associated with chorea.

Tics, a third category in this hyperkinetic movement disorder group, have not been consistently associated with specific neuropathologic lesions of the basal ganglia.

In contrast, hypokinetic movement disorders are characterized by akinesia (lack of movement), bradykinesia (slow movement), and/or rigidity. Parkinson disease is the best understood movement disorder. Parkinson disease results from impaired dopaminergic transmission from the substantia nigra (in the midbrain) to the striatum. This may be caused either pharmacologically (e.g., by phenothiazines), by toxin exposure (e.g., 1-methyl-4-phenyl-1,2,3,6-tetrahydropyridine [MPTP]), or by cell loss in the region of the substantia nigra.

Dystonia occurs when the patient spontaneously and uncontrollably assumes an unusual, fixed posture that lasts from seconds to minutes. Radiographic studies of patients with hemidystonia, in whom symptoms are confined to one side of the body, have implicated the putamen, globus pallidus, or the thalamic target regions of the globus pallidus (Marsden et al. 1985).

Chorea and athetosis

This group of disorders presents with quick, jerk-like movements (chorea) that can at times seem to flow into the writhing snake-like movements of athetosis. Some of these disorders have dystonic movements as well. Ataxia-telangiectasia (AT; discussed later in this chapter) should be in the differential diagnosis of an individual with chorea, since the choreoathetoid movements of AT are as prominent as the ataxia. Some of the more frequent disorders seen in children with choreoathetosis are described below.

Sydenham chorea

Sydenham chorea (St. Vitus dance) was first described by Sydenham in 1684. It was recognized as the major neurologic manifestation of rheumatic fever a century later. St. Vitus was originally designated as "protector" of the faithful from the dancing manias of the Middle Ages. St. Vitus later lost his protector status when his name became synonymous with the chorea of acute rheumatic disease (Park & Park 1990). Rheumatic fever, an inflammatory disease that may affect heart, joint, central nervous system (CNS), and subcutaneous tissue, follows a group A β-hemolytic streptococcal pharyngitis. The chorea is characterized by quick, uncoordinated motions (often occurring unilaterally), whereas the athetosis is writhing in nature. Hypotonia and emotional lability are also characteristics of this disorder. The symptoms are often short-lived (typically regress over a period of weeks to months), but can be quite debilitating.

Experimental evidence suggests that Sydenham chorea is due to an autoimmune response. Serum immunoglobulins from patients with Sydenham chorea binds to caudate and subthalamus brain tissue in direct proportion to the clinical severity of the chorea (Husby et al. 1976; Swedo 1994). Cross-reactivity occurs between these CNS tissues and the bacteria, because serum-binding activity can be abolished by preabsorption with group A streptococcal membranes. Antibasal ganglia autoantibodies that cross-react with streptococcal, caudate, and subthalamic nuclei antigens can be identified by Western immunoblotting and immunofluorescence in both acute and persistent Sydenham chorea (Church et al. 2002). Recent evidence of increased cytokines and interleukins suggest that cell-mediated mechanisms may also be involved (Church et al. 2003; Teixeira et al. 2004).

MRI studies may be normal or may show an increased signal intensity on T2-weighted images in the basal ganglia or cerebral white matter after symptoms appear (Kienzle et al. 1991; Robertson & Smith 2002). Signal abnormalities may occur contralateral to the affected extremities in children with hemichorea, and gradually resolve after the movements cease.

The onset of Sydenham chorea is usually subtle, beginning with clumsiness, restlessness, fidgetiness, and fatigue. The abnormal movements begin in the face. Unlike Huntington disease, Sydenham chorea affects the upper extremities more than the lower extremities, and the distal muscles are more affected than the proximal. Speech is dysarthric, and patients may even become mute. Onset occurs between 5 and 15 years of age, and the gender ratio is about 50:50 until puberty, when females become affected twice as often as males. There may be a positive family history for rheumatic fever. The chorea can lag behind the etiologic streptococcal infection by 1–6 months, so antistreptococcal titers may be negative (Ayoub & Wannamaker 1966).

The physical signs associated with Sydenham chorea are summarized in Table 12.1.

Chorea is most often generalized, but one out of five patients has hemichorea (Nausieda et al. 1980). Hemiparesis, seizures, or EEG abnormalities may occur rarely. Psychological disturbances may occur before, during, or after the onset of the illness. These manifestations include emotional lability, nightmares, poor attention span, and obsessive-compulsive symptoms (Swedo 1994).

Up to one-third of patients who present with chorea, but no other signs of rheumatic fever, will even-

Table 12.1 Physical signs associated with Sydenham chorea

Sign	Explanation
Milkmaid's grip	Inability to maintain a sustained handgrip contraction
Darting tongue	Inability to maintain tongue protrusion
Pronator sign	External rotation of the hands when arms are held over head
Choreic hand	So-called dishing hand or spoon hand
"Hung up" deep tendon reflexes	Evoked choreic movement when deep tendon reflexes (e.g., knee jerk) are elicited, resulting in a slow return to original position
Pendular knee jerks	Antagonist hypotonia
Diffuse hypotonia	Floppy muscular tone
Abnormal speech	Indistinct, jerky, explosive, and irregular speech

tually develop rheumatic heart disease. If other manifestations of rheumatic fever occur at any time, the risk of heart disease is greatly increased (Aron et al. 1965).

The course of the disease is *subacute*. Often chorea and associated findings disappear by 1–6 months, and invariably are gone by 2 years. About 20% of patients develop a second episode of chorea, usually within 2 years of the first attack (Nausieda et al. 1983, Demiroren et al, 2007).

Uncomplicated Sydenham chorea is usually a benign, self-limited disorder of the CNS, although minimal neurologic sequelae may remain. Mild motor abnormalities, such as choreiform movements, hypotonia, intention tremor, and impaired fine and gross motor abilities, have been found 20 years after the initial episode (Bird et al. 1976; Nausieda et al. 1983). Psychiatric symptoms are more frequent in patients evaluated two or three decades after the onset of Sydenham chorea (Freeman et al. 1965).

Commonly prescribed drugs—such as phenytoin, female sex hormones, thyroid hormones (which sensitize postsynaptic striatal dopamine receptors), decongestants (sympathomimetic or anticholinergic), and *d*-amphetamine—may induce chorea at low doses in patients with a previous history of Sydenham chorea. Nausieda and colleagues (1983) found dopaminergic hypersensitivity (adverse choreic reactions to these drugs) in about half of patients who had had Sydenham chorea an average of 22 years earlier. These patients also had elevations in their Minnesota Multiphasic Personality Inventory scores, indicative of a potential for psychotic thought processes. These findings are consistent with the notion of chronic hypersensitivity of the dopaminergic system with effects on both motor and mental function in some patients following episodes of Sydenham chorea.

Treatments for Sydenham chorea have included bed rest, diazepam, haloperidol, pimozide, carbamazepine, valproate, and baclofen, but their efficacy has not been well established. A recent study showed an improvement in chorea with prednisone (Paz et al. 2006). Plasma exchange or intravenous immunoglobulin (IVIG) also appears to be effective (Garvey et al. 2005). Because of the high incidence of associated serious heart disease, penicillin or other antibiotic prophylaxis is indicated until at least adulthood, and during childbearing years (Table 12.2).

Table 12.2 Sydenham Chorea

Discriminating features
- Chorea

Consistent features
- Generalized chorea
- Subacute in onset
- Usually chorea disappears by 2 months

Variable features
- Insidious onset
- Distal more affected than proximal
- Hemichorea
- Mental and emotional disturbances
- Recurrence within 2 years in 20% of cases

Huntington disease

Huntington disease is an autosomal dominant neurodegenerative disease, the result of a trinucleotide (CAG) expansion in the gene Huntingtin on chromosome 4 (4p16.3) (Huntington Disease Collaborative Research Group 1993), which encodes a protein known as huntingtin, found throughout the brain. Individuals with the disease generally have more than 39 CAG repeats, with normal being less than 20. Repeats over 80 are often associated with the juvenile form. Complete (100%) penetrance has been described with CAG repeats of greater than 42, whereas only some with CAG repeat lengths of 36–41 showed signs or symptoms within a normal lifespan (Brinkman et al. 1997).

The CAG expansion occurs during meiosis. Children tend to have a larger expansion (and therefore worse disease) than their parents. The size of the expanded CAG repeat is inversely associated with the age of onset of the disease (Brinkman et al. 1997). However, only 70% of the variation in the onset of Huntington disease is accounted for by repeat size (Djousse et al. 2003; Li et al. 2003). Recent evidence is that the unexplained variation is strongly heritable, suggesting that several other genes modify the age of onset (Li et al. 2003).

The tendency of CAG repeats to expand from generation to generation underlies *genetic anticipation*, a worsening of the disease in subsequent generations, and paternally derived CAG repeats seem more unstable (Ranen et al. 1995).

The juvenile form is more likely to be inherited from the father. Juvenile-onset Huntington disease, with onset at or before 10 years of age, accounts for about 5% of reported cases (Jervis 1963; Osborne et al. 1982). The onset, presentation, and course of Huntington disease differ in juveniles and adults.

Adult-onset Huntington disease may present as (a) abnormal movements, especially chorea; (b) intellectual decline and dementia; (c) emotional instability; or (d) some combination of the foregoing. The course is slowly progressive and unaffected by current treatment. Juvenile-onset Huntington disease most often presents with rigidity (the Westphal variant), speech defects, intellectual abnormalities, chorea or choreoathetosis, and tremor (Markham & Knox 1965; Hansotia et al. 1968; Gonzalez-Alegre & Afifi 2006). Cerebellar signs and seizures are also frequent. In contrast to patients with adult-onset Huntington disease, seizures occur in up to

50% of children; the seizures are either grand mal or grand mal in combination with absence, myoclonic, astatic, or photosensitive seizures. The juvenile-onset disease progresses about twice as rapidly as the adult-onset version, with an average duration of 9.3 years (Osborne et al. 1982). Table 12.3 presents a comparison of juvenile- and adult-onset Huntington disease.

The pathologic findings include atrophy of the corpus striatum and, in contrast to adult-onset cases, severe gliosis of the globus pallidus and cerebellar atrophy. Involvement of the vestibular nuclei and the lateral corticospinal tracts has also been described. The damage to the globus pallidus has been proposed to be responsible for the prominence of rigidity in children (Byers & Dodge 1967).

Genetic testing is now available through direct mutation analysis using polymerase chain reaction (PCR) testing to estimate the number of CAG repeats. Children under the age of 18 years are generally not tested unless symptomatic.

Computed tomography (CT) scan and MRI may show atrophy of the caudate nuclei, which often precedes clinical symptoms (Terrence et al. 1977; Sax & Menzer 1977). In mild Huntington disease, atrophy of putamen may be detected before obvious changes in the caudate (Harris et al. 1992), especially in children (Harris et al. 1999). In early to mid stages, morphometric MRI studies show volume reduction in almost all brain structures, including total cerebrum, total white matter, cerebral cortex, caudate, putamen, globus pallidus, amygdala, hippocampus, brainstem, and cerebellum (Rosas et al. 2003). In children, cerebellar atrophy may be seen. Positron emission tomographic (PET) scans show decreased glucose use in the caudate and putamen, which appears even earlier than the tissue loss demonstrable by CT (Kuhl et al. 1982; Antonini et al. 1996).

Concern has been raised regarding the potentially damaging psychological effects of presymptomatic testing for this devastating disease. However, studies show that 75–80% of people at risk for Huntington disease wish to know this information in order to cope, plan, and prepare for the future (Koller & Davenport 1984). Specific guidelines are available for the testing of patients at risk (Hersch et al. 1994).

Table 12.3 Comparison of juvenile and adult-onset Huntington disease

Symptoms of juvenile-onset	Symptoms of adult-onset
Rigidity	Chorea
Speech disorder	Dementia
Behavioral abnormality	Emotional effects
Seizures	
Cerebellar signs	
Inheritance from father in 90%	Inheritance from mother in 55–70%

Pearls and Perils

Disorders Presenting with Chorea, Athetosis, or Both

- Persistence of choreic movements over a 6-month period is uncommon in Sydenham chorea.
- In the assessment of a child who presents with chorea and a positive family history distinguishes Huntington and benign familial chorea from Sydenham chorea.
- Magnetic resonance imaging (MRI), metabolic studies, and drug screening tests should be considered in all children with a new acute-onset movement disorder.

Management consists of symptomatic treatment and genetic counseling. The chorea may respond to such dopamine receptor blockers as haloperidol, dopamine depletors such as tetrabenazine (Huntington Study Group 2006), or benzodiazepines. Medical management of comorbidities such as depression, anxiety, or obsessive-compulsive disorder (OCD), and supportive management by members of a multidisciplinary team is important.

Benign hereditary chorea

This condition was initially described in 1967 by Haerer and associates. It is characterized by the early onset of nonprogressive chorea and is not associated with intellectual deterioration. Lack of progression of the chorea and the absence of dementia distinguishes it from Huntington disease. The persistence of involuntary movements for many years distinguishes this condition from Sydenham chorea. A history of familial occurrence makes the diagnosis of a choreic form of cerebral palsy unlikely.

The abnormal movements usually have their onset early, during infancy or childhood, and are often first noted when the child begins to walk. The gait of children with the syndrome is noticeably more lurching and halting than that of other children learning to walk. The abnormal movements show little or no progression after the initial presentation. In adulthood, the movements may persist or decrease (Mahajnah et al. 2007). The severity of the choreic movements varies from mild jerking of the extremities to gross sudden jerks that interfere with ambulation and writing. As with other individuals with movement disorders, the chorea is aggravated by tension and anxiety. Some patients suffer varying degrees of dysarthria, the severity of which may be related to the extent of the chorea. The involuntary movements impair smooth air production during speech.

Affected children are often delayed in walking and may present to a physician for evaluation of delayed motor milestones (Wheeler et al. 1993). Cognitive and academic skills may be impaired; however, progressive dementia is not a feature of this disorder. One kindred was assessed for intellectual function; affected members were noted to have lower verbal intelligence and greater deficits in verbal abstract concept formation than unaffected family members (Leli et al. 1984). Some affected children have significant difficulty in learning to write legibly due to the severity of the involuntary movements.

This condition is the result of mutations in the *TITF-1* (thyroid transcription factor-1) gene (Breedveld et al. 2002).

No medication has been consistently effective in relieving the abnormal movements of these patients. It was discovered serendipitously that the movements were lessened by steroids in one instance (Robinson & Thornett 1985). Some of our patients felt better while on short-term courses of haloperidol or other dopamine receptor blockers. Genetic counseling, occupational and speech therapy, and educational guidance are important management measures (Table 12.4).

Table 12.4 Benign familial chorea

Discriminating features
- Nonprogressive chorea
- No intellectual deterioration or dementia
- Persistence of involuntary movements for many years

Consistent features
- Family history; autosomal dominant
- Early onset
- Lurching walk

Variable features
- Dysarthria
- Mildly impaired cognitive skills

Kernicterus

Bilirubin encephalopathy (kernicterus) is caused when brain tissue is exposed to toxic levels of free (unbound) unconjugated bilirubin. The clinical features of bilirubin encephalopathy range from severe to mild. The severity of bilirubin encephalopathy depends on the amount and duration of bilirubin exposure, the maturational state of the exposed brain, and factors that favor the net transfer of bilirubin into brain tissue, such acidosis and hypoalbuminemia. Most newborns with elevated bilirubin who receive phototherapy or exchange transfusion will not develop kernicterus (Newman et al. 2006).

Autopsies of infants with severe bilirubin toxicity reveal the pathologic syndrome of kernicterus with bright yellow staining of fresh brain tissue and neuronal necrosis of the basal ganglia, hippocampus, and brainstem nuclei, including oculomotor, cochlear, and inferior colliculi (Gerrard 1952; Malamud 1961).

Kernicterus is mistakenly believed to be a disease of the past, owing to the decline of its best-known cause, Rh disease of the newborn. However, the prevalence of kernicterus in newborns with other conditions (e.g., prematurity, low birth weight, and associated conditions) is a continuing concern (Gartner et al. 1970), particularly in the preterm population. Recent reports of kernicterus in term and near-term infants due in part to early discharge of newborns from hospitals (Brown & Johnson 1996; Johnson et al. 2002; Braveman et al. 1995; Seidman et al. 1995; Maisels & Newman 1998) have prompted new warnings to hospitals in the United States and a new Practice Parameter on Hyperbilirubinemia from the American Academy of Pediatrics (2004).

Kernicterus in current usage refers to both the clinical as well as the neuropathologic syndrome. The clinical symptoms of bilirubin toxicity can be classified into acute and chronic bilirubin encephalopathy. Acute bilirubin encephalopathy in a neonate initially manifests with lethargy, decreased feeding, poor suck, and may include variable abnormal tone (hypotonia and/or hypertonia). As toxicity evolves, high-pitched cry, the "setting sun" sign, hypertonia, retrocollis, and opisthotonos occur and may progress to fever, seizures, and death.

Laboratory evidence ranges from prolonged brainstem auditory evoked potential (BAEP) interwave intervals I–III and I–V and decreased amplitude waves III and V, to absent BAEPs, which may improve with exchange transfusion (Wennberg et al. 1982; Nwaesei et al. 1984). The MRI shows acute abnormalities in the globus pallidus and subthalamic nucleus (Penn et al. 1994; Johnston & Hoon 2000; Govaert et al. 2003).

After the first year of life, infants who survive significant bilirubin toxicity gradually develop the syndrome of chronic post kernicteric bilirubin encephalopathy.

Chronic bilirubin encephalopathy is characterized by (a) a movement disorder consisting mainly of dystonia and/or athetosis, but also including spasticity and hypotonia; (b) auditory dysfunction consisting of deafness or hearing loss and auditory neuropathy or dyssynchrony; (c) oculomotor impairments especially impairment of upgaze; and (d) dental enamel hypoplasia of the deciduous teeth. The extrapyramidal abnormalities are the most striking feature of this syndrome, occurring in over 90% of patients with severe neonatal jaundice (Perlstein 1960). Athetosis is the principal manifestation, involving all limbs, but usually with the upper limbs affected more than the lower. Abnormal swallowing, phonation, and facial movements are also present, and chorea, ballismus, dystonia, and less often, tremor or rigidity may occur. In some cases, the extrapyramidal abnormalities may be apparent only during attempted skilled movements.

In the "athetoid" cerebral palsy due to kernicterus, the dystonia does not usually lead to fixed postures and contractions, and sparing of cortex and subcortical white matter tracts usually results in normal intelligence. However, specific learning disorders and abnormal sensory or sensorimotor integration may occur from involvement of auditory pathways, and proposed sensorimotor integration areas of globus pallidus integration may occur from involvement of auditory pathways (Boecker et al. 1999).

The less severe type of bilirubin encephalopathy may produce subtle cognitive disturbances, neurologic abnormalities, and hearing loss (Hyman et al. 1969; Odell et al. 1970; Johnson & Boggs 1974; Naeye 1978; Rubin et al. 1979), and may occur in premature infants without marked hyperbilirubinemia (Connolly & Volpe 1990). Choreoathetosis and impaired upgaze are uncommon findings in this group of patients—about 60% having hearing loss as their only manifestation (Bergman et al. 1985). Measures of free bilirubin—that is, unconjugated bilirubin that is not bound to albumin—predict these outcomes better than conventional total or conjugated bilirubin (Odell et al. 1970; Johnson & Boggs 1974) (Table 12.5).

Athetotic cerebral palsy

Cerebral palsy refers to a set of static motor impairment syndromes that occur from insults acquired before, at, or immediately after birth. Extrapyramidal disorders are rarely observed before the end of the first year of life, possibly because the pyramidal tracts, which are necessary for the expression of movement disorders, have not yet fully myelinated. One-fifth of children with static encephalopathy caused by developmental defect or a brain injury acquired in the perinatal period develop movement disorders (Lagregran 1981). Both athetoid and dystonic forms of cerebral palsy have been identified, primarily in full-term infants (Kuban & Leviton 1994). Chorea or choreoathetosis may also occur. Pyramidal tract signs (spasticity, paresis) are usually seen in combination with the movement disorder. Oromotor difficulties, speech dysarthria, and drooling are particularly prominent in this group.

In some cases of athetotic cerebral palsy, no etiology is discovered. In a few cases, calcifications of the basal ganglia are seen on CT scans (Billard et al. 1989). In one study, abnormalities in the basal ganglia, thalamus, and/or white matter were seen on MRI imaging of 14 of 16 children with athetotic cerebral palsy (Yokochi et al. 1991). The association of prematurity, hypoxia, ischemia, acidosis, and subependymal and intraventricular hemorrhage with increased susceptibility to bilirubin neurotoxicity may explain the frequent intermingling of pyramidal and extrapyramidal symptoms.

Two causes of athetoid, dystonic CP have now been recognized, hypoxia–ischemia and bilirubin neurotoxicity (kernicterus, see earlier section for description). In hypoxia–ischemia, areas of abnormal, hyperintense MRI signal are identified in the putamen, thalamus, and motor strip, whereas in kernicterus, hyperintense signal are seen in the globus pallidus and, occasionally, subthalamus (Penn et al. 1994; Johnston & Hoon 2000; Govaert et al. 2003). Although perinatal adverse events are frequently seen in this group (Himmelmann et al, 2007), metabolic disorders should be suspected when no other causes are identified.

Table 12.5 Bilirubin encephalopathy

Discriminating features
- Unconjugated hyperbilirubinemia

Consistent features
- Athetosis
- Impairment of upgaze
- Hearing loss

Variable features
- Dental enamel hypoplasia
- Impaired extraocular movements
- Dysarthria

Postpump chorea

Postpump chorea occurs in about 1% of children who undergo open cardiac surgery. The chorea begins 3–12 days after surgery, and may be either transient or permanent. Imaging studies reveal diffuse atrophy. Many patients have additional cognitive deficits. During surgery, affected patients seem to have spent more time on the pump, and at temperatures under 36°C, compared to unaffected controls (Medlock et al. 1993). Other authors have hypothesized that hypothermia and respiratory alkalosis during the rewarming period may contribute to this insult (Curless et al. 1994).

Systemic illness involuntary movements

Chorea and other movement disorders are occasionally associated with systemic illness, presumably by altering basal ganglia function through a variety of mechanisms, such as hypoperfusion of subcortical vascular watershed regions secondary to ischemia, cytotoxic or inflammatory reactions, or vasculopathy caused by infections or autoimmune processes (Cardoso 2004).

Chorea associated with systemic diseases such as systemic lupus erythematosus and Henoch-Schönlein purpura may resemble Sydenham chorea (Herd et al. 1978). Chorea may be a manifestation of hyperthyroidism or its treatment, hypocalcemia, or hypoparathyroidism with cerebral calcification, processes that may influence neurotransmitter balance in the basal ganglia (Janavs and Aminoff 1998). Infections such as *Mycoplasma pneumoniae* (Beskind & Keim 1994), Epstein-Barr virus (Tachi et al. 1993), or HIV (Cardoso 2004) have also been associated with the onset of chorea. In patients with severe preexisting brain damage, valproate may also provoke choreiform movements (Lancman et al. 1994). Conditions that increase estrogen concentration, such as the taking of oral contraceptives or pregnancy, may be associated with chorea (Nausieda et al. 1979).

Chorea may also be sequelae of brain injury caused by head trauma or vascular disease. Various chronic, progressive, metabolic, and neurodegenerative disorders of childhood may be associated with chorea. These include infantile Leigh syndrome, Pelizaeus-Merzbacher disease, Lesch-Nyhan disease, juvenile Niemann-Pick disease, ataxia-telangiectasia, and glutaric aciduria. Tumors of the basal ganglia are very rarely a cause of chorea, but should be considered in cases of unilateral chorea, even though other conditions are much more likely. Thus—in addition to the taking of clinical and family histories—a physical examination; tests such as serum amino acids, urine organic acids, blood measurements of lactate and pyruvate, uric acid, calcium, phosphorus, and thyroid and parathyroid hormones; screening tests for connective tissue disorders such as lupus; lysosomal enzyme assays; and neuroradiologic imaging studies, especially MRI, may be useful.

Dystonia

Dystonia, as a symptom, is characterized by slow, sustained contortions of axial and appendicular muscles producing twisting, often repetitive movements and abnormal positions and postures; it is found in a number of disorders. Dystonia is a result of coactivation of antagonistic groups of muscles and the lack of reciprocal inhibition. The differential diagnosis of disorders that present with chronic and progressive dystonia include torsion dystonia, NBIA, and metabolic disorders such as glutaric aciduria. However, more than one type of abnormal movement may regularly occur in specific disorders. Wilson disease and torsion dystonia may manifest tremors as well as dystonic symptoms. The nature, course, and association of other types of movements, along with the presence or absence of significant dementia, provide significant differential diagnostic information.

DYT1, Torsion dystonia

Torsion dystonia (formerly dystonia musculorum deformans) is a familial disorder transmitted as an autosomal dominant trait with incomplete penetrance. One major gene for torsion dystonia has been found to lie on chromosome 9q34, *DYT1*; however, the frequency of detecting a *DYT1* mutation without a family history of dystonia is less than 6%. *DYT1* encodes a protein called torsinA, and the defect deletes a glutamate residue from the protein. Additional gene loci can be causative (Németh 2002).

The average age of onset is 10 years, although it varies from 1 to 40 years of age. The initial major symptom is dystonic posturing of the leg (in DYT1) or axial muscles (in non-DYT1 patients), particularly the neck muscles, thus starting as a focal dystonic disorder. In some cases, torticollis or another focal dystonia is the only manifestation of the disorder. Initial symptoms may be misdiagnosed as hysteria. Many other patients will have a variably progressive course in which dystonia affects other axial and limb muscles, resulting in segmental or generalized dystonia with contortions of the trunk, appendicular dystonia, and tortipelvis. Peripheral injuries may precipitate dystonia in the genetically predisposed: In one study of 104 patients, 17% had a history of injury within days or up to 12 months before the onset of dystonia, which began in the injured part of the body before becoming generalized (Fletcher et al. 1991). Dysphonia may develop in some cases. Mental retardation is not a consistent associated finding. There is no convincing evidence of a decreased lifespan in individuals with torsion dystonia (Table 12.6).

The diagnosis is based on clinical findings, and laboratory studies help exclude the secondary forms of dystonia. Currently, genetic testing for a *DYT1* mutation in conjunction with genetic counseling is recommended for patients with onset before 26 years of age (Bressman et al. 2000).

Management of the patient with torsion dystonia requires attention to the physical and emotional aspects of the disorder. The patient with generalized dystonia needs support from members of a multidisciplinary team, including physicians, counselors, and physical and occupational therapists. No medication provides dramatic relief of the symptoms. L-Dopa has had limited success in

Table 12.6 Torsion dystonia

Discriminating features
- Dystonia
- Familial

Consistent features
- Commonly autosomal dominant or recessive
- Dystonic posturing of the neck and axial muscles
- Abnormality of *DYT1* gene

Variable features
- Can be X-linked recessive
- Dysphonia

Pearls and Perils

Disorders Presenting with Dystonia

- Chronic progressive dystonia is a symptom complex that may be seen in children with a number of movement disorders. Treatable diseases such as dopa-responsive dystonia and Wilson' disease should be carefully ruled out.
- As in other neurodegenerative diseases, extraneural tissue may provide supporting histologic evidence of neurodegeneration with brain iron accumulation (NBIA) when the presence of sea-blue histiocytes and cytosomic inclusions can be demonstrated.
- Early dystonia may be misinterpreted as a hysterical mannerism.

controlling dystonia. High doses of anticholinergics (trihexyphenidyl) have been successful in some patients and are well tolerated in children. If the symptoms of dystonia are paroxysmal, then patients may respond to phenytoin or carbamazepine. Diazepam has been recommended but has not been universally beneficial. Recent experience has shown that deep brain stimulation of the internal globus pallidus is over 70% effective for the primary generalized dystonias (Cif et al. 2003).

Neurodegeneration with brain iron accumulation

Neurodegeneration with brain iron accumulation is a heterogeneous group of disorders differentiated by clinical, radiographic, and molecular features (Hayflick 2003). The autosomal recessive disorder known as pantothenate kinase-associated neurodegeneration (PKAN) accounts for most patients diagnosed with NBIA and is caused by mutations in the gene encoding pantothenate kinase 2 (PANK2; Hayflick 2003). PKAN is characterized by dystonia and pigmentary retinopathy in children, speech and neuropsychiatric defects in adults, and a specific "eye of the tiger" abnormality on MRI of the brain (Hayflick 2003; Hayflick et al. 2003).

The clinicopathologic findings were initially described by Hallervorden and Spatz in 1922, who found pathologic amounts of iron stored in the globus pallidus and reticular zone of the substantia nigra of five siblings. The term *Hallervorden-Spatz disease* has been replaced by NBIA due to the subsequent unethical activities of these German neuropathologists (Hayflick et al. 2003; Shevell 2003). The clinical features include occurrence at a young age, a motor disorder of the extrapyramidal type, dementia, and a progressive course. The pathologic features are symmetric lesions of the globus pallidus and pars reticulata of the substantia nigra with loss of myelinated fibers and neurons, dissemination of round nonnucleated swollen axons (spheroids) in the CNS, and accumulation of iron-containing pigments in the affected regions (Dooling et al. 1974).

The onset of symptoms typically occurs by 10 years of age. A small number of cases may begin in adulthood. Posturing or movement abnormalities are the most frequent presenting symptoms. These changes lead to gait disorders. Motor symptoms include rigidity, dystonic posturing, choreoathetoid movements, and tremors. Dysarthria is present in most of the cases. The deep tendon reflexes tend to be hyperactive and the toe reflexes upgoing. Progressive intellectual deterioration (dementia) is often present, and the rate of its progression is variable. Seizures may occur (Hayflick et al. 2003).

In a recent genetic, clinical, and radiographic delineation of this disorder, 123 patients were classified as having either classic disease (66 patients) or atypical disease (57 patients). In the classic disease, symptoms were early-onset, with 88% before 6 years of age. The disease was rapidly progressive, manifested by dystonia progressing to severe disability by 20 years of age, and the MRI indicated high iron content in the basal ganglia. Atypical disease included patients with extrapyramidal dysfunction and radiographic evidence of iron accumulation in the basal ganglia, had a later onset, and a more slowly progressive course.

In *classic* NBIA or PKAN disease, early dystonia often involved the cranial and limb musculature. Acanthocytosis was found in 8%, 68% had clinical or electroretinographic evidence of retinopathy, only 3% had optic atrophy, and 85% became nonambulatory within 15 years after onset.

Clinical features of *atypical* NBIA and PANK2 mutations were heterogeneous, with patients older at onset (mean about 14 years), extrapyramidal defects were less severe and more slowly progressive, and retinopathy was less common. Speech difficulties, palilalia, and dysarthria were often a presenting or early feature, in contrast to no speech difficulties in patients with the classic disorder (Hayflick et al. 2003). *PLA2D6* mutations may account for some of these atypical NBIA patients (Morgan et al. 2006).

The nearly pathognomonic MRI abnormality, is the "eye-of-the-tiger" sign, which consists of bilateral areas of hyperintensity within a hypointense medial globus pallidus on T2-weighted images. A striking correlation is found between the presence of the "eye of the tiger" on the MRI and the presence of PANK2 mutations in patients (Hayflick et al. 2003). In addition, no mutation-negative patients with NBIA had the eye-of-the-tiger sign; MRIs from these patients showed only a region of hypointensity in the medial globus pallidus (Table 12.7).

Extraneural evidence of the disease can be found when the presence of sea-blue histiocytes is demonstrated

Table 12.7 Neurodegeneration with brain iron accumulation (NBIA)

Discriminating features
- Symmetric pathologic lesions of the globus pallidus and pars reticularis of the substantia nigra
- Autosomal recessive

Consistent features
- Occurs at young age
- Extrapyramidal motor disorder; rigidity, dystonia, choreoathetosis, and tremor
- Dementia
- Progressive course
- MRI findings of cortical atrophy, "eye-of-tiger" abnormality

Variable features
- Abnormal electroencephalograph (EEG), visual evoked potentials (VEP)
- Sea-blue histiocytes and cytoplasmic inclusions in lymphocytes
- Seizures
- Increased radioactive uptake of iron in basal ganglia
- Late (adult) onset

in the bone marrow cells and cytoplasmic inclusions of circulation lymphocytes (Swaiman et al. 1983; Zupanc et al. 1990) in children with NBIA.

Supportive and symptomatic therapy should be provided to children and their families. Emotional support and genetic counseling are important components of the management program. Systemic administration of iron chelators does not lower CNS iron in NBIA. Baclofen and trihexyphenidyl may help to relieve some of the extrapyramidal symptomatology of disabling dystonia and spasticity, and patients generally do not benefit from L-dopa (Hayflick 2003). Deep brain stimulation has benefited some patients (Castelnau et al. 2005).

DYT5, Dopa-responsive dystonia

Dopa-responsive dystonia is also called *progressive dystonia with diurnal variation* or *Segawa syndrome*. It is caused by mutations or deletions in the guanosine triphosphate cyclohydrolase 1 (*DYT5*) gene responsible for conversion of guanosine triphosphate to tetrahydrobiopterin (BH4), an essential cofactor for tyrosine hydroxylase, which in turn is the rate-limiting enzyme for dopamine synthesis. This is an autosomal dominant disorder with variable penetrance and variable expressivity. Abnormalities of tyrosine hydroxylase and another autosomal dominant (DYT14) variant have been described (Furukawa 2006) to cause similar symptoms.

Symptoms begin in childhood, usually before the age of 10 years, with dystonic manifestations and respond rapidly to L-dopa (Nygaard & Duvoisin 1986). Females are more frequently affected than males by at least a 2:1 ratio. A patient's presenting sign is often a gait disorder, with dystonia of the legs or with equinovarus posturing of a foot. As the disorder progresses, dystonia becomes more generalized and features of parkinsonism may appear. Flexor and extensor posturing of the upper extremities and trunk musculature may occur. Parkinsonian features include cogwheel rigidity, bradykinesia, and tremors. The deep tendon reflexes are often brisk, with extensor toe responses. Diurnal variation, in which symptoms become more severe during the day and improve after sleeping, is a prominent feature especially noted in the cases reported from Japan (Segawa et al. 1976), although some do not experience these fluctuations (Table 12.8).

The diagnosis is based on clinical assessment, cerebrospinal fluid (CSF) studies, and genetic testing. Cerebrospinal fluid homovanillic acid, 5-hydroxyindoleacetic acid, and biopterin levels are low. Autopsy studies have revealed poorly pigmented cells in the substantia nigra (Yokochi et al. 1984) and a reduction in tyrosine hydroxylase, without the dramatic cell loss seen in juvenile parkinsonism (Rajput et al. 1994). Pharmacologic challenge with low-dose L-dopa separates dopa-responsive dystonia from idiopathic torsion dystonia and the secondary dystonias, and it is recommended that an empiric trial of levodopa be considered in any child with dystonia.

The reduction of dystonic and parkinsonian features after the administration of L-dopa is rapid and marked. Function is often normalized within a day of initiation of medication. Small dosages of medication sometimes result in dramatic changes. Dosages should be individualized. Control with L-dopa is sustained, in some cases for more than 10 years.

DYT11, Myoclonic dystonia

Myoclonus-dystonia is an autosomal dominant movement disorder caused by mutations or deletions in the

Table 12.8 Progressive dystonia with diurnal variation (dopa-responsive dystonia)

Discriminating features
- Progressive dystonia
- Diurnal variation

Consistent features
- Gait disorder
- Marked and rapid response to L-dopa
- Caused by mutations in guanosine triphosphate cyclohydrolase 1 (DYT5)

Variable features
- Brisk deep tendon reflexes
- Posturing

ε-sarcoglycan gene (Zimprich et al. 2001). Essential myoclonus is also affected by this same gene.

The clinical features include myoclonus that typically involves the neck and arms, with mild and sometimes focal dystonia. Obsessive-compulsive features may also be seen (Cassim 2003). Epilepsy may be an uncommon feature (Foncke et al. 2003).

Symptoms are improved with alcohol and propranolol. One patient was successfully treated with deep brain stimulation (Cif et al. 2004).

Focal dystonias

Focal dystonia is a descriptive rather than etiologic term. Focal dystonias express themselves when the eyes screw shut (blepharospasm), the jaw is forced open or shut (oromandibular dystonia), the neck is twisted (torticollis), or the arm adopts a posture of hyperpronation with flexed wrist and extended fingers, particularly during the act of writing (writer's cramp). Professional musicians are known to develop their own peculiar cramps or dystonic reactions. Although many of these syndromes are more typical in adults, occasionally focal dystonias can be seen in children. Some of the primary dystonias first present as a focal dystonia (Marsden 1986). In some series, up to 30% of people with "focal dystonia" carry an abnormal *DYT1* (Spinella & Sheridan 1994). Other genes causing focal dystonia include *DYT6*, *DYT7*, *DYT13*, and *PANK2* (Németh 2002).

Most of the focal dystonias respond poorly to medications (Marsden 1986). Local injection of botulinum toxin, a neuromuscular blocking agent, is effective therapy for temporary relief of focal dystonias (American Academy of Neurology 1994). Occasionally these injections may have the side effect of local weakness; however, the dystonia is typically improved.

Other genetic forms of dystonia

DYT2 is an autosomal recessive form of dystonia that can be seen in Ashkenazi families (Moretti et al. 2005). DYT3, X-linked recessive dystonia-parkinsonism, known as *lubag*, is typically seen in adults and is endemic in the Philippines; it may be caused by mutations in TATA-binding protein-associated factor 1 gene (*TAF1*; Makino et al. 2007). DYT4, DYT6, and DYT7 refer to autosomal dominant torsion dystonias whose specific genes have not been delineated. DYT8, DYT9, and DYT10 are associated with paroxysmal movement disorders. DYT12 is a rapid onset of parkinsonism and dystonia occurring in childhood or adulthood, caused by mutations in the *ATP1A3* gene (Brashear et al. 2007). DYT13 is associated with focal dystonia in a single family (see Németh 2002 for review).

Tremor

Tremor can be defined as an involuntary, rhythmic oscillation. Tremor may be worse with trying to maintain a posture or with action, as in essential tremor, or worse at rest as in a parkinsonian tremor. The presence or absence of other symptoms and signs helps to differentiate the various conditions.

Essential tremor

Benign familial or essential tremor is the most common persistent childhood tremor. Essential tremor is a monosymptomatic disorder. The mean age of onset is 7 years. The tremor primarily involves the arms. It may involve both a postural tremor and an action tremor. Tremor is absent at rest. The characteristic tremor is rapid (5–8 Hz) and exacerbated by stress, anxiety, and antigravity posture. Characteristically, the tremor in adults responds dramatically to alcohol. There is a positive family history in about 70% of cases (Louis et al. 2001) (Table 12.9).

This can be inherited as an autosomal dominant disorder, with approximately 5% of cases presenting in childhood. A positive family history is present in about 50% of patients. The pathophysiology is unknown in hereditary cases. However, there may be as yet unidentified environmental factors that contribute to the tremor (Louis 2001).

The condition is not usually debilitating, although slow progression with prolonged plateaus may occur. Propranolol (1–3 mg/kg/day), or primidone (starting at 25 mg at bedtime, titrating up to a dose of 250 mg/day) may be therapeutically useful in some cases. Other medications

Pearls and Perils

Childhood Tremor

- Benign essential tremor is the most common persistent tremor in childhood.
- Stress and fatigue will increase tremor in benign familial or essential tremor.
- Shuddering attacks in infancy and childhood should prompt a careful history for the presence of familial tremor.
- "Wing-beating tremor," in which arms are abducted and elbows flexed, suggests Wilson disease.
- A Kayser-Fleischer ring (a brown to yellow to green discoloration in the Descemet membrane at the limbus of the iris) is pathognomonic of Wilson disease. This can be seen more readily in persons with blue eyes. It is definitively diagnosed by slit-lamp examination.

Table 12.9 Benign familial tremor

Discriminating features
- Intention or postural tremor
- Most often affects the hands and arms
- Autosomal dominant

Consistent features
- Positive family history
- Worse after caffeine ingested and with stress; better after alcohol ingestion

Variable features
- Shuddering

such as benzodiazepines, gabapentin, and topiramate may also be helpful in select patients (Pahwa & Lyons 2003).

Psychogenic tremor

Psychogenic tremor usually is apparent when the child has a tremor that has a variable frequency, amplitude, and axis. It is often distractible. Surface EMG recordings are often useful to characterize the tremors and demonstrate this variability (Kenney et al. 2007).

The patient who presents with psychogenic tremor frequently also may have anxiety or a posttraumatic stress disorder.

The treatment in children should be supportive rather than confrontational. The patient often wishes to resolve these problems, but doesn't have the ability to do so. Antianxiety agents can be useful. A benzodiazepine such as clonazepam can be useful if the symptoms are intermittent, or an antianxiety agent such as fluoxetine can be used if the symptoms are persistent. Working with a psychologist will also be helpful to the patient (see Schrag and Lang 2005, for review of topic).

Infantile movements

Chin trembling occurs in infants, and is characterized by episodes of involuntary quivering of the chin. These episodes can be induced by emotional stimuli. The episodes are hereditary, possibly as an autosomal dominant disorder. The frequency decreases with age (Danek 1993; Grimes et al. 2002).

Head rolling or head tremor can also present in young children between the ages of 5 and 10 months. Patients with this "yes-yes" or "no-no" tremor have an otherwise normal neurologic examination and laboratory studies. A family history of tremor or shuddering spells can be obtained in some children. Spontaneous remission occurs (DiMario 2000).

Spasmus nutans is a benign syndrome of infancy that consists of a triad of head nodding, pendular nystagmus, and a head tilt. Spontaneous remissions of the head nodding typically occur by 2 years of age, although some cases persist up to 6 years of age (Doummar et al. 1998). Subclinical nystagmus may still persist until 5–12 years of age (Gottlob et al. 1995). There have been case reports of spasmus nutans being associated with an optic chiasm or third ventricle glioma; however, the prevalence of tumors in spasmus nutans is estimated to be less than 2% (Arnoldi & Tychsen 1995).

Shuddering spells

Shuddering spells may start during infancy and continue during early childhood. The episodes appear as a "shudder" or a shivering movement, lasting for seconds, and without producing loss of consciousness. The shuddering attacks may be precipitated by emotional stimuli and disappear with time. There may be a family history of essential tremor (Vanasse et al. 1976).

These attacks are often confused with epileptic seizures. When severe, propanolol has been useful in attenuating the episodes (Barron & Younkin 1992).

Wilson disease

Hepatolenticular degeneration, or Wilson disease, results in the deposition of copper in the CNS, liver, cornea, and other organs. Ninety-five percent of patients with Wilson disease will have low ceruloplasmin levels. However, the gene for Wilson disease, *ATP7B*, encodes a copper-transporting ATPase, and not ceruloplasmin (Thomas et al. 1995). The reduced or absent function of *ATP7B* leads to decreased liver excretion of copper into the bile, and this in turn leads to increased hepatic accumulation of copper.

Pearls and Perils

Wilson Disease

- Wilson disease is rare and has no specific early manifestations. Physicians should think of Wilson disease when confronted with children with unexplained hepatic dysfunction or disease, hepatomegaly, acute hemolysis, acute dystonia, and recent onset of school or behavioral problems.
- Wilson disease is not a cause of mental retardation.
- A golden-brown Kayser-Fleischer ring near the limbus of the eye is seen only by slit-lamp examination until late in the course. Kayser-Fleischer rings are more frequent in neurologic or psychiatric forms of the disease.
- Most patients with Wilson disease have a low serum ceruloplasmin and an increased concentration of loosely bound, nonceruloplasmin copper in the serum.

After the liver has been saturated with copper, the elevated copper enters the bloodstream and results in copper deposition in other tissues, including the brain.

Patients may present with hepatic, neurologic, or psychiatric symptoms. Dystonia is a common presentation in young children. Dysarthria, intention tremor, and a rigid-akinesia syndrome are other findings. The onset of neurologic symptoms is often rapid, presenting with tremor, coarse "flapping," or fine rhythmic tremor, whereas in adults the onset is usually insidious. Half of patients are symptomatic by age 15 years, and rarely do patients present before the age of 6 years. Cerebellar and pseudobulbar signs, such as drooling, difficulty in swallowing, and dysarthria often occur. Rigidity develops later in the course of the disease. Dementia is not prominent in juvenile presentations. A Kayser-Fleischer ring (a brown to yellow-green discoloration in the Descemet membrane at the limbus of the iris) is frequently seen.

Early diagnosis and treatment of Wilson disease may prevent permanent neurologic damage. Because it is treatable, the diagnosis of Wilson disease should be considered in all children with new onset of tremor or dystonia. A search for low ceruloplasmin levels is a good initial screen for this disease. However, ceruloplasmin levels are subject to false-positive and false-negative results. Twenty-four-hour urinary copper excretion or measurement of serum non–ceruloplasmin-bound copper concentration are helpful to confirm the diagnosis. In cases in which the diagnosis is in doubt, hepatic parenchymal copper concentration can be measured (Roberts & Schilsky 2003).

Treatment with the chelating agent penicillamine, trientine, and/or zinc can result in symptomatic improvement. Dietary restriction of copper and pyridoxine are also useful. Liver transplantation can also be considered for select cases (see El-Youssef 2003, for review).

Secondary causes of tremor

Hyperthyroidism is associated with tremor that is rapid, mainly involves the extremities, and is more prominent with the arms outstretched. Tremor secondary to hyperthyroidism can be diagnosed by appropriate thyroid function tests. Drugs, such as the β-adrenergic agonists, valproic acid, lithium, heavy metals, alcohol, and "street drugs" can all produce tremor. The tremor stops when the drug is withdrawn, or (as in the case with valproate) when the levels of the drug are decreased. Finally, up to 45% of severely head injured children will manifest a tremor within the first 18 months after injury (Johnson & Hall 1992).

Tics

Tics are rapid, brief involuntary movements. Tics can be primarily motor such as eye blinking or facial grimacing, or the tics can be vocal such as throat clearing or sniffing. Transient tic disorder is defined by tics that last for at least 4 weeks but less than a year in duration. Motor or vocal tics that persist over 1 year are defined as a chronic tic disorder. Patients with Tourette syndrome will have multiple motor and vocal tics that persist for longer than a year. Transient tic disorder and chronic motor tics may be part of a spectrum with Tourette syndrome, since all three disorders may be seen within the same family (Kurlan et al. 1988).

Tics are common in children. Up to 5% of all children will experience a single transient tic lasting a few weeks to months (Solomon 1991). In a classroom situation, 6% of regular students and 26% of special education students were observed to have tics during the school day (Kurlan et al. 1994). Often, these involuntary movements are manifested in only one muscle group and occur transiently.

Tourette syndrome

Gilles de la Tourette syndrome (TS) is a disorder characterized by the early onset (2–15 years of age) of chronic motor and vocal tics. The tics involve multiple motor groups and will vary in intensity, waxing and waning over a period of months to years. Patients often acknowledge a premonitory urge before the tic. The motor tics may be simple or complex, with manifestations changing over time. Eye blinking and facial grimacing may occur in one period, more complex movements in the next. Vocal tics include simple sniffling sounds, barking, grunting, and throat-clearing sounds, and also more complex echolalia and coprolalia. However, coprolalia (explosive production of obscene words) is uncommon in children with TS (Table 12.10).

Tics may appear in preschool or early grade school years, and they have an average age of onset of 6 years. Often, tics seem to increase in severity during childhood,

Pearls and Perils

Tics

- Children with attention-deficit/hyperactivity disorder (ADHD) on stimulant medications should be monitored for the onset of tics.
- Because of the high incidences of behavioral disorders in children with Tourette syndrome (TS), psychological or psychiatric consultation may be helpful.
- Tourette syndrome, chronic motor tics, ADD or ADHD, and obsessive-compulsive disorder may be commonly seen within the same family.

Table 12.10 Tourette syndrome

Discriminating features

- Motor and vocal tics greater than 1 year in duration
- Involves multiple motor groupings
- Waxing and waning of symptoms
- Onset before 18 years

Consistent features

- ADD or ADHD in 70% of patients
- Obsessive compulsive features
- Response to dopamine receptor antagonists

Variable features

- Coprolalia is unusual
- Remission in late adolescence or early adulthood in some patients

reaching a peak period of severity at 10 years of age. Many patients will show fewer tics, or a complete disappearance of tics, by the time they reach late adolescence or early adulthood (Erenberg et al. 1987). The improvements in tic disability with age do not appear to relate to medication use, as many patients never treated with medications will often show improvements (Pappert et al. 2003).

The lifetime prevalence of TS is estimated to be 1% (Robertson 2003). Tourette syndrome is probably inherited as an autosomal dominant with incomplete penetrance and variable expressivity. There are likely modifier genes that affect expression (Paul 2001). Although evidence suggests a strong genetic contribution, nongenetic factors (such as a history of prematurity, anxiety, head injury, infections, medications) also play a role in the expression of tics.

Medications can effectively reduce the symptoms of TS. However, the management of these children can be quite complex. Typical target symptoms for treatment include the tics, problems with attention, OCD, anxiety, depression, oppositional behavior, and learning disabilities. The severity of the symptoms and the extent to which these symptoms affect the development, self-image, and performance of the child in school and at home should be addressed. Parents need to be educated about the disorder and counseled about its possible transmission. To reduce the frequency of the tics, several medication groups have been used. Often patients are started on an α-2-adrenergic agonist, such as clonidine. It is started at 0.05 mg/day and slowly titrated to 0.15–0.3 mg/day. Tiredness and hypotension are dose-limiting side effects. Neuroleptics may be the most effective group of medications for the control of the tics. Older-generation neuroleptics such as haloperidol or pimozide are now being replaced with the "atypical antipsychotics" such as risperidone, olanzapine, and ziprasidone. These atypicals are also efficacious and may have an advantage of producing a lower rate of tardive dyskinesia (Budman et al. 2001; Gilbert et al. 2004; Sallee et al. 2000). Risperidone may be started at 0.5 mg/day, and titrated up to 3 mg/day. Weight gain is a significant problem. The concurrent use of nizatidine may attenuate the neuroleptic-induced weight gain (Atmaca et al. 2003). Other agents, including baclofen, some anticonvulsants (topiramate and levetiracetam), benzodiazepines, pergolide, and tetrabenazine have been used less frequently to treat patients with TS. In the future, deep brain stimulation may show promise in severe cases (Temel & Visser-Vandewalle 2004; Servello et al. 2008).

Over half of the children with this syndrome may have symptoms of attention deficit disorder (ADD), obsessive-compulsive symptoms, or other behavioral disorders. Typically, the attentional problems are evident before the onset of the tics. The use of stimulant medications (methylphenidate and dextroamphetamine) may be associated with the first appearance of, or an increased incidence of, tics. However, a recent multicenter clinical trial showed a benefit of stimulants on both attention and tics (Tourette Syndrome Study Group 2002). Tricyclics, such as desipramine, may be a useful alternative for the treatment of attentional symptoms and impulsivity in Tourette syndrome (Singer et al. 1995). Atomoxetine has also been used to improve attention in patients with tics. Early experience seems to suggest that atomoxetine does not aggravate the tic frequency. Anxiety or obsessive-compulsive symptoms can also be quite troubling and may respond to selective serotonin reuptake inhibitors or cognitive behavioral therapy (Miguel et al. 2003).

The pathogenesis of this syndrome is incompletely understood. A number of neurotransmitter alterations have been implicated. The dramatic response of symptoms to dopamine receptor-blocking agents like haloperidol suggests a dopaminergic involvement. Noradrenergic mechanisms have been implicated because symptoms of the syndrome are reduced after the administration of clonidine, a drug that inhibits noradrenergic functioning. Mutations in the Slit and Trk-like 1 (*SLITRK1*) gene has been associated with Tourette syndrome in a minority of patients (Abelson et al. 2005). However, more information is needed to adequately understand these complex mechanisms.

Pediatric autoimmune neuropsychiatric disorder

As early as 1929, it was noted that some children with OCD and/or tics have symptom exacerbations triggered by group A β-hemolytic streptococcal (GBHS) infection or other infections (Garvey et al. 1999; Singer 1999). A proposed mechanism is that the GBHS triggers antibodies that cross-react with the basal ganglia of genetically susceptible hosts, leading to OCD and/or tics (Garvey et al. 1998).

In PANDAS, symptom onset of tics or OCD is believed to be triggered by GABHS infection or pharyngitis. In addition to tics and OCD, many of the patients described in the literature have emotional lability, separation anxiety, nighttime fears and bedtime rituals, cognitive deficits, oppositional behaviors, and motor hyperactivity (Swedo et al. 1998). However, abrupt tic onset or an exacerbation of tics associated with a streptococcal infection (11%) or any infection (18%) is not uncommon in patients with tic disorders (Singer et al. 2000). Serum autoantibodies also do not differentiate between patients diagnosed with PANDAS or Tourette syndrome (Singer et al. 2005).

One controlled study of penicillin prophylaxis failed to prevent either the exacerbation of symptoms or the frequency of infections (Garvey et al. 1999). An open label trial of plasma exchange has failed to show benefit in a group of five patients with OCD without streptococcal exacerbations (Nicolson et al. 2000). In contrast, either plasma exchange or IVIG benefits the symptoms of patients with severe infection-triggered exacerbations of OCD or tic disorders (Perlmutter et al. 1999). Since these studies have limited controls and utilize highly select populations, many authors suggest that treatment be given to patients only as part of controlled double-blind protocols (Singer 1999).

To date, PANDAS is a controversial hypothesis rather than a proven clinical disorder. Clinical diagnostic criteria have not yet proven to be reliable nor valid. Similarly, there are no convincing data for the routine use of immunologic or antibiotic therapy in patients with tics (Kurlan 2004).

Stereotypies

Stereotypies occur in normal children as well as in children who are delayed in their development or autistic. These movements are repetitive, nonpurposeful, rhythmic, and the child can exert some degree of volitional control over the movements. Common examples can include head banging, rocking, jumping, or flapping of the hands and arms. Often they occur more frequently when the child is excited or bored. In the nonautistic child with normal intelligence, the stereotypies may also be associated with obsessive-compulsive symptoms and perfectionism (Niehaus et al. 2000).

The movements can be transient, or they may persist for years. The movements are resistant to either behavioral therapy or to medications. An occasional child may respond to a neuroleptic or a selective serotonin reuptake inhibitor.

Myoclonus

Myoclonic movements are sudden, brief, shock-like, and involuntary. These movements can be the result of muscle contractions (positive myoclonus) or inhibitions (negative myoclonus). Myoclonus is a sign that can be seen in a variety of neurologic conditions. For instance, myoclonus may be seen in a patient after a severe hypoxic–ischemic injury. Myoclonus may also be seen in neurodegenerative diseases, such as neuronal ceroid lipofuscinosis. Myoclonic movements may also have an epileptic etiology, and an EEG should be considered in a patient who shows a new onset of daytime myoclonus. In contrast, most children will exhibit sleep myoclonus, a totally normal movement. This occurs as the child is falling asleep or just prior to awakening (Butler 1992).

Opsoclonus-myoclonus-ataxia

The rare syndrome of opsoclonus-myoclonus-ataxia (OMA) has generated great interest because of its association with neuroblastoma. It consists of the sudden onset of myoclonus, opsoclonus ("dancing eyes"), and ataxia in infants. It appears in the literature with the names *myoclonic encephalopathy of infancy*, *Kinsbourne syndrome*, *infantile polymyoclonia*, and *dancing eyes syndrome* (Kinsbourne 1962; Lott & Kinsbourne 1986). A comparison of OMA with myoclonic epilepsy is shown in Table 12.11.

The syndrome may be idiopathic, viral, or neuroblastoma-related. Idiopathic and neuroblastoma-related OMA may be distinct entities, or may represent immunologic reactions of varying effectiveness against neuroblastoma formation. In the published literature, the incidence of neuroblastoma associated with OMA is about 50%; however, because of a selection bias in favor of reporting cases associated with neuroblastoma, the true incidence of associated neuroblastoma is probably much lower (Lott & Kinsbourne 1986).

Patients with opsoclonus-myoclonus generate an immune response against a variety of brain antigens

Pearls and Perils

Myoclonus

- Myoclonic movements occur commonly in sleeping infants and are frequently misinterpreted as seizures.
- Predominantly front-to-back head movements, with the head appearing like a doll's head on a spring, occur in the "bobble head doll" syndrome, which should prompt a search for neuroblastoma and for third-ventricle cyst, dilatation, or tumor.
- The occurrence of myoclonus with abnormal eye movements (opsoclonus) and ataxia should prompt an investigation for a neuroblastoma.

Table 12.11 Opsoclonus-myoclonus-ataxia versus myoclonic epilepsy

Criteria	Opsoclonus-myoclonus-ataxia	Myoclonic epilepsy and infantile spasms
Character of myoclonus	Asymmetric, arrhythmic, asynchronous	Bilateral, symmetric, synchronous, rhythmic
Dependence on stimuli	Induced by voluntary movement	Not induced by movement
Electroencephalograph	Normal	Abnormal (hypsarrhythmia, atypical absence)

(Connolly 1997; Pranzatelli 1992). It is probable that neuroblastoma (or viral antigens) and the cerebellum are joint targets of an immunologic attack. In adults with paraneoplastic OMA, some patients develop antibodies to the RNA-binding protein Nova-1 (Jensen et al. 2000). To date, this antibody has not been found in the childhood version of OMA. Other as yet unidentified antibrain antibodies can be seen in childhood cases of OMA (Antunes et al. 2000).

Onset usually occurs between the ages of 6 and 18 months but can occur at up to 36 months of age. The onset of myoclonus is acute, often occurring after a nonspecific respiratory or gastrointestinal illness, and reaches maximal intensity in 2–7 days. The myoclonic movements are intense and brief, with continual shock-like muscular contractions, irregularly timed, and of variable amplitude. They are widely distributed across muscle groups, asymmetric, increased by startle, present at rest, and abolished only by deep sleep. Rarely, choreoathetosis may also be seen.

Abnormal eye movements (opsoclonus) temporally unrelated to the myoclonus consist of rapid (up to eight displacements or rotations per second), irregular, conjugate ocular movements, mainly horizontal but also vertical and diagonal. The eye movements are exacerbated by the same stimuli as the myoclonus, and some authors consider opsoclonus to be the ocular equivalent of myoclonus.

Patients may also exhibit cognitive and mood changes as well, which persist past the myoclonic stages of this illness (Klein et al. 2007).

When OMA is associated with a neuroblastoma, neurologic symptoms may occur months before a tumor if found. Fifty percent of reported tumors are localized to the thorax. Imaging of the chest has the highest diagnostic yield, followed by abdominal films. Urinary catecholamines are rarely diagnostic. Electroencephalogram is normal. Anti-Hu antibodies were seen in 10 of 64 patients with neuroblastoma, but were not specific for the development of OMA (Antunes et al. 2000).

Success of treatment ranges from complete recovery in 3 months to persistence over several years, and the latter course is more frequently noted. Incomplete recovery may be followed by relapse related to infection or discontinuation of effective therapy. Most cases show a remarkable response to adrenocorticotropic hormone (ACTH) or corticosteroid therapy. Usually 20–40 units/day of ACTH, or 5–20 mg/day of prednisolone have been needed for therapeutic benefit, with the dose titrated downward to a level below which symptoms appear. Rituximab, an anti-CD20 monoclonal antibody, is also being used (Pranzatelli et al. 2006).

More than half of patients are left with sequelae: mental retardation, dysarthria, learning disabilities, or attention deficit hyperactivity disorder (ADHD). Patients with neuroblastoma have slightly less serious sequelae. Neuroblastoma associated with myoclonic encephalopathy has a more favorable prognosis for survival than neuroblastoma without the neurologic syndrome (Altman & Bachner 1976; Klein et al. 2007).

Paroxysmal movement disorders

Some movement disorders only occur paroxysmally or intermittently. Paroxysmal movement disorders are characterized by sudden attacks of involuntary movements of the body without loss of consciousness. The movements may be choreic, athetotic, tonic, dystonic, or ataxic. They may be unilateral or bilateral. There is no loss of awareness during the episode. Paroxysmal movement disorders may be classified into (a) paroxysmal kinesigenic choreoathetosis, (b) nonkinesigenic paroxysmal dyskinesia, (c) acquired forms of paroxysmal movement disorders, with neurologic disorders or metabolic disorders, and (d) familial periodic ataxia.

The differentiation of paroxysmal dyskinesia and tonic seizures induced by movements is not always readily discernible. Some cases of paroxysmal choreoathetosis are initially misdiagnosed as seizures. In reflex epilepsy, when the seizures are induced by movements, the differentiation may be particularly difficult. The state of consciousness is the most helpful distinguishing feature. When alteration or loss of consciousness occurs, the episode is more consistent with seizures. However, it may be necessary to obtain an EEG during the attack to confirm the diagnosis.

Paroxysmal kinesigenic dyskinesia

A frequently reported familial paroxysmal movement disorder is the kinesigenic one, in which the episodes are precipitated by movement. The abnormal movements may be dystonic, choreic, athetotic, ballistic, or mixed forms of movement occurring unilaterally or bilaterally (Goodenough et al. 1978). Dystonia is generally the predominant symptom. Diagnostic criteria include an identified trigger for the attacks (sudden movements), short duration of attacks (<1 minute), lack of loss of consciousness or pain during attacks, antiepileptic drug responsiveness, exclusion of other organic diseases, and age at onset between 1 and 20 years (Bruno et al. 2004). The lower limbs may be primarily affected. Individuals with these episodes have noted the ability to abort some of the attacks by various maneuvers. Occasionally an aura of tightness or other vague sensation occurs prior to the episode.

The precipitating movement is often a brisk and sudden event, such as a quick head turn or suddenly moving the leg. Attacks may be induced in the examination room by having the individual hop in place on one foot for a short period, or perform other movements that the patient reports to induce the problem.

The attacks usually start in childhood and may increase in frequency during adolescence. The episodes may decrease in frequency in the early adult years (Goodenough et al. 1978). Spontaneous remission can occur (Table 12.12). The neurologic examination and history are otherwise normal. Electroencephalograms obtained during the episode are normal. There have been no consistent pathologic findings at autopsy. When the diagnosis is uncertain, video recordings of the event may provide additional diagnostic information.

An autosomal dominant mode of inheritance with incomplete penetrance is described by a number of authors. Sporadic cases have been reported. However, a woman previously described as a sporadic case had a daughter 10 years later who not only inherited the disorder, but was more severely affected (Bird et al. 1978). Two separate loci on chromosome 16 have been proposed for this entity, but the causative genes have not been found. A third locus may exist as well (Spacey et al. 2002; Lotze & Jankovic 2003). Patients may also exhibit these symptoms secondary to other underlying neurologic disorders, such as a previous history of kernicterus, encephalitis, trauma, or multiple sclerosis (Blakeley & Jankovic 2002).

Table 12.12 Paroxysmal kinesigenic dyskinesia

Discriminating features
- Movement-induced paroxysmal episodes

Consistent features
- Induced by specific movements
- Brief duration of episodes
- Choreoathetotic, dystonic, tonic, or mixed forms
- Dramatic response to anticonvulsant medication
- No EEG changes during episode
- Often involve the lower extremities

Variable features
- Often positive family history

The response to anticonvulsant medication is dramatic in most instances. Phenytoin or carbamazepine are the medications most commonly prescribed. The serum concentration necessary for control of the attacks is lower than that employed when phenytoin is prescribed for seizure control (Wang & Chang 1985). Other anticonvulsants used include phenobarbital, valproic acid, primidone, levetiracetam, lamotrigine, and clonazepam. Some cases have responded to medications not ordinarily used for seizure control (e.g., L-dopa).

Nonkinesigenic paroxysmal dyskinesia

Nonkinesigenic paroxysmal dyskinesia, initially described in 1940, occurs less frequently than the kinesigenic form (Mount & Reback 1940).

The attacks in many of the cases begin in infancy; a smaller number of patients do not exhibit attacks until adulthood. The paroxysmal attacks have been manifested as choreoathetotic or dystonic movements. They are often bilateral and may involve the face and laryngeal muscles or extremities. Episodes invariably last longer than 5 minutes and can last for more than an hour. The attacks can occur daily, or the patients may go for months without one. The attacks are not precipitated by movement. More commonly, episodes are induced by intake of alcohol, coffee, tea, fatigue, hunger, or emotion. The attacks may be relieved by a short period of sleep in some patients (Jarman et al. 2000). As in the kinesigenic form, no loss of consciousness occurs during the attack. Muscle stiffness without involuntary movement may be a forme fruste of this disorder (Matsuo et al. 1999).

Nonkinesigenic paroxysmal dyskinesia is clearly transmitted through an autosomal dominant mode of inheritance with linkage to chromosome 2q (Fouad et al. 1996). As in the kinesigenic form, more males are affected than females. Routine laboratory studies, including EEGs during the attacks, have been normal. There have been no pathologic findings in the CNS. Mutations in the myofibrillogenesis regulator 1 gene has been found in multiple families (Lee et al. 2004).

Unlike the kinesigenic form, the frequency of the attacks has not been reduced by many different anticonvulsants. Benzodiazepines have been an effective therapeutic agent in eliminating or significantly reducing the frequency of the episodes (Lance 1977; Mayeux & Fahn 1982). Alternate-day oxazepam therapy provided sustained relief of the attacks in another study (Kurlan & Shoulson 1983), as did acetazolamide (Mayeux & Fahn 1982) or Neurontin (Chudnow et al. 1997) (Table 12.13).

Table 12.13 Nonkinesigenic paroxysmal dyskinesia

Discriminating features
- Paroxysmal episodes of choreoathetosis or dystonia
- Not induced by movement
- Autosomal dominant

Consistent features
- Typically has an early onset
- Episodes of long duration
- Inconsistent response to medication
- May involve the face or arms

Variable features
- Adult onset

Paroxysmal exertional dystonia

In this disorder, patients have attacks precipitated by continuous exercise such as walking or running. Stress and cold may also be precipitating factors. The episodes last minutes to hours in duration, often involving the lower limbs, although it may spread to other body parts. The attacks are frequently unilateral (Lance 1977; Demirkiran & Jankovice 1995; Bhatia et al. 1997).

The onset occurs in childhood or as a young adult. There have been families reported with an autosomal dominant pattern of inheritance, but many cases are sporadic. Exertional cramping without dystonia may also occur in family members (Kurlan et al. 1987). This has been also associated with the myofibrillogenesis regulator 1 gene (Bruno et al. 2007).

Clonazepam, levodopa, carbamazepine, trihexyphenidyl, and acetazolamide have been tried as therapy (Demirkiran & Jankovice 1995; Bhatia et al. 1997).

Acquired forms of paroxysmal movement disorders

Acquired forms of paroxysmal disorders occur in association with an underlying disease and are not the result of a genetic defect. Underlying processes include trauma, multiple sclerosis, stroke, endocrinopathies, or a history of CNS infection. The nature of the involuntary movements during the attacks can be similar to that in the kinesigenic or nonkinesigenic form of paroxysmal movement disorders (Blakeley & Jankovic 2002).

Paroxysmal movement disorders, particularly in children diagnosed with a static encephalopathy, are often misdiagnosed as seizures or hysteria. Because of their length, the episodes can be very painful and distressing to patients, families, and teachers. The paroxysmal episodes that occur in individuals with a static encephalopathy syndrome often begin in childhood (Rosen 1964). The attacks are usually brief, measured in minutes; however, in a number of cases the attacks have lasted for hours (Erickson & Chun 1987). Neurologic examination reflects the findings of the past encephalopathy. Some individuals have signs of spasticity or hemiparesis; others are severely hypotonic or have persistent choreoathetosis. Electroencephalograms during the episode are no different than those recorded during the interictal period. The response to anticonvulsants is variable. Botulinum toxin injections may also be helpful in select cases.

The paroxysmal episodes of patients with multiple sclerosis are primarily flexor spasms (Miley & Forster 1974). Because of the intensity, the attacks are often painful. They may be the initial symptoms of multiple sclerosis. The attacks are short, lasting minutes, and frequently stop after 1 or 2 months of symptoms. They respond to anticonvulsants.

Paroxysmal choreoathetotic episodes occur in individuals with endocrine diseases such as hyperparathyroidism (Arden 1953), thyrotoxicosis (Fischbeck & Layzer 1979), and diabetes during periods of hypoglycemia (Newman & Kinkel 1984).

Nocturnal paroxysmal dystonia

These complex motor attacks arise abruptly during sleep, especially during non-rapid eye movement (REM) sleep. The typical patient displays attacks lasting 15 seconds to 2 minutes in length. There may be a sudden opening of the eyes, followed by dystonic postures or by disordered violent movements. The episodes may occur several times during the night. Nocturnal paroxysmal dystonia may respond to carbamazepine, but not to other agents (Montagna 1992). These attacks often represent a form of seizure activity, and this can be verified by overnight video EEG recording.

Ataxia

Ataxia may be caused by a heterogeneous group of diseases. Patients with recessively inherited errors of metabolism such as Hartnup disease, Leigh disease, and maple syrup urine disease may intermittently be ataxic. Individuals with acquired diseases could possibly manifest ataxia as part of the clinical spectrum. Stroke or mass lesion can present with ataxia when the lesions involve the posterior fossa. Acute onset of ataxia, particularly when other focal neurologic signs are present, warrants consideration of an MRI or CT scan. Some peripheral neuropathies, especially those occurring in families, also present with ataxia, either because the underlying disease directly affects cerebellum, or because of posterior column damage (and loss of position sense input). Medications can cause ataxia, and not infrequently patients taking anticonvulsants will become ataxic at higher levels of these medications.

Weakness can also appear as indistinguishable from ataxia (Stumpf 1985; 1987).

Acute cerebellar ataxia

Acute cerebellar ataxia (ACA) most often presents as a sudden disturbance of gait and balance. Although the ataxia of gait is the most prominent sign, appendicular ataxia and nystagmus also occurs.

Acute cerebellar ataxia usually develops days to weeks after a viral illness, particularly chickenpox. In the largest series (Connolly et al. 1994), 26% of patients had chickenpox, 3% had Epstein-Barr virus infection, 49% had other viral illnesses, 19% had no prodrome, and 3% developed ACA after immunizations. Other preceding infections include measles, mumps, herpes simplex virus, coxsackievirus, echovirus, poliovirus, *Mycoplasma pneumoniae*, and *Legionella pneumophila*.

Acute cerebellar ataxia usually occurs in children between 2 and 5 years of age and is rare in adolescents and adults. Epstein-Barr virus infection and immunizations are the most common causes in these older patients (Connolly et al. 1994). Some ataxia is seen in all children who have ACA, and 20–50% of patients are unable to walk. Finger dysmetria is seen in two-thirds of these children but is strikingly mild compared with the gait ataxia (Connolly et al. 1994). Nystagmus was present in less than 20% of Connolly's (1994) patients Transient behavioral alterations and school difficulties are seen in at least one-third of children with ACA.

Laboratory studies reveal a mild CSF pleocytosis. Neuroimaging studies are typically normal, although occasionally abnormal signal can be seen in the cerebellum.

Given the variety of antecedents, it is likely that a common immunoinflammatory process mediates ACA. Antineuronal antibodies to triosephosphate isomerase follow Epstein-Barr virus infection (Uchibori et al. 2005). CSF pleocytosis occurs in 25–50% of children, almost always with a lymphocytic predominance (Connolly et al. 1994). The CSF IgG index is elevated in 50% of these children, and oligoclonal bands are present in 10–17%.

Ninety percent of children will completely recover from the ataxia, typically within the first few months after the onset of disease. Supportive therapy is needed. One-fifth of children experience transient behavioral or intellectual problems (see Connolly et al. 1994, for extensive review). In rare cases without complete recovery, atrophy of the cerebellar hemispheres or other conditions, such as cerebellar tumor, OMA, or intoxication should be expected (Table 12.14).

Table 12.14 Acute cerebellar ataxia

Discriminating features
- Acute onset of ataxia

Consistent features
- Follows viral infection
- Typically occurs in young children
- Recovery over the first few months

Variable features
- CSF pleocytosis
- Abnormalities on MRI scan

Ataxia-telangiectasia

Ataxia-telangiectasia (AT) is a multisystem disease, affecting both the nervous and immune systems. Soon after beginning to walk, these children present with a progressive ataxia, as well as choreoathetotic movements of their extremities. Typically, also a loss of deep tendon reflexes, dysarthria, and an oculomotor apraxia occurs. In addition to their neurologic symptom, these children will also show prominent telangiectasias that can be most obviously seen in the conjunctiva and skin. These children become wheelchair-bound during their second decade.

The gene responsible for AT, called *ATM*, is a kinase that may be involved in cell cycle control, DNA repair, and prevention of programmed cell death (Savitsky et al. 1995). *In vitro*, the cells derived from AT patients have defective DNA repair capability when exposed to irradiation. Heterozygotes for the AT gene (about 1% of the general population) may be at increased risk for cancer, particularly female breast cancer.

Care should be taken to avoid radiographs in these patients, since their cells are hypersensitive to ionizing radiation. Neuroimaging shows atrophy of the cerebellar hemispheres and vermis These patients also have nearly a 100-fold increased risk for malignancy, and they should be carefully monitored for malignancies. Heterozygotes for the AT gene will carry nearly a sevenfold risk of increased malignancies (Swift et al. 1987).

Serum studies reveal a decrease in the IgA and IgE levels and elevated α-fetoprotein levels. α-Fetoprotein levels are highly elevated, although difficult to interpret prior to the age of 2 years. The diagnosis is often a challenge to make before the age of 5 years, and many children will experience symptoms for several years before a definitive diagnosis is made.

The treatment is supportive. Infections can be treated with antibiotics and IVIG. Live-virus vaccines should not be used after the diagnosis of AT is made. Genetic counseling should be provided for families carrying this autosomal recessive disorder.

Prognosis is poor, and the progression is relentless. Children lose the ability to walk independently in their second decade. Death may occur in adolescence or early adulthood due to malignancy or pulmonary infection.

Consider Consultation When...

- The child has a family history of chorea or dystonia.
- The symptoms of a child suspected of having Sydenham chorea continue for more than 2 months.
- Dystonia involves the legs and/or is progressive.
- Tremor is associated with rest or with an increase in muscle tone.
- The symptoms of ataxia have no defined cause and are persisting over 1 month.

Table 12.15 Episodic ataxia

Discriminating features
▶ Periodic episodes of ataxia or vertigo
▶ Autosomal dominant
Consistent features
▶ Difficulty walking during ataxia or vertiginous attacks
▶ Precipitated by physical or emotional stress
▶ Cerebellar signs on neurologic examination
▶ Responds to acetazolamide
Variable features
▶ Cerebellar degeneration

Episodic ataxia

The syndrome of episodic ataxia (EA) results in episodes of vertigo and ataxia, often triggered by stress, fatigue, or exercise. Episodic ataxia has been called by a variety of other names, including *periodic ataxia*. It was initially described in 1946 (Parker 1946). Since that time, multiple families have been reported. It is an autosomal dominantly inherited disorder. Episodic ataxia type 1 (EA-1) is caused by mutations in the potassium channel gene *KCNA1*, whereas episodic ataxia type 2 (EA-2) is caused by mutations in the calcium channel gene *CACNA1A* (Baloh & Jen 2002).

The episodes usually begin in infancy or childhood, but infrequently may start in adulthood (Tibbles et al. 1986). The attacks of cerebellar incoordination are characterized by paroxysmal bouts of ataxia, dysarthria, and nystagmus. The frequency is variable; episodes may occur daily or may be separated by weeks or months. The duration of the episodes may be brief, but more often the episodes last for hours and sometimes days. Ataxia of the trunk and extremities is frequently so severe during the episodes that the patient cannot stand without assistance. Speech becomes dysarthric and difficult to understand, although receptive language function remains intact. Vertical or horizontal nystagmus may be present during the attack.

Slight cerebellar signs are often noted during interim neurologic examination. Horizontal and sometimes vertical nystagmus and mild ataxia on finger-to-nose and heel-to-shin testing are typical findings. Although some authors found no progressive neurologic involvement, others reported a slow progression of ataxia. EA-1 is more likely to have interictal myokymia and EA-2 often has interictal nystagmus (Jen 2000).

CT and MRI studies are usually unremarkable in young children; however, in individuals whose symptoms persist over a prolonged period, neuroimaging will frequently reveal cerebellar atrophy, especially of the vermis.

Acetazolamide in many cases completely eliminates or greatly reduces the number of episodes within 24 hours of its administration (Griggs et al. 1978). Some patients on medication have remained attack-free for many years. Other authors report a less complete response to this drug. Anticonvulsants such as phenytoin and phenobarbital have no effect on these paroxysmal attacks (Table 12.15).

Additional resources

The website "We Move" is a not-for-profit organization that maintains an up-to-date pediatric section, "Kids Move" (http://www.wemove.org/), that provides current information for both physicians and patients. Many of the disorders discussed in this chapter are discussed in depth at this website.

CHAPTER 13

Infections of the Central Nervous System

Amisha Malhotra, William E. Bell, and Frederick W. Henderson

Outline

Bacterial infections of the central nervous system

Acute bacterial meningitis

Acute bacterial meningitis, in most cases, is a septic-borne, rapidly progressive infection that occurs in an anatomic area of impaired host resistance. This local physiologic immunodeficiency is because cerebrospinal fluid (CSF) contains very low contents of immunoglobulins and complement compared to plasma, components required for effective phagocytosis and intracellular bacterial killing. For this reason, eradication of bacteria in CSF requires the attainment of high levels of bactericidal antibiotics within the CSF.

Pyogenic meningitis can affect patients of any age but, among children, the disorder has a decided predisposition to occur in the younger age groups, including the neonate and those younger than 4 years of age. Currently, the most common causes of bacterial meningitis in the neonatal period are group B *Streptococcus* and *Escherichia coli* followed less often by *Listeria monocytogenes*. In older infants and children, *Streptococcus pneumoniae* and *Neisseria meningitidis* now account for the great majority of cases. Peak incidence of meningococcal meningitis is under age 2 years and that of pneumococcal meningitis is under age 4 years.

Childhood vaccination strategies have markedly altered the epidemiology of pediatric bacterial meningitis over the decades. Before 1990, *Haemophilus influenzae* type b meningitis was the most common cause of bacterial meningitis in children. Since the introduction of the vaccine in 1988, the incidence of invasive disease has decreased by 99%. The heptavalent pneumococcal vaccine recommended for routine administration in infants since 2000 has made a substantial impact on the incidence of invasive pneumococcal infections in children.

It is now known that the inflammatory reaction to invading bacterial organisms is not primarily from the pathogens themselves. Bacterial cell death within the CSF, as well as in the systemic circulation, leads to release of endotoxins: lipopolysaccharide from gram-negative bacteria and teichoic acid-peptidoglycans from gram-positive organisms. These substances stimulate the production from macrophages, monocytes, and brain-cell elements of cytokines, which activate the complement cascade and result in meningeal and meningovascular inflammatory responses. Cytokine-induced meningeal inflammation provokes a CSF cellular response, whereas that affecting the microvasculature of the brain and CSF alters the blood–brain barrier, increasing vascular permeability and causing brain swelling. The degree of CSF pleocytosis and vascular inflammation has been found to correlate with the magnitude of cytokine production. The recognition that cytokine production can be curtailed by the administration of corticosteroids given before or at the time of initiation of antibiotic therapy has led to the consideration of dexamethasone use in patients over 1 month of age with acute pyogenic meningitis. Except for certain unusual instances with rapid onset of high-grade cerebral swelling, this therapeutic approach remains controversial and was studied most extensively only in infants with *H. influenzae* meningitis.

Table 13.1 Characteristic cerebrospinal fluid (CSF) findings in meningitis

CSF findings	Normal	TB	Viral	Bacterial
Cells	0	10–500	0–500	5–10,000
Differential	—	polys→monos	polys→monos	polys
Protein (mg/dL)	15–45	>150 (elevated)	20–50 (normal)	20–400 (normal/↑)
Glucose (mg/dL)	50–75	20–50 (normal/↓)	30–80 (normal/↓)	<20 (low) (<20–40)*

*CSF-to-serum ratio <0.6

Clinical manifestations of bacterial meningitis are outlined in the following sections and are more determined by age of the affected infant or child than the causative organism. Except in the neonate, fever is customary. In all age groups, the illness tends to result in decline in responsiveness unless treatment is begun early. Lethargy is often preceded by headache, vomiting, confusion, and disorientation. Seizures occur in up to 50% of cases of meningitis and can be the first suggestive event in the febrile infant or child. Although brain swelling usually rapidly becomes a component of the illness, well-established papilledema is not usually found and, if present, suggests an alternative diagnosis. Meningeal signs, including neck stiffness, Kernig signs, and Brudzinski sign, are not usually found in neonates but begin to be common signs in infants beyond a few months of age with acute meningitis.

The indication for CSF examination is determined by the clinical suspicion from history and physical examination. In the neonate, it is often on the basis of signs of bacterial sepsis, especially when complicated by seizures, lethargy, or a full fontanel. On gross observation, infected CSF may range from clear to purulent. Characteristic CSF abnormalities with pyogenic meningitis include a neutrophilic pleocytosis, reduced glucose content, and increase in the protein level. Meningitis in older children or adults caused by *L. monocytogenes* has been notable for the occasional occurrence at a lymphatic pleocytosis and a normal CSF glucose content. Table 13.1 shows typical CSF findings seen in children and adults with meningitis caused by either bacteria, viruses, or tuberculosis, as compared to normal values. Preliminary antibiotic therapy can alter the CSF abnormalities, although not usually to the degree that precludes establishing the diagnosis of meningitis. A controversial issue concerns the need in older children for neuroimaging before lumbar puncture when signs of meningitis include those indicative of intracranial hypertension. Certain findings listed in Table 13.2 warrant preliminary computed tomography (CT) scanning, although in many other cases performing a lumbar puncture as soon as possible is highly desirable.

Table 13.2 Indication for computed tomography (CT) examination before lumbar puncture in a child suspected of pyogenic meningitis

- Papilledema
- Dilated or poorly reactive pupils
- Focal (simple partial) seizures
- Hemiparesis
- Bradycardia
- Decerebrate posturing
- Tonic attacks
- Immunosuppressive disease
- Bradycardia or hypertension with neck flexion

Neonatal meningitis

Bacterial meningitis in the first month after birth is considered separately from that occurring later in infancy and childhood because the predisposing factors are different, the clinical signs of the illness are different, and the causative organisms are usually different. Except for lethargy and the common occurrence of seizures, the clinical signs in the neonate with pyogenic meningitis reflect the presence of sepsis, present in almost all with neonatal meningitis. Temperature instability, poor feeding, vomiting, irritability, and respiratory abnormalities are hallmarks of neonatal bacteremia. The association with meningitis is usually documented by CSF examination in the infant suspected or known to be septic. As noted earlier, meningeal signs, including neck stiffness and Kernig sign, are not usually seen in the neonate but begin to correlate with meningeal inflammation later in infancy. Fullness of the anterior fontanel in the septic neonate suggests the possibility of meningitis but is often not present, at least early in the illness. In the infant with signs indicative of sepsis, the occurrence of a seizure should immediately indicate the probability of meningitis.

Group B *Streptococcus* (*S. agalactiae*) is the most common cause of neonatal meningitis in this country, followed by *E. coli* and other gram-negative pathogens. Less common causes include *L. monocytogenes*, *Salmonella* sp., and *Citrobacter koseri*, the latter being complicated by periventricular abscess formation in the majority of cases (Table 13.3).

Table 13.3 Most common causes of bacterial meningitis from birth to 4 weeks

- Group B *Streptococcus*
- *Escherichia coli*
- *Listeria monocytogenes*
- *Klebsiella species*
- *Proteus species*
- *Pseudomonas aeruginosa*
- *Citrobacter koseri*
- *Salmonella species*

Group B *Streptococcus* neonatal infection occurs in two clinical forms. The early-onset form is more common and describes onset of illness between birth and age 7 days, with most showing overwhelming signs of infection with respiratory distress, cardiovascular collapse, and neutropenia within hours after birth. The early-onset form is caused by vertical transmission from the maternal anogenital tract. Meningitis is found in about 20% of such cases. The late-onset form has onset of illness between 7 and 90 days after birth and usually presents with clinical evidence of meningitis, most often between 2 and 4 weeks of age. Unlike infants with the early-onset form, those who present later do not usually experience severe respiratory compromise, although many have intense signs of CNS infection. In only about 50% of late-onset cases is the organism derived from the mother. Studies by Sundell and colleagues in 2000 suggest that the more virulent early-onset form of illness with prominent respiratory compromise is due to an exotoxin termed CM101, liberated from group B *Streptococcus*, which binds to immature pulmonary vascular receptors. Rapid maturation of pulmonary vascular receptors after 1 week of age supposedly explains the less severe septic components of the late-onset form of the illness. As a result of maternal screening with vaginal and anal cultures at approximately 36 weeks of gestation, with intrapartum penicillin given to culture-positive mothers, the incidence of early-onset group B *Streptococcus* invasive disease in the neonate has sharply decreased from 2–4 per 1,000 live births in 1993 to 0.61 per 1,000 in 1998. Factors that predispose to neonatal invasive disease with group B *Streptococcus* include a heavy inoculum of the fetus at delivery with organisms from the maternal anogenital tract, low birth weight and obstetrical complications, and deficiency of maternal type-specific antibodies directed against group B *Streptococcus*.

Among gram-negative enteric bacilli causing neonatal meningitis, *E. coli* is the most common offender. In older children and adults, *E. coli* is well known as a cause of meningitis complicating neurosurgical procedures, following open craniocerebral injuries, and in the immune compromised. Low-birth-weight sick neonates requiring persistent intubation or those with indwelling intravascular catheters are also susceptible to sepsis and meningitis with *Pseudomonas aeruginosa*, *Klebsiella* sp., *Proteus* sp., *Serratia marcescens*, as well as *Candida* sp., a yeast-phase fungus.

Escherichia coli meningitis can present soon after birth but most neonates become symptomatic near the end of the first week after birth or 1–2 weeks later. In perhaps 20% of cases of *E. coli* meningitis in the neonate, a predisposing cause will be apparent, including urinary tract malformations, neurosurgical closure of an open neural tube defect, necrotizing enterocolitis, or complicating sepsis in a child with galactosemia or hereditary tyrosinemia. Usual presenting manifestations are seizures, lethargy, poor feeding, vomiting, and temperature instability. Blood leukocyte counts are variable, some being elevated and others being suppressed and associated with thrombocytopenia. Cerebrospinal fluid is diagnostic in the majority of the cases. Blood cultures are frequently positive, and urine culture may reveal the same organism. Among a large series of neonates with gram-negative bacillary meningitis, Unhanand and colleagues (1993) found a case fatality rate of 17%. Among survivors, 61% had long-term sequelae such as seizures, deafness, long-tract signs, visual loss, developmental and mental retardation, and hydrocephalus.

Haemophilus influenzae type B meningitis

Following the widespread use of *H. influenzae* conjugate vaccine in early infancy in 1990, the incidence of invasive disease, including meningitis, caused by this organism declined by well over 95%. Prior to that time, *H. influenzae* type B accounted for approximately 70% of all cases of acute pyogenic meningitis in children. The disease is now rarely seen in large medical centers but, before effective immunization given in early infancy, the peak age at occurrence of the illness was 6–9 months and the great majority occurred before age 3 years. Most cases would begin with fever and irritability for 1–3 days, when vomiting, lethargy, seizures, and variable neurologic signs evolve, indicating blood-borne CSF invasion. Less often, the illness is more fulminating, with rapid evolution of high fever, deep coma, respiratory compromise, evidence of consumption coagulopathy and shock, and rapidly progressive intracranial hypertension. Meningitis can be complicated by pneumonia, otitis media, or suppurative pericarditis. In 5–8% of cases, either septic or reactive arthritis will be found. About 30% of children with *H. influenzae* meningitis will have the illness complicated by sterile subdural effusion that resolves spontaneously in most cases. Infected subdural effusions or subdural empyemas are less common but more symptomatic and require surgical drainage.

Haemophilus influenzae was originally highly sensitive to ampicillin until 1974, when ampicillin-resistant strains emerged and eventually became common. Thereafter, cefotaxime became the standard mode of therapy. Most studies revealed that *H. influenzae* meningitis had a mortality of about 3%, and neurologic sequelae would occur in over 30% of survivors, with hearing loss being the single most common deficit.

Meningococcal meningitis

Invasive meningococcal infections have been categorized as primarily meningitis in presentation or primarily in the form of meningococcemia. Schuchat and colleagues (1997) state that, in all age groups, about 48% of cases of meningococcal disease present predominantly as meningitis and 48% are manifested with signs of meningococcemia. In 3%, pneumonia is the primary form of illness. In this review, the overall case fatality rate was 11%. Among those presenting as meningococcal meningitis, the fatality rate was 3%, whereas those in the meningococcemia group had a case fatality rate of 17%. Among persons with fulminating meningococcemia with early onset of hypotension and purpura fulminans, the case fatality rate is considerably higher.

At least 13 serogroups of *N. meningitidis* have been described with most human infections being caused by serogroups A, B, C, Y, and W-135. Serogroup A has been known since the early 20th century to cause periodic epidemics of meningococcal disease, occurring roughly at intervals of 8–12 years. Serogroup A is now infrequent in the United States but continues to be a serious public health problem in sub-Saharan Africa and Asia. Most cases of meningococcal disease in the United States are caused by serogroups B or C and occur sporadically or in localized outbreaks. Serogroups Y and W-135 are less common causes of invasive disease and are better known as causes of pneumonia.

Invasive disease with *N. meningitidis* has two peaks in age incidence. The first is among infants younger than 2 years of age who commonly lack protective antibodies. The second affects adolescents and young adults. These illnesses can occur any time of year but are more frequent in late winter and early spring. During winter months, 5–10% of the population have nasopharyngeal colonization with *Neisseria* sp., most being nonpathogenic strains. Of those colonized with pathogenic *N. meningitidis*, on infrequent occasions organisms become transferred from the mucosal surface to the vascular compartment, and invasive disease follows in some fashion. Presentation of meningococcal meningitis, like that with other common offenders, is usually with abrupt onset of fever, chills, and headache, soon followed by lethargy, confusion, and the development of meningeal signs. Approximately 60–70% will develop skin lesions, sometimes initially with a maculopapular rash but more characteristically with multiple petechial lesions indicative of either vascular wall disruption due to infectious vasculitis or thrombocytopenia. In some, the illness will rapidly resolve with antibiotic therapy, while others will experience rapidly progressive disease reflecting sepsis, endotoxemia with consumption, and hypotension leading to shock and multiple organ failure.

Among children presenting with meningococcemia, most will exhibit petechiae and, when fulminant, the rash may proceed to purpura fulminans, which can be associated with systemic hypotension, shock, and multiple organ failure with visceral hemorrhages. This condition is called the Waterhouse-Friderichsen syndrome and, although adrenal hemorrhage along with hemorrhage in other organs is commonly found at autopsy, the fulminate nature of the illness is due to massive endotoxemia with consumption coagulopathy. Acquired protein C and protein S deficiency appears to play a role in the severity of the coagulopathy and may be a component of the illness amenable to treatment.

Diagnosis of invasive meningococcal disease is often suspected clinically when fever occurs with a petechial rash, with or without meningitis. Because of the potential for invasive meningococcal disease to progress rapidly within hours after onset of first symptoms, intravenous antibiotic treatment should be started as soon as possible. When the illness is suspected on the basis of fever and the characteristic rash, if transport to a medical facility will require more than a short time period and if CSF examination cannot be done locally, treatment should be initiated before transport even though this might diminish the value of subsequently obtained specimens for culture. Etiologic diagnosis is confirmed by cultures of blood, CSF, and urine. Latex agglutination can also be useful where available. In children with meningitis, Gram stain shows intracellular gram-negative diplococci in most. Cerebrospinal fluid may be cloudy or purulent and includes findings typical of acute bacterial meningitis in the majority. Exceptions do occur and, in a large series of pediatric meningococcal meningitis cases reported by Wong and co-workers (1989), CSF that was ultimately culture positive for meningococci in 11% did not have a neutrophilic pleocytosis and had normal CSF glucose contents and negative Gram stains. It is probable that the CSF specimens in these atypical cases were obtained soon after entrance of bacteria from blood into CSF and before an inflammatory reaction could occur. Infants with meningococcal meningitis are more likely to have sequelae than are adolescents. Findings early in the illnesses that predict a poor or fatal outcome include neutropenia, hypothermia, hypertension or shock, and evidence of coagulopathy including purpura fulminans.

Penicillin is the antibiotic of choice for treatment of meningococcal disease. Isolates in this country have been found to be sensitive to penicillin, although decreasing sensitivity to penicillin has recently been found in some other countries. For children intolerant to penicillin, cefotaxime or ceftriaxone can be used. Antibiotic therapy is usually given for 5–7 days, and management of complicating features such as endotoxic shock, thrombocytopenia, cardiac or respiratory compromise, and the indications for corticosteroids, requires intensive care and consultation with the appropriate medical specialties.

Household members and those with close contact with the infected person are at high risk for development of meningococcal disease and are advised to receive prophylactic therapy, ideally within the first 24 hours of diagnosis of the index case. Rifampin, ciprofloxacin, and ceftriaxone are all appropriate medications to be used for this purpose.

Currently, two meningococcal vaccines are licensed in the United States for use in children and adults against serogroups A, C, Y, and W-135. The preferred vaccine for individuals over 10 years of age is the conjugate vaccine, which is recommended for routine immunization of all preadolescents (11–12 years old) and high-risk individuals. It is not licensed for use in children under 2 years of age, so routine immunization is not recommended for this age group. However, the polysaccharide meningococcal vaccine is available for use in children 2–10 years of age who are at high risk for development of meningococcal disease. Those considered at high-risk for developing meningococcal disease include persons with functional or anatomic asplenia, those with terminal complement or properidin deficiency, those in disease outbreak situations, military recruits, college dormitory freshmen, and travelers going to or residing in certain endemic regions, such as sub-Saharan Africa.

Streptococcus pneumoniae meningitis

Streptococcus pneumoniae is a gram-positive diplococcus that is now considered to be the leading cause of pyogenic meningitis in infants and children. Among the common cases of bacterial meningitis in children, pneumococcus causes the highest mortality and provokes the most abundant meningeal inflammatory response. The mortality rate of pneumococcal meningitis occurring in infants and children is generally stated to be approximately 10% and is higher when the illness occurs in early infancy. Pneumococcal meningitis in children has its highest incidence in the first 4 years of life, indicative of the common occurrence and high bacterial density of nasopharyngeal colonization at this age. By age 2 years, the majority of children have had at least one occasion of nasopharyngeal colonization with this organism. Invasive pneumococcal infections have only rarely been described in the first days after birth, but infrequent cases occur between 2 and 4 weeks of age, probably by vertical transmission from the mother.

Most cases of *S. pneumoniae* meningitis occur in previously normal children. Studies suggest that about 10–15% of cases occur in children with a predisposing factor, which includes functional or anatomical asplenia, sickle cell disease, agammaglobulinemia, and intracranial CSF fistula. In approximately 70% of children who develop meningitis and who have posttraumatic or congenital defects associated with CSF rhinorrhea or otorrhea, *S. pneumoniae* will be the cause. In addition, the pneumococcus is the most common cause of community-acquired pneumonia in children and in adults, the most common cause of acute otitis media and sinusitis, and by far the most common cause of "occult bacteremia" in infancy, an illness with fever without localizing signs that sometimes will be complicated by localized disease if not treated.

Aspects of pneumococcal meningitis suggestive of a poor prognosis include young age of onset, a very low CSF glucose content and a markedly elevated CSF protein, coma, respiratory distress, shock and seizures early in the course of the illness, and its development in the asplenic patient, which is frequently associated with a fulminating septic course, with or without meningitis.

A major factor that has affected the management of children with pneumococcal meningitis has been the rapid rise in penicillin-resistant strains in the past decade. Decreased susceptibility to cephalosporins is also on the rise. Although penicillin resistance has been found in a high percentage of isolates in many foreign countries, the incidence of resistant strains continues to vary from community to community in this country. It is sufficiently prevalent, however, to account for the therapeutic use of vancomycin in combination with cefotaxime or ceftriaxone as initial therapy for unspecified bacterial meningitis in children over 1 month of age until identification and sensitivities of the isolated pathogen are obtained. The concern of the possibility of antibiotic resistance in the pneumococcus has led to the common practice of repeating the CSF examination after 48 hours of treatment if the organism is then known to be a nonsusceptible strain and if clinical signs have not improved or have worsened.

Two types of pneumococcal vaccines are currently available in the United States. Heptavalent pneumococcal vaccine is U.S. Food and Drug Administration (FDA)-approved for routine immunization of children beginning at 2 months of age, and it provides protection against seven of the most common pneumococcal strains that cause invasive disease in children. Following its availability in 2000, the vaccine has already had a substantial impact on the occurrence of pneumococcal disease, with an 80% reduction in invasive pneumococcal infections in children under 2 years of age. The 23-valent polysaccharide vaccine is still available and licensed for use in older children and adults at risk for pneumococcal invasive disease.

Treatment of acute bacterial meningitis

The best chance of a favorable outcome among infants and children with acute pyogenic meningitis is with the initiation in the early stage of the illness of high-dose, intravenous bactericidal antibiotics. In most cases, antibiotics will be started before the causative organism is isolated. The current recommendations for selection of antimicrobials are outlined in Table 13.4. In the neonate, ampicillin is included because some strains of *E. coli* remain sensitive to the drug and because *L. monocytogenes* is resistant to cephalosporins. Should group B streptococcus be proven to be the cause, either ampicillin, with or without an aminoglycoside, or penicillin is usually chosen. With less common enteric bacilli CSF infections, changes in the regimen will be determined by in vitro sensitivity studies. In those over 1 month of age, vancomycin is now included, since the pneumococcus has become the most common isolate from CSF and is now known to have a significant rate of increased resistance to penicillin. Invasive meningococcal infections are treated with single-drug therapy with penicillin or with cefotaxime or ceftriaxone.

Control of fever, control of seizures, control of increased intracranial pressure, and fluid and electrolyte management are additional important aspects of care of the infected child. Among children with meningitis who are not dehydrated, a modest reduction in the fluid volume administered in the first 24 hours of treatment can be useful relative to cerebral edema. When clinical signs or laboratory findings suggest vascular volume depletion, not less than maintenance fluid needs must be given. It is critical to maintain vascular volume to protect tissue and cerebral perfusion during an acute febrile illness, especially so in more severe cases in which cerebral autoregulation may be disturbed.

Use of dexamethasone to diminish cytokine production, thereby curtailing the inflammatory response, has become a popular topic in the past decade but remains controversial. In children, most studies evaluating the effect of dexamethasone have been among young children with *H. influenzae* meningitis. Early studies did show that their use reduced the inflammatory response and decreased the incidence of sequelae, especially hearing loss. It is generally agreed that if dexamethasone is to be used, it should be given before or at the time of initiation of antibiotics. Concerns of the possible adverse effects of dexamethasone in children with meningitis include their possible adverse effect on neutrophil phagocytic function as well as the possibility of decreasing penetration of antibiotics, especially vancomycin, into CSF. If one chooses to use dexamethasone, the dose for this purpose is 0.6 mg/kg/day given in four divided doses for the first few days of the treatment regimen.

Table 13.4 Empirical antibiotic therapy for unspecified bacterial meningitis

Under Age 1 Month
- Cefotaxime or ceftriaxone
- Ampicillin

Over Age 1 Month
- Vancomycin
- Cefotaxime or ceftriaxone

Recurrent bacterial meningitis

Recurrent attacks of bacterial meningitis are not common but certainly not rare, and the underlying cause can be identified in most, as outlined in Table 13.5. The majority are secondary to an abnormal communication between the external environment and the CSF. Specific localization of the defect can often be difficult and requires help from consultants in neurosurgery and ear-nose-throat medicine in many instances, for both diagnosis and treatment. The most common causes are traumatic injuries with dural lacerations through frontal or ethmoidal sinuses, the base of the skull, or the tegmen tympani of the temporal bone, leading to CSF leakage into the middle ear. The next most common causes are congenital defects, especially at the cribiform plate, with or without a basilar encephalocele, and, as infectious complication of a ventricular shunt for hydrocephalus. Congenital dermal sinuses that penetrate into the CSF can be located along the midline in the occipital region or anywhere along the spine. A dermal sinus is suspected in any child with recurrent meningitis not secondary to craniocerebral trauma and without CSF rhinorrhea. Dermal

Table 13.5 Causes of recurrent bacterial meningitis in children

- Posttraumatic craniocerebral injuries
- Postsurgical defects with dural lacerations
- Ventricular shunt infections
- Congenital defects
  - Basal encephaloceles
  - Congenital defects of the cribiform plate
  - Congenital inner ear defects
  - Congenital dermal sinuses
  - Neuroenteric fistula
- Chronic increased intracranial pressure
- Empty sella syndrome
- Parameningeal suppurative foci
- Immunosuppression and late complement component deficiencies

sinus presents as a small, midline orifice in the skin often surrounded by a surface capillary hemangioma or a tuft of hair. A dermal sinus in the occipital region sometimes terminates in a posterior fossa dermoid, a non-neoplastic lesion that predisposes to bacterial meningitis due to transmission of bacteria via the dermal sinus into the CSF or to aseptic meningitis secondary to spontaneous leakage of material from the dermoid into the CSF.

Additional causes of abnormal CSF communications include erosion of the skull base from chronic increase in intracranial pressure, the empty sella syndrome, and post-neurosurgical dural defects, especially as a complication of pituitary surgery by a transnasal, transsphenoidal approach. Congenital defects affecting the inner ear, such as the Mondini defect with a perilymphatic fistula through the oval window or a malformation affecting the stapes footplate, which allow CSF and perilymph to be transmitted into the middle ear, likewise can cause recurrent meningitis. These conditions are suspected in a child with unilateral deafness, sometimes with episodes of ataxia or vertigo, who develops acute pyogenic meningitis.

Cerebrospinal fluid rhinorrhea is a finding indicative of an intracranial defect predisposing to recurrent meningitis and can present almost immediately after cranial injury or a neurosurgical operative procedure or can be delayed for weeks, months, or even years thereafter. Nasal discharge of CSF is often abundant when the dural laceration is anteriorly placed but may be scanty or absent when the source is from inner ear pathology, in which case CSF is transmitted into the middle ear, down the Eustachian tube, and into the posterior nasopharynx where the majority may be swallowed. Should the injury or pathology disrupt the tympanic membrane, CSF otorrhea will occur. It cannot accurately be documented that the clear fluid dripping from the nostrils is CSF by testing the fluid for glucose by dipstick methods or by testing for chloride content, as these substances can be similar in fluid generated by the nasal mucosa or in tears. That the fluid *is* CSF can sometimes be shown by the presence of B-transferrin on protein electrophoresis.

Precise localization of a CSF fistula is highly desirable before surgical correction is undertaken. Numerous techniques have been proposed, and the least invasive methods are usually first attempted. High-resolution CT is useful for defects anteriorly along the cribiform plate, and especially for temporal bone fractures and congenital defects, including the Mondini defect. Conventional magnetic resonance imaging (MRI) and also MRI cisternography performed with heavily weighted T2 sequences can be helpful in the demonstration of abnormal CSF communications. Additional studies sometimes resorted to include CT cisternography with iohexal as a contrast agent and intrathecal radioactive technetium with placement of cotton pledgets in the nostrils. The latter, when positive, indicates that CSF is gaining entrance into the nasal region but does not specifically localize the site of pathology. Both are invasive techniques and are only considered when other methods have failed.

With intracranial CSF leaks causing bacterial meningitis, about 80% are caused by *S. pneumoniae.* Other causative organisms include the meningococcus, *Haemophilus* sp., and *Staphylococcus aureus.* With intraspinal defects such as dermal sinuses, meningitis is more often caused by gram-negative bacilli or *S. aureus. Staphylococcus aureus* meningitis in a child without a ventricular shunt or immunosuppression is so unusual that it should always provoke a search for a neurocutaneous fistula such as a dermal sinus.

The use of prophylactic antibiotics during the investigation to find the site of a CSF leak is controversial. Most do not recommend their use because the effectiveness has not been proven, and they may lead to the occurrence of meningitis from resistant organisms. Dural lacerations with CSF fistulae from basilar skull fractures heal spontaneously within days to weeks in the majority. Cerebrospinal fluid leaks that accompany congenital defects—including those with cribiform plate defects, anterior encephaloceles, inner ear anomalies, or congenital dermal sinuses—are expected to persist until surgically corrected. Meningitis complicating an acquired intracranial CSF fistula can occur within days after the injury or surgical procedure or can be delayed for years. For this reason, the history from any patient with meningitis, and especially recurrent meningitis, should include questions pertaining to possible previous craniofacial injuries, history of deafness, and whether CSF rhinorrhea has been observed.

Recurrent meningitis caused by *N. meningitidis* is an infrequent but well-established disorder associated with hereditary late complement deficiency, predominantly C5 through C8. It is estimated that about 1% of persons with their first attack of invasive meningococcal disease have this familial deficiency. The condition should be suspected and searched for by complement measurement when a child or adolescent has acute meningococcal meningitis and there is a history of a previous attack with the same organism in a direct family member remote in time from the current patient's illness. It should also be considered when one has repeated attacks of meningococcal invasive disease. The mean age of onset of meningococcal infection with this familial disorder is approximately 15 years, thus considerably later than the mean age of onset of meningococcal meningitis in immunologically normal children. Clinical features and CSF findings are similar to those without late complement deficiencies, although in most, the illness is less severe, sequelae are milder, and mortality rate is lower. It has been proposed that the lesser intensity of meningococcal disease in persons with deficiency of late complement components is indicative of a more abundant inflammatory response with greater immune attack on peripheral blood cells and vascular endothelium in complement-normal persons. Patients identified to have predisposition to invasive meningococcal disease due to late complement component deficiencies are maintained on prophylactic penicillin and are also given meningococcal vaccine.

Cerebrospinal fluid shunt infection

In the mid-1960s, ventriculoperitoneal (VP) shunts largely supplemented ventriculoatrial (VA) shunts for CSF diversion in persons with hydrocephalus. This was mainly because of the diverse complications of VA shunts, such as pulmonary vascular microemboli and immune-mediated glomerulonephritis, among others. Although the incidence of shunt infection is approximately the same with the two types of shunts, bacteremia is common with VA shunt infection and occurs only occasionally with VP shunt infections. Most workers claim the incidence of VP shunt infection is about 10% with the initial insertion of the shunt, but the rate increases with subsequent shunt reinsertions required after prior shunt infection. With modifications in the perioperative technique and meticulous attention to sterility in the operating room, Choux and colleagues (1992) in France found that postoperative shunt infections could be reduced to less than 1%. There have been many published trials with the use of perioperative prophylactic antibiotics; however, their benefit as a method to reduce the incidence of shunt infection remains controversial. Most published protocols for shunt placement do advocate the use of perioperative antibiotics at the time of CSF shunt placement.

The majority of shunt infections occur within 2 months of placement and some occur within days after operation. Approximately 70% of CSF shunt infections are caused by *Staphylococcus* sp. with *S. epidermidis* being much more common than *S. aureus*. The high incidence of these organisms plus *Propionibacterium acnes* among cases with infected shunts indicates that most such infections stem from the skin of the patient or less often from the gloved hand of operating room attendants. Airborne bacilli in the operating room may account for some, whereas others, especially gram-negative bacillary shunt infections, evolve from intestinal perforation by the distal end of the shunt. *Enterococcus faecalis* has become an additional important cause of CSF shunt infection.

The clinical signs of an infected shunt are quite variable and can range from subtle to dramatic and rapidly progressive. As a generalization, signs are usually less intense when shunt infection is caused by *S. epidermidis* and more severe when caused by the more virulent *S. aureus*. Gram-negative bacillary shunt infections usually give rise to recognizable signs of CNS infections and definite evidence of infection on CSF examination. The most common clinical findings associated with VP shunt infection include some combination of fever, irritability, lethargy, poor feeding, vomiting, and abdominal pain or tenderness. Definite meningeal signs are not usually found. Shunt failure often, but not always, will accompany shunt infection and will lead to signs of intracranial hypertension in some. In others, fever and acute onset of abdominal signs indicative of peritoneal inflammation will represent the presenting signs of an infected VP shunt. Infrequently, an obvious wound infection on the scalp or erythema along the scalp portion of the shunt tube will indicate the probability of an infected shunt.

When suspected, diagnosis of an infected shunt is on the basis of abnormal CSF findings, although these also can be variable. With *S. epidermidis* shunt infections, the CSF cellular response is usually minimal to mild and the CSF Gram stain is often negative. Reduced CSF glucose content and a positive culture of ventricular fluid are generally more indicative of this infection. Both *S. aureus* and gram-negative bacillary shunt infections are likely to reveal more striking ventricular fluid abnormalities. Unlike those with *S. epidermidis* shunt infection, those caused by gram-negative organisms will have positive CSF Gram strains in the majority of cases. Thus, with few exceptions, when a child has clinical evidence of a VP shunt infection and the CSF reveals few cells and a negative Gram stain, it can be assumed that the causative pathogen will be *S. epidermidis*.

Although recognition of the possibility of an infected VP shunt is often a responsibility of the pediatrician, its management is the domain of the neurosurgeon. In most cases, the infected shunt must be removed. Temporary external ventricular diversion with a ventricular cannula is often resorted to as a measure to control intracranial pressure during the time period required for eradication of the infection with intravenous antibiotics. Most antibiotics used for VP shunt infections will only gain entrance into the CSF in the presence of meningeal inflammation. Because ventriculitis/meningitis associated with shunt infections, especially those caused by *S. epidermidis*, is usually associated with minimal meningeal inflammation, the effect of antibiotic therapy in eradicating the infection is often sluggish. Most workers recommend either nafcillin or vancomycin for *Staphylococcus* sp. shunt infection, depending on in vitro sensitivity studies, sometimes in combination with an aminoglycoside or rifampin with vancomycin. When *Staphylococcus* sp. shunt infection relapses or is found to be intractable with intravenous antibiotics, vancomycin is sometimes administered by intraventricular injection.

Intracranial abscesses

Intracranial abscesses occur within the brain parenchyma or in the epidural or subdural spaces. Brain abscesses have become less common in children in recent years as a result of the more aggressive treatment of acute otitis media, the decrease in occurrence of chronic mastoiditis, and the earlier correction of congenital cyanotic heart lesions. The widespread use of CT and MRI neuroimaging techniques have enhanced earlier diagnosis of cerebritis and abscess within the brain. Brain abscess is usually a single localized cerebral lesion that not uncommonly is multiloculated. Multiple abscesses are less common but are the rule when brain abscesses complicate meningitis caused by *C. koseri* in neonates or in early infancy.

The initiating event leading to brain abscess formation is a site of localized bacterial infection in brain parenchyma, called *cerebritis*. The affected area undergoes necrosis over 1–3 weeks in most cases, with the eventual formation of a localized purulent collection that provokes a surrounding fibrotic response referred to as a *capsule*. Once the encapsulated abscess has developed, the area becomes surrounded by a wide zone of edema readily seen in CT or MRI and which contributes to the mass effect of the infectious process. This evolution of the development of a brain abscess is now classified into stages: early cerebritis, late cerebritis, early capsule formation, and late capsule formation. Each stage has different MRI findings and, to some extent, different modes of therapy.

Numerous factors predispose to brain abscesses in children, as outlined in Table 13.6. In 10–20% of cases, no obvious predisposing cause can be identified. Currently, the most common predisposing causes in infants and children include bacterial sepsis, penetrating cranial injuries, chronic immunosuppression associated with disease, treatment of disease, and organ transplantation. Although less common than in past years, conditions with chronic oxygen desaturation, such as congenital cyanotic heart disease and pulmonary arteriovenous malformations, remain as contributing factors for the development of brain abscesses.

Brain abscesses can occur anywhere in the brain, including the brainstem, but most are found in the cerebral hemispheres. Their location is largely determined by the site of the primary, causative infection. Brain abscess complicating suppurative sinusitis is usually found in the frontal lobe, resulting from extension of bacteria via veins from the sinuses or cavernous sinus to the brain. Abscess secondary to otitis media or mastoiditis is commonly localized to the temporal lobe or the cerebellar hemisphere. Otogenic infection can also give rise to epidural empyema on the same side. With cyanotic heart disease, the favored location of brain abscess is at the cortical–white matter junction in the distribution of the middle cerebral artery. These conditions with chronic cyanosis and compensatory hyperviscosity give rise to areas of cerebral microinfarction, and the right-to-left shunting allows entrance of bacilli to the systemic circulation bypassing the normal filtering effect of the pulmonary circulation.

Table 13.6 Predisposing factors associated with brain abscesses in children

- Congenital cyanotic heart disease
- Suppurative sinusitis
- Chronic otitis media and mastoiditis
- Dental infections
- Penetrating cranial injury
- Immunocompromising conditions
- Large animal bites to the cranium
- Complication of acute pyogenic meningitis
- Pulmonary arteriovenous fistula

The symptoms and signs of a brain abscess in infants and children are quite variable and depend upon numerous factors including the size and the location of the lesion, the degree of intracranial hypertension, and the presence or absence of bacterial sepsis. A single, small abscess in the anterior frontal or posterior parietal lobe may be associated with few clinical signs except, perhaps, fever and headache. The classically described syndrome with symptoms and signs of increased intracranial pressure, localized neurologic signs such as seizures or hemiparesis, and signs of infection including fever and leukocytosis is diagnostically important when present but is found mainly when the disorder is in an advanced state. Headache is the most common symptom in older children, whereas hemiparesis can be expected if the abscess is located in the posterior frontal or anterior parietal region. Papilledema is found in only 25–50% of cases. Seizures are estimated to occur in 40–50% of cases with cerebral hemisphere brain abscesses. Seizures are of greatest localizing value when they are simple partial in type. Cerebellar brain abscesses tend to have a more uniform clinical presentation with ataxia, nystagmus, and features indicative of obstructive hydrocephalus with headache, vomiting, and lethargy. Children with pyogenic brain abscesses in any location generally have blood leukocytosis to some degree although fever is more variable.

Brain abscesses in neonates or in early infancy are infrequent complications of bacterial sepsis or meningitis. Most are caused by gram-negative bacilli including *Proteus* sp., *Salmonella* sp., or *C. koseri*. Usual clinical features include fever or temperature instability, poor feeding, vomiting, lethargy, seizures, and rapid enlargement of the head circumference. On occasion, an infant septic in the first week of life will seemingly remain well until 2–6 weeks of age when found to have abnormal head enlargement, usually with leukocytosis. Neuroimaging will show multiple brain abscess lesions provoked by gram-negative bacilli. *Citrobacter koseri* septic infection in the neonate has a strong predilection for invasion of the CNS, and up to 80% of infants with neonatal meningitis caused by this organism have been found to have periventricular brain abscesses. Although meningitis in these infants is septic-borne, the parenchymal abscesses are believed to be the result of ependymal necrosis with transmission of *Citrobacter* sp. bacilli directly from the ventricle into the adjacent brain tissue.

In older infants, children, and adolescents, the bacterial organisms that cause brain abscesses are legion and are determined to some extent by the primary source of the infection. With abscess resulting from penetrating head injuries, *S. aureus* is the most common offender. When septic-borne, or when brain abscess develops secondary to dental, sinus, or middle ear infection, they are often polymicrobial, sometimes with both aerobic and anaerobic organisms. In addition to many aerobic and anaerobic bacterial pathogens, brain abscess can be caused by a variety of other infectious agents. Tuberculous brain abscess and abscesses caused by *Toxoplasma gondii* have become lesions seen in patients with AIDS. Multiple cerebral microabscesses sometimes complicate systemic *Candida* sp. infections in sick premature infants. Fungal brain abscess, including those induced by *Histoplasma capsulatum* and *Blastomyces dermatitidis*, are seen primarily in immunosuppressed patients. Chronically ill and immunosuppressed persons are also susceptible to brain abscesses caused by *Nocardia* sp., a gram-positive bacterium susceptible to sulfa antibiotics. *Aspergillus* sp. brain lesions in immunocompromised persons are more often in the form of hemorrhagic granulomas rather than abscess.

When brain abscess is suspected in any age group, lumbar puncture for CSF examination is assumed to be contraindicated because of the danger of provoking internal herniation. Neuroimaging with CT, MRI, or both, and performed both without and with contrast enhancement, is highly accurate for the identification and localization of intracranial abscesses. MRI is superior for brainstem and cerebellar lesions and generally provides more information regardless of the location of the lesion. The findings on MRI vary depending on whether the process is in the early cerebritis stage or in the more advanced encapsulated stage. In the stage of cerebritis, T1 weighted MRI usually shows an area of hypointensity which, with contrast enhancement, reveals a bright signal either heterogeneously or diffusely. When the abscess is encapsulated, the T1 MRI with enhancement demonstrates a hypointense central area surrounded by a hyperintense capsule that has a smooth contour and that is thinner on the medial, ventricular margin than elsewhere. The area of surrounding edema remains hypointense on the enhanced T1 image.

Treatment of a brain abscess in most cases consists of a combination of intravenous antibiotics, methods to control intracranial hypertension, and surgical drainage of the abscess. Certain select cases can be managed with antibiotic therapy alone when the lesion is believed to be in the cerebritis stage or if the abscess is relatively small and without a significant degree of mass effect upon the ventricular system. Conservative treatment is also sometimes chosen in a child with uncorrectable coagulation abnormalities. The value of dexamethasone as a method to control intracranial hypertension with a brain abscess is controversial. If clinical evidence plus neuroimage findings indicate that intracranial hypertension is marginal, corticosteroids should be avoided. If pressure signs are marked, the benefits of dexamethasone in dosage of 0.6 mg/kg/day (up to 40 kg body weight) probably outweigh the disadvantages. Intravenous mannitol in periodic doses of 0.5 g/kg given over 15–20 minutes can also be considered if there are signs of impending herniation.

Various antibiotic regimens have been recommended before the causative organism is recovered. One regimen often selected pending surgery is a combination of vancomycin, ceftriaxone, and metronidazole. Once the causative organism is found, the antibiotic regimen is altered accordingly. The goal of surgical therapy is to remove the purulent exudate to the extent possible and to prevent the major, life-threatening complications of a brain abscess such as internal herniation and spontaneous perforation of the abscess into the adjacent lateral ventricle, which can precipitate fulminating meningitis (Table 13.7).

Osteoplastic craniotomy under general anesthesia for total excision of a brain abscess has become less popular in recent years. CT-guided aspiration via a burr hole has become the more common surgical approach and is believed to be equally effective when compared to total excision. When multiple abscesses of variable size are found, some will elect to aspirate the larger lesions, thus providing decompression and also yielding a specimen for culture. The remaining smaller lesions hopefully will respond to antibiotic therapy.

Epidural and subdural abscesses are managed in a similar fashion. These lesions also have multiple possible causes in children including sinusitis, middle ear and mastoid infections, and postmeningitic and postsurgical complications. Subdural empyema usually presents with impressive symptoms including those of infection and those of cortical irritation. Headache, lethargy, fever, seizures, and focal neurologic deficits are commonly described in persons with subdural empyema. Intracranial epidural abscess is usually less dramatic in regard to clinical findings although this is variable depending on its size

Table 13.7 Dangers of brain abscess

- Internal herniation
- Spontaneous perforation into ventricle
- Complication of sepsis, when present
- Complication of prolonged antibiotic therapy

and the virulence of the causative pathogen. Nontraumatic subdural abscess has a close association with suppurative sinusitis and most occur in the frontal region in adolescents or young adults. MRI is the preferred diagnostic image to identify these lesions.

Viral infections of the central nervous system

Herpes virus infections

Neonatal herpes simplex virus infection

Although intrauterine transmission of herpes simplex virus (HSV) can occur, 85–90% of neonatal HSV disease occurs following viral transmission during labor and delivery. Postnatal transmission from infectious contacts during the first 3–4 weeks of life can also result in severe infant disease and appears to account for the remainder of perinatal cases. HSV-2 is the cause of approximately 75% of HSV disease during the first month of life. The risk of maternal–infant transmission of HSV ranges from 30% to 50% for infants of mothers with primary genital infection at the time of delivery. Transmission rates are less than 5% for the infants of immune mothers with recurrent symptomatic virus shedding at delivery. Approximately 50% of mothers of infants with HSV disease have not experienced recognizable genital HSV disease. Premature birth (<37 weeks gestation) is overrepresented among children with neonatal HSV infection, occurring in about 35% of cases.

There are three syndromes of neonatal HSV infection: (a) skin–eye–mouth involvement only (SEM), (b) CNS disease without disseminated infection, and (c) disseminated infection with or without CNS disease. In multicenter clinical trials, the three syndromes are approximately equally represented. Most infants with neonatally acquired HSV infection develop clinical illness between 3 and 21 days of age. Children with isolated CNS disease have a mean age of onset approximately 4 days later than children with disseminated infection or SEM infection. The age of onset of postneonatal HSV encephalitis overlaps temporally with CNS disease acquired at or near the time of delivery. Thus, infants with postneonatal HSV encephalitis can have disease onset between 4 and 8 weeks of age. The neonatal HSV disseminated multiorgan system syndrome rarely occurs beyond 3 weeks of age. Central nervous system infection occurs in about 50% of neonatal HSV cases. Of children who initially appear to have disease limited to SEM, between 15% and 20% will develop CNS involvement. Between 50% and 70% of children with the disseminated HSV disease have CNS infection. Central nervous system invasion may occur by viremic spread in children with multiorgan system infection or by neural spread in infants with isolated CNS disease. Central nervous system disease may be manifest clinically as lethargy, progressive obtundation, seizures, or focal neurologic deficits including hemiparesis or quadriparesis. Alternatively, infants with destructive disease detected by CNS imaging may occasionally demonstrate only minor clinical signs of CNS dysfunction (Table 13.8).

Table 13.8 Herpes simplex encephalitis

Perinatal herpes simplex virus (HSV) infection
- Most children become symptomatic between 3 and 28 days of age.
- CNS involvement in up to 70% of cases overall
  - Skin, eye, mouth: 33%
  - Disseminated: 33%
  - Isolated CNS: 33%
- Identification of HSV infection by culture or polymerase chain reaction (PCR) testing of specimens from eye, respiratory tract, skin lesions, rectum, urine, blood
- Diagnosis of central nervous system (CNS) involvement by HSV PCR on cerebrospinal fluid (CSF) and CNS imaging
- Treatment: acyclovir: 60 mg/kg/day divided every 8 hours for 3 weeks

Herpes simplex virus encephalitis beyond the perinatal period
- Accounts for approximately 25% of sporadic viral encephalitis
- HSV PCR testing on CSF is diagnositic method of choice
- Fronto-temporal involvement (unilateral or bilateral) by CNS imaging
- Treatment: acyclovir 45–60 mg/kg/day divided every 8 hours for 2–3 weeks

Rapid clinical recognition of neonatal HSV has remained elusive. In clinical trials, the diagnosis of HSV infection has been delayed beyond 5 days of the onset of clinical disease in about 40% of patients. All skin vesicles and mucosal ulcers observed during the first month of life should be studied for HSV. Fever or temperature instability occurs in most infants with disseminated or CNS disease, although fever is present as a first manifestation in just over 50% of cases. Regardless, when fever occurs during the first month of life, HSV disease must be entertained. Pneumonia, hepatitis, and disseminated intravascular coagulation (DIC) are prominent components of the disseminated disease syndrome. Any ill infant with seizures, obtundation, or focal neurologic findings should prompt evaluation for HSV infection. Diagnosis is established using virologic and molecular (polymerase chain reaction [PCR]) techniques. Viral cultures should be obtained of any skin vesicles or mucosal ulcers. In addition, cultures of the oropharynx, conjunctivae, stool, and CSF (approximately 20% positive with CNS disease) should be performed. Polymerase chain reaction on CSF is approximately 95% sensitive for detecting CNS infection. Polymerase chain reaction is also applicable to vesicle or throat swab specimens and to plasma in disseminated disease. Intravenous acyclovir (60 mg/kg/day) divided every 8 hours is the treatment of choice. The potential for benefit is maximum when therapy is initiated as early in the course of clinical disease as possible. For children with CNS infection, treatment should be given for 21 days, and the HSV PCR test on CSF should have been shown to have converted to negative by repeat testing during the third week of treatment. In recent clinical trials, death has continued to occur in close to 50% of acyclovir-treated infants with disseminated disease. In treated children with CNS disease only, mortality is 15% or less with antiviral therapy; however, moderate to severe neurodevelopmental impairment occurs in about 45% of these children. Concern continues regarding recrudescent CNS disease following neonatal antiviral treatment. Recurrences of skin lesions are characteristic of many infants surviving neonatal HSV. Whether CNS reactivation may be occurring together with or apart from skin exacerbations has not been defined. Oral acyclovir effectively suppresses skin recurrences in most infants. Its role in controlling hypothesized subclinical CNS reactivation is the subject of ongoing study.

Herpes simplex virus encephalitis and meningitis in children and adults

HSV is the single most common cause of sporadic, endemic encephalitis in adults and children. HSV is implicated in about 10% of the 20,000 cases of encephalitis that occur annually in the United States, and represents 25% of cases for which an etiology can be defined. HSV-1 accounts for more than 90% of cases of HSV encephalitis (HSE) beyond the first month of life. In adults, HSE is predominantly the result of reactivation of latent infection in cranial sensory ganglia. In children, HSE can occur during primary HSV infection or as a consequence of viral reactivation. At younger ages, the likelihood that HSE is occurring in association with primary HSV infection is increased. Primary HSV infection with associated encephalitis may or may not include other evidence of overt HSV disease (skin vesicles, conjunctivitis, pharyngitis, gingivostomatitis). Primary genital HSV-2 infection can be associated with HSV aseptic meningitis, and this syndrome may recur. HSV-2 is probably the predominant cause of recurrent, benign, aseptic, "Mollaret" meningitis. Patients with encephalitis (including brainstem encephalitis) associated with HSV-2 have been described, but are uncommon. In typical adult HSE, disease onset is usually subacute with signs and symptoms of CNS dysfunction emerging and progressing over a 2- to 4-day period. However, rapid progression to coma can occur. Dysphasia is a common early manifestation before progressive obtundation has become predominant. Most patients are febrile. Seizures often occur during the first 4 days of disease. Focal motor abnormalities are also observed early in the illness. Characteristic CT abnormalities of inflammation and hemorrhagic necrosis predominantly localized to the infero-medial fronto-temporal region are observable about 4 days into the illness. MRI is usually informative earlier. Electroencephalograph (EEG) abnormalities are highly prevalent in HSE and generally provide evidence of localization of pathology to the fronto-temporal distribution. The EEG pattern of periodic lateralizing epileptiform discharges (PLEDs) is characteristically associated with HSE. However, other conditions also cause the abnormality and PLEDs occur in only about 60% of HSE cases. Diagnosis of HSE is usually established using CSF PCR. The sensitivity and specificity of the test is over 95%, when performed by evperienced personnel. Occasionally, first CSF specimens may be PCR-negative in HSE. In these circumstances, inflammatory cell counts and protein concentrations are usually normal or near normal. Repeat PCR in 3–4 days has usually provided informative results in true HSE cases; and CSF indices are usually abnormal by the second CSF examination. Children and adults of all ages with acute onset of encephalopathy should be investigated for infectious and inflammatory causes unless an alternative diagnosis is rapidly established. After CNS imaging, samples of CSF should be obtained for bacterial, viral, mycobacterial, and fungal culture. Cerebrospinal fluid should be submitted for HSV and enteroviral PCR, and CSF should be stored frozen for subsequent microbiological, molecular, serological, or biochemical testing. Treatment for possible HSV encephalitis should be instituted with acyclovir, 45 mg/kg/day divided every 8 hours. The standard duration of therapy is 2 weeks in adults as opposed to 3 weeks in neonates, as stated earlier. Demonstration of negative CSF PCR results before terminating antiviral therapy is recommended (Table 13.8).

Cytomegalovirus

Before the advent of HIV-associated immunodeficiency, cytomegalovirus encephalitis was essentially restricted to infants with congenital cytomegalovirus (CMV) infection. Approximately 1% of infants are infected with CMV in utero, as demonstrated by culturing urine on the first day of life. Most infants with in utero CMV infection are the offspring of seropositive mothers who experienced either reactivation of latent CMV during pregnancy or occasionally acquisition of infections with new CMV strains during pregnancy. Regardless, most of these infants are clinically well at birth. The most important clinical and neurologic manifestation of these infections is sensorineural hearing loss, which can be established at birth or which may develop progressively during the first year of life. Infants of nonimmune mothers who acquire primary CMV infection during pregnancy are at risk for developing overt congenital cytomegalovirus inclusion disease (CID) in utero. These infants manifest disease at birth. The principal components of the CID syndrome include intrauterine growth failure, CNS disease (microcephaly, periventricular leukomalacia, periventricular calcifications, cerebral cysts, sensorineural deafness), chorioretinitis, hepatitis, leukopenia, and thrombocytopenia. The neurodevelopmental prognosis for children with CMV-associated microcephaly is typically bleak. Sensorineural hearing loss, although frequently established at birth, can progress during the first year of life. A recent clinical trial of ganciclovir therapy of infants with symptomatic CID with CNS involvement demonstrated a beneficial effect of antiviral treatment on hearing loss progression. The congenital CID syndrome is usually readily recognized clinically. Substantiation of the virologic etiology can be obtained by viral culture of urine, stool, respiratory tract secretions, or CSF. PCR for CMV DNA is positive in blood and CSF in children with overt CNS disease. The CMV IgM antibody test has a sensitivity of only 60% and should not be relied upon solely for diagnosis of disease. Proof of congenital infection requires isolation of the virus from urine, stool, respiratory tract secretions, or CSF obtained within 3 weeks of birth. Differentiating between intrauterine and peri-/postnatal infection is difficult later in infancy. Risk factors for primary CMV infection during pregnancy include young maternal age and exposure to day care–attending children excreting CMV. Postneonatal CMV encephalitis occurs only in patients with marked immunodeficiency, most often related to HIV infection. CMV can be a cofactor in HIV encephalopathy.

Human herpes virus 6

Human herpes virus 6 (HHV6) is the predominant cause of roseola infantum, an acute febrile exanthematous disease of infants and toddlers. The roseola rash occurs in no more than 20% of children with primary HHV6 infection; the remainder of infections are usually discovered among children with acute febrile illnesses. Typically, the fever is high-grade and abrupt in onset. Given the occurrence of this highly febrile infection in infants and toddlers, it is not surprising that HHV6 infection is associated with febrile seizures, which occur in approximately 20% of infected, febrile children. When PCR for HHV6 has been performed on CSF specimens of children with HHV6 infection, fever, and seizures, the CSF PCR for HHV6 has been positive in about 40% of cases. It remains unclear whether direct viral invasion of the CNS contributes to the pathogenesis of seizures during HHV6 infection. Evidence for more extensive CNS disease during HHV6 infection is rare in immunocompetent children or adults. In contrast, HHV6 meningoencephalitis has been repeatedly observed in bone marrow transplant recipients, and occasionally in solid organ transplant patients and persons with HIV immunodeficiency (including children). Congenital HHV6 infection has also been identified in neonates with seizures.

Arbovirus encephalitis

Three Flaviviruses (West Nile virus, Saint Louis encephalitis virus, and Powassan virus), three Togaviruses (α virus group: Eastern equine, Western equine, Venezuelan equine), and three Bunyaviruses (LaCrosse, Jamestown Canyon, and Snowshoe Hare) cause encephalitis in residents of North America. For travelers, European and Asian tick-borne encephalitis and Japanese encephalitis (Flaviviruses) are potential concerns. Until the arrival of West Nile virus in North America in 1999, Saint Louis encephalitis and LaCrosse virus accounted for most cases of vector-borne encephalitis in the United States. West Nile virus has spread rapidly and progressively across the United States since 1999. Globally, Japanese encephalitis virus far surpasses all other agents as causes of infection and disease.

LaCrosse virus

LaCrosse virus, a member of the California virus serogroup, has been recognized as an endemic cause of childhood encephalitis in the United States since its identification in 1965. The CDC recorded 2,776 laboratory-confirmed cases between 1966 and 2000, an average of 75 cases per year. Ninety percent of cases were identified in seven states: Ohio, Wisconsin, West Virginia, Minnesota, Illinois, Indiana, and Iowa. Smaller numbers of cases were documented along the Appalachian mountain range from New York to Georgia. Illness occurs predominantly between June and October, with a broad peak in incidence during July through September. The virus is sustained in the treehole mosquito (*Aedes triseriatus*) population by transovarial transmission. Children 3–15 years of age are affected predominantly, with an excess of illness among males. Illness severity ranges from headache and nausea (with classification as aseptic meningitis) to disorientation, seizures (40–60%), focal neurologic deficits (15–25%), obtundation, and cerebral edema (15%). Approximately 50% of patients will need to be placed in an intensive care unit for an average of 3–4 days, but the death-to-case ratio is less than 5%. After initial recovery from the more severe phase of illness, approximately 15% of children have demonstrable neurologic deficits. Among children more severely affected during acute illness, long-lasting neurodevelopmental dysfunction may occur in up to 30%. The CSF white cell count ranges from normal to 500 cells, with a median of approximately 75 cells/mm^3 and 60% mononuclear. Cerebrospinal fluid protein is rarely elevated substantially and glucose is normal. The peripheral white count can be slightly elevated to between 15,000 and 20,000 cells/mm^3 with a PMN fraction of 65–85%. Periodic lateralizing epileptiform discharges (PLEDs) have been observed in up to 15% of patients. CT scanning is rarely revealing except in patients with diffuse brain edema. MRI findings have not been reported from a large case series, but cortical lesions, including fronto-temporal abnormalities similar to those characteristic of HSE (Table 13.7) have been described in several case reports. Culture of CSF for LaCrosse virus is rarely positive, although brain biopsy tissue can yield the etiologic agent. Serologic testing provides confirmation of the specific diagnosis. Serum LaCrosse virus specific IgM is diagnostic during acute illness. Cerebrospinal fluid IgM can also be of diagnostic value. If an initial sample is IgM negative, IgM seroconversion can be demonstrated within 1 week. Testing of paired sera (acute illness with convalescent serum 3–4 weeks later) for changes in concentrations of IgG antibody identifies the remainder of proven cases with negative IgM responses. PCR testing of CSF is also available.

Eastern equine encephalitis

Eastern equine encephalitis (EEE) is endemic in the coastal states from the Gulf Coast to New England. Mosquitoes prevalent in swamplands harbor the virus, which is maintained in a mosquito to bird to mosquito cycle. The infected vectors attack man infrequently; thus, human cases are uncommon. Approximately 5–15 sporadic cases are confirmed annually, with occasional small outbreaks. Persons of all ages are susceptible to the encephalitic manifestation. Eastern equine encephalitis is typically a severe illness, with a death-to-case ratio that averages 35%. Moderate to severe residual neurologic impairment occurs in about 35% of survivors. The illness begins as a flu-like syndrome with fever and malaise. Central nervous system involvement is usually manifest between the second and fifth days of illness with headache, stiff neck, confusion, somnolence, focal neurologic findings, or seizures. There is rapid progression to coma in most patients (90%), typically within 2–3 days of the appearance of CNS disease. Seizures occur in 50% of cases, focal weakness in 40%, and cranial nerve palsies in 25%. Deaths usually occur during the second or third week of coma. Among survivors with mild to moderate sequelae, the median duration of coma is 5 days. Cerebrospinal fluid examination reveals a median leukocytosis of 370 cells/mm^3 with 70% neutrophils at first examination. Median CSF protein is 97 mg/dL and glucose is normal. Electroencephalographs show diffuse slowing with disorganization of background activity. MRI reveals multifocal brain injury most apparent on T2-weighted images and usually present within 3 days of the onset of neurologic findings. Lesions are concentrated in the basal ganglia and thalami, but abnormalities can also be observed in the brainstem, cortex, and periventricular regions. Diagnosis is serologic, with the IgM capture antibody test useful for diagnosis during the acute illness and paired acute/convalescent serologies demonstrating changes in concentrations of virus-specific IgG antibody.

West Nile virus

West Nile virus, a flavivirus, is a member of Japanese encephalitis serogroup that includes Japanese, Saint Louis, Murray Valley, and Kunjin encephalitis viruses. The virus is maintained in nature in a cycle involving *Culex* sp. mosquitoes and birds and is transmitted to man by mosquitoes. Since there is an early viremic phase of infection, disease has also been transmitted by blood transfusion, organ donation, and from mother to fetus in utero. West Nile virus was first introduced into the northeastern United States in 1999, when symptomatic human infections were recognized simultaneously with unusually high rates of death among crows. Seroepidemiologic research has consistently demonstrated that meningoencephalitis is manifest in approximately 1 in 100–150 infected persons and that approximately 1 in 5 infected persons develops a febrile flu-like (fever, malaise, achiness) illness without CNS disease. Since its introduction, the virus has spread progressively across the country, with increasing numbers of cases annually. In 2003, over 8,900 symptomatic West Nile virus infections were documented and registered with 45 different state health departments and the CDC. Meningoencephalitis accounted for 30% of laboratory-confirmed infections, while West Nile fever was diagnosed in most of the remainder. Two-hundred five deaths occurred, presumably concentrated among those with encephalitis, yielding an encephalitis death-to-case ratio near 10% (range 5–15%, increasing with age). In 2003, the largest numbers of infections were identified in the Plains states and states on the eastern slope of the Rocky Mountains. However, disease continued to occur with substantial frequency in the upper Midwest into the mid-Atlantic states. A broad incidence peak occurs between mid-July through late September; however, illness has been encountered as late as December. The incubation period ranges from 4 to 16 days. West Nile fever is a summer flu-like syndrome with headache, malaise, myalgia, arthralgia, and occasionally macular rash lasting 3–6 days. Central nervous system disease usually emerges between days 2 and 5 of fever. The aseptic meningitis-to-encephalitis ratio is approximately 1:2 among those with CNS involvement. Being over 50 years old is the major risk factor for development of encephalitis. Persons 50–60 years old are 10 times more likely to experience CNS disease than younger persons, while those over 80 years of age are 40 times more likely to manifest encephalitis. Although West Nile infections are equally common in children and adults, children under 16 years old probably account for no more than 5% of encephalitis cases. Although disordered cerebration is common, coma develops in only 15% of cases. Seizures are also relatively uncommon. Development of localized, marked, polio-like muscle weakness occurs in approximately 50% of West Nile encephalitis cases. Weakness or paralysis usually involves the extremities rather than cranial nerves. Pathologic findings occur in the brain, brainstem, and spinal cord. MR imaging demonstrates abnormalities in patients with the most severe clinical illness, possibly up to one-third of encephalitis patients. Involvement of the basal ganglia, thalami, and substantia nigra has been prominent in reported cases. The findings are similar to those observed in Japanese encephalitis virus disease. Polymerase chain reaction on blood or spinal fluid has a sensitivity between 30% and 50%. Therefore, diagnosis is usually established with IgM capture antibody testing on spinal fluid or serum. The IgM test is positive within the first 4 days of illness in approximately 75% of cases and in more than 90% of cases by the eighth day of disease. The IgM and IgG enzyme-linked immunosorbent assay (ELISA) tests cross-react among the flaviviruses. The plaque-reduction neutralization test is virus specific.

Saint Louis encephalitis

Prior to the advent of West Nile virus infection, St. Louis encephalitis virus had caused the largest outbreaks of arboviral disease in the United States. Over 4,000 cases were recorded between 1966 and 2000, but close to 2,000 of these cases occurred in 1975. Fewer than 20 cases were documented annually between 1991 and 2000. Disease has been concentrated in the Ohio River valley, south central states, Florida, Texas and California. St. Louis encephalitis is maintained in nature in *Culex* mosquitoes and small birds, particularly sparrows. The clinical expression of St. Louis encephalitis has many similarities to West Nile virus infection. In St. Louis encephalitis, encephalitis occurs in approximately one in 300 infected persons, and the risk of encephalitis increases progressively with age. However, among persons with proven symptomatic infection encephalitis is manifested by over 50% in all age groups. Marked muscle weakness is not nearly as common in St. Louis encephalitis cases as in West Nile disease. Pathologic changes are concentrated in the brainstem, midbrain, and thalamus, as in West Nile virus and Japanese encephalitis. Cerebrospinal fluid findings are characteristic of viral meningoencephalitis with leukocyte counts ranging from 10 to 200 cells/mm3 with progressive predominance as disease progresses. Cerebrospinal fluid protein is rarely over 200 mg/dL and glucose is routinely normal. The death-to-case ratio ranges from 8% to 20% and is strongly and directly age related. Diagnosis is by IgM capture ELISA using CSF or serum, and specific species confirmation with virus-specific neutralization tests.

Paramyxoviruses

The paramyxoviruses include agents with substantial neurotropism. These include rubeola (measles), mumps, and a recently identified zoonotic infection of Southeast Asia caused by the Nipah virus.

Measles

Control of measles by immunization with live-attenuated measles virus vaccine has almost eliminated wild-type measles and measles-virus CNS disease from the United States. When wild-type virus was endemic, viral and postviral meningoencephalitis occurred in 1:1000 measles cases with a death-to-case ratio of 10–30% and long-lasting neurodevelopmental sequelae in approximately 30% of survivors. Prior to effective immunization, measles was the most important cause of acquired mental retardation in the United States. Since virus cultures of CSF in measles encephalitis were rarely positive, there has been debate regarding the importance of viral invasion of the CNS in disease pathogenesis. However, molecular techniques (PCR) that might have more readily demonstrated direct viral CNS invasion were not available when disease was prevalent. The capacity of measles virus to invade the CNS is proven in subacute sclerosing panencephalitis (SSPE). It is also possible that measles is tropic for endothelium of CNS vessels and that this is of importance in disease expression. Regardless of the extent of direct viral invasion of the CNS during acute measles, immunologic mechanisms almost certainly have a prominent role in the pathogenesis of measles encephalomyelitis. The measles encephalitis syndrome usually emerges during the period of exanthem and within 8 days of illness onset. Seizures occur in over 50% of cases and coma in close to one-third. Long-lasting sequelae include recurrent seizures, paresis, and cognitive impairment. Measles is diagnosed by isolation of the virus from respiratory secretions or by antibody testing.

Subacute sclerosing panencephalitis is a persistent measles virus infection of the CNS caused by a defective, mutated measles virus that lacks the M protein believed to be necessary to bring about release of the virus from its intracellular location, thus giving rise to progressive degenerative neuronal pathology. The disease occurs in approximately 1 in 100,000 measles cases, and the incubation period is approximately 5–7 years. Measles during infancy carries a higher risk for SSPE. The clinical expression of SSPE includes insidious-onset progressive mental deterioration with behavioral changes, motor incoordination, myoclonic jerks, and speech impairment. The illness progresses relentlessly over 6–9 months to dementia, stupor, and decorticate rigidity. Measles-specific antibody titers are extremely high in serum and CSF.

Mumps

Mumps was the single most common cause of viral meningoencephalitis in children in the United States until the development of effective immunization. Aseptic meningitis and mild meningoencephalitis are the most frequent complications of mumps in healthy children occurring approximately 5 days into the mumps syndrome. Fever, headache, vomiting, lethargy, and nuchal rigidity are the most common manifestations of CNS involvement in mumps. Seizures occur in approximately 15% of cases, and disease progresses to delirium in no more than 5–8%. Death during the acute encephalitic phase is rare, but can occur. Recovery is usually complete. It is possible that acquired aqueductal stenosis may follow mumps virus infection. The CSF shows typical findings of aseptic meningitis with mononuclear pleocytosis of approximately 250 cells/mm^3, with mild elevation in protein and normal glucose. Specific diagnosis is by isolation of mumps virus from respiratory secretions; the virus is also isolated from CSF inpatients with meningoencephalitis. Testing of acute and convalescent sera for mumps antibody provides serologic confirmation of illness etiology.

JC virus

Progressive multifocal leukoencephalopathy (PML) is a chronic CNS papovavirus infection that occurs exclusively among persons with severely impaired immune function including genetically determined immunodeficiencies, organ transplantation, lymphoproliferative malignancies, and HIV infection. Exposure to JC virus is common. By young adulthood, close to 90% of healthy persons have serologic evidence of prior infection. Progressive multifocal leukoencephalopathy is probably the result of reactivation of latent JC virus infection in CNS microglial cells in the setting of profound immune compromise. Plaques of demyelination show infected microglia at their peripheral advancing edge. The clinical syndrome is one of the insidious onset of weakness, cognitive impairment, and speech dysfunction in most individuals. Patients may also present with ataxia or symptoms suggestive of mass lesions. Central nervous system JC virus infection does not cause fever. The CSF examination may show slightly increased protein concentration but otherwise is unremarkable. CT and MRI studies demonstrate nonenhancing lesions. The disease progresses relentlessly to coma over 6–9 months in many instances. However, the course of illness may extend over a substantially longer period in persons with less severe immunodeficiency. Diagnosis is by CSF PCR, with a sensitivity close to 90%. Progressive multifocal leukoencephalopathy can coexist with other brain diseases in severely immunosuppressed patients. Thus, there remains a role for brain biopsy in defining the causes of brain lesions in such patients. Successful control of HIV infection with antiviral drugs can halt PML progression. Reducing immunosuppression in organ transplant recipients may halt PML progression but does not reverse established disease.

Enteroviral infections

The enteroviruses include the polioviruses, Coxsackie viruses, and echoviruses, and more recently identified serotypes numbered sequentially including enteroviruses 68 through 72. All enteroviruses exhibit neurotropism to variable degrees. Enterovirus CNS disease encompasses the range from aseptic meningitis to encephalitis to flaccid paralysis. Most cases of aseptic meningitis occurring in summer months in temperate climates are attributed to non-polio enteroviral disease.

Enterovirus 71

Enterovirus 71 (EV 71) was first isolated from a child with aseptic meningitis in 1969. The virus appears to circulate endemically in many populations, as the prevalence of seropositivity among adults can be as high as 60%. Small clusters of severe CNS disease were recognized sporadically after the virus was first isolated. Major outbreaks of infection with high rates of severe CNS disease, frequently accompanied by fatal pulmonary edema, have occurred in central Europe in the 1970s and in Australia and Southeast Asia in the 1990s. The virus causes the hand-foot-mouth disease (HFMD) syndrome in approximately 25% of infected persons, and the occurrence of this syndrome permits recognition of major outbreaks. In the 1998 outbreak in Taiwan, over 125,000 cases of HFMD were documented over a 9-month period of time. Although many enteroviruses can cause HFMD, EV 71 was responsible for approximately 60% of cases during the 1998 Taiwan outbreak. Within the outbreak, over 400 cases of severe disease were encountered; EV 71 was implicated in 80%. Severe disease occurred most often in children less than 5 years, who accounted for 90% of mortality. The highest death-to-case ratio occurred in children 6–12 months of age. Encephalitis occurred in 75% of severe EV 71 cases, and was associated with pulmonary edema (considered probably neurogenic) in close to one-half of encephalitis patients. Pulmonary edema also occurred in absence of clinical encephalitis. Aseptic meningitis occurred in five of 78 patients and acute flaccid paralysis in only one instance.

Severe neonatal enterovirus infection

Life-threatening perinatal enterovirus infections due to Coxsackie and echoviruses may develop during the first 2 weeks of life. In most instances, infection is acquired by viremic spread from the mother who has developed infection during the last days before delivery. Infection can also be transmitted to the infant as a result of contact with infectious maternal body fluids at the time of delivery. Nursery outbreaks with infant–infant and infant–staff–infant transmission have occurred on multiple occasions. Severe neonatal disease is not restricted to maternal–infant viremic transmission cases. A multisystem infection occurs in the neonate with meningoencephalitis, myocarditis, hepatitis, and a multiorgan failure sepsis-like syndrome. The Coxsackie B viruses are most often implicated in the meningoencephalitis/myocarditis presentation. Fulminant hepatic necrosis dominates the clinical expression of the most severe cases of neonatal echovirus 11 infection. Overall, aseptic meningitis or meningoencephalitis occurs in about 50% of perinatal enterovirus infections. Survival usually depends on the severity of myocarditis, hepatitis, or the associated sepsis-like syndrome.

Polioviruses

The polioviruses include three serotypes, all with neurotropic potential. Paralytic poliomyelitis occurs in approximately 1–2% of persons with primary wild-type poliovirus infection, whereas aseptic meningitis without paralytic involvement occurs in a similar percentage. Over 90% of infected persons are asymptomatic. Central nervous system disease can occur at any age, but the risk of CNS manifestations increases with age. The hallmark of poliovirus pathogenesis is tropism for anterior horn cells of the spinal cord and brainstem with consequent flaccid paralysis of innervated muscle groups. When infection was highly endemic, most adults were immune and paralytic disease occurred most frequently in infants and young children. With improved sanitation and reduced transmission of infection during childhood, an increasing fraction of older children and adults were nonimmune and susceptible to infection and paralytic disease. Tonsillectomy during asymptomatic infection increases the risk of bulbar disease. Pregnant women are at increased risk of severe infection. Intramuscular injections of diptheria-tetanus-pertussis (DTP) vaccine increase the risk of paralysis in the injected extremity. Infection can be transmitted to the infant in utero throughout pregnancy. When maternal disease occurs during the several days before delivery, the infant typically develops poliomyelitis between days three and ten of life. In postneonatal polio, symptoms of CNS disease that may or may not progress to paralysis include signs of aseptic meningitis together with diffuse muscle spasm that may be emphasized in the paraspinous muscles and hamstrings. Changes in superficial and deep tendon reflexes (loss of cutaneous reflexes followed by accentuation then loss of deep tendon reflexes) herald the emergence of paralysis. Marked paralysis may develop over a very short time interval or be spread over several days. Typically, motor involvement is asymmetrical. With involvement of the intercostal muscles, diaphragm, and pharyngeal musculature, respiratory insufficiency is common. Prevention is with inactivated trivalent polio vaccine. Vaccination has been very successful in eradicating polio in the United States, with the last case of indigenous polio diagnosed in 1979. However, global outbreaks still occur and vaccination strategies for eradication by the World Health Organization (WHO) and its partners are underway.

Fungal infections of the central nervous system

Fungi that cause human disease occur as yeast forms such as *Candida* sp. and *Cryptococcus neoformans*, and filamentous or mycelial forms as is true of *Aspergillus* sp. and the *Phycomycetes*. Dimorphic fungi exist in the mycelial phase in nature but revert to yeasts or spherules in tissue. Among the dimorphic fungi are *Histoplasma capsulatum*, *Blastomyces dermatitides*, and *Coccidioides immitis*. With the exception of *Candida* sp. infections, which are a common problem in sick, low-birth-weight neonates, serious invasive fungal infections are not common among otherwise normal children. Those predisposed to invasive fungal infections usually are immunosuppressed, especially children following bone marrow transplantation and with hematologic malignancy. Chronic granulomatous disease predisposes to infection with catalase-positive bacteria and fungi. Patients with AIDS are at risk of developing *C. neoformans* meningitis, an opportunistic infection much more often seen in adults than in children. Regardless of the underlying immunocompromising condition, neutropenia, use of corticosteroids, and persistent antibiotic therapy increases the risk of invasive fungal infections.

Candida sp. and *Aspergillus* sp. account for the majority of serious fungal infections in children. Other fungal species are less common and include those caused by members of the genus *Phycomycetes*, which cause the disease known as mucormycosis.

The type of tissue pathology in the CNS will vary with different fungal organisms. *Aspergillus* sp. and the *Phycomycetes* have a strong predisposition to invade vascular structures, leading either to hemorrhagic granulomas or ischemic infarctions. *Candida* sp. classically cause cerebral microabscesses, whereas *Cryptococcus* and *Coccidioides immitis* result in chronic granulomatous meningoencephalitis when CNS invasion occurs.

Aspergillus sp. rank second only to *Candida* as causes of fungal disease in immunosuppressed patients. The primary infection is acquired by respiratory inhalation, with dissemination to various organs, including the brain. Neurologic infection with *Aspergillus* is mainly in the form of multiple granulomas with surrounding edema. The lesions are frequently hemorrhagic and can be solitary or multiple. Central nervous system aspergillus is difficult to eradicate with amphotericin B, with or without intraconazole, and has a high mortality rate.

Histoplasmosis has its highest incidence in the Mississippi and Ohio valley regions and is usually asymptomatic or manifests with flu-like respiratory infection, with eventual spontaneous resolution, but often leaving multiple punctate calcific lesions in the lungs. Although benign fungal dissemination is common in infected, immunocompetent persons, symptomatic disseminated histoplasmosis is seen largely in persons with AIDS or other immunocompromising disease. Neurologic histoplasmosis is usually associated with a chronic granulomatous meningitis.

Blastomyces dermatitides is widespread in nature, with primary infection occurring in the lungs. It is now known that symptomatic blastomycotic pneumonia can either progress to chronic pulmonary disease or can resolve spontaneously. When dissemination occurs from the lungs, spread is usually to skin or to skeletal structures. Neurologic infection can result from direct epidural extension from adjacent skull or vertebral osteomyelitis. Blood-borne spread can also bring about a chronic granulomatous basilar meningitis.

Coccidioidomycosis is endemic in the southwestern part of this country and has its highest incidence in the San Joaquin Valley in California. *Coccidioides immitis* is a normal inhabitant in dry soil and is acquired by transmission in dust. Respiratory inhalation of the fungus is associated with asymptomatic infection in 60%. Most of the remainder of cases are in the form of a transient respiratory illness and less often as chronic pulmonary disease. In less than 1% of pulmonary infections, the disease is disseminated to skin, bone, ocular structures, or to the meninges, where it produces a chronic, indulent granulomatous meningoencephalitis. The CSF with meningeal infection shows a mixed cellular pleocytosis, reduced glucose content, marked elevation of CSF protein, and specific IgG antibodies determined by complement-fixation testing. Tissue examination reveals coccidioidal spherules containing endosporins with Grocott-Gomori staining. Coccidioidal meningitis in children is infrequent in endemic areas but is an intractable, debilitating disease poorly responsive to treatment. Hydrocephalus often complicates the illness, and the morbidity and mortality are high. Fluconazole is the mainstay of therapy for CNS disease. Amphotericin B is recommended for severe and progressive non-CNS disease as well as for CNS disease not responsive to fluconazole, and it usually requires intrathecal administration.

Cryptococcus neoformans is the most common fungal cause of granulomatous meningitis in otherwise healthy adults but is unusual in children. The infection is acquired by inhalation of yeast-phase fungus from the environment. The primary respiratory illness is often asymptomatic or not recognized as a potentially serious illness. When dissemination occurs, it is usually to the meninges, where it causes an infection with first symptoms usually being headache and mental status changes without fever or meningeal signs. These signs can progress gradually but sometimes will persist for weeks before advancing. Vomiting, lethargy, ataxia, localized neurologic signs, and papilledema eventually emerge. Diagnosis is established by CSF examination, which usually shows a limited cellular response and a positive test for cryptococcal polysaccharide antigen. India ink preparation is usually positive in AIDS patients with the illness, but much less so in previously normal persons. Cerebrospinal fluid culture will be positive in most. The organism is seen with proper stains as a round or oval encapsulated yeast. Cryptococcal meningitis now is a widely recognized complication in persons with AIDS and can be seen in HIV-positive persons without significant immunosuppression. Intensive antifungal therapy will eradicate the infection in over 80% of cases, although relapses can occur and are frequent in AIDS patients. Amphotericin B in combination with flucytosine or fluconazole is indicated for initial therapy.

Mucormycosis is an invasive fungal infection resulting from members of the class Zygomycetes (Phycomycetes). The name of the disease stems from the fact that most cases are caused by members of the order Mucorales, and specifically by the genus *Rhizopus*. The illness occurs almost entirely among persons who are immunosuppressed or have conditions with persisting or chronic acidosis such as chronic renal failure or diabetes mellitus. It is far more frequent in adults than in children. Primary pneumonia or disseminated disease is seen mainly among persons with leukemia or lymphoma. The most widely recognized form is known as rhinocerebral mucormycosis, a distinctive fungal disease that follows hyphal invasion of the nasal and paranasal sinus mucosa. Fungal invasion of the vascular endothelium in these areas leads to ischemic tissue injury, resulting in black necrotic lesions in the nose and sinuses. The orbit may be invaded, resulting in proptosis and rapid visual loss. Spread of infection to the cavernous sinus compounds the illness when intracavernous invasion of the carotid artery causes carotid thrombosis and ischemic cerebral infarction. The child then develops hemiparesis with other neurologic signs. The resulting brain injury is mainly ischemic but fungal hyphae without surrounding inflammation can be found in the area, especially within and adjacent to cerebral arterioles. Mucorales hyphae are identified on hemolysin-eosin (H&E) and Grocott-Gomori methanamine silver stains as broad, nonseptate structures with right-angle branching and which accept stains in irregular fashion along the hyphal structure. Rhinocerebral mucormycosis, like the disseminated form, was once considered to be uniformly fatal, although with intensive antifungal therapy and hyperbaric oxygen treatments, the rhinocerebral form of illness can occasionally be overcome. The logic of hyperbaric oxygen therapy stems from the prominent role of ischemia due to fungal vascular invasion causing tissue injury. It is believed that this form of treatment increases oxygen delivery to damaged tissues.

Candida species central nervous system infections

Candida sp. are the most common members of the fungi that cause invasive disease and CNS disease in infants and children. Such infections are seen almost entirely in very-low-birth weight neonates, in children with immunocompromising conditions, and, less often, as a complication of surgical procedures associated with compromise of mucosal barriers. The factors that predispose to *Candida* infections are outlined in Table 13.9. Most infections are caused by *C. albicans*, although in recent years there has been a relative increase in serious infections by other species including *C. tropicalis*, *C. krusei*, and *C. parapsilosis*. *C. glabrata*, previously termed *Torulopsis glabrata*, has in some series become the second most common invading offender among the *Candida* sp.

Infants weighing less than 1,500 g account for most cases of disseminated candidiasis in the neonate, with the organism acquired either by vertical transmission from the maternal anogenital tract or by horizontal transmission from the environment. Disseminated neonatal candidiasis gives rise to a septic-like condition and closely resembles bacterial sepsis. Tissue dissemination can be to multiple organs, resulting in hepatosplenic infection, septic arthritis or osteomyelitis, endophthalmitis, meningitis, and infrequently, to the heart with endocarditis or an intracardiac fungal mass.

The most common presenting signs among premature neonates with generalized candidiasis are shown in Table 13.10. Bacterial sepsis in the neonate more characteristically is associated with hypothermia, whereas fever is more often found with *Candida* sepsis. In a large series of neonates with disseminated *Candida* sp. infections, Fernandez and colleagues (2000) found that 25% were associated with *Candida* meningitis. The clinical signs in those with meningitis are mainly those of septic and disseminated infection with evidence of meningitis found by CSF examination. Cerebrospinal fluid abnormalities in infants with *Candida* meningitis resemble those with bacterial meningitis, with reduced glucose levels and elevated protein content, although the cellular reaction is usually much less intense, and mixed pleocytosis or lymphocytic cellular responses are more common with *Candida* meningitis. In the low-birth-weight neonate, *Candida* sp. CNS infection is usually meningitic in type, with or without parenchymal brain lesions and, as a result, the CSF is usually abnormal. Yeast are rarely seen in CSF by staining methods, although CSF and blood cultures are generally positive. Growth of the fungus is slow and may not become evident for 3–4 days. In older children with CNS *Candida* sp. infections, the pathology is more often that of multiple cerebral microabscesses that are readily seen on enhanced MRI examination. Unless some of the lesions are located close to the brain surface, the CSF can be unrevealing.

Table 13.9 Predisposing factors for invasive *Candida* sp. infections

- Immunosuppressive conditions
- Low-birth-weight neonate
- Damaged mucosal surfaces
- Neutropenia
- Antibiotic therapy
- Corticosteroid therapy
- Indwelling vascular catheters
- Hyperalimentation and lipid infusions
- Mechanical ventilation

Table 13.10 Common presenting signs of disseminated candidiasis in the very-low-birth-weight neonate

- Respiratory compromise
- Abdominal distention
- Poor peripheral perfusion
- Metabolic acidosis
- Hyperthermia

Vascular invasion with *Candida* sp. in the neonate will sometimes result in a hepatosplenic syndrome in which the liver rapidly enlarges and becomes tender or with joint involvement with acute arthritis, which resembles acute bacterial septic arthritis. Aspiration of joint fluid or tissue samples from any infected tissue will reveal *Candida* yeast as pseudohypae; elongated structures consisting of stacks of single yeast cells and stained with H&E or Grocott-Gomori methanamine silver stain.

Although there is a definite case fatality rate in neonates with disseminated *Candida* sp. infections, it is difficult to assign mortality specifically to the fungal infection in most because the illness occurs in a sick infant usually with indwelling vascular catheters and multiple other medical problems. The infection can usually be eliminated with amphotericin B, which is used as the sole, initial method of therapy by most. Nearly all species of Candida are susceptible to amphotericin B, with the exception of *C. lusitaniae*. In older infants and children, flucytosine can be co-administered with amphotericin for *C. albicans* infections involving the CNS if enteral administration is feasible. Lipid preparations of amphotericin may be used if significant nephrotoxicity or clinical failure is observed with conventional amphotericin. Certain *Candida* sp. are also sensitive to fluconazole, which has been successfully used in eradicating candidemia.

Parasitic diseases of the central nervous system

Parasitic infections seen in the United States that affect the CNS are mainly toxoplasmosis, cysticercosis, and primary amoeba meningoencephalitis. Very unusual cases of *Toxocara canis* encephalitis complicating visceral larval migrans have been described and recently, malaria has been observed with increasing frequency. Many parasitic conditions (Table 13.11) affect the nervous system in tropical and developing nations, most of which can now be seen in this country, either among returning travelers or in immigrants from regions endemic for a particular disease. Rapid transportation by air and frequent foreign travel have made it important that these illnesses, generally considered to be exotic and rare, be known to caregivers in this country.

An illness called *eosinophilic meningitis* is endemic in Hawaii and other Pacific regions, as well as in Southeast Asia. It also occurs in the Caribbean and Jamaica, thus, close to U.S. borders. Eosinophilic meningitis is caused by a nematode, *Angiostrongylus cantonensis*, with an incubation period of 2–3 weeks. Human infection follows consumption of raw snails that harbor the larvae. Following penetration of intestinal vascular structures, larvae are transported to CSF and, on dying, provoke an eosinophilic reaction that results in headaches, believed to be symptomatic of intracranial hypertension. Fever occurs in some with the illness but most remain afebrile. Cerebrospinal fluid is clear to hazy, contains 100–1,000 white blood cells per milliliter, of which 20–70% are eosinophils. Detection of specific antibodies by ELISA or Western blot is sometimes used for specific diagnosis. Much less often, this illness will present with more dramatic encephalitic signs. There is no specific treatment, and spontaneous resolution is expected in 3–4 weeks. Corticosteroids have been found to provide symptomatic relief in some but do not shorten the duration of the illness.

Paragonimiasis, sparganosis, coenurosis, trypanosomiasis, and schistosomiasis are further examples of parasitic CNS infections that are endemic to tropical/subtropical areas of the world and rarely seen in the United States. However, they should be considered in patients who have resided in or travelled to endemic parts.

Table 13.11 Classification of some of the parasites that can cause central nervous system disease

Protozoa
- *Entamoeba histolytica*

Sporozoa
- *Plasmodium sp.*
- *Leishmania sp.*
- *Trypanosoma sp.*

Amoebae
- *Naegleria fowleri*
- *Acanthamoeba sp.*
- *Balamuthia mandrillaris*

Coccidia
- *Toxoplasma gondii*
- Nematodes (roundworms)
- *Trichinella spiralis*
- *Angiostrongylus cantonensis*
- *Gnathostoma spinigerum*
- *Toxocara canis*

Cestodes (tapeworms)
- *Taenia solium*
- *Echinococcus granulosa*
- *Taenia multiceps* (formerly *Multiceps multiceps*)
- *Spirometra mansonoides*

Trematodes (flukes)
- *Paragonimus westermanni*
- *Schistosoma sp.*

Modified from Garcia 1999.

Congenital toxoplasmosis

Toxoplasma gondii is a parasite with worldwide distribution, and it infects a wide variety of warm-blooded small and large animals. Cats are the definitive host. The parasite exists in three forms, including the oocyst excreted in feces of infected animals; the trophozoite, which is the proliferative form in tissue; and toxoplasma cysts, the chronic latent stage found in tissues. Humans become infected with the parasite by consumption of undercooked or raw meat or from oocysts found in cat litter, especially from farm-residing cats that have greater access to infected small rodents than do urban domestic cats.

Most primary infections with toxoplasmosis in children or adults are asymptomatic or with mild flu-like illnesses and, thus, are not identified. When the illness is symptomatic, it causes an Epstein-Barr virus (EBV)-negative mononucleosis syndrome with fever, erythematous rash, and diffuse lymphadenopathy but without pharyngitis, typical of EBV-induced infectious mononucleosis.

Fetal infection resulting in congenital toxoplasmosis represents the most common parasitic infection with CNS implications in this country; it occurs when a mother acquires her primary infection with the organism during pregnancy. According to Wong and Remington (1994), untreated primary infection late in the first trimester is transmitted to the fetus in approximately 10%; in the second trimester, fetal infection occurs in 30%; and in the third trimester, fetal infection occurs in 60%. Among neonates with congenital toxoplasmosis, approximately 80% are asymptomatic at birth. Of the 20% of neonates who are symptomatic, 10% will exhibit severe multiorgan involvement and 10% will have milder expressions of disease (Table 13.12).

Severe neonatal toxoplasmosis can be manifested by jaundice, hepatosplenomegaly, maculopapular rash, thrombocytopenia, chorioretinitis, and toxoplasmic en-

Table 13.12 Summary of congenital toxoplasmosis

Incidence is 1 in 1,000 live births
▶ 70–90% of infected neonates are asymptomatic at birth
▶ 85% of asymptomatic infected infants later develop neurologic or ophthalmologic sequelae
▶ 10% of infected neonates have severe illness
▶ Spiramycin given to mothers with primary infection during pregnancy may decrease fetal transmission and/or severity of sequelae

cephalitis, more often with hydrocephalus than with microcephaly, and frequently with intracranial calcifications seen on CT. Cerebral calcific densities are usually diffuse and punctate but can be found in a periventricular location, more characteristic of congenital CMV encephalitis. Hydrocephalus is usually secondary to intraventricular obstruction and in most is associated with a markedly elevated CSF protein, often of sufficient degree to render the CSF a xanthochromic appearance. Most severe neonatal infections with multiorgan involvement result from primary maternal infections early in pregnancy. When maternal toxoplasmosis occurs in the last trimester, almost all infected neonates are asymptomatic.

Of the 70–90% of congenitally infected but asymptomatic and untreated neonates, about 85% will subsequently develop signs of the disease later in infancy or in childhood. Macular chorioretinitis with visual loss is the most common and sometimes the only sign of inflammation. Other features that commonly emerge are sensorineural deafness, global developmental delay, specific neurologic deficits, and recurrent seizures. Abnormal progressive head enlargement can be delayed for weeks or months after birth.

Serologic diagnosis of congenital toxoplasmosis is complex, in part because specific maternal IgG antibodies will be transplacentally transferred to the fetus and can persist for 6–12 months before becoming undetectable. In addition, most infected neonates do not generate specific IgM antibodies. The lack of sensitivity of the IgM assay is the reason why most authors recommend an assay for specific IgA antibodies as well. Polymerase chain reaction amplification is used to detect *T. gondii* DNA in body fluids and tissues and has been successfully used to diagnose congenital, ocular, cerebral, and disseminated toxoplasmosis. Polymerase chain reaction performed on amniotic fluid has revolutionized the diagnosis of fetal *T. gondii* infection by enabling an early diagnosis to be made, thereby avoiding the use of more invasive procedures on the fetus.

Spiramycin is a macrolide antibiotic that remains an investigational drug in this country but can be made available upon request (see *Red Book*, American Academy of Pediatrics, 2006). Studies in France have shown that spiramycin given soon after primary infection in pregnancy will reduce transmission of *T. gondii* from mother to fetus by 60%. In addition, maternal therapy may decrease the severity of sequelae in the fetus once congenital infection has occurred. Studies by McAuley and colleagues (1994) have demonstrated the decided benefits of treatment of the congenitally infected neonate with pyrimethamine and sulfadiazine. Prolonged treatment is necessary, and the regimen should be directed and monitored by one familiar with the use and complications of these drugs.

In addition to the congenital infection, toxoplasmosis is well known to be an opportunistic infection in cell-mediated immune deficiency states, especially AIDS. As such, the illness does occur in children but is far more common in adults. In AIDS patients, cerebral toxoplasmosis is said to occur in about 15% and is the most common opportunistic infection associated with this condition. It is also the most common cause of multiple ring-enhancing mass lesions in AIDS, being far more common than primary cerebral lymphoma.

Meningoencephalitis caused by free-living amoeba

Clinicians are generally familiar with brain abscess possibly occurring with infection with *Entamoeba histolytica* but less so with the CNS infections caused by the so-called free-living amoeba (Table 13.13). These parasites cause two distinctive types of neurologic infection, each with different clinical patterns and epidemiologic features, as reviewed by Ma and co-workers (1990) and Schumacher and co-workers. (1995). The free-living amoeba have a worldwide distribution and are found in water, soil, and elsewhere in the environment. Central nervous system infections in either form are poorly responsive to therapy and most cases have been fatal.

Table 13.13 Central nervous system infections caused by free-living amoeba

Naegleria fowleri
▶ Primary amoebic meningoencephalitis
▶ Acute purulent meningitis
▶ A water-borne infection
***Acanthamoeba* sp.**
▶ Subacute or chronic granulomatous encephalitis
▶ Most in immunosuppressed patients
▶ Usually with focal neurologic signs
▶ Cerebrospinal fluid lymphocytic pleocytosis
Balamuthia mandrillaris
▶ Subacute or chronic granulomatous encephalitis
▶ Previously normal or immunosuppressed patients
▶ No known effective therapy

Primary amoebic meningitis is caused by *Naegleria fowleri* and usually affects adolescents and young adults. It is a rare disorder, with most cases in the United States having occurred in Virginia, the Carolinas, and Florida. The organism is acquired from the warm water of lakes, ponds, and poorly kept private swimming pools. Portal of entry is across the nasal mucosa to the olfactory nerves and to the olfactory bulbs embedded in CSF. Infection within the olfactory structures rapidly leads to hemorrhagic necrosis and explains the occasional early complaint of disturbance of smell and taste sensations. Once in CSF, the parasite provokes a fulminating purulent meningitis that is usually initially assumed to be bacterial meningitis. Symptoms begin 3–6 days after exposure to contaminated water, with headache, vomiting, and fever being the first complaints, followed by rapid decline in consciousness. Meningeal signs appear early in the illness. Generalized brain swelling is visualized on neuroimaging, with collapsed ventricles and effacement of the perimesencephalic and quadrigeminal cisterns. Cerebrospinal fluid is purulent, under markedly elevated pressure, and contains a neutrophilic pleocytosis with reduced glucose content and a striking increase in the protein content. Diagnosis of infection with *N. fowleri* is suspected when acute, rapidly progressive meningitis occurs within a week after swimming in warm water and with purulent but aseptic meningitis. The illness progresses so rapidly that serologic tests are of no help diagnostically. A fresh CSF specimen may reveal motile amoebic trophozoites with Giemsa or Wright stains. If not, meningeal biopsy will demonstrate trophozoite structures about the size of macrophages and clustered in a perivascular distribution. Recommended treatment includes intravenous and sometimes intrathecal amphotericin B, usually in combination with rifampin. It is usually a fatal illness, although there are reports of recovery with early initiation of therapy.

Subacute or chronic granulomatous amoebic meningoencephalitis is caused by *Acanthamoeba* species and has been described more often in immunosuppressed or debilitated adults than in children. The organism enters the respiratory tract from environmental sources, and CNS infection follows hematogenous spread from the lungs. The clinical illness evolves slowly over weeks, usually with low-grade fever and signs of focal or multifocal neurologic dysfunction. Parenchymal brain lesions are necrotizing and granulomatous, containing multinucleated giant cells and with evidence of vascular invasion by the parasite. The site of the mass lesions and whether solitary or multiple determines the neurologic signs. Cerebrospinal fluid abnormalities consist of a lymphocytic pleocytosis and diagnosis in vivo is determined by brain biopsy. The infection has not been found to be responsive to any therapeutic regimen. A similar illness has recently been recognized with *Balamuthia mandrillaris*, a similar soil parasite previously assumed to be nonpathogenic. Unlike infection with *Acanthamoeba* species, that with *Balamuthia mandrillaris* can occur in previously normal persons as well as in the immunosuppressed patient. Treatment is quite difficult since the organism is unresponsive to many available agents; however, combination therapies with antifungal and antibacterial agents have been successfully used in a few documented cases.

Cerebral cysticercosis

Infection with *Taenia solium*, the pork tapeworm, presenting as asymptomatic carriage or as cysticercosis, is widespread in the world, especially in Mexico, Central and South America, Africa, Southeast Asia, and many central European nations. Cysticercosis is not rare in the United States and is primarily seen in immigrants from endemic zones. The intestinal tapeworm is acquired by humans by ingestion of undercooked pork infected with *T. solium*.

Human cysticercosis is acquired by ingestion of *T. solium* eggs through fecal–oral contact with a person infected with the pork tapeworm, via contaminated food or water, or autoinoculation. The eggs hatch in the intestine, resulting in the larval stage, which penetrates the intestinal wall to be transported by blood or lymphatics to various tissues throughout the body, including the CNS. When the CNS is affected, the parasite becomes encapsulated within a cystic lesion, which will contain the scolex. The live, encysted parasite provokes little inflammatory reaction and remains clinically dormant until death of the organism occurs, which then elicits a brisk inflammatory response with local cerebral edema and irritation of adjacent structures. The adjacent edema can be extensive and associated with headaches and seizures. Less often, intracranial localization of the encysted parasite will be within the ventricular ependyma and, if in the aqueduct or fourth ventricle, it will lead to obstruction and hydrocephalus. In others, the degenerative process of the encysted parasite remains asymptomatic; months or years later, the lesions will shrink in size and become densely calcified. This stage may also remain asymptomatic but is usually recognized when, with the occurrence of seizures, neuroimaging is obtained. Calcific lesions are most prominent at the cortical–white matter junction and in the chronic stage are not surrounded by edema. Lesions may be few in number or dozens can be observed.

Diagnosis of cerebral cysticercosis can be made in most cases on the basis of history, exposure in an endemic area, and from findings on neuroimaging. In the stage when dying parasites leads to cerebral edema, T2 weighted MRI will reveal the degree of edema and will usually show an encysted area containing the scolex. In the chronic stage, multiple cerebral punctate calcific lesions are best seen with CT. Regardless of the stage of illness, blood eosinophilia is not usually present, although occasionally eosinophils may be found in CSF. Antibody assays that test for specific antibodies to *T. solium* in serum and CSF are also available.

Treatment in the acute, inflammatory stage of cysticercosis is with albendazole in a childhood dose of 15 mg/kg/day for 7–10 days. Many experts will also administer corticosteroids during the treatment regimen because drug-induced death of remaining parasites can be expected to add to the cerebral swelling. Treatment of patients with single parenchymal cysts is controversial. When the disease is identified in the chronic stage by finding multiple punctuate calcific lesions mainly at the cortical–white matter junction and without adjacent edema, antiparasitic therapy is not indicated.

Spirochaetal diseases of the central nervous system

The best-known spirochaetal infections that can be associated with neurologic involvement include Lyme disease, leptospirosis, and congenital syphilis. Lyme disease is the most common tick-borne infection in the United States, and a wide variety of nervous system manifestations have been described with this condition.

Leptospirosis is not common in the United States; because most infections are mild and symptoms nonspecific, the majority resolve without diagnostic identification. It is one of the less common causes of acute, infectious, aseptic meningitis in children or adults but should be kept in mind because of possible treatment implications. Leptospirosis is a zoonotic infection acquired by humans from water contaminated by the urine of infected animal species, such as dogs, pigs, cattle, raccoons, rats, mice, and other small rodents. The organism enters the host's bloodstream across abraded areas of skin or mucosal surfaces. Following an incubation period that varies from 7 to 21 days, the most common presentation of leptospirosis is a self-limited febrile illness with malaise, myalgia, headache, diarrhea, conjunctivitis, and a maculopapular rash in some. During the first week of leptospirosis, leptospires commonly enter CSF but do not provoke an inflammatory reaction. After 1–3 weeks of illness, a small percentage of patients will develop clinical signs of acute aseptic meningitis, which represents a meningeal immune response to the previously present leptospires in CSF. The CSF shows a mononuclear pleocytosis with an elevated protein content in most. Serologic diagnosis of leptospirosis requires the demonstration of a fourfold rise in serum antibodies over time by use of the leptospira agglutination test. Leptospires can sometimes be isolated from blood and CSF during the first week of illness or from urine thereafter; however, isolation of the organism is technically difficult and sensitivity of culture as a diagnostic method is low. Treatment of leptospirosis when the illness is mild is usually with oral doxycycline. With more severe illness requiring hospitalization, intravenous penicillin is recommended.

Congenital syphilis is largely a preventable disease by treatment of infected women during pregnancy who are in the primary or secondary stage of the illness. Neonates with congenital syphilis are usually asymptomatic at birth but within days to weeks develop the characteristic rash, nasal discharge, adenopathy, hepotosplenomegaly, and skeletal lesions, all representative of the transplacentally transmitted secondary stage of the illness. Central nervous system infection in an infected young infant is identified by CSF examination, including the venereal disease reference laboratory (VDRL) test or the rapid plasma reagin (RPR) test. Tertiary neurosyphilis in older children with general paresis or tabes dorsalis as late complications of untreated congenital syphilis is now mainly a matter of historical interest.

Lyme disease

Lyme disease in the United States is caused by *Borrelia burgdorferi* and is widely distributed, although most infections are acquired in northeastern states, in the upper Midwest, and in northern California. Studies by Steere (2001) indicate that about 15,000 cases of Lyme disease are reported each year, resulting in the disease being the most common vector-borne illness in the United States. Lyme disease is usually transmitted by the nymph stage of the tick vector, whose natural host is the white-tailed deer and with reservoir in mice. In the northeastern and midwest United States, *Ixodes scapularis* is the tick vector for Lyme disease, whereas *I. pacificus* is the tick vector in the western part of United States.

Symptoms and signs of Lyme disease can be variable, largely depending on whether it is adequately treated in the early stage. Lyme disease affects mainly the skin, central and peripheral nervous systems, the heart, and the joints. The clinical illness is divided into three stages: early localized, early disseminated, and late disease.

Early localized disease is characterized by a large, annular, erythematous skin lesion called *erythema migrans*, which appears at the site of the tick bite. Over 80% of persons who acquire Lyme disease will develop erythema migrans, which is usually associated with transient flu-like symptoms, with fever, malaise, and myalgia.

Early disseminated disease can emerge within weeks to months after the illness is acquired, and in 15% of patients manifests with multiple erythema migrans. These lesions reflect spirochetemia with cutaneous dissemination. Fevers, myalgias, headache, conjunctivitis, and fatigue can also be seen in this stage. Other manifestations of this stage that can occur with or without the rash involve the musculoskeletal, cardiac, and/or nervous system. Among untreated infected children, arthritis can occur in up to 50% of patients; 10% develop CNS disease presenting as cranial nerve palsies (especially of the seventh nerve) or lymphocytic meningitis. Cardiac involvement, although rare in children, can occur in 5–10% of untreated children and manifests with atrioventricular (AV) conduction defects or mild myocarditis

Late disease reflects an inflammatory reaction of the joint synovia and is most commonly characterized by recurrent arthritis usually affecting the large joints, especially the knees, occurring months after the infection is acquired. Peripheral neuropathy or CNS disease occurs rarely in late disease. Late disease is uncommon in children who have been treated with appropriate therapy in the early stage.

Diagnosis of Lyme disease rests on a compatible clinical picture along with positive serologic tests. A two-step approach is recommended for the diagnosis of *B. bergdorferi* infection. Initially, a screening test for serum antibodies is performed via ELISA, followed by a more specific Western immunoblot if the ELISA is positive. Serologic responses are customarily delayed in the initial stage of the illness, but after 4–6 weeks IgG antibody titers are expected to rise. Steere (2001) has pointed out that in some, IgM antibodies may persist for months or years, decreasing its value as an indicator of recent infection. Polyermase chain reaction has been useful for testing synovial fluid for *Borrelia* DNA in the early phases of arthritis but has not been consistently reliable on CSF specimens in persons suspected to have Lyme neuroborreliosis, except in those with acute aseptic meningitis.

Antibiotic treatment of Lyme disease is complex and will be determined by the age of the patient and the organs affected. Erythema migrans and early dissemination in nonpregnant patients and those over 8 years of age are treated with doxycycline given orally for 14–21 days. For children younger than 8 years and during pregnancy, amoxicillin is recommended. Lyme disease complicated by neurologic or cardiac involvement is generally treated with intravenous ceftriaxone for 2–4 weeks. Lyme arthritis can usually be managed with doxycycline although, when intractable, intravenous ceftriaxone may be required.

Neurologic manifestations in Lyme disease have been estimated to occur in 10–20% of cases (Table 13.14). A commonly encountered pattern of neurologic disease is its occurrence with multilevel involvement or its development coincident to myocardial inflammation with AV conduction abnormalities. Multilevel neurologic disease is suspected in a child with simultaneous occurrence of facial nerve paralysis and aseptic meningitis or peripheral neuropathy with acute myelitis, encephalitis, or acute optic neuritis. Lymphocytic aseptic meningitis and acute facial paralysis are the most common neurologic complications in children. Aseptic meningitis can be relapsing with this infection and is associated with headache, mild neck stiffness, and CSF pleocytosis. Lyme disease can cause optic disc abnormalities, with acute optic neuritis associated with unilateral or bilateral visual loss. Papilledema reflecting increased intracranial pressure can be provoked by encephalitis, encephalopathy, or an ill-defined but postulated disturbance of CSF outflow at the level of the arachnoid granulations. A late-onset form of Lyme neuroborreliosis is referred to as *Lyme encephalopathy*, in which chronic cognitive and behavioral abnormalities predominate. The CSF does not show an inflammatory response in this condition although intrathecal production of antibodies has been found. The pathogenesis of this unusual complication in children with Lyme disease remains unclear.

Table 13.14 Neurologic manifestations of Lyme disease

- Acute or subacute aseptic meningitis
- Facial paralysis
- Acute optic neuritis and other cranial neuropathies
- Meningoencephalitis
- Acute transverse myelitis
- Acute cerebellar ataxia
- Peripheral neuropathies
- Increased intracranial pressure syndrome
- Lyme encephalopathy

Rickettsial infections

Rocky Mountain spotted fever

Rickettsia rickettsiae causes a tick-borne bacterial infection that is endemic in certain parts of the United States. The highest numbers of cases occur in the central Atlantic states (North Carolina, South Carolina, Virginia) and Oklahoma. Lower rates of infection occur from New England through the Gulf Coast states and into the Midwest. The organism is maintained in nature by transovarial transmission in ticks. In the eastern United States *Dermacentor variabilis* (dog tick) is the principal vector but *Ambylomma americanum* (Lone Star tick) has an important role, as well. In the western United States, *Dermacentor andersonii* (wood tick) is the vector. Infection is transmitted to man by adult ticks, which must remain attached for approximately 6 hours. Most infections occur between mid-April and October, with a peak in May and June. However, infections have occurred as late as December in warmer climates. The organism is an obligate intracellular pathogen that is tropic for vascular endothelial cells. Thus, the illness is a consequence of a multiorgan bacterial vasculitis. Disease onset occurs 2–8 days after the tick bite with the appearance of fever, headache, general malaise, and myalgia. Rash, which eventually occurs in 90% of cases, usually appears between the second and fifth days of illness. A maculopapular rash begins on the wrists and ankles and spreads centrally and distally. Individual lesions of the rash progress to petechiae and purpura with disease progression. The death-to-case ratio without treatment is 25%; fatalities usually occur between days 8 and 12 of illness. Headache occurs in most infected persons early in the course of illness and, as the disease progresses, symptomatic CNS infection emerges beginning after 4–5 days of clinical illness. Central nervous system manifestations progress from lethargy to confusion, obtundation, and coma. Focal paresis may occur. CT or MRI findings include infarction, brain edema, and meningeal enhancement, all consequences of CNS vasculitis. Death rates are high when CNS disease is severe enough to result in neuroimaging changes. Central nervous system disease usually occurs in the setting of readily recognizable disease (rash, thrombocytopenia, multiorgan system involvement, history of tick exposure); however, Rocky Mountain spotted fever should be considered within the differential diagnosis of all encephalitic illnesses occurring in endemic areas. As indicated earlier, cases can occur outside the season of highest risk. The disease is effectively treated with doxycycline, which is the drug of choice. Diagnosis is usually made serologically. Elevated concentrations of antibody are not observed during the first 6 days of illness when decisions about antibiotic therapy must be made to ensure a satisfactory clinical outcome. Clinicians should not consider early antibody data to have any meaningful negative predictive value. Seroconversion can be demonstrated as early as day 9–11 of illness, but more routinely during the second through fourth weeks after illness onset.

Ehrlichiosis

Human monocytic (*Ehrlichia chafeensis*) and granulocytic (*Anaplasma phagocytophila*) ehrlichioses both occur in the United States. Monocytic ehrlichiosis is most prevalent in the south Atlantic and south Central states into the Plains states. Granulocytic ehrlichiosis occurs predominantly in the upper Midwest into the northeast and upper Atlantic regions. The etiologic agents of ehrlichiosis are intracellular bacteria transmitted to humans via the tick vector. Monocytic ehrlichiosis is transmitted predominantly by *Amblyomma americanum*, while granulocytic disease is spread by *I. scapularis*, the vector of *B. burgdorferi* (Lyme disease). Clinical symptoms are similar to Rocky Mountain spotted fever with fever, malaise, headache, and myalgia. A mild maculopapular rash occurs in approximately one-third of patients but has no distinguishing characteristics. Typical laboratory findings of leukopenia (1,500–3,000), thrombocytopenia (20,000–30,000), and elevated AST/ALT (150–400) are usually demonstrable. Without antibiotic treatment, severe disease will develop in approximately 15–20% of patients. In these patients, CNS involvement with typical manifestations of lethargy, impaired cognition, and obtundation are common. Spinal fluid shows a mild mononuclear pleocytosis in up to 15% of patients. Death occurs in about 5% of untreated, symptomatic patients with monocytic ehrlichiosis and in 10% with granulocytic disease. Tetracyclines are the treatment of choice and the only proven effective therapy. Diagnosis is usually established serologically.

Mycobacteria infections

Tuberculosis

Mycobacterium tuberculosis

Tuberculosis (TB) accounts for significant morbidity and mortality in children and adolescents worldwide, with a majority of cases occurring in developing nations. Childhood TB accounts for only 2–7% of TB cases in developed nations, compared with 15–40% of cases in developing countries. The epidemiology of TB in the United States has undergone substantial changes in the past two decades. With a rise in cases in the late 1980s and 1990s due to multiple factors including the HIV epidemic, increase in foreign immigration, and dismantling of national TB control programs, there is now a steady decline. Since 1993 to 2006, there has been an approximately 50% decline in childhood TB cases from a rate of 2.9 cases per 100,000 persons to 1.3 cases per 100,000 persons. However, TB is still a problem; the majority of cases in the United States occur in the eastern, southern and western regions, including Alaska and Hawaii, with a disproportionate burden of disease among younger children, racial and ethnic minorities, and foreign-born persons.

As in adults, more than 98% of infections in children occur when *M. tuberculosis* organisms enter the lungs via inhalation of infectious aerosolized droplets. The majority of children with *M. tuberculosis* infection have silent pulmonary infection with no signs, symptoms, or radiographic abnormality. Progression of infection within the lung is the most common manifestation of primary TB disease and usually presents as enlargement of the affected regional lymph node. Progression of disease beyond the lungs occurs most frequently in younger children. Meningeal TB develops after hematogenous dissemination of *M. tuberculosis*, usually with 3–6 months of initial infection. Meningitis develops when caseating lesions on the cerebral cortex invade the meninges and disseminate into the subarachnoid space. Tuberculous meningitis is the most severe complication of TB disease and is usually fatal without treatment. It accounts for 2.1% of pediatric cases of TB.

The clinical presentation of meningeal TB can be rapid or gradual. Rapid progression usually occurs in young children and infants, who may be symptomatic for a few days before the onset of hydrocephalus, seizures, or cerebral edema. Often, the course is indolent, with symptoms presenting 1–4 weeks before diagnosis. The most common presenting symptoms are high-grade fever, vomiting, lethargy, headache, and seizures. The clinical course can be divided into three stages: stage I: nonspecific symptoms with no focal neurologic findings; stage II: nonspecific symptoms with neurologic findings, such as nuchal rigidity, cranial nerve abnormalities, Kernig or Brudzinski signs; and stage III: marked decrease in mental status with neurologic findings, such as coma, hemiplegia, posturing.

Risk factors for poor outcome are associated with stage III disease at the time of admission, young age (<3 years), miliary disease, or delay in initiation of treatment.

Diagnosis and rapid confirmation of TB meningitis is difficult since the tuberculin skin test can be nonreactive in up to 40% of cases and chest radiographs can be normal in up to 50% of patients. Cerebrospinal fluid findings include a leukocyte cell count range from 10 to 500 cells/mm^3 with a lymphocytic predominance, although polymorphonuclear cells can predominate early in the disease. The CSF glucose level is usually between 20 and 40 mg/dL, and CSF protein levels are elevated (>150 mg/dL) (Table 13.1). Positivity of CSF acid-fast bacillus (AFB) stain or culture correlates directly with the quantity of CSF sampled: with 10 mL of CSF, the AFB stain yields a positive result in up to 30% of cases and the culture result is positive in up to 70% of cases. Isolation of the TB organism is very important since treatment is dependent on sensitivity of the bacillus to anti-TB medications. In addition to CSF AFB culture, a full workup, including pulmonary evaluation, is suggested to help isolate the organism. Investigation of adult contacts is important to identify adult sources of infection. Cranial CT and MRI can also be helpful in the diagnosis of TB meningitis. Although the CT scan can be normal in early disease, basilar enhancement with communicating hydrocephalus, signs of cerebral edema, and focal ischemia are helpful clues in making the diagnosis.

Treatment of meningeal TB requires therapy with multiple antituberculous drugs for 6 months. Most experts recommend a 2-month regimen with four drugs taken daily, followed by daily or twice-weekly isoniazid and rifampin to complete the course. However, individual regimens may vary depending on the susceptibility of the *M. tuberculosis* organism. Directly observed therapy (DOT) is the recommended treatment modality for compliance.

With effective treatment regimens, the mortality rate is less than 10%; however, meningitis still causes significant long-term morbidity such as mental retardation, seizure disorders, and hemiparesis. The prognosis of TB meningitis correlates closely with the clinical disease stage at the time of initiation of effective therapy. Most patients with stage I disease have an excellent outcome, whereas most survivors of stage III have permanent disabilities.

Tuberculomas, presenting as space-occupying lesions, are yet another manifestation of CNS TB disease that are usually seen in children under 10 years of age. A typical lesion is single, infratentorial, and located at the base of the brain. The most common symptoms are headache, fever, and seizures. Most cases occur in developing nations and are rare in North America. However, appearance of tuberculomas during effective treatment of CNS TB is a paradoxic phenomenon. This development does not indicate failure of therapy but is likely due to an inflammatory or immunologic reaction. Most cases are treated with steroids and continuation of TB therapy.

CHAPTER 14

Vascular Disease in Infants and Children

Richard H. Haas and Jennifer Armstrong-Wells

Outline

- Arterial ischemic and hemorrhagic stroke in the newborn
- Infant, child, and adolescent ischemic disease
- Metabolic stroke
- Cerebral veins and sinuses
- Intracranial hemorrhage in infancy and childhood

Cerebrovascular events in adults are common and are generally well explained by established risk factors, which include hypertension, diabetes mellitus, and atherosclerosis. Similar events in children have traditionally received less clinical and investigative attention because of their perceived rarity. The World Health Organization (WHO) defines stroke as "A clinical syndrome of rapidly developed clinical signs of focal or global disturbance of cerebral dysfunction lasting greater than 24 hours or leading to death with no obvious cause other than of vascular origin." Recently, there has been increased recognition of childhood stroke and other forms of cerebrovascular disease in infancy and childhood. Retrospective epidemiologic studies have reported an incidence of 2.3 pediatric strokes per 100,000 children per year in California (Fullerton et al. 2003) and 2.6 in Cincinnati, where intracerebral hemorrhage accounted for a surprising 58% of cases (Broderick et al. 1993). The ready availability of magnetic resonance (MR) and computed tomographic (CT) neuroimaging techniques has allowed easier confirmation of the diagnosis and etiology. A prospective high-ascertainment study using these imaging modalities in Dijon, France reported a much higher incidence of 13 strokes per 100,000/year in children younger than 16 years of age excluding the neonatal period (Giroud et al. 1995). The incidence and etiology of neonatal cerebrovascular events varies depending on gestational age but accounts for significant morbidity and mortality, particularly in premature infants. An incidence of neonatal arterial ischemic stroke of 93 per 100,000 was reported from the Canadian Registry (Andrew et al. 2001). In the same study, cerebral sinovenous thrombosis occurred in 41 per 100,000 newborns per year. The majority of pediatric stroke patients survive the acute insult, with survival increasing by 58% in the United States between 1979 and 1998 (Fullerton et al. 2002), yet many are left with residual disability (Gordon et al. 2002). Thus, the importance of this condition is related more to its high prevalence, in contrast to adult cerebrovascular disease, which has a higher incidence but generally a shorter survival time.

In this chapter, prenatal and perinatal periods are grouped together and considered separately from later childhood lesions. For each group, ischemic and hemorrhagic lesions are discussed separately.

Arterial ischemic and hemorrhagic stroke in the newborn

Ischemic injury in the premature infant

The premature brain is anatomically different from that of term infants. One of the most striking differences is the presence of the germinal matrix in the region of the basal ganglia, with its network of fragile vessels that are prone to hemorrhage. Second, the reduced degree of autoregulation in the cerebral vasculature in the premature infant, particularly in the context of hypoxic–ischemic encephalopathy, contributes to hemorrhage. A third important developmental factor is the extreme vulnerability to anoxic and free-radical injury of immature oligodendroglia in the white matter, leading to a predisposition to periventricular leukomalacia (PVL), which is infrequent at term (Volpe 2001a).

Periventricular leukomalacia lesions are usually symmetric and are located adjacent to the lateral ventricles and represent necrosis of cerebral white matter. The lesions vary in degree and size. This region is vulnerable owing to its location in the border zone areas between major cerebral arteries. The lesions occur predominantly in premature infants who have survived several days or more and have had severe systemic illness, such as cardiorespiratory dysfunction or sepsis. Periventricular leukomalacia is the main cause of brain injury in the premature infant. The three major etiologic factors are (a) incomplete development of the vascular supply to the white matter, (b) a maturation-dependent impairment of cerebral blood flow regulation, and (c) a window of extreme vulnerability of immature oligodendroglia to free-radical injury (Volpe 2001a). The most common clinical correlate to PVL that evolves outside of the neonatal period is spastic diplegia, as the fibers from the motor cortex to the leg course closest to the lateral ventricle. Periventricular leukomalacia has a characteristic appearance on computed tomography (CT) in late infancy and childhood. Because the white matter is deficient, the lateral wall of the lateral ventricle has a scalloped contour, and the gray matter at the depth of the sylvian fissure nearly touches the ventricular wall (Flodmark et al. 1987). Magnetic resonance imaging (MRI) with diffusion weighting is the preferred imaging modality for the detection and definition of severity and extent of PVL acutely (Bozzao et al. 2003), with fluid attenuated inversion recovery (FLAIR) also effective in the neonatal period (Iwata et al. 2004).

Ischemic injury in the term infant

Labor and delivery is a high-risk period for CNS insults; immaturity of cerebral vasculature and autoregulation, along with white matter vulnerability, also contribute to vascular disease in the term infant. Hypotension and anoxia are the major causes of ischemic disease in the term infant (hypoxic–ischemic encephalopathy). Perinatal stroke is increasingly recognized as a risk factor for cerebral palsy, congenital hemiparesis, and subsequent behavioral, cognitive, and language problems (Koelfen et al. 1995; Trauner et al. 2001; Wu et al. 2004).

Key Clinical Questions

- Is there unexplained encephalopathy with one or more of the following signs: hypotonia, apnea, bradycardia, lethargy?
- Are focal or generalized seizures present?
- Do CT or MRI findings suggest ischemia?

It has long been recognized by pathologists that some congenital brain injuries are the result of cerebrovascular events that occur during gestation. Anencephaly, hydranencephaly, and some porencephalic cysts have either a distribution or pathologic features suggestive of a vascular pathogenesis. The arterial border zone location of some lesions suggests that infarcts were related to circulatory failure. All of these cases are recognized as prenatal in origin. Recently, some families have been identified with porencephaly, intracranial hemorrhages, and genetic disorders of collagen synthesis (Gould et al. 2005; Gould et al. 2006).

The clinical importance of focal and multifocal ischemic infarcts has acquired new emphasis in recent years as a result of the improved survival of neonates and the availability of newer imaging methods. Criteria for dating perinatal strokes lesions are evolving. Diffusion- and perfusion-weighted MRI of acute lesions can assist in timing of the insult (Wardlaw & Farrall 2004). Infarcts in neonates have a greatly accelerated rate of clearing of necrotic tissue and early calcification compared with later-onset lesions. In isolated case series, cerebral infarcts, excluding venous infarcts and PVL, occurred in at least 5.4% of autopsied neonates (Barmada et al. 1979), and cerebral hemorrhages were found in at least 26% of asymptomatic neonates (Looney et al. 2007). Both clinical and pathologic series usually show perinatal cerebral infarcts are more commonly left-sided (Golomb et al. 2004; Lee et al. 2005; Trauner et al. 1993); this left-sided preference is also seen with perinatal hemorrhagic stroke (Armstrong-Wells et al. 2008).

Because of the paucity of population-based studies, little is known of the true prevalence and risk factors for perinatal stroke. Focal infarcts can be seen in a variety of systemic disturbances. However, a specific etiology is not demonstrable in most perinatal cases of focal ischemia, and many cases are multifactorial. However, although it was previously believed that birth trauma and anoxia were major causes of perinatal ischemia, new studies have illuminated other risk factors. Maternal factors, such as infertility, preeclampsia, and chorioamnionitis, have been associated with perinatal arterial ischemic stroke (Lee et al. 2005; Wu et al. 2003). Neonatal infections, such as sepsis and meningitis, are also associated with newborn stroke. Up to 30% of autopsies in neonates with meningitis show infarcts, many of which are hemorrhagic (Friede 1973), although this number may be decreasing with earlier antibiotic treatment. Congenital heart defects have been strongly associated with ischemic stroke in children, as well as in neonates. Placental abnormalities may also contribute to perinatal arterial ischemic stroke. Maternal or fetal thrombophilia resulting in hypercoagulability causes abnormality of the placental vasculature, placental infarctions, and vessel thrombosis, which can result in perinatal stroke (Chabrier & Buchmuller 2003).

Consider Consultation When...

- A cerebral infarction is diagnosed or suspected.
- Neonatal seizures occur.

Perinatal infarcts occasionally are due to amniotic fluid embolization. Maternal cocaine abuse has been associated with both ischemic and hemorrhagic infarction (Chasnoff et al. 1986).

Hematologic factors have been weakly associated with perinatal stroke. Those suggested are factor V Leiden mutation or protein C deficiency (Kurnik et al. 2003), elevated homocysteine or increased lipoprotein-(a) (Govaert et al. 2000; Hogeveen et al. 2002), or maternal anticardiolipin antibodies and lupus anticoagulant (Andrew et al. 2001). However, most reports of prothrombotic states are observational and without convalescent titers, making interpretation difficult.

The germinal matrix has largely disappeared by 36 weeks gestation, so hemorrhage from this site is unusual; however, intracranial hemorrhage may be an underrecognized etiology for congenital hemiparesis and cerebral palsy. Like perinatal arterial ischemic stroke, perinatal hemorrhagic stroke was thought to be due mainly to birth trauma and brain contusion. Although birth trauma most likely is associated with perinatal subdural hematomas, in contemporary studies, intracerebral and subarachnoid hemorrhages were not associated with birth trauma (Looney et al. 2007; Sandberg et al. 2001). In a recent nested case-control study, it was found that fetal distress and postmaturity were strong predictors for intracerebral hemorrhage (Armstrong-Wells et al. 2008).

Although less common than perinatal arterial ischemic stroke, cerebral sinovenous thrombosis is an increasingly recognized cause of neonatal stroke. Neonatal dehydration, systemic infection, thrombophilia, and hypoxia have been associated with neonatal sinovenous thrombosis (deVeber & Andrew 2001). Chorioamnionitis and extracorporeal membrane oxygenation were common associations of neonatal sinovenous thrombosis in one recent study (Wu et al. 2002).

Signs and symptoms

Clinical presentation of perinatal arterial ischemic or hemorrhagic stroke, as well as sinovenous thrombosis, may include encephalopathy, seizures, hypotonia, apnea, and bradycardia, without focal neurologic deficits. Focal seizures are seen, but sometimes may only be apparent on electroencephalogram (EEG). With prenatal vascular lesions, hemiparesis almost always spares the face. The neurologic examination in the neonatal period, reflecting primarily brainstem function, is usually of no localizing help, even in extensive cortical strokes, and many newborns may have a normal examination in the newborn period (Table 14.1).

The infant with a prenatal lesion most often presents with developmental abnormalities at 6–12 months of age. This usually presents as asymmetry of motor function (early hand preference, asymmetric persistent grasp reflex, or asymmetric parachute reflex), or other developmental delay. Even when an infant has a known cerebral infarct, his development and examination may be normal for several months or years. The reasons for such delay of symptoms and signs, and for their failure to occur in some cases, are not well understood. Infants with damage confined to the basal ganglia may not present with dystonia or choreoathetoid symptoms until the second year of life or later. The frequency of cerebral palsy was found to be 76 in 111 children with perinatal stroke (68%) (Golomb et al. 2008). It is also important to realize that 50% of children showing motor dysfunction at 1 year of age may be normal by 7 years, especially if the earlier involvement was not severe (Nelson & Ellenberg 1982). Language and cognitive development are usually good following unilateral focal pre- or perinatal lesions. However, subtle deficits are seen that generally mirror the findings in adults with acquired left and right hemisphere strokes. The plasticity of the immature nervous system mitigates the traditional adult deficit pattern in interesting ways. Children with congenital left lesions tend to have more grammatical language problems until age 5–7 years, when they catch up. Children with congenital right lesions tend to have mild but persistent spatial difficulties (Stiles et al. 2008). Additionally, special neglect may persist (Trauner et al. 2001; Trauner 2003).

Seizures are the other major presenting symptom of perinatal cerebral infarcts (Clancy et al. 1985; Laugesaar et al. 2007; Lee et al. 2005; Ment et al. 1984), as well as in perinatal hemorrhagic stroke (Armstrong-Wells et al. 2008; Laugesaar et al. 2007; Sandberg et al. 2001). In neonates with sinovenous thrombosis, seizures occur in 71% (deVeber & Andrew 2001) and were the presenting

Table 14.1 Prenatal and perinatal ischemic disease

Discriminating features
- Focal infarction on computed tomography (CT) or magnetic resonance imaging (MRI)

Consistent features
- Hemiparesis or persistent motor asymmetries by the first year of life

Variable features
- Focal seizures in the neonatal period
- Focal electroencephalograph (EEG) abnormalities
- Cognitive and language delays after the first year of life

Pearls and Perils

Prenatal and Perinatal Ischemic Disease

- Persistent focal seizures in the neonate suggest infarction.
- Electrographic status epilepticus may be due to perinatal infarction.
- Seizures are a common feature of sinovenous thrombosis.
- The neurologic examination is usually nonfocal in neonatal stroke.
- Facial sparing in an infant with hemiparesis suggests a prenatal onset.
- The development of early hand preference (younger than 1 year of age) suggests dysfunction of the contralateral cerebral hemisphere.
- Noncerebral conditions that might mimic a prenatal or perinatal stroke include spinal cord injury, brachial plexus injury, and hypoplasia of the depressor angularis oris muscle.

feature in 57% (Wu et al. 2002). Persistent focal seizures in the term newborn, in the absence of infectious or metabolic etiologies, suggest that a stroke has occurred.

Diagnostic studies

Ultrasound and, often, noncontrast CT or MRI scans of the head are needed to recognize a recent infarct, hemorrhage, or other focal lesion (Figure 14.1). However, ultrasound may miss areas of infarction, and CT scan delivers high radiation to the developing neonatal brain. Therefore, MRI is the preferred imaging study, but may be limited by center availability. Diffusion- and/or perfusion-weighted MR imaging allows detection of acute areas of ischemia (Wardlaw & Farrall 2004), and MR angiography/venography can assist in the identification of arteriovenous malformations and sinovenous thrombosis. Limited information is available about the safety or yield of transfemoral angiographic studies; they are rarely performed and should be performed only at experienced pediatric medical centers.

If the injury is old, neuroimaging may reveal either a unilateral enlarged ventricle or an area of porencephaly, usually in the distribution of the middle cerebral artery.

In both groups—those with focal seizures and those with focal neurologic dysfunction—one should seek the etiologic factors described in the discussion of pathophysiology. In many cases the cause will not be identified; in many others more than one etiologic factor is present, producing a combination of interacting causes. Further diagnostic workup for perinatal arterial ischemic stroke, as well as sinovenous thrombosis, includes a complete prothrombotic workup. Evaluation of coagulopathy is needed in cases of perinatal hemorrhagic stroke, especially if an ongoing bleed is suspected. Transthoracic echocardiogram can help identify undiagnosed congenital heart defects associated with perinatal arterial ischemic stroke. Ongoing radiologic evaluation may be needed to evaluate the progression of sinovenous thrombosis, and also should be obtained for any change in neurologic examination for any of the stroke etiologies. If no cerebral lesion is found on CT or MRI, careful examination and

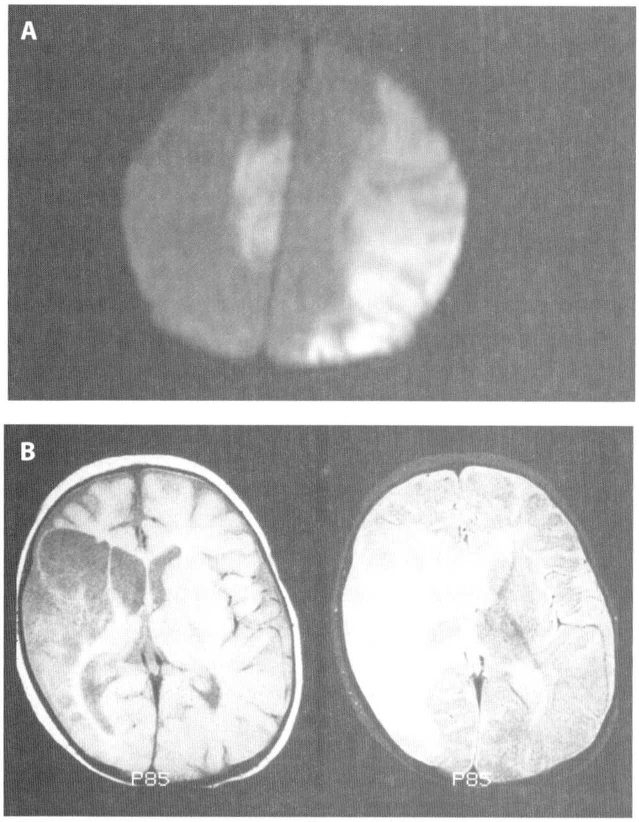

Figure 14.1 (A) Acute neonatal stroke in a term infant with an unremarkable labor and delivery presenting with a generalized seizure at 3 hours of age. The placenta showed an umbilical vein varix with an organized thrombus supporting the likely embolic origin of these ischemic strokes through a patent foramen ovale. This child later developed a hemiparesis and infantile spasms. The diffusion-weighted axial MRI at 8 hours of age shows restricted diffusion in the left middle cerebral artery distribution and in the right parasagittal area supplied by the right anterior cerebral artery. Time-of-flight MR angiogram shows lack of flow in the left middle cerebral artery (not shown). (B) A child who presented at 5 months of age with infantile spasms that responded to ACTH. At 15 years of age she has a left hemiparesis predominantly involving the upper extremity with mild learning disability and rare generalized tonic–clonic seizures. The brain axial MRI shows cystic encephalomalacia in the right middle cerebral distribution appearing as decreased signal on T1 and bright signal on T2 weighting indicating an old infarct.

localization to exclude a spinal cord process may require a spinal MRI. Peripheral nerve damage (that is, a brachial plexus injury) should be considered but is usually differentiated clinically from central lesions.

If a motor deficit of cerebral origin or seizures is recognized in the first year or two of life, and there is no indication of acute onset or acquired etiology, careful clinical follow-up to detect progressive diseases is essential. The workup includes MRI scan for structural lesions, EEG for functional lesions, and consideration of metabolic studies if no clear etiology is identified.

Treatment

Supportive therapy is the mainstay of neonatal stroke treatment. Thrombolytic agents such as tissue plasminogen activator (TPA) are not well studied in children; due to the possible increased risk of hemorrhage and unclear physiologic dosing in neonates it is rarely used. Progression of clot may be treated with heparin to prevent further neurologic deficit. Antiplatelet therapy, such as aspirin, is also not well studied in children and is not generally used in neonates in the United States. Although controversial, patients homozygous for methylene tetrahydrofolate reductase (MTHFR) mutation or with elevated homocysteine may be treated with folate. Recurrent seizures should be treated with anticonvulsants, at least over the short term. Daily head circumference should be monitored and neurosurgical consultation obtained as needed.

Although recurrent infarcts are rare in neonates (Fullerton et al. 2007), neonatal stroke is a profound risk factor for subsequent motor and cognitive impairment. Involvement of the basal ganglia and posterior limb of the internal capsule are associated with worse motor outcomes (Mercuri et al. 1999). All children with perinatal stroke should have close follow-up and early institution of physical, occupational, and language therapy if deficits emerge.

Hemorrhage

Intraventricular hemorrhage (IVH) is the major type of intracranial hemorrhage in the premature newborn. It originates from rupture of fragile blood vessels within the subependymal germinal matrix (Figure 14.2). The magnitude of this problem relates to direct correlation of IVH with the degree of prematurity, the improved survival rates for increasingly premature infants, and the persistent high rate of prematurity.

Intraventricular hemorrhage lesions are usually graded on radiologic criteria as follows (Papile et al. 1978a; Volpe 1995):

- *Grade I.* Subependymal (germinal matrix) only
- *Grade II.* Intraventricular blood with no ventricular dilatation

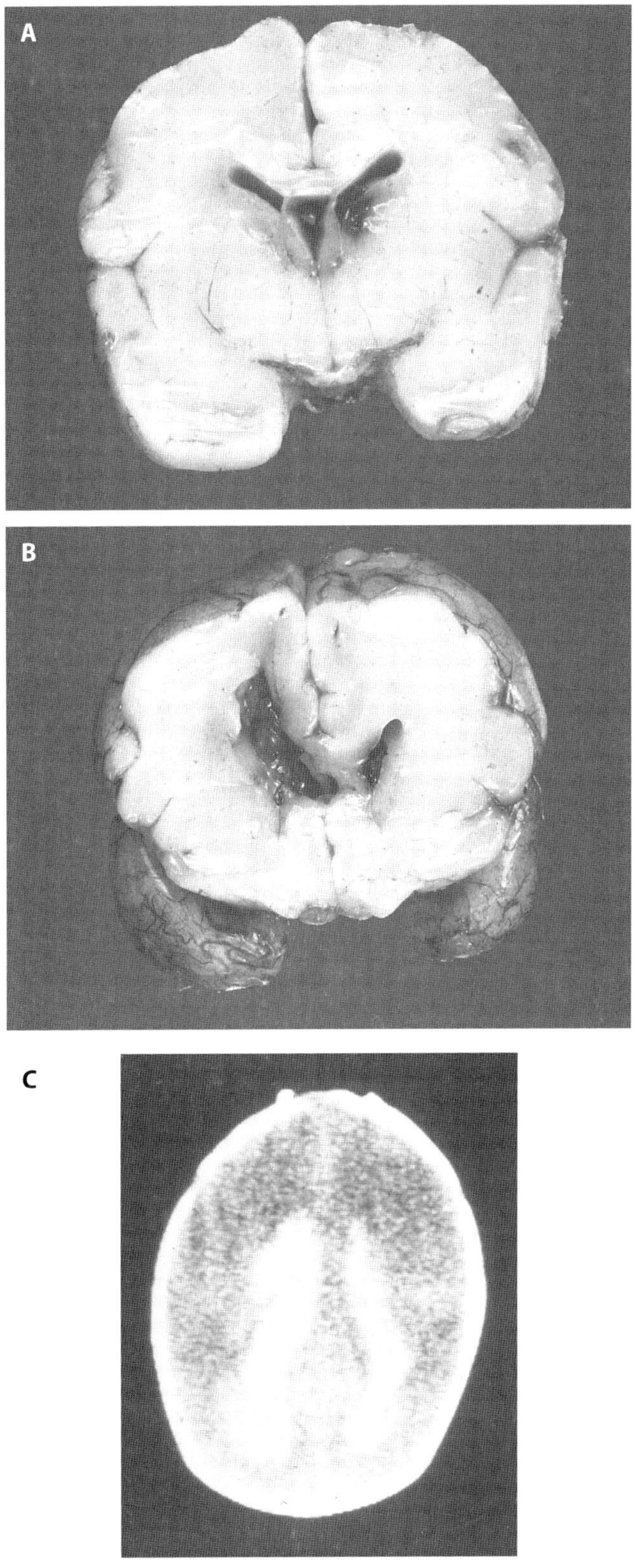

Figure 14.2 Pathological specimen of unilateral grade IV intraventricular hemorrhage in a preterm infant: (A) left-sided germinal matrix hemorrhage; (B) bilateral intraventricular hemorrhage with parenchymal hemorrhage on the right; (C) axial noncontrast head CT scan showing bilateral grade IV intraventricular hemorrhage in a different case.

- *Grade III.* Intraventricular blood with ventricular dilatation
- *Grade IV.* Intraventricular blood with ventricular dilatation plus parenchymal hemorrhage.

Grade IV IVH has been shown in a very meticulous pathology study to not involve parenchymal hemorrhage as much as ventricular extension into infarcted periventricular tissue. The pathology showed ependyma around the blood, including large, irregularly shaped hemorrhage (Paneth et al. 1990).

The forebrain germinal matrix is the source of cortical neurons in the first two trimesters and of supporting glial cells in the final trimester. Late in gestation, major changes occur. At this time, the germinal matrix is most prominent at the thalamostriate groove at the head of the caudate nuclei and is the most common site for hemorrhage. The matrix gradually decreases in size until it is nearly completely involuted by term, which helps explain why IVH is not a significant problem in the term infant. The majority of hemorrhages arise from the choroid plexus.

Histopathologically, germinal matrix hemorrhage is associated with primary or secondary infarcts, edema, parenchymal extension beyond the germinal matrix, rupture of overlying ependyma, and intraventricular blood clots. As a consequence, the germinal matrix is destroyed and approximately 15% of neonates with IVH develop unilateral hemorrhagic infarction in the periventricular white matter. Studies indicate that such hemorrhage represents venous infarction rather than extension of the IVH (Volpe 2001b). Later evolution of the lesions produces porencephaly in up to two-thirds of long-term survivors of grades III and IV hemorrhages. These multicystic or confluent areas result from associated leukomalacia and infarction.

The majority of neuropathologic studies support the view that most cases of parenchymal hemorrhage in grade IV IVH are due to ischemic hemorrhagic infarction, presumably as a result of impairment of venous drainage (deVries et al. 2001). The hemorrhages follow the medullary veins in the periventricular white matter and are most marked at the confluence of the veins adjacent to the ventricular angle (Gould et al. 1987; Volpe 2001b). These findings are supported by Doppler flow studies, MR spectroscopy (MRS), and MRI (Counsell et al. 1999; Dean & Taylor 1995; Toft et al. 1997).

The pathogenesis of IVH is multifactorial and involves intravascular, vascular, and extravascular factors (Volpe 1995). Intravascular factors are those that regulate blood pressure, volume, and flow. Vascular factors involve the vulnerable microvascular complex that comprises the germinal matrix. Extravascular factors are those referable to the space surrounding the germinal matrix capillaries, specifically the fragile and gelatinous supporting structures.

The risk of IVH increases with low Apgar scores, vaginal delivery, prolonged labor, blood pressure fluctuations, intrapartum hemorrhage, sepsis, coagulopathies, and rapid infusion of colloid. Defective or pressure-passive regulation of cerebral blood flow is a major risk factor (Lou & Friis-Hansen 1979); therefore, prevention of fluctuations in cerebral blood flow velocity is important. Extracorporeal membrane oxygenation (ECMO) has been associated with risk of IVH, with those infants of younger postconceptual age being the most at risk (Hardart et al. 2004). In a study of 74 term neonates exposed antenatally to cocaine, methamphetamine, or cocaine and a narcotic, 35% had IVH on ultrasonography (Dixon & Bejar 1989). Many cases are complicated by traumatic or hypoxic events at birth; however, in 25–50% of affected infants, no identifiable predisposing cause is found.

Intraventricular hemorrhage occurs in the first 3 days of life in 90% of cases. It is present by the end of the first postnatal day in 35–50% (Rumack et al. 1985). There are three clinical profiles, depending in part on the gestational age and on the general condition of the infant. The least common but most dramatic is a catastrophic presentation. An abrupt deterioration characterized by coma, posturing, seizures, fixed pupils, and apnea occurs in a previously stable neonate. Concurrent with this may be a falling hematocrit, metabolic acidosis, bradycardia, hypotension, and a bulging anterior fontanel. More common is a saltatory presentation, in which clinical deterioration occurs subacutely over several hours. This was highly associated with the development and subsequent abrupt decompression of a pneumothorax, the frequency of which has dramatically decreased with improvements in the respiratory management of premature infants. Most common is a clinically silent presentation, in which despite careful clinical assessment, no changes are noted. There can also be considerable overlap between the clinical profiles of premature infants with and without IVH. A valuable sign is an unexplained fall in hematocrit or failure to rise after transfusion. Although clinical signs, such as decreased tracking, abnormal popliteal angle, and decreases in tone or motility, are correlated with IVH in infants under 36 weeks gestation (Dubowitz et al. 1981), these symptoms are nonspecific. Less than 50% of IVH in premature neonates can be identified on the basis of clinical findings alone.

Diagnostic studies

Because of its bedside accessibility, ultrasound is the mainstay of diagnosis and follow-up for both IVH and its consequences. All high-risk babies should be routinely scanned at 3–4 days of age and at any time suggestive symptoms occur. Once IVH has been diagnosed, subsequent scans provide information on the evolution of the

Table 14.2 Intraventricular hemorrhage

Discriminating features
- Demonstration of the hemorrhage with head ultrasound or computed tomography (CT) scan

Consistent features
- Prematurity (in germinal matrix hemorrhage)
- Associated with hypoxia and ischemia or major cerebrovascular disturbance
- Blood in brain parenchyma and/or ventricles on CT scan

Variable features
- Associated parenchymal damage from periventricular leukomalacia, hemorrhagic infarction, or hematoma

hemorrhage, the development of hydrocephalus, the effect of treatment, and the development of encephalomalacia or porencephaly. Ultrasound has the advantages of having no ionizing radiation, being relatively cost-effective, and being easily portable (Table 14.2).

CT is preferred if subdural hematoma or acute hemorrhage in a cortical or superficial location is suspected. It can identify skull fractures and the outer table fracture of a cephalohematoma. As discussed earlier, MRI with diffusion weighting and FLAIR imaging is the best imaging method for infarction. Emergency MRI scans are not readily available in most centers, and the complexities of transport, monitoring, and ventilation of sick neonates limit its usefulness. High-resolution CT carries a significant radiation dosage (Huda et al. 2004) but its ready availability to the sick neonate, speed (resulting in a short time out of the neonatal unit), utility in the imaging of acute hemorrhage, and increasingly higher definition result in its continued usage. Electroencephalograph is helpful in detecting subclinical and subtle seizures and also has prognostic importance; amplitude-integrated EEG (aEEG) or cerebral function monitoring (CFM) are also gaining importance as diagnostic tools. Spinal fluid examination is poorly discriminating for IVH but is often important to evaluate the possibility of bacterial meningitis. The characteristic cerebrospinal fluid (CSF) profile in IVH is many red blood cells and elevated protein, followed by xanthochromia and a depressed glucose. In full-term infants with unexplained IVHs, laboratory evaluation should include platelet count, prothrombin and partial thromboplastin times, imaging to evaluate for cerebral venous thrombosis, and screening for illicit drugs in both the mother and baby.

Consider Consultation When...

- An infant is found to have intraventricular hemorrhage. Neurologic and neurosurgical evaluation and follow-up are needed.

Treatment

Clarification of the pathogenesis of IVH continues, and new approaches to reducing occurrence and improving outcome have resulted (Goddard-Finegold & Mizrahi 1987; Ment et al. 2004). Birth-related hypoxic–ischemic insult, impaired autoregulation of cerebral blood flow, and many secondary effects of these factors contribute. The best method of treatment is prevention. Prenatal intervention includes identifying women at high risk for premature delivery and providing appropriate care and education. When premature delivery appears inevitable, transporting the mother to a high-risk perinatal center and administering tocolytic agents and glucocorticoids are useful measures. Postnatal administration of phenobarbital, vitamin E, indomethacin, and fresh-frozen plasma have also been advocated to reduce the risk of IVH but remain investigational. Use of neuromuscular paralytics in ventilator-dependent infants has been shown to minimize erratic fluctuation in cerebral blood flow, hence minimizing incidence and severity of IVH. The goals of avoiding hypoxia, hypertension, rapid volume expansion, seizures, and excessive use of heparin in intravascular catheters are now often obtainable and remain important even after IVH has occurred. Studies vary on the effect of surfactant on IVH. Most studies have shown the incidence and severity of IVH to be either reduced or unchanged.

Severe IVH (grade III/IV) has declined with improvements in preterm infant care, with an incidence in infants weighing less than 1,500 g of 18% in 1987–1988 and 11% since 1993, but still accounts for significant morbidity and mortality (Fanaroff et al. 2003). The most recent reports do not demonstrate further improvement in IVH incidence in the last decade, although exact comparison between studies is difficult because study groups are of different gestational ages and birth weight and use different grading scales. In the Danish nation-wide study for 1994–1995, the incidence of grade III–IV IVH in survivors of less than 28 weeks' gestation or birth weight of less than 1,000 g was 10% (Kamper et al. 2004). The EPIPAGE study of nine regions in France in 1997 reported that, for gestational ages of 22–32 weeks, white matter damage was present in 22% and IVH, diagnosed by ultrasound, in 9% without ventricular dilatation and 3% with ventricular dilatation (Larroque et al. 2003). A New Zealand national study reported an incidence in 1998–1999 of grade II–III IVH in infants weighing less than 1,000 g of 9% and grade IV of 3% (Darlow et al. 2003). Indomethacin treatment in less than 1,250-g birth-weight infants significantly reduces IVH by 2.5 times in males (Ment et al. 2004); adoption of this approach should improve IVH incidence in the future.

All groups are at high risk for posthemorrhagic hydrocephalus, 35% of which will require shunting. This may be either obstructive at the fourth ventricle or aqueduct, or communicating due to occlusion of the arachnoid granulations responsible for CSF absorption over the surface of the brain. The management of posthemorrhagic hydrocephalus is complex because of clinical variables, limitations of the data available for individual patients, and limited knowledge of the risks and benefits of various approaches. Ventricular dilation spontaneously resolves in 65% of neonates. In the remaining 35%, dilation occurs rapidly (5%) or slowly (30%). A ventriculoperitoneal shunt may be placed if hydrocephalus is severe. Many infants with less severe hydrocephalus, if monitored with daily ultrasound examinations, have resolution of the problem without need for a shunt. Similar efficacy has been reported in a limited number of patients treated with acetazolamide (maximal dose 100 mg/kg/day) and furosemide (1 mg/kg/day) (Shinnar et al. 1985). An international study subsequently found no benefit to the combination treatment, and 24% of the combination treated infants developed nephrocalcinosis (1998). It is unknown if acetazolamide alone is beneficial. With serial lumbar punctures or acetazolamide treatment, close surveillance for the development of progressive hydrocephalus is essential. Having a high clinical suspicion of developing hydrocephalus is of the utmost importance, and daily head circumference measurements are a must in all infants.

Neurologic outcome

The long-term neurologic prognosis is clearly linked to the grade of IVH, presence of hydrocephalus, and degree of parenchymal involvement; however, multiple other factors also play a role. Short-term mortality is about 20% and occurs largely with grades III and IV lesions (McGuinness & Smith 1984). Progressive ventricular dilatation occurs in approximately half of the babies with IVH (usually 1–3 weeks following the hemorrhage), more often with grades III and IV hemorrhage, and in only 10% of grade I cases.

The long-term outcome for infants with IVH is one of markedly increased incidence of all major neurologic handicaps. Follow-up studies in 2003 confirm a 75% survival, with 70% of survivors developing mental retardation (Ment et al. 2005). Morbidity depends most on the degree of associated parenchymal injury. In cases complicated by periventricular hemorrhagic infarction or PVL, the evidence of severe neurologic sequelae approaches 90%. On the other hand, in infants with grade II IVH, 75% of infants have normal intellectual and motor development. Survivors of grades I and II IVH do not clearly have a worse outcome than similar-weight babies without IVH (Ment et al. 1985).

Infant, child, and adolescent ischemic disease

In this section, our approach to arterial and venous ischemic disease is etiologic and anatomic. Localizing information can often be obtained from the history and examination, as well as from neuroimaging. The ready availability of CT and MRI technologies allows a diagnosis of even small ischemic and hemorrhagic strokes in adults and children. Many of these would have remained unsuspected clinically. Incidence and prevalence figures produced in the past originate largely from clinical data and may underestimate the true incidence of childhood stroke.

Thrombotic occlusions of the carotid artery or branches of the middle cerebral artery are the most frequently documented causes of stroke in children. Over the 20-year period 1979–1998, analysis of the National Center for Health Statistics database revealed 244 deaths per year in the United States in children less than 20 years of age (Fullerton et al. 2002). Boys had an increased risk of death from subarachnoid and intracranial hemorrhage but not from ischemic stroke. Ischemic strokes accounted for 26% of deaths, with hemorrhagic strokes and subarachnoid hemorrhage accounting for 74%. Between 1979 and 1998 the death rate from stroke in children declined from 5.5 per million to 2.3 per million. The mortality from childhood stroke is fortunately low, and therefore the prevalence of this condition is far higher than the mortality figures suggest. Incidence of stroke in childhood determined in recent U.S. retrospective studies is 2.3 per 100,000/year (Fullerton et al. 2003). The Canadian Registry found an incidence of ischemic stroke alone of 7 per 100,000/year (deVeber 2003) and a prospective high-ascertainment study from France reported a total stroke incidence of 13 per 100,000/year, with 8% ischemic and 5% hemorrhagic (Giroud et al. 1995). Earlier retrospective studies found hemorrhagic stroke (subarachnoid hemorrhage and parenchymal hemorrhage) to account for 22–56% of pediatric stroke cases (Broderick et al. 1993; Earley et al. 1998; Lanthier et al. 2000).

The two basic pathophysiologic mechanisms involved in an ischemic stroke, regardless of age, are thrombosis and embolization. In adults, hypertension, diabetes mellitus, atherosclerosis, cardiac arrhythmias, and valvular abnormalities are the common underlying risk factors for stroke. However, in childhood, the potential etiologies are more variable and numerous. The pathophysiologic mechanisms are not always well understood.

Cardiac disorders

In most early series of pediatric stroke patients, congenital cyanotic heart disease is frequently identified as a predisposing factor for stroke. Tetralogy of Fallot and transposition of the great vessels account for most of the defects. The incidence of stroke in this population is 4%, and 75% occur within the first 2 years of life. Potential mechanisms of stroke include hyperviscosity due to polycythemia, diminished oxygenation, paradoxic emboli from right-to-left cardiac shunting, and emboli from vegetations secondary to valvular disease. Other abnormal structural defects predisposing to emboli include atrial myxoma, cardiac rhabdomyoma, cardiomyopathies, bacterial endocarditis, rheumatic heart disease, and prosthetic valves. Cardiac arrhythmias, particularly atrial fibrillation, also predispose to embolic phenomena. In a recent retrospective study of 212 children presenting with a first ischemic stroke, 22% had cardiac abnormalities but intracardiac thrombus was only identified in two cases (Ganesan et al. 2003).

Infectious disorders

A variety of infectious processes can lead directly to stroke. Meningitis in particular can produce intense basilar inflammation, locally damaging vessels in the circle of Willis and the anterior and posterior circulations. Pharyngitis, cervical adenitis, tonsillitis, sinusitis, retropharyngeal abscess, and tonsillectomy are all reported precursors of internal carotid artery thrombosis. The mechanism is thought to be local inflammation of the arterial wall. Less commonly, cat-scratch fever, ophthalmic herpes zoster, viral encephalitis (herpes simplex, Coxsackie virus A9, rubella), and *Mycoplasma* infections have been associated with cerebrovascular disease. The mechanism is again believed to be related to vasculitis with subsequent thrombosis. Acquired immunodeficiency syndrome (AIDS) is now responsible for an increasing number of exotic systemic and central nervous system (CNS) infections, which may produce embolic occlusion. Chickenpox is a major risk factor for childhood stroke. A recent British retrospective review of 212 patients admitted to a tertiary care pediatric hospital found a history of varicella zoster infection in the previous year in 18% (Ganesan et al. 2003). A prospective cohort study of 70 consecutive children with arterial ischemic stroke found a threefold increase in preceding varicella infection in the previous 12 months suggesting that varicella zoster infection accounts for one-third of childhood acute ischemic stroke (Askalan et al. 2001). These children also have a twofold increase in recurrent ischemic stroke and transient ischemic attacks. The most recent data shows that 30% of patients with varicella angiitis have no CSF pleocytosis and in 50% both large and small vessels are involved, with 97% showing abnormal MR or CT findings (Nagel et al. 2008).

Hematologic disorders

A variety of hematologic causes lead to arterial ischemic disease in children, although venous occlusion and hemorrhagic events may also occur in the same disease processes. Hyperviscosity syndromes (polycythemia vera, hyperleukocytosis [acute leukemia], and thrombocytosis [rarely]) can lead to arterial occlusion. Hemoglobinopathies, the prototype of which is sickle cell disease, are often complicated by stroke. The frequency of stroke in sickle cell disease is between 5% and 10%, with the median age of first stroke at 7 years of age. Recurrence occurs in up to 90%, most within 3 years. The Baltimore-Washington Cooperative Young Stroke Study reported an incidence of stroke in sickle cell disease in children ages 1–14 years as 285 per 100,000/year (Earley et al. 1998). Autopsy studies have revealed multifocal infarcts of various ages involving both large and small vessels. More recently MRI studies have shown a high incidence of vasculopathy and stroke in even asymptomatic sickle cell patients. Silent infarction (asymptomatic MR finding) was found in 35% of 185 patients with sickle cell disease studied at St. Jude's Hospital (Steen et al. 2003). This raises the question of the need for transfusion therapy in the asymptomatic patient. Patients on chronic transfusion protocols require chelation therapy. Use of ultrasound Doppler has been shown by the Stroke Prevention Trial in Sickle Cell Anemia (STOP) to be a useful screening tool for children with sickle cell disease at risk for stroke (Adams et al. 2004). Transfusion therapy is the mainstay for treatment of CNS symptomatic sickle cell disease; however, iron overload and transfusion reactions can limit its utility. Treatment with hydroxyurea, which stabilizes sickle hemoglobin, has been shown to decrease new stroke and recurrent stroke with efficacy similar to transfusion, preventing increases in Doppler velocities (Lefevre et al. 2008), and is advocated by consensus as an important treatment (Brawley et al. 2008). Nitric oxide (NO) resistance occurs in sickle cell disease, and inhaled NO has been suggested as a treatment (Wood et al. 2008). Bone marrow transplantation offers a potential cure. An excellent review discusses the management of sickle cell disease (Claster & Vichinsky 2003). Patients with hemoglobin SC disease and hemoglobin S-thalassemia are also at increased risk but tend to have milder courses. Patients with sickle cell trait are not at risk, although there have been rare reports of strokes occurring in this population (Greenberg & Massey 1985).

There has been a recent recognition of hypercoagulable states; some are genetically determined, some associated with autoimmune disorders, and some found to be independent of an underlying disease. Antithrombin III, protein C, and protein S are naturally occurring anticoagulants that have deficiencies that are inherited as autosomal recessive traits (Camerlingo et al. 1991). Homozygosity causes severe systemic disease, often with stroke. Affected patients are prone to both venous and arterial thrombosis. Heterozygosity is a predisposing factor to stroke. Acquired deficiencies of these proteins occur in various systemic diseases, particularly in liver disease and malignancies. The presence of antiphospholipid antibodies, which include the lupus anticoagulant and the anticardiolipin antibody, also predisposes the patient toward thrombotic events (Olson et al. 1994). These are found in 50% of children with systemic lupus erythematosus (SLE), but also in children with other autoimmune disorders and in some individuals without any apparent systemic disease. The presence of recurrent thrombosis and antiphospholipid antibodies in patients without features of lupus is called "the primary antiphospholipid syndrome." Thrombocytopenia and recurrent spontaneous abortions are important features of this syndrome. Recurrent thromboembolism occurred on follow-up in 3.3% of neonatal arterial stroke patients. Testing in pediatric patients should include C-reactive protein, factor V Leiden, lipoprotein-(a), prothrombin G20210A, protein C, protein S, and antithrombin. A guide to laboratory testing for the hypercoagulable state is available (Rahemtullah & Cott 2007). In five of seven cases of recurrent thromboembolism, prothrombotic risk factors, including the MTHFR C677T mutation, elevated lipoprotein-(a), hyperhomocysteinemia, or protein C deficiency, were involved in the recurrence (Kurnik et al. 2003).

Autoimmune disorders

Systemic vasculitic diseases may involve the CNS. Vasculitic damage to the arterial wall results in the development of local thrombi and the potential for occlusion and embolization. Small arterioles are generally involved in this process, but larger vessels may also be damaged. Both carotid and vertebrobasilar arterial distributions may be affected. In the case of SLE, neurologic involvement is seen in over 50% of patients. Arterioles are predominantly involved in this disease, with the production of microinfarcts leading to cortical atrophy. However, steroid treatment of these disorders may cause reversible shrinkage simulating atrophy. Polyarteritis nodosa, Wegener granulomatosis, Henoch–Schönlein purpura, ulcerative colitis, Kawasaki syndrome, and the dermatomyositis and polymyositis complex have had rare associations with childhood ischemic stroke. Takayasu disease ("pulseless disease") causes a large vessel vasculitis, affecting the aorta and its major branches. It, too, has been linked to childhood stroke, and occurs primarily in Asian teenage women. An idiopathic angiitis may involve only the CNS without systemic evidence of inflammation. Small or medium and large vessels may be affected. The patients with small-vessel involvement tend to present with chronic headache with focal seizures, or defects of mood or cognition in some. MRI scans typically have gadolinium-enhancing focal T2 signal hyperintensities that may simulate tumors. Patients with large-vessel involvement typically present with acute stroke. Immunosuppressive therapy should be initiated rapidly in these conditions (Lanthier et al. 2001). Central nervous system vasculitis in children has recently been reviewed (Elbers 2008).

Mechanical and toxin-related disorders

Trauma to the neck predisposes an individual to carotid thrombosis and dissection. This can be a blunt injury to the neck, intraoral trauma (for example, falling with a pencil in the mouth), or trauma to the cervical spine (for example, diving and trampoline injuries and contact sports). Cervical spine trauma and anomalies can lead to a vertebrobasilar occlusion. The vertebral artery is vulnerable to injury as it passes through the vertebral foramina. Arterial dissection was identified in 6.6% of 212 children presenting with arterial ischemic stroke (Ganesan et al. 2003) and in 15% of young adults with acute ischemic stroke (Williams et al. 1997). Dissection should be considered in any pediatric stroke patient and in cases with transient focal deficit, especially when vascular risk factors are absent. Even minimal trauma can, rarely, cause dissection. Diagnosis usually requires standard transfemoral arteriography or magnetic resonance angiography (MRA).

Emboli may be introduced into the cerebrovascular system by several different mechanisms. Fat emboli occur 12–24 hours after long-bone fractures. Iatrogenic causes include emboli from indwelling central venous catheters, fat emboli from parenteral nutrition, and accidental air emboli following thoracic surgery. A cardiac right-to-left shunt must be present for emboli to find their way to the cerebral circulation.

Various drugs, both illicit and legally prescribed, have been linked to ischemic and hemorrhagic strokes. Cocaine and crack cocaine, phencyclidine, lysergic acid (LSD), and amphetamines predispose an individual to vascular injury via hypertension and vasospasm, and may induce a vasculitic picture. Stroke following cannabis use has been described. Illegal drug use was noted in 12.1% of young adults with stroke in the Baltimore-Washington Young Stroke Study. Phenylpropanolamine, a legal stimulant that until recently was found in many over-the-counter cold medications, has been reported to induce a similar pathologic picture. Corticosteroids may cause endothelial hyperplasia and increase platelet adhesiveness. Birth control pills have been causally implicated in unexplained strokes in women, and contribute to stroke risk in teenage girls. Current pills, with lower doses of estrogen, are thought to have a much lower risk.

Primary vascular disorders

Despite increasingly sophisticated diagnostic technology, many children with strokes have no recognizable cause. They are assumed to have a primary vascular disorder.

Acute infantile hemiplegia refers to a condition in a young, previously healthy child with sudden hemiplegia, fever, coma, and seizures. Alternating hemiplegia of childhood also primarily affects young children. It is characterized by repeated attacks of abnormal eye movements and dystonic episodes followed by hemiplegic spells and autonomic disturbances, with gradual motor and mental deterioration (Mikati et al. 2000). Fibromuscular dysplasia is a systemic arterial disease primarily affecting middle-aged adults, which affects predominantly the renal arteries. When the internal carotid arteries are involved, aneurysms, thrombosis, and emboli may occur. Pathologically, fibrosis is present in the media, with associated hyperplasia of the intima or adventitia. Migraine-related stroke, although rare among all migraineurs, has been reported (Rossi et al. 1990). Conversely, migraines were causally implicated in as many as 25% of "idiopathic" strokes in young adults (Broderick & Swanson 1987).

Moyamoya disease (Suzuki & Takaku 1969) is characterized by an angiographic picture of progressive, occlusive disease involving unilateral or bilateral supraclinoid carotid arterial occlusion and the development of a fine web-like collection of abnormal anastomotic vessels at the base of the brain, particularly involving the circle of Willis (Figure 14.3). The name comes from the Japanese for "puff of smoke" describing the angiographic appearance of the abnormal vascular network. This disorder is usually bilateral. but initial motor and sensory symptoms in childhood (hemiparesis, involuntary movements, sensory impairment) are often unilateral. Headache is common, and seizures may be problematic. Mental retardation is a frequent outcome in moyamoya disease. The majority of cases are idiopathic; 10% are familial. Familial cases have been linked to chromosomes 6 and 17, with linkage to 3p24–26 found in Greek and Japanese families (Zafeiriou et al. 2003) and with polymorphisms found in tissue inhibitors of metalloproteinase genes at these sites (Kang et al. 2006). Adults more frequently present with sudden intracranial hemorrhage. Several associated conditions have been reported: post-irradiation therapy, neurofibromatosis, tuberous sclerosis, sickle cell disease, and Down syndrome (Pearson et al. 1985). Surgical treatment is available, utilizing a variety of methods to bypass stenotic or occluded vessels. Superficial temporal artery-middle cerebral artery anastomosis is an effective procedure but technically difficult in children under the age of 2 years.

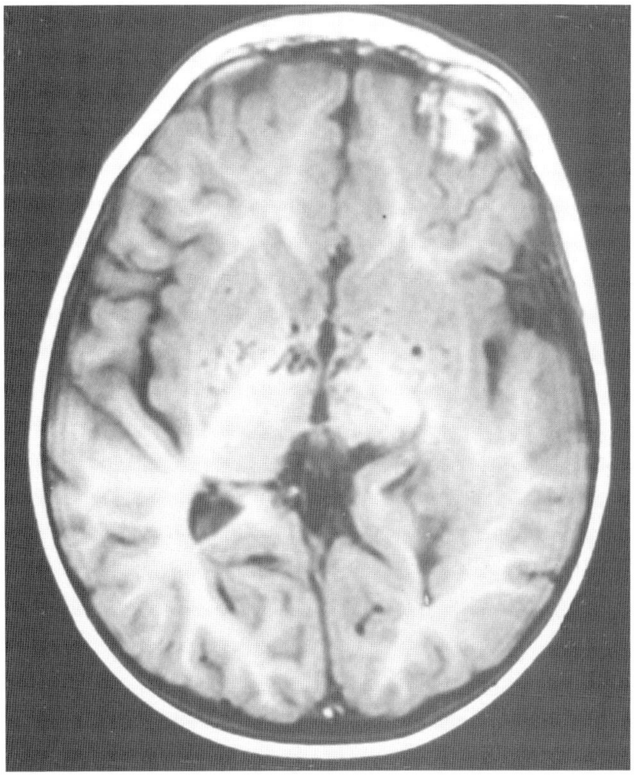

Figure 14.3 Moyamoya in a 16-month-old boy with seizures. Axial T1-weighted MRI image at the level of the basal ganglia shows multiple low signal intensity punctate areas in the lentiform nuclei bilaterally. These represent collateral vessels from the lenticulatostriates vessels. Incidently noted is the presence of heterotopic gray matter adjacent to the posterior portion of the left lateral ventricle. (Courtesy of Dr. Rosalind Dietrich.)

Hypoxic–ischemic injury

Hypoxic–ischemic injury is the most common cause of more widespread ischemic brain injury in childhood. Causal events include cardiorespiratory arrest, asphyxia, near-drowning, and hypotension. Damage tends to be widespread and bilateral, although preexisting variations in collateral blood supply may result in asymmetric lesions. Areas of the brain particularly susceptible to damage are those with a border zone or terminal end-arterial supply. Medial hemisphere infarctions occur in the border zone between the anterior and middle cerebral artery distributions, typically clinically affecting primarily the arms. Occipital infarcts producing cortical blindness are a common result of ischemia at the boundary of the middle and posterior cerebral artery distributions. Multiple rounded infarcts, which tend to be symmetric, are often found scattered throughout gray and white matter in these circumstances. The basal ganglia are largely supplied by the distal portions of small perforating arteries originating at the anterior portion of the circle of Willis, producing additional sites of enhanced susceptibility to hypoxic ischemic change.

Signs and symptoms

Patients with cerebral emboli typically present acutely with a sudden loss of neurologic function. Thrombi may present in a subacute fashion, with prodromal transient ischemic attacks or a stuttering course. There may be considerable overlap, and it may not be possible to distinguish an embolic event from a thrombotic event by clinical criteria alone. Signs and symptoms depend on the location and size of the occluded vessel, as well as the age of the patient. Children have anterior circulation strokes much more commonly than posterior strokes, and the left hemisphere is affected more often than the right.

Two-thirds of children present with an acute hemiplegia. Seizures, lethargy, or coma may complicate presentation. Prodromal self-limited episodes of hemiparesis are experienced in 25% of patients. Medical attention is often sought for these transient events but cerebrovascular disease is not usually considered at that time. The remainder present with a more indolent course noted over several weeks. A profound motor weakness (initially flaccid and later becoming spastic) is the most striking presentation, although some very young children have no clinical manifestations of major arterial occlusive disease. Pathologic early hand preference is commonly the presenting complaint. In these cases, the potential for recovery is so great that children may be seen without major deficit months or years after an ischemic event, despite large areas of brain infarction. Clinical signs may not be identified until brain maturation reaches a stage that allows for the expression of the clinical deficit.

Sensory symptoms and signs often accompany hemiplegia and may include visual field loss and loss of sensation in affected limbs. These signs are usually unilateral. Speech often becomes slurred (dysarthria), and language involvement is often seen when the language-dominant hemisphere is involved. Receptive and expressive dysphasias, as well as difficulty with reading, writing, and naming objects, may be demonstrated in older children. When arterioles or small arteries are involved in a thrombotic or embolic process, symptoms and signs are often subtle. This is particularly the case if the "silent" areas of the brain, such as the posterior parietal lobes or the frontal lobes, are involved. If only the vertebrobasilar system is involved, the child can present with any combination of brainstem, cerebellar, and occipital lobe dysfunction. Symptoms may include drowsiness, ataxia, vertigo, and visual loss. Signs may include eye movement disorders including internuclear ophthalmoplegia, and are referable to cranial nerves III, IV, and VI or their central connections. Ataxia and cerebellar or bulbar dysarthria are common in brainstem ischemia. Long-tract motor signs and sensory loss may occur. Respiratory abnormalities, including apnea, apneustic breathing, hyperventilation, and gasping or ataxic breathing patterns, may be seen. Children with large brainstem infarcts are usually comatose.

Diagnostic studies

The evaluation of a child with an acute deficit due to focal cerebral ischemia has two components. The first is to distinguish an ischemic event from other processes that might mimic it. The differential diagnosis of an acute focal loss of neurologic function in a child is listed in Table 14.3. Once an infarct is confirmed, the second component is to identify the underlying cause in hopes of preventing a recurrence.

As in all of medicine, nothing can replace a detailed history and physical examination including past medical, social, and family histories. Emphasis on the family history should include premature coronary and cerebrovascular disease suggestive of hyperlipidemia, unexplained thrombotic events suggestive of metabolic or hypercoagulable disorders, and migraines. Social history should include inquiries regarding drug and alcohol abuse, and risk factors for human immunodeficiency virus (HIV). Other potentially important historical items that might be overlooked include recent head or neck trauma (even mild),

Table 14.3 Differential diagnosis and discriminating features of acute focal loss of neurologic function

Condition	Discriminating features
Focal cerebral ischemia	History, neurologic examination, neuroimaging
Primary intracerebral hemorrhage	Neuroimaging
Traumatic epidural or subdural hematoma	Neuroimaging, neurologic examination, history
Subarachnoid hemorrhage	History, cerebrospinal fluid (CSF) studies, neuroimaging
Cerebral abscess	History, fever, neuroimaging
Epilepsy: Postictal Todd paralysis or a focal inhibitory seizure	History, neuroimaging without stroke, electroencephalograph (EEG)
Brain tumor (via hemorrhage, infarction, herniation, or hydrocephalus)	History, neuroimaging
Focal encephalitis	History, EEG, neuroimaging, CSF
Complicated migraine	History, family history, transient signs, normal neuroimaging
Acute demyelinating encephalomyelitis (ADEM)	History, neurologic examination, CSF, magnetic resonance imaging (MRI)
Alternating hemiplegia of infancy	History, neurologic examination, unrevealing diagnostic evaluation
Multiple sclerosis	History, neurologic examination, MRI, CSF studies
Malingering/conversion disorder	History, neurologic examination, exclusion of organic disease

migraine headaches, recent viral infection, and systemic signs such as rashes, arthralgias, fevers, and weight loss. A careful general examination includes the skin (in an attempt to locate rashes that might suggest an autoimmune disorder, stigmata of neurocutaneous syndromes, intravenous (IV) needle tracks, and evidence of systemic emboli) and particularly the cardiovascular system. The head and neck should be carefully auscultated for bruits. A thorough neurologic examination should always be performed and documented.

The MRI scan is the most sensitive method for detecting small or early ischemic lesions. Diffusion-weighted imaging is particularly useful early in the course (Soul et al. 2001). Posterior fossa and brainstem lesions are much more reliably seen on MRI than on CT. CT scanning, however, is more readily available and more suitable for seriously ill patients. It will detect most hemorrhagic and many ischemic lesions. However, a CT scan may not reveal ischemic changes for the first 12–24 hours following a stroke and may need to be repeated or followed up with an MRI scan.

The timing and role of cerebral angiography is controversial. It can be of value in localizing pathology, excluding arteriovenous malformations, and establishing prognosis. However, because of its invasiveness, associated risks, and possible need for general anesthesia, the physician should carefully consider the risk-to-benefit ratio before proceeding. Early angiography is generally recommended in cases of unexplained subarachnoid hemorrhage or recent trauma and if a surgically remediable lesion is likely. Regardless of timing, such a procedure should always be performed in a medical center with considerable pediatric experience. Magnetic resonance angiography and CT angiography (CTA) are noninvasive methods that have been growing in acceptance. Resolution of these newer methods is constantly improving but still lags behind traditional transfemoral angiography, especially in viewing small vessels, but it serves as a screen of the intracranial vasculature and images large vessels well. Magnetic resonance angiography or CTA can delay or avoid the need for a cerebral angiogram.

Identifying the underlying etiology in a child with a stroke may be a very simple process in some cases or can be a challenging and frustrating task in others. In a child known to have a predisposing cause or systemic illness such as congenital heart disease, meningitis, or sickle cell disease, the extensive evaluation suggested in Table 14.4 is not necessary. However, if preliminary evaluation fails to reveal a definitive cause, further testing is mandatory. Laboratory testing should be individualized to each patient. An organized, systematic approach is best. However, despite an extensive evaluation, Schoenberg and colleagues

Table 14.4 Investigative studies for systemic disease in cerebral ischemia

Disorder	Test
Infection, leukemia, polycythemia, thrombocytosis	Complete blood count, differential, platelet count
Meningitis, encephalitis with hemorrhage	Cerebrospinal fluid (CSF) analysis, magnetic resonance imaging (MRI) scan
Hemoglobinopathies	Sickle prep, hemoglobin electrophoresis
Vasculitis and autoimmune diseases	Erythrocyte sedimentation rate, C-reactive protein (CRP), antinuclear antibody, antineutrophil cytoplasmic antibodies (ANCA), rheumatoid factor, VDRL, complement profile, magnetic resonance angiography (MRA), angiography
Renal disease (hemolytic uremic syndrome), renal causes of hypertension, systemic vasculitis, diabetes mellitus	Blood urea, creatinine, electrolytes, calcium, phosphorus, glucose, urinalysis
Coagulopathies, disseminated intravascular coagulation (DIC), hypercoagulable states, thrombophilias	Prothrombin time, partial thromboplastin time, fibrin split products, platelet count, factor V Leiden, protein C and S (functional and immunologic assay) antithrombin III, antiphospholipid antibody (lupus anticoagulant, anticardiolipin antibody)
Cardiac source for emboli	Electrocardiogram (EKG), chest x-ray study, blood cultures, echocardiogram (transesophageal/contrast), Holter monitor
Homocystinuria, amino and organic acid disorders	Plasma amino acids and acyl-carnitine profile, urine organic acids
Mitochondrial encephalopathy, MELAS	Lactate (plasma and CSF), MRI and MR spectroscopy, mitochondrial DNA studies, muscle biopsy
Dyslipoproteinemias	Lipid profile (triglycerides, high-density lipoproteins, low-density lipoproteins), apolipoproteins A1 and B
Drug abuse	Urine toxicology

(1978) found that one-third of childhood strokes remain unexplained, leaving parents and physicians confounded. With current advances in understanding of the pathophysiology, with comprehensive evaluation and newer brain imaging techniques 15% of cases have no identified stroke risk factor (Lanthier et al. 2000). Transesophageal and saline contrast echocardiograms have increased the cardiologist's ability to detect subtle structural defects that are overlooked on transthoracic studies. Full evaluation for thrombophilias requires a panel of diagnostic testing, but hypercoagulable states may be difficult to diagnose because of the complexity of the involved pathways, often requiring hematologic consultation to evaluate effectively. Recognition of the potential importance of homocysteine, lipid, and mitochondrial disorders is important (see later section on metabolic strokes).

Treatment

The acute treatment of cerebral ischemia is largely supportive and requires an intensive care unit setting. Attention to oxygenation, fluid and electrolyte status, seizures, and infections is critical. If an underlying systemic disorder is identified, it is treated to reduce the risk of recurrence. Thus an aggressive diagnostic approach to evaluation is important for prevention of future episodes.

Cerebral edema is maximal over the first 72 hours. Initially, edema is cytotoxic, although a vasogenic component occurs after 2–3 days, following breakdown of the blood–brain barrier. Edema is usually effectively managed with hyperventilation and fluid restriction. In general, the use of steroids and osmotic agents is not indicated. However, in cases with progressive deterioration, mannitol (0.25–0.5 g/kg IV, repeated every 4–6 hours) and dexamethasone (0.5 mg/kg IV, repeated 0.25 mg/kg every 8 hours) may be used. However, mannitol may lead to rebound increase in intracranial pressure (ICP), and dexamethasone has not been proved to have clinical benefit. Hypertonic saline (7.2%) may be a useful treatment for intracranial hypertension in stroke (Forsyth et al. 2008).

The use of anticoagulation in ischemic stroke is controversial and places the child at risk for hemorrhage. It may be indicated in the presence of a continuing source of emboli or evolving thrombotic stroke. It is contraindicated in hemorrhagic infarct and uncontrolled hypertension. Long-term anticoagulation with warfarin has been advocated in deficiencies of proteins C and S and antithrombin III and in the presence of antiphospholipid antibodies (Khamashta & Hughes 1995). Low-dose aspirin, as an antiplatelet drug, is a consideration for patients when recurrent stroke is a concern, although controlled studies in children have not been performed. In patients with sickle cell disease, strokes should be initially treated with an exchange transfusion and then with a chronic transfusion protocol to maintain sickle hemoglobin at less than 20–30% (Wilimas et al. 1980). As discussed earlier, prophylactic transfusion in patients at high risk of stroke is advocated. Early thrombolytic therapy with IV tissue plasminogen activator (TPA) is recommended routinely in the United States in adults who present within the first several hours after an acute occlusive event (Lyden et al. 2001). Such approaches might be reasonable with children, although children with stroke rarely present for urgent treatment within the 3- to 6-hour window recommended for thrombolytic therapy. The time to diagnosis of stroke in one recent survey averaged 36 hours (Gabis et al. 2002). Preliminary investigative studies are also being performed on several cytoprotective agents. These include voltage-regulated calcium channel antagonists, N-methyl-o-aspartate channel antagonists, free-radical inhibitors, gangliosides, and opiate antagonists. Until lay and medical education succeeds in increasing awareness of the symptoms of stroke in childhood there will be few opportunities for early intervention.

Rehabilitation through aggressive physical, occupational, and speech therapy appropriate to the deficits is essential for all patients. Behavioral problems and learning disabilities may become apparent on returning to school, and children may require neurocognitive testing and counseling.

The outcome following a childhood stroke is dependent on numerous variables: the type of stroke, the location of the lesion, and the underlying etiology (Table

Pearls and Perils

Infant, Child, and Adolescent Ischemic Disease

- In infants, the symptoms and signs of cerebral ischemia may be subtle. A high index of suspicion is needed.
- Neuroimaging studies may be needed to diagnose small ischemic lesions and define the extent of larger lesions. Computed tomography (CT) scan may not reveal ischemic changes for the first 12–24 hours following a stroke and may need to be repeated or followed up with magnetic resonance imaging (MRI). MRI or CT should be obtained in all cases.
- A history of previous transient neurologic deficit suggests the possibility of complicated migraine, seizures, hysteria, or, rarely, demyelinating disease.
- In children, as in adults, transient ischemic attacks may be a prodrome to an ischemic stroke.
- Delay in the identification of underlying disease may allow recurrent ischemic episodes.
- Anticoagulation should be used only after very careful consideration and then only in cases with clear evidence of continued risk for continuing thrombosis or embolization.

Table 14.5 Infant, child, and adolescent ischemic disease

Discriminating features

- Focal infarction on computed tomography (CT) or magnetic resonance imaging (MRI)

Consistent features

- Children with cerebral ischemia lose neurological function in ischemic areas of brain. This loss may be temporary or permanent. It may not be detectable clinically or by neuroimaging. Thus there are no consistent features of cerebral ischemia.

Variable features

- Headache
- Focal seizures
- Predisposing disease
- Clinical presentation of brain ischemia ranges from very subtle changes in mentation to gross motor deficit with or without coma
- Small lesions may not be seen on neuroimaging studies. CT scanning may miss early ischemia and often cannot detect abnormality when lesions are isodense 1 week after the ischemic event. MR diffusion and perfusion weighted imaging are best for early identification of ischemic stroke

14.5). The prognosis after a cerebral ischemic event in childhood is thought to be better than for adults. The plasticity of the developing brain is one reason for the improved outcome. Although survival is expected in almost all patients, residual deficits persist in the majority (Schoenberg et al. 1978). Recovery from hemiparesis follows the same pattern in children and adults; recovery of the ability to walk occurs faster and more completely, whereas recovery of the fine movements of the hand occur over a longer period of time. Although there may be residual motor deficits, early-onset unilateral focal stroke has a good prognosis for cognitive outcome but subtle residual findings such as hemispacial neglect may persist (Trauner 2003). The prognosis for language and cognition is less good with bilateral cortical injury.

Metabolic strokes

Many serious metabolic disorders produce cortical infarction, which is often multifocal. In lactic acidemia, the organic acidemias, and hyperammonemic states, cerebral ischemia and infarction may occur, particularly during episodes of severe metabolic decompensation. Several inborn errors of metabolism have strong associations with childhood strokes.

Basal ganglia infarction is often seen in disorders of oxidative metabolism such as Leigh disease, methylmalonic and propionic acidemias, glutaric aciduria, and molybdenum cofactor deficiency or sulfite oxidase deficiency. Stroke-like episodes in a nonvascular distribution are seen in mitochondrial cytopathies and in particular in mitochondrial myopathy and encephalopathy with lactic acidemia and stroke-like episodes (MELAS). Fabry disease and carbohydrate glycoprotein deficiency syndromes are storage disorders associated with stroke. Disorders of lipid metabolism continue to generate interest. As in adults, high-density lipoproteins (HDLs) are considered to be protective to vascular endothelial cells, whereas low-density lipoproteins (LDLs) are thought to be toxic. Although hypercholesterolemia is a known risk factor for adult coronary and cerebrovascular disease, its effect is long term. Although lipid-induced arteriopathy begins in childhood, stroke and coronary artery disease from this cause are adult phenomena. Progeria, familial hypoalphalipoproteinemia, Tangier disease, and several other familial forms of hypercholesterolemia are conditions associated with stroke in children and young adults.

Homocystinemia

Elevated blood homocysteine levels can result from homozygous or heterozygous mutations and are very common in the adult stroke, peripheral artery disease, and coronary artery disease populations. Folate supplementation is thought to decrease the risk (Boushey et al. 1995). Homocystinuria, an autosomal recessive condition due to one of several enzyme deficiencies, may present as a thrombotic syndrome. In its homozygous form, this error of methionine metabolism is associated with a marfanoid body habitus, lens dislocation, and mental retardation. High levels of homocysteine lead to endothelial damage and increased platelet aggregation. Homozygosity for the thermolabile tetrahydrofolate reductase gene tMTHFR was found in 18 of 119 children presenting with a first arterial ischemic stroke, and seven other children had high homocysteine levels. Thus 25% of children with ischemic arterial strokes had a risk of homocystinemia (Ganesan et al. 2003). Young adults heterozygous for homocystinuria are also at increased risk (Boers et al. 1985; Clarke et al. 1991). Such patients may respond to dietary changes and supplementation with vitamin B_6, vitamin B_{12}, or folic acid.

Mitochondrial myopathy, encephalopathy, lactic acidosis, and stroke-like episodes

The phenotype of MELAS was recognized as a distinctive syndrome in 1984 (Pavlakis et al. 1984). The majority of cases are due to a pathogenic mitochondrial DNA mutation in one of the leucine tRNAs, A3243G. Like most mitochondrial disorders MELAS is a multisystem disorder with short stature, cardiac, and renal and gastrointestinal (GI) dysfunction commonly seen. Diabetes and deafness are the most common manifestations. Basal ganglia disease is often present, with calcification often noted. Stroke-like episodes in nonvascular distributions are common, in particular in the occipital lobes, producing cortical blindness. These lesions are to some extent reversible, and diffusion-weighted MRI suggests an element of cytotoxic edema (Wang et al. 2003); in addition, there is also a likely vasogenic component due to oxidative phosphorylation failure in the endothelium.

Organic acidemias and fatty acid oxidation defects

Propionic and methylmalonic acidemias are classical organic acid disorders and both are associated with "metabolic strokes" affecting the basal ganglia. The etiology of these strokes is not thought to be vascular but rather is the result of mitochondrial failure impacting a particularly vulnerable part of the CNS. In propionic acidemia, these lesions may progress to hemorrhagic infarction with fatal outcome (Haas et al. 1995). In methylmalonic acidemia, acute metabolic decompensation may be associated with acute basal ganglia metabolic strokes, and diffusion-weighted MRI can discriminate acute from chronic lesions (Burlina et al. 2003).

Fatty acid oxidation defects may produce basal ganglia strokes, as well as more widespread atrophy and white matter disease. Glutaric aciduria type 2 is due to a deficiency of electron transfer factor (ETF) or, in the more severe form, the ETF dehydrogenase enzyme. As in other forms of mitochondrial disease, the presumed mechanism is localized mitochondrial failure coupled with the accumulation of toxic metabolites. Patients may present with an athetoid cerebral palsy picture due to these lesions.

Hypoglycemia

Profound symptomatic hypoglycemia may produce stroke. Surprisingly, lesions are often unilateral despite the generalized nature of the insult. Insulin-dependent diabetics are most prone to this complication, but it occurs in sepsis and hepatic failure. Hypoglycemia may complicate metabolic decompensation in a number of metabolic inborn errors, in particular glycogen storage diseases and disorders of fatty acid oxidation. Patients often present with obtundation, sympathetic overactivity (tachycardia, sweating, dilated pupils), and focal or generalized seizures. Urgent diagnosis and treatment of hypoglycemia with IV 25% dextrose is necessary, and prompt treatment may limit brain damage. If there is a possibility of Wernicke encephalopathy, intravenous thiamine 250 mg should be administered with glucose.

Fabry disease

In Fabry disease, an X-linked lysosomal storage disorder, glycosphingolipid storage occurs due to deficiency of alpha-galactosidase. Ceramide trihexoside is the storage material, and it is found predominantly in vascular endothelium (intima and media) in multiple organs. This leads to stroke, painful neuropathy, coronary artery occlusion, and renal failure. Patients also have characteristic nonblanching clusters of small, dark, vascular, reddish skin lesions—*angiokeratomata*—and may develop cataracts. Untreated affected males have a mean age of stroke at 34 years, showing T2 hyperintense lesions on MRI in 100% of cases older than 54 years (Crutchfield et al. 1998). Less commonly, females can be symptomatic as manifesting carriers. There may be a positive family history. Onset of symptoms of the neuropathy is in the teenage years or earlier, with complaints of pain in the hands and feet. Strokes affect the posterior circulation predominantly (70%) with small perforating arteries in the anterior circulation another common site. It is important to make the diagnosis of this disease, as effective treatment with enzyme replacement is now available. Patients are also treated prophylactically with antiplatelet agents.

Cerebral veins and sinuses

The cerebral veins and sinuses provide the major drainage pathway of intracranial blood and sites of CSF reabsorption. A thrombosis involving these structures leads to increased ICP by interfering with the outflow of blood and CSF. Specific clinical syndromes occur depending on which vessels are obstructed. Sinovenous thrombosis is most common in infancy and in the neonate. In 160 consecutive children with sinovenous thrombosis enrolled in the Canadian Pediatric Ischemic Stroke Registry, 43% were neonates and 54% were younger than 1 year old. A prothrombotic state was present in 41%, an acute systemic disease in 54%, with bacterial systemic infection in 9%. Chronic systemic disease was present in 36%, dehydration in 25%, and head and neck infection in 18% (deVeber & Andrew 2001).

The pathophysiologic mechanisms affecting the cerebral venous system can be divided into those related to local infection of the head or neck and "primary" cerebral venous or dural sinus occlusions, which usually occur in a child with a systemic illness.

Many of the previously discussed systemic diseases that cause arterial occlusion also affect the venous system. The most common cause of dural sinus thrombosis is dehydration, especially hypernatremic dehydration. This is a problem generally occurring in infants and young children with acute gastroenteritis. Such children are often hypotensive and acidotic, compounding the ischemic insult. Hematologic causes include hemoglobinopathies (particularly sickle cell disease) and hypercoagulable states. As noted earlier, deficiency of pro-

Pearls and Perils

Cerebral Veins and Sinuses

- Severe headache with a rapid deterioration in consciousness is a common presentation of extensive cerebral venous or dural sinus thrombosis.
- An urgent computed tomography (CT) scan helps exclude other causes and may confirm the diagnosis. Early radiologic study is important if the diagnosis is to be confirmed.
- An urgent magnetic resonance imaging (MRI) scan provides the best noninvasive test for cerebral venous or dural sinus thrombosis, but risks of transport and difficulties with patient monitoring in the scanner may be contraindications for MRI in sick and unstable patients.
- Urgent treatment of the precipitating cause and of raised intracranial pressure is essential.
- Anticoagulation therapy has risks and is generally contraindicated in patients with hemorrhage.
- Prolonged seizures, hypoxia, or hypotension increase the cerebral insult.

tein C, its cofactor protein S, and antithrombin III can lead to arterial occlusion; however, venous thrombosis is more common. This tends to be seen in older children and adolescents heterozygous for these proteins. Homozygous deficiency of protein C presents in the newborn with purpura fulminans. Genetic thrombophilias were present in four out of seven neonates with sinovenous thrombosis. Three had factor V Leiden heterozygosity and one had MTHFR homozygosity (Wu et al. 2002). Acquired protein S and antithrombin III deficiency are sometimes associated with L-asparaginase therapy, the nephrotic syndrome, and protein-losing enteropathy. Children with cyanotic congenital heart disease are at increased risk for cerebral venous thrombosis, accounting for 5% of cases (deVeber & Andrew 2001), primarily owing to increased viscosity due to polycythemia and diminished oxygen transport. Oncologic causes of venous thrombosis include direct invasion of cerebral veins and dural sinuses with tumor cells. Both primary CNS tumors and secondary tumors, particularly neuroblastomas, can cause thrombotic complications. Venous thrombosis may complicate radiotherapy for neoplasms. Hyperleukocytosis from leukemia can lead to sludging of blood in the venous system and subsequent infarcts. The primary inborn error of metabolism linked to venous thrombosis is homocystinuria. Infections of the head or neck adjacent to veins or dural sinuses may involve the wall of the vessel and produce local inflammation and thrombosis. The most common cause of cerebral vein thrombosis is purulent meningitis. Cortical vessels running through the subarachnoid space are particularly susceptible to injury in meningitis. Stroke from venous thrombosis is a major cause of neurologic sequelae in meningitis, and small cortical strokes may be missed unless searched for by MRI. Meningitis can produce major ischemic injury.

Trauma may produce local venous or dural sinus damage, leading to thrombosis. Infection secondary to trauma produces an additional risk of thrombosis. Infectious causes of dural sinus thrombosis are usually close to the site of infection. Otitis media and mastoiditis may cause lateral sinus thrombosis. Facial soft tissue, periorbital, paranasal, or frontal sinus infections may produce cavernous sinus thrombosis. Infectious sagittal sinus thrombosis usually arises from retrograde spread from dural sinuses involved in a head or neck infection. In these hemorrhagic infarctions, edema is often more marked than with arterial occlusive disease, and thus raised ICP is a common problem. The edematous phase can last for several days and presents a major management challenge. Neuronal and glial necrosis occurs in the infarcted area, and ultimately macrophages remove necrotic material, leaving a cystic cavity.

Generalized or extensive cerebral vein or dural sinus thrombosis is usually rapidly fatal. In neonates, the usual presentation is nonfocal, with seizures in 71%, encephalopathy, often with a decreased level of consciousness in 36%; however, 29% had focal neurologic signs (deVeber & Andrew 2001). The older child presents with a rapidly evolving encephalopathic picture (90%) consisting of confusion, headache, irritability, seizures (48%) (deVeber & Andrew 2001), and increasing lethargy as the ICP rises. Localized thrombosis of cerebral veins or dural sinuses can produce more focal CNS signs. Depending on the vessels involved, various clinical syndromes can occur. The most dramatic constellation of signs arises from cavernous sinus thrombosis, which is

Key Clinical Questions

- Has sinovenous thrombosis been considered in the differential for a deterioration in neurologic status?
- Has sinovenous thrombosis been considered in an infant or older child, particularly if seizures are present? Such patients will deteriorate as intracranial pressure increases and should be monitored in an intensive care unit.
- Has magnetic resonance imaging (MRI) scanning included MR angiography in any child with a possible diagnosis of sinovenous thrombosis?
- Have plasma homocysteine and a comprehensive evaluation for thrombophilias been carried out in confirmed cases of sinovenous thrombosis?

fortunately rare. Impaired drainage of the ophthalmic veins and direct involvement of cranial nerves III, IV, V (first division), and VI lead to a chemosis, exophthalmos, unilateral fixed-dilated pupil, ptosis, decreased facial sensation, strabismus with a severe headache, and eye pain. Sagittal sinus thrombosis and the resultant impairment of parasagittal cortical venous drainage tend to produce bilateral cortical signs, seizures, and deepening coma. Lateral sinus thrombosis impairs venous drainage from the ipsilateral cerebellum and occipital lobe, producing visual field loss and ataxia along with headache. Because the right lateral sinus is often larger than the left, a right-sided thrombosis is more likely to be clinically evident. Thrombosis of the sagittal sinus or lateral sinus may lead to a generalized increase in ICP. When otitis media or mastoiditis leads to such a scenario, the term *otitic hydrocephalus* has been applied.

Diagnosis of cerebral vein or dural sinus thrombosis is usually difficult. Only in the case of cavernous sinus thrombosis are there discriminant symptoms and signs. Differential diagnosis includes toxic and metabolic causes of coma, viral encephalitis, bacterial meningitis, and cerebral abscess, as well as the various causes of intracranial hemorrhage. Lumbar puncture reveals raised pressure, and CSF will often be xanthochromic or blood-tinged.

Neuroimaging studies are warranted (Table 14.6). Because of the tendency for occluded veins and sinuses to recanalize, studies must be carried out early, preferably within 48 hours. With CT scanning, hemorrhagic infarctions are seen adjacent to the venous thrombosis, and edema is usually obvious. A ring or delta sign on CT scanning occurs when IV contrast material surrounds the thrombosis. MRI with MRA is the study of choice. A dural sinus thrombosis is seen as an area of high signal intensity on the T-weighted image, which replaces the normally low-signal sinus.

Table 14.6 Cerebral veins and sinuses

Discriminating features

- History of gradual deterioration helps discriminate between arterial ischemia and cerebral venous or dural sinus thrombosis
- Cerebral edema is often severe in venous infarction
- Neuroimaging studies provide the best confirmatory test

Consistent features

- Location and extent of both cerebral venous thrombosis and dural sinus thrombosis determine the physical findings
- Headache is generally present
- Raised intracranial pressure is usual

Variable features

- Focal findings may be seen in localized cerebral vein or dural sinus thrombosis
- Usually irritability, lethargy, and generalized symptoms of pressure are seen
- In some patients, fluctuating neurologic signs are found

Consider Consultation When...

- An infant or child with gastroenteritis develops seizures, irritability, or decreased level of consciousness.
- A febrile child develops acute headache.
- Signs or symptoms of raised intracranial pressure (vomiting, bradycardia, hypertension, sixth or third nerve palsy, decreased conscious level) develop in a child with systemic illness.

A good outcome can occur in isolated sinus thrombosis if ICP is controlled. Treatment is thus primarily supportive and directed at control of intracranial pressure, cerebral edema, seizures, and the predisposing cause of the thrombosis, whether it is local infection or a systemic disorder such as dehydration. In acute and extensive thrombosis, dexamethasone (0.25–0.5 mg/kg IV, then 0.25 mg/kg every 8 hours) for 3–4 days then gradually tapered may be helpful in controlling edema. A pressure bolt or ventricular catheter allows accurate ICP monitoring and may be useful. Mannitol is generally to be avoided, particularly in patients who are dehydrated, because it may lead to further thrombosis. Antibiotics are initially given empirically. In patients with raised ICP, repeated lumbar puncture may save vision and should not be delayed if visual impairment is present or if there is any concern that medical therapy is not working. Use of anticoagulants has been controversial. Because hemorrhage is often present, use of anticoagulants is generally contraindicated. Yet, in one study of adult patients, the majority of heparin-treated patients made a complete recovery (Rousseaux et al. 1985). The use of anticoagulants has not been established in childhood; however, in patients who are clinically deteriorating despite symptomatic treatment, IV heparin is an option (Solomon et al. 1970), and subcutaneous low-molecular-weight heparin may be considered. The benefits of anticoagulation may outweigh the risks in such cases. In a prospective pediatric study of unfractionated heparin in 65 children, of which 13 of the subjects were newborns, no significant bleeding occurred (Andrew et al. 1994).

Intracranial hemorrhage in infancy and childhood

Outside of the neonatal age group, the incidence of childhood intracranial hemorrhage is similar to that of ischemic infarction. In the Baltimore-Washington Cooperative Young Stroke Study, 18 children with ischemic infarction and 17 with intracerebral hemorrhage were identified (Earley et al. 1998). Children with intraparenchymal and subarachnoid hemorrhage (SAH), similar to adults, typically present dramatically, with the sudden onset of severe headache, vomiting, meningismus, and progressive neurologic deterioration. Hemorrhage may occur following a primarily ischemic event due to any of the previously mentioned causes (hemorrhagic conversion) or can occur because of an underlying vascular abnormality, such as an aneurysm or vascular malformation. Other less common conditions also deserve consideration. Trauma, a common cause of intracranial hemorrhage, is discussed elsewhere in the text.

Although 5–7% of the population develops an intracranial arterial aneurysm of 2 mm or larger by the time of death, aneurysms are very rare in children. There is a slight predominance in boys (1.5:1 male-to-female ratio). Most present after 10 years of age, although they rarely may be observed in infancy.

Intracranial aneurysms

Intracranial aneurysms can be divided into three types: congenital, traumatic, and infectious, which occur in the proportions of 75%, 15%, and 10%, respectively, during childhood. Childhood aneurysms are more variable and more peripheral in location when compared with those in adults. Most (85%) are located in the anterior circulation, particularly at the bifurcation of the internal carotid artery and in the anterior cerebral artery–communicating artery complex, although the most common site varies from study to study. Cerebral arteriovenous aneurysms were reported in 35% of 17 neonates presenting with massive cardiomegaly in the first 10 days of life (Kachaner et al. 1977). Multiple lesions are rare and raise the possibility of bacterial aneurysms from infected emboli.

The main histopathologic features are abnormalities of the elastica and media portions of the arterial wall, with inflammatory changes in infectious cases. Unlike in adults, saccular, fusiform, or irregular aneurysms are less common. A clot is usually present in some portion of the lumen. A mural defect responsible for hemorrhage can often be found. Perivascular and extensive subarachnoid blood is the rule. Traumatic aneurysms are less common in children, occurring mainly in adolescence. Ninety percent are located in the anterior circulation, predominately on the anterior cerebral artery and its branches. Their pathogenesis is presumed to be due to arterial wall damage following closed head injuries.

Infectious aneurysms comprise 2–5% of all intracranial aneurysms. They may be separated into true mycotic aneurysms (fungal) and the much more common bacterial aneurysms (usually staphylococcal). Infectious aneurysms have a far higher relative incidence in children than in adults. They occur in children with congenital heart disease involving bacterial endocarditis and less commonly are seen as a complication of a local infection, such as meningitis or sinusitis. The mortality rate is as high as 18%.

Intracerebral hemorrhage complicates aneurysmal SAH in 25–50% of cases. Although vasospasm complicates SAH in 30% or more of children, it does not seem to affect the outcome as it does in adults. Most studies indicate that the majority of aneurysms (up to 95%) are asymptomatic until they rupture. The sudden onset of a severe headache (often described by the patient as "the worst headache of my life"), associated with focal neurologic deficits and frequently followed by diffuse cerebral dysfunction of mild to profound extent, represents a clinical picture as characteristic in children as in adults (Table 14.7). A retrospective history of headache is present in 20%. Because some children bleed at the time of or soon after head trauma of variable severity, aneurysm may not be considered and may be missed on head CT scan. Vasospasm, or obliteration of the aneurysm may compromise detection. Mass effect from enlarging giant aneurysms has been described as producing progressive lower cranial nerve, brainstem, and oculomotor nerve dysfunction, as well as hydrocephalus owing to aqueductal compression. Seizures may occur early if the bleeding occurs near the cerebral cortex but are uncommon except in infancy. Blood spilling into the subarachnoid spaces causes meningismus, fever, leukocytosis, nausea, and vomiting. Examination may show nuchal rigidity, alteration of consciousness, and focal deficits referable to cranial nerves or any portion of the cerebrum or brainstem. Bruits are rare. Retinal hemorrhages can occur. Although ICP is generally elevated and the fontanel reflects this in infants, papilledema is uncommon. If the patient is seen early, progression of these findings is frequent, may be very rapid, and is of ominous significance.

Giant aneurysms (>25 mm) represent 5% of aneurysms if all ages are considered; however, in childhood, they represent up to one-third of aneurysms often

Table 14.7 Aneurysms

Discriminating features

- Neuroradiologic demonstration of the aneurysm on computed tomography (CT) with contrast or magnetic resonance imaging (MRI)
- Confirmation with MR angiography (MRA) or cerebral angiogram

Consistent features

- Symptoms or signs of acute subarachnoid hemorrhage (SAH)

Variable features

- Antecedent headache (20% of patients)
- Focal cerebral ischemia secondary to vasospasm

Pearls and Perils

Aneurysms

- Consider associated medical conditions in children with aneurysms.
- Unusual severe, sudden-onset headache in children deserves evaluation.
- Prognosis for a child with an aneurysm is better than that for an adult with similar involvement.
- Consider infectious aneurysm if lesions are multiple and/or congenital heart disease is present.
- An unruptured aneurysm may produce a mass effect.
- An aneurysm or other vascular anomaly should be considered in any child with unexplained subarachnoid hemorrhage (SAH) or intraparenchymal hemorrhage.
- If the clinical picture suggests a SAH and the computed tomography (CT) scan is normal, a lumbar puncture should be performed.

presenting in the first year of life with mass effect, seizures, and hydrocephalus.

Cerebral aneurysms have been associated with several medical conditions. Genetically acquired disorders include the autosomal dominant adult form of polycystic kidney disease (more rarely, the childhood autosomal recessive form), Ehlers-Danlos syndrome, Marfan syndrome, pseudoxanthoma elasticum, tuberous sclerosis, and Klinefelter syndrome. Other conditions include fibromuscular dysplasia and coarctation of the aorta. The association of aneurysms with cysts and malformations, such as agenesis of the corpus callosum, suggests a developmental basis for some aneurysms.

Diagnostic studies

Early recognition is important, and hemorrhage is most readily first demonstrated by CT. However, a CT scan might not detect the hemorrhage if the amount of intracranial blood is small or the study is delayed until several days after the bleed. MR with FLAIR is more sensitive than CT for detection of SAH. Five percent of CT scans will be normal if performed on the first day of a SAH. If the study is delayed to the third day, this number increases to 25% owing to rapid reabsorption of blood. Hence, if the clinical picture strongly suggests SAH, and the CT is normal, CSF analysis for xanthochromia or red blood cells should be performed. A CT scan with contrast will detect lesions larger than 15 mm, whereas the resolution of the MRI is sufficient to detect 3- to 5-mm aneurysms. CT angiography is another noninvasive option. An MRA or CTA is performed followed by catheter angiography if needed.

MRA is a noninvasive option; however, its resolution for small vessels is still below that of the cerebral angiogram, which remains the gold standard. The angiogram provides the diagnosis and the basis for planning surgery, and is optimally performed in medical centers with expertise in pediatric neuroradiologic and neurosurgical procedures. The timing of the initial studies is based first on the need to establish a diagnosis in an acutely ill child in whom the differential diagnosis includes not only aneurysm and arteriovenous malformation but also neoplasm, meningitis, hemorrhagic encephalitis, hemorrhagic infarction, and trauma. Additionally, the timing, especially of angiography, should be related to the total management approach to the lesion, in coordination with the neurosurgical consultant. Factors to be considered are time since bleeding, condition of the patient, medical therapy modalities, and preferred time of surgery. A common current approach in cases arriving within 24 hours of the event is early angiography, with subsequent management planned thereafter. In the case of unruptured aneurysms, this study helps define the prognosis, because the probability of rupture increases with size. Interventional radiography treatments are available for smaller lesions; however, surgery is generally indicated if the diameter is greater than 10 mm because of the high risk of a fatal hemorrhage.

In many ways more difficult for the physician is the approach to the unfounded anxiety that parents have about the possibility of an unruptured aneurysm, particularly in children with chronic headaches. This fear is often based on the occurrence of rupture in an acquaintance or a relative and is precipitated by a severe headache in the child. The associated conditions listed earlier should be considered. Barring evidence for these, or a family history of aneurysm, CTA or MRA can be deferred. Clearly, in most cases, reassurance rather than MRA or angiography is appropriate. A brain MRI scan may be indicated in some cases of chronic headache, primarily to exclude tumor. Reports of familial occurrence of aneurysms are rare.

Improved treatment of ruptured aneurysms appears to have lowered mortality, particularly in the first 24 hours. However, 40–60% of adult patients still die or survive significantly disabled. The functional survivors are predominantly from the early-diagnosis group hospitalized in a neurologic center. Children do better than adults

Key Clinical Questions

- Is urgent pediatric neurosurgery available? If not stabilize and arrange transfer to a specialized pediatric neurosurgical unit.
- Is magnetic resonance angiography (MRA) and angiography urgently available?
- Is there evidence of possible infected embolism?

Consider Consultation When...

- A child presents with sudden onset severe headache or coma.
- Meningismus is found with red cells in the cerebrospinal fluid (CSF).
- Head computed tomography (CT) scan shows subarachnoid blood.

when operated on early, and there is a greater risk of rebleeding if not surgically treated (Wojtacha et al. 2001). The patient's level of consciousness on admission is the most important predictor of survival. Surgical mortality for clipping is less than 10%. In one series of 33 children, surgical mortality was 3%, and 80% of patients had no deficit except on psychometric testing (Heiskanen & Vilkki 1981). Given the high mortality from rebleeding, early surgery is usually indicated for alert patients. Authors disagree about the benefit of surgery for the moribund child. The good results in children from aneurysm clipping raise the question of the role of endovascular detachable coil treatment by interventional radiology in children. In adults, the International Subarachnoid Aneurism Trial has shown that this procedure has a lower morbidity and mortality than surgery (Molyneux et al. 2002). In the case of an asymptomatic unruptured aneurysm, studies have also revealed a 1–2% risk of rupture per year. The cumulative rate of rupture was 35% at 15 years (Yasui et al. 1996). Lesions greater than 5 mm are believed to have an increased risk. In experienced centers, the rate of mortality and morbidity in resecting such lesions approximates 5%. Hence any patient with a life expectancy of greater than 3 years should benefit from intervention.

Treatment

Treatment advances include endovascular detachable coil treatment, the care of intracranial hypertension, supportive intensive care, and prevention of rebleeding by surgical means. The treatment of vasospasm continues to be controversial. No controlled studies have demonstrated benefit from use of antifibrinolytic agents (aminocaproic acid) and calcium-channel blockers (nimodipine) in children with SAH. Bacterial aneurysms are treated with prolonged courses of antibiotics continued for 4–6 weeks. Half will resolve and one-third will decrease in size using this approach. Intervention is indicated if the aneurysm is unchanged or larger on repeat angiogram.

Vascular malformations

Four major types of congenital vascular malformations exist: arteriovenous malformations (AVMs), venous angiomas, cavernous angiomas, and capillary telangiectasia. Arteriovenous malformations, in which there is a direct connection of arteries and veins, most frequently produce clinical symptoms, with 10% manifesting in the first decade.

Pathophysiology

Vascular malformations vary greatly in location, size, number of arteries, character of the abnormal vessels, and changes over time. All consist of a mixture of normal and abnormal blood vessels. Fibrosis, inflammation, and gliosis surround the lesions, and calcification within the malformation are common. The most common lesion is the AVM "proper." In this lesion, one (60%) or several arteries drain directly into venous channels, without intervening capillaries. Both the arteries and the veins may be either enlarged, normal, or anomalous vessels. Locations are parietal in 30% of patients, frontal in 17%, occipital in 10%, temporal in 10%, and in the basal ganglia in 16%. Specimens show unsuspected old hemorrhage in 10% of cases.

Venous angiomas are the most common asymptomatic vascular malformation and are present in 2.6% of persons coming to autopsy (Sarwar & McCormick 1978), more than four times the incidence of AVMs. They are pathologically distinct, and consist of a convergence of multiple venous channels into a single anomalous draining vein. Up to 20% may calcify. Cavernous angiomas are malformations in which large, venous channels form a complex mulberry-like meshwork. No intervening brain parenchyma is present. These lesions are frequently multiple, and various parts of the CNS, as well as other organs (retina, liver, kidneys, or skin), may be affected. They occur predominantly in frontal and parietal regions and are much less frequent than AVMs. A significant familial incidence has been reported, compatible with an autosomal dominant trait (Rigamonti et al. 1998). Capillary telangiectasias are much smaller than any of the malformations mentioned earlier and occur in the posterior fossa (pons and medulla) and in the subependymal region in the cerebral hemispheres. A hemorrhage in these areas can be catastrophic.

Cryptic vascular malformations are sometimes found on pathologic examination. They are hypothesized when a patient presents with intracerebral hemorrhage and/or SAH, but angiogram, surgical specimen, or autopsy fail to demonstrate a specific lesion. Patients with AVMs may present with acute intracranial hemorrhage, ischemia, seizures, or a bruit. Arteriovenous malformations are occasionally discovered incidentally or during evaluation of extensive cutaneous hemangiomas.

Signs and symptoms

If a primary SAH occurs, the signs and symptoms are the same as for aneurysms—that is, severe headache with meningeal signs. If it is intraparenchymal, focal neurologic signs develop, often with increased ICP. For either type of hemorrhage, symptoms at presentation may be sudden and catastrophic or gradually progressive, or they may fluctuate (Table 14.8). Seizure is the first symptom in one-third of AVMs, and 50% of adult patients with AVMs have seizures preoperatively with a reduction by half after surgery (Thorpe et al. 2000). Other series have reported 89% of patients were seizure-free postoperatively (Piepgras et al. 1993). Of patients presenting with seizure, 20–70% hemorrhage before their AVM is diagnosed. In children, presentation with seizures is less frequent than in adults (21%), and surgery seems more effective at seizure control when γ-knife surgery is employed (Gerszten et al. 1996). Headache is a symptom in 70% of cases, and altered state of consciousness is present in 35%. Ischemia may result from a distal thrombotic infarction, in which case it may produce focal signs. A "steal" syndrome can produce ischemia of variable degree, with reversible dysfunction, but at times resulting in infarction of deprived areas. After bleeding, vasospasm may produce ischemia.

Many children with intracranial AVMs have bruits heard over the head; however, bruits are common in children without vascular malformations, especially in those with heart murmurs. Occasionally they are reported by the child. The vast majority are not due to AVMs. Bruits over the great vessels of the neck, which are particularly common, are usually modified by turning the head in various directions, and rarely indicate pathology. Conversely, bruits heard in infants younger than 4 months are almost always associated with AVMs regardless of the presence of cardiac murmurs (Cohen & Levin 1978).

Cavernous angiomas typically present with seizures, headaches, and intracranial hemorrhage in adults. Venous angiomas and capillary telangiectasias are usually asymptomatic but may have a presentation similar to AVMs. Seldom are either of these associated with bruits.

Diagnostic studies

CT scan with contrast usually reveals the abnormality. However MRA is more sensitive and specific. Recently susceptibility-weighted MRI has been shown to be particularly useful in the diagnosis of AVMs (Tong et al. 2008). Cerebral angiography not only confirms the diagnosis of AVM, but also defines major feeding and draining vessels—a step critical in deciding therapeutic options. If the hemorrhage is recent, angiography may fail to reveal the malformation, either because the lesion was obliterated by the hemorrhage, vasospasm, or clotting within the malformation.

Table 14.8 Arteriovenous malformations

Discriminating features
- Radiologic demonstration, angiography

Consistent features
- None

Variable features
- Occurrence of headache, seizure, bruit, signs and symptoms of hemorrhage
- Neurologic symptoms and signs depending on size and location of lesions
- Natural history and surgical risks

Pearls and Perils

Arteriovenous Malformations (AVMs)

- Bruits over AVMs may be limited to a 1-cm diameter spot on the skull; one may have to search to find the spot.
- Most neck and cranial bruits in children are of no significance. However, bruits heard in infants younger than 4 months are almost always associated with AVMs.
- It is easy to confuse the clinical manifestations and cerebrospinal fluid (CSF) findings of aseptic meningoencephalitis with traumatic tap on the one hand and subarachnoid hemorrhage (SAH), especially from AVM, on the other. Care to observe the color of spun CSF for the presence or absence of xanthochromia and to compare red and white blood cell counts in two tubes usually prevents this error.
- It is easy to confuse the presentation of AVM with seizures or stroke with the occurrence of other symptoms from other etiologies. This again emphasizes the need for thorough workup in cerebrovascular disease of childhood.
- Seizures with encephalopathy are possible with bleeding AVM.
- Signs of SAH or focal deficit may be due to parenchymal hemorrhage with bleeding AVM.
- AVMs which have not bled are usually clinically silent.
- Venous angiomas are usually benign

Treatment

The mortality rate in patients with the first bleed from an AVM is 5–25%, and the morbidity rate is 50%. Rebleeding occurs in 25–50% of patients, with a higher mortality rate of 28–41%. The risk of rupture in incidentally discovered AVM is 3–4% per year, with a 1% annual risk of death. Smaller lesions (diameter less than 3 cm) have a higher risk of rupture because of higher feeding arterial pressure (Spetzler et al. 1992). Surgery gives excellent results in selected cases, with a low rate of morbidity or mortality. Conservative treatment has a high long-term risk: roughly 20% mortality, 30% of patients disabled, and 11% of patients with moderate dysfunction in variable follow-up periods in reported series;

however, recent data confirm that the risk of rupture in AVMs that have not bled is lower than previously thought, questioning the need for surgery in these patients (Hartmann et al. 2007)

Initially, treatment is supportive: maintaining oxygenation and the airway, monitoring of fluid and electrolyte balance, and administration of steroids if herniation is threatened. Surgical approaches vary from occlusion of feeding arteries to total excision, and both strategies may be implemented in stages. Interventional neuroradiology with embolization aiming to occlude feeders is an option. A flexible approach that includes combinations of methods has been advocated (Stein & Wolpert 1980a; 1980b). For small, surgically inaccessible locations, stereotactic γ-radiation is relatively safe and effective.

Unruptured venous angiomas should be considered incidental lesions that do not require surgical intervention. These malformations have a low risk of bleeding. Removal has resulted in venous infarcts, because these lesions often provide the primary venous drainage for the adjacent brain. In the rare instance of associated hemorrhage, a cavernous angioma or other source of hemorrhage should be sought. In two studies, the risk of rupture in cavernous angiomas was found to be 0.25–0.7% per year (Del et al. 1991; Robinson et al. 1991). Outcome in both studies was uniformly good. Hence surgical resection is not recommended unless recurrent hemorrhages occur or there is progressive neurologic deterioration or intractable seizures.

Vein of Galen malformation

Vein of Galen malformations are the most common AVM presenting in the neonatal period, comprising 63% of such malformations presenting before 6 months of age. They result from a direct connection between the carotid or vertebral arteries and the vein of Galen. The vein of Galen is enlarged due to high pressure and in some cases is malformed.

Signs and symptoms

A patient with a vein of Galen malformation can present in one of three ways depending on the size of the malformation and blood flow. The largest lesions present in the neonate with high-output congestive heart failure due to massive shunting of blood flow. On examination, a systolic heart murmur, a wide arterial pulse pressure, a loud cranial bruit, hepatomegaly, tachycardia, and respiratory distress are noted. The shunt may produce a cerebral steal syndrome sufficient to produce cerebral ischemia.

Older infants with smaller shunts may present with hydrocephalus, dilated scalp veins, bruits, seizures, and hemorrhage. Hydrocephalus is a result of aqueductal compression by the malformation. Much less common is presentation in later life with headaches and signs typical of an intracranial bleed.

Diagnosis

Diagnosis depends on proper clinical suspicion when faced with unexplained congestive heart failure in the setting of a cranial bruit. Ultrasound of the head may reveal the malformation, which should then be confirmed by MRI or CT. Angiography aids in planning therapy.

Treatment

Treatment options are limited. Neonates are usually in a fragile cardiovascular state, rendering surgery difficult. Congestive heart failure is treated with digoxin and diuretics. Surgical outcome traditionally has been poor. At major pediatric centers, staged procedures involving selective embolization and microsurgical techniques have been more effective.

Other intracranial hemorrhages in childhood

Intracerebellar hemorrhage is similar to posterior fossa subdural hematoma in newborns in regard to predisposing factors and the clinical picture; however, neurologic outcome is much poorer. Clinical features indicating a significant cerebral insult may lead to discovery of this lesion. Recent reports and personal experience indicate that, even with no specific therapy, the outcome can be good (Koch et al. 1985) (Table 14.9).

Any bleeding disorder may cause intracranial hemorrhage, which can be subarachnoid, subdural, or intracerebral. Primary processes include sickle cell disease and those conditions that are associated with coagulopathy, primarily the hemophilias and idiopathic thrombocytopenic purpura. In hemophilia, 25% of patients have an intracranial hemorrhage; 40% of deaths and 10% of all bleeding episodes involve intracranial bleeds. Secondary

Pearls and Perils

Other Intracranial Hemorrhages in Childhood

- Always consider the possibility of child abuse. The history is usually factitious, and there may be no external sign of trauma because of impact with padded surfaces. Retinal hemorrhages, if present, are a strongly suggestive sign.
- Consider both encephalitis and various causes of intracerebral hemorrhage when multifocal dysfunction and multiple lesions on imaging are present.
- Transfer the patient with intracranial hemorrhage to a neurosurgical center.

Table 14.9 Other intracranial hemorrhages in childhood

Discriminating features
- Results of neuroimaging studies
- Laboratory tests for the various underlying medical conditions

Consistent features
- These conditions have a predisposing traumatic or medical basis

Variable features
- Size of hematoma or amount of cerebral damage, even in apparently similar circumstances
- Early clinical course in cases with life-threatening lesions

causes include hepatic dysfunction, disseminated intravascular coagulopathy (DIC), thrombocytopenia (platelet count <20,000), hemorrhagic disease of the newborn (due to vitamin K deficiency), and various hypercoagulation states, including those in dehydration of infancy, diabetic ketoacidosis (Atluru 1986), collagen vascular diseases, dysproteinemias, parasitic infections, poststreptococcal glomerulonephritis, and moyamoya disease.

Bleeding into neoplasms occurs at all ages and should always be considered in the differential diagnosis of an intraparenchymal hemorrhage, particularly in adults. Abuse of sympathomimetic drugs such as phenylpropanolamine, cocaine, and amphetamines has also been associated with intracranial hemorrhage. Intraventricular hemorrhage has been reported in infants born to cocaine- and methamphetamine-abusing mothers (Dixon & Bejar 1989). Cocaine causes intracranial aneurysms in young patients, which may bleed (Nanda et al. 2000).

Separate mention should be made of the potential confusion, clinically and on imaging studies, of hemorrhage in necrotizing encephalitis, particularly that due to herpes simplex virus, as opposed to bleeding from vascular lesions or other causes listed earlier. In addition to a careful history and physical examination, MRI, CSF analysis, and EEG are the most useful early diagnostic tests for encephalitis.

Pearls and Perils

Spinal Cord Vascular Disease

- In acute spinal cord syndromes, treatable causes of cord compression must be urgently excluded with magnetic resonance imaging (MRI) or myelography.
- If there is subarachnoid hemorrhage and no cause can be found on cerebral angiography, a spinal arteriovenous malformation (AVM) should be considered.
- A segmental cutaneous angioma over the spine should raise suspicion of a spinal vascular malformation.

Spinal cord vascular disease

Pathophysiology

In theory, the spinal cord is susceptible to the same systemic disorders that produce vasculitis and thrombosis in cerebral arteries. In practice, however, spinal cord ischemia is rare in childhood. This may in part be due to the extensive blood supply of the spinal cord. The anterior and posterior spinal arteries have a limited anastomosis and are supplied by several arterial branches at various levels of the cord. The anterior two-thirds of the spinal cord is supplied largely from branches of the anterior spinal artery. The levels of maximal susceptibility to generalized ischemia lie at arterial border zones, usually located at the lower cervical and lower thoracic levels of the spinal cord. Tumor and arteriovenous malformation are the most common lesions causing cord ischemia. Cord compression or vascular steal reduces the blood supply, resulting in ischemia. Sickle cell disease has been reported with thrombosis of spinal cord vessels (Rothman & Nelson 1980). Severe scoliosis can compromise flow in the anterior spinal artery, but actual cord ischemia is rare in scoliotic patients. Traumatic lesions to the spinal cord generally produce contusion without arterial or venous thrombosis, although epidural and subdural hematomas can produce cord ischemia by vascular compromise. Iatrogenic causes of spinal cord ischemia are important but fortunately rare. Umbilical artery catheterization in the newborn is associated with a significant risk of aortic, iliac, and femoral artery thrombosis. In some of these infants, the arterial supply to the spinal cord is in jeopardy. Surgery for aortic coarctation is associated with symptoms of cord ischemia in some patients. Usually this ischemia is reversible, but some patients are left with irreversible cord infarction.

Signs and symptoms

The clinical signs of spinal cord ischemia depend on the level of the lesion. Initially, a cord shock syndrome is seen at and below the level of the lesion. Later, this evolves into

Key Clinical Questions

- Is there loss of neurologic function below the level of the lesion? A sensory level may be identified.
- Is pain present? Pain is a common manifestation of both acute and chronic lesions. This is an uncommon symptom in childhood and should trigger a high index of suspicion for spinal cord pathology.

Consider Consultation When...

- A child presents with an acute focal neurologic deficit.
- The etiology of an apparent cerebrovascular event cannot be readily identified.
- A child with a recent hemorrhage or ischemic stroke has progressive neurologic deterioration.

upper motor neuron signs of spasticity below the level of the lesion, with flaccidity and areflexia confined to the level of the cord infarction itself. A dermatomal level of sensory loss may be present. Bladder and bowel function is often affected, with urinary retention most common. The anterior spinal artery syndrome is characteristic, with loss of anterior cord function and preservation of the dorsal column functions of vibration and joint position sense.

Diagnosis and treatment

Diagnosis of spinal cord ischemia in childhood is made when signs of partial or complete ischemic damage to the cord appear and a predisposing cause is apparent. Cord ischemia is usually a sudden event, although a more stuttering progression of symptoms and signs may be seen, and clinical presentation may be delayed for some hours (Lenn 1977). Causes of spinal cord compression and ischemia, including AVM, tumor, abscess, or transverse myelitis, must be identified. MRI provides an excellent view of the spinal cord without bony artifact, but CT myelography is still necessary in selected cases.

Treatment is supportive. Early use of high-dose corticosteroids decreases spinal cord edema and may significantly improve outcome, depending on the etiology. Hypotension, which may further damage the ischemic cord, must be avoided. An organized spinal cord injury protocol should be instituted at once. Urinary retention requires catheterization. Early passive and later active physical therapy is important to prevent joint contractures and improve residual function. The prognosis depends on the extent and duration of the ischemic insult.

A spinal cord syndrome due to a vascular malformation is rare in childhood. Venous angiomas are the most common vascular malformation of the spinal cord but are usually asymptomatic. In childhood, the cervical region is the most common site for an AVM.

Half of the lesions are intramedullary, 20% are extramedullary, and 30% are mixed. Associated skin lesions have been described in 20–35% of cases, consisting of a port wine stain or the cutaneous manifestations of Osler-Weber-Rendu disease, Klippel-Trenaunay syndrome, familial hereditary cutaneous hemangioma, or Cobb syndrome (Barek et al. 1982). When a spinal AVM and cutaneous hemangioma are both present (20–30% of cases), they are in the same dermatome in almost half the cases. Spontaneous spinal epidural hematomas have been attributed to cryptic vascular malformations (Posnikoff 1968).

Spinal vascular malformations

Spinal vascular malformations may present acutely or insidiously. Acute presentation due to SAH may occur with sudden motor impairment, which includes severe local back pain that may radiate. Pain and paresthesias follow a dermatomal pattern. However, the majority of patients present with a slowly progressive spastic paraplegia and bowel and bladder dysfunction. Pain is a common feature in this group. A bruit over a spinal AVM is rare.

Diagnosis and treatment

Spinal cord AVMs are difficult to document. CT alone is not useful. MRI and MRA are often diagnostic. If the AVM is localized to the dura, a myelogram may be the only revealing study. Myelography demonstrates some abnormality in almost all spinal AVMs but often does not discriminate the nature of the lesion. Treatment options for intraspinal vascular malformations are similar to those for intracranial malformations.

Acknowledgments

The authors would like to thank their coauthors on previous versions of this chapter, Harry S. Abram, MD and Nicholas J. Lenn, MD, who are major contributors to this work. Dr. Rosalind Dietrich generously provided many MR and CT figures.

Annotated bibliography

Chabrier S, Buchmuller A. Editorial comment—specificities of the neonatal stroke. *Stroke* 2003;34:2892–2893.
An interesting two-page discussion of current issues in neonatal stroke.

Claster S, Vichinsky EP. Managing sickle cell disease. *BMJ* 2003;327:1151–1155.
A comprehensive but readably brief review of the complications and current treatment of sickle cell disease.

Counsell SJ, Rutherford MA, Cowan FM, Edwards AD. Magnetic resonance imaging of preterm brain injury. *Arch Dis Child Fetal Neonatal Ed* 2003;88:F269–274.
A comprehensive overview of MR neuroimaging techniques and the application to preterm brain injury. This paper is the product of experience with one of the few MR scanners located within a tertiary care neonatal unit, the Hammersmith Hospital, London.

deVeber G. Risk factors for childhood stroke: Little folks have different strokes! *Ann Neurol* 2003;53:149–150.
An authoritative, brief overview of risk factors for childhood stroke provided by one of the chief investigators in the Canadian Pediatric Ischemic Stroke Study Group.

Earley CJ, Kittner SJ, Feeser BR et al. Stroke in children and sickle-cell disease: Baltimore-Washington Cooperative Young Stroke Study. *Neurology* 1998;51:169–176.

A report on one of the largest U.S. pediatric stroke epidemiology studies.

Gordon AL, Ganesan V, Towell A, Kirkham FJ. Functional outcome following stroke in children. *J Child Neurol* 2002;17: 429–434.

An outcome report on the long-term effects of childhood stroke on affected children and their parents and families.

Roland EH, Hill A. Germinal matrix-intraventricular hemorrhage in the premature newborn: Management and outcome. *Neurol Clin* 2003;21:833–851, vi–vii.

An authoritative review on the current state of IVH management and outcome.

Stiles J, Reilly J, Levine S, Nass R. Prenatal stroke: Effects and outcomes. In: Yeates KO, Ris MD, Taylor G, Pennington B, eds. *Pediatric neuropsychology: Research, theory, and practice.* New York: Guilford, 2008.

An up-to-date review of current knowledge about outcomes of prenatal stroke.

Tong KA et al. Susceptibility-weighted MR imaging: A review of clinical applications in children. *AJNR* 2008;29(1):9–17.

A review of a new MR technique particularly useful for the evaluation of vascular disease in infants and children.

Volpe JJ. Neurobiology of periventricular leukomalacia in the premature infant. *Pediatr Res* 2001a;50:553–562.

An excellent comprehensive review article on PVL etiology and prevention.

Volpe JJ. *Neurology of the newborn*, 5th ed. Philadelphia: Elsevier, 2008.

The best authoritative comprehensive text on neonatal neurology, with in-depth discussions of prenatal, perinatal cerebrovascular disease in preterm and term infants.

Wu YW et al. Perinatal stroke in children with motor impairment: A population-based study. *Pediatrics* 2004;114(3): 612–619.

A large population-based case control study identifying preeclampsia and IUGR as risk factors for perinatal arterial stroke.

CHAPTER 15

Inborn Errors of Metabolism I: Neurologic Degenerative Diseases

Paul Maertens

Outline

- Polioencephalopathies
- Leukoencephalopathies
- Corencephalopathies
- Spinocerebellopathies
- Diffuse encephalopathies

Neurodegenerative diseases with onset in utero, infancy, childhood, or adolescence make up a sizable portion of the practice of pediatric neurology. Our knowledge of the incidence of such disorders is inexact and varies from one reporter to the next. This variation is explained in part by lack of consensus on progression, the major feature of neurodegenerative diseases. Most would agree that progression is characterized by a subacute or chronic clinical course. A normal, early psychomotor development is observed in most patients. In some patients with degenerative disease beginning in utero, significant clinical and pathologic features are present at birth, leading to the erroneous diagnosis of static dysgenetic encephalopathy (e.g., Zellweger syndrome). The early phase of normal development is usually followed by a phase of developmental slowing. In some conditions, duration of this phase is so long that diagnosis of cerebral palsy is mistakenly suspected (e.g., Pelizaeus-Merzbacher disease). After developmental slowing, most patients reach a plateau phase before entering a phase of deterioration leading to death. One exception to these rules is Rett syndrome, which starts with a phase of deterioration followed by another phase of slow development or plateau. Our understanding of mechanisms responsible for these various patterns of presentation in neurodegenerative disorders is still fragmentary.

This chapter is organized as an overview of some of the more characteristic neurologic degenerative diseases encountered in pediatric neurology, presented in the manner suggested by Dyken and Krawiecki in 1983. These authors used an anatomopathologic classification in which progressive neurodegenerative illnesses are organized into five subtypes according to clinical phenomena and pathologic features that are most characteristic for a group of illnesses. In the polioencephalopathies, the clinical and pathologic features are maximum in the cerebral cortex. In the corencephalopathies, there is more obvious involvement of the subcortical gray matter including structures of the basal ganglia, thalamus, and midbrain. In the leukoencephalopathies, there is a prominent involvement of the subcortical and/or periventricular white matter. In the spinocerebellopathies, the clinical and pathologic features are maximum in the cerebellum, spinal cord, and sometimes medulla and pons, regardless of whether gray or white matter is affected. In the diffuse progressive encephalopathies, clinical and pathologic studies fail to characterize a maximum central nervous system (CNS) involvement. In this chapter, the discussion will be limited to the most common genetic disorders leading to various progressive encephalopathies.

Although no curative therapy is available for most neurodegenerative diseases, palliative therapy (diet, vitamins, anticonvulsant) may sometimes delay or prevent neurodegeneration. Supportive therapy (physical therapy, gastrostomy, splinting, bracing, communication devices) should be provided to individual patients and their families (or caregivers) to improve individualized care. Preventive therapy includes genetic counseling and prenatal diagnosis. The only permanent solution for all genetic neurodegenerative disease is gene therapy. To be a candidate for gene therapy, patients must be asymptomatic or only show early signs of the illness. It is, therefore, important to develop new methods to aid predicting the clinical course in a newly diagnosed patient. The continual progress in this area makes a prediction of the ultimate success of this modality of treatment possible.

Polioencephalopathies

The progressive polioencephalopathies are either primary, resulting from an intrinsic metabolic defect of the cerebral cortex neurons (including mitochondrial DNA repair defects) or secondary to infection (e.g., subacute sclerosing panencephalitis), autoimmune disease (e.g., Rasmussen encephalitis), or recurrent metabolic insults (e.g., glucose transport protein deficiency). This discussion is limited to some inherited polioencephalopathies. Common clinical features are intellectual deterioration, epilepsy, progressive spasticity, and progressive sensory impairment. Peripheral neuropathy is not a feature of any polioencephalopathies except for Niemann-Pick syndrome.

Neuronal ceroid-lipofuscinoses

The neuronal ceroid-lipofuscinoses (NCLs) are a group of lysosomal disorders characterized by neurologic symptoms of polioencephalopathy and intralysosomal accumulation of waxy, autofluorescent lipopigments composed of ceroid and lipofuscin within neurons and other cells in the body (Table 15.1). In all forms of NCL, a disruption of lysosome function occurs that results in neuronal apoptosis and autophagic stress leading to cerebral and cerebellar cortical atrophy. The accumulation of lipopigments in extraneural cells such as lymphocytes, sweat gland epithelial cells, vascular endothelial cells, and skeletal muscle has no effect on their survival and causes no visceral involvement. This group of conditions is clinically, pathologically, genetically, and biochemically heterogeneous. Clinically, each specific syndrome is defined by age of onset of first neurologic impairment and rapidity of the clinical course, resulting in progressive specific neurologic signs and symptoms. Pathologically, ultrastructural analysis of peripheral blood, skin biopsy, conjunctival biopsy, rectal biopsy, or muscle biopsy shows osmophilic cytosomes that are delimited by a single membrane and are characteristic of the neuronal ceroid lipo-

Pearls and Perils

- Diagnosis of late infantile neuronal ceroid-lipofuscinoses (NCL) should be entertained in any infant or toddler who was previously normal, develops some seizures, and shows no etiology for seizures after extensive workup.
- Diagnosis of juvenile NCL should be entertained in any young school-age child who develops poor vision without refractive error.
- If the presentation and course are chronic and if behavioral and visual symptoms are present, it is probably Batten disease (chronic juvenile NCL).
- Look at the retina for the most important diagnostic feature in Batten disease.
- If the disease is acute with seizures, it is probably Bielschowsky disease (acute late-infantile NCL).
- The presence of early incoordination and abnormal electroencephalogram (EEG) are the most important clinical features of Bielschowsky disease.
- Pathologic reports on tissues studied by electron microscopic methods may be misleading owing to lack of experience in searching for the bodies and naïveté in recognizing them.
- In some rare cases of NCL, pure autism, pure pervasive psychosis, and pure cerebellar ataxia are prominent, but NCL accounts for a minute fraction of these syndromes.

Key Clinical Questions

- *Did you have your child checked by the ophthalmologist?* Eyeglasses do not improve the visual defect and examination of the retina most often demonstrates specific changes suggestive of NCL.

Table 15.1 Subacute diabetic neuropathies

Discriminating features
- Vacuolar or avacuolar osmophilic cytosomes in lymphocytes, conjunctiva, skin, rectum, muscle, and brain
- PPT1, TTP1, or cathepsin D deficiency in CLN1, CLN2, or CLN10, respectively.
- Mutations in CLN1, CLN2, CLN3, CLN5, CLN6, CLN7, CLN8, or CLN10 gene.

Consistent features
- Waxy, yellow type of optic atrophy
- Peripheral retinitis pigmentosa
- Abnormal ERG

Variable features
- Progressive dementia
- Seizures, myoclonia
- Ataxia
- Early blindness
- Mental changes (disruptive behavior, psychosis, neurosis)
- Basal ganglia symptoms
- Rett-like symptoms (hand wringing)

PPT1, protein palmityl thioesterase; TTP1, tripeptidylpeptidase fuscinoses. The morphology of the cytosomes varies in each NCL type. Four cytosomes define various forms of NCL: fingerprint (FP) cytosomes, curvilinear (CL) cytosomes, granular osmophilic deposits (GROD), and rectilinear cytosomes (RL). Genetically, all NCLs are autosomal recessive traits except for the rare families with the adult autosomal dominant form of Kufs disease. Eight genes have been identified and sequenced (*CLN1*, *CLN2*, *CLN3*, *CLN5*, *CLN6*, *CNL7*, *CLN8*, and *CLN10*). Studies are still in progress to identify other genetic defects in various forms of NCL and in other patients with atypical clinical course (Wisniewski et al. 2001). Several mutations, including point mutations, deletions, or nucleotide duplication, have been identified for most CLN genes. All mutations in an individual CLN gene predict the presence of specific cytosome(s). For example, all *CLN1* mutations are associated with GROD profiles. The most common mutations in an individual CLN gene predict a specific clinical phenotype with characteristic clinical features and specific age of onset. However, other mutations of the same individual CLN gene can result in a different clinical phenotype. For example, point mutations in *CLN1* result in the classic acute infantile Finish syndrome (NCL1). In countries other than Finland, other mutations in the same gene cause NCL phenotypes with a later age of onset and protracted disease progression: the subacute late infantile syndrome, the chronic juvenile syndrome, or even the adult-onset variant. Biochemically, storage material identified in each condition varies. Biochemically, storage material in lysosomes is heterogeneous, consisting of the sphingolipid activator proteins A and D, various lipids, and other proteins in most forms of NCL. Subunit C of mitochondrial adenosine triphosphate (ATP) synthase has a propensity for self-aggregation in various forms of NCL, except for the infantile disease (CLN1) and the neonatal disease (CLN10). Enzyme testing on fibroblasts or white blood cells is available for CLN1 and CLN2. CLN1 is characterized by a deficient lysosomal palmitoyl-protein thioesterase 1 (PPT1) activity (Vesa et al. 1995), an enzyme that removes long-chain fatty acids from cysteine residues in S-acylated proteins. The classic acute late-infantile NCL (CLN2) results from a deficiency in lysosomal tripeptidyl peptidase 1 (TPP1), a peptidase that removes three amino acids from a small protein (Wisniewski et al. 2001). More recently, the lysosomal aspartyl proteinase cathepsin D activity has been shown to be deficient in congenital NCL (CLN10) fibroblasts (Siintola et al. 2006). Most of the other NCL types are caused by defects in endosomal membrane proteins that are mislocalized to the lysosomal compartment.

The NCLs are the most common neurodegenerative diseases of childhood, with an estimated incidence of 1–7 per 100,000 (Rider & Rider 1988). The clinical presentation of NCL is dependent on the specific syndrome represented (Dyken 1988). The most commonly encountered form of NCL is the acute late-infantile type of NCL (LINCL) or Bielschowsky disease. In this variety, the onset of the disease occurs between 2 and 4 years of age. Initial symptoms are overwhelmingly of seizures of a wide variety. If a seizure is not the first complaint, progressive psychomotor regression is encountered. In rare cases, sudden onset of incoordination as frank ataxia is seen. These early symptoms often occur together. The course is dramatically downhill, so that within months the patient is often nonambulatory if not bedridden. In this condition, mental and motor regression has been so severe that visual failure is often unnoticed. The retinal picture is similar to the findings in juvenile NCL or Batten disease (see later section) if the disease has become well developed. In the early stages, however, the retina may be normal, only to be characterized within weeks by severe pigmentary disturbances. Laboratory findings are also variable depending on the stage of the disease. The electroencephalograph (EEG) is almost always severely abnormal and of an epileptogenic type, especially early in the course or at the onset of the disease. Evoked potential studies may show an early exaggerated response, which is replaced by poor or absent responses later. The electroretinograph (ERG) may also be absent. Brain computed tomography (CT) scans and magnetic resonance imaging (MRI) may show atrophic changes more readily than in Batten disease, even early in the course. These changes are especially located in the cerebellum and brainstem. Cerebrospinal fluid (CSF) analysis may be normal.

Within the NCLs, the late infantile-onset forms (LINCL) are the most heterogeneous. Pathohistologic studies of the lymphocytes reveal excessive vacuolization of lymphocytes in most cases, except in the Finnish variant. Ultrastructurally, each form of LINCL is characterized by specific cytosomal morphologies (Table 15.2). For example, the classic LINCL is associated with curvilinear bodies. Diagnosis of the classic LINCL is confirmed by demonstration of a deficient activity of the lysosomal tripeptidylpeptidase (TPP1) in skin fibroblasts or white blood cells. In other forms of LINCL, TPP1 activity is normal. If skin biopsy reveals GROD inclusions, PPT1 activity should be tested. Decision for which gene to test depends first on results of PPT1 and TPP1 activities. Molecular analysis for *CLN2* mutations (classic LINCL) is indicated if TPP1 activity is low and testing for *CLN1* mutations is indicated if PPT1 activity is low (Bonsignore et al. 2006). If diagnosis of LINCL is suggested by ultrastructural analysis and PPT1 and TPP1 activities are normal, molecular analysis for variants of LINCL should include testing of other known NCL genes like *CLN5* (Finnish variant), *CLN6* (Lake variant), and *CLN8* (Turkish variant) (Siintola et al. 2007).

The next most common type of NCL has been described as chronic juvenile NCL (JNCL) or Batten disease (CLN3). As the descriptive name implies, onset is usually

Table 15.2 Neuronal ceroid-lipofuscinoses

Subtype (gene)	Major clinical features	Prominent morphologic features
Acute form		
Congenital NCL (CLN10)	Microcephaly, seizures, spasticity	Granular (GROD)
Infantile (classic) (CLN 1)	Motor dysfunction, seizures	Granular (GROD)
Late infantile (classic) (CLN 2)	Seizures	Curvilinear (CV)
Late infantile (Finnish) (CLN 5)	Motor dysfunction, seizures	FP without vacuole
Late infantile (Lake) (CLN 6)	Seizures, myoclonus, visual loss	Mixed but no vacuole
Late infantile (Turkish) (CLN 7)	Seizures or ataxia, visual loss	FP without vacuole in lymphocyte, mixed
Late infantile (Turkish) (CLN8)	Seizures, ataxia, visual loss	FP without vacuole in lymphocyte, GROD, CV
Late infantile (CLN10)	Blindness, motor difficulties, seizures	GROD
Chronic forms		
Juvenile (classic) (CLN 3)	Early visual loss, dementia	FP with vacuole in lymphocytes
Juvenile (atypical) (CLN9)	Early visual loss, dementia	FP with vacuole in lymphocytes
Juvenile (Northern) (CLN8)	Seizures, ataxia, late or no visual loss	FP, RL, CV
Juvenile (atypical) (CLN1)	Learning failure, visual loss later	GROD
Juvenile (atypical) (CLN10)	Blindness, dementia	GROD
Adult (dominant with seizures)	Seizures, myoclonia	Mixed
Adult (recessive with dementia) (CLN1 or ?)	Dementia (motor loss)	Mixed

FP, fingerprint profiles; RL, rectilinear profiles; GROD, granular osmophilic deposits; CV, curvilinear bodies

during a period between 4 and 12 years of life and takes on a chronic course. Initial symptoms are usually visual failure, behavioral reaction, speech disturbances (frequent echolalia), or intellectual failure. These symptoms are slowly progressive, usually over a period of years. Within this framework, neurologic symptoms owing to slowly pyramidal and extrapyramidal dysfunction are seen. Seizures are at first uncommon but later become much more frequent. Early clinical diagnosis can often be made by the typical retinal picture, which shows an early attenuation of retinal vessels, macular degenerative changes, patches of retinal atrophy, and a so-called waxy yellow type of optic atrophy. Later, minimal peripheral retinitis pigmentosa may be seen. Because the disease is slowly progressive, a monophasic staging process can be identified over years of follow-up. The ERG is consistently attenuated or absent. The results of the neuroimaging investigations show, in advanced cases, diffuse cerebral atrophy. In classic JNCL, pathohistologic examination reveals blood lymphocytes, which are excessively vacuolated even on light microscopy. Within the vacuoles highly characteristic osmophilic cytosomes are identified, with the so-called fingerprint profile predominating. Ultrastructural examination of conjunctiva and skin biopsy shows similar inclusions. Cases of classic JNCL result from *CLN3* mutations. In rare instances, no *CLN3* mutation is found in JNCL patients with vacuolated lymphocytes. The gene of *CLN9* remains unknown (Schulz A et al. 2006). In other JNCL variants, no vacuoles or storage material is seen in peripheral lymphocytes. If ultrastructural analyses of other tissues reveal GRODs, testing of the lysosomal PPT1 activity in the blood should be considered before ordering *CLN1* mutation screening (Mazzei et al. 2002). If PPT1 activity is normal and skin biopsy also reveals GROD inclusions in nonmyelinated Schwann cells of skin biopsy, cathepsin D fibroblast activity may be reduced, and *CLN10* mutations should be considered (Steinfeld et al. 2006). In other rare JNCL variants without lymphocyte vacuoles, skin biopsy shows curvilinear bodies. Lysosomal TPP1 activity in the blood should be tested before ordering screening for *CLN2* mutation (Sleat et al. 1999). If TPP1 activity is normal, screens for *CLN5* (Pineda-Trujillo et al. 2005) and *CLN8* mutations (Striano et al. 2007) should be considered.

All other types of NCL are less common and can be summarized by differences in their clinical course, age of onset, morphologic picture, and genetics. An acute-infantile form of the disease (NCL1) was described by Finnish workers (Santavuori-Haltia syndrome) in 1975. This syndrome deviates from the other acute NCL disorders by occurring within the first 2 years of life and by a rapidly downhill course characterized by severe seizures (simple or complex partial) or myoclonia, severe mental-motor regression, and blindness. Aggressive behaviors and irritability are frequently reported. By the age of 2, funduscopic examination reveals a brownish discoloration of the macula, retinal degeneration, and optic atrophy. By 3 years of age, electrophysiologic studies demonstrate abnormal ERGs, abolished visual evoked responses, and frequently a markedly suppressed EEG with disappearance of eye opening/closing reaction. MRI shows severe progressive brain atrophy. The ultramorphologic picture is quite different in NCL1 (Santavuori-Haltia syndrome). Granular osmophilic deposits are the characteristic electron microscopic cytosomes and rarely are the other electron microscopic cytosomes encountered. Vacuolated lymphocytes are not found in peripheral blood smear. Pathologic reaction is characterized by a more severe atrophic picture, more signs of acute cellular destruction, and a severe, almost diagnostic, macrophagocytosis. Definite diagnosis is currently based on measurement of the PPT1 activity in amniotic fluid, chorionic villi, leukocytes, lymphoblasts, or fibroblasts.

Another rare variety of NCL is represented by the chronic adult-onset form of the disease (Kufs disease) (NCL4). Most cases display an autosomal recessive mode of inheritance, with only a few families reported to have a dominant transmission (sometimes referred to as Boehme or Parry disease). There are at least two distinguishable clinical subtypes of this disease. Type A is characterized by progressive myoclonic seizures followed years later by dementia. Type B is characterized by early dementia with or closely followed by prominent motor symptoms. The motor features are usually either a pure cerebellar syndrome or a pure basal ganglion deterioration. It is important to emphasize that NCL4 shows no retinal disturbance. In families, the subtypes show homotypism (same characteristics) and homochronism (same onset and course). In the uncommon instances when this disorder has been studied, granular cytosomes have been identified ultrastructurally in the lymphocytes. A skin biopsy is the least invasive diagnostic approach, demonstrating membrane-bound GRODs and/or sporadic fingerprint profiles (FP) without membrane-bound vacuoles. Pathologic study of the CNS shows less striking storage. The class type of lipofuscin, which is seen in the aging process, is encountered but is the least diagnostic cytosome, whereas the presence of mixed (membrane-bound GRODs, rectilinear and curvilinear) profiles in association with fingerprint cytosomes without membrane-bound vacuoles is diagnostic. In most cases, the underlying molecular defects in Kufs disease remain unknown. In rare instances, enzyme testing on fibroblasts or white blood cells reveals a deficient lysosomal PPT1 activity and the molecular analysis reveals *CLN1* mutations (van Diggelen et al. 2001).

The chronic juvenile "Northern epilepsy" form of NCL (NCL8), or progressive epilepsy with mental retardation (EPMR), belongs to the group of NCLs due to the presence of intraneuronal accumulation of cytoplasmic autofluorescent granules and identification of curvilinear bodies and GRODs on ultrastructural analysis. The infantile and early childhood periods are normal. The youngsters develop epilepsy (generalized tonic–clonic seizures, complex partial seizures) between 5 and 10 years of age. Mental regression is most rapid when epileptic activity is most pronounced. As seizure activity decreases in adulthood, mental deterioration slows down. Behavioral problems such as inattentiveness, restlessness, disobedience, irritability, and insomnia are frequently encountered. It is not until middle age, however, that gait and station disturbances become so obvious that a progressive neurologic disease is first considered in the differential diagnosis. Then patients develop definite cerebellar symptoms and signs, consisting of both truncal and appendicular involvement. Ataxia, dyssynergia, dysmetria, dysdiadochokinesis, scanning speech, and nystagmus may develop. Hyperreflexia is common throughout the course of the disease, even early in the course. The retina does not show the typical picture believed to be diagnostic of NCL, although vague ocular abnormalities have been seen. These usually represent the retinal picture that can be seen in severe refractive errors and are not diagnostic of retinal NCL. Progression of neurologic symptoms is slow, covering a period of many years. The slow progression is out of proportion to the course in all the other syndromes of NCL. Life expectancy frequently exceeds 50 years. Neurophysiologic studies are nonspecific and depend on the stage of the illness. MRI shows in early adulthood cerebellar and brainstem atrophy. No vacuolated lymphocytes are found in the peripheral smear. Ultrastructural study of skin shows accumulation of a wide variety of GRODs, with atypical curvilinear and rectilinear bodies. All the patients with Northern epilepsy are homozygous to one missense mutation (Arg-24-Gly) in *CLN8*. *CLN8* testing confirms the diagnosis. In contrast, the Turkish and Italian patients (other mutations) suffer from a more severe course, with retinal degeneration and clinical features that overlap with the classical *LINCL* and *JNCL* variants.

Congenital NCL represents the earliest-onset and the most aggressive form of the NCLs, leading to congenital microcephaly with overriding sutures, receding forehead, and low-set ears (Siintola et al. 2006). Deceleration of head growth already begins during the third trimester and jerky fetal movements may be interpreted as myoclonic seizures. Spasticity is congenital. Status epilepticus and respiratory insufficiency are noted soon after birth. Death occurs in early infancy. Autopsy shows extreme brain atrophy with complete disorganization of the neurons in the cerebral cortex, and loss of Purkinje cells and inner granule cells in the cerebellum. Most cells of the CNS are loaded with autofluorescent storage bodies, showing the granular ultrastructure of GRODs. Cathepsine D staining is absent in paraffin-embedded brain specimens. A truncating cathepsin D (*CTSD*) gene mutation underlies congenital NCL.

There has been no consistent beneficial therapy in any of the NCLs. Antioxidant treatment programs using vitamin E, vitamin C, D-L-methionine and butylated hydroxytoluene, or vitamin E and selenium in large dosages have shown some promise in arresting progression, especially in the chronic forms of the disease, but have been ineffective in the acute forms. Enzyme replacement therapy is presently under investigation for the acute infantile and late-infantile NCL. Human CNS stem cells may be an alternative therapy. Key features of the NCLs are summarized in Tables 15.1 and 15.2.

Gaucher disease

Gaucher disease is a group of autosomal recessive, lysosomal storage disorders characterized by the accumulation of an extremely insoluble sphingolipid, glucocerebroside (glucosylceramide), in *Gaucher cells*, the hallmarks of the disease (Table 15.3). Gaucher cells are found in most tissues (but not skin) and are characterized by one or multiple central or eccentric small nuclei and a large lipid-filled "wrinkled tissue paper" appearance. On electron microscopy, membrane-bound inclusions (Gaucher bodies) are filled with "tubules" composed of 10–12 fibrils that spiral the entire length of the tubule. Skin abnormalities such as disorganized lamellar membranes within the stratum corneum interspersed with amorphous nonlamellar microclefts suggest a poor neurologic outcome (Holleran et al. 2006). In the vast majority of cases, the enzyme required for lysosomal degradation of glucocerebroside, glucocerebrosidase is deficient (Beutler & Saven 1990). Mutations in the GBA gene, encoding for glucocerebrosidase and located on chromosome 1q21, do not predict the individual clinical phenotype (Park et al. 2003). Other variants lack the glucosylceramide activator protein, saposin C. Mutations in the saposin C coding region of the prosaposin (PSAP) gene, mapped to chromosome 10, have been reported in patients with Gaucher-like disease (Schnabel et al. 1991; Tylki-Szymanska et al. 2007). Gaucher disease is the most frequently reported lysosomal storage disease, with an incidence in Ashkenazi Jews of about 1 in 2,500 births.

Table 15.3 Gaucher disease

Discriminating features
- Gaucher cells in bone marrow and other tissues, except skin
- Glucocerebrosidase deficiency in leukocytes, serum, and skin

Consistent features
- Hepatosplenomegaly

Variable features
- Anemia
- Fractures
- Cirrhosis
- Pinguicula
- Spasticity
- Opisthotonos
- Horizontal oculomotor apraxia
- Myoclonic seizures
- Ataxia
- Mental retardation
- Cranial nerve involvement

Pearls and Perils

Gaucher disease

- The neurologic triad—strabismus, trismus, and retroflexion of the head—and its association with hepatosplenomegaly are suggestive of type II Gaucher disease.
- Patients with type II or type III disease have no clinical or neurophysiologic signs of peripheral nerve involvement.
- Gaucher cells from bone marrow aspirate must be differentiated from foam cells seen in Niemann-Pick disease. Gaucher cells are commonly multinucleated and their cytoplasm has a "wrinkled tissue paper" appearance. Gaucher cells are not found in the skin.
- Cells that can be mistaken for Gaucher cells are found in patients with unusually rapid turnover in the marrow, e.g., those with leukemia, thalassemia, or multiple myeloma (who do not have Gaucher disease).
- Gaucher bodies are only occasionally seen in neurons.
- Caution is advised in recommending splenectomy.

Gaucher disease has been divided into three clinical phenotypes, according to the presence and severity of neurologic symptoms. One single phenotype is usually seen among affected siblings of one family. Type I disease (neonatal or adult type), the most common phenotype, is a non-neuronopathic chronic disorder characterized by splenomegaly with hypersplenism, pulmonary involvement, and skeletal changes. Type II disease (infantile type) is an acute neuronopathic disorder characterized by hepatosplenomegaly and neurologic symptoms by 6 months of age. Brainstem abnormalities are responsible for stridor, difficulty in sucking and swallowing, apneic episodes, and bilateral fixed strabismus or oculomotor apraxia. Retroflexion of the head is an early sign, probably due to laryngomalacia and hypotonia of pharyngeal muscles. Corticospinal signs are common. A profound psychomotor deterioration occurs. Seizures are uncommon. Most patients die before 2 years of age in a vegetative state.

Type III disease (juvenile type) is a rare subacute neuronopathic disorder characterized by hepatosplenomegaly, hypersplenism, and slowly progressive neurologic deterioration beginning between early childhood and adult life. The most common neurologic manifestations are seizures and mental deterioration (Nishimura et al. 1980). Progressive myoclonic epilepsy may become severe and interfere with all activities. Mental deterioration may

Key Clinical Questions

- *Is there any Ashkenazi Jewish ancestry?*
  In a Jewish infant presenting with early strabismus, generalized hypertonia, opisthotonic posturing, and difficulty in swallowing, Gaucher disease should be suspected. Although the incidence of Gaucher disease is high in Ashkenazi Jews, the disease is not restricted to this population. In any case, abdominal exam should be performed looking for organomegaly. In the non-Jewish population, children frequently present later in life with difficulties tracking moving objects.

range from mild memory deficits to severe global dementia. Other neurologic abnormalities may include spasticity, ataxia, dystonia, parkinsonism, and supranuclear gaze disorders (slow saccades, saccadic palsies, vertical oculomotor apraxia). Death may occur between the second and fourth decade.

Ancillary laboratory findings on the serum may include elevation of acid phosphatase and angiotensin-converting enzyme. Cerebrospinal fluid is usually normal. Bone marrow aspirate can be used to demonstrate Gaucher cells. The finding of sulfatides in urine suggests a prosaposin deficiency (see metachromatic leukodystrophy, described in the next section). In most cases, diagnosis of Gaucher disease is established by direct assay of glucocerebrosidase activity in leukocytes, skin fibroblasts, or amniocytes. Genetic analysis of GBA or PSAP genes confirms diagnosis. Prognostic information and genetic counseling are now possible by DNA analysis with techniques that use the polymerase chain reaction (PCR) technique. The presence of the N370S mutation predicts the absence of neuropathic disease. Patients homozygous for the mutation at nucleotide 1448 of nuclear DNA are very likely to have neuronopathic disease, whereas the presence of even a single allele for the mutation at nucleotide 1226 appears to protect against the occurrence of neuronopathic disease (Beutler 1991).

Splenectomy is advisable when hypersplenism develops. However, total splenectomy is followed by a high mortality from sepsis, an increase in bone involvement with osteolytic changes within a few months of surgery, and rapid deterioration of the neurologic status in patients with type II or type III diseases. Intravenous enzyme replacement therapy using recombinantly produced glucocerebrosidase is successful in improving outcome, even in neuronopathic cases (Vellodi et al. 2001). Chemical *chaperone therapy*, using small-molecule drugs that improve the enzyme trafficking from the endoplasmic reticulum to the lysosome, is beneficial in some variants. Substrate reduction therapy using N-butyl deoxynojirimycin, an inhibitor of glucosylceramide synthase, has been suggested in non-neuronopathic cases.

GM_2 gangliosidoses

The GM_2 gangliosidoses are autosomal recessive neuronal lipidoses in which lysosomal catabolism of a glycosphingolipid, GM_2 ganglioside, in the neurons of the cerebral cortex is deficient, leading to progressive mental and motor deterioration. The cell body of neurons is distended by abnormal lipids, leading in rapidly progressive forms of the disease to megalencephaly. Neuronal storage also involves the cerebellum and anterior horn cells of the brainstem and spinal cord. Outside the CNS, neuronal storage is found in the ganglion cells and amacrine cells of the retina, spiral ganglia of the inner ear, spinal ganglia, autonomic ganglia, and neurons of the myenteric plexus. Neuronal storage progressively results in death of nerve cells. Electron microscopy of the stored material in all forms of GM_2 gangliosidoses demonstrates a great number of round or oval laminated membrane-bound structures. Three forms of cytosomes are described: concentric, compound, and zebra bodies. In concentric bodies, the lamellae are arranged concentrically, with a homogeneous or firmly granular zone in the center. In compound bodies, several outer concentric layers surround an inner zone filled with straight elements. In zebra bodies, a dense, double-layer, oval shell is filled with flat layers.

GM_2 gangliosides accumulate when the activity of hexosaminidase A, a heteropolypeptide made of two α and two β subunits, is deficient or when the GM_2 activator protein is deficient. GM_2 gangliosidosis with hexosaminidase A deficiency can result from mutations in one of the gene encoding either the α-subunit (HexA) on chromosome 15q23 (producing Tay-Sachs disease or type I GM_2 gangliosidosis variants) or the β-subunit (HexB) on chromosome 5q13 (producing Sandhoff disease or type II GM_2 gangliosidosis variants). In Sandhoff disease, hexosaminidase B, a polypeptide made of four β-subunits, is also deficient. GM_2 gangliosidosis with partial or no hexosaminidase A deficiency may result from mutations in the GM_2 activator protein (GM_2A) gene on chromosome 5q32-33 (producing type III GM_2 gangliosidosis).

The three types of GM_2 gangliosidosis, infantile, juvenile, and adult, differ by age of onset and clinical course. The infantile, acute form (Tay-Sachs and Sandhoff diseases) is characterized by an early onset of symptoms. Infants appear normal at birth and develop normally, except for irritability and an exaggerated startle response, which does not attenuate with stimulus repetition. Seizures may start early and are unprovoked. Various major and minor seizures occur; some seizures may begin with inappropriate laughter (gelastic seizures). By 6 months of age, psychomotor retardation becomes apparent. After 6 months of age, motor weakness becomes obvious with flaccid paralysis, hyporeflexia, and hypotonia. Visual acuity deteriorates. The characteristic cherry-red (black) spot results from the accumulation of lipids within the macular bipolar ganglion cells, with the formation of a white halo that surrounds the fovea, which retains its color (red or black depending on the race) as rod and cone cells do not accumulate lipids. Cortical blindness usually occurs by the end of the first year. After 1 year of age the symptoms progress, and the hyporeflexia and hypotonia give way to generalized spastic paralysis with hyperreflexia and opisthotonos. The child becomes progressively deaf. The occipitofrontal circumference increases at an abnormal rate because storage of ganglioside and glial proliferation enlarges the brain. Feeding difficulties, owing to ineffective swallowing, leads to progressive weight loss and cachexia. Late in the disease, a state of decerebrate rigidity is reached. The patient usually expires from a respiratory infection before the age of 5 years. Tay-Sachs disease (infantile type I GM_2 gangliosidosis), Sandhoff disease (infantile type II GM_2 gangliosidosis), and GM_2 activator protein deficiency (infantile type III GM_2 gangliosidosis) are clinically similar (Okada et al. 1972). Mild hepatosplenomegaly and skeletal deformities, when present, are characteristic of Sandhoff disease but less severe than those seen in type I GM_1 gangliosidosis.

Juvenile subacute GM_2 gangliosidosis has an onset between 2 and 6 years of age and progresses more slowly than the infantile GM_2 gangliosidosis. Spinocerebellar ataxia, dysarthria, and loss of speech are frequently the initial symptoms. Dysphagia tends to appear later in the illness. During the first decade, progressive psychomotor deterioration is accompanied by increasing spasticity and development of seizures. Dementia is a universal feature but frequently is not apparent during the first years of the illness. Movement disorders, such as choreoathetosis, dystonia, and oculogyric crisis, may occur early or late in the course of the disease. Often, a progressive spasticity, leading to a decerebrate rigidity, is reported. Seizures are not always present. Cherry-red spots are uncommon and not well defined when they are present. Blindness occurs late in the disease. Megalencephaly does not develop. Death occurs up to 10 years from the onset of clinical symptoms (Meek et al. 1984). Some juvenile patients with onset in childhood have a protracted course with long survival into adulthood.

The onset of adult chronic GM_2 gangliosidosis is variable. Presenting symptoms include dementia, psychosis, progressive muscle weakness with atrophy (with clinical course similar to that of Kugelberg-Welander disease), seizures, ataxia, dystonia, rubral tremor, and supranuclear ophthalmoplegia, either alone or in various combinations. A slow, progressive ataxia with dysarthria is not always present. Intellectual function is normal or mildly impaired. Seizures rarely occur. Funduscopic examination is frequently normal (Harding et al. 1987).

Key Clinical Questions

- *Is there any Ashkenazi Jewish ancestry?*
  If an infant presents a decreased visual attentiveness, progressive head enlargement, and sudden jerks with extension of four extremities in reaction to sharp noises, Tay–Sachs disease should be suspected. Although the incidence of Tay-Sachs disease is high in Ashkenazi Jews, the disease is not restricted to this population. In any case, a funduscopic exam should be performed looking for cherry-red spots.

Cerebrospinal fluid is usually unremarkable. Urinary excretion of oligosaccharides containing N-acetylglucosamine and mannose has been observed in Sandhoff disease (Sewell 1980). The diagnosis of GM_2 gangliosidoses is confirmed by enzyme assay of HexA and HexB in serum, separated white blood cells, fibroblasts, or amniotic cells. Assays for HexA and HexB employing synthetic substrates (sulfated or nonsulfated) are generally sufficient to diagnose defects in α or β chains. However, mutations in the β subunit leading to heat-labile HexB may be misdiagnosed. Furthermore, this assay procedure cannot diagnose the GM_2 activator deficiency or HexA mutations resulting in a decreased responsiveness to activator protein. In such cases, identification of storage material in rectal biopsy may be helpful, although more complicated tests are needed (Gravel et al. 1991; Raghavan 1985). Molecular DNA-based diagnostic techniques should be carried out, as mutations leading to infantile, juvenile, and adult GM_2 gangliosidosis can be distinguished at the molecular level. Prenatal diagnosis of Tay-Sachs disease can be accomplished in high-risk pregnancies. Discriminating

Table 15.4 Tay-Sachs disease

Discriminating features

- Hexosaminidase A deficiency in serum and fibroblasts

Consistent features

- Exaggerated startle response
- Cherry-red spot

Variable features

- Nystagmus
- Megalencephaly
- Hypotonia (early) and hyperreflexia (late)
- Hyporeflexia (early) and hyperreflexia (late)
- Difficulty swallowing
- Seizures
- Deafness
- Blindness

Table 15.5 Sandhoff disease

Discriminating features
- Oligosaccharides in urine
- Hexosaminidase A and B deficiency in serum and fibroblasts

Consistent features
- Exaggerated startle response
- Cherry-red spot

Variable features
- Nystagmus
- Megalencephaly
- Hypotonia (early) and opisthotonos (late)
- Hyporeflexia (early) and hyperreflexia (late)
- Difficulty swallowing
- Seizures
- Deafness
- Blindness
- Splenomegaly
- Bony deformities

features in the diagnosis of Tay-Sachs and Sandhoff disease are listed in Tables 15.4 and 15.5.

Extensive genetic counseling and prenatal diagnosis have reduced the incidence of GM_2 gangliosidoses in Ashkenazi Jews. Most cases today are in families that do not have identifiable risk factors. Management of patients with GM_2 gangliosidoses is entirely supportive. Stem cell transplant may prove helpful if used early.

Menkes disease

Menkes disease is an X-linked recessive disorder of copper transport due to a deficiency in the extrahepatic transmembrane copper-transporting ATPase, a glycoprotein normally localized in mitochondria and Golgi apparatus (Vulpe et al. 1993). This enzyme transports copper from the cytoplasm of extrahepatic cells into the mitochondria and Golgi system. Most of the symptoms of Menkes disease can be explained by copper deficiency and secondary defects of copper-dependent enzymes. For instance, decreased lumbar CSF 3-methoxy-4-hydroxyphenylglycol (MHPG), the metabolite of norepinephrine, is explained by copper-dependent β-dopamine-hydroxylase deficiency.

Key Clinical Questions

- Do you know of any other boy in your family who had intractable seizures, never had a haircut, and died in infancy?

Pearls and Perils

Menkes kinky hair syndrome

- The bone changes in Menkes syndrome are easily confused with those seen in maltreated babies and the tendency for subdural hematoma to occur in this disorder adds to the risk of confusion of the two entities. Wormian bones are present in early life.
- Early diagnosis may be difficult because bony changes, hair abnormalities, and serum copper and ceruloplasmin may be normal in the very early neonatal period. In neonates with a positive family history, demonstration of an increased uptake of copper in skin fibroblasts may allow early diagnosis. Similarly, diagnosis may be achieved by demonstrating an increased uptake of copper in amniotic fluid cells in fetuses.
- Menkes disease is an X-linked autosomal recessive disorder.
- A cherubic face, hypopigmentation, and frequent uncontrolled seizures in a young infant with progressive brain atrophy is not unique to Menkes disease as it is also seen in sulfite oxidase deficiencies (primary or secondary to molybdenum cofactor deficiency). Diagnosis of sulfite oxidase deficiencies is suggested when the sulfite dipstick test on fresh urine turns pink. Ectopic lenses typical of sulfite oxidase deficiencies is a late finding (Johnson & Duran 2001).

The illness is characterized clinically by seizures, psychomotor retardation, failure to thrive, connective tissue findings, hypopigmentation, and peculiar hair. These babies are often born prematurely. The diagnostic features of neonates with Menkes disease are subtle: feeding difficulties, temperature instability, jaundice. The characteristic alterations in the hair are usually absent. Inguinal hernia and diathesis recti abdominus may be present. Many acquire head control and responsive smile. Truncal hypotonia, progressive spasticity of the limbs, psychomotor delay, and/or convulsions (partial, generalized, myoclonic) are usually reported by 2–4 months of age. The hair is hypopigmented, lusterless, and short with a steely texture. Pili torti and trichorrhexis nodosa are seen under light microscopy. Pudgy cheeks, sparse eyebrows, and depressed nasal bridge with micrognathia give these patients a cherubic appearance (Figure 15.1). The skin is hypopigmented, hyperextensible, and joints are hypermobile. The bones are osteoporotic, with flared long-bone metaphyses, and there may be wormian bones on skull x-rays. The blood vessels are tortuous and elongated, with irregular lumen (Figure 15.2). Diverticula of the bladder are common. Progressive deterioration leads to spastic quadriparesis with clenched fists and leg scissoring, while

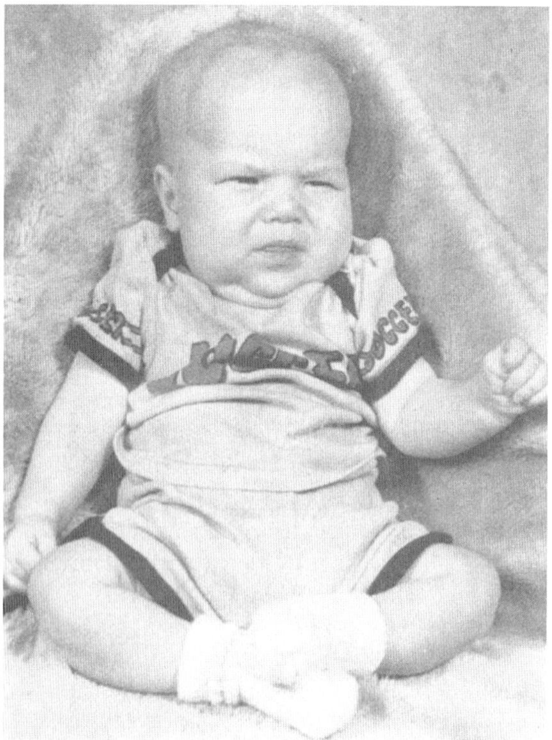

Figure 15.1 In this 7-month-old boy, the diagnosis of Menkes disease was suggested by the cherubic expression of the facies (pudgy cheeks); short, sparse, and hypopigmented hair; clenched fists; and truncal hypotonia. Seizures were first reported at 3 months of age.

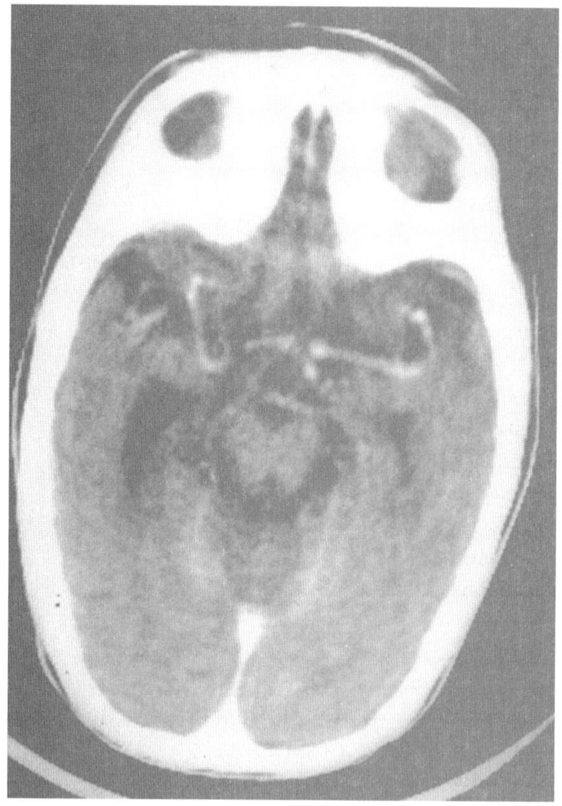

Figure 15.2 Contrast-enhanced computed tomography scan of the head showing brain atrophy with enlargement of the ambient cistern and tortuous middle cerebral arteries in a 2-year-old boy with Menkes syndrome who presented at 1 month of age with inguinal hernia and at 6 weeks of age with seizures, failure to thrive, and unusual hair.

axial muscles remain hypotonic. Blindness with optic atrophy is associated with vertical and horizontal nystagmus. Death occurs between 6 months and 3 years of age, often from recurrent urinary tract infections.

A milder phenotype has been reported (Danks 1988; Westman et al. 1988). These patients present with cerebellar ataxia, developmental delay, loose skin, lax joints, and typical hair changes. Bladder diverticula, bone changes, and arterial changes are milder. Survival may extend into adulthood.

The "occipital horn syndrome" (or X-linked cutis laxa or Ehlers-Danlos syndrome type IX) is characterized by tissue and bony abnormalities, including hyperelastic skin, easy bruisability, bladder diverticula, hyperextensible joints, marked arterial tortuosity, and skeletal anomalies, as well as chronic diarrhea (defect in bowel motility). Typical radiologic features include ossified occipital exostosis, a "hammer-like" extension of the lateral end of shortened clavicles, and a waxy outline of the cortex of most long bones (Sartoris et al. 1984). Neurologic features may include congenital myopathy, psychomotor retardation, and seizures since early childhood. In adulthood, generalized muscular atrophy and mental retardation have been reported (Wakai et al. 1993). There is no microcephaly. The hair appears to be normal.

In classical Menkes disease, mild Menkes disease, and occipital horn syndrome, laboratory studies typically reveal low serum copper and ceruloplasmin levels. Copper transport is affected in all tissues except the liver. In most cells (except liver), when copper is available, normal uptake occurs with reduced efflux, hence, the increased copper accumulation in gut mucosa and renal tubular cells. Intestinal absorption of copper is poor. An increased uptake and an impaired efflux of copper in cultured skin fibroblasts is characteristic of various forms of extrahepatic transmembrane copper-transporting ATPase deficiency. Mild Menkes disease and occipital horn syndrome are allelic with the classic Menkes disease (Table 15.6).

Parenteral administration of copper histidinate is the treatment of choice for Menkes disease. This readily corrects the serum and liver copper levels but does not restore the levels of all copper-dependent enzymes in other organs (Danks & Cartwright 1973). In particular, restoration of normal brain copper has not yet been achieved. Decreased lumbar CSF MHPG persists after parenteral copper therapy. At best, patients with Menkes

Table 15.6 Menkes disease

Discriminating features
- Cherubic pudgy face, hypopigmented skin, and pili torti
- Low serum copper
- Low ceruloplasmin
- Low cerebrospinal fluid 3-methoxy-4-hydroxyphenylglycol
- Increased uptake but reduced efflux of copper in cultured skin fibroblasts
- Defects of extrahepatic transmembrane copper-transporting ATPase gene

Consistent features
- X-linked recessive
- Brittle, sparse, and coarse hair
- Hyperextensibility of skin
- Pallor of skin
- Ligament laxity
- Psychomotor retardation
- Myopathy

Variable features
- Chronic diarrhea
- Osteoporosis
- Fracture of long bones and ribs
- Subdural hematoma
- Anemia
- Hemochromatosis
- Seizures
- Bladder diverticula
- Recurrent bladder infections
- Hypo/hyperthermia

disease who have been treated with copper histidinate soon after birth are at the lower end of the normal range intellectually and have some residual features of the disease in hair and connective tissues. Therapeutic intervention with copper histidinate in occipital horn syndrome has a marginal effect, perhaps due to the higher susceptibility of lysyl oxidase to copper deficiency.

Alpers syndrome

Alpers syndrome, or progressive infantile poliodystrophy, is a heterogeneous group of autosomal recessive, X-linked, or maternally inherited (in the case of mitochondrial DNA point mutation) (Uusimaa et al. 2002) disorders characterized by psychomotor deterioration, convulsions, myoclonus, hypotonia or spasticity, cerebellar ataxia, involuntary movements, visual disturbances, and abnormal respiration. Liver dysfunction and exacerbation during infections are consistent features. Two distinct categories can be defined. In the first group, a defect of selenium metabolism results in liver dysfunction and abnormal hair (Ramackers et al. 1994). In the second group, various defects of energy metabolism are reported. Those include defects in the citric acid cycle (Gabreels et al. 1984), pyruvate carboxylase (Atkin et al. 1979), pyruvate dehydrogenase (Robinson et al. 1987), nicotinamide-adenine dinucleotide (NADH) dehydrogenase (complex I) (Tulinius et al. 1991), and cytochrome c oxidase (complex IV) (Prick et al. 1983). Alpers syndrome has also been associated with point mutations of mitochondrial DNA (Uusimaa et al. 2002) and mitochondrial DNA depletion due to mutations in the nuclear-encoded mitochondrial DNA polymerase (POLG) gene (Naviaux et al. 1999), Twinkle (C10ORF2) gene (Sarzi et al. 2007), or ribonucleotide reductase (RRM2B) gene (Bourdon et al. 2007).

> **Key Clinical Questions**
>
> - *Do you have videotapes showing your child before and after the onset of the visuomotor regression?*
>   Review of videotapes will allow the physician to recognize the progressive nature of the microcephaly, the rapid retrogression of developmental milestones and the characteristics of myoclonic seizures.

Clinically, three forms of the syndrome have been recognized according to age of onset: neonatal form, infantile form, and juvenile form. The neonatal form may present at birth with joint limitations, micrognathia, cryptorchidism, pulmonary hypoplasia, and intrauterine growth retardation suggesting fetal akinesia (Frydman et al. 1993). Micropenis and hypospadias have been described in patients with NADH dehydrogenase (complex I) deficiency and cytochrome c oxidase (complex IV) deficiency. Features reminiscent of fetal alcohol syndrome can be seen in pyruvate dehydrogenase E_1 α-subunit deficiency. Most infants appear lethargic and floppy. Microcephaly is mild at birth and worsens with age. Refractory neonatal convulsions, swallowing difficulties, and pneumonia complicate the clinical course. Occasional features include cardiomyopathy and the de Toni-Fanconi-Debré syndrome. Most patients die before 2 years of age from respiratory arrest or liver failure. The infantile form has its onset before 2 years of age with recurrent vomiting, failure to thrive, hypotonia, and developmental delay, typically following a short period of normal development. Intractable seizures appear weeks or months later, often acutely. Other manifestations may include ataxia, involuntary movements, myoclonus, and blindness. Hair may become depigmented and brittle. Microcephaly and spasticity appear late in the illness. Some instances of terminal jaundice have been described. Most patients die between 3 and 4 years of age. The rare juvenile form has its onset in childhood with migraines, convulsions, and visual impairment. Later myoclonus, spasticity, choreoathetosis, and dementia are progressive. Death results from uncontrollable seizures.

The EEG is variable, yet often shows diffuse abnormalities with low-voltage background and numerous multifocal paroxysmal discharges. Visual evoked potentials are frequently abnormal. Nerve conduction studies and electromyograms (EMGs) are usually normal. Repeated CT scans of the head document progressive cortical atrophy. Basal ganglia calcification is seen in juvenile cases (Shapira et al. 1975). T_2-weighted MRI of the brain may show decreased signal of the thalamus (Figure 15.3). Liver dysfunction is an early manifestation in most cases, and biochemical evidence of liver disease may precede the onset of seizures. The CSF proteins are usually normal. An elevated blood and/or CSF lactate and lactate/pyruvate ratios may be found intermittently in some patients. Diagnosis of Menkes disease should be excluded. Selenium deficiency and glutathione peroxidase deficiency have been demonstrated in some patients (Ramacker et al. 1994).

Alpers syndrome is associated with characteristic neuropathologic lesions. The brain is small, with a striking cerebral cortical atrophy. Histology demonstrates neuronal degeneration and loss, astrocytic gliosis, spongiosis, microglial proliferation, and capillary proliferations. These changes are most severe in the striate calcarine cortex. Neuronal loss can also be seen in the cerebellum and to less extent in the basal ganglia. Alzheimer type II astrocytes are often present in the basal ganglia. White matter is relatively spared. Liver biopsy may show microvesicular fatty infiltration, necrosis of hepatocytes, inflammation, and cirrhosis (Narkwick et al. 1991) (Table 15.7). In Alpers syndrome, the inexorable progress of liver involvement may be accelerated by anticonvulsant therapy, particularly valproate (Bicknese 1992). Selenium therapy may be beneficial in improving seizure control and preventing liver dysfunction. A more definite therapy awaits discovery of underlying genetic defects.

Table 15.7 Alpers syndrome

Discriminating features
- Spongiosis, neuronal loss, and astrocytosis which progress down through the brain cortex

Consistent features
- Intractable seizures with myoclonus
- Liver dysfunction

Variable features
- Clinical evidence of liver disease
- Failure to thrive
- Developmental delay
- Ataxia
- Hypotonia
- Progressive spasticity
- Blindness and optic atrophy
- Microcephaly (late)
- Peripheral neuropathy

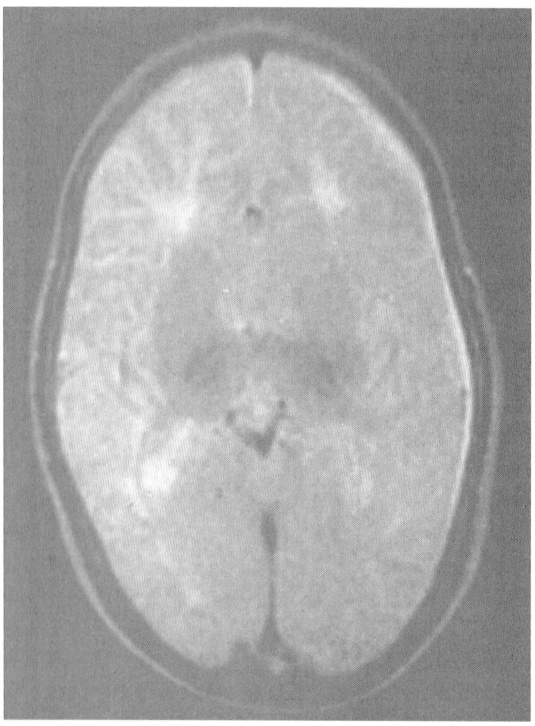

Figure 15.3 Magnetic resonance imaging of the brain (SE 2100/100) showing low signal in thalami (suggesting iron deposits) and cortical atrophy in a 15-month-old girl with Alpers syndrome.

Niemann-Pick disease

Niemann-Pick disease is a heterogenous group of autosomal recessive lysosomal storage disorders characterized by the accumulation of varying amounts of the phosphosphingolipid sphingomyelin in certain tissues. It is also frequently characterized by neurodegeneration, in which neuronal loss and glial proliferation follow neuronal ballooning and vacuolization. On bone marrow biopsy, Niemann-Pick foam cells and/or sea-blue histiocytes are found in various types of the disease. Two groups of sphingomyelinoses differ pathologically, biochemically, genetically, and clinically.

Pathologically, in group I diseases, foam cells are large macrophages 20–90 μm in diameter. The abundant pale cytoplasm is filled with lipid droplets, fairly uniform in size and highly refractile. On electron microscopy, Niemann-Pick cells are filled with membrane-bound vacuoles containing loosely packed lamellae. Skin biopsy is not helpful diagnostically. In group II disease, foam cells are filled with nonuniform lipid droplets with less birefringence than in type I. In skin biopsy, the intravesicular ac-

> **Pearls and Perils**
>
> **Niemann-Pick disease**
>
> - Niemann–Pick cells can very easily be distinguished from Gaucher cells. Foam cells resembling those seen in Niemann-Pick disease are also observed in Wolman disease, Tay-Sachs disease, Batten disease, sea-blue histiocyte syndrome, generalized gangliosidosis (infantile GM_1 gangliosidosis type I), and chronic granulomatous syndrome of childhood.
> - Peripheral neuropathy may be demonstrated by neurophysiologic studies and nerve biopsy in Niemann-Pick A (NPA) and NPB forms of the disease.
> - Infants with the NPA form of Niemann-Pick disease are typically emaciated with a protuberant abdomen. Finding a macular cherry-red spot excludes the diagnosis of Wolman disease.
> - Type II Niemann-Pick disease (NPC and NPD) should be suspected in patients with supranuclear ophthalmoplegia, dystonia, and splenomegaly. No funduscopic abnormality is found in those patients.
> - Splenomegaly is never severe enough to require splenectomy.

cumulation of unesterified cholesterol is demonstrated in the dermal fibroblasts by their bright punctated fluorescence after probing with filipin, a cholesterol-binding antibiotic. Ultrastructurally, osmiophilic pleomorphic oligolamellar inclusions in dermal fibroblasts and perivascular histiocytes are observed.

Biochemically, in group I disease, a striking increase in sphingomyelin content is found in most organs. Sphingomyelinase activity is severely reduced. In patients with no residual activity (type A), sphingomyelin brain content is increased; in contrast, patients with residual catalytic activity (type B) maintain a normal sphingomyelin brain content. In group II, there is a regional variability of sphingomyelin storage. In this group of patients, sphingomyelinase activity is either partially deficient (NPC) or normal (NPD). Esterification of exogenous low-density

> **Key Clinical Questions**
>
> - *Did the child have a prominent abdomen, jaundice, and/or feeding difficulties in early infancy?*
>   If those features are absent, ask if the child has difficulties going down the stairs. This symptom resulting from vertical supranuclear ophthalmoplegia is rarely seen in other childhood neurodegenerative diseases.

lipoprotein (LDL)-derived cholesterol is impaired in skin fibroblasts, whereas cholesteryl ester synthesis from endogenous cholesterol is normal. The primary defect in type II disease disrupts cholesterol trafficking out of the Golgi and interferes with its subsequent utilization (Langmade et al. 2006; Vance 2006).

Genetically, mutations causing group I diseases have been described in various populations in the acid sphingomyelinase gene (SMPD1) on chromosome 11p15 (Simonaro et al. 2002). The majority of patients with the NPA form have Ashkenazi Jewish ancestry. Mutations leading to NPA phenotype are more severe (small deletions, nonsense or catalytical missense) than the one leading to NPB (extracatalytical missense). Group II is genetically heterogenous. In the vast majority of patients (with NPC or NPD phenotype), mutations of *NPC1* on chromosome 18q11 reduce the level of NPC1 protein, a post-lysosomal membrane permease belonging to one of the superfamilies of efflux pumps. In a minority of cases, mutations of *NPC2* on chromosome 14q24 reduce levels of HE1 protein, a soluble lysosomal cholesterol-binding protein that interacts with NPC1 protein (Millat et al. 2001). HE1 protein levels are increased in patients with *NPC1* mutations (Blom et al. 2003).

Clinically, the hepatosplenomegaly is massive in group I patients. NPA disease, or acute infantile Niemann-Pick disease, is the most common form of the disease. This acute neurovisceral form is characterized by hepatosplenomegaly and severe early neurologic involvement. Feeding difficulty, failure to thrive, and organomegaly are usually evident by 6 months of age. Psychomotor regression with loss of reactivity to the environment and postural hypotonia become evident by age 1 year. Seizures sometimes occur, but not as frequently as in Tay-Sachs disease. An atypical cherry-red spot is noted in most patients by 12 months of age. Some patients have clinical symptoms and pathologic findings of a peripheral neuropathy. With time, the child becomes apathetic, blind, and deaf. Pupils become unresponsive to light. Death usually occurs before the fourth year of life.

NPB disease, or chronic juvenile Niemann-Pick disease, is a rare visceral or neurovisceral disorder characterized by organomegaly, diffuse infiltration of the lungs, and occasionally a decreased nerve conduction velocity. Ocular changes such as macular halo, granular pigmentation, and gray discolorations of the macula do not interfere with vision. Most patients are free of neurologic symptoms until adulthood, although mental changes and extrapyramidal signs may appear during adolescence. Most patients survive until late adulthood, where some develop parkinsonism.

Hepatosplenomegaly is variably present in group II patients. NPC disease can be classified into three major phenotypes according to the age of onset of neurologic symptoms: early infantile, late infantile, and juvenile forms. In the acute early infantile form, a transient cholestatic jaundice with hepatosplenomegaly and biliary atresia is associated with hypotonia and a rapid neurologic deterioration. In the subacute late infantile form, the patients usually seem normal until 2 years of age; psychomotor deterioration with ataxia, dysarthria, dysphagia, and drooling is slow. Hepatosplenomegaly is less prominent. Most patients belong to the chronic juvenile form, also known as dystonic juvenile lipidosis. Cognitive and behavioral difficulties frequently precede the onset of motor problems. Dystonia or choreoathetosis may be a presenting complaint. Dystonia starts distally and gradually becomes generalized. Some patients may never develop visceromegaly. Most patients develop mental retardation, ataxia, dysarthria, spasticity, seizures (generalized tonic, clonic, and myoclonic), and supranuclear vertical gaze paresis leading to difficulties negotiating stairs. Gelastic cataplexy has been observed in some subjects. Death usually occurs before 15 years of age.

NPD disease, or chronic adult Niemann-Pick disease, also called Nova Scotia variant (Vethamany et al. 1972), is a rare neurovisceral disorder characterized by a protracted course, mild organomegaly, and late onset of neurologic abnormalities (ataxia, seizures, vertical supranuclear ophthalmoplegia, intellectual deterioration), which may begin in adulthood (Elleder et al. 1983a).

In the NPA and NPB forms of Niemann-Pick disease, assessment of nerve conduction velocities may provide evidence of peripheral nerve involvement. The ERG may show marked reduction of responses at a time when visual evoked potentials are only slightly abnormal. In NPA disease, slit lamp examination may reveal corneal and lenticular opacifications. In both NPA and NPB disease, chest radiography frequently shows diffuse bilateral interstitial infiltrates. CT scan of the head may be consistent with cerebral atrophy.

Blood chemistry may reveal some degree of liver disease. High-density lipoprotein (HDL) cholesterol is low in NPB. Bone marrow examination reveals Niemann-Pick foam cells and/or sea-blue histiocytes in various types of Niemann-Pick disease. Sea-blue histiocytes are seen in NPA and type II diseases with Wright-Giemsa stain. In addition to the bone marrow, foam cells and sea-blue histiocytes can be found in most organs (e.g., peripheral nerves, retina, spleen, liver, lungs). An accurate diagnosis of the NPA and NPB forms of Niemann-Pick disease is achieved by demonstrating a profound deficiency of sphingomyelinase activity in peripheral leukocytes, cultured fibroblasts, or cultured amniotic fluid cells. Diagnosis of NPC and NPD does not rely on measurement of sphingomyelinase activity, as it is frequently normal. Instead, the diagnosis of NPC and NPD requires not only the demonstration of an impaired esterification of LDL-derived cholesterol in the fibroblasts, but also the evidence of intralysosomal accumulation of unesterified cholesterol using filipin staining. Final diagnosis is confirmed by linkage analysis and sequence analysis of the mutated genes (Table 15.8).

Table 15.8 Niemann-Pick disease

Discriminating features
- Vertical supranuclear ophthalmoplegia
  - Type 1: Sphingomyelinase deficiency in fibroblasts and leukocytes
  - Type 2: Impaired cholesterol esterification and cholesterol accumulation in cultured fibroblasts after low-density lipoprotein (LDL) cholesterol and evidence of intralysosomal accumulation of unesterified cholesterol

Consistent features
- Hepatosplenomegaly
- Sea-blue or foamy histiocytes in bone marrow

Variable features
- Failure to thrive
- Psychomotor delay
- Peripheral neuropathy
- Atypical cherry-red spot
- Vertical oculomotor apraxia
- Seizures
- Ataxia
- Dystonia
- Spasticity
- Interstitial pulmonary infiltration

Of the various therapeutic approaches, intracerebral transplantation of mesenchymal stem cell-mediated gene therapy and exogenous recombinant protein replacement have attracted interest for the management of NPA and NPB, whereas pregnane X receptor (PXR) activation appears promising for the management of NPC and NPD (Langmade et al. 2006).

Glucose transport protein deficiency

Glucose transport protein deficiency is an autosomal dominant, progressive polioencephalopathy characterized by infantile seizures, developmental delay, and progressive microcephaly. Biochemically, the disorder has been shown to result from a defective glucose transport across the blood–brain barrier, resulting in persistently low CSF glucose concentration in the absence of systemic hypoglycemia or CNS infection. The glucose transport protein, GLUT-1, is deficient in membranes of erythrocytes and brain capillary endothelial cells, which do not respond to insulin. Few individuals diagnosed with glucose transport protein deficiency have an affected parent. Disease-provoking mutations in the SLC2A1 gene encoding GLUT-1, located on the short arm of chromosome 1 (De Vivo et al. 1995), have been found in 80% of the patients (Wang et al. 2005).

Key Clinical Questions

- *Do symptoms of coordination problems and poor motor performance fluctuate during the day, and do you occasionally see staring spells accompanied by loss of tone?* Such patients may benefit from a ketogenic diet.

Most patients appear healthy at birth, and early motor development seems to be normal. Seizures of different types start in infancy in most patients. Nonconvulsive seizures with loss of muscle tone are the most prominent clinical type. In addition, patients may have recurrent episodes of ataxia, dystonia, headache, unresponsiveness, or limpness. Patients display fluctuations in the motor performance throughout the day. Seizures are usually resistant to traditional anticonvulsants. Early recognition and prompt treatment with a ketogenic diet improve seizure control and neurologic outcome. Ketone bodies provide an alternative source of energy to the brain when supplies of glucose available to the brain are limited. Untreated, varying degrees of psychomotor retardation become evident in the first year of life. Patients may develop evidence of spasticity with or without athetoid dystonia. Cognitive and language development are frequently delayed. Hyperactive and aggressive behavior may be additional findings when diagnosis is not made. Acquired microcephaly is an inconsistent finding (De Vivo et al. 1991, 1994).

Most interictal EEGs and neuroimaging studies, including CT scans and MRI of the brain, are normal. The ictal EEG typically shows generalized paroxysmal 2–2.5 Hz spike-wave discharges (Boles et al. 1999). Blood glucose is normal. A low CSF glucose concentration (<45 mg/dL), together with normal or low CSF lactate concentrations suggests the diagnosis. The kinetic studies of red blood cell (RBC) glucose uptake are used as a physiological measure of the glucose transport protein integrity. The patients' RBC glucose uptake values represent approximately 50% of the parents' values. Similarly, the patients' RBC membrane immunoreactivity for GLUT-1 is approximately 50% of the parents' values by Western blot technique (Miller 1971) (Table 15.9).

Pearls and Perils

- Low cerebrospinal fluid (CSF) glucose in the absence of central nervous system infection or hypoglycemia can be seen in mitochondrial disorders as well as in glucose transport protein deficiency; however, in mitochondrial disorders, CSF lactate is markedly elevated (6.03 ± 0.54 mM/L) if CSF glucose is low (<45 mg/dL).
- Patients responding to ketogenic diets should be suspected of having glucose transport protein deficiency.
- Patients with mental retardation and fluctuating ataxia should be assessed for GLUT-1 deficiency even when they don't have epilepsy (Overweg-Plandsoen et al. 2003).

Table 15.9 Glucose transport protein deficiency

Discriminating features

- Low CSF/blood glucose (0.33 ± 0.01) (Normal: 065 ± 0.01) while normal cell count and normal cerebrospinal fluid lactate (<1.1 mM/L
- Kinetic studies of red blood cell glucose uptake

Consistent features

- Fluctuation of neurologic symptoms/disability through the day
- Delayed motor and mental development
- Resolution of seizures and motor fluctuation with ketogenic diet

Variable features

- Seizures in infancy
- Microcephaly
- Spasticity
- Dystonia
- Paroxysmal fatigue, limpness, ataxia, palsy unresponsiveness, or autonomic myoclonus
- Sleep disturbance, nocturnal myoclonus
- Emotional outbursts
- Fluctuating cognition

Leukoencephalopathies

The progressive leukoencephalopathies result either from a primary genetic defect of myelin metabolism (primary leukodystrophies) (Table 15.10) or from glial cell damage by infectious conditions (AIDS encephalopathy, progressive multifocal encephalopathy), immune or inflammatory phenomena (multiple sclerosis, X-linked adrenoleukodystrophy), DNA repair defects (Cockayne syndrome), poststress cytoprotective defects (vanishing white matter disease), or metabolic conditions resulting in the accumulation of toxic metabolites interfering with glial cell function and differentiation (nonketotic hyperglycinemia, Zellweger syndrome, Hurler disease, Pearson syndrome, glutaric aciduria) (Table 15.11).

This section discusses the primary leukodystrophies with known metabolic defects, listed by age of onset in Table 15.12. The progressive leukoencephalopathies are characterized clinically by motor manifestations that include spasticity, weakness, pyramidal tract signs, and cerebellar signs. Involuntary movements are prominent in

Table 15.10 Primary leukoencephalopathies

Disorder	Chromosome	Peripheral nerve involvement	Metabolic defect
Pelizaeus-Merzbacher disease	X	–	Proteolipid protein (PLP) synthesis
Metachromatic leukodystrophy	22 or 10	+	Arylsulfatase A or sphingolipid activator protein B
Multiple sulfatase deficiency	3	+	Formylglycine generating enzyme
Krabbe disease	14	+	β-Galactocerebrosidase
X-linked adrenoleukodystrophy (ALD)	X	+	ALD-peroxisomal membrane protein synthesis
Alexander disease	17	–	Glial fibrillary acid protein
Canavan disease	17	–	Aspartoacylase

Pelizaeus-Merzbacher disease. Cognitive and behavioral deterioration are often late and overshadowed by motor disability. Seizures are absent or appear late in the course (except in some cases of adrenoleukodystrophy). Macrocephaly with startle response to sound, irritability, and incessant crying is a frequent sign in Canavan disease, Alexander disease, and Krabbe disease. Peripheral neuropathy is a feature of Krabbe disease, metachromatic leukodystrophy, and some forms of adrenoleukodystrophy. High protein in the CSF is found in metachromatic leukodystrophy, Krabbe disease, and adrenoleukodystrophy.

Metachromatic leukodystrophy

Metachromatic leukodystrophy (MLD), or sulfatide lipidosis, is a heterogeneous group of autosomal recessive lysosomal storage disorders. The biochemical defect has been localized in the catabolism of a sphingolipid, sulfatide, which is a normal constituent of myelin and cellular membranes. In MLD, sulfatide is stored in the lysosomes of the oligodendrites and Schwann cells, as well as in many somatic tissues. The metachromasia, for which the disorder is named, results from a shift of blue stains toward red in tissues containing sulfatide. Mutations of at least three genes result in MLD. The most common disease-producing mutations occur in the ARSA gene encoding for arylsulfatase-A (ASA) and assigned to the long arm of chromosome 22 (22q13) (Hors-Cayla et al. 1979). Arylsulfatase-A mutations fall into two groups that correlate with clinical phenotype. Group I mutations produce no enzyme activity and no immunoreactive protein, producing the late infantile form of MLD. Group II mutations generate small amounts of immunoreactive protein and low levels of functional enzymes. Individuals homozygous for type II mutation develop the adult form of MLD. Heterozygotes with type I and II mutations develop the juvenile form of MLD. Mutations within the saposin B region of the prosaposin (PSAP) gene on chromosome 10 (Inui et al. 1985) have resulted in MLD due to loss of sphingolipid activator protein activity. The multiple sulfatase deficiency gene that regulates in the endoplasmic reticulum the post-translational processing of all the sulfatases (SUMF1 for sulfatase modifying factor 1) has been mapped to chromosome 3p26 and encodes a formylglycine-generating enzyme (FGE) (Cosma et al. 2003).

In the United States, the incidence of all forms of metachromatic leukodystrophy is estimated to be 1 in 100,000 births, although the true incidence may be higher because many cases remain undiagnosed.

Clinically, at least four forms of metachromatic leukodystrophy can be distinguished. The late-infantile form is the most frequent. The first clinical symptoms begin insidiously in the second year of life. Abdominal pain may be the presenting symptom. The clinical picture

Table 15.11 Secondary leukoencephalopathies

Disorder	Chromosome	Peripheral nerve involvement	Metabolic defect
Zellweger syndrome	8	+	Peroxisomal assembly factor
Nonketotic hyperglycinemia	9 (glycine decarboxylase)	–	Glycine cleavage system (4 proteins)
Hurler disease	4	–	L-Iduronidase
Glutaric aciduria type I	19	–	Glutaryl-CoA-dehydrogenase
Cockayne disease	5 and 10	+	DNA repair
Vanishing white matter disease	12, 14, 1, 2, 3	–	Cytoprotection during stress
Mitochondrial leukodystrophy	?	±	Respiratory chain enzymes

Table 15.12 Age of onset of progressive leukoencephalopathies and leukodystrophies

Early infancy (before 12 months)
- Infantile Krabbe disease
- Canavan disease
- Alexander disease
- Pelizaeus-Merzbacher disease
- Vanishing white matter disease

Early childhood (1–5 years)
- Metachromatic leukodystrophy
- Late infantile forms of Krabbe disease
- Vanishing white matter disease

Late childhood and adolescence (5–15 years)
- X-linked adrenoleukodystrophy
- Juvenile metachromatic leukodystrophy
- Juvenile Krabbe disease
- Vanishing white matter disease

Adulthood
- Metachromatic leukodystrophy (ataxia, dementia)
- Krabbe disease
- Adrenomyeloneuropathy
- Vanishing white matter disease

Pearls and Perils

- Detection of large amounts of urinary sulfatides is essential for diagnosis. Urine should be kept at 4°C for collection.
- Low arylsulfatase-A in asymptomatic persons may be seen in two situations. Presymptomatic cases of metachromatic leukodystrophy excrete excessive amounts of urinary sulfatide. Normal amounts of sulfatide are found in pseudoarylsulfatase-A deficiency.
- Arylsulfatase-A is not always low in metachromatic leukodystrophy. Assay of arylsulfatase-A in intact cells and detection of large amounts of sulfatide in the urine allow diagnosis of saposin B deficiency.
- Arylsulfatase-A deficiency is deficient in multiple sulfatase deficiency, a rare autosomal recessive metachromatic leukodystrophy associated with combined features of mucopolysaccharidoses, X-linked ichthyosis, and X-linked chondrodysplasia punctata.
- CT scan and MRI of the head typically demonstrate mild enlargement of the ventricles and demyelination bilaterally, with the maximum at the anterior and posterior poles of the ventricles.

is characterized by progressive motor losses and dysfunction. Motor symptoms characteristically occur early and are more prominent than seizures and mental deterioration. A frequent early problem is a gait disorder with unsteadiness. Within months, this leads to the loss of the ability to walk and stand. Decrease in deep tendon reflexes occurs in the early stage, as the peripheral neuropathy worsens and is later replaced by hyperreflexia. Bilateral extensor toe responses occur early and persist. Speech deteriorates as a result of dysarthria and aphasia. Ataxia and truncal instability become obvious. Intermittent pain is a manifestation of peripheral neuropathy. Nystagmus is present. Optic atrophy and a grayish discoloration of the macula are occasionally observed. Hypotonia is progressively replaced by rigidity and spasticity. Megalencephaly is frequently noted. Most children are bedridden by age 3 years. All meaningful contact with the surroundings is progressively lost. An opisthotonic posture with flexion of the arms, equinovarus posture, and scissoring of the legs is present in later stages of the illness and may last for a few months to several years.

The juvenile form has its onset between age 4 and 10 years. The majority of cases develop during the first years of school with bradykinesia and poor school performance. Daydreaming, confusion, or emotional lability may be seen early. Unsteadiness of gait, usually owing to pyramidal system involvement, may occur. Extrapyramidal dysfunction, as suggested by postural abnormalities, rigidity, and tremor may also develop. Seizures occur in more than half of the patients. Deep tendon reflexes are usually increased. The rate of deterioration is usually slower and more variable than in the late-infantile form. Patients may not be bedridden until 5–50 years after symptoms begin.

The adult form has its onset any time after puberty. Initial symptoms consist of personality and mental changes. Such symptoms are often misdiagnosed as attention deficit disorder, schizophrenia, or manic-depressive illness. Seizures are rarely the presenting symptom. Movement disorders, ataxia, and paresis appear later. There are usually no clinical signs of peripheral neuropathy. In the final stage, the patient is mute, blind, bedridden, and unresponsive.

A rare variant of MLD combines features of the mucopolysaccharidosis with X-linked ichthyosis, X-linked chondrodysplasia punctata, and those of MLD. It is now called *multiple sulfatase deficiency*. The mucopolysaccharidosis-like features include a mild gargoylism (facial changes with depressed bridge of the nose), hydrocephalus, growth retardation, limitation in extension of the elbows, radiologic changes of chondrodysplasia punctata, hepatosplenomegaly, heart defects, and deafness. Corneal opacities do not occur. Ichthyosis, when present, develops at an early age. In general, presymptomatic development is less advanced than that of late-infantile metachromatic leukodystrophy. Most children never achieve normal gait or speech. Neurologic regression follows the pattern of late-infantile MLD. By the age of 5, the child is profoundly retarded with quadriplegia, pseudobulbar paralysis, and optic atrophy.

A number of laboratory tests may reinforce a clinical suspicion of metachromatic leukodystrophy. Cerebrospinal fluid studies may show an elevated protein concentration. Nerve conduction studies may demonstrate slow nerve conduction velocities or an increase in duration and number of potential components. In the adult form, nerve conduction studies and CSF proteins may be normal while EEG abnormalities are diffuse and nonspecific. Multimodality, evoked potentials may reveal a latency prolongation or loss of evoked potential components that is dependent on the type of metachromatic leukodystrophy (late infantile, juvenile, or mucosulfatidosis) and on the duration of the disease. MRI is more sensitive than CT scan and allows earlier recognition and more precise characterization of areas of brain demyelination (Figure 15.4). When multiple sulfatase deficiency is suspected, additional clinical laboratory tests should include skeletal x-ray series for evidence of chondrodysplasia punctata and examination of the peripheral blood smear for the characteristic lymphocytic storage vacuoles called Alder-Reilly granules.

The diagnosis of MLD is confirmed by demonstrating excess excretion of sulfatide in urine and by assay of arylsulfatase-A in leukocytes or skin fibroblasts (Table 15.13). All patients with MLD excrete large amounts of sulfatide in the urine. Most patients with MLD have, on cell-free preparations (e.g., serum, urine), a profound deficiency of arylsulfatase-A regardless of the age of onset. However, intact cells in culture are able to express subtle variations in their ability to clear sulfatide, giving a biochemical basis for variation in the age of onset in MLD. Low arylsulfatase-A activity in the cell homogenates of asymptomatic persons does not always indicate a diagnosis of MLD. Some are healthy individuals with pseudoarylsulfatase-A deficiency who excrete normal amounts of urinary sulfatide. Excessive amounts of sulfatide are, however, found in the urine of presymptomatic patients. In a rare variant, arylsulfatase-A activity in all homogenates is normal, whereas large amounts of sulfatide are found in the urine. The molecular basis for this variant is a deficiency of saposin B, required for in vivo sulfatide catabolism. These patients present clinically with the features of juvenile MLD and show arylsulfatase-A activity in cultured fibroblasts that is in the heterozygous range but can be enhanced to normal levels by the action of the activator protein. Sulfatide loading shows deficient turnover in cultured fibroblasts. In multiple sulfatase deficiency, mucopolysacchariduria and oligosacchariduria are associated with sulfatiduria. In multiple sulfatase deficiency, not only is lysosomal arylsulfatase-A deficient, but also other lysosomal sulfatases acting in the catabolism of glycosaminoglycans (deficient in mucopolysaccharidoses type II, IIIA, IIID, IVA, and VII), as well as non-lysosomal sulfatases such as steroid sulfatase (defi-

Table 15.13 Metachromatic leukodystrophy

Discriminating features
- Metachromasia of peripheral nerves
- Large amount of sulfatides in urine
- Arylsulfatase deficiency in fibroblasts or white blood cells (type I & II)

Consistent features
- Mental deterioration
- Ataxia
- Extensor toe signs
- Reduced or absent sensory action potential

Variable features
- Hypotonia (early) and spasticity (late)
- Deep tendon reflexes decreased early and increased late
- Strabismus
- Visual impairment
- Psychiatric symptoms
- Extrapyramidal dysfunction
- Seizures (rarely)
- Elevated cerebrospinal fluid proteins
- Slow motor conduction velocity
- Mucopolysaccharidosis-like symptoms (rarely)

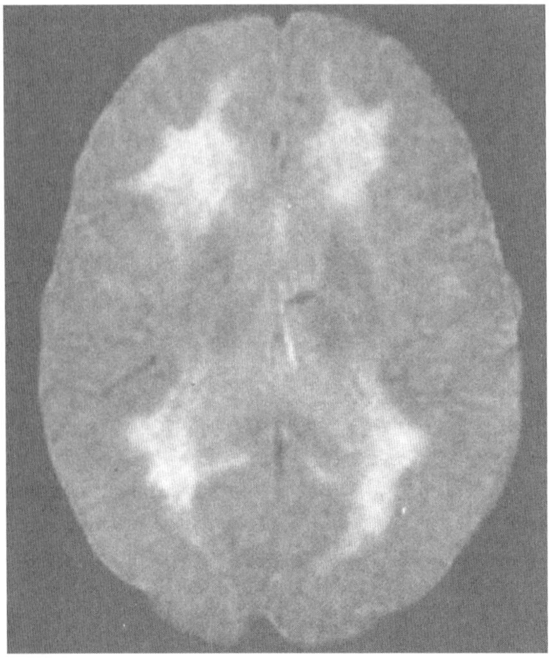

Figure 15.4 Magnetic resonance image of the brain (SE 2100/100) showing bilateral, symmetric, homogeneous, and diffuse elevation of the signal intensity throughout the deep hemispheric white matter (sparing U fibers) in a 3-year-old girl with metachromatic leukodystrophy.

cient in X-linked ichthyosis) and arylsulfatase E (deficient in X-linked chondrodysplasia punctata). At the genetic level, analysis of ASA, prosaposin, and SUMF1 genes is now possible. Prenatal diagnosis of different forms of MLD can be accomplished.

Metachromatic leukodystrophy is a systemic disease affecting not only the CNS and peripheral nervous system (PNS), but also other organs such as kidneys (renal tubular epithelium), gallbladder, liver, pancreas (islets of Langerhans), adrenal cortex, ovaries, and testes. The reticuloendothelial system is never affected. In the PNS, segmental demyelination occurs.

Treatments have been unsuccessful in correcting the progression of MLD. Bone marrow transplantation has produced only limited success. Although it is expected to yield better results if performed at the presymptomatic stage, further clinical trials are needed to establish its value. Multiple sulfatase deficiency is expected to respond to enzyme replacement therapy.

X-linked adrenoleukodystrophy

X-linked adrenoleukodystrophy (ALD) is the most common peroxisomal disorder (incidence of 1:20,000–1:100,000), with impaired β-oxidation of straight-chain lipids, characterized by adrenal insufficiency and neurologic disturbances. Tissues and body fluids of patients with X-linked ALD contain abnormally high levels of unbranched and saturated, very-long-chain fatty acids (VLCFA), particularly hexacosanoate (C26:0). The peroxisomes are unable to form the normal coenzyme A (CoA) derivative of VLCFA. The adrenoleukodystrophy (ALD) gene has been mapped to the terminal segment of the long arm of the X chromosome (Xq28 locus). The ALD gene product is a peroxisomal membrane protein that belongs to the ATP-binding cassette family of transporters. It has been postulated that a deletion or point mutation in ALD results in a defective transport of the peroxisomal acyl CoA synthetase to its site of activity (Ligtenberg et al. 1995).

The clinical forms of X-linked ADL have been classified according to age of onset, gender, and presenting clinical symptoms. Neurologic manifestations vary considerably, even among members of the same family. The most common form presents in boys during childhood, with Addison disease without neurologic symptoms. The primary adrenocortical insufficiency leads to skin hyperpigmentation, intermittent vomiting, and fatigue. The interval between the onset of adrenal insufficiency and neurologic disability is variable. Some patients may remain neurologically intact until adulthood, while others develop cerebral ALD or adrenomyeloneuropathy before or without adrenal insufficiency. Adrenal insufficiency is extremely rare in symptomatic females.

Childhood cerebral ALD, the second most common form of X-linked ALD, is an inflammatory encephalomyelopathy characterized by onset in boys between 4 and 10 years of age of an overt neurologic disability. The classic childhood form is characterized by behavioral, intellectual, and motor changes. Hyperactivity, withdrawal, aggressive outbursts, learning difficulties, poor memory, gait disturbances, speech difficulties, poor coordination, and impaired vision and hearing are the most common presenting symptoms. Other less common neurologic symptoms include seizures, incontinence, headaches, and tics. The disease runs a relentless, rapidly progressive course lasting between 1 and 9 years. The motor examination shows signs of upper motor unit involvement with continuing progression to quadriparesis. Signs of peripheral nerve dysfunction are never prominent. Visual disturbances include homonymous hemianopia, visual

Pearls and Perils

X-Linked adrenoleukodystrophy

- Clinical and laboratory signs of adrenal insufficiency may precede onset of childhood cerebral X-linked adrenoleukodystrophy.
- There are no clinical signs of peripheral neuropathy in childhood X-linked adrenoleukodystrophy, and nerve conduction velocities may be normal despite pathologic involvement.
- Magnetic resonance imaging (MRI) is often pathognomonic in childhood adrenoleukodystrophy. The finding of a unilateral lesion or lesions without a perilesional enhanced rim does not exclude childhood cerebral adrenoleukodystrophy.
- Except during addisonian crisis, plasma cortisol values are normal. A provocative adrenal stimulation with adrenocorticotropic hormone (ACTH) is usually required to demonstrate the diminished adrenal reserve.
- In X-linked adrenoleukodystrophy, the cerebrospinal fluid may show pleocytosis and local production of immunoglobulin G.
- Until recently, the eponym, Schilder disease, was used to describe various progressive leukoencephalopathies characterized by massive, bilateral, diffuse demyelination, more prominent in the occipital regions, and displaying histologic features of multiple sclerosis (anisomorphic gliosis and perivascular inflammatory reaction). Schilder's three cases represent three different conditions: the 1912 case probably represents a subacute (or chronic) diffuse encephaloclastic disorder, a variant of multiple sclerosis; the 1913 case probably represents X-linked adrenoleukodystrophy; and the 1924 case probably a postinfectious encephalomyelitis. The three conditions are easily differentiated using appropriate laboratory studies.

agnosia, and loss of visual acuity. Optic atrophy eventually occurs in all patients. Seizures, when present, are focal or multifocal. Duration of the illness is short. Death frequently occurs within the first 15 years of life. Childhood cerebral ALD is rare in females and seems to have a slower progressive course.

The adolescent cerebral ALD is a rare form of X-linked ALD characterized by onset of neurologic disability between ages 11 and 21 years. The neurologic deterioration is rapid, leading to dementia, spastic quadriparesis, and vegetative state months to years after onset of symptoms. This syndrome is extremely rare in girls (Hershkovitzet al. 2002).

The adult cerebral ALD is a rare phenotype seen in both sexes. These patients have no sign of spinal cord involvement and develop psychotic symptoms or focal neurologic signs from the early 20s to the 50s.

Adult onset adrenomyeloneuropathy (AMN) is the most common phenotype, accounting for 45% of all cases. Neurologic problems, at least initially, are due to noninflammatory axonopathy without inflammatory brain involvement. Predominant neurologic manifestations begin in the second or third decade with resulting progressive spastic paraparesis, distal sensory loss, stiffness or weakness of legs, sphincter disturbances, and sexual impotence. Symptoms show slow progression, sometimes over decades. Symptoms are usually mild to moderate in females. About half of all patients eventually also develop an inflammatory myeloencephalopathy that becomes severely progressive in about 10–20% of patients with AMN. Some men have hypogonadism with azoospermia and hypotestosteronism.

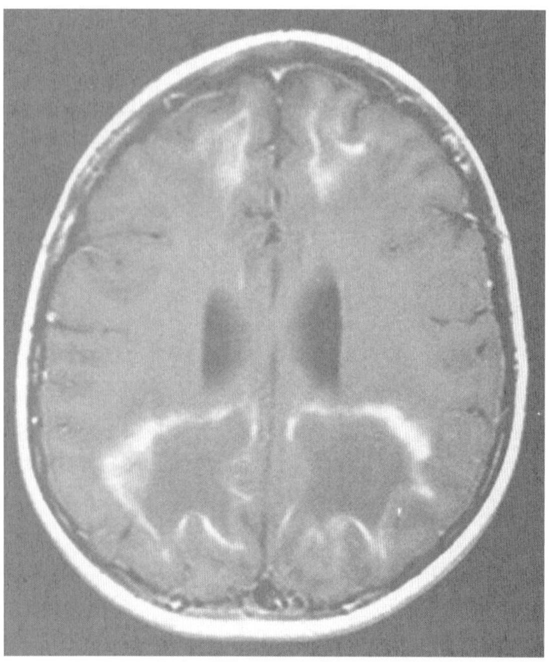

Figure 15.5 Contrast-enhanced magnetic resonance image of the brain (SE 650/16) showing bilateral, symmetric low-signal inactive lesions of the subcortical white matter with typical parieto-occipital localization associated with enhancing active periphery zone of high signal in a 9-year-old boy with X-linked adrenoleukodystrophy.

Key Clinical Questions

- *Does your son have intermittent vomiting and a darkening skin complexion even in unexposed skin?*
  Addison disease should be suspected. In such patient plasma very-long-chain fatty acid (VLCFA) levels should be requested.

Recent experience has shown that MRI is superior to CT scan in demonstrating CNS involvement in X-linked ALD. In the childhood cerebral form of ALD, MRI shows symmetric high-signal areas in the parieto-occipital white matter extending to subcortical regions on T2-weighted images. Gadolinium-enhanced MRI shows accumulation of contrast material in regions undergoing demyelination (Figure 15.5). The prognostic significance of mild MRI abnormalities in asymptomatic patients remains uncertain. In AMN, nerve conduction studies often suggest a mixed neuropathic pattern of both multifocal demyelination and axonal loss. Nerve conduction studies can help identify preclinical AMN without neurologic disability.

Except during addisonian crisis, serum electrolyte levels and plasma cortisol values are normal. Baseline adrenocorticotropic hormone (ACTH) values may be elevated. A provocative adrenal stimulation is required in most cases to demonstrate the diminished adrenal reserve. The CSF proteins are frequently elevated in the childhood form. Diagnosis of X-linked ALD is suggested by assays of VLCFA in plasma, red blood cells, white cells, and cultured skin fibroblast phospholipids. Concentrations of the VLCFA, tetracosanoic (C24:0), and hexacosanoic (C26:0) acids, and the ratios of C24:0/C22:0 and C26:0/C22:0 are increased. The defects are confined to saturated VLCFA. (In neonatal ALD, both monounsaturated and saturated VLCFA are elevated.) Analysis of ALD gene is now possible (Ligtenberg 1995) (Tables 15.14 and 15.15).

Pearls and Perils

- Male patients with adrenomyeloneuropathy (AMN) should be monitored for adrenal insufficiency and steroid replacement therapy should be initiated as necessary. Females with AMN are not at risk for adrenal insufficiency.

Table 15.14 X-Linked adrenoleukodystrophy (childhood)

Discriminating features
- Increased very-long-chain fatty acids in plasma
- Peroxisomal lignoceroyl-CoA ligase deficiency
- ALD gene mutations

Consistent features
- Male
- Adrenal insufficiency (clinical or subclinical)
- Higher cortical function
- Visual impairment with optic atrophy
- Abnormal gait with pyramidal tract signs
- Magnetic resonance imaging of brain shows occipito-parietal white matter disease with perilesional enhancement

Variable features
- Cerebrospinal fluid (CSF) pleocytosis; intrathecal production of γ-globulins
- Elevated CSF protein
- Skin hyperpigmentation
- Seizures
- Incontinence
- Ataxia

Hormonal substitution may be necessary to correct adrenal insufficiency, but this therapeutic approach does not influence the progression of the neurologic symptoms. Specific therapy for X-linked ALD is under investigation. Flavanoid therapy has recently been suggested (Morita 2007). Plasmapheresis should probably be initiated early after onset of neurologic symptoms. Bone marrow transplant appears beneficial in patients with minimal neurologic involvement.

Table 15.15 X-Linked adrenomyeloneuropathy (adulthood)

Discriminating features
- Elevation of very-long-chain fatty acids in plasma
- Peroxisomal lignoceroyl-CoA ligase deficiency
- ALD gene mutations

Consistent features
- Male (occasional female)
- Spastic paraparesis
- Distal polyneuropathy
- Adrenal insufficiency in males

Variable features
- Skin hyperpigmentation
- Hypogonadism
- Sphincter disturbances
- Behavior changes
- Dementia
- Cerebellar
- Focal central syndromes
- Psychosis

Krabbe disease

Krabbe globoid cell leukodystrophy, or galactosylceramide lipidosis, is an autosomal recessive lysosomal storage disease resulting from a defect in the catabolism of a sphingolipid galactocerebroside (or galactosylceramide). This lipid is exclusively a constituent of myelin and thus accumulates in Schwann cells and oligodendrocytes. Globoid cells, containing membrane-bound dense linear or curved tubular profiles, are pathognomonic in the CNS but are not seen in the PNS. The characteristic metabolic defect in various forms of Krabbe disease is a deficiency in galactocerebroside β-galactosidase, which is involved in the catabolism of galactocerebroside. Mutations of the galactosylceraminidase gene (GALC) on chromosome 14q31 can affect various portions of the structural gene. The one affecting the central domain is more likely to cause a severe phenotype, whereas those occurring in the N- or C-terminus predict a milder phenotype (Furuya et al. 1997). Mutations in the saposin A coding region of the prosaposin (PSAP) gene on chromosome 10 are responsible for a Krabbe-like phenotype (Spiegel et al. 2005). In Sweden, the incidence is about two cases per 100,000 births. In a large Druze isolate in Israel, incidence has been found to be as high as 6 in 1,000 births.

Krabbe disease has been divided into two clinical subgroups according to age of onset of neurologic symptoms. Most cases are of the infantile form. The clinical onset of the disease usually occurs between 3 and 6 months of life, although a few cases with earlier (neonatal variant) or later onset have been reported. Usually, during the first months of life, the infants have a normal development. From the onset, the course of disease is steadily progressive and can be divided into three stages.

Pearls and Perils

- The head circumference is usually normal in Krabbe disease, although hydrocephalus may occur.
- There is no visceromegaly and no cherry-red spot.
- Peripheral neuropathy and elevation of cerebrospinal fluid protein are constant findings in infantile Krabbe disease. Those findings need not be present for the diagnosis of late-onset Krabbe disease.
- Galactocerebroside-β-galactosidase should always be assayed with natural substrates.

Stage I is characterized by intermittent fever, hyperirritability, feeding difficulties, and stimulus-sensitive, tonic extensor spasms. At the same time, stagnation in motor and mental development is noted. Seizures may occur. In stage II, rapid and severe motor and mental deterioration develops. There is marked hypertonicity with opisthotonus, scissoring of the legs, flexion of the arms, and clenching of the fists. Deep tendon reflexes are hyperactive. Optic atrophy is common, and pupillary response to light may be compromised. There are no cherry-red spots. The child remains small and may display macrocephaly. There is no visceromegaly. Various seizures (irregular myoclonic seizures, infantile spasms, major tonic–clonic seizures) frequently occur. Stage III is the "burn-out" stage. The infant is decerebrate and has no contact with the surroundings. Deep tendon reflexes are depressed. Most patients die of an intercurrent infection or bulbar paralysis before 2 years of age, although a protracted course has been observed in rare cases.

The second clinical subgroup is late-onset Krabbe disease. In most patients, the clinical manifestations appear between the ages of 2 and 6 years, although later onset has been described. The most common presenting complaint is rapidly failing vision, together with gait difficulties. The failure of vision is caused by cortical blindness with optic atrophy. Gait difficulties may be caused by hemiparesis, paraparesis, progressive cerebellar ataxia, or acute polyneuropathy. Rare individuals may first present at school age with dementia or psychotic traits. Despite the variable presentation of the disease, the clinical picture progressively becomes more uniform and is dominated by dementia, cortical blindness with optic atrophy, and spastic quadriparesis. Death usually occurs 1–3 years from the onset of symptoms, although a protracted course also occurs.

CT scan of the head early in the course of infantile Krabbe disease may be normal. Later, nonenhanced CT scan may show high signal lesions in the thalami, body of the caudate nuclei, corona radiata, and cerebellum. Low attenuation in the periventricular white matter appears in the intermediate stage and, in the third stage, cerebral atrophy involves both gray and white matter. Hydrocephalus may be an additional finding. In late-onset Krabbe disease, CT of the head shows nonspecific enlargement of the lateral ventricles and low attenuation around the frontal horns. An enhancing rim may be observed between the demyelinated white matter and unaffected arcuate fibers. MRI in infantile Krabbe disease may show, on T2-weighted images, symmetric high-signal lesions in the white matter of the centrum semiovale and low-signal lesions in the thalamus and brainstem. At later stages, atrophy can been seen (Figure 15.6). In late-onset Krabbe disease, symmetric confluent hyperintense lesions in the peritrigonal region are associated with atrophy of the splenium of the corpus callosum. Small hyperintensity lesions can also be seen in the posterior limb of the internal capsule. There is no rim enhancement with gadolinium diethylenetriamine pentaacetic acid (DTPA) in late-onset Krabbe disease.

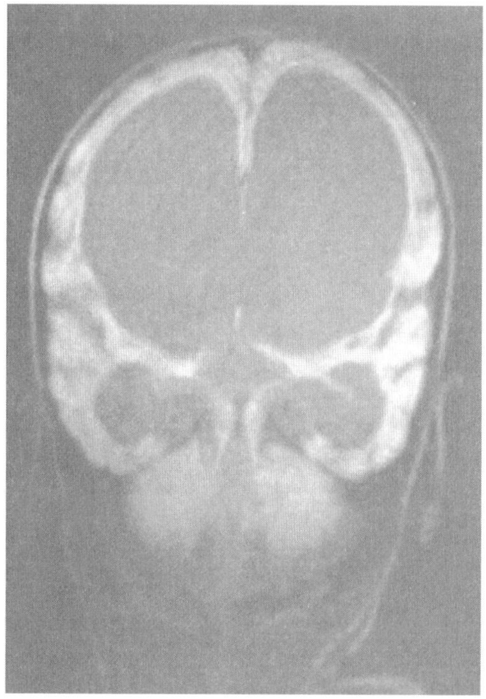

Figure 15.6 Magnetic resonance image of the brain (SE 1585/40) showing hydrocephalus ex vacuo in a 6-year-old boy with stage III Krabbe disease.

In the first stage of infantile Krabbe disease, the CSF protein is already elevated. The electrophoretic pattern may be diagnostically helpful in that albumin and α_2-globulin levels are elevated and β_1- and γ-globulin levels are decreased. This pattern persists throughout the course of the disease. Assays of galactoceroside β-galactosidase in white cells, serum, or cultured fibroblasts with the use of appropriate natural glycolipid substrates provide the means for antemortem diagnosis. When the enzyme β-galactosidase is assayed with synthetic substrates, no deficiency is found. This differentiates Krabbe disease from GM_1 gangliosidosis, in which galactocerebroside β-galactosidase activity is normal, but β-galactosidase assayed with synthetic substrates is deficient (Table 15.16). Defi-

Key Clinical Questions

- *Did your infant present an increased irritability with sudden episodes of posturing in response to minor stimuli with arching of the back, extension of the lower extremities, flexion of the upper extremities, and fisting?*
  The exam fails to show organomegaly.

Table 15.16 Krabbe globoid cell leukodystrophy

Discriminating features
- Galactocerebroside-β-galactosidase deficiency in leukocytes and fibroblasts
- Globoid cells in white matter (brain biopsy)

Consistent features
- Increased cerebrospinal fluid (CSF) proteins
- Abnormal electrophoretic pattern of CSF proteins
- Extensor toe signs

Variable features
- Spasticity
- Psychomotor retardation
- Irritability
- Spasticity, hyperextension
- Hyperreflexia (early) and hyporeflexia (late)
- Blindness (with optic atrophy)
- Deafness
- Failure to thrive
- Macrocephaly
- Ataxia
- Focal motor deficits

ciency of galactocerebroside β-galactosidase may be equally severe in both infantile and late-onset cases, although considerable residual activity is sometimes found in late-onset form. Genetic studies confirm diagnosis and occasionally predict clinical course. Prenatal diagnosis of Krabbe disease may be achieved.

Treatment at this time is limited to allogenic hematopoietic stem cell transplantation that appears to slow the progression of the disease and improve MRI. The use of stem cells and viral vectors to transduce transplantable cells is still under investigation (Krivit et al. 1999).

Spongy degeneration of the central nervous system or Canavan-Van Bogaert-Bertrand disease

Spongy degeneration of the CNS or Canavan-Van Bogaert disease is an autosomal recessive leukoencephalopathy characterized by megalencephaly, axial hypotonia, peripheral spasticity, and optic atrophy. The peripheral myelin is spared. The spongy appearance of the brain results from excessive fluid accumulation in astrocytes. Neurons are spared. The biochemical basis of Canavan-Van Bogaert disease is a deficiency in aspartoacylase, an enzyme playing a role in central myelin synthesis. The incidence of Canavan disease in the Ashkenazi Jewish population is expected to be 1:5,000 births. In that population, three point mutations (E285A, Y231X, and A305E) of the aspartoacylase (ASPA) gene on the chromosome 17p account for most cases (Feigenbaum et al. 2004). In the non-Jewish population, more than 20 disease-producing mutations have been reported (Zeng et al. 2002). Some mutations (D249V) lead to a congenital disease, whereas other mutations (R71A) predict a milder phenotype (Velinov et al. 2008).

Pearls and Perils

- Symmetrical areas of putaminal hypodensities can be seen in head computed tomography (CT) scan in some cases before the appearance of subcortical leukodystrophy.
- A spongy degeneration similar to that seen in Canavan-Van Bogaert disease may be seen in some amino acidopathies (e.g., maple syrup disease, phenylketonuria, nonketotic hyperglycinemia, arginosuccinic aciduria), organic aciduria (e.g., 3-hydroxy-methylglutaryl-CoA-lyase deficiency), mitochondrial disorders (e.g., Kearns-Sayre syndrome), infections (e.g., Creutzfeldt-Jakob disease), and intoxications (e.g., triethyltin). These conditions are easily distinguishable from Canavan-Bogaert-Bertrand disease on clinical and pathological grounds.
- Macrocephaly, a characteristic feature of Canavan disease, can also be found in Alexander disease, metachromatic leukodystrophy, Krabbe disease (some cases), glutaric acidemia type I, Tay-Sachs disease (late), mucopolysaccharidosis, and disorders of glycoprotein metabolism.
- The proton magnetic resonance (MR) spectroscopy shows high levels of N acetylaspartate (NAA) in the white matter. High NAA levels are also seen in patients with Salla disease, an inherited lysosomal disorder characterized by accumulation of sialic acid and in Pelizaeus-Merzbacher disease (Takanashi et al. 2002).

Three forms of Canavan-Van Bogaert disease have been described. The infantile form is the most common. Visual attentiveness and smiling are usually noted during early development. An increasing head circumference crossing percentile lines, not explained by hydrocephalus is frequently the first clinical sign. Between 2 and 4 months of age, decreased motor activity, hypotonia, and poor head control are noted. Clinical course is variable. Deterioration is frequently rapid, leading to axial hypotonia and peripheral spasticity. Some hyperreactivity is precipitated by auditory, visual, and tactile stimuli. Severe spasticity with pseudobulbar palsy and visual loss is seen in the terminal stage. Optic atrophy is demonstrated by funduscopic exam. Seizures, usually generalized tonic–clonic type, occur in about 50% of patients. Death usually occurs in the first decade from aspiration pneumonia. The congenital form is characterized by macrocephaly at birth and severe hypotonia leading to death shortly after birth. The juvenile form is characterized by slower progression of symptoms and normal head size. Gross and fine motor developments are slightly delayed. Dysarthria is frequently noted. The disorder is characterized by a protracted course, prolonged survival until adulthood, and mental retardation with a phenotype mimicking extrapyramidal cerebral palsy. Progressive cerebellar syndrome and mental deterioration followed by generalized spasticity, seizures, and visual loss occur in adolescence or adulthood.

Diagnosis is suggested by neuroimaging, which shows symmetrical subcortical white matter changes (Table 15.17). Symmetric involvement of the striatum may precede appearance of white matter changes. Later in the course of the illness, diffuse atrophy is found. Nerve conduction studies and EMG are normal. Somatosensory, visual, and brainstem auditory evoked potentials are abnormal. Spinal fluid frequently reveals elevation of CSF proteins. High concentrations of N-acetylaspartate (NAA) are found in plasma, urine, and CSF, analyzed by gas chromatography-mass spectrometry. Proton magnetic resonance spectroscopy (MRS) of the brain white matter shows very high levels of NAA relative to other metabolites such as creatine, phosphocreatinine, and choline. Aspartoacylase activity in fibroblasts of individuals with Canavan-Van Bogaert disease is absent or reduced. DNA analysis can be carried out on blood from the proband and the parents. Prenatal diagnosis combines measurements of NAA with DNA analysis. Gene therapy using a virus-based gene transfer is under investigation. Acetate supplementation may have therapeutic benefits (Kirmani et al. 2002). Symptomatic support includes nutritional therapy and generous use of antiepileptic drugs and antibiotics.

Table 15.17 Canavan-Van Bogaert disease

Discriminating features

- Urinary excretion of large amounts of N-acetylaspartic acid
- High N-acetylaspartic acid signal by proton magnetic resonance spectroscopy
- Aspartoacylase deficiency in skin fibroblasts
- Mutations of aspartoacylase gene on chromosome 17

Consistent features

- Macrocephaly
- Hypotonia progressing to spasticity
- Lack of peripheral neuropathy

Variable features

- Generalized seizures (late)
- Dysphagia
- Optic atrophy
- Leukodystrophy on neuroimaging
- Dystonia

Key Clinical Questions

- *Is there any Ashkenazi Jewish ancestry or are the parents of the child closely related?*
  The diagnosis of Canavan disease should be considered if the disease presents in early infancy with poor head control, early hypotonia, and a progressive head enlargement.

Pelizaeus-Merzbacher disease

Pelizaeus-Merzbacher disease (PMD) is a slowly progressive X-linked orthochromatic leukodystrophy sparing the PNS. Oligodendrocytes fail to deposit myelin due to decreased production of its chief protein, proteolipid protein (PLP). The PLP gene has been mapped to the human chromosome Xq22 region. In about 30% of patients, who present with a connatal phenotype of PMD, there is a point mutation in the coding portion (exons) of the PLP gene resulting in the apoptosis of maturing oligodendrocytes. In patients with classic PMD, duplications of genomic fragments containing the entire PLP gene, as well as deletions or specific point mutations in one of several exons, result in an abnormal myelin compaction without oligodendrocyte death. Mutations of the extra-

Pearls and Perils

Pelizaeus-Merzbacher disease (PMD)

- Early onset stridor in association with abnormal eye movements in a newborn infant should suggest the possibility of connatal PMD.
- Some individuals affected with PMD may present with clinical and electromyographic features suggestive of neonatal spinal muscular atrophy.
- Recurrence of an apparent athetoid cerebral palsy in several males of a family following a maternal lineage should raise the suspicion for PMD. In some families an occasional female is found to have the disease (Hodes et al. 1993).
- In some patients, feeding difficulties and failure to thrive are so severe that child neglect may be mistakenly suspected.
- An autosomal recessive inheritance has been seen in some families presenting features of Pelizaeus-Merzbacher disease. A peripheral neuropathy accompanies central dysmyelination. Mutations in the gap junction protein 2 (GJC2) encoding a connexin have been found in some families (Uhlenberg B et al. 2004).

exonic PLP gene sequences or of another unknown nearby gene could be involved in rare families (Boespflug-Tanguy et al. 1994). The PLP mutations have also been associated with X-linked spastic paraplegia 2, an allelic disorder with progressive spasticity and weakness in the lower extremities.

Clinical PMD is characterized by onset in infancy or early childhood of abnormal eye movements (slow irregular, roving eye movements interspersed with occasional rotating searching motions) coexisting with head nodding reminiscent of spasmus nutans. The infants are usually floppy early on and have significant psychomotor delay. Most patients never learn to sit, stand, or walk. As the child matures, bilateral pyramidal tract signs, athetosis, choreiform movements, facial grimacing, ataxia, intention tremor, recurrent vomiting, and feeding difficulties become apparent. Speech, when present, is slow. Optic atrophy is a frequent but not early feature of the disease and is usually recognized by 6 years of age. Some patients have seizures of the generalized tonic–clonic, partial motor, or myoclonic type. The disease often progresses to cause death in childhood or adolescence, although some patients survive until the sixth decade.

The onset of the disease in the first 3 months of life has been reported by several investigators and is referred to as the *connatal variant*. Laryngeal stridor due to floppy vocal cords has been observed in these patients. Optic atrophy can be identified early. Some individuals may present with clinical features suggestive of neonatal spinal muscular atrophy (Kaye et al. 1994). The connatal form has a severe course, leading to death in infancy or childhood. X-linked spastic paraplegia type II, resulting from a point mutation in the PLP gene, may have its onset between the toddler years and early teens. The disease progresses slowly without dementia. Some patients develop a dysarthria, nystagmus, and ataxia in the upper extremities. Optic atrophy is sometimes seen.

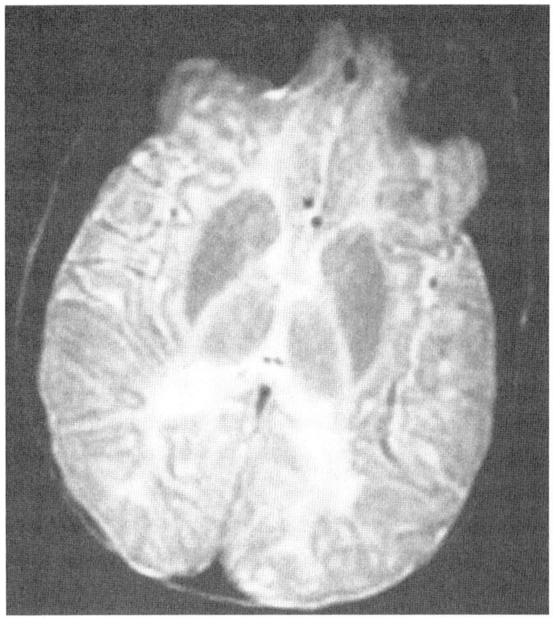

Figure 15.7 MRI of the brain (SE 200/90) showing paucity of white matter in a 2-year-old boy with Pelizaeus-Merzbacher disease.

Table 15.18 Pelizaeus-Merzbacher disease (PMD)

Discriminating features
- Mutation in the PLP gene
- Symmetrical and homogeneous inversion of the myelin signal on MRI of brain; thin corpus callosum

Consistent features
- Abnormal eye movements
- Oscillatory motions of the head
- Psychomotor deterioration
- Male (rarely female)
- Normal nerve conduction velocities

Variable features
- Stridor
- Optic atrophy
- Bilateral pyramidal tract signs
- Choreoathetosis
- Vomiting
- Ataxia
- Seizures
- Muscle atrophy
- Spastic paraplegia

Spinal fluid studies are noncontributory. Nerve conduction velocities and muscle biopsy are normal, but EMG changes suggestive of spinal muscular atrophy may be present in infancy. Abnormalities of evoked potential responses are nonspecific indicators of central white matter disease. CT scan of the head is usually normal in the early stages of the disease and nonspecific in the late stages, showing abnormalities such as diffuse atrophy. MRI of the brain in the early stages reveals symmetrical and homogenous inversion of the signals between white matter and gray matter in T1- and T2-weighted images (Table 15.18). The amount of white matter is decreased, and the corpus callosum is thin (Figure 15.7). Definite diagnosis is established by mutation analysis.

Neuropathologic examination may reveal cerebral and cerebellar atrophy and poor demarcation between gray and white matter. Amidst widespread dysmyelination, perivascular islets of myelin are frequently spared, a characteristic of Pelizaeus-Merzbacher disease also found in Cockayne syndrome. In the connatal form, a complete absence of myelin sheaths is present. Nerve cells and axons tend to be preserved. No involvement of the peripheral nerves is found. Treatment of Pelizaeus-Merzbacher disease is symptomatic.

Alexander disease

This degenerative disorder is a primary genetic disorder of astrocytes, characterized pathologically by the presence in astrocytes of cytoplasmic eosinophilic hyaline bodies, called *Rosenthal fibers*. Rosenthal fibers result from overproduction of the glial fibrillary acid protein GFAP, an intermediate filament protein. Alexander disease has been shown to result from multiple mutations in the GFAP gene on chromosome 17 (Brenner et al. 2002). In all patients, the GFAP mutations are dominant. The parents are usually normal, and the disorder arises de novo from a spontaneous dominant heterozygous mutation or from germinal mosaicism in cases with early onset. In adults, milder mutations are autosomal dominant (Rodriguez et al. 2001).

Clinically, three forms are distinguished by age of onset. The rare neonatal form is characterized by early, often intractable, multifocal seizures, hydrocephalus due to aqueductal stenosis by the propagation of astrocytes. These astrocytes contain excessive amounts of eosinophilic cytoplasmic material, lack of developmental maturation, and elevated CSF protein content (Springer et al. 2000).

The most frequent form of Alexander syndrome is the infantile form, which has an average onset at 6 months of age. However, onset may occur at any time from shortly before birth to as late as 2 years of age. The average duration of disease is 2–3 years, but it can vary from a few months to several years. Predominant psychomotor retardation exists initially, and progressive spasticity and seizures develop in the context of megalencephaly, with or without frank hydrocephalus (Li et al. 2005).

In the juvenile form, which is much less common than the infantile form, onset usually occurs between 7 and 14 years of age, and the duration is approximately 8 years. Bulbar and pseudobulbar dysfunction predominates, with dysphagia, dysarthria, nystagmus, ptosis, full facial palsy, and tongue atrophy (Seil et al. 1968). Generalized spasticity and weakness may also occur, but unlike the severe mental retardation characteristic of the infantile form, mentation tends to remain intact. The adult form of Alexander syndrome has an early stuttering clinical course mimicking multiple sclerosis and characterized by blurred vision, pyramidal tract signs, cerebellar signs, dysarthria, and dysphagia. Other reported neurologic manifestations include severe atrophy of medulla, and spinal cord atrophy and palatal and ocular myoclonus (Martidis et al. 1999).

CT changes include low attenuation in the deep cerebral white matter, most extensively in the frontal lobes and subependymal regions. The ventricles are variably enlarged. There is inconsistent abnormal enhancement of the caudate nuclei, anterior columns of the fornix, optic radiations, and periventricular areas. MRI reveals bilateral and symmetrical white matter changes most prominent frontally. Cystic cavitation may be seen within the white matter.

Since the types of Alexander disease are phenotypically distinct, the differential diagnosis varies by age. If one encounters an infant with chronically developing megalencephaly or macrocephaly with mild regression in psychomotor milestones in the absence of any other obvious cause, Alexander syndrome is a highly probable diagnosis. Juvenile leukoencephalopathy must be considered in children and multiple sclerosis in adults. Diagnosis is suggested by the demonstration of Rosenthal fibers in subpial zone, around the blood vessels, and along the ventricles in brain biopsy or at autopsy. DNA analysis of the GFAP gene confirms the diagnosis (Table 15.19).

Key Clinical Questions

- *Do you know of any boy, on the maternal side of the family, who presented in infancy with abnormal eye movements, head shaking, and feeding difficulties?*
  The disease is slowly progressive with early hypotonia and involuntary movements.

Pearls and Perils

- Peripheral nerves sparing and macrocephaly are typical features of Alexander disease. These features are not specific, as they are also seen in Canavan disease.

Table 15.19 Alexander disease

Discriminating features
- Mutation in the GFAP gene

Consistent features
- Rosenthal fibers on brain biopsy
- Large head
- Psychomotor deterioration
- Normal nerve conduction velocities

Variable features
- Nystagmus
- Bilateral pyramidal tract signs
- Dysphagia
- Dysarthria
- Seizures
- Muscle atrophy

Key Clinical Questions

- *Is the developmental regression accompanied by a rapid head growth?*

No specific therapy is available for Alexander syndrome. Much supportive care, however, is necessary and includes good nutrition and generous use of antibiotics and antiepileptics. Despite these measures, the prognosis for infants and children with this disease at present is poor.

Corencephalopathies

The progressive corencephalopathies are characterized clinically by progressive, and sometimes intermittent, extrapyramidal signs such as dystonia, dyskinesia, choreoathetosis, and parkinsonism. Progressive corencephalopathies are insidious and inherited. They differ from acute corencephalopathies, which are usually acquired and nonprogressive (e.g., opsoclonus myoclonus, Sydenham chorea, hyperthyroidism, kernicterus, methemoglobinemia, hypoparathyroidism), and tardive dyskinesia (each discussed elsewhere). The age of onset of progressive corencephalopathies depends on etiology (Table 15.20). The discussion in this section is limited to Rett syndrome, ataxia telangiectasia, Leigh syndrome, and Wilson disease.

Table 15.20 Causes of progressive corencephalopathies

First year of life

- Phenylketonuria due to biopterin synthesis or recycling deficiencies (Naylor et al.1987; Scriver et al.1987)
- Pelizaeus-Merzbacher syndrome
- Leigh syndrome
- Aromatic L-amino acid decarboxylase deficiency (Hyland et al. 1988)

Early childhood (1–5 years)

- Glutaric aciduria type I
- Lesch-Nyhan syndrome
- Ataxia telangiectasia
- Rett syndrome
- Leigh syndrome

Late childhood or juvenile (>5 years)

- Segawa disease
- Wilson disease
- Dystonia musculorum deformans
- Huntington disease
- Neurodegeneration with brain iron accumulation (NBIA)
- Leigh syndrome
- Folate and cobalamin homeostasis defects

Rett syndrome

Rett syndrome is a virtually female-limited, X-linked dominant disorder characterized by a catastrophic loss of language, social, and voluntary hand function with stereotyped hand-washing movements, following normal development for 5–18 months. The mapping of Rett gene to human Xq28 led to the discovery that mutations in the methyl-CpG-binding protein 2 gene (MECP2), a widely expressed transcriptional repressor with affinity for a subset of methylated genes (Amir 1999). Rett syndrome is the most common cause of severe mental impairment in girls, with a prevalence of 1 per 10,000. Rett syndrome is almost always sporadic, originating on the paternal chromosome. Only 1% of Rett cases are familial, originating in a female carrier suffering only from learning disability. *MECP2* mutations have been identified in 80% of sporadic cases and 50% of familial cases. The same *MECP2* mutations that produce the classic Rett syndrome in girls lead to a severe neonatal encephalopathy with hypotonia, apnea, seizures, and early death in the affected males unless the mutations are mitigated by partial or complete Klinefelter karyotype or by a somatic mosaicism, in which cases males present a classic Rett syndrome phenotype. Some other *MECP2* point mutations are asymptomatic in girls, whereas boys may present a nonspecific X-linked mental retardation phenotype (Shahbazian & Zhogbi 2002). Mutations in the CDKL5 gene on Xp22 produce a severe Rett variant with early infantile onset of seizures (Li et al. 2007).

Rett syndrome exists in a classic and in variant forms. In its classical form, birth and early development are normal. Four clinical stages have been suggested by Hagberg. Stage I, a phase of stagnation, is characterized by the appearance of early signs in infancy (5–18 months of age). Hypotonia with increased joint mobility is a frequent early symptom. Subtle abnormal signs such as facial

Key Clinical Questions

- *Did you have to hold the hands of your baby to take a baby picture because she was constantly bringing her hands to her mouth instead of reaching for objects?*
  Classically, stereotypic movements of the hands, bruxism, motor apraxia, dystonic posturing, and cognitive regression appear later.

Pearls and Perils

- The diagnosis of Rett syndrome is excluded if microcephaly is present at birth, if there is an obvious brain dysfunction in early infancy, or if the patient is a male.
- In both infantile autism and Rett syndrome, interaction with social environment is poor; smiling and laughing may occur without apparent reason, and stereotypic movements are found. In infantile autism, elaborate actions and behaviors are possible. Rett syndrome is differentiated from infantile autism by the developmental history, the presence of acquired microcephaly, a specific constellation of neurological signs, the inability to organize purposeful activities, and the poverty of the stereotypies.
- In both Rett syndrome and neuronal ceroid-lipofuscinoses (NCL; e.g., infantile atypical type), hand stereotypes and loss of hand use may be present. In Rett syndrome, retinopathy and ultrastructural changes pathognomic of neuronal ceroid-lipofuscinosis are absent.
- Some children with Rett syndrome may have wounds on their hands or fingers. In contrast with Lesch-Nyhan syndrome where the lesions result from self-injurious activity, those seen in Rett syndrome result from long-lasting wetting of the hands.
- In both Rett syndrome and tuberous sclerosis, stereotyped hand movements, severe mental retardation and seizures suggestive of Lennox-Gastaut syndrome may occur. Diagnosis of tuberous sclerosis is suggested by depigmented skin lesions, normal head circumference, and tuberous lesions on computed tomography (CT) scan or magnetic resonance imaging (MRI) of brain.
- In both Rett syndrome and happy puppet syndrome of Angelmann, unmotivated laughing, jerking, apraxic gait and limb movements, and microcephaly are reported. However, stereotypic hand movements characteristic of Rett syndrome do not occur in Angelmann syndrome. Angelmann syndrome is nonprogressive.
- Fragile-X syndrome may be misdiagnosed as Rett syndrome when stereotypic hand movements, poor eye contact, and poor social interaction occur. A large head and a relatively long face with prominent ears and jaw should suggest diagnosis of Fragile-X syndrome.

grimacing, increased movements of the hands and tongue, locomotion changes (refusal to put feet to the ground), and equilibrium delay (lack of parachute response) are frequently noted. Head size fails to increase normally. Most girls learn to walk and say a few words. Stage II, a phase of regression, is characterized by loss of acquired hand skills and speech, fluctuating attention, and appearance of intense involuntary movements (between 13 and 36 months of age). Involuntary movements are particularly prominent following emotional stimuli. Excessive flapping, wringing, and patting movements are intermingled with choreiform movement and dystonic postures. Hand mouthing, tongue pulling, teeth grinding (back teeth), squinting, and jerky trunk movement increase in intensity. Emotional withdrawal is accompanied by diminished eye contact. Time spent in handling objects decreases markedly. Hands and feet remain small and cold. Gait is apraxic.

The girls look apprehensive when change of position is involved. Irregular breathing is frequently noted during wakefulness. Sleep difficulties with inappropriate laughter or screaming develop. Appetite is increased with good swallowing but decreased chewing. Seizures usually start at the end of stage II. Complex partial, atypical absence, generalized tonic–clonic, atonic, or myoclonic seizures occur in 70–80% of the patients. Stage III, or pseudostationary phase, is characterized by some resemblance of reawakening. Patients may become more communicative and regain some of their gross motor skills. Single words can be uttered in the right context when the girls are highly motivated. However, their previous range of speech is never regained. Girls may learn eye pointing to communicate their preferences. Some girls demonstrate bloating due to extreme air swallowing. Vomiting and constipation are common. Weight loss may be extreme. With increasing age, neurogenic scoliosis, and peroneal muscular atrophy become more severe. Stage IV, or late motor deterioration, is characterized by a progressive spasticity and scoliosis leading to loss of ambulation between 4 and 31 years of age. Survival may extend past the third decade. The main causes of death are cardiorespiratory arrest and acute peritonitis.

Four Rett variant phenotypes have been described. The most common is the form fruste Rett variant. These patients fulfill most criteria for Rett syndrome but head size may be normal and some finger skills or some speech may be preserved. The early seizure onset variant of Rett syndrome is the next most common variant. In these patients, the early onset of seizures blurs the phenotypes throughout stages I to III. Congenital Rett variant is characterized by slow development in the first months of life. Late childhood regression variant is characterized by normal head circumference and gradual loss of acquired speech and fine motor skills in late childhood.

The brain may show a number of abnormalities, none of which is diagnostic of Rett syndrome. The EEG becomes progressively abnormal. During stage II, repetitive high-amplitude spike and slow wave discharges (focal, multifocal, or generalized) are seen consistently during sleep. Other epileptic discharges are also present in many cases. In stage III, the epileptic discharges are less frequent, and the normal EEG morphology of sleep disappears. Bursts of irregular waves appear against a flat background. In stage IV, seizure activity may persist, and slowing of the cortical background is found during wakefulness. Sensory evoked potentials in advanced Rett syndrome indicate involvement of the dorsal column and spinothalamic tracts. Investigation may show peripheral neuropathy in advanced cases. Brain weight is decreased by 10–15%, with greater loss of gray matter in comparison to white matter, and reduced volume of the caudate nucleus and midbrain (Russ et al. 1993). Single-photon emission CT (SPECT) has indicated a frontal lobe and brainstem hypoperfusion. Metabolic studies have been consistently normal, although a disturbance of mitochondrial phosphorylation can be found (Dott et al. 1993; Matsuishi et al. 1994). Electron microscopy of pyramidal neurons from the frontal cortex have shown large-appearing mitochondria, abundant ribosomal content, and some lipofuscin granules (Cornford et al. 1994) (Table 15.21).

The treatment remains symptomatic. Physical, occupational, and other therapies maintain and maximize function of girls with Rett syndrome. Drugs like L-dopa and haloperidol have no effect and may increase stereotyped hand movements and screaming. L-carnitine appeared effective in improving social interaction in a girl with advanced Rett syndrome (Plioplys & Kasnicka 1993). It has been speculated that Rett syndrome patients may benefit from an early dietary intervention with betaine and folic acid to increase the supply of labile methyl groups to the brain. Surgical inventions, which may be lifesaving in selected patients, include gastrostomy and spinal fusion. Sympathectomy may improve peripheral circulation.

Table 15.21 Classic Rett syndrome

Discriminating features

- Loss of language and social skill combined with loss of voluntary hand function and hand stereotypies.
- *MECP2* mutations

Consistent features

- Female sex
- Normal head circumference at birth, acquired microcephaly
- Normal early development
- Bruxism
- Small and cold feet
- Late failure to thrive
- Progressive dystonia, scoliosis

Variable features

- Bloating, vomiting, constipation
- Seizures
- Overbreathing with stimulation
- Electroencephalogram abnormalities
- Peripheral neuropathy of later onset

Subacute necrotizing encephalomyelopathy of Leigh

Subacute necrotizing encephalomyelopathy (SNE) of Leigh is an inherited neurodegenerative syndrome with an episodic or chronic clinical course characterized by

Pearls and Perils

Leigh syndrome

- Patients with Leigh syndrome who exhibit in addition dermatitis and/or stridor should be suspected of having biotinidase deficiency. In biotinidase deficiency, neurologic symptoms frequently occur in the absence of aciduria and metabolic acidosis.
- The findings of low thiamine levels in blood and cerebrospinal fluid of patients with suspected Leigh syndrome suggest the diagnosis of beriberi (Wyatt et al. 1987).
- The clinical feature that usually leads to the diagnosis of subacute necrotizing encephalomyelopathy (SNE) is the severe and rapid onset in infancy of variable neurologic signs, among which respiratory involvement, eye findings, and cranial nerve signs are most suggestive.
- Radiolucencies in the thalamus, basal ganglia, and tegmentum of the brainstem are frequently seen in SNE. A normal computed tomography (CT) scan does not exclude the diagnosis of SNE.
- Leigh syndrome has clinical, biochemical, and pathologic features similar to other mitochondrial encephalomyopathies.
- Familial bilateral striatal necrosis closely resembles Leigh syndrome with a relatively nonprogressive course. Familial bilateral striatal necrosis may be maternally inherited (acute onset) with mitochondrial DNA point mutations at base pairs FBSN 3308, LHON 11696, LHON 14459, and LHON 14596, which encode for subunits of the complex I (Thyagarajan et al. 1995) or autosomal recessive (insidious onset) (Basel-Vanagaite et al. 2006).
- The Mohr-Tranebjaerg syndrome is an X-linked disorder associated with small mitochondrial DNA deletions and due to a defect in TIMMSA gene encoding the deafness-dystonia protein (DDP1), a component of the mitochondrial-protein-import machinery in the intermembrane space. Patients present in early childhood with sensorineuronal hearing loss and progressive dystonia associated with spasticity, mental deterioration, and cortical blindness (Roesch et al. 2002).

ataxia, involuntary movements, hypotonia, and brainstem dysfunction. Several different defects of pyruvate and mitochondrial oxidative metabolism have been reported in association with Leigh syndrome. Inheritance of Leigh syndrome is heterogeneous. Leigh syndrome can result from both mendelian (please refer to Table 15.47) and mitochondrial (maternally inherited) mutations (see Table 15.46). Pathologically, Leigh syndrome characteristically exhibits bilateral and symmetrical areas of demyelination with vascular proliferation and neuronal sparing in the putamen and brainstem.

Clinically, three syndromes can be distinguished, according to age of onset. The neonatal form presents initially with disorders of sucking and swallowing, and respiratory difficulties (e.g., Ondine curse) (Seitz et al. 1984). Later, other symptoms of brainstem dysfunction (aberrant eye movements, facial weakness) and severe motor delay are recorded. Death occurs early. The classic infantile form presents at an age of less than 2 years and often less than 1 year. Early psychomotor development is usually normal. The early course is usually rapid. Symptoms are made worse by intercurrent infection or a carbohydrate-rich diet. Presenting complaints may include progressive psychomotor slowing, weakness, ataxia, feeding and swallowing difficulties, vomiting, poor weight gain, decreased alertness, poor visual fixation, myoclonic jerks, or generalized convulsions (Pincus 1972). On examination, clinical features that lead to the diagnosis are respiratory involvement, eye findings, and other cranial nerve signs. Respiratory irregularities, a central hyper/hypoventilation syndrome, or central apnea are remarkable. Eye findings may include nystagmus, strabismus, profound saccadic/slowing, ptosis, ophthalmoplegia, optic atrophy, and atypical pigmentary degeneration of the retina (Sedwick et al. 1984). Retinal pigmentary degeneration is present in about 40% of patients with maternally inherited Leigh syndrome (Santorelli et al. 1994). Other cranial nerve signs may include deafness, dysphagia, and facial weakness. Less specific neurologic signs may include axial hypotonia, spasticity, dystonia, choreoathetoid movements, and varying degrees of ataxia (Campistol et al. 1986). Deep tendon reflexes may be increased or decreased. Some patients are unusually hirsute. Other occasional features include cardiomyopathy and the renal de Toni-Fanconi-Debré syndrome of tubular renal acidosis. If nephrotic syndrome results in widespread edema, diagnosis of coenzyme Q10 (CoQ_{10}) deficiency should be considered (Lopez et al. 2006). Death is the final outcome, occurring often rapidly within the course of a few weeks or months. However, remissions followed by further exacerbations are sometimes seen, and the child may live several years.

A rare juvenile form of the disease has also been described (Grunnet et al. 1991). The course of the illness is often characterized by an insidious onset in childhood, leading to neurologic defects, such as mild spastic paraparesis, ataxia, exercise intolerance, nystagmus, visual impairment, and Parkinson-like features. Children with Leigh disease are usually below normal weight and height. After a long quiescent period, the illness terminates acutely or subacutely during the second decade. The terminal stage is characterized by a rapid deterioration to coma and marked respiratory depression.

The results of electrophysiologic studies change with time and vary from patient to patient. Motor nerve conduction velocities may be slow. The EEG may show a generalized slowing of background activity, sometimes superimposed with epileptogenic features. Brainstem auditory evoked potentials and visual evoked potentials may be abnormal. The ERG may suggest diffuse retinal dysfunction.

Neuroradiologic investigations are particularly helpful in the diagnosis of Leigh syndrome. Cranial MRI is much more sensitive in detecting lesions than CT scan (Figure 15.8). Hyperintensive lesions on T2-weighted images with symmetric involvement of the basal ganglia and brainstem, with predominant involvement of the putamen, are highly suggestive of Leigh syndrome (Table 15.22). Abnormalities of the subcortical white matter can occur.

The main biochemical findings are intermittent metabolic acidosis with elevation of lactate/pyruvate ratios in the blood and CSF. An increase in blood alanine is

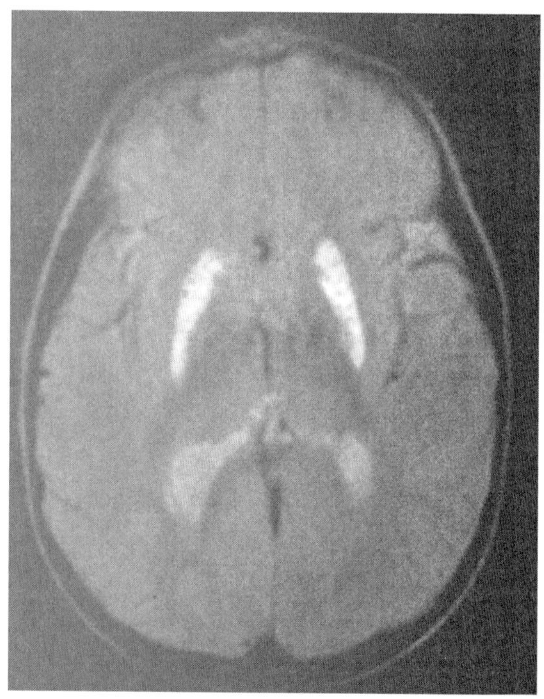

Figure 15.8 Magnetic resonance image of the brain (SE 2100/100) showing increased signal in the caudate nucleus and putamen of a 5-year-old boy with autopsy-proven Leigh syndrome and cytochrome oxidase deficiency.

Table 15.22 Subacute necrotizing encephalopathy of Leigh

Discriminating features

- Intermittent clinical course with periods of worsening triggered by intercurrent illness
- Symmetric lesions of putamen and brainstem (hyperintense on magnetic resonance imaging and hypodense on computed tomography)

Consistent features

- Elevated plasma and cerebrospinal fluid lactate and pyruvate during exacerbation
- Symmetric foci of partial necrosis with associated capillary proliferation and relative sparing of neurons in putamen, brainstem, and posterior columns of spinal cord
- No dementia

Variable features

- Variable inheritance
- Fulminant (intermittent) or slowly progressive course
- Variable age of onset
- Signs of brainstem dysfunction (respiratory, ocular motility, or swallowing disturbances)
- Movement disorder (dystonia, myoclonus, choreoathetosis, parkinsonism)
- Hypotonia or spasticity
- Spasmus nutans
- Visual impairment
- Peripheral neuropathy with elevated cerebrospinal fluid proteins
- Seizures
- Ragged red fibers in striated muscles
- Cardiac and renal involvement
- Failure to thrive

also frequent. The absence of metabolic acidosis between acute episodes does not exclude the diagnosis of SNE. Cerebrospinal fluid protein may be elevated. Diagnosis of biotinidase deficiency, if suspected, is established by measuring biotinidase activity in the serum included in the neonatal screen in some states in the United States.

Muscle and skin biopsy are often necessary to establish biochemical diagnosis. Pyruvate carboxylase and pyruvate dehydrogenase activity are best measured in tissue fibroblasts. At the time of muscle biopsy, histochemistry, electron microscopy, and oxidative phosphorylation enzymology should be performed. Ragged red fibers or striated muscles are almost never identified by light microscopy. Ultrastructural examination frequently shows discrete mitochondrial changes, such as increased size, bizarre shape, and disoriented cristae (Wyatt et al. 1987). Mitochondria should be immediately isolated for oxidative phosphorylation biochemistry. Deficiencies of complex I (NADH dehydrogenase), complex II (succinate dehydrogenase), complex III (cytochrome bc1), complex

Key Clinical Questions

- *Does the child have a history of relapsing–remitting episodes of unsteadiness, cognitive decline with floppiness, respiratory abnormalities, and difficulties moving the eyes?* Most children display a lactic acidosis during exacerbations.

IV (cytochrome oxidase), and complex V (ATP synthase) of the mitochondrial respiratory chain have been reported, and several genes have been sequenced. At the time of muscle biopsy, a small portion of muscle is placed in liquid nitrogen for mitochondrial DNA testing. Muscle should be screened for the most common mitochondrial DNA point mutations (associated with neuropathy, ataxia, and retinitis pigmentosa syndrome [NARP], mitochondrial encephalomyopathy, lactic acidosis, and stroke-like episodes syndrome [MELAS], and myoclonic epilepsy and ragged red fiber [MERRF]) and mitochondrial DNA depletion. Ubiquinone content in muscle should be measured (Lopez et al. 2006). If an X-linked inheritance is suspected, the PDH $E_1\alpha$ gene should be sequenced. Immunoblot techniques using anti-Surf1 antibodies are useful in detecting SURF1 defects in patients with Leigh disease associated with cytochrome oxidase deficiency.

Treatment of Leigh syndrome is palliative and symptomatic, as in diffuse mitochondrial encephalomyopathies. Children with Leigh syndrome due to pyruvate dehydrogenase complex deficiency can be helped by thiamine and a ketogenic diet (Di Rocco et al. 2000). Riboflavin may be beneficial in patients with NDUFV1 deficiency. Biotin supplementation is suggested in rare patients with biotinidase deficiency. Early therapeutic intervention with CoQ_{10} prevent neurologic deterioration when CoQ_{10} deficiency is suspected.

Wilson disease

Please refer to Chapter 12 for information on this disorder.

Ataxia telangiectasia

Ataxia telangiectasia (AT) is an autosomal recessive disorder of nuclear DNA repair. The ataxia telangiectasia mutated (ATM) kinase gene, on chromosome 11q22–23, acts like a glue that holds chromosome pieces together. After ionizing radiation, it is essential in rejoining of the repaired breaks with the unaltered segment of the same chromosome. The ATM gene prevents breaks on one chromosome joining to another. The ATM gene is also essential in mature B cells for antigen-driven immunoglobulin gene diversification: ATM allows the efficient rejoining of breaks between the gene segment encoding the so-called constant region of antibody molecules and the segment undergoing gene somatic hypermutation and class switch recombination (Reina-San-Martin et al. 2004). AT has a prevalence of approximately 2 per 100,000. More than 200 distinct mutations have been reported associated with AT. Most AT patients are compound heterozygous for various mutations. More than 95% of patients fail to make the ATM protein as detected by immunoblotting of cell line extracts (Becker-Catania et al. 2000).

Clinically, AT is characterized by onset in childhood of progressive neurologic symptoms, various immunologic deficiencies, premature aging, an increased frequency of cancers, endocrine abnormalities, and oculocutaneous telangiectasias. The clinical spectrum of AT is very wide (Table 15.23). Neurologic symptoms are the usual presenting complaint. In severe cases, cerebellar ataxia has its onset in infancy or childhood. Ataxia is predominantly truncal with "swaying movements" of the head and trunk while sitting, walking, or standing. Dysarthria usually develops simultaneously to the ataxia. Nystagmus is present on lateral gaze. Romberg sign is negative. All modalities of sensation are intact. A mild choreoathetosis frequently accompanies ataxia. Difficulty in initiating voluntary eye movements (oculomotor apraxia) is characteristic of AT (Baloh et al. 1978) even in the earliest stages. Most children learn to ambulate and show no progression in their motor symptoms until school age. In the earliest stages, cognitive development usually remains normal. Pyramidal signs are absent. In adolescence, ataxia, which was truncal earlier, involves the limbs, with incoordination and intention tremor. Myoclonic jerks, particularly on intention, may result in frequent falling and make the patient nonambulatory.

Other patients with AT who have a relatively benign course and prolonged survival may present in adolescence or early adulthood with extrapyramidal involvement, spinocerebellar ataxia, or spinal muscular atrophy. The extrapyramidal signs include difficulties in initiating movements; dull, expressionless facies as in Parkinson disease;

Table 15.23 Ataxia telangiectasia

Discriminating features
- Immune deficiencies and oculomotor apraxia
- Defects of AT gene and chromosomal instability radiosensitivity

Consistent features
- Cerebellar atrophy
- Elevated serum carcinoembryonic antigen (CEA) and alfa-fetoprotein
- Defects of humoral and cellular immunity
- No pyramidal signs or symptoms

Variable features
- Cerebellar ataxia
- Spinocerebellar ataxia
- Choreoathetosis
- Spinal muscular atrophy
- Microcephaly
- Sinopulmonary infections
- Malignancies
- Early aging of skin and hair
- Telangiectasia
- Elevated liver enzymes

Pearls and Perils

Ataxia telangiectasia

- Ataxia telangiectasia should be considered in the etiologic diagnosis of ataxic or athetoid cerebral palsy (when onset is infantile).
- Ocular and skin telangiectasias are not always present in ataxia telangiectasia.
- Slow viscous eye movement and absent optokinetic nystagmus are present in most patients with ataxia telangiectasia. Similar eye movements are a feature of two ataxia-oculomotor apraxia syndromes (AOA): AOA1 due to aprataxin deficiency (APTX gene on chromosome 9) and AOA2 due to senataxin deficiency (SETX gene on chromosome 9). Both syndromes are characterized by a progressive cerebellar ataxia with peripheral axonal neuropathy and lack systemic symptoms. They do not share the extra-neurologic features of AT (immune deficiency, chromosomal instability, and hypersensitivity to x-rays) AOA1 can be associated with coenzyme Q10 deficiency (Le Ber et al. 2007). In AOA2, elevated serum alpha-fetoprotein levels are seen.
- Neurologic presentation is highly variable and progressive (cerebellar ataxia, spinocerebellar ataxia, spinal muscular atrophy, dystonia, choreoathetosis, and/or parkinsonism).
- The severity of the neurologic features is not directly related to the severity of the systemic symptoms.
- Ataxia telangiectasia-like disorder due to mutations in the meiotic recombination 11A gene (MRE11A on chromosome 11q21) presents with early onset, slowly progressive ataxia but is easily distinguishable from classic ataxia telangiectasia as extra-neurologic features such as telangiectasias, raised alfa-fetoprotein, and reduced immunoglobulin levels are usually absent. Cellular features of such patients are similar to those seen in classic ataxia telangiectasia and include chromosomal instability with increased levels of chromosome breaks in peripheral blood lymphocytes and increased sensitivity to ionizing radiation (Fernet et al. 2005).

> **Key Clinical Questions**
>
> ▶ *Has your child been hospitalized for recurrent pneumonia, and is there a family history of breast cancer?*
> Patients with ataxia telangiectasia frequently suffer from sinopulmonary infections. In addition, the ataxia telangiectasia carrier has a shortened lifespan and an elevated risk of breast cancer.

slow eye movement; stooping posture; drooling; and seborrheic dermatitis. Smile is delayed and protracted. Rigidity is usually absent. Dystonic posturing of the fingers is frequent. In the predominant spinocerebellar form, there is diminution and even loss of position and vibratory sense. Romberg sign is positive. Plantar responses are usually flexor in contrast to Friedreich ataxia (Barbieri et al. 1986) (see Table 15.24). In the predominant spinal muscular atrophy variant, patients show generalized muscle weakness with marked distal atrophy and gross fasciculations of muscles. Flexion contractures of the fingers and bilateral foot drop are present (Goodman et al. 1969). Spinocerebellar ataxia and spinal muscular atrophy may develop simultaneously (Rosen & Harris 1987) in AT.

Non-neurologic features have a variable age of onset. Telangiectasias, dilations of venous capillaries, are usually evident by age 6 years. Some patients, however, lack telangiectasias (Willems et al. 1993). Telangiectasias are usually symmetrical, appearing initially on the bulbar conjunctiva and later on exposed areas of the skin (nasal bridge, eyelids, ears, lobes, antecubital and popliteal areas, flexor folds of the neck, and mucosa of nose and mouth). Telangiectasias are frequently in the liver and in elderly patients, in the CNS. They are rarely associated with hemorrhage, unlike the telangiectasias of Osler-Rendu-Weber disease. Skin and hair show premature aging (Smith & Conerly 1985). Bodily growth and sexual development are frequently retarded. There is a strong tendency to develop sinopulmonary infections and malignancies, the two leading causes of early death. Fifteen percent of patients with AT die from malignancies, particularly lymphomas and lymphocytic leukemia. Primary carcinomas of the stomach, liver, ovary, salivary glands, oral cavity, breast, and pancreas have also been reported (Morrell et al. 1986).

Half the patients with AT have mild elevation in liver enzymes. More than 50% of patients display glucose intolerance. The most constant biochemical markers of AT are elevated serum levels of alfa-fetoprotein (AFP) and carcinoembryonic antigen (CEA). Immunological deficiency is very common, but its pattern is highly variable. Defects in both humoral and cellular immunity have been described. About 75% of patients with AT have an absence or extreme deficiency of serum IgA, and 80% manifest extreme immunoglobulin (Ig)E deficiency. IgG2 and IgG4 may be deficient or absent. Autoimmune phenomena are common in AT. Forty-five percent of AT patients show one or more autoantibodies to muscle, mitochondria, bile canaliculi, basement membrane, thyroglobulin, parietal cells, and even IgG. Impaired function of T lymphocytes is suggested by delayed rejection of skin grafts and cutaneous anergy to delayed hypersensitivity skin testing. In vitro, T lymphocytes show a poor response to T-cell mitogens and a defective cytotoxic response to viral pathogens (Waldmann et al. 1982). T-cell levels are usually low while B-cell levels are normal or elevated. γ/δ T-cell levels are usually elevated. Cytogenetic abnormalities are frequently found in AT patients and include a variety of chromosomal aberrations reflecting a general "chromosomal instability." They are less frequent in young children and are not commonly observed in fibroblasts. Colony in vitro assay (irradiation of colony formation of lymphoblastoid cells) is a very sensitive test. Mutation analysis is useful to confirm the clinical diagnosis.

Presently, no specific treatment has been found to halt the progression of the disease. Avoidance of undue exposure to sunlight is recommended. Radiologic procedures should be limited. The use of radiation therapy in conventional doses is contraindicated. Radiomimetic agents such as bleomycin, actinomycin D, and cyclophosphamide should be avoided. Immunotherapy may decrease the frequency and severity of infections. Trihexyphenidyl may improve dystonia and parkinsonism. Propranolol may improve ataxia.

Spinocerebellopathies

Spinocerebellopathies are a heterogeneous group of inherited neurologic disorders characterized by variable degrees of degeneration of the cerebellum, brainstem, and spinal cord. The PNS may be involved. An autosomal dominant pattern of inheritance is characteristic of adult onset in spinocerebellar ataxia. An earlier childhood onset occurs in subsequent generations of dominantly inherited spinocerebellar ataxia (Zoghbi & Balladio 1995). This phenomenon, known as *anticipation*, is due to an increased number of an unstable trinucleotide repeats in the affected gene. An autosomal recessive pattern of inheritance is seen in most childhood-onset spinocerebellar ataxia (Table 15.25). Not every progressive spinocerebellopathy is due to a genetic defect. Nutritional, toxic, and immune causes are discussed in other chapters.

Spinocerebellar ataxia and vitamin E deficiency

Vitamin E deficiency is a significant cause of spinocerebellar ataxia and/or neuropathy. Most disorders causing

Table 15.24 Differential diagnosis of childhood slowly progressive spinocerebellopathies

Type	C*	Age of onset	Ataxia	Sensory	Dtr	Babinski	Muscle	Mental	Eye	Heart	Other
IOSCA	10	Infancy	Severe	Moderate and late	Absent	+	Hypotonia	Late	Ptosis, optic atrophy, ophthalmoplegia	No	Hypogonadism athetosis, seizures, hearing loss
RL	17	Infancy	Moderate	Mild	Absent	+	Atrophy (legs)	Normal	Normal	No	Pes cavus
SLO	7	Infancy	Severe	Moderate	↓	+	Hypotonia	Abnormal	Ptosis, cataract	Congenital defects	Failure to thrive, malformations
FA	9	1st decade	Severe	Moderate	↓ in LE	+	Atrophy (legs)	Normal	Normal	Cardiomyopathy	Pes cavus
BKS	4	1st decade	Severe	Moderate	↓	+ late	Atrophy (legs)	Normal	Degenerative retinopathy	Rare cardiomyopathy	Pes cavus
Refsum	10	1st decade	Severe	Severe	↓	+	Atrophy	Normal	Degenerative retinopathy	Hypertrophic cardiomegaly	Pes cavus, deafness, ichthyosis
AVED	8	1st or 2nd decade	Severe	Moderate	↓	+	Late atrophy	Normal	Cataract,	Normal retinopathy	Pes cavus, scoliosis
NARP	M*	1st decade or later	Mild	Mild	↑-early ↓-late	+	Proximal weakness	Deterioration	Degenerative retinopathy	No	Seizures
SCD		1st or 2nd decade	Moderate	Paresthesia	↓	+	Weakness and atrophy (legs)	Frequent deterioration	Macular changes	No	Microcephaly, seizures
CDG	16	1st decade or later	Moderate	Mild	↑-early ↓-late	+	Weakness and atrophy (legs)	Deterioration	Retinopathy, strabismus	Pericarditis, hypertrophic cardiomegaly	Skeletal deformity
AT	11	1st decade	Severe	Mild	↓-late	–	Atrophy (late)	Late deterioration	Slow eye movements	No	Telangiectasia, immune deficiency
AOA1	9	1st decade	Severe	Mild	↓-late	–	Atrophy (late)	Mild	Slow eye movements		Dystonia
MS	5	1st decade	Moderate truncal	Mild	↑-early ↓-late	+ in 50%	Atrophy (legs)	Deterioration	Cataracts (congenital)	No	Skeletal deformity, short stature
CX	2	2nd decade	Mild-early	Mild-early	↑	+	Later	Deterioration, early at times	Cataracts, retinopathy	Myocardial infarction	Tendon xanthomas, fractures, diarrhea

IOSCA, infantile onset spinocerebellar ataxia; C*, abnormal chromosome; RL, Roussy-Levy syndrome; M*, mitochondrial DNA; SLO, Smith-Lemli-Opitz; FA, Friedreich ataxia; BKS, Bassen-Kornzweig syndrome; AVED, ataxia with isolated vitamin E deficiency; NARP, neuropathy, ataxia, retinitis pigmentosa syndrome; SCD, subacute combined degeneration; CDG, carbohydrate deficiency glycoprotein; AT, ataxia telangiectasia; AOA1, early-onset ataxia with oculomotor apraxia; MS, Marinesco-Sjögren; CX, cerebrotendinous xanthomatosis.

Table 15.25 Spinocerebellar ataxia caused by vitamin E deficiency

Discriminating features
- Vitamin E deficiency

Consistent features
- Spinocerebellar ataxia
- Vibratory sense loss

Variable features
- Peripheral neuropathy
- Decreased myotatic reflexes in LE
- Retinopathy
- Cataract
- Myopathy
- Steatorrhea
- Weight loss, failure to thrive
- Facial dysmorphism
- Hepatomegaly
- Jaundice
- Acanthocytosis

vitamin E deficiency produce a chronic steatorrhea (Bassen-Kornzweig syndrome, hypobetalipoproteinemia, cystic fibrosis, celiac disease, intestinal lymphangiectasia, a_1-antitrypsin deficiency, Wilson disease, biliary atresia, and defects of bile acid synthesis). Ataxia with isolated vitamin E deficiency is not associated with steatorrhea (Table 15.25).

Bassen-Kornzweig syndrome

Bassen-Kornzweig syndrome (BKS), or abetalipoproteinemia, is an autosomal recessive inherited disorder of lipoprotein metabolism characterized by steatorrhea, hypocholesterolemia, hypertriglyceridemia, lack of all apo B-containing lipoproteins (chylomicrons, very-low-density lipoprotein [VLDL], LDL), hematologic changes, and progressive neurodegeneration with cerebellar ataxia, degenerative retinitis pigmentosa, and peripheral neuropathy. Biochemically, the disorder is caused by an absence of microsomal triglyceride transfer protein (MTTP). The MTTP gene locus is on chromosome 4q24. Both point mutations and deletions in the MTTP gene are responsible for abetalipoproteinemia (Ohashshi et al. 2000; Xiao Ping et al. 1999).

The infant with BKS is usually normal at birth. Failure to thrive and abdominal distention, along with steatorrhea, are the first symptoms in infancy. Endoscopy reveals a yellow discoloration of the duodenum, and jejunal biopsy is generally pathognomonic, showing extensively vacuolated mucosal cells packed with lipid droplets. The earliest neurologic findings are hypotonia and the loss of deep tendon reflexes at an early age. Neurologic symptoms typically develop toward the end of the first decade of life as a spinocerebellar degenerative disorder. Position and vibratory sensation are lost, and a positive Romberg sign typical of sensory ataxia can be elicited. Clinical evidence of pyramidal tract lesions usually appears later. Weakness and muscle atrophy are progressive. Most subjects are unable to walk by their mid-20s. Pes cavus and scoliosis are common findings. Athetosis has been observed. Some degree of mental retardation may become apparent in 20% of the patients. Behavioral and cognitive changes may occur. Degeneration of the retina may develop during infancy, but more often it occurs later. Pigmentary retinopathy is a constant finding. Reduced electroretinographic amplitudes precede visual decline. Oscillating, vertical, horizontal, and dissociated nystagmus are concomitant with the progressive loss of vision. Ophthalmoplegia may result from both supranuclear and nuclear involvement.

Laboratory findings suggestive of BKS include a very low plasma concentration of cholesterol (<100 mg/mL) and triglycerides (<30 mg/mL), and acanthocytosis of the peripheral erythrocytes. (Acanthocytes are crenated red blood cells of normal size exhibiting spiny processes of various sizes in thick smears. Their formation is attributed to changes in the lipid composition of erythrocyte membranes.) Severe anemia may occur. Hyperoxaluria is one consequence of fat malabsorption. Vitamin E is undetected in the serum of symptomatic patients. The diagnosis of BKS depends on the confirmation of the absence of apoprotein B.

Treatment consists of providing a low-fat diet, supplementing the fat-soluble vitamins A and K, and pharmacologic doses (100–200 mg/kg/day) of standard vitamin E preparations. Much smaller doses of a-tocopherol acetate (50 mg/kg/day) inhibit progression of neurologic symptoms (myopathy, neuropathy, ataxia) more rapidly. Some regression of neurologic symptoms may also be seen.

Hypobetalipoproteinemia

Hypobetalipoproteinemia is an autosomal dominant inherited disorder of lipoprotein metabolism characterized by hypocholesterolemia with low levels of LDL and with a number of mutations resulting in the synthesis of truncated apoprotein B. The apoprotein B gene locus is on chromosome 2q24.

The condition is usually asymptomatic in simple heterozygotes except for reduced levels of plasma LDL. Compound heterozygotes and homozygotes may show steatorrhea, hematologic manifestations, and neurologic signs and symptoms similar to Bassen-Kornzweig syndrome (Scott et al. 1979). These conditions differ from abetalipoproteinemia by identification of truncated apoproteins.

Treatment for the homozygotes and compound heterozygotes is the same as for BKS. In simple heterozygotes, restriction of fat is initiated when malabsorption and oxalate urolithiasis are present.

Steatorrhea

Steatorrhea caused by disorders other than BKS or hypobetalipoproteinemia (e.g., cystic fibrosis, celiac disease, intestinal lymphangiectasia, biliary atresia) may result in variable neurologic symptoms, including spinocerebellar degeneration, proprioceptive loss, areflexia, weakness, delayed motor and cognitive development, ophthalmoplegia, and retinal pigmentation. The clinical progression of neurologic symptoms is variable and depends on the etiology (Table 15.26).

Vitamin E deficiency is common in unsupplemented patients with cystic fibrosis, but rarely causes a spinocerebellar degeneration (Sokol et al. 1989). Disorders that interfere with biliary excretion—bile acid synthesis defects (Clayton 1995), Alagille syndrome (Alagille et al. 1987), Aagenaes syndrome (Åagenes 1974), and peroxisomal disorders—are not only frequently complicated by steatorrhea, vitamin E deficiency, and other fat-soluble vitamin deficiencies (Rosenblum et al. 1981), but also may result in copper retention with subsequent lenticular degeneration (Danks 1991). Disorders of biliary excretion frequently present in infancy with pruritus.

Table 15.26 Causes of vitamin E deficiency

Chronic pancreatic insufficiency
- Cystic fibrosis

Reduced intestinal bile salt concentration
- Liver disease: α1 antitrypsin deficiency
  - Wilson disease
- Biliary atresia
- Cholesterol synthesis defects:
  - Deficient bile synthesis
    - Smith–Lemli–Opitz syndrome
    - 3-β hydroxy C27 steroid dehydrogenase/isomerase deficiency
    - 3-oxo steroid 5 β-reductase deficiency
  - Peroxisomal disorders

Chronic intestinal mucosal absorption defects
- Celiac sprue (gluten-induced enteropathy)
- Short bowel syndrome
- Bassen-Kornzweig disease
- Hypobetalipoproteinemia
- Lymphatic obstruction
- Whipple disease
- Intestinal lymphangiectasia

Familial isolated vitamin E deficiency

Pearls and Perils

- Areflexia is not present in all patients with vitamin E deficiency.
- Ophthalmoplegia may be found in fat malabsorption but is not a feature of isolated vitamin E deficiency.
- Smith-Lemli-Opitz syndrome should be distinguished from peroxisomal disorders.
- Very-long-chain fatty acids are normal in Smith-Lemli-Opitz syndrome.
- Ataxia with isolated vitamin E deficiency (AVED) differs from Friedreich ataxia by the absence of cardiomyopathy and diabetes and by the occasional presence of head titubation or dystonia.

Smith-Lemli-Opitz syndrome

The Smith-Lemli-Opitz syndrome (SLOS) is an autosomal recessive disorder of cholesterol biosynthesis characterized by an extremely variable phenotype ranging from minor anomalies to life-threatening congenital anomalies (Table 15.27). The patients have an elevated 7-dehydrocholesterol-to-cholesterol ratio or high 7-dehydrocholesterol level by gas chromatography. The disorder has been shown to result from a microsomal 7-dehydrocholesterol reductase deficiency (Shefer et al. 1994). Over 70 mutations in the DHCR7 gene (locus on chromosome 11q12-q13) have been described. The incidence of this disorder has been estimated to be 1:20,000 births.

The facial features are pathognomic with microcephaly, a narrow high forehead, ptosis, low-set posteriorly rotated ears, broad anteverted nares, inner epicanthal folds, micrognathia, and often alveolar ridging. Y syndactyly of the second and third toes is typically seen. Hypospadias, cryptorchidism, or more severe genital abnormalities (ambiguous genitalia) are common in males. Other visceral malformations involving the brain, heart, and respiratory, genitourinary, and gastrointestinal

Key Clinical Questions

- *Does your child have chronic diarrhea with vomiting and failure to thrive?*
  If there is steatorrhea, ataxia with isolated vitamin E deficiency (AVED) is unlikely. AVED should be considered in the differential diagnosis of Friedreich ataxia.

Pearls and Perils

- In patients with combined degeneration of the spinal cord, signs suggestive of Friedreich ataxia are always accompanied by mental changes or developmental delay.
- If there are signs of stomatitis or atrophic glossitis, an inborn error of cobalamin absorption should be suspected.
- Megaloblastic anemia, the hallmark of cobalamin deficiency, may be absent in errors of folate and cobalamin metabolism.
- Homocystinuria and homocystinemia are consistently seen in all patients.
- Defects of adenosylcobalamin synthesis are not associated with subacute combined degeneration. Such patients have a severe methylmalonic acidemia and no homocystinuria.

systems have been associated with a high infantile mortality. Less severely affected patients may have early feeding difficulties. Global developmental delay occurs universally among affected patients. Speech does not develop. Most children with SLOS have some variant form of autism.

Treatment of SLOS consists of HMG-CoA reductase inhibitors (simvastatin) and providing cholesterol, bile acids, and fat-soluble vitamins, except for vitamin D.

Ataxia with isolated vitamin E deficiency

Ataxia with isolated vitamin E deficiency (AVED) is an autosomal recessive neurodegenerative disease due to free radical damage and characterized by spinocerebellar ataxia with peripheral neuropathy. Ataxia with isolated vitamin E deficiency results from a defect in liver cells of a-tocopherol transfer protein (aTTP) (Afif Hentati et al. 1985). The aTTP incorporates the a-tocopherol form of vitamin E into VLDL. This leads to a vitamin E deficiency, which occurs in the absence of steatorrhea. The AVED locus has been mapped to chromosome 8q13 (Doerflinger et al. 1995).

Clinically, patients with AVED have a normal early development. Some patients develop an intention tremor, head titubation, and impaired vibratory sensation in childhood, whereas others remain asymptomatic until adulthood. Proprioreceptive loss, weakness, gait disturbances, kyphoscoliosis, and pes cavus develop later. Areflexia and dysarthria are not present in all patients. An extensor plantar response is generally found in the lower extremities. Head titubation is reported in 28% of patients, and dystonia is present in 13% of patients. Ophthalmoplegia is not a feature of isolated vitamin E deficiency. Visual impairment and retinitis pigmentosa have been reported in some families (Benomar et al. 2002).

Key Clinical Questions

- *Is there any sign of mental decline?*
  Dementia frequently accompanies other signs of myelopathy and peripheral neuropathy.

Table 15.27 Smith-Lemli-Opitz syndrome

Discriminating features
- Y-shaped two- to three-toe syndactyly
- Typical face with ptosis, epicanthal folds, short nose, and small chin
- Elevated levels of dehydrocholesterol or elevated 7-dehydrocholesterol-to-cholesterol ratio
- Mutations in the 7-dehydrocholesterol reductase (DHCR7) gene

Consistent features
- Moderate to severe mental retardation
- Autism spectrum disorder
- Congenital microcephaly with large metopic suture
- Congenital malformations/anomalies
- Failure to thrive; early feeding difficulties

Variable features
- Hypocholesterolemia
- Age of onset and presenting symptoms
- Intrauterine growth retardation
- Abnormal visceral development (especially kidneys, liver, heart, and lungs): megacolon, pyloric stenosis or gastrointestinal malrotation, renal cysts, ureteral duplication, hepatomegaly, endocardial cushion defect
- Hypotonia
- Cerebral dysgenesis with agenesis or hypoplasia of the corpus callosum, cerebellar hypoplasia, holoprosencephaly, frontal lobe hypoplasia, cortical migration defects
- Choanal atresia, low-set ears, micrognathia, broad alveolar ridge, cleft palate
- Sacral dimple, scoliosis, short neck
- Postaxial polydactyly
- Cryptorchidism or hypospadias in males and labial hypoplasia in females, short proximally placed thumbs, transverse palmar crease
- Seizures
- Cataract, retinal degeneration
- Chondrodysplasia punctata
- Skin hypersensitivity to ultraviolet light due to hypervitaminosis D (Acosta 1995)
- Polyneuropathy

Pearls and Perils

Smith-Lemli-Opitz syndrome (SLOS)

- Mildly affected individuals may have only minor physical abnormalities with a phenotype mimicking autism spectrum disorders.
- The presence of Y-shaped two- to three-toe syndactyly or skin ultraviolet light hypersensitivity in a child with borderline intellectual functioning, speech delay, behavioral stereotypies (impulsivity, aggression, and sensory hyperreactivity), sleep difficulties, and/or autism should prompt consideration of SLOS.
- Severe cases can be life-threatening and involve profound mental retardation and major physical abnormalities. The phenotype in such cases resembles that of peroxisomal biogenesis disorders. Biochemical testing allows correct diagnosis.

Diagnosis of AVED is suggested by low-fasting serum vitamin E concentrations, absence of steatorrhea, normal lipoprotein electrophoresis, and normal intestinal absorption of vitamin E, as demonstrated by oral vitamin E tolerance test (OVETT). An accelerated decline of serum tocopherol after the OVETT peak represents the effects of the liver clearing the circulating chylomicron remnant containing tocopherol, combined with a failure to adequately secrete tocopherol into hepatic-derived lipoproteins (Sokol et al. 1988). Red blood cell morphology is normal. Genetic diagnosis can now be achieved.

Treatment with 800–900 IU/day of oral DL-a-tocopherol normalizes vitamin E status and stabilizes or improves neurologic status.

Subacute combined degeneration of the spinal cord

In children, subacute combined degeneration of the spinal cord may result from a familial malabsorption of cobalamin (congenital intrinsic factor deficiency or cubilin deficiency) (Aminoff et al. 1999; Yang et al. 1985), an inadequate dietary intake (Maclean & Graham 1980), a congenital cobalamin transport defect (transcobalamin II deficiency) (Hall 1992), or inborn errors of folate and cobalamin metabolism (Beckman et al. 1987; Carmel et al. 1988; Clayton et al. 1986; Dillon et al. 1974; Shinnar & Singer 1984). The human gene for methylene-tetrahydrofolate reductase has been localized to chromosome 1p36.3 (Goyette et al. 1994). Defects of adenosylcobalamin synthesis are not associated with combined degeneration.

The clinical features of this disorder vary with age of onset and underlying metabolic defect. Classically, sensory signs are combined with motor signs. The presenting symptoms are usually paresthesias in the lower extremities. Loss of proprioception and vibratory sensation lead to a sensory ataxia and positive Romberg sign. The motor signs include loss of strength, spasticity, and extensor plantar responses. Deep tendon reflexes may be diminished. Disturbances of sphincter function are uncommon. Mental and personality changes are frequent. Visual impairment may occur. Funduscopic examination may reveal a hypopigmented perimacular zone surrounded by a hyperpigmented ring (Goyette et al. 1994). In severe cases, lethargy, feeding difficulties, and seizures are the usual presenting symptoms. Head growth may be delayed (Beckman et al. 1987; Clayton et al. 1986). Parkinsonism has been reported in 5,10-methylenetetrahydrofolate reductase (Clayton et al. 1986). Some children, however, may only have a mild developmental delay (Carmel et al. 1988).

Serum vitamin B_{12} level is lower in nutritional deficiency or malabsorption, but normal in inborn errors of folate and cobalamin metabolism. Homocystine is increased and methionine reduced in the plasma. Homocystinuria with methylmalonic aciduria is found in defective cytosolic processing of hydroxocobalamin (cobalamin C and D disorders) (Shinnar & Singer 1984), in severe nutritional B_{12} deficiency, and in defective B_{12} absorption. Homocystinuria without methylmalonic aciduria suggests impaired function of methionine synthase (Carmel et al. 1988) or 5,10-methylenetetrahydrofolate reductase (Beckman et al. 1987; Clayton et al. 1986). Megaloblastic anemia, the hallmark of cobalamin deficiency, is also seen in hereditary folate malabsorption and functional methionine synthase deficiency (cobalamin E and G disorders). The Schilling test shows a cobalamin

Table 15.28 Subacute combined degeneration of spinal cord

Discriminating features
- Bilateral symmetric paresthesia starting in lower extremities followed by weakness

Consistent features
- Homocystinuria
- Sensory ataxia
- Spasticity

Variable features
- Mental changes
- Seizures
- Microcephaly
- Involuntary movements (tremor, chorea, myoclonus, parkinsonism)
- Visual impairment due to optic neuropathy
- Demyelinating polyneuropathy
- Megaloblastic anemia
- Methylmalonic academia

Pearls and Perils

Subacute combined degeneration

- Copper deficiency myelopathy presents with features indistinguishable from combined degeneration. In copper deficiency, dysfunction of the methylation cycle is caused by deficiency of two copper-dependent enzymes: methionine synthase (also cobalamin-dependent) and S-adenosylhomocysteine hydroxylase (not cobalamin-dependent) (Winston and Jaiser 2008).
- Symptoms of subacute spinal degeneration can be obscured by peripheral neuropathy or mental changes.

malabsorption in inborn errors of cobalamin absorption and transcobalamin II deficiency (Table 15.28).

Early diagnosis and treatment may be the only way to prevent permanent neurologic damage. Methylenetetrahydrofolate reductase deficiency is very resistant to treatment, but some response has been seen with methionine, folates, and betaine. Betaine in conjunction with hydroxocobalamin has been effective in treating patients with cobalamin C disorder and methionine synthase deficiency. Treatment with reduced folates has been successful in hereditary folate malabsorption and inadequate dietary intake.

Carbohydrate-deficient glycoprotein syndrome

Carbohydrate-deficient glycoprotein (CDG) syndrome is a newly described group of autosomal recessive disorders of glycoprotein glycosylation characterized by posttranslational defects in the addition of carbohydrates to the amide group of selected asparagine residues of glycoproteins before their transfer into the rough endoplasmic reticulum (Yamashita et al. 1993). Patients with N-glycosylation disorders have a cathodal shift of their serum transferrin isoelectrofocusing (IEF) profile. In CDG I, the hypoglycosylation of the high-mannose type lysosomal enzymes causes a cellular mis-sorting, with targeting of the lysosomal enzymes to the secretory pathway and deficient uptake in the lysosome. Plasma levels of lysosomal enzymes are elevated. Storage lysosomes containing hypoglycosylated glycoproteins are found in hepatocytes. In CDG II, there is no defect in the sorting of lysosomal enzymes. Plasma lysosomal enzymes are not elevated, and no abnormal lysosomal inclusion is seen in hepatocytes. Thus far, 12 enzyme defects have been identified (Jaeken 2003). The most common is CDG Ia due to phosphomannomutase (PMM) deficiency. The gene has been mapped to chromosome 16p13, and multiple mutations have been reported in the sequenced gene.

Clinically, most patients present in infancy with prominent neurologic symptoms such as hypotonia, muscular weakness, psychomotor retardation, strabismus, and failure to thrive. In childhood, cerebellar ataxia and mental retardation (mild to severe) may be associated with retinitis pigmentosa and axonal peripheral neuropathy involving particularly the lower limbs, suggesting, in these latter cases, a diagnosis of neuropathy, ataxia, and retinitis pigmentosa syndrome (NARP; described in the next section). Acquired microcephaly is seen in 50% of patients. Some patients may walk unaided. Most attend special schools. In adolescence and adulthood, ataxia and mental retardation remain stable while lower extremity weakness and atrophy increase slowly. Multivisceral involvement is suggested in younger patients by mild to moderate hepatomegaly, diarrhea, vomiting, and failure to thrive, and in older patients by hypogonadism and skeletal abnormalities (kyphoscoliosis, extensor defects of the joints, pigeon breast deformity). Relative specific symptoms of CDG Ia, including dysmorphic features (prominent forehead, large ears and jaw, thin upper lip), inverted nipples, and lipocutaneous abnormalities (prominent fat pads on buttocks and thighs), are occasionally absent. In addition to these chronic symptoms, the patient may present acutely at any age with stroke-like episodes, seizures, and cerebral hemorrhage. Most patients

Pearls and Perils

Carbohydrate-deficient Glycoprotein (CDG) Syndromes

- CDG syndrome is an infantile autosomal recessive form of olivopontocerebellar atrophy with remarkable systemic manifestations involving the liver and kidney. CDG syndrome is a hepatocerebellorenal syndrome that should not be confused with hepatocerebrorenal syndrome of Zellweger.
- Abnormalities of transferrin and other glycoproteins similar to CDG syndrome are reported in untreated galactosemia, chronic alcoholism, and hemolytic uremic syndrome.
- CDG may mimic mitochondrial diseases. Early screening for CDG may be helpful in preventing an unnecessary muscle biopsy.
- Relatively specific symptoms of CDG Ia include dysmorphic features, inverted nipples, and abnormal fat pads. Such features are not always present.

Key Clinical Questions

- *Are there signs of a multisystemic disease in this child with cerebellar atrophy, hypotonia, cognitive decline, and peripheral neuropathy?*

with this syndrome have been reported to survive into early adulthood. Some patients with a more severe multivisceral involvement succumb in the neonatal period from severe hepatocellular failure, protein-losing enteropathy, proximal tubular proteinuria, pericardial and pleural effusions, or hypertrophic cardiomyopathy.

CT and MRI of the brain show varying degrees of cerebellar and brainstem hypoplasia. The EEG is usually unremarkable. Nerve conduction velocities are decreased in virtually all patients. Nerve biopsy shows absence of myelin sheaths and the presence of multivacuolar myelinoid-bodies in Schwann cells. Abnormalities of the electroretinogram are present in the majority (Andréasson et al. 1991). The CSF analysis may transiently show increases of protein content. Liver dysfunction is frequently suggested by elevated aspartate aminotransferase (AST) and alanine aminotransferase (ALT). Liver biopsy consistently shows the presence in hepatocytes of lysosomal vacuoles containing membranous myelin-like inclusions. Kupffer cells are normal or show signs of cholestasis. Low serum levels of thyroxine-binding globulin, haptoglobulin, albumin, apoliprotein B, cholesterol, and coagulation factors (factor XI, antithrombin III, and protein C) have been reported repeatedly. Serum lysosomal enzymes are consistently elevated in CDG I patients. Deficiencies of transferrin sialylation may be detected quantitatively by carbohydrate-deficient transferrin analysis or qualitatively by IEF. Phosphomannomutase activity is preferably measured in leukocytes, as patients with a mild presentation may show a high residual activity in their fibroblasts. Screening for mutations in the PMM2 gene has shown that most patients are compound heterozygous (Table 15.29).

Treatment is symptomatic. The pathologic characteristics of this syndrome are (a) hepatic micronodular cirrhosis, (b) renal microcysts affecting exclusively tubules and sparing glomerular spaces, and (c) olivopontocerebellar atrophy with sparing of the cerebrum. Ultrastructural examination of the Purkinje cells reveals dendrite expansions containing membranous cytoplasmic body-like inclusions (Chang et al. 1993).

Table 15.29 Carbohydrate-deficient glycoprotein syndrome

Discriminating features
- Inverted nipples

Consistent features
- Mental retardation
- Liver dysfunction
- Cerebellar ataxia (olivopontocerebellar atrophy)
- Peripheral neuropathy
- Elevation of carbohydrate-deficient transferring

Variable features
- Stroke-like episodes
- Lipocutaneous abnormalities
- Pericardial and other effusions
- Retinitis pigmentosa
- Epilepsy

Friedreich ataxia

Friedreich ataxia is an autosomal recessive progressive neurodegenerative disease characterized by early age of onset of a spinocerebellar ataxia with corticospinal tract signs and areflexia. Skeletal deformity and hypertrophic cardiomyopathy are additional features. At the cellular level, the syndrome is caused by the death of neurons with long axons. The gene locus is on chromosome 9q13–9 (Duclos et al. 1994). The incidence of Friedreich ataxia is approximately 1:50,000 individuals. Clinical heterogeneity among family members is common, with some family members exhibiting only extraneural findings. The syndrome is caused primarily by a deficiency in frataxin, small mitochondrial matrix protein that binds to Fe^{2+} (like ferritin), decreases the rate of oxidation of Fe^{2+}, and promotes the iron export to the cytosol. Frataxin deficiency results in mitochondrial iron accumulation, enhancing the sensitivity of mitochondria to oxidative stress and leading eventually to free radical–mediated cell death. Frataxin deficiency is caused primarily by expansion of a trinucleotide (66–1800 GAA triplets) in the first intron of the frataxin gene (Adinolfi et al. 2002). Friedreich ataxia is the most frequent nuclear encoded mitochondrial encephalopathy.

The onset of Friedreich ataxia is anywhere between 4 and 20 years of age. Peak age of onset is 12 years. The usual presenting symptoms are weakness, gait instability, and difficulty with running. Postexertional cramps and aching in the legs are occasionally reported. If the patient is examined at this stage, ataxia is found to be worse in the legs than in the arms. Tandem walking and standing on one leg for more than a few seconds are impossible. Position sense and vibration sense are impaired in the lower limbs. Romberg sign is usually present. The patellar reflexes are absent. Few patients with Friedreich ataxia have preserved lower limb deep tendon reflexes (Harding 1981). Bilateral extensor toe signs are easily elicitable. Pes cavus and kyphoscoliosis are early findings. As the child grows older, the ataxia progresses, with arm dysfunction and dysarthria occurring later. Intention tremor of the upper extremities becomes evident. Muscle weakness predominantly involves the distal muscles and is mild compared with that seen in the hereditary motor and sensory neuropathies. Distal muscle wasting tends to appear and may result in a mild atrophy of peroneal muscles. Diagnosis of Roussy-Levy syndrome should be considered if abdominocutaneous reflexes are abolished or if peroneal muscle wasting is severe. Claw deformity of the hand is sometimes present in Friedreich ataxia. Speech becomes dysarthric and slurred, and gradually evolves into

Pearls and Perils

Friedreich ataxia

- In many cases of hereditary motor and sensory neuropathy type I (HMSN I, the Roussy-Levy variant of Charcot-Marie-Tooth disease), features of spinocerebellar degeneration may include dysarthria, limb and gait ataxia, nystagmus, areflexia, pes cavus, extensor plantar responses, and sensory changes. HMSN I can be distinguished from Friedreich disease by virtue of its autosomal-dominant inheritance, its benign course, its early onset before 2 years of age, and its severely reduced motor conduction velocities.
- Hyporeflexia, Romberg sign, extensor plantar response, cerebellar ataxia, and loss of position and vibration sense in the first decade are the hallmarks of Friedreich ataxia. A clinical syndrome similar to Friedreich ataxia is seen in vitamin E deficiency. This condition is associated with pigmentary retinal degeneration, which is absent in Friedreich ataxia. In ataxia telangiectasia, peripheral sensory degeneration is a secondary factor that exacerbates the ataxia of cerebellar origins during the second decade.
- In Refsum disease, there is no extensor plantar response, and pigmentary degeneration of the retina is a prominent feature.
- In tabes dorsalis, there is no peripheral neuropathy.
- Clinical features of B12-deficient polyneuropathy are somewhat similar to those of Friedreich ataxia. A megaloblastosis and methylmalonic aciduria are typical of B12 deficiency.
- An atypical form of neuronal ceroid-lipofuscinoses (NCL) with juvenile ataxia predominating can be distinguished by hyperreflexia in NCL and hyporeflexia in Friedreich ataxia. An atypical spinocerebellar degeneration with hyperreflexia is also found in juvenile GM2 gangliosidosis.
- Adrenomyeloneuropathy may present as a spinocerebellar syndrome.
- Leigh syndrome may present as a spinocerebellar syndrome that can be distinguished from Friedreich ataxia if its course is intermittently progressive and if eye involvement is present.
- A computed tomography (CT) scan of the head is usually normal in Friedreich ataxia (cerebellar atrophy is demonstrated in Marinesco-Sjögren-Garland syndrome and ataxia telangiectasia).
- An echocardiogram permits recognition of heart disease in Friedreich ataxia before the onset of cardiac symptoms.
- Friedreich ataxia should be suspected in patients with spastic paraparesis of undetermined etiology, especially when there is neurophysiologic evidence of a sensory axonal neuropathy.

a severe scanning staccato type of speech. Head titubation is sometimes observed. By the end of the third decade of life, most patients are wheelchair-bound or bedridden. Bladder dysfunction may manifest at any time during the illness. Symptoms of spastic bladder are most common. Ophthalmologic findings more frequently include horizontal nystagmus (Harding 1981) and optic atrophy (Geoffroy et al. 1976). Higher cortical functions remain intact until later stages of the illness. Cardiac arrhythmia or congestive heart failure are major complications (Hewer 1968). Diabetes mellitus has been reported in 20% of patients (Finocchiarro et al. 1985). The mean age of death is 30 years. Somatosensory evoked potentials are impaired in all patients regardless of the duration or the severity of the illness. The features of Friedreich ataxia are outlined in Table 15.30.

The motor conduction velocity of peripheral nerves is usually normal. Sensory nerve conduction, however, is practically absent in the lower limbs, and considerably slowed in the upper. On EMG, fasciculation and an impaired interference pattern indicate denervation. Patients with Friedreich ataxia have no or only minor abnormalities on cranial CT scan. MRI of the spine may be helpful in assessing spinal cord atrophy. The CSF is usually normal.

Table 15.30 Friedreich ataxia

Discriminating features
- Weakness in lower extremities and extensor plantar responses
- Trinucleotide GAA repeat expansion of frataxin gene

Consistent features
- Ataxia of limbs
- Decreased or absent vibratory sense
- Abnormal echocardiogram and electrocardiogram
- Normal or mildly slow motor nerve conduction velocity
- Absent or reduced sensory nerve potentials
- Impaired somatosensory evoked potentials

Variable features
- Absent myotatic reflexes in lower extremities (distal first)
- Muscle atrophy and weakness (distal)
- Truncal ataxia
- Dysarthria
- Loss of position sense
- Cramp and aching in legs
- Pes cavus and kyphoscoliosis
- Claw hands
- Optic atrophy
- Nystagmus
- Cranial nerve palsies, neurosensory hearing loss
- Intellectual difficulties
- Seizures
- Palpitation or shortness of breath
- Diabetes mellitus

Key Clinical Questions

- *Does your child complain of shortness of breath or palpitations?*
  Although heart disease is frequently asymptomatic, shortness of breath is reported in 40% of patients and palpitation in 10%.

Laboratory investigation reveals an abnormal glucose tolerance test in about 40% of cases, and an abnormal insulin response to glucose in more than 60% of cases (Finocchiaro et al. 1985). Abnormalities of mitochondrial enzymes are frequently found (Sorbi et al. 1989). However, no specific metabolic defect or enzyme deficiency has been found to date. Dunn and Dolman (1969) reported a case resembling atypical Friedreich ataxia with a fluctuating course and elevated serum lactate and pyruvate levels. Subacute necrotizing encephalomyopathy of Leigh was diagnosed at autopsy. Vitamin E levels should be obtained in order to exclude one of the few treatable causes of spinocerebellar degeneration. Documentation of cardiomyopathy confirms the diagnosis of Friedreich ataxia. The best early indicators of myocardial involvement appear to be the presence of EKG and echocardiographic (ECG) abnormalities (Salih et al. 1990). In most patients, EKG shows inverted T-waves. Echocardiography demonstrates concentric hypertrophy of the ventricles in 60% of patients or asymmetric septal hypertrophy in 30% of patients. A molecular diagnosis of Friedreich ataxia can be made by demonstration of homozygosity for the GGA repeat expansion in the frataxin gene by PCR.

No treatment halts the progression of the disease. Free radical scavengers such as idebenone (5 mg/kg/day divided into three doses) have been shown to decrease the rate of neurologic decline and improve the cardiomyopathy (Rustin et al. 1999). Congestive heart failure secondary to cardiomyopathy is generally treated with digitalis and diuretics. Increased taurine intake and administration of calcium channel blockers have been suggested to prevent the progression of cardiomyopathy. Scoliosis should be observed before deciding on surgical intervention in order to assess the rate of progression of the deformity, because in some patients the deformity may remain mild throughout the course of the illness.

Neuropathy, ataxia, and retinitis pigmentosa (NARP) syndrome

Neuropathy, ataxia, and retinitis pigmentosa (NARP) syndrome is a maternally inherited multisystem disorder characterized by development delay, retinitis pigmentosa, ataxia, and proximal weakness. The disease is associated with mitochondrial DNA (mtDNA) point mutations at base pair 8993, causing a substitution of a thymidine by a guanine in the gene coding for the subunit 6 of ATP synthase (Holt et al. 1990). More than 20 families have been published with this mutation (Tatuch et al. 1992). These families have shown similar clinical features and marked intrafamilial variability. Clinical phenotypes such as "cerebral palsy," Kearns-Sayre syndrome, and Leigh syndrome may coexist with NARP in the same family. The Leigh syndrome phenotype is seen in patients with abundant (above 90% of the mtDNA) mtDNA mutation (see Table 15.31).

Pearls and Perils

Neuropathy, ataxia, and retinitis pigmentose (NARP) syndrome

- Ragged red fibers are not essential for diagnosis of neuropathy, ataxia, and retinitis pigmentosa syndrome (NARP).
- Recurrence of cerebral palsy in multiple family members should raise suspicion for NARP.
- A maternal mode of inheritance is always seen in NARP.
- NARP can mimic Kearns-Sayre syndrome when progressive external ophthalmoplegia and cardiac conduction defects are clinical features.
- Maternal relatives of NARP patients may present with Leigh syndrome.

Table 15.31 Neuropathy, ataxia, and retinitis pigmentosa syndromes

Discriminating features
- Proximal neurogenic muscle weakness
- Retinitis pigmentosa
- Adenosine triphosphate (ATP) synthase (complex V) dysfunction due to mitochondrial DNA point mutation (heteroplasmic T-to-G transversion at nucleotide pair 8993)

Consistent features
- Axonal neuropathy (sensory > motor)
- Ataxia (sensory)

Variable features
- Leigh syndrome
- Cardiomyopathy
- Convulsion
- Learning difficulties, mental retardation, or dementia
- Muscle wasting and weakness
- Short stature
- Kearns-Sayre syndrome

Key Clinical Questions

- *Does the mother, her sister, or the maternal grandmother suffer or have children suffering from migraine-like headache, seizures, night blindness, proximal weakness, unsteady gait, cerebral palsy, dementia, or cardiomyopathy?* If no family member is found, examination of the maternal retina may reveal an asymptomatic retinitis pigmentosa.

Symptoms associated with the NARP mutation are highly variable. Some individuals are hypotonic from birth and have a psychomotor retardation. Microcephaly can be an occasional feature (Fryer et al. 1994). These individuals frequently carry the diagnosis of cerebral palsy. Other individuals present intermittent episodes of drowsiness, ataxia, and hyperventilation suggesting a diagnosis of Leigh syndrome. Other individuals have a normal early development. By school age or early adulthood, they develop a dysarthria, a progressive limb and gait ataxia, and night blindness. Deep tendon reflexes are frequently decreased. Babinski signs are extensor. Sensory examination reveals decreased position sense and a positive Romberg sign. There is frequently a progressive loss of peripheral and sometimes central vision. Ophthalmologic examination reveals a retinitis pigmentosa with "bone spicule" and optic atrophy. Even asymptomatic individuals may show a retinal degeneration. Seizures, dementia, and proximal muscle weakness with wasting are other variable features. A cardiomyopathy is seen in some individuals (Fryer et al. 1994). Long-term outcome remains unknown.

Lactic acid and pyruvate in blood and CSF are usually normal (unless patient presents as a severe phenotype reminiscent of Leigh syndrome). Brain CT and MRI may disclose brainstem and cerebellar atrophy (Holt et al.1990). Electroretinogram may show attenuated responses. Nerve conduction velocities suggest an axonal sensorimotor neuropathy (low amplitude motor and/or sensory responses). The EEG may show a slow background and paroxysmal activity. Analysis of blood usually shows the NARP point mutation.

Muscle biopsy may show ragged red fibers on Gomori trichrome or signs of chronic denervation. Ultrastructural studies may show large mitochondria with abnormal branching cristae. Polarographic analysis of isolated muscle mitochondria shows ATP synthase (complex V) deficiency (Di Mauro 1993). The NARP point mutation is more easily detected in muscle than blood.

Refsum disease

Refsum disease (or heredopathia atactica polyneuritiformis) is a rare autosomal recessive peroxisomal disorder of branched-chain lipid metabolism characterized biochemically by accumulation of phytanic acid in body fluids and tissues. Phytanic acid is a fatty acid derived from phytol, a component of the chlorophyll molecule. It cannot be synthesized endogenously; therefore, the only source is diet. Pristanic acid, the end-product of phytanic acid's a-oxidation, is not elevated in Refsum disease (Table 15.32). It has been shown that the phytanic acid accumulation is due in most cases to a deficiency of the peroxisomal phytanoyl-CoA α-hydroxylase (PAHX). The sequence of *PAHX* is known and localized on chromosome 10p13. Both point mutations and deletions have been described in the *PAHX* associated with Refsum disease (Mukherji et al. 2001).

Clinically, Refsum disease is characterized by progressive onset in first or second decade of the fairly consistent neurologic clinical tetrad. First, nyctalopia is due to retinitis pigmentosa. Second, spinocerebellar ataxia is due to posterior column myelin loss and loss of neurons in granular layer. Third, bilateral distal muscle weakness, atrophy, and sensory disturbance are due to

Table 15.32 Refsum disease

Discriminating features
- Anosmia
- Early-onset pigmentary degeneration of the retina with night blindness
- Elevated phytanic acid levels in blood with normal α-hydroxyphytanic and pristanic acid levels
- Phytanic oxidase deficiency in fibroblasts

Consistent features
- Decreased motor and sensory nerve conduction
- Hyporeflexia (ankle)
- Distal muscular atrophy
- Ataxia (sensory and cerebellar)
- Chronic progressive sensorimotor polyneuropathy: hypertrophic demyelinating neuropathy with onion bulb formation
- Elevated cerebrospinal fluid proteins
- Normal intelligence
- No pyramidal tract signs

Variable features
- Age of onset and presenting symptoms
- Neural hearing loss
- Anosmia
- Cataracts
- Cardiomyopathy
- Ichthyosis
- Bony changes
- Renal tubular involvement
- Enlarged palpable peripheral nerves
- Improved with dietary restriction

Pearls and Perils

Refsum disease

- Infantile-onset Refsum disease should be distinguished from "infantile Refsum disease" (see Peroxisomal disorders). Infantile-onset Refsum disease is not associated with hepatomegaly. The accumulation of phytanic acid in plasma is due to a defective hydroxylation of phytanic acid; therefore, there are normal plasma levels of α-hydroxyphytanate and pristanate in infantile-onset Refsum disease. Plasmalogen synthesis is normal.
- Mutations in the PEX7 gene (normally causing rhizomelic chondrodysplasia type I) are found in some rare patients with noninfantile Refsum phenotype (van den Brink et al. 2003). Such patients with pseudo-Refsum disease have a decreased plasmalogen synthesis in their skin fibroblast, whereas in classic Refsum disease plasmalogen synthesis is normal.
- Childhood-onset Refsum disease should be distinguished from Friedreich ataxia. Generally, the plantar responses are flexor or absent in childhood-onset Refsum disease. Dysarthria is not found in Refsum disease. Night blindness, anosmia, deafness, ichthyosis, and elevated cerebrospinal fluid protein are not found in Friedreich ataxia.
- Mental deterioration, seizures, and pyramidal and extrapyramidal signs and symptoms are not features of Refsum disease.
- Some patients with Refsum disease may present with a clinic picture resembling that of relapsing or chronic polyneuropathy, or Guillain-Barré syndrome. Other patients present with a neurologic disorder resembling other hypertrophic neuropathies (e.g., Charcot-Marie-Tooth disease or Dejerine-Sotos syndrome). A pigmentary degeneration of the retina distinguishes Refsum disease.
- The clinical course of Refsum disease may be improved by dietary restriction of phytanic acid.

chronic progressive sensorimotor polyneuropathy. Fourth, elevated CSF protein concentration is due to inflammatory neuropathy. Other clinical features of Refsum disease may include anosmia, sensorineural hearing loss, cataracts, cardiac arrhythmias, skeletal malformations, and dermatologic manifestations such as palmar hyperkeratosis and ichthyosis. Dysarthria, dementia, and epilepsy are not features of the illness. Age of onset of symptoms is highly variable. An early onset of the disease does not necessarily indicate a particularly poor prognosis. Onset of symptoms is usually insidious. The sensorimotor neuropathy is slowly progressive, although, early symptoms may have an acute or subacute presentation that mimics Guillain-Barré syndrome or chronic inflammatory demyelinating polyneuropathy. The acute or subacute presentations are usually

Key Clinical Questions

- *Do you suffer from difficulties walking in the dark and/or did you lose your sense of smell?*

caused by rapid weight loss due to stress, infection, surgery, or pregnancy.

Most patients with classical Refsum disease are normal during the first few years of life. However, congenital skeletal malformations are recorded in more than half of the patients (Skjeida et al. 1987). The most common finding appears to be bilateral shortening or elongation of the metatarsal bones, particularly the third and fourth. Other common skeletal malformations include symmetrical epiphysial dysplasia of large joints and pes cavus.

Neurologic examination in Refsum disease reveals decreased or absent deep tendon reflexes. Muscle weakness and atrophy affects the distal parts of the limbs. Romberg sign is positive. Vibration and position senses are impaired distally, more than superficial sensory modalities. Intension tremor is seen. The plantar responses are indifferent or flexor.

Ophthalmologic manifestations of Refsum disease include retinal changes, lenticular opacities, myosis, and nystagmus. Retinal changes are variable. Some patients present the typical "bony spicules" of retinitis pigmentosa. In others, the pigmentation appears as fine, small granules giving a "salt and pepper" appearance to the retina. In some cases, areas of retinal depigmentation associated with attenuation of the retinal vessels and prominence of the choroid vasculature have been described. The optic disks are slightly yellowish. Night blindness and constriction of the visual field result from retinopathy. Cataract has been described in one-third of the cases, usually of the posterior subcapsular kind. Miosis may occur because of high lipid levels in the iris or as a consequence of a generalized dysautonomia. Nystagmus appears more frequently in children.

In Refsum disease, nonspecific EKG changes are found. Sudden death among patients with Refsum disease has been reported in children as well as adults. Sudden death has been related to cardiomyopathy. Half the untreated patients have died before the age of 30 years from sudden death or respiratory failure.

Electrophysiologic studies may reveal markedly reduced motor and sensory nerve conduction velocities. Electromyography may show evidence of denervation. The ERG shows reduction or complete absence of rod and cone responses. The EEG is normal in most cases.

Laboratory findings suggestive of classic Refsum disease include increased CSF protein content without a corresponding increase in the number of cells (albuminocytologic dissociation), and increased plasma phytanic acid level (normally less than 0.3 mg/100 mL). Accumulation of phytanic acid cannot be considered diagnostic for Refsum disease, as this acid has also been elevated in patients with peroxisomal disorders, such as neonatal adrenoleukodystrophy, Zellweger syndrome, infantile Refsum disease, and chondrodysplasia punctata (rhizomelic type)/pseudo-Refsum disease due to *PEX7* mutations. Normal plasma levels of a-hydroxyphytanate and pristanate differentiate Refsum disease from peroxisomal disorders other than rhizomelic chondrodysplasia punctata type I. The demonstration of a deficient activity of the phytanic acid oxidase and phytanoyl-CoA hydroxylase in skin fibroblasts does not differentiate Refsum disease from rhizomelic chondrodysplasia type I. Measurement of plasmalogen synthesis in cultured fibroblast is necessary for the differential diagnosis: in Refsum disease it is normal, whereas in rhizomelic chondrodysplasia puncta type I/pseudo-Refsum disease it is decreased. Mutation analysis of *PAHX* in most cases confirms the diagnosis.

A restricted dietary intake of phytanic acid is achieved by avoiding fats obtained from herbivores (e.g., milk, beef, rabbit), fish, pork, and green vegetables. It is important to maintain sufficient caloric intake to avoid release of phytanic acid from body stores. Vitamin and mineral supplementation is required. Carefully supervised dietary restriction can lower the plasma phytanic acid levels in a few weeks, with a concomitant improvement in peripheral nerve conduction, muscle strength, and skin abnormalities. In patients with severe exacerbations of symptoms, plasmapheresis reduces plasma phytanic acid levels rapidly, reversing most clinical symptoms. Central neurologic damage, however, is permanent (Lundberg et al. 1972).

Spinocerebellar ataxia with neuropathy, dysarthria, and ophthalmoparesis

Spinocerebellar with sensory neuropathy, dysarthria, and ophthalmoparesis (SANDO) is a recessive phenotypically heterogenous syndrome (refer to Table 15.33) resulting from mitochondrial dysfunction due to mutations in two nuclear-encoded genes essential for mitochondrial DNA maintenance: polymerase-γ gene 1 (POLG1 on chromosome 15) and chromosome 10 open reading frame 2 gene (C10ORF2). Skeletal muscle biopsy typically shows multiple mitochondrial DNA deletions.

Table 15.33 Spinocerebellar ataxia with neuropathy, dysarthria, and ophthalmoparesis (SANDO)

Discriminating features

- Chronic progressive external ophthalmoplegia
- Dysarthria
- Sensory axonal neuropathy
- Mutation in the nuclear-encoded DNA polymerase-gamma (POLG1) or chromosome 10 open reading frame 2 (C10ORF2) genes

Consistent features

- Spinocerebellar ataxia
- Areflexia, hypotonia
- Cerebellar atrophy or cerebellar white matter signal changes

Variable features

- Age of onset (infantile to adult)
- Athetosis in childhood
- Ptosis
- Optic atrophy
- Seizures or migraine
- Muscle atrophy
- Multiple mitochondrial DNA deletions
- Scoliosis
- Hypogonadism
- Hearing loss and dysarthria
- Gastrointestinal paresis and weight loss
- Myoclonus
- Elevated cerebrospinal fluid proteins

Pearls and Perils

- The clinical symptoms are very similar to those found in mitochondrial encephalomyopathies.
- Distinguishing features are normal growth pattern and lack of mitochondrial abnormalities in muscle biopsies.

Clinically, most patients present in early adulthood with gait disturbance, distal muscle weakness, paresthesias in the lower extremities, hyporeflexia, and dysarthria. Bilateral ptosis and ophthalmoplegia may suggest diagnosis of recessive chronic progressive external ophthalmoplegia (CPEO). Other patients have symptoms of mitochondrial neurogastrointestinal encephalopathy (MNGIE). Cerebrospinal fluid proteins can be elevated. Diagnosis of spinocerebellar ataxia with epilepsy (SCAE) is suggested in patients with a similar disorder preceded by juvenile onset of migraine or seizures (status epilepticus) (Van Goethem et al. 2004; Winterthunon et al. 2005).

In the Finnish population, a more severe variant called infantile onset spinocerebellar ataxia (IOSCA) is characterized by acute or subacute infantile onset of ataxia. In addition to ataxia, the clinical examination reveals loss of deep tendon reflexes, hypotonia with pes planus, athetoid movements of hands and face and, on occasion, ptosis. By school age, ophthalmoplegia with only convergence persisting and loss of speech due to

Key Clinical Questions

- *Does the patient have Finnish ancestry?*
  Most patients with infantile onset spinocerebellar ataxia (IOSCA) originate from Finland.

hearing loss are diagnosed. Babinski sign appears with the progression of the disease. In adolescence, most patients become wheelchair-bound. Proprioception and kinesthetic sensation are impaired. Progressive atrophy of thighs, legs, and distal hand muscles occurs. Scoliosis may appear. Optic atrophy is demonstrated on funduscopic exam. Myoclonus and seizures are late manifestations (Nikali et al. 2005). The height of the patients is normal. Hypogonadism is an occasional feature.

Slowing of sensory nerve conduction velocities occurs early. Latencies of somatosensory evoked potentials are also frequently delayed. In older patients, moderate slowing of motor nerve velocities, delayed latencies of visual evoked potentials, and abnormal EEG are additional findings. Neuroimaging studies may show cerebellar atrophy or bilateral cerebellar white matter lesions. The main pathologic features are sensory axonal neuropathy (with severe loss of large myelinated fibers) and progressive spinocerebellar atrophy. Treatment is still purely supportive.

Diffuse encephalopathies

In this section, the discussion will be limited to peroxisomal disorders, mitochondrial encephalopathies, Lafora disease, and cerebrotendinous xanthomatosis. This group of disorders is obviously heterogeneous. Common clinical features are dementia, seizures, involuntary movements, and ataxia.

Peroxisomal disorders

Peroxisomes are single membrane subcellular organelles with important function in cellular catabolic and anabolic processes. Catabolic peroxisomal function involves various oxidases that produce hydrogen peroxide (H_2O_2). Peroxisomes have the ability to decompose H_2O_2 via catalase, which is present in high concentration in peroxisomes. Peroxisomes also contain superoxide dismutase and glutathione peroxidase (Singh et al. 1994), suggesting importance of this organelle in free radical metabolism. Peroxisomes are the site of the oxidation of various fatty acids such as VLCFAs, long-chain dicarboxylic acids, and side chains of cholesterol (important in synthesis of bile acids). Peroxisomes also catabolize pipecolic acid (an intermediate in lysine catabolism) and polyamines. Anabolic peroxisomal functions include certain steps in plasmalogen (an ether phospholipid), bile acids, steroid hormones, and isoprenoid biosynthesis (cholesterol, dolichols, coenzyme Q, squalene, farnesylated proteins, and the isoprenoid moiety of heme-a).

Peroxisomal disorders have a frequency of 1 per 5,000 births. Peroxisomal disorders can be subdivided into two categories (Table 15.34): the disorders of peroxisomal biogenesis or assembly (class 1) and disorders involving a single peroxisomal enzyme (class 2).

Class 1 disorders are characterized pathologically by a reduced number of peroxisomes (disorders of peroxisomal biogenesis) or by the finding of ghost peroxisomes (disorders of peroxisomal assembly). Biochemically, class 1 disorders are characterized by the concomitant loss of activity in both membrane (plasmalogen synthesis) and matrix peroxisomal enzymes. As a result, the hallmark of class 1 disorders is the concomitant decrease in plasmalogen synthesis with multiple biochemical abnormalities such as the increased plasma VLCFA, phytanic acid, and trihydroxy-cholestanoic acid (THCA). Clinically, most class 1 disorders are not separate disease states but represent phenotypes differing in their severity with Zellweger syndrome (the most severe), infantile Refsum disease (the least severe), and neonatal adrenoleukodystrophy (NALD) (of intermediate severity). Rhizomelic chondrodysplasia punctata type I and rare cases of Refsum-like disease are the only class 1 disorders that represent a separate disease state. Genetically, the class 1 disorders are transmitted in an autosomal recessive mode of inheritance. Since the genetic heterogeneity was elucidated in 1989 (Roescher et al. 1989), complementation studies have shown that class 1 disorders can be classified in at least 13 complementation groups (Table 15.35). Class 1 disorders result from mutations in PEX genes. The PEX genes encode peroxins, proteins involved in and necessary for peroxisomal biogenesis or assembly. The absence of detectable peroxisome is seen exclusively in patients with Zellweger syndrome and results from defects in

Pearls and Perils

Peroxisomal disorders

- Analysis of very-long-chain fatty acids is a highly reliable test to establish whether one is dealing with a peroxisomal disorder. Normal very-long-chain acids do not exclude a peroxisomal disorder.
- Peroxisomal morphology is frequently abnormal in peroxisomal disorders. However, a normal morphology does not exclude a peroxisomal disorder.

Table 15.34 Classification of peroxisomal disorders

Defect	Disorder	Enzyme defect	Peroxisomes	VLCFA	Phytanic	Pristanic	THCA	Plasmalogen
Class 1 peroxisomal biogenesis or assembly	Zellweger syndrome	Generalized defect	Absent/ghosts	Increased	Increased	Increased	Increased	Decreased
	Infantile Refsum	Generalized defect	Ghosts	Increased	Increased	Increased	Increased	Decreased
	Neonatal ALD	Partial defect	Ghosts	Increased	Normal	Normal	Normal	Decreased
	RCDP type 1	Partial defect	Ghosts	Normal	Increased	Increased	Increased	Decreased
	Pseudo-Refsum	Partial defect	Ghosts	Normal	Increased	Increased	Increased	Decreased
Class 2 single enzyme defect	RCDP type 2	DHAP-AT	Normal	Normal	Normal	Normal	Normal	Increased
	RCDP type 3	Alkyl-DHAP synthase	Normal	Normal	Normal	Normal	Normal	Increased
	X-linked ALD	ALDP	Normal	Increased	Normal	Normal	Normal	Normal
	Pseudo-neonatal	Acyl CoA-oxidase ALD	Large	Increased	Normal	Normal	Normal	Normal
	Pseudo-Zellweger syndrome	Bifunctional enzyme	Normal or large	Increased	Increased	Increased	Increased	Normal
	Refsum-like protein X	Sterol carrier	Normal	Normal	Increased	Increased	Normal	Normal
	LDMN	AMARC	Normal	Normal	Increased	Increased	Increased	Normal
	Classic Refsum	Phytanoyl hydroxylase	Normal	Normal	Increased	Normal	Normal	Normal
	Mevalonic aciduria	Mevalonate kinase	Normal	Normal	Normal	Normal	Normal	Normal

ALD, adrenoleukodystrophy; DHAP-AT, dihydroxyacetone phosphate acyltransferase; DHAP-S, dihydroxyacetone-phosphate synthase; RCDP, rhizomelic chondrodysplasia punctata; THCA, trihydroxy-cholestanoic acid; VLCFA, very-long-chain fatty acids; LDMN, leukoencephalopathy with dystonia and motor neuropathy; AMACR, α-methylacyl-CoA racemase

Table 15.35 Categories of peroxisomal biogenesis or assembly disorders

CG KG	CG J	Protein	Gene	Chromosome	Phenotype
1	E	ABC protein (AAA ATPase)	PEX1	7q21-q22	ZS, NALD, IRD
2		PTS-1 receptor	PEX5	12p13.3	ZS, NALD, IRD
3		Ring finger membrane protein (PXMP)	PEX12	17q21.1	ZS, NALD, IRD
4 (6)	C	ABC protein (PAF-2)	PEX6	6p21.1	ZS. NALD, IRD
7 (5)	B	Ring finger membrane protein	PEX10	1p36	ZS, NALD, IRD
8	A	Interacts with PEX1–PEX6 complexes	PEX26	22q11.2	ZS, NALD, IRD
9	D	"Chaperone"	PEX16	11p12-p11.2	ZS
10	F	Ring zinc finger membrane protein (PXMP)	PEX2	8q21.1	ZS, IRD
11	R	PTS-2 receptor	PEX7	6q21	RCDP, PRD
12	G	Anchor for Pex19	PEX3	6q23-q24	ZS
13	H	Docking site for PTS-1	PEX13	2p15	ZS, NALD
14	J	"Chaperone"	PEX19	1q22	ZS
15	K	Interacts with PTS-1 and PTS-2	PEX14	1p32	ZS

CG, complementation group; KG, Kennedy-Greiger; J, Japanese; PEX, peroxine; PAF, peroxisomal assembly factor; PTS, peroxisomal targeting signal.

"chaperone" proteins lacking peroxisomal targeting signals (PTS) but required for proper assembly of membrane vesicles before targeting of all peroxisomal membrane proteins (PMP). These "chaperone" proteins, including peroxin 3 (chromosome 6q23–24), peroxin 16 (chromosome 11p12-p11.2), and peroxin 19 (chromosome 1q22), are essential for peroxisomal biogenesis. Ghost peroxisomes may result from targeting defects of newly synthesized peroxisomal proteins or from defects in the process of peroxisomal matrix enzyme import. Matrix and membrane protein targeting requires the presence of either peroxin 5 (chromosome 12p13), which acts as receptor for the proteins containing the peroxisomal targeting signals 1 (PTS1), or the presence of peroxin 7 (chromosome 6q21), which acts as receptor for PTS2. Mutations of at least eight other genes encoding peroxins result in defects of the peroxisomal protein import (Matsumoto et al. 2003). The prevalence of peroxisomal biogenesis disorder is estimated to be 1:50,000 with PEX1 mutations associated with about 65% of all cases. *PEX6*, *PEX10*, *PEX12*, and *PEX26* mutations account for another 25% of the cases.

Disorders involving a single peroxisomal enzyme (class 2) are characterized by a normal morphology and number of peroxisome, and in most cases, by a normal plasmalogen synthesis. A single peroxisomal enzyme is deficient, and therefore metabolic abnormalities are selective, involving in general only one metabolic pathway. However, when the deficient peroxisomal enzyme is necessary for the normal function of multiple metabolic pathways, the finding of multiple metabolic derangements may suggest a PBG disorder: bifunctional enzyme deficiency is associated with VLCFA and THCA, and presents with the clinical phenotype of "pseudo-Zellweger." Class 2 disorders can result from a defect in the transport of the enzyme to its site of action or from a structural defect (deletion, point mutation) of the gene encoding for the enzyme. For example, X-linked ALD results from a defect in the transport of the peroxisomal acyl CoA synthetase. Large deletion of the peroxisomal acyl CoA synthetase gene produces the pseudo-NALD phenotype (Fournier et al. 1994).

At least nine different disorders affecting the nervous system result from a single peroxisomal enzyme defect. Elevation of VLCFAs is seen in X-linked ALD, pseudo-NALD, and pseudo-Zellweger syndrome. Elevated phytanic acid is seen in Refsum disease. Elevation of pristanic acid and of the pristanic-to-phytanic acid ratio is seen in pseudo-Refsum and leukoencephalopathy with dystonia and motor neuropathy (LDMN).

Patients with peroxisomal encephalopathies have various signs and symptoms depending on the severity and complexity of biochemical defect(s) resulting from a specific mutation. In neonates, the most common neurologic findings are seizures, hypotonia, generalized weakness, feeding difficulties, and blindness. Multisystem involvement is common as suggested by dysmorphic features, short stature, cataract, glaucoma, hepatomegaly, diarrhea, and bleeding tendencies. In infants of more than 6 months of age, neurologic features are psychomotor retardation, seizures, and visual and hearing impairment. Systemic findings include hepatomegaly, osteoporosis, ichthyosis, and hyperpigmentation of skin. In children, ataxia, developmental regression, peripheral neuropathy, behavior changes, speech difficulties, deafness, loss of vision and hearing, and spastic quadriparesis are common neurologic findings. Systemic findings include nausea, vomiting, hyperpigmentation of skin, and ichthyosis. In adults, spastic paraparesis, ataxia, peripheral neuropathy, dementia, deafness, and visual loss are frequently seen with minimal systemic manifestation. However, cardiac arrhythmia can result in sudden death. X-linked ALD (see White matter diseases) and Refsum disease (see Spino-cerebellopathies) will not be discussed in this section.

Cerebrohepatorenal syndrome of Zellweger

Zellweger syndrome is characterized by typical dysmorphic features and cerebrohepatorenal involvement (Figures 15.9 and 15.10). Multiple gene defects can result in Zellweger phenotype. The appearance of newborns with Zellweger syndrome is characteristic of the following: the forehead is broad; the supraorbital ridges and bridge of the nose are flat; the anterior fontanelle is large with splitting of the metopic suture; the eyes may show bilateral glaucoma with corneal clouding, cataracts, and retinal pigmentary degeneration; the mouth is triangular with the upper lip shaped like an inverted V; the infants generally show micrognathia, high-arched palate, and full cheeks; ears are low-set with abnormal pinna; clitorimegaly, hypospadias, and undescended testes are common features; neck webbing may be noted; and limbs may display simple transverse palmar creases, syndactyly, camptodactyly, clubfeet, and stippled chondral calcifications of the patella and acetabulum.

Early onset of cerebral involvement may be indicated by a history of paucity of intrauterine movements and polyhydramnios. At birth, respiration is spontaneous but apneic episodes may occur. Sucking and swallowing difficulties necessitate gavage feedings. The infants are paretic and severely hypotonic. Deep tendon reflexes are difficult to elicit. Seizures of various types are frequent. Psychomotor development is limited. Hepatomegaly is nearly a constant finding. Postnatal weight gain is poor. Bleeding tendency, osteopenia, retinal pigmentary degeneration, and poor wound healing are caused by fat-soluble vitamin deficiency. Jaundice may develop before death. Most patients die within the first 3 months of life.

Small subcapsular renal cysts are a constant finding and can be detected by abdominal ultrasound. Skeletal x-rays may show osteoporosis or scattered calcified stippling in the patellar areas, acetabular synchondrosis, and proximal epiphyses of femur and humerus. The epiphyses are generally spared but may be retarded in development.

Neuroimaging may show cysts in the subependymal region of the germinal matrix, hypoplasia of corpus callosum, gyral malformations, hypomyelinization, and cerebellar hypoplasia. The ERG is grossly abnormal. The EEG demonstrates seizure activity.

Laboratory studies in Zellweger syndrome show low serum cholesterol (due to mevalonate kinase deficiency), high serum iron levels with low iron-binding capacities (due to a derangement in the reduction and delivery of ferric iron

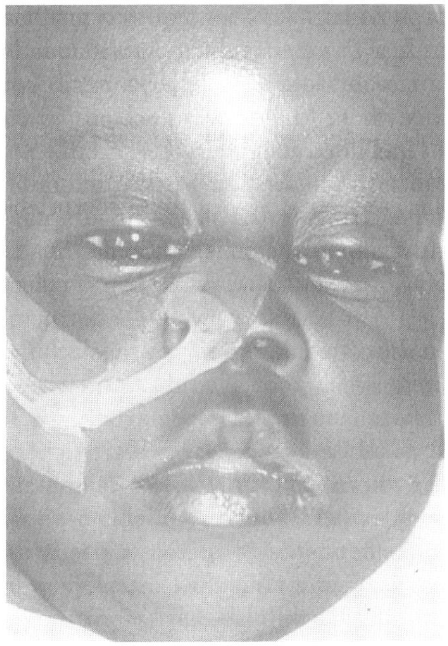

Figure 15.9 Characteristic facial features, such as flat supraorbital ridges, high forehead, ptosis, epicanthal folds, depressed nasal bridge, short anteverted nose, tented mouth, and micrognathia, in a 2-month-old girl with Zellweger syndrome who has to be gavage fed.

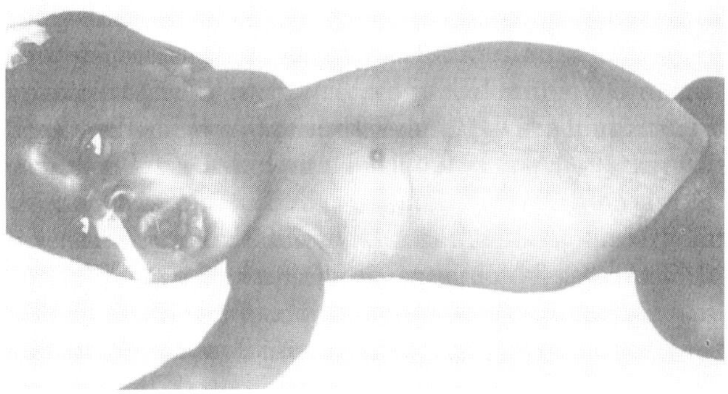

Figure 15.10 In this 2-month-old girl, the diagnosis of Zellweger syndrome was suggested by a generalized muscle wasting and weakness with bifacial involvement, hyporeflexia, and severe hypotonia with frog-leg position. In addition, the liver was enlarged and multiple dysplastic features were noted.

Key Clinical Questions

- *Did your baby appear more premature than expected for the gestational age?*
  The premature appearance of a newborn with Zellweger syndrome is suggested by the posture, poor activity and feeding difficulties, head shape, and inspection of genitalia.

in transferrin to the ferrous iron in heme), and microcytic nonhemolytic anemia. A functional deficiency of the adrenal cortex may be evidenced by ACTH stimulation. There is liver (elevated liver enzymes, hyperbilirubinemia, and abnormal bile acids in blood and urine) (Van Eldere et al. 1987) and kidney (nonspecific aminoaciduria) involvement. Pipecolic acid is typically found in the plasma and urine. Very-long-chain fatty acids (C26:0 and C26:1) are elevated in plasma, body fluids, and tissues with increased C26:C22 and C24:C22 ratios. Other biochemical markers suggesting diagnosis include an elevation of plasma phytanic acid and pristanic acid, and an elevation of plasma/urine dihydroxycholestanoic acid and trihydroxy-cholestanoic acid. In addition, C16 and C18 plasmalogens are severely diminished in the erythrocyte membranes (Fauler 1994; Wanders et al. 1986, 1994).

Table 15.36 Cerebrohepatorenal syndrome of Zellweger

Discriminating features

- Characteristic facies with flat/shallow supraorbital ridges
- Multiple defects of peroxisomal functions; dihydroxyacetone phosphate acyltransferase deficiency in fibroblasts; pipecolic aciduria and acidemia; elevated very-long-chain fatty acids in serum and plasma; abnormal bile acid metabolites; abnormal plasmalogen synthesis
- Disorder of peroxisomes biogenesis: no or ghost peroxisomes in liver and renal tubular epithelia
- Mutations in *PEX1, PEX2, PEX3, PEX5, PEX6, PEX10, PEX12, PEX13, PEX14, PEX16, PEX19*, or *PEX26*

Consistent features

- Seizures
- Hypotonia
- Widely patent fontanelles and sutures
- Hepatomegaly
- Failure to thrive
- Subcapsular renal cysts
- Nonspecific aminoaciduria
- Cerebral dysgenesis with dysmyelination, disordered lamination of cerebral cortex, Purkinje cell heterotopias and inferior olive dysplasia

Variable features

- Cataracts, retinitis pigmentosa, glaucoma, cloudy cornea
- Congenital heart lesions
- Cryptorchidism or clitoromegaly
- Limb abnormalities
- Calcific stippling of epiphysis and patellae
- Redundant skin on the neck
- Osteoporosis
- Jaundice
- Gastrointestinal bleeding
- Elevated serum iron and total iron-binding capacity
- Hypoglycemia
- Vitamin E, A, D, and K deficiency

Pearls and Perils

Cerebrohepatorenal syndrome of Zellweger

- Zellweger syndrome and Smith-Lemli-Opitz syndrome share similar facial features except for the flat supraorbital ridges, which are only seen in disorders of peroxisomal biogenesis.
- Zellweger syndrome should be suspected in newborns with craniofacial dysmorphism, seizures, and hypotonia. Cataracts and hepatomegaly may not be present at birth.
- Renal cysts and subependymal cysts may be demonstrated by ultrasound.
- X-rays of the lower extremities may demonstrate osteoporosis and/or chondral calcifications, most marked in the patellas.
- Laboratory findings typical of Zellweger syndrome include (a) hyperpipecolic acidemia, (b) elevated levels of plasma C26 very-long-chain fatty acids and elevated C26:0/C22:0 ratio, (c) elevated levels of urine C27 bile acid intermediates, (d) sometimes elevated levels of plasma branched-chain fatty acids (phytanic acid), and (e) deficient erythrocyte plasmalogen associated with deficient fibroblasts plasmalogen synthesis (deficient dihydroxyacetone phosphate acyltransferase activity).
- Diagnosis of peroxisomal biogenesis defect is proven by absence of catalase immunostain in the fibroblasts proving the absence of peroxisomes.

Pathologic changes occur in the liver, kidney, and nervous system. The liver is large, cirrhotic, and dysgenetic. The kidneys show dysgenetic parenchyma and small subcapsular cysts. No peroxisomes can be recognized in the liver and kidneys. The brain shows macrogyria, polymicrogyria, hypoplasia of the corpus callosum, bilateral subependymal cysts in the area of the head of the caudate nuclei, and olivary dysplasia (Table 15.36).

Treatment with oral plasmalogen normalizes erythrocyte plasmalogen levels and may result in clinical improvement. Bile acid therapy may reduce burden on cholesterol synthesis and help fat-soluble vitamin absorption. Supplementation with Ω-3 fatty acids, coenzyme Q10, vitamin E, vitamin K, and vitamin A may be beneficial. Replacement of adrenal steroids should be considered, particularly under stress.

Infantile Refsum disease

Infantile Refsum resembles Zellweger syndrome but with milder muscular hypotonia and fewer feeding difficulties.

Key Clinical Questions

Infantile Refsum

- *Did you have your child's hearing tested?*
  All patients with infantile Refsum syndrome have a sensorineuronal hearing loss. Most patients are floppy at birth, show mild dysmorphic features, acquire the ability to walk, and remain severely retarded but stable until mid-teens. In patients with possible Usher syndrome (retinitis pigmentosa and congenital deafness) examination of plasma very-long-chain fatty acids and branched-chain fatty acids is recommended (Raas-Rothschild et al. 2002).

Pearls and Perils

- Protracted diarrhea with low cholesterol levels appears during the first months of life in infantile Refsum syndrome.
- Patients with infantile Refsum syndrome can survive until adolescence or adulthood.
- Neurosensory hearing loss and elevation of phytanic acid differentiate infantile Refsum from X-linked adrenoleukodystrophy (ALD).
- Mental retardation and elevation of very-long-chain fatty acids differentiate infantile Refsum from Refsum disease.

Patients have minor dysmorphic features, such as simian creases, pectus excavatum, redundant skin folds in the neck, epicanthal folds, low-set ears, flattened facial profile, high arched palate, undescended testes, and/or contractures. Most patients learn to walk, although gait may be ataxic and broad-based. Diarrhea and vomiting with mild hepatomegaly, weight loss, and failure to thrive may precede onset of neurologic symptoms. Bilateral ptosis and generalized hypotonia are frequently observed during the first year of life. Between 6 and 36 months of age, neurologic deterioration leads to progressive hearing loss, poor vision, nystagmus, and severe mental retardation. Late in the course of the illness, seizures and increased spasticity dominate the clinical picture. A prolonged survival into the second and third decade is the rule.

X-rays of long bones demonstrate osteoporosis in the absence of chondrodysplasia punctata. No renal cysts are found by abdominal ultrasound. CT scan of brain may show atrophy or subdural hematoma. MRI demonstrates leukodystrophy. ERG is extinguished and visual evoked potential shows only feeble responses. Nerve conduction studies may be normal or demonstrate a polyneuropathy (Poll-Thé et al. 1987) (for biochemical features see Table 15.37). Therapeutic trials suggest that a phytanic acid–restricted diet, fat-soluble vitamin supplementation, and bile acid therapy may be beneficial in selected patients.

Table 15.37 Infantile Refsum

Discriminating features
- Elevated phytanic, hydroxyphytanic, and pristanic levels
- Deficiencies in the enzymes related to plasmalogen synthesis
- Disorder of peroxisomal biogenesis: no peroxisomes in liver and renal tubular epithelia
- Mutations in *PEX1*, *PEX2*, *PEX5*, *PEX6*, *PEX12*, or *PEX26*

Consistent features
- Early systemic symptoms: hepatomegaly, failure to thrive, hypocholesterolemia
- Hypotonia
- Minor dysmorphic features
- Late neurologic deterioration with deafness, retinitis pigmentosa, microcephaly, severe mental retardation
- No aminoaciduria
- Dihydroxyacetone phosphate acyltransferase deficiency in fibroblasts
- Elevated very-long-chain fatty acids, pipecolic acid and bile acid intermediates

Variable features
- Seizure
- Polyneuropathy
- Subdural hematoma
- Vitamin K-responsive coagulation defects
- Hyperbilirubinemia
- Spasticity
- Vitamin E deficiency

Neonatal adrenoleukodystrophy

In NALD dysmorphic features are less striking and more variable than in Zellweger syndrome, including midfacial hypoplasia with depressed nasal bridge, epicanthal folds, ptosis, short philtrum, prominent forehead, and abnormal ears (Figure 15.11). In addition, patients may have simian creases and/or cryptorchidism. Some infants appear severely ill at birth with hypotonia, stridor, poor respiratory efforts, and seizures whereas others appear near normal at birth. Half are macrocephalic at birth. NALD patients show initial, slow psychomotor development, rarely advancing beyond mental age of 12 months. Some may walk and say a few words. Hypotonia is the rule before regression sets in. Hearing and vision are frequently impaired. Cataract and retinopathy are common. Hepatomegaly, when present, is mild.

Severe growth retardation is usually noted by 2 years of age. Some patients develop subdural hematoma.

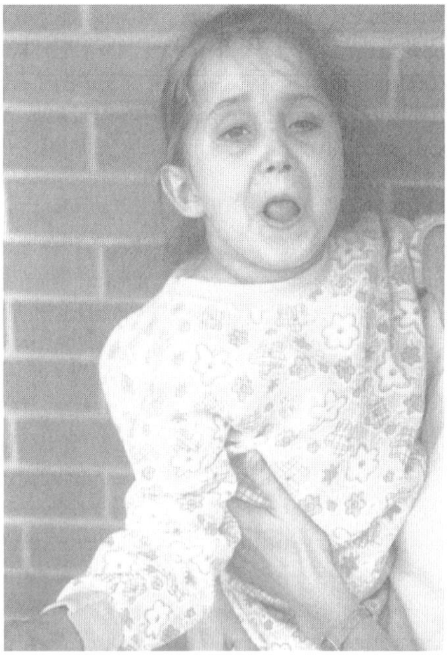

Figure 15.11 In this 12-year-old girl, the diagnosis of neonatal adrenoleukodystrophy was suggested by a loss of acquired motor skills, unusual facial features, and generalized muscle wasting and weakness with bifacial involvement, truncal hypotonia, and limb spasticity. There was no hepatomegaly.

The age at which regression begins varies from 12 months to more than 7 years of age (Kelly et al. 1986). Intention tremor, ataxia, hyporeflexia, and sensory defects develop while truncal hypotonia persists. Survival into the second decade has been reported. If not present neonatally, seizures usually develop during the degenerative period.

X-rays of long bones demonstrate osteoporosis but no sign of chondrodysplasia punctate. No cysts are found on renal ultrasound. MRI of the brain demonstrates a leukodystrophy. The ERG is extinguished. Brainstem auditory evoked responses are abnormal. Nerve conduction studies may demonstrate polyneuropathy.

Hypocholesterolemia, vitamin E deficiency, vitamin D deficiency, and clotting factor deficiencies are frequently demonstrated. Most patients have subnormal adrenal cortical response to ACTH stimulation. The CSF may show elevation of proteins. Saturated VLCFAs (C26:0) are usually elevated while mono-unsaturated C26:1 VLCFAs are normal (Kelly et al. 1986). The C26:C22 ratio is increased. Extremely low levels of docosahexanoic acid (DHA) are found (Martinez et al. 1993). Pipecolic acid may be normal or elevated. Plasmalogen may be normal or decreased (Sakai et al. 1986). Dihydroxyacetone phosphate acyltransferase (DHAP-AT) activity in fibroblasts may be normal or decreased. Peroxisomes are usually presenting but decreased in liver (Table 15.38). It has been suggested that docosahexanoic (DHA) deficiency causes visual and brain dysfunction. Therapy with pure DHA ethyl ester appears to produce good results (Martinez et al. 1993).

Table 15.38 Autosomal recessive neonatal adrenoleukodystrophy (NALD)

Discriminating features
- Increased very-long-chain fatty acids (C26:0) and low C26:C22 ratio8
- Deficiencies in the enzymes related to plasmalogen synthesis
- Disorder of peroxisomal biogenesis: decreased number and size of liver peroxisomes
- Mutations in *PEX1, PEX5, PEX6, PEX10, PEX12, PEX13*, or *PEX26*

Consistent features
- Autosomal recessive
- Hypotonia and hyporeflexia
- Failure to thrive
- Psychomotor retardation
- Dysmorphic features less severe than in Zellweger syndrome
- Osteoporosis
- Abnormal brain auditory evoked response
- Normal phytanic and bile acids
- Dihydroxyacetone phosphate acyltransferase (DHAP-AT) normal or decreased
- Abnormal central myelination on magnetic resonance imaging

Variable features
- Enlarged liver and impaired liver function
- Adrenal insufficiency
- Pigmentary retinal disturbances
- Cataracts
- Nystagmus
- Ataxia
- Seizures
- Deafness
- Subdural hematoma

Pearls and Perils

- Perilesional enhancement usually does not occur in neonatal adrenoleukodystrophy (NALD) but is typically seen in X-linked adrenoleukodystrophy (ALD).
- NALD may be misdiagnosed as cerebral palsy in patients who show little or no progression of symptoms.

Rhizomelic chondrodysplasia punctata type I

Rhizomelic chondrodysplasia punctata (RCDP) type I is characterized clinically by short limb dwarfism, affecting especially the proximal parts of the limbs (rhizomelic

Key Clinical Questions

- *Did your infant make any maturation gains after 1 year of age?*
  Most infants with neonatal adrenoleukodystrophy (NALD) are floppy and poor feeders at birth. Dysmorphic features are mild. Maturation is slow, reaching a plateau phase around 1 year of age. The plateau phase may last several years. The phase of regression is frequently heralded by seizures.

shortening of knees and hips), dysmorphic facial features, congenital cataract, contractures of knees and hips, profound psychomotor retardation, spastic quadriparesis, and epilepsy. Dysmorphic facial features include depressed bridge of the nose, flat supraorbital ridge, upturned nostrils, short nose, hypertelorism, epicanthal folds, high arched palate, and long philtrum. The anterior fontanel is large with an open metopic suture. The head is small. External ears are dysplastic. Neck and proximal limbs are short. Hands may exhibit camptodactyly with abnormal palmar creases. Chest is long and narrow. Intrauterine growth retardation is the rule. The eyes may show corneal changes and evidence of cataract formation (70%). Skin changes, such as those observed in ichthyosiform erythroderma, are demonstrated in about 25% of patients (Bodian 1966). Other malformations may include pulmonary stenosis (Gray et al. 1992) and laryngeal atresia (Storm & Fassa 1991). Sucking is poor, leading to failure to thrive. In 40% of patients, recurrent infections in infancy cause death in the first year of life. A milder phenotype mimicking noninfantile Refsum disease has been described in some patients presenting congenital cataract.

Radiologic abnormalities include punctate stippling of epiphyses at the knees, hips, elbows, shoulders, and vertebrae visible in late infancy. CT scan and MRI of the brain show cortical and subcortical atrophy (Williams et al. 1991). The EEG may demonstrate seizure activity

Pearls and Perils

Rhizomelic chondrodysplasia punctata

- Rhizomelic chondrodysplasia punctata should not be confused with autosomal recessive (multiple sulfatase deficiency) and X-linked recessive (defect in arylsulfatase E) nonrhizomelic chondrodysplasia punctata. The recessive nonrhizomelic chondrodysplasia punctata shares with rhizomelic chondrodysplasia punctata the evidence of ichthyosis, deafness, and progressive neurodegeneration (see Metachromatic leukodystrophy). There is no limb shortening but instead hypoplasia of distal phalanges is noted.
- Rhizomelic chondrodysplasia punctata (autosomal recessive) should not be confused with X-linked dominant chondrodysplasia punctata (Conradi-Hünermann syndrome). In rhizomelic chondrodysplasia punctata, the limbs are short proximally and bilaterally and both genders are affected. In Conradi-Hünermann syndrome, limb shortening is asymmetrical and not always proximal. This disorder of cholesterol biosynthesis is lethal in males. Cataract is sectorial. In severely affected individuals, bilateral findings may mimic rhizomelic chondrodysplasia. Diagnosis is confirmed by measuring the plasma concentration of sterols and assay of sterol-8-isomerase.
- Plasmalogen biosynthesis defects are found in all cases of rhizomelic chondrodysplasia punctata. If plasma phytanic acid is elevated, suspect *PEX7* defects. If plasma phytanic acid is normal, suspect rarer isolated defects of peroxisomal bile acid synthesis.
- *PEX7* mutations may cause a noninfantile Refsum phenotype. A deficiency in plasmalogen synthesis is consistently found.

Table 15.39 Rhizomelic chondrodysplasia punctata

Discriminating features
- Rhizomelic dwarfism
- Elevated phytanic acid and pristanic acid
- Deficiencies in the enzymes related to plasmalogen synthesis
- Disorder of peroxisomal biogenesis (complementation group 11): abnormal peroxisomes
- *PEX7* defects

Consistent features
- Dysmorphic features
- Failure to thrive
- Psychomotor delay
- Contractures
- Absent hepatomegaly liver dysfunction & malabsorption
- Cataract
- Normal very-long-chain fatty acids and bile acids
- Not associated with dysmyelination or neuronal migration defects

Variable features
- Microcephaly
- Corneal clouding
- Retinopathy
- Stippled calcifications of epiphyses
- Ichthyosis
- Epilepsy
- Laryngeal atresia
- Pulmonary stenosis

(Gray et al. 1992). The ERG is grossly abnormal. Brainstem auditory evoked responses may be delayed. Ultrasound fails to show renal cysts.

Plasma phytanic acid level in RCDP is equal to that seen in classic Refsum disease. Plasma VLCFAs, bile acids, and pipecolic acid levels are normal. Plasmalogen synthesis in cultured fibroblasts is deficient, distinguishing RCDP from classic Refsum disease. Hepatocytes lack peroxisomes or contain an increased number of large, irregularly shaped peroxisomes (Heymans et al. 1986) (Table 15.39). Molecular analysis of the PEX7 gene (chromosome locus 6q22-q24) is available. Present treatment consists of palliative orthopedic care, cataract removal, and dietary restriction of phytanic acid.

Pseudo-neonatal adrenoleukodystrophy

Pseudo-neonatal adrenoleukodystrophy (pseudo-NALD) is an autosomal recessive isolated defect of peroxisomal acyl-CoA oxidase, the first enzyme of β-oxidation system, resulting in a phenotype mimicking NALD. Dysmorphic features when present may include hypertelorism, depressed nasal bridge, low-set ears, and polydactyly (Suzuki et al. 1994). Profound hypotonia and areflexia are present at birth. Intrauterine growth retardation is the rule. Early-onset seizures and slow psychomotor development are the rule. Some patients walk and say a few words. Hearing and vision are impaired. Age of death is variable up to 5 years of age.

Plasma VLCFAs are elevated while bile acid intermediates, pristanic acid, and phytanic acid levels are normal. DHAP-AT activity in skin fibroblasts is normal (Poll-Thé et al. 1988). In some patients a large deletion of the acyl-CoA oxidase gene is found, whereas other cases probably result from a point mutation (Suzuki et al. 1994). This disorder is associated with enlarged hepatic peroxisomes (Table 15.40).

Table 15.40 Pseudo-neonatal adrenoleukodystrophy (NALD)

Discriminating features
- Elevated plasma very-long-chain fatty acid levels
- Normal plasmalogen synthesis
- Large peroxisomes in liver
- Peroxisomal acyl-CoA oxidase deficiency

Consistent features
- Slow development precedes regression
- Seizures
- Visual and hearing impairment
- Survival up to 5 years of age
- Normal bile and phytanic acid levels

Variable features
- Facial dysmorphic features
- Retinal degeneration

Key Clinical Questions

- *Was there any perinatal complication?*
  Both pseudo-neonatal adrenoleukodystrophy (NALD) and pseudo-Zellweger clinically present with neonatal seizures and hypotonia, mimicking perinatal asphyxia. Plasma very-long-chain fatty acids are elevated, and fibroblast plasmalogen synthesis is normal in both conditions. The clinical course and urine bile acid intermediates differentiate the two syndromes

Pseudo-Zellweger syndrome

Pseudo-Zellweger syndrome results from a group of autosomal recessive, isolated defects of peroxisomal β-oxidation that affect either bifunctional enzyme or peroxisomal thiolase, resulting clinically in a phenotype mimicking Zellweger syndrome (Table 15.41) (Goldfischer et al. 1986; Suzuki et al. 1994).

Table 15.41 Pseudo-Zellweger syndrome

Discriminating features
- Elevated very-long-chain fatty acid and bile acid intermediates
- Normal plasmalogen synthesis
- Abundant peroxisomes in liver
- Peroxisomal bifunctional enzyme deficiency

Consistent features
- Severe hypotonia
- Minimal development progress
- Seizures
- Visual and hearing impairment
- Brain dysplasia
- Death in infancy or early childhood

Variable features
- Facial dysmorphic features
- Hepatomegaly
- Osteopenia
- Stippled patella
- Renal microcysts
- Bleeding tendency
- Adrenal insufficiency
- Ventricular septal defect
- Retinitis pigmentosa

Trihydroxycholestanic acidemia

Trihydroxycholestanic acidemia is an autosomal recessive isolated defect of peroxisomal bile acid metabolism due to trihydroxycholestanoic acyl-CoA oxidase deficiency presenting with progressive ataxia in the second or third year of life (Christensen et al. 1990; Vanhove et al. 1993). Patients are hypotonic without deep tendon reflexes, and hearing is impaired. Biochemical studies show an accumulation of di- and trihydroxycholestanoic acid in urine.

Rhizomelic chondrodysplasia punctata type II and type III

Rhizomelic chondrodysplasia punctata type II is caused by an isolated defect of peroxisomal DHAP-AT, whereas type III results from an isolated defect of peroxisomal alkyl-DHAP synthase (alkyl-DHAP synthase) (Wanders et al. 1994). Rhizomelia may be absent. Mental retardation, hypotonia, and stippled epiphysis are consistent features. Cataract and skin changes are consistently seen. In all forms of RCDP plasma, VLCFAs are normal and plasmalogen synthesis in fibroblasts is decreased. In RCDP variants, unlike classic RCDP type I, phytanic acid metabolism is normal, and liver biopsy shows mature peroxisomes. The diagnosis is confirmed by measurement of the specific enzyme activity in cultured skin fibroblasts.

Refsum-like disorder

See Table15.42.

Table 15.42 Refsum-like disorder

Discriminating features
- Minimal elevation of phytanic acid
- Pristanic acid, and dehydrocholic acid (DHCA) and/or trihydroxycholestanoic acid (THCA) are elevated
- Peroxisomal 2-methylacyl-CoA racemase deficiency

Consistent features
- Onset in childhood of fat malabsorption

Variable features
- Juvenile or adult onset
- Retinopathy
- Leukoencephalopathy
- Learning disability
- Spastic paraparesis
- Seizures
- Sensorimotor neuropathy in adults
- Seizures
- Ataxia with involvement of posterior columns and pyramidal tracts

Table 15.43 Leukoencephalopathy with dystonia and motor neuropathy

Discriminating features
- Minimal elevation phytanic acid
- Elevated pristanic acid, and slightly elevated dehydrocholic acid (DHCA) and/or trihydroxycholestanoic acid
- Abnormal bile acids in urine with increased excretion of C-27 bile alcohol glucuronides (similar to cerebrotendinous xanthomatosis)
- Peroxisomal sterol carrier protein X

Consistent features
- Leukoencephalopathy

Variable features
- Adult onset
- No retinopathy
- Learning disability
- Dystonia, stutter
- Sensorimotor neuropathy
- Hyposmia
- Hypoacousia

Leukoencephalopathy with dystonia and motor neuropathy

See Table 15.43.

Mevalonic aciduria

Mevalonic aciduria is an autosomal recessive disorder of peroxisomal cholesterol and nonsterol isoprene biosynthesis associated clinically with two clinical phenotypes that may overlap. The subacute classic neurologic form is characterized by psychomotor retardation, hypotonia, failure to thrive, recurrent crisis with fever, and gastrointestinal symptoms. The chronic "systemic" form is a hyperimmunoglobulin D (hyper IgD) and periodic fever syndrome. The human gene for mevalonate kinase has been localized to chromosome 12q24 (Schafer et al. 1992). Compound heterozygosity can result in mevalonic aciduria.

Pearls and Perils

- Mevalonate kinase deficiency can be seen in peroxisomal biogenesis disorders such as Zellweger syndrome.
- Mevalonic aciduria should be suspected in patients with visual impairment and development delay anytime there is a history of recurrent inflammatory crisis. Some patients survive into adulthood.

Key Clinical Questions

- *Does your child with unsteady gait have developmental delay and failure to thrive and appear susceptible to infections?*
  In such a child, look for unusual facial features, cataract, hepatomegaly, and cerebellar hypoplasia. Organic acids should be tested in the urine.

Patients with subacute neurologic mevalonic aciduria consistently present in infancy with psychomotor retardation and failure to thrive. Dysmorphic features such as microcephaly, dolichocephaly, frontal bossing, hypertelorism, down-slanted eyes, large fontanels, hypoplasia alae nasi, low-set ears, and syndactyly have been reported in some patients (Mancini et al. 1993; Hoffman et al. 1993). Typically, noninfectious recurrent crisis characterized by fever, diarrhea, and vomiting develop in most patients. These episodes are accompanied by arthralgia, edema, morbilliform rash, lymphadenopathies, hepatomegaly, hypotonia, lethargy, and seizures. Severely affected patients die in infancy. A cardiomyopathy with heart block may develop in some patients. Survivors have a mild mental retardation, sometimes accompanied by hypotonia and cerebellar ataxia. Cataract is found in half of the patients.

The hyperimmunoglobulin D (hyper IgD) and periodic fever syndrome (HIDS) is an autoinflammatory disease beginning in infancy and characterized by life-long recurrent episodes of fever not triggered by infection (every 4 to 6 weeks) accompanying signs and symptoms such as headache, abdominal distress, erythematous rash, aphthous ulcers, arthralgia, and lymphadenopathies. Most patients have no neurologic symptom, although some patients exhibit mild to severe mental retardation, cerebellar ataxia, and a progressive blindness due to tapetoretinal degeneration and cataract. Seizures have been reported in two cases. Survival to adulthood is common (Simon et al. 2004).

Bone age and skull suture closure are frequently delayed. Brain imaging demonstrates cerebral and cerebellar vermis atrophy. White and gray matter signals are normal. Nerve conduction velocities and EMG are normal. The EEG findings are variable.

Blood cholesterol is normal or low. A deficiency in plasma ubiquinone-10 (Q_{10}) is demonstrated in plasma of patients who develop a cardiomyopathy, hypotonia (Hübner et al. 1993), and cerebellar atrophy. The excretion of fat in the feces, when present, results from a deficient synthesis of bile acids (Gibson et al. 1993). Liver enzymes may be normal or elevated. Anemia and increased sedimentation rate can be found during recurrent crisis. Hyperimmunoglobulinemia D and elevated sedimentation rate are found in patients with HIDS. Urinary excretion of leukotriene E_4 is elevated in most patients (Mayatepek et al. 1993).

Table 15.44 Mevalonic aciduria

Discriminating features
- Recurrent "inflammatory" crisis with fever of unknown origin
- Mevalonic aciduria
- Mevalonic kinase deficiency

Variable features
- Cataract
- Tapetoretinal degeneration
- Mental retardation
- Failure to thrive
- Myopathy with elevated creatine kinase
- Cerebellar atrophy
- Cardiomyopathy
- Dysmorphic features
- Seizures
- Headache
- Coenzyme Q10 deficiency
- Hyper IgD

The diagnosis can be made readily by analysis of urine organic acids, which demonstrate mevalonic aciduria. Plasma levels of mevalonate are also elevated, although the elevation may only be transient in patients with episodic fever. Mevalonate kinase deficiency is proven by assay of the enzyme in fibroblasts or lymphocytes (Table 15.44).

Treatment with lovastatin, an inhibitor of hydroxy methyl glutaryl CoA reductase, to reduce mevalonate production, may exacerbate symptoms. Supplementation with cholesterol, coenzyme Q10, and vitamins E, D, and A may be beneficial. Corticosteroid therapy prevents death during clinical crisis. Therapy inhibiting interleukin (IL)-1 activity by using a recombinant human IL-1 receptor antagonist (anakinra) has been successful in reducing and preventing inflammatory signs and symptoms.

Diffuse mitochondrial encephalomyopathies

The mitochondrial encephalomyopathies are hereditary neurodegenerative disorders characterized by multiple features indicating dysfunction of mitochondrial aerobic oxidative metabolism: elevated levels of lactate and pyruvate in the blood and CSF, alteration of mitochondrial morphology in various tissues, and diminished activity of oxidative mitochondrial enzymes (Table 15.45).

The mitochondrial encephalomyopathies are clinically, biochemically, and genetically heterogeneous. Many mitochondrial encephalomyopathies have been discussed in various sections of this chapter based on the most

Table 15.45 Mitochondrial encephalomyopathies

Discriminating features
- Defective mitochondrial oxidative phosphorylation due to defective nuclear or mitochondrial DNA

Consistent features
- Increased lactate in areas of brain involved by acute process (by proton magnetic spectroscopy)
- Increased lactate in the blood after exercise or glucose loading test

Variable features
- Ragged red fibers in muscles
- Histochemical changes
- Morphological changes of mitochondria
- Elevated lactate and pyruvate in cerebrospinal fluid

prominent neuropathologic features. Menkes disease and Alpers disease are examples of polioencephalopathies Leigh syndrome, familial bilateral striatal necrosis (BFSN), Mohr-Tranebjaerg syndrome (MTS), and Wilson disease are corencephalopathies. Neuropathy, ataxia, and retinitis pigmentosa (NARP) syndrome; sideroblastic anemia spinocerebellar ataxia (ASAT); spinocerebellar ataxia with neuropathy, dysarthria, and ophthalmoparesis (SANDO); and Friedreich ataxia are spinocerebellopathies. In this section, seven diffuse mitochondrial encephalopathies will be discussed. It has been demonstrated that the nature of a given clinical syndrome depends not so much on the exact oxidative enzyme that is defective, but rather on the degree to which flux through oxidative pathways is impaired. Therefore, affected individuals within a single kindred may display different clinical syndromes (e.g., Leigh and NARP; Leigh being seen in the most severely affected individuals). Similarly, in different kindreds, the same mitochondrial biochemical defect may lead to various clinical syndromes. Additionally, the same clinical syndromes can be caused by various biochemical defects. Organs other than the brain and muscle are frequently involved. Systemic involvement may result in renal tubular, cardiac, pancreatic, and bone marrow dysfunction, endocrinopathy, neuropathy, hearing loss, and retinopathy.

The mitochondrial encephalomyopathies can result from nuclear gene defects (mendelian inheritance) or abnormal mitochondrial DNA. Nuclear gene defects may result in mutations in the genes encoding the structural components of the respiratory chain (e.g., ND genes in Leigh syndrome), the genes required for the mitochondrial protein importation (TIMM8A gene in Morh-Tranebjaerg syndrome), the genes required for the assembly of active complexes (SURF-1 gene in Leigh syndrome), the genes required for transport of protein cofactors (ATP7B gene, encoding the Golgi and mitochondrial hepatic transmembrane copper-transporting ATPase, in Wilson disease), and the genes required for the intramitochondrial cofactor homeostasis (FRDA gene in Friedreich ataxia). In addition, mitochondrial DNA defects may result from abnormalities in communication between nuclear and mitochondrial genome. Mitochondrial DNA "depletion," a quantitative alteration in mitochondrial DNA, results from a defective nuclear-encoded protein controlling mitochondrial replication (deoxyguanosine kinase gene in lethal infantile mitochondrial disease of Boustany). Qualitative alterations in mitochondrial DNA, such as multiple mitochondrial DNA "deletions," result from defective nuclear-encoded proteins required for maintenance (ANT1 gene, an ADP/ATP carrier protein in CPEO or thymidine phosphorylase gene in mitochondrial neurogastrointestinal encephalopathy) and repair (mitochondrial DNA polymerase gene in autosomal dominant CPEO) of mitochondrial DNA. Other qualitative alterations, such as mitochondrial "deletions" and duplications, are sporadic. Mitochondrial DNA point mutations are always maternally inherited due to exclusive maternal transmission of mitochondrial DNA. Mitochondrial DNA point mutations are homoplastic when intracellular mitochondrial DNA is purely mutant. Such mutations are, of necessity, only mildly deleterious and affect structural genes of the respiratory chain. Mitochondrial DNA point mutations are heteroplasmic when mixed populations of mutant and normal mitochondrial DNA coexist in each cell. Such mutations frequently affect tRNA. The patient's clinical symptoms and survival depend on the amount of normal mitochondrial DNA present in each tissue. Most tRNA gene mutations are functionally recessive, as the critical mutation threshold in affected tissues has to exceed 70–90% to become symptomatic (Sacconi et al. 2008). The neurologic syndromes associated with abnormal mitochondrial DNA are summarized in Table 15.46. Mitochondrial encephalopathies due to nuclear DNA mutations are summarized in Table 15.47.

One of the most encouraging aspects of this group of diseases is the fact that preventive/palliative therapy can be achieved if the basic pathophysiology is understood. Prevention of exacerbation can be achieved simply by rapid treatment of infections and fever and avoidance of fasting and strenuous exercise. Frequent or continuous feeding during the night and/or high caloric intake may be necessary to avoid catabolic state. Drugs that inhibit mitochondrial protein synthesis (tetracyclines, chloramphenicol), sequestrate carnitine (valproic acid), and inhibit respiratory chain (barbiturate, phenytoin) should be avoided. Other palliative therapeutic measures include removal of toxic products, reduction of the load of substrate presented to the mutant enzyme, coenzyme supplementation at pharmacologic levels, replacement of products (important intermediates in metabolism) that are missing due to enzyme deficiencies,

Table 15.46 Neurologic syndromes associated with abnormal mitochondrial DNA

Syndrome	Abnormal mitochondrial DNA	Inheritance
MELAS	Heteroplasmic point mutations in genes encoding $tRNA^{Leu}$ (MTTL1: 3243, 3260, 3271, 3291, 3308; MTTL2:), $tRNA^{Gln}$ (MTTQ: 4336), $tRNA^{Phe}$ (MTTF: 583), $tRNA^{His}$ (MTTH: 12147), $tRNA^{Lys}$ (MTTK: 8356), $tRNA^{Ser}$ (MTTS1: 7512; MTTS2: 12207), $tRNA^{Val}$ (MTTV)	Maternal
	Heteroplasmic point mutations in genes encoding complex I (ND1: ; ND5: 12770, 13042, 13045, 13084, 13513; ND6: 14453)	Maternal
	Deletion/duplications	Sporadic
	No defect (defects of mitochondrial oxidative metabolism)	Nuclear
MERRF	Heteroplasmic point mutations in genes encoding $tRNA^{Leu}$ (MTTL1: 3243, 3256), $tRNA^{Phe}$ (MTTF: 611), $tRNA^{His}$ (MTTH: 1247), $tRNA^{Lys}$ (MTTK: 8344, 8356) $tRNA^{Ser}$ (MTTS1: 7512), $tRNA^{Ser}$ (MTTS2: 12207)	Maternal
	Heteroplasmic mutation in the gene encoding complex I (ND5:13042)	Maternal
CPEO/KSS	Heteroplasmic point mutations in genes encoding $tRNA^{Leu}$ (MTTL1: 3243, 3249, 3251, 3273; MTTL2: 12315, 12420), $tRNA^{Tyr}$ (MTTY: 5877, 5885), $tRNA^{Gln}$ (MTTQ: 4366), $tRNA^{Ala}$ (MTTA: 5628), $tRNA^{Asn}$ (MTTN:5703, 5692), RNA^{Ile} (4285, 4298), RNA^{Lys} (8342)	Maternal
	Sporadic	
	Multiple deletions	Nuclear
NARP	Heteroplasmic point mutations encoding complex V (8993, 8851, 9176)	Maternal
Leigh	Heteroplasmic point mutations in genes encoding $tRNA^{Lys}$ (MTTK: 8344), $tRNA^{Val}$ (MTTV: 1624), $tRNA^{Trp}$ (MTTW: 5537), $tRNA^{Leu}$ (MTTL1: 3243), $tRNA^{Ser}$ (MTTS2: 12207)	Maternal
	Maternal	
	Depletion (complex II: SUCLA2)	Nuclear
	No defect (defects of mitochondrial oxidative metabolism)	Nuclear
FBSN	Homoplasmic or heteroplasmic point mutations in genes encoding complex V (8851, 9176), complex I (ND6: 14459, 14596, 11696)	Maternal
	No defect	Nuclear
LHON	Homoplasmic or heteroplasmic point mutations in genes encoding complex I (ND4: 11778; ND1: 3460, 3733, 4171; ND6:14484, 14495, 14459, 14482, 14498, 14568, 14596; ND2: 4640, 4917, 5244; ND5: 12484, 13708, 13730), complex III (cyt b: 15257, 15812), complex IV (CO1: 7444;CO3: 9438, 9804), complex V (8851, 8993, 9176)	Maternal
MNGIE	$tRNA^{Lys}$ (MTTK: 8313), tRNATrp (MTTW: 5532)	Maternal
	Partial depletion/multiple deletions	Nuclear
DIDMOAD	Multiple deletions	Nuclear
LIHRMD	Heteroplasmic point mutation (15923, 15924)	Maternal
Depletion	Nuclear	
Alpers	Heteroplasmic point mutation in COX II (7706)	Maternal

MELAS, mitochondrial encephalomyopathy with lactic acidosis and stroke-like episodes; MERRF, myoclonic epilepsy with ragged red fibers; CPEO, chronic progressive external ophthalmoplegia; KSS, Kearns-Sayre syndrome; NARP, neurogenic muscle weakness, ataxia, retinitis pigmentosa; FBSN, familial bilateral striatal necrosis, LHON, Leber hereditary optic neuroretinopathy; MNGIE, mitochondrial myopathy, peripheral neuropathy, gastrointestinal, and encephalopathy disease; DIDMOAD, diabetes insipidus, diabetes mellitus, optic atrophy, deafness (Wolfram); LIHRMD, lethal infantile hepatocerebral mitochondrial DNA depletion syndrome.

and pharmacologic therapy. Detoxification strategies are summarized in Table 15.48.

Restricting dietary precursors decreases production of toxic metabolites. A low-carbohydrate, high-fat diet (essentially a ketogenic diet) is effective in preventing lactic acidosis in patients with deficiency in the El subunit of pyruvate dehydrogenase complex, whereas a high-carbohydrate diet has favorable effect in the deficiency of the E3 subunit of pyruvate dehydrogenase complex and pyruvate dehydrogenase phosphatase deficiency.

Coenzyme supplementation at pharmacologic levels should be tried (Table 15.49). Sodium succinate is a product that is favorably replaced in MELAS and CPEO. Corticosteroids have been reported to be effective in MELAS.

Mitochondrial encephalomyopathy, lactic acidosis, and stroke-like episodes syndrome

Mitochondrial encephalomyopathy, lactic acidosis, and stroke-like episodes (MELAS) syndrome is a maternally inherited or sporadic, progressive, neurodegenerative disease that is characterized by migraine headaches, focal neurologic defects, and focal or generalized

Table 15.47 Mitochondrial encephalopathies due to nuclear DNA mutations

Syndrome	Gene function	Chromosome
MELAS	Mitochondrial DNA polymerase (POLG1)	15q25
CPEO with multiple	Adenine nucleotide translocator 1 (Ant1)	4q35
mtDNA deletions	Mitochondrial DNA polymerase gamma (POLG1 POLG2)	15q25, 17q
	Twinkle (C10ORF2)	10q23
	Mitochondrial DNA instability (OPA1 gene)	3q28
MNGIE	Thymidine phosphorylase (multiple mitochondrial DNA deletions)	22q13.32-qter
	Mitochondrial DNA polymerase (POLG1)	15q25
MSMA	Thymidine kinase 2 (mitochondrial DNA depletion)	16q22
LIHRMD	Deoxyguanosine kinase (mitochondrial DNA depletion)	2p13
	MPV17	2p23-p21
	Twinkle (C10ORF2)	10q24
	Mitochondrial DNA polymerase-γ (POLG1)	15q25
DIDMOAD	WS1	4p16
SANDO	Mitochondrial DNA polymerase-γ (POLG1)	15q25
	Twinkle (C10ORF2)	10q24
ADOA	Mitochondrial DNA instability (OPA1 gene)	3q28
Leigh	Complex I – NDUFV1, NDUFS1,	11q13, 2q33
	NDUFS3, NDUFS4	11p11.11, 5q11
	NDUFS7, NDUFS8	19q13, 11q13
	Complex II – flavoprotein subunit (SDH2)	5p15
	Complex II – iron-sulfur protein (SDH1)	1p35–36
	Complex III _ BCS1L (assembly)	2q33
	Complex IV – COX10, COX15, copper transport (SCO2)	17p12, 10q22,
	Assembly genes (SURF-1, LRPPRC)	22q13, 9q34, 2p
	Pyruvate dehydrogenase (PDH-E1α, PDH-E3)	Xp22, 7q31, 8q22
	Succinyl-CoA synthase (SUCLA2)	13q
	Mitochondrial protein synthesis (Elongation factor G1)	3q25
	Coenzyme Q10 synthesis (PDSS2)	6q21
FBSN	Nucleoporin (NUP62)	19q13
DDS	TIMMSA gene encoding a component of the mitochondrial-protein import machinery	Xq22
Friedreich	Frataxin, Fe transport	9q13
ASAT	Iron transport (ABC7)	Xq13
AD HSP 13	Mitochondrial matrix chaperonin HSP60	2q24-q34
AD HSP 31	REEP1 (function?)	2p12
AR HSP7	Paraplegin, mitochondrial metalloprotease with ATPase associated activities	16q24.4l
Wilson	Hepatic transmembrane copper ATPase, Cu transport	13q14.3-q21.1
Menkes	Extrahepatic transmembrane copper ATPase, Cu transport	Xq13.33
Alpers	Mitochondrial DNA polymerase-γ (POLG1)	15q25
	Ribonucleotide reductase (RRM2B)	8q23
	Twinkle (C10ORF2)	10q24
ECOQD	Coenzyme Q10 synthesis (PDSS1, PDSS2,	10p12, 6q21
	CoQ2)	4q21,
	Chaperone-like protein (CABC1)	1q42

CPEO, chronic progressive external ophthalmoplegia; MNGIE, mitochondrial myopathy, peripheral neuropathy, gastrointestinal, and encephalopathy disease; MSMA, myopathy and spinal muscular atrophy; LIHRMD, lethal infantile hepatocerebral mitochondrial DNA depletion syndrome; DIDMOAD, diabetes insipidus, diabetes mellitus, optic atrophy, deafness (Wolfram); SANDO, spinocerebellar ataxia, sensory neuropathy, dysarthria and ophthalmoparesis; ADOA, autosomal dominant optic atrophy (Kjer); FBSN, familial bilateral striatal necrosis; DDS, deafness-dystonia dementia syndrome of Mohr-Tranebjaerg; ASAT, X-linked sideroblastic anemia with ataxia; HSP, hereditary spastic paraplegia; ECOQD, encephalopathy with ataxia/ seizures and coenzyme Q deficiency.

Table 15.48 Detoxification strategies in mitochondrial encephalomyopathies

Drugs	Dosage	Route	Conditions
Dichloroacetate	15–150 mg/kg/day	IV/PO	Lactic acidosis
Coenzyme Q10	4.3 mg/kg/day	PO	Complex I or II deficiency
Phytonadione	0.36 mg/kg/day	PO	Complex III deficiency
Menadione	1.1–1.5 mg/kg/day	PO	Complex III deficiency
Ascorbic acid	57 mg/kg/day	PO	Complex III deficiency
Idebenone	5 mg/kg/day	PO	Mitochondrial disorders
L-Carnitine	50–300 mg/kg/day	PO/IV	Mitochondrial disorders
Lipoic acid M	10–50 mg/kg/day	PO/IM	Respiratory chain defects
Vitamin E	200–400 mg/kg/day	PO	Respiratory chain defects

seizures. Lactic acidosis is an inconsistent feature. Many cases of MELAS have been reported to be associated with isolated deficiency of NADH dehydrogenase (complex I) activity (Koya et al. 1988). Maternal inheritance is suggested by detection of mitochondrial DNA point mutations encoding for mitochondrial RNA. In sporadic patients combining features of MELAS and Kearns-Sayre syndrome (KSS), mitochondrial deletions can be found (Zupanc et al. 1991).

Patients with MELAS syndrome are usually asymptomatic in infancy and have normal early development. Most patients are short. Some patients display muscle weakness, fatigability, and myalgia before the onset of central neurologic dysfunction. Chronic asthma may be an unusual presentation of MELAS (Shanske et al. 1993). Central neurologic symptoms begin between infancy and young adulthood. The mitochondrial angiopathy may manifest early in the skin as purpura (Horiguchi et al. 1991). Most patients have recurrent epileptic seizures, which are partial or generalized. Myoclonic seizures are uncommon. Attacks of prolonged migraine headaches with vomiting are prominent in some patients. In the wake of headaches or partial seizures, patients may abruptly develop stroke-like episodes. Episodes of cortical infarction lead to the gradual decline of motor, sensory, and mental functioning.

There is usually a history of bilateral hemiparesis with corticospinal tract signs, dysarthria, visual impairment with hemianopia, and decline in cognitive function. Patients progressively become bedridden, quadriparetic, deaf, blind, and demented. A progressive myoclonic epilepsy can be seen late in the course of the illness. Ocular signs and symptoms may include posterior subcapsular cataract, bilateral ptosis, chronic external ophthalmoplegia, diffuse choroidal atrophy, atypical pigmentary retinopathy with macular involvement, and optic atrophy (Rummelt et al. 1993). Myocardial involvement may produce mitral regurgitation (Suzuki et al. 1993), hypertrophic or dilated cardiomyopathy (Inui et al. 1992), and cardiac conduction defects, including ventricular arrhythmias, pre-excitation syndromes, and cardiac conduction block (Ciafaloni et al. 1992). Renal involvement may result in nephrotic syndrome (Inui et al. 1992) or renal tubular dysfunction (Ciafaloni et al. 1992). Endocrine involvement may include diabetes mellitus, pituitary dwarfism, and hypothyroidism (Inui et al. 1992). Death usually occurs within a few years from onset.

Table 15.49 Coenzyme therapy in mitochondrial encephalomyopathies

Drugs	Dosage	Route
Biotin	10–50 mg/day	PO
Thiamine	150–300 mg/day	PO/IV
Riboflavin	30–300 mg/day	PO/IV
Pyridoxine	50–500 mg/day	PO/IV
Hydroxocobalamin	1–10 mg/day	IV/IM

Laboratory findings of MELAS syndrome are variable. Most patients present with elevations of lactate and pyruvate in the blood and CSF. However, lactic acidosis may be intermittent, and glucose tolerance tests may fail to produce lactic acidemia (Breningstall & Lockman 1988). The CSF proteins may be elevated (Shapira et al. 1975). Mitochondrial DNA point mutation analysis should evaluate 3243, 3271, and 3252 MELAS point mutations in blood. Patients with MELAS syndrome may develop autoantibodies, such as rheumatoid factor and antimitochondrial antibodies (Shapira et al. 1990). Cardiac abnormalities can be shown on chest x-ray study, EKG, and ECG. Electromyogram and nerve conduction studies may be normal or show various myopathic and neuropathic patterns (Breningstall & Lockman 1988). The EEG may show focal or diffuse slowing with or without epileptogenic potentials. Neuropathology demonstrates infarct-like lesions in the cortex and subcortical white matter, and mitochondrial abnormalities are found in the endothelial cells and smooth muscle cells of blood vessels.

Pearls and Perils

- Approximately 80–90% of MELAS patients have a point mutation in the mitochondrial gene encoding for the $tRNA^{Leucine(UUR)}$, either at the base pair 3243 or at base pair 3271.
- Patients suffering from recurrent migrainous strokes and progressive dementia should be tested for mitochondrial DNA point mutations. Most patients with hemiplegic migraine do not have a defect in mitochondrial DNA.
- Cardiac manifestations of MELAS are major determinants of prognosis.
- Most patients with MELAS have elevated blood lactate concentrations, but it may be intermittent, and is not mandatory for diagnosis of MELAS.
- Computed tomography scan and magnetic resonance imaging of the brain are less sensitive than single-proton emission CT (SPECT) scan in visualizing stroke-like episodes in the early stages of the illness.
- The absence of ragged red fibers does not exclude MELAS.
- MELAS point mutations are maternally inherited. Maternal relatives of MELAS patients may be normal or may have migraine, deafness, diabetes mellitus, limb-girdle myopathy, cardiomyopathy, or other mitochondrial encephalomyopathy (chronic progressive external ophthalmoplegia, Leigh syndrome).

The strokes in MELAS can be seen as hypoperfusion by SPECT even when MRI and CT are normal (Satoh et al. 1991).

CT scan of the head may show hypodensity and swelling of the cerebral cortex in multiple vascular tortuousities with a predilection for parieto-occipital regions. Sequential scans may show resolution and subsequent reoccurrence of the abnormal areas. Calcifications or hypodensities of the basal ganglia are found in some patients. Gyriform enhancement can be demonstrated on contrast studies (Allard et al. 1988). Some patients may show multifocal white matter hypodensities (Fujii et al. 1990). In advanced cases sulcal and ventricular prominence is present. In one patient with infantile-onset MELAS syndrome the author found diffuse white matter calcifications (Figure 15.12) (Maertens et al. 1988). MRI of brain reveals the lesions more distinctively and precisely than CT scan. Lesions have high signal intensities on T2-weighted MRI (Figure 15.13). MRI may reveal cerebellar lesions that could not be detected on CT scan

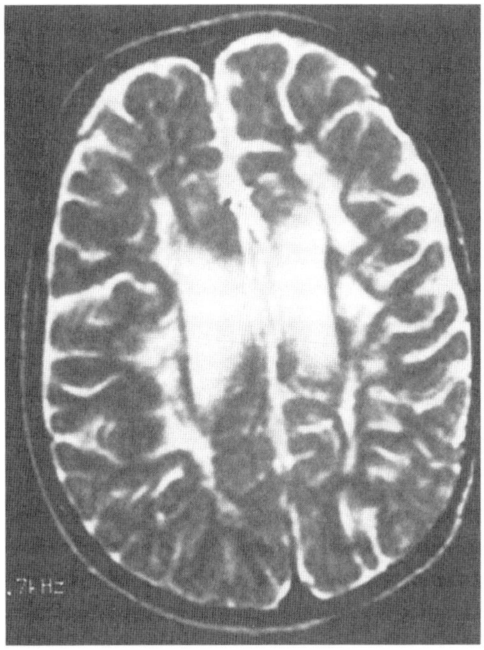

Figure 15.12 Noncontrast computed tomography scan of the brain showing diffuse brain atrophy with white matter calcifications in the pons and the frontal white matter in a 23-month-old girl with MELAS and cytochrome oxidase deficiency.

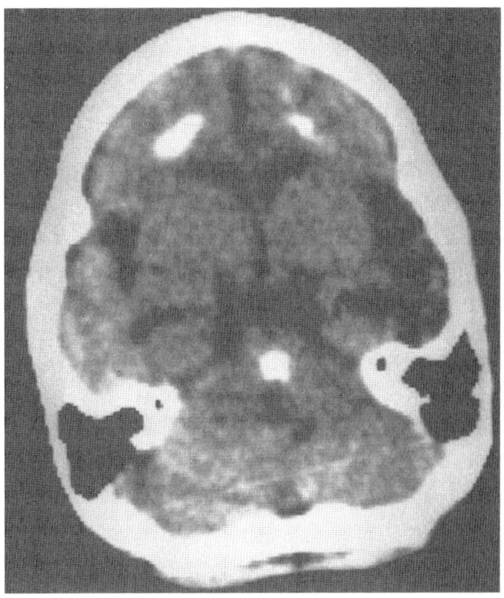

Figure 15.13 Magnetic resonance image of the brain (SE 3000/80) showing bilateral, asymmetric, irregular areas of high signal involving both gray and white matter in an 18-year-old woman with MELAS.

Key Clinical Questions

- *Does anyone on your mother side of the family have a history of hemiplegic migraine, cerebral palsy, epilepsy, weakness, hearing loss, or diabetes?*

Table 15.50 Mitochondrial encephalomyopathy, lactic acidosis, and stroke-like episodes

Discriminating features
- Migraines or convulsions associated with stroke-like episodes of transient hemiparesis or hemianopsia
- Point mutation of mitochondrial DNA (or mitochondrial DNA deletion in patients combining MELAS and Kearns-Sayre syndrome phenotype)

Consistent features
- Maternal inheritance

Variable features
- Lactic acidosis
- Cortical blindness
- Short stature
- Hearing loss
- Gastrointestinal symptoms
- Dementia
- Muscular atrophy and weakness/proximal
- Hypertrophic or dilated cardiomyopathy
- Renal dysfunction
- Endocrine dysfunction
- Ophthalmoplegic findings
- Dystonia, late myoclonus
- Ragged red fibers

(Fujii et al. 1990). Proton MR spectroscopy shows high lactate levels in the affected areas of the brain (Barkovich et al. 1993).

Muscle biopsy is particularly useful in reaching morphologic, biochemical, and genetic diagnosis of MELAS syndrome. Ragged red fibers are observed in some patients. Ultrastructural studies may reveal aggregates of mitochondria, which may contain paracrystalline bodies. Muscle biopsy should be performed in individuals showing MELAS phenotype and negative blood testing for point mutation analysis (Table 15.50). Treatment of MELAS syndrome is palliative and symptomatic.

Myoclonic epilepsy and ragged red fiber

Myoclonic epilepsy and ragged red fiber (MERRF) disease is a maternally inherited disease characterized by progressive myoclonic epilepsy, mitochondrial myopathy with ragged red fibers, and slowly progressive dementia (Fukuhara et al. 1991; Rosing et al. 1985). Elevations of lactate and pyruvate in the blood and CSF suggest an oxidative phosphorylation defect. Biochemical analysis has revealed deficient activity of complex I and IV in most pedigrees (Bindoff et al. 1991; Wallace et al. 1988). Maternal inheritance is suggested by the detection of mitochondrial DNA point mutations encoding for mitochondrial tRNA.

Pearls and Perils

- Approximately 80–90% of myoclonic epilepsy and ragged red fiber (MERRF) patients have a point mutation in the gene encoding for the $tRNA^{Lysine}$ gene, either at the base pair 8344 or at base pair 8356.
- Ragged red muscle fibers are not invariably found in MERRF disease.
- MERRF point mutations are maternally inherited. Maternal relatives of MERRF patients may be normal or have a mild, partial clinical syndrome.
- MERRF syndrome causes progressive myoclonus epilepsy. Other conditions causing progressive myoclonus epilepsy include Lafora disease, neuronal ceroid-lipofuscinoses, Gaucher disease, Unverricht-Lundborg syndrome, Huntington disease, and cherry-red spot myoclonus syndrome.

The onset of symptoms ranges from late childhood to adulthood. Typically MERFF patients have normal early development, although the most severely affected individuals have pes cavus at birth and deafness in childhood. The cardinal triad of symptoms is myoclonus, spinocerebellar ataxia, and convulsions. The onset of this triad is between 5 and 42 years of age. Myoclonus involves the neck, trunk, and proximal portions of limbs, and is not associated with loss of consciousness. These involuntary movements are triggered by attempted postures and actions, emotional reactions, or photic and auditory stimulation. They disappear at rest and during sleep. Spinocerebellar ataxia leads to dysarthria, intention tremor, and gait ataxia. Myoclonic epilepsy and other forms of seizures are frequent. Various other findings less commonly seen in this syndrome include muscle weakness associated with easy fatigability and muscle wasting (Lance & Evans 1984), dementia (Rosing et al. 1985), hearing loss (Lance & Evans 1984), accumulation of lipomas (Holme et al. 1993), short stature, sleep apnea with respiratory failure (Byrne et al. 1985), and stroke-like episodes (McKelvie et al. 1991). Typically patients with MERRF syndrome do not have ophthalmoplegia, retinal pigmentary degeneration, or heart block. However, optic

Key Clinical Questions

- *Is there any sign of deafness?*
  Deafness is common and should suggest the diagnosis. Other suggestive features include diabetes, short stature, migraine, and fatigue.

neuropathy, ophthalmoparesis with ptosis, retinopathy, and diabetes have been associated with MERFF 8356 mutation (Moraes et al. 1983).

Elevation of lactate and pyruvate levels in the blood and CSF is commonly intermittent. Mitochondrial DNA analysis should evaluate 8344 and 8356 MERRF point mutations in blood. However, replicative segregation of leukocyte and platelets may create false-negative values. The EEG may show generalized spike-wave discharges. Photic stimulation may induce 2- to 5-Hz diffuse spike-wave epileptiform activity of posterior predominance or even a photomyoclonic response. Giant visual evoked potentials are usually demonstrated (Roger et al. 1992). Imaging studies of patients with MERRF are nonspecific. Some patients may present with intracerebral calcification on CT scan (Fukuhara et al. 1983). MRI of the brain almost always demonstrates cerebellar atrophy (Iwanga et al. 1992).

Although patients with MERRF generally have ragged red fibers on muscle biopsy, some individuals with progressive myoclonic epilepsy and ataxia without ragged red fibers show the MERRF mitochondrial DNA point mutation. Muscle biopsy, however, is useful in demonstrating mitochondrial oxidative phosphorylation defects and allowing a detailed mitochondrial DNA analysis (Table 15.51).Treatment of MERRF is no different from that of other mitochondrial encephalomyopathies.

Table 15.51 Myoclonic epilepsy and ragged red fiber (MERRF)

Discriminating features
- Myoclonus
- Ragged red fibers
- Mitochondrial myopathy with defects of mitochondrial oxidative metabolism and point mutation of mitochondrial DNA

Consistent features
- Epilepsy, generalized
- Cerebellar ataxia
- Maternal inheritance

Variable features
- Short stature
- Dementia
- Hearing loss
- Peripheral neuropathy
- Pes cavus
- Optic atrophy
- Retinitis pigmentosa
- Ophthalmoplegia
- Diabetes
- Stroke-like episodes
- Lipoma
- Cardiomyopathy with Wolf-Parkinson-White syndrome

Kearns-Sayre syndrome and chronic progressive external ophthalmoplegia

Kearns-Sayre syndrome (KSS) and CPEO are sporadic, autosomal dominant, or maternally inherited neurodegenerative disorders. Kearns-Sayre syndrome is characterized by onset before 20 years of age of ophthalmoplegia (paralysis of eye muscles), ptosis (droopy eyelids), atypical retinitis pigmentosa, mitochondrial myopathy, and one of the following: cardiac conduction defect, cerebellar syndrome, or a CSF protein elevated above 100 mg/dL (Rowland 1983). Individuals whose symptoms are less severe and present in childhood or adolescence with extraocular muscle weakness with ptosis are classified as having CPEO. CPEO is often accompanied by limb weakness, dysphagia, or dysarthria (mitochondrial myopathy). Patients with an intermediate disorder, less severe than KSS and more severe than CPEO, are referred to as having CPEO Plus. CPEO Plus patients have complex and variable clinical manifestations. Kearns-Sayre syndrome and CPEO Plus may overlap with other mitochondrial encephalopathies because CPEO has been seen in patients with otherwise typical

Pearls and Perils

- Chronic progressive external ophthalmoplegia (CPEO) can be associated with mitochondrial encephalomyopathy, lactic acidosis, and stroke-like episodes syndrome (MELAS), myoclonic epilepsy and ragged red fiber (MERRF), and, mitochondrial myopathy, peripheral neuropathy, gastrointestinal, and encephalopathy disease (MNGIE).
- Edrophonium testing should not be performed in Kearns-Sayre syndrome (KSS) due to the risk of arrhythmia. Patients presenting with external ophthalmoplegia frequently undergo edrophonium chloride testing to rule out myasthenia gravis. Ptosis in CPEO does not respond to edrophonium testing.
- Blood for mitochondrial deletions is frequently negative in KSS. Muscle is the tissue of choice for the evaluation of the mitochondrial genome. If no mitochondrial DNA rearrangement/deletion is found, mitochondrial DNA point mutations should be considered.
- Kearns-Sayre patients should be followed carefully with serial electrocardiogram and Holter monitoring. At the first indication of a serious conduction defect, a pacemaker should be placed.
- KSS patients typically have a higher proportion of mitochondrial DNA deletion in more tissues than do CPEO patients.

MELAS syndrome (Fang et al. 1993), MERFF (Silvestri et al. 1993), and mitochondrial neurogastrointestinal encephalomyopathy (MNGIE) (Threlkeld et al. 1992). Biochemical analysis of blood and biopsied skeletal muscles suggest deficiencies in oxidative phosphorylation in most patients with CPEO or KSS.

Genetic analysis suggests heterogeneity. KSS, CPEO Plus, and CPEO cases have been associated with various defects of mitochondrial DNA. The great majority of KSS and CPEO cases are due to spontaneous mitochondrial DNA rearrangements (combinations of duplications and deletions), which are not inherited. Despite extensive heterogeneity in deletion size and breakpoint positions, the two origins of the mtDNA replication are spared, thus defining two areas in which mitochondrial deletions occur. Over 90% of the deletions occur in the large arc and can remove 9–50% of mitochondrial genome. One-third of all KSS/CPEO patients harbor the same deletion. Approximately 6% of CPEO cases have multiple mitochondrial DNA deletions in all tissues and show most often an autosomal dominant inheritance pattern. Although, an autosomal recessive inheritance can also be seen. At least three genes are known to cause the autosomal dominant CPEO: adenine nucleotide translocator 1 (Ant1, chromosome 4), DNA polymerase (POLG, chromosome 15) and Twinkle (C10orf2, chromosome 10) (Lewis et al. 2002). Those KSS or CPEO patients who have no mitochondrial DNA deletion are likely to have a mitochondrial DNA point mutation. Maternal inheritance of CPEO is suggested by discovery of a mitochondrial DNA point mutation in variable amounts in various tissues of some patients. Patients with one or more mitochondrial DNA point mutation present with combined features of Kearns-Sayre disease or CPEO with features of MELAS (Fang et al. 1993) and MERRF syndromes (Silvestri et al. 1993). All the mutations seen in patients with CPEO or KSS alter or remove one or more mitochondrial tRNA genes. The result is a defect in the synthesis of proteins necessary for oxidative phosphorylation.

The presenting manifestations of KSS are frequently the same as diseases such as Pearson syndrome (a disorder presenting in infancy with a unique combination of bone marrow and pancreatic exocrine dysfunction) (Bernes et al. 1993), renal tubular acidosis (Mori et al. 1991), and Lowe syndrome (congenital cataract, hypotonia, mental retardation, and progressive renal tubular dysfunction) (Moraes et al. 1991). Before 20 years of age, most patients develop a combination of ophthalmoplegia, ptosis, retinal degeneration, and heart block or cerebellar ataxia. The KSS may also include signs and symptoms of myopathy, hearing loss, pyramidal and extrapyramidal dysfunction, seizures, and dementia. Kearns-Sayre syndrome has also been associated with a variety of endocrine and metabolic disorders, in particular short stature, gonadal failure, hypothyroidism, hypoparathyroidism, and hyperaldosteronism (Harvey & Barnett 1992). Patients with KSS may deteriorate rapidly and die from heart block or brainstem dysfunction.

The clinical features of sporadic chronic progressive external ophthalmoplegia are restricted to eye and proximal muscles without other organ involvement. Rarely, weakness becomes severe. CPEO Plus may combine features of MELAS, MERRF, MNGIE, and KSS. Patients with autosomal CPEO may present during the second decade with symptoms other than ptosis and ophthalmoplegia. Those symptoms vary greatly between and within families and may include dysarthria, depression, mental retardation, sensory ataxic neuropathy, deafness, exercise intolerance, muscle pain, gastrointestinal dysmotility, cardiac conduction defects, and hypogonadism. Four patterns of retinal degeneration are encountered in KSS and CPEO Plus: (a) generalized, (b) "salt and pepper," (c) "bone spicule," and (d) complete atrophy of choroid and sclera (Herzberg et al. 1993).

Elevated blood lactate and pyruvate are frequently found at rest or after exercise in patients with CPEO or KSS. Renal tubular dysfunction can be suggested by hypermagnesemia, hypophosphatemia, hypocalcemia, hypokalemia, glycosuria, and aminoaciduria. Endocrine abnormalities are suggested by impaired glucose tolerance, insufficient rise of growth hormone following administration of growth hormone-releasing hormone, insufficient rise of follicular-stimulating hormone (FSH) after administration of gonadotrophin-releasing hormone, and/or abnormal parathyroid and thyroid hormone. Electrocardiogram assesses severity of conduction disturbances. The CSF frequently reveals elevated protein (>100 mg/dL) in KSS. Blood studies for mitochondrial DNA deletions or point mutation may be negative.

Kearns-Sayre syndrome is associated on CT scans with cortical and white matter atrophy, hypodensity of the cerebral and cerebellar white matter, and variable hypodensity or calcification of the basal ganglia (Kendall 1992). MRI scans show T2 prolongation in the deep gray matter nuclei, particularly the thalamus and globus pallidus, and patchy white matter involvement (Demange et al. 1989). Proton MR spectroscopic evaluation shows large increases in lactate/creatinine and large decreases in N-acetylaspartate/creatinine in central brain regions (Matthews et al. 1993).

Muscle biopsy is particularly useful in establishing diagnosis of KSS or CPEO, demonstrating ragged red fibers on Gomori-trichrome stain and dissociation in en-

Key Clinical Questions

- *Is the ophthalmoplegia associated with retinal degeneration?* In that case one should suspect Kearns-Sayre syndrome.

Table 15.52 Kearns-Sayre syndrome

Discriminating features
- Ophthalmoplegia, progressive
- Ptosis
- Pigmentary retinal degeneration
- Mitochondrial DNA deletions, duplication, or partial mutation

Consistent features
- Proximal muscle weakness
- Onset before age 20 years
- Lactic acidosis
- Ragged-red fibers

Variable features
- Elevated cerebrospinal fluid protein
- Cerebellar ataxia
- Cardiac conduction defect
- Short stature
- Sensorineural deafness
- Neuropathy
- Mental retardation
- Endocrinopathy
- Renal tubulopathy
- Corneal clouding
- Pyramidal/extrapyramidal symptoms
- Dysphagia
- Sporadic, dominant, recessive, or maternally inherited
- Pearson syndrome

zyme activity on oxidative stains (e.g., low cytochrome oxidase stain, strong succinic dehydrogenase stain) of the same fibers. Electron microscopy not only confirms the presence of supranumary mitochondria, but also demonstrates that some are enlarged, and the cristae of their inner membranes disordered or simplified, with paracrystalline "parking lot" inclusions in their matrix. Biochemical analysis demonstrates partial impairments in a variety of biochemical reactions, all of them related to oxidative phosphorylation metabolism.

Mitochondrial DNA analysis allows detection of mitochondrial deletions or deletions/duplications by Southern blotting. Mitochondrial DNA point mutation analysis should be considered if the Southern blot analysis is normal. In patients with autosomal inheritance and mitochondrial DNA deletions, the ANT1, POLG, and Twinkle genes should be sequenced. Patients without mitochondrial DNA deletion or rearrangement should be evaluated for heteroplasmic mitochondrial DNA point mutation in the following tRNA genes: $tRNA^{Lys}$ (MERRF 8344), $tRNA^{Leu\,(UUR)}$ (MELAS 3243), $tRNA^{Leucine(CUN)}$ (CPEO 12308, 12311 and 12315), $tRNA^{Tyrosine}$ (CPEO 5877), $tRNA^{Cysteine}$ (CPEO 5814), $tRNA^{Asparagine}$ (CPEO 5692 and 5703), and $tRNA^{Isoleucine}$ (CPEO 4285 and 4298) (Tables 15.52 and 15.53).

Table 15.53 Chronic progressive external ophthalmoplegia

Discriminating features
- Progressive external ophthalmoplegia
- Ptosis
- Mitochondrial deletions and point mutations

Consistent features
- Ragged-red fibers

Variable features
- Myopathy
- Mitochondrial encephalomyopathy, lactic acidosis, and stroke-like episodes (MELAS) syndrome,
- Myoclonic epilepsy and ragged red fiber (MERRF)
- Mitochondrial myopathy, peripheral neuropathy, gastrointestinal, and encephalopathy disease (MNGIE)
- Features of Kearns-Sayre syndrome (KSS)
- Sporadic, dominant, recessive, or maternally inherited

Mitochondrial neurogastrointestinal encephalomyopathy

Mitochondrial neurogastrointestinal encephalomyopathy (MNGIE) (Hirano 1994) is characterized clinically by progressive ophthalmoparesis, including ptosis, mitochondrial myopathy, peripheral neuropathy, gastrointestinal dysmotility, and progressive encephalopathy. The disorder is frequently associated with multiple mitochondrial DNA deletions and has similarities to CPEO and Kearns-Sayre syndrome. The condition is most frequently autosomal recessive (Nishino et al. 1999; Van Goethem et al. 2003) but can be sporadic (Maniura-Weber et al. 2004) (Tables 15.46 and 15.47).

Age of onset ranges between 2 and 30 years of age. The initial symptoms are gastrointestinal or ocular. Diarrhea, malabsorption, nausea, vomiting, and weight loss with normal pancreatic function are the most frequent gastrointestinal symptoms. The most common ocular feature is progressive external ophthalmoparesis, including

Key Clinical Questions

- *Is the ophthalmoplegia associated with gastrointestinal symptoms?*
  In that case one should suspect mitochondrial myopathy, peripheral neuropathy, gastrointestinal, and encephalopathy disease (MNGIE) instead of chronic progressive external ophthalmoplegia (CPEO) or Kearns-Sayre syndrome (KSS).

Pearls and Perils

- Both Kearns-Sayre syndrome and mitochondrial myopathy, peripheral neuropathy, gastrointestinal, and encephalopathy disease (MNGIE) present with external ophthalmoplegia and are associated with multiple mitochondrial DNA deletions. MNGIE can readily be identified by assay of plasma levels of thymidine.
- Some patients with mitochondrial point mutation in mitochondrial tRNA glycine (CIP 10006) and tRNA serine (CIP 12258) genes present clinically with a chronic intestinal pseudo-obstruction associated with a chronic progressive external ophthalmoparesis mimicking MNGIE syndrome.
- Chronic progressive external ophthalmoplegia (CPEO) and gastrointestinal dysmotility can also be seen in some patients with multiple mitochondrial DNA deletions (e.g., mutation in POLG gene).

ptosis. Limb weakness is frequently associated with areflexia. Most patients have a thin body habitus. Voice may be nasal. Short stature and hearing loss are less common findings. Mental functions are usually preserved in early stages of the illness. Visual acuity may be decreased. Seizures may occur in sporadic cases. Survival into adulthood is common.

MRI of the brain may show signs of leukoencephalopathy. Nerve conduction studies and EMG studies are consistent with a diffuse sensorimotor neuropathy. Gastrointestinal tract studies show delayed gastric emptying, decreased duodenal motility, and, in some patients, gastrointestinal pseudo-obstruction. Electrocardiogram reveals heart block in a third of the patients. Lactic acidosis suggests a mitochondrial impairment in 60% of patients. The CSF protein can be elevated. Plasma thymidine level is increased more than 20-fold in MNGIE patients with thymidine phosphorylase gene mutations (Nishino et al. 1999). Muscle biopsy shows, in most cases, multiple mitochondrial DNA deletions. In sporadic cases, heteroplasmic mitochondrial point mutations are found (Maniura-Weber et al. 2004) (Table 15.54).

Table 15.54 Mitochondrial neurogastrointestinal encephalomyopathy

Discriminating features
- Progressive external ophthalmoplegia and ptosis
- Gastrointestinal symptoms with abdominal distension and weight loss
- Mutations in thymidine phosphorylase (TP) or POLG1 gene
- Multiple mitochondrial DNA deletions or tRNA point mutations

Consistent features
- Sensorimotor neuropathy (90%)
- Normal cognition
- Ragged red fibers

Variable features
- Hearing loss
- Short stature
- Hypo/hyperreflexia
- Ataxia
- Limb weakness and atrophy
- Retinopathy
- Heart block
- Elevated cerebrospinal fluid protein
- Lactic acidosis
- Leukoencephalopathy if TP mutation
- Elevated thymidine plasma levels if TP mutation

Leber hereditary optic neuropathy

Leber hereditary optic neuropathy (LHON) is a maternally inherited form of central visual loss due to apoptotic death of retinal ganglion cells and optic nerve degeneration. Leber hereditary optic neuropathy affects predominantly men (80% of cases) and occurs acutely or subacutely in adolescence or early adulthood (Newman et al. 1991). Although LHON is predominantly an ocular disease, patients can have a detectable deficiency of NADH dehydrogenase (complex I) in muscle (Larsson et al. 1991). Maternal inheritance is suggested by detection of mitochondrial DNA point mutations in affected patients and asymptomatic relatives. More than 90% of LHON families have a heteroplasmic mitochondrial DNA point mutation in four genes encoding subunits of the NADH dehydrogenase (complex I): LHON 3460 (ND1 subunit), LHON 11778 (ND4 subunit), and LHON 14484 and 14459 (ND6 subunit). All the pathogenic mutations, including all the rare mutations seen in other maternal pedigrees, encode subunits of respiratory chain complex I.

Clinically, the onset of visual loss is in the second or third decade. The vision loss begins in the central visual field with loss of color vision. Both eyes are usually affected within weeks to months. Tobacco and alcohol may

Key Clinical Questions

- *Does the patient have a bilateral, painless, progressive central visual loss?*
  Funduscopic exam shows nonedematous disk elevation and peripapillary telangiectasia. The diagnosis is unlikely if eye movements are painful or papilledema is present.

Pearls and Perils

- Maternal relatives of Leber hereditary optic neuropathy (LHON) patients may present in infancy or childhood with bilateral putaminal necrosis and severe dystonia, corticospinal tract dysfunction, and extrapyramidal rigidity. Diagnosis of neurodegeneration with brain iron accumulation (NBIA) or Leigh syndrome is sometimes made.
- Posterior column dysfunction and peripheral neuropathy are not uncommon in some patients with LHON presenting with ataxia, tremor, amyotrophy, and sensory loss.
- Blood for mitochondrial point mutation is all you need for LHON diagnosis. Muscle biopsy is not necessary.
- A multiple sclerosis-like illness is sometimes seen in LHON.

Table 15.55 Leber hereditary optic neuropathy

Discriminating features
- Visual impairment
- Optic nerve hyperemia acutely followed by optic nerve pallor

Consistent features
- Male preponderance
- Peripapillary telangiectasia
- mtDNA point mutations

Variable features
- Ataxia (spinocerebellar)
- Dystonia
- Amyotrophy
- Peripheral neuropathy
- Multiple sclerosis
- Dementia (rare)
- Spastic paraparesis
- Autonomic disturbances
- Pseudobulbar syndrome
- Cardiac dysrhythmia
- Short stature
- Hearing loss

precipitate visual loss. Recovery of vision has been reported in some patients after many months or years. Asymptomatic individuals and acutely affected patients frequently have peripapillary telangiectasia (Nikoskelainen et al. 1983). Optic atrophy is a late sequela in patients who fail to recover vision.

In some patients, there is evidence of neurologic involvement. Neurologic symptoms may be the only manifestation in some individuals of a LHON kindred or may precede visual decline. Some individuals may present with pediatric-onset dystonia associated with bilateral striatal necrosis mimicking neurodegeneration with brain iron accumulation (Larsson et al. 1991) or Leigh syndrome (Jun et al. 1994). Patients present with gait disturbance, pseudobulbar signs, and impaired intelligence. Other individuals develop a spinocerebellar syndrome with prominent ataxia, hypotonia, and weakness (Wilson 1963). A multiple sclerosis–like illness has been reported in other patients (Keller-Wood et al. 1994).

Autonomic nervous system involvement may manifest by vasomotor lability, excessive perspiration, and constipation (Wilson 1963). A pseudobulbar syndrome with poor voluntary tongue movements, and incoordination of swallowing may be observed in terminal stages of the illness. Intellectual impairment and sensorineural hearing impairment occur. Evidence that the disorder is a multisystem disease includes the findings of short stature, variable myopathic features, and cardiomyopathy (Rose et al. 1970). Several mitochondrial DNA point mutations have been shown to be associated with LHON.

Serum lactate and pyruvate are usually normal. Neurophysiologic studies are useful in confirming neurologic phenotype in LHON Plus patients. CT scan of the head may reveal low density in the putamina. T1-weighted MR scan may show low intensity in the pallidonigral system. The EKG may show in some families a pre-excitation syndrome with prolonged QT interval.

In affected individuals, analysis of mitochondrial DNA should be performed on blood looking for LHON 11778, LHON 14484, and LHON 3460 in pedigrees without neurologic symptoms and LHON 11696, LHON 14596, and LHON 14459 in pedigrees with pediatric-onset dystonia associated with bilateral strial necrosis. If analysis on blood sample is negative, muscle biopsy for oxidative phosphorylation studies and mitochondrial DNA point mutation analysis should be obtained (Table 15.55). Treatment of LHON is symptomatic and palliative. A new therapeutic approach, such as the lowering of blood thymidine concentration, is suggested by the knowledge of the basic metabolic defect.

Lethal infantile mitochondrial DNA depletion hepatocerebral syndrome

Lethal infantile mitochondrial DNA depletion hepatocerebral syndrome (LIMDHCS) is an autosomal recessive neurodegenerative disease characterized by onset in infancy of a myopathy associated with multisystem involvement and progressive mental deterioration. Affected tissues in all patients show respiratory chain defects involving cytochrome oxidase (complex IV) alone or in connection with NADH dehydrogenase (complex I) or succinate cytochrome c reductase (complex III) or both. LIMDHCS is caused in most cases by tissue-specific depletions of the mitochondrial DNA (Figarella-Branger et

Pearls and Perils

- Lethal infantile hepatocerebral mitochondrial DNA depletion syndrome should be differentiated from benign reversible muscle cytochrome c oxidase deficiency. A mitochondrial DNA depletion and multisystem involvement are characteristic of lethal infantile mitochondrial disease.
- A mitochondrial DNA (mtDNA) depletion can be seen as a secondary phenomenon in succinyl-CoA synthetase deficiency (*SUCLA2* mutation) and inherited disorders of propionate metabolism. An encephalomyopathy mimicking Leigh syndrome is typically associated with methylmalonic aciduria in such patients.
- Alpers syndrome due to nuclear C10ORF2, RRM2B, or POLG1 gene mutations is characterized by an encephalomyopathy with seizures associated with a mitochondrial DNA depletion.

Table 15.56 Lethal infantile mitochondrial DNA depletion hepatocerebral syndrome

Discriminating features
- Early progressive liver failure due to micronodular cirrhosis
- Depletion of the mtDNA in liver and muscle
- Mutations in the deoxyguanosine kinase, C10ORF2, POLG1, or MPV17 genes

Consistent features
- Cytochrome oxidase deficiency and other variable defects of respiratory chain
- Muscles with proliferation of enlarged mitochondria
- Hypotonia and weakness
- Respiratory failure
- Lactic acidosis

Variable features
- Renal dysfunction
- Liver dysfunction
- Cardiac dysfunction
- Progressive encephalopathy

al. 1992). This disorder is caused by mutations in the nuclear-encoded mitochondrial deoxyguanosine kinase (DGUOK) gene (Tadiboyina et al., 2005), MPV17 gene (Spinazzola et al. 2006), POLG1 (Kollberg et al. 2006), or C10ORF2 (Sarzi et al. 2007).

LIMDHCS patients appear clinically normal at birth. The mean age of onset of symptoms is 3 weeks. The infants present with feeding difficulties, failure to thrive, profound weakness, and severe hypotonia. Respiratory failure soon occurs. Extraocular muscles are spared. The clinical picture deteriorates progressively. Most children become lethargic and present with myoclonic seizures. Death occurs during infancy from cardiac arrest.

Lactic acidosis is usually severe. Hepatic dysfunction may be prominent (Figarella-Branger et al. 1992). Renal dysfunction with proximal tubule abnormalities is suggested by a generalized amino aciduria or the de Toni-Debré-Fanconi syndrome (Zeviani et al. 1985). Central nervous system involvement is suggested by elevated CSF protein levels (Heiman-Patterson et al. 1982), abnormal EEG with diffuse slow waves (Zeviani et al. 1985) and paroxysmal discharges (Tritschler et al. 1992), and abnormal neuroimaging studies with delayed myelination (Tritschler et al. 1992). A dilated or hypertrophic cardiomyopathy is found late in the course of the illness (Figarella-Branger et al. 1992).

Key Clinical Questions

- *How long does it take for your baby to empty his bottle and does your infant act as if out of breath while eating?*
  In a floppy infant, episodic tachypnea associated with feeding difficulties should suggest the diagnosis.

Muscle biopsy shows abundant ragged red fibers with markedly decreased cytochrome oxidase activity by histochemistry. Ultrastructural studies show a massive mitochondrial proliferation with lipid and glycogen accumulation. Mitochondria are enormous and abnormally shaped but no paracrystalline inclusions are seen. The presence of DNA depletion has been documented by quantitative Southern blot hybridization analysis, by in situ hybridization of affected muscle sections with mtDNA probes, and by immunohistochemistry of affected muscle sections using anti-DNA antibodies. Knowledge of the mutation responsible for LIMDHCS makes the prenatal diagnosis feasible (Table 15.56). No treatment has improved outcome.

Encephalomyopathy with coenzyme Q 10 deficiency

Encephalomyopathy with CoQ_{10} deficiency is a group of autosomal recessive disorders characterized by encephalomyopathy and coenzyme Q10 deficiency. Measurement of respiratory-chain enzyme activity in muscle and fibroblasts shows decreased activities of complex I+II and II+III that are repaired by decylubiquinone supplementation. Muscle biopsy may show ragged red fibers with prominent lipid accumulation in patients with primary CoQ_{10} deficiency. Muscle CoQ_{10} level is typically severely (>50%) decreased. Mutations in genes regulating CoQ_{10} synthesis are responsible for most cases of these treatable encephalomyopathies (Table 15.48). Sec-

Key Clinical Questions

- *Are neurologic symptoms improved by coenzyme Q10 therapy?*

ondary CoQ_{10} deficiency has been reported in patients with autosomal recessive progressive ataxia with cerebellar atrophy due to apraxatin deficiency (Quinzii et al. 2005). Primary CoQ_{10} deficiency has at least three clinical presentations depending on the severity of systemic and neurologic symptoms and age of onset.

An early infantile-onset encephalomyopathy (Lopez et al. 2006; Mollet et al. 2008; Rötig et al. 2000) is characterized in neonates by hypotonia, nystagmus, and optic atrophy followed by early onset of intractable seizures. Later, in some patients, dystonia, ataxia, and dysphagia may suggest diagnosis of Leigh syndrome. A diagnosis of MELAS is suggested by recurrent stroke-like episodes followed by developmental regression. A rapidly progressive nephrotic syndrome is seen in most infants.

A childhood-onset encephalomyopathy (Ogasahara et al. 1989; Quinzii et al. 2006) is characterized by normal early development and slowly progressive cerebellar ataxia with acquired cerebellar atrophy. In some families, mental regression, Hoffman sign, and pyramidal signs are commonly seen (Lagier-Tourenne 2008). In other families, seizures dominate the clinical picture. Exercise intolerance and slowly progressive myopathy involving axial and proximal limb muscles are occasionally reported. Episodes of recurrent rhabdomyolysis can follow seizures or infections. Axonal neuropathy is occasionally reported. Renal dysfunction does not occur.

A milder phenotype (Mollet et al. 2007) is characterized by normal early development followed by early deafness, optic atrophy, and mild mental retardation. Boulimia is associated with overgrowth syndrome with macrocephaly. Areflexia suggests a peripheral neuropathy. Obesity, livedo reticularis, and valvulopathy are additional features (Table 15.57).

Pearls and Perils

- Cerebellar ataxia with variable central nervous system involvement (seizures, mental deterioration, and/or spasticity) can improve with coenzyme Q 10 (CoQ_{10}) supplementation even if it is a secondary phenomenon. In such cases, muscle biopsy shows very low CoQ_{10} levels, but neither ragged red fibers nor lipid storage are seen. Such cases may result from defects such as Apraxatin gene mutations.
- Nephrotic syndrome in an infant with Leigh syndrome suggests diagnosis of primary CoQ_{10} deficiency.
- Exercise intolerance may be an isolated feature in primary CoQ_{10} deficiency.

Table 15.57 Encephalomyopathy with coenzyme Q10 deficiency

Discriminating features
- Clinical response to CoQ_{10}
- Coenzyme Q10 deficiency in muscle
- Mutations in the COQ2, PDSS1, PDSS2, CABC1 genes

Consistent features
- Progressive ataxia with cerebellar atrophy
- Lipid droplets in muscles
- CII +CIII deficiency repaired by decylubiquinone
- Ragged-red fibers

Variable features
- Nephrotic syndrome
- Deafness
- Spasticity, hypotonia
- Mental retardation
- Intractable epilepsy, myoclonus
- Optic atrophy, nystagmus
- Areflexia/ hyperreflexia
- Hypogonadism, obesity
- Lactic acidosis
- Exercise intolerance

Mildly elevated plasma lactate and lactate-to-pyruvate ratios are frequently observed. Pathologic elevations of plasma lactate levels with standardized exercise are reported in some patients. Elevated creatine phosphokinase (CPK) and myoglobulinuria are occasionally seen after exercise or during infection. Proteinuria is a feature of most severely affected patients. Brain imaging may show cerebellar atrophy, diffuse cerebral atrophy, stroke-like lesions, and/or putaminal necrosis.

Treatment with oral ubidecarenone (5 mg/kg/day) results in a substantial clinical improvement, in most cases.

Lafora disease

Lafora disease is an autosomal recessive disorder of the cytoplasmic protein degradation (ubiquitine-proteasome system) leading to an impaired degradation of glycogen and characterized by the presence of cytoplasmic polyglucosan inclusions known as Lafora bodies in most tissues, including the brain. Lafora disease is caused by mutations in *EPM2A* encoding laforin, a dual-specificity phosphatase, or in *EPM2B* encoding malin, an ubiquitin ligase (Shuchi et al. 2007). Both genes are encoded on chromosome 6. Other yet unidentified gene loci are likely.

Key Clinical Questions

- *Did you notice a rapid cognitive decline and erratic fragmentary myoclonic jerks since the onset of the epilepsy?*

There are two forms of Lafora disease. The classic juvenile form, first described by Unverricht in 1891, begins between 6 and 19 years of age (mean, 11 years). The first manifestations are decreased scholastic performance, behavior disorders, or seizures (Van Heycop Ten Ham 1974). Generalized seizures are initially nocturnal. Partial simple seizures with visual manifestations may constitute the aura of generalized seizures (Rapin 1986). Absence and drop attacks may also occur. Myoclonic jerks appear insidiously during the following months, characteristically arrhythmic, asymmetrical, segmental, or fragmentary, and variable in intensity, becoming almost constant. The face is frequently involved. Myoclonic jerks are spontaneous or stimulus sensitive but are not induced by movements. Oscillatory eye movements contribute to visual deterioration. Swallowing and speech difficulties become severe. In the limbs, flexor muscles are more affected. Within 1 or 2 years of the onset of seizures, dementia develops. Pyramidal, cerebellar, and extrapyramidal manifestation (parkinsonian rigidity, choreoathetosis) appear after a variable delay. Death occurs within 2–10 years as a result of heart failure, liver failure, or aspiration pneumonia.

The more protracted adult, or Lundborg variety, begins between the ages of 17 and 20 years. Grand mal seizures are the first manifestation. Myoclonic jerks and dementia are slowly progressive, and death usually occurs after the age of 40 years.

Early in Lafora disease, the EEG has spike-wave activity superimposed on slow background. Generalized myoclonic seizures may be induced by photic stimulation. With progression, all patients develop fast-frequency polyspike waves. In the terminal phase, the EEG is totally disorganized. No enzymatic defect has been identified so far.

Pearls and Perils

- Lafora disease, a progressive myoclonus epilepsy associated with mental decline, ataxia, and occasional visual impairment, should be differentiated from other progressive degenerative disorders with myoclonic epilepsies.
- Diagnosis is readily established by axillary skin biopsy: presence of cytoplasmic periodic acid-positive inclusions, Lafora bodies, in apocrine or eccrine sweat glands. The lack of mutations in *EPM2A* or *EPM2B* does not exclude the diagnosis.

Table 15.58 Lafora disease

Discriminating features
- Lafora bodies in cytoplasm of neurons and sweat gland duct cells
- Mutations of *EPM2A* or *EPM2B*

Consistent features
- Polymyoclonia
- Generalized epilepsy
- No or minimal action myoclonus
- Photomyoclonic or photoconvulsive response to photic stimulation on electroencephalogram
- Cognitive deterioration
- Onset between 10 and 20 years

Variable features
- Dementia
- Ataxia, dysarthria
- Choreoathetosis, rigidity, spastic quadriplegia
- Focal seizures arising from occipital regions

The ketogenic diet is being investigated in clinical trials. This low-carbohydrate diet has the promise of reducing intracellular polyglucosan buildup. Active-site chaperone therapy is under investigation in the animal model (Table 15.58).

Cerebrotendinous xanthomatosis

Cerebrotendinous xanthomatosis (CTX) is an autosomal recessive disorder of mitochondrial bile acid biosynthesis leading to diffuse tendinous xanthomatosis, juvenile cataracts, and multiple progressive neurological manifestations. Other possible manifestations include recurrent bone fractures, pes cavus, and arteriosclerosis (Beringer et al. 1993). The disorder is caused by an almost complete lack of activity of the mitochondrial cytochrome P-450 sterol 27-hydroxylase enzyme, which catalyzes the first steps in bile acid biosynthesis. The gene of sterol 27-hydroxylase has been mapped to chromosome 2 (Beringer et al. 1993) and mutations identified (Kim et al. 1994).

Key Clinical Questions

- *Is there a family history of cataract, dementia, ataxia, or seizures, and does anyone have tendon xanthomas?* Demonstration of a high cholestanol serum level suggests the diagnosis.

Pearls and Perils

- The slowly progressive nature of the disease and the nonuniformity of the clinical manifestation even within each cerebrotendinous xanthomatosis (CTX) family may preclude early clinical diagnosis.
- CTX should be suspected if there is no hypercholesterolemia in the presence of tendon xanthoma.
- CTX, although extremely rare, is a treatable neurodegenerative disorder.

The symptoms may develop during the first and second decades of life and become severe with increasing age, leading to profound disability. The first symptoms occur in early childhood, with developmental delay and chronic diarrhea. Toward the end of the first decade, the diagnosis of CTX should be suspected in patients with unexplained juvenile cataracts and juvenile-onset painless grayish swellings (xanthoma) along the course of Achilles, triceps, or finger extensor tendons with multiple progressive neurologic symptoms that are variable within each CTX family. The latter include behavioral abnormalities, mental deterioration, mild cerebellar ataxia, pyramidal dysfunction, and seizures. Retinitis pigmentosa can occur. With advancing age, spasticity, ataxia, and parkinsonism become more severe, speech becomes more difficult, and signs of peripheral neuropathy with loss of pain and vibratory sensation become noticeable. Death usually results from pseudobulbar paralysis between the fourth and sixth decade.

Laboratory studies show normal serum cholesterol and elevated serum cholestanol levels and altered urine bile acid composition.

MRI of the brain shows, in the T2-weighted images, hyperintense signals in the cerebral and cerebellar white matter associated with the hypointensity of the dentate nuclei. The CSF proteins are elevated. Peripheral nerve conduction velocities are slightly decreased. A definitive

Table 15.59 Cerebrotendinous xanthomatosis

Discriminating features
- Achilles tendon xanthoma and normal serum cholesterol levels
- Lack of sterol 27-hydroxylase activity in skin fibroblasts
- Analysis of genomic DNA

Consistent features
- Elevated cholestanol level
- Abnormal bile acids in urine with increased excretion of C-27 bile alcohol glucuronides

Variable features
- Cataract and retinopathy
- Tendon xanthoma of extensor tendons of fingers, elbow, and patella
- Pes cavus
- Mental retardation
- Dementia
- Ataxia
- Seizures
- Peripheral neuropathy
- Motor paresis

Consider Consultation When ...

- An apparent cerebral palsy is transmitted to multiple family members following a maternal lineage. Pelizaeus-Merzbacher disease and Menkes disease should be suspected if only males are affected. When both sexes are affected mitochondrial encephalopathy is likely.
- An apparent cerebral palsy is associated with intractable seizures and dysmorphic features or cerebral dysgenesis (suggesting a mitochondrial disorder or peroxisomal disorder).
- An infant develops a macrocephaly, startle response to stimuli and ocular symptoms. Etiologic workup and management are demanding.
- A patient develops progressive neurologic signs and symptoms such as psychomotor deterioration, acquired microcephaly, spasticity, seizures, myoclonias, myoclonic epilepsy, complicated migraine, ataxia, movement disorder, ophthalmoplegia, ptosis, dysarthria, stridor, loss of speech, dysphagia, visual impairment, deafness, peripheral neuropathy, muscle weakness, and hypotonia. Such progressive neurologic deterioration may present alone or in association with mental regression, behavior disturbances, stereotyped agitation, personality and mood changes, or psychiatric abnormality. Mental deterioration may precede neurologic decline.
- A patient develops obvious extra-neurologic signs and symptoms before neurologic or mental deterioration occurs. Screening the appropriate neurodegenerative disease may allow early diagnosis and appropriate management. For example, if a school-aged child develops a progressive visual failure, screening for Batten disease is achieved by ordering a detailed retinal examination before ordering ultrastructural studies of the lymphocytes. If a male patient develops Addison disease, he should be screened for adrenoleukodystrophy by ordering very-long-chain fatty acids, and careful neurologic examination may reveal a slight neurologic involvement. If an infant develops chronic diarrhea associated with malabsorption, hypocholesterolemia, and osteopenia, vitamin E levels should be monitored.

diagnosis is obtained from the identification of low cholesterol 27-hydroxylase activity in fibroblast (Skrede et al. 1986). The detection of the specific mutation in each family is important to definitely confirm the diagnosis (Table 15.59).

Treatment with chenodeoxycholic acid (15 mg/kg/day) with 3-hydroxy 3-methyl glutaryl coenzyme A (HMG-CoA) reductase inhibitor such as pravastatin or simvastatin (10–40 mg/day) should normalize blood cholestanol levels without increasing risk for atherosclerosis. When treated early, when neurologic disability is mild, a number of patients show reversal of their neurologic symptoms. If treatment is delayed until the appearance of severe neurologic deficits, the deficits are irreversible (Peynet et al. 1991).

Annotated bibliography

Neuronal ceroid-lipofuscinoses

Dyken P. Neuronal ceroid-lipofuscinoses. In: Swaiman K, Wright F, eds. *The practice of pediatric neurology*. St. Louis: Mosby; 1982: 902–914.
An excellent description of the neuronal ceroid-lipofuscinoses.

Gaucher disease

Beutler E, Grabowski GA. Gaucher disease. In: Scriver CR et al., eds. *The metabolic and molecular basis of inherited disease*. New York: McGraw-Hill; 1995:2641–2670.
An updated and comprehensive review of Gaucher disease.

GM_2 gangliosidoses

Gravel RA, et al. The GM_2 gangliosidoses. In: Scriver CR et al., eds. *The metabolic and molecular basis of inherited disease*. New York: McGraw-Hill; 1995:2839–2879.
An excellent and updated review of GM_2 gangliosidoses.

Menkes disease

Menkes JH. Kinky hair disease: Twenty-five years later. *Brain Dev* 1988;10:77–79.
An excellent review of key features of Menkes syndrome.

Niemann-Pick disease

Pentchev PG, et al. Niemann-Pick disease type C: A cellular cholesterol lipidosis. In: Scriver CR et al., eds. *The metabolic and molecular basis of inherited disease*. New York: McGraw-Hill; 1995:2625–2639.
An excellent updated review of type in Niemann-Pick disease.

Schuchman EH, Desnick RJ. Niemann-Pick disease types A and B: Acid sphingomyelinase deficiency. In: Scriver CR et al., eds. *The metabolic and molecular basis of inherited disease*. New York: McGraw-Hill; 1995:2601–2624.
The best review available on Niemann-Pick disease type I.

Metachromatic leukodystrophy

Kolodny EH, Fluharty AL. Metachromatic1eukodystrophy and multiple sulfatase deficiency: sulfatide lipidosis. In: Scriver CR, et al., eds. *The metabolic and molecular basis of inherited disease*. New York: McGraw-Hill; 1995:2693–2739.
An excellent and well-updated review.

X-Linked adrenoleukodystrophy

Moser HW, Smith KD, Moser AB. X-linked adrenoleukodystrophy. In: Scriver CR, et al., eds. *The metabolic and molecular basis of inherited disease*. New York: McGraw-Hill; 1995:2693–2739.
An excellent and well-updated review.

Alexander disease

Der Perng M, Su M, Wen SF, et al. The Alexander disease-causing glial fibrillary protein mutant, R416W, accumulates into Rosenthal fibers by a pathway that involves filament aggregation and the association of alpha B-crystallin and HSP27. *Am J Hum Genet* 2006;79:197–213.
An excellent and well-updated review.

Canavan-Van Bogaert disease

Beaud AL, et al. Aspartoacylase deficiency (Canavan disease). In: Scriver CR, et al., eds. *The metabolic and molecular basis of inherited disease*. New York: McGraw-Hill; 1995:4599–4605.
The diagnosis of Canavan disease is suggested by acetylaspartaturia.

Pelizaeus-Merzbacher disease

Zoghbi HY, Ballabio A. Pelizaeus-Merzbacher disease. In: Scriver CR, et al., eds. *The metabolic and molecular basis of inherited disease*. New York: McGraw-Hill; 1995:4481–4585.
Extrapyramidal signs are prominent in Pelizaeus-Merzbacher disease.

Rett syndrome

Hagberg B. Rett syndrome: Clinical and biological aspects. *Clin Dev Med* 1993;127:1–120.
An excellent and complete review of Rett syndrome.

Subacute combined degeneration of the spinal cord

Jaeken J, Stibler H, Hagberg B. The carbohydrate-deficient glycoprotein syndrome. A new inherited multi-systemic disease with severe nervous system involvement. *Acta Paediatr Scand* 1991(Suppl 1)375:5–71.
An updated and detailed review.

Friedreich ataxia

Ulku A, Arnc N. Friedreich's ataxia: A clinical review of 20 childrens' cases. *Acta Neurol Scand* 1988;17:493–497.
An excellent review. Women with Friedreich ataxia have a significantly better prognosis than men.

Refsum disease

Steinberg D. Refsum disease. In: Scriver CR, et al., eds. *The metabolic and molecular basis of inherited disease*. New York: McGraw-Hill; 1995:2351–2369.
An excellent review.

Krabbe disease

Suzuki K, Suzuki Y, Suzuki K. Galactosyle-mide lipidosis: Globoid-cell leukodystrophy (Krabbe's disease). In: Scriver CR, et al., eds. *The metabolic and molecular basis of inherited disease*. New York: McGraw-Hill; 1995:2671–2692. *An excellent review.*

Encephalomyopathy with coenzyme Q10 deficiency

DiMauro S, Quinzii CM, Hirano M. Mutations in coenzyme Q19 biosynthetic genes. *J Clin Invest* 2007;117: 587–589. *An excellent and well-updated review.*

CHAPTER 16

Inborn Errors of Metabolism II: Disorders of Purine and Amino Acid Metabolism

William L. Nyhan

Outline

Lesch-Nyhan syndrome

Lesch-Nyhan syndrome is due to an inborn error in the metabolism of purines, leading to substantial interference with central nervous system (CNS) function and bizarre, compulsive, and aggressive behavior (Table 16.1). Affected children appear normal at birth and usually develop normally for the first 6–8 months. They almost always have impressive quantities of urate crystals, which look like orange or yellow sand, in their diapers, and they may have hematuria, urinary tract stones, or infections early in life. However, in most instances the first signs of disease are neurologic. Patients who have been sitting well begin to lose this ability. They develop opisthotonic posturing, which persists intermittently as a regular feature of the disease. Muscle tone gradually increases, and in the established phenotype, the child is spastic. Involuntary movements are characteristic; they may be choreic, athetoid, or dystonic. Involuntary movements and spasticity may be evident before the first birthday. Most patients are mentally retarded, but the degree of motor disability is usually greater than the degree of intellectual impairment. None of these patients is able to walk or even to sit unsupported, but virtually all learn to talk, and they all appear to comprehend much of what is said to them.

The most striking feature of the behavior is self-mutilation through biting. Biting usually begins with the arrival of teeth, but age of onset of the abnormal behavior is highly variable. It may begin after several years. A hallmark feature is loss of tissue about the lips. There may be partial amputations of the tongue or fingers, and most patients have had some self-induced injury to the fingers. However, the self-mutilating activity is not limited to biting; it is limited only by the patient's disability. Patients also injure others, or try to. There is no abnormality in sensation.

Hyperuricemia is a regular feature of the disease. Its clinical consequences of gouty arthritis, urate nephropathy, urinary tract calculi, and tophaceous deposits may be prevented by treatment with allopurinol. Most untreated patients have died of renal failure by 10 years of age.

The diagnosis depends on the demonstration of virtually absent activity of the enzyme hypoxanthine-guanine phosphoribosyltransferase (HGPRT). The assay can be performed on erythrocytes, and the normal enzyme is stable during shipment at ambient temperatures. The blood should not be frozen. The companion enzyme adenine phosphoribosyltransferase (APRT) is often run as a control on conditions of shipment. In patients with Lesch-Nyhan syndrome, the activity of this enzyme is increased, usually to 150% of normal.

The gene for Lesch-Nyhan syndrome is on the long arm of the X chromosome and is usually fully recessive. Clinical illness is usually expressed only in the male.

Table 16.1 Lesch-Nyhan syndrome

Discriminating features
- Complete deficiency of HPRT

Consistent features
- Hyperuricemia
- Uricosuria
- Mental retardation
- Spasticity
- Choreoathetosis, dystonia
- Self-mutilation

Variable features
- Convulsions
- Hematuria
- Urinary tract stones
- Urinary tract infections
- Tophi
- Urate nephropathy
- Vomiting

However, there have now been six females with the disease, so testing for HGPRT should not ignore a female with the phenotype. The enzyme is expressed in cultured amniocytes and chorionic villus samples. Prenatal diagnosis has been accomplished using either. The human gene for HGPRT has been cloned, and a considerable number and variety of mutations have been identified. Once the mutation in a family is known, mutational analysis is the most convenient method for prenatal diagnosis and carrier detection.

The differential diagnosis includes an enlarging spectrum of disorders caused by variants of the HGPRT enzyme that are deficient in activity but not as deficient as the Lesch-Nyhan enzyme. At one end of the spectrum are patients with hyperuricemia and gout or renal stone disease and no abnormalities of the CNS. In others, however, the degree of deficiency is so severe that they look neurologically like patients with Lesch-Nyhan syndrome; but these patients have normal, or nearly normal, intelligence, and their behavior is normal. The recognition of this neurologic syndrome of HGPRT deficiency makes it important to screen more broadly among patients diagnosed as having cerebral palsy rather than solely among patients demonstrating self-mutilation. The deficiency can readily be detected by the assay of erythrocytes. On the other hand, the reliable distinction of these patients from classic Lesch-Nyhan patients, which may be very important for prognosis in a patient diagnosed sufficiently early so that he may be either premutilative or nonmutilative, requires the assay of cultured fibroblasts.

Some patients with hyperuricemia and uricosuria and normal HGPRT levels have abnormal phosphoribosylpyrophosphate synthetase levels. One of our patients also had severe deafness, some developmental retardation, and absent lacrimal glands.

Allopurinol is the treatment of any of the overproduction hyperuricemias of childhood. Patients often require larger doses than adults with gout. The goal is to keep the serum uric acid level at less than 3 mg/dL. Thereafter it may be useful to monitor the excretion of xanthine, hypoxanthine, and uric acid, optimally to avoid urinary tract calculi. Many patients are less stiff, especially in the morning, if treated with diazepam (Valium). Operative or other orthopedic treatment directed at dislocation of the hips is not effective. The only treatments effective for the self-mutilative behavior are physical restraint and the removal of teeth.

Pearls and Perils

Lesch-Nyhan Syndrome

- If the patient can walk it is in virtually all cases not Lesch-Nyhan syndrome.
- Reports on hyperuricemic patients from the routine clinical laboratory may be misleading because the accepted normal ranges given are for populations of adult males in whom hyperuricemia is common. A child with a serum uric acid level of 5 mg/dL is hyperuricemic, but the laboratory will not flag the sample as such. There may also be perils in the assay of urinary urate because it is a favorite food for contaminating microorganisms. Therefore, it is best to conduct this assay on fresh or freshly frozen urine in a local laboratory.
- A small number of efficient excreters displays a normal level of uric acid in the blood.

Purine nucleoside phosphorylase deficiency

Deficiency of purine nucleoside phosphorylase (PNP), like deficiency of adenosine deaminase, leads to severe combined immunodeficiency. In this disorder T-cell function is

Pearls and Perils

Purine Nucleoside Phosphorylase Deficiency

- The importance of early diagnosis cannot be overemphasized; in the presence of a suitable sibling donor, this otherwise fatal disease is curable by bone marrow transplantation.

always impaired, whereas B-cell function may be normal or somewhat impaired. There is an associated lymphopenia and deficiency of thymic function. T-lymphocyte–mediated immunity is markedly deficient. Skin tests for delayed hypersensitivity are negative, and lymphocytes do not respond to phytohemagglutinin. As a consequence, affected patients have frequent life-threatening infections. Most have died of infection. One patient developed vaccinia gangrenosa following vaccination against smallpox. Malignant neoplasms have also been observed, as has autoimmune hemolytic anemia.

Two of the earliest patients described had mild mental retardation and spastic tetraparesis. Another patient had a mild intention tremor. It has now been recognized that surviving patients with virtually complete deficiency of PNP may have more severe neurologic features. Five siblings from two families had severe developmental retardation and spastic tetraparesis. Spastic diplegia and behavioral abnormalities were reported in another patient. Patients with PNP deficiency may be suspected in the laboratory by the presence of hypouricemia and an associated low level of uric acid excretion in the urine. Nevertheless, they overproduce purines and excrete large amounts of inosine and guanosine in the urine. Concentrations of deoxyguanosine triphosphate (deoxy GTP) accumulate intracellularly.

The molecular defect in PNP can be demonstrated in erythrocytes and leukocytes, as well as other cells; most severely affected patients have essentially no detectable activity.

Purine nucleoside phosphorylase deficiency is inherited in an autosomal recessive fashion. Heterozygotes display activity of PNP that is intermediate between the activities of patients and controls. Prenatal diagnosis should be possible. The human PNP gene has been cloned, and the mutation has been defined in a number of patients.

The disease can be cured by bone marrow transplantation. Improvement has been reported using repeated erythrocyte transfusions.

Phenylketonuria

Phenylketonuria (PKU) is an inborn error in the metabolism of phenylalanine that causes severe mental retardation. The metabolic defect also interferes with pigment development. Affected individuals are always less deeply pigmented than their relatives, and they are often blonde and blue-eyed. However, the only significant effect of the disease is that on the brain. Untreated patients usually have IQ levels of less than 30.

Early symptoms include irritability and vomiting severe enough to have led to surgery for pyloric stenosis. An eczematoid rash may occur on the face, but this is not commonly seen. A characteristic odor, which is that of phenylacetic acid, has been variously described as mousey, wolf-like, musty, or barny.

Neurologic findings in addition to severe mental retardation are found in about two-thirds of patients. About half of these have subtle findings, such as some hypertonicity or an upgoing toe, but some patients may have severe spastic paraplegia. Some are microcephalic. Purposeless hand posturing, rhythmic rocking, and tremors of the hands may be present. Hyperkinetic activity, uncontrollable temper, and other behavioral problems are common. Seizures occur in about one-fourth of the patients, predominantly in those most severely retarded. Electroencephalogram (EEG) abnormalities have been described in approximately 80% of patients. The computed tomography (CT) or magnetic resonance imaging (MRI) scan may reveal cortical atrophy.

Pearls and Perils

Phenylketonuria (PKU)

- Mental retardation caused by PKU should be preventable in developed countries through programs of routine neonatal screening, definitive diagnosis, and the early institution of dietary therapy.
- Infants now go home from the hospital so soon after birth that patients with PKU may be missed because the patient has not been receiving protein long enough to experience a diagnostic rise in the concentration of phenylalanine.
- Physicians can avoid this problem by the routine determination of phenylalanine in blood at the first office visit after neonatal discharge from the hospital.

Table 16.2 Phenylketonuria

Discriminating features
- Deficient hepatic phenylalanine hydrolase
- Elevated plasma phenylalanine
- Depressed plasma tyrosine

Consistent features
- Mental retardation
- Diminished pigment
- Phenylpyruvic aciduria
- Phenyllactic aciduria
- Phenylacetic aciduria
- Phenylacetylglutamine in urine

Variable features
- Vomiting
- Eczematoid rash
- Odd odor
- Restriction fragment length polymorphism

The neuropathology of PKU consists of a delay in myelination in the CNS. Thus autopsies carried out in childhood have revealed dysmyelination in the subcortical white matter. These findings are absent in patients studied after 21 years of age. Patients with PKU accumulate large amounts of phenylalanine in body fluids and convert some of this phenylalanine to intermediates, such as phenylpyruvic acid, phenyllactic acid, phenylacetic acid, and phenylacetylglutamine. The disease was first discovered because of the green color that results from the reaction of ferric chloride with phenylpyruvic acid. The optimal method for the detection of PKU is the analysis of the blood for phenylalanine. This technique has been adapted to the assay of spots of dried blood on filter paper and has permitted the development of universal neonatal screening programs that now are the rule in all developed countries of the world. In this way, patients are detected before the development of brain damage and treated with diets restricted in phenylalanine (Table 16.2).

The enzymatic defect in PKU is in the enzyme phenylalanine hydroxylase, which catalyzes the conversion of phenylalanine to tyrosine. It is expressed only in the liver. The gene has been cloned and mapped to chromosome 12. A number of different mutations have been identified in the phenylalanine hydroxylase gene. Two mutations that express no enzyme activity or cross-reactive material account for about half of the patients with PKU in the best-studied northern European Caucasian population.

Treatment of PKU is accomplished by restriction of dietary intake of phenylalanine. This strategy has been successful in the prevention of the clinical manifestations of the disease when instituted in the neonatal period, as a result of case finding in siblings of previous patients or through a program of routine neonatal screening.

The objective is to keep plasma concentrations of phenylalanine under 300 µmol/L. Preparations such as Phenex (Ross) XCAnalog-Maximaid (SHS), Phenylade (Applied Nutrition), and Phenylfree (Mead Johnson) make long-term treatment economically feasible and palatable. Dietary therapy readily lowers levels of phenylalanine in the blood, and phenylpyruvic acid and its metabolic products disappear.

The management of infants on a low-phenylalanine diet is demanding. All infants require a certain amount of phenylalanine, including those with PKU, for whom the minimal requirements are similar to those of normal infants. Patients with PKU often vomit or refuse feedings, and infections may complicate the altered metabolic state. Management should be directed by a clinician with experience with the problem and access to facilities for accurate determination of serum concentrations of phenylalanine. If phenylalanine is restricted below levels required for growth, catabolism results and levels of phenylalanine increase. Hypoglycemic convulsions and death can occur. The optimal time for termination of dietary therapy is unclear. It was once customary to stop the diet at 5 years of age, but recent experience has indicated that discontinuation of dietary treatment at 6 years of age may lead to a reduction in IQ. The rigidity of dietary restriction is relaxed in the teenage years. In a woman with PKU contemplating childbearing, it is preferable to begin any diet restriction prior to the onset of pregnancy and to continue with frequent monitoring of levels of phenylalanine throughout gestation. The advent of therapy with tetrahydrobiopterin (BH4 Kuvan) may permit less stringent dietary restrictions in some patients; 10–20 mg/kg is the dose studied thus far.

Abnormalities in the metabolism of biopterin

Abnormalities in the metabolism of biopterin result in a group of disorders that have variously been referred to as *malignant hyperphenylalaninemia* or *atypical phenylketonuria*. These disorders result from abnormalities in the synthesis of tetrahydrobiopterin, the cofactor for the phenylalanine hydroxylase reaction, or from defective recycling of the cofactor (Table 16.3).

Initially, most children were identified because of progressive neurologic degeneration in those thought to have PKU because of a positive neonatal screening test, and managed with good dietary control of the blood levels of phenylalanine. Now children are being detected earlier by testing for biopterin defects in those with hyperphenylalaninemia detected by screening programs.

In the fully developed phenotype, the patient is hypertonic, often severely, and has extensor posturing or episodic opisthotonos. Convulsions may occur as early as 3 months of age. Myoclonic seizures are common. Deep tendon reflexes are exaggerated and a Babinski sign is present. Patients are difficult to feed. They have problems with their secretions and commonly drool. The pa-

Pearls and Perils

Abnormalities in the Metabolism of Biopterin

- Everyone with a positive neonatal screen for phenylalanine does not have phenylketonuria (PKU). Some have benign hyperphenylalaninemia, and a few have defects in biopterin metabolism. In the absence of early recognition and effective therapy, the effects of defective biopterin metabolism on the nervous system are profound.

Table 16.3 Abnormalities in the metabolism of biopterin

Discriminating features
- Defective activity of dihydropteridine reductase
- Evidence of deficient synthesis of tetrahydrobiopterin

Consistent features
- Hyperphenylalaninemia
- Degenerative neurologic disease
- Convulsions
- Spasticity

Variable features
- Rigidity
- Tremors
- Dystonic movements

tient appears expressionless or drowsy and may have tremors or dystonic movements. The intelligence may deteriorate progressively to the range of profound retardation. CT or MRI scan reveals cerebral atrophy, and ultimately the patient is microcephalic. Death usually supervenes in childhood.

Concentrations of phenylalanine in the blood are elevated. The levels are sometimes more like those in atypical hyperphenylalaninemia than in classic PKU. Worrisome is the fact that these disorders can occur, at least in infancy, without elevation of the serum concentration of phenylalanine, as documented in one patient diagnosed early because of an affected sibling.

Ultimately, of course, levels of phenylalanine should rise, because tetrahydrobiopterin is the cofactor required for activity of phenylalanine hydroxylase. Defects have been noted in the synthesis of biopterin at the initial guanosine triphosphate (GTP) cyclohydrolase step and later in the formation of the reduced biopterin itself. The syndrome also results when there is a deficiency of dihydropteridine reductase occurs, which catalyzes the recycling of tetrahydrobiopterin from the inactive quinonoid oxidation product of the phenylalanine hydroxylase reaction. Tetrahydrobiopterin is also the cofactor for the hydroxylation of tryptophan and tyrosine. Deficiency in this compound interferes with the synthesis of serotonin, dopamine, and norepinephrine.

The diagnosis of these disorders is generally made by analysis of urinary pterins and the activity of dihydropteridine reductase in dried blood spots. The cDNA for dihydropteridine reductase has been cloned and localized to chromosome 4p15.3. The GTP-cyclohydrolase deficiency can be documented on assay of lymphocytes, and the cDNA has been cloned. Mutations have been identified in the genes for dihydropteridine reductase, GTP cyclohydrolase, 6-pyruvoyltetrahydropterin synthase, and 4a-carbinoxamine dehydratase.

These disorders are all autosomal recessive. Heterozygote detection is possible in dihydropteridine reductase deficiency by assay of the enzyme. Prenatal diagnosis should be possible by enzyme assay. In any of these diseases, mutational analysis provides a method for earlier detection and prenatal diagnosis.

Treatment is by the administration of tetrahydrobiopterin, 5–hydroxytryptophan, and dihydroxyphenylalanine (DOPA), the precursors of biogenic amines.

Defects in the GTP cyclohydrolase also cause DOPA-responsive dystonia. This disease can also be caused by deficiency of tyrosine hydroxylase. Those with defects in the GTP cyclohydrolase are heterozygotes, and they do not have hyperphenylalaninemia. Penetrance is such that some are asymptomatic, whereas others have severe dystonia, with childhood onset and oculogyric crises. Patients have been identified with severe DOPA-responsive dystonia, who have mutations on both alleles of the cyclohydrolase gene. A striking aspect of this syndrome, in either its autosomal dominant or recessive forms, is a rewarding clinical response to low doses of levodopa.

Maple syrup urine disease

Maple syrup urine disease (MSUD) is an inborn error in the metabolism of the branched-chain amino acids that is fatal in the neonatal period in a majority of patients. Even those diagnosed promptly and treated carefully may die in infancy. The survivors are often retarded in mental development. The metabolic abnormality is very profound. This is a strong argument for programs of neonatal screening, but even in those states in which screening programs exist for MSUD, it is not uncommon to find a patient severely ill by the time the initial positive result becomes known.

In MSUD, leucine, isoleucine, and valine are not effectively catabolized because of a defect in their common

Pearls and Perils

Maple Syrup Urine Disease

- The characteristic maple syrup, or caramel, odor can be detected in urine, skin, or hair and may be very striking but may not be detected at all, especially in very ill patients who may not have ingested protein for days.
- It has not been possible to detect MSUD prenatally by analysis of the amino acids of amniotic fluid.
- A pitfall was reported in an infant in whom prenatal assay of the enzyme was normal but who went on to develop typical elevations of amino acids in the blood.

branched-chain ketoacid decarboxylase. The activity of this enzyme and its deficiency in MSUD are readily demonstrable in leukocytes and in cultured fibroblasts by assay of the conversion of ^{14}C leucine to $^{14}CO_2$.

Infants with MSUD appear well at birth, but symptoms begin within 24 hours to 5 days of life, with feeding difficulty or irregular respirations. There is progressive loss of vigor and the Moro reflex. Symptomatic hypoglycemia may occur. Characteristically, these patients develop convulsions, opisthotonos, and generalized muscular rigidity with or without intermittent flaccidity. Coma may be profound. Death usually occurs following the development of decerebrate rigidity. On CT or MRI scan, cortical atrophy may be seen, along with hypodense myelin. This finding is consistent with the defective myelinization that has been observed at autopsy (Table 16.4).

The name of the disease derives from the odor of the urine, which is reminiscent of maple syrup. The branched-chain amino acids are present in high concentration in the blood and urine, and so are their ketoacid analogs. Diagnosis is best made by the quantitation of the amino acids of the blood plasma. Ketoacids may be recognized in the urine by the yellow precipitate that forms on the addition of 2,4-dinitrophenylhydrazine.

Milder forms of the disorder occur, representing less complete deficiencies of the decarboxylase enzyme. Patients with some of these enzyme variants have been referred to as having *intermittent branched-chain ketoaciduria* because of the intermittent occurrence of the symptoms. The enzyme abnormality is always present, just as in classic MSUD. Ataxia and repeated episodes of lethargy may progress to coma in patients with or without mental retardation. The episodes may be precipitated by infection, surgery, or anesthesia. A variant form of the disease has been described that is responsive to the administration of thiamine.

Table 16.4 Maple syrup urine disease

Discriminating features

- Deficiency of branched-chain ketoacid decarboxylase

Consistent features

- Elevated concentrations of leucine, isoleucine, and valine
- Positive dinitrophenylhydrazine test of urine
- Branched-chain ketoaciduria

Variable features

- Maple syrup odor of urine
- Mental retardation
- Spasticity
- Opisthotonos
- Coma
- Convulsions
- Hypodense cerebral myelin

All of the forms of branched-chain ketoaciduria are transmitted as autosomal recessive traits. The enzyme has three protein components, designated E_1, E_2, and E_3. Mutations have been identified in the E_1 decarboxylase enzyme and in the E_2 protein. In the Mennonite population, in which the abnormal gene is very common, the mutation is a T to A change in the E_1a subunit.

The enzyme is expressed in cultured amniocytes. The disorder has been detected prenatally in a number of affected fetuses. In addition, methods have been developed for rapid, accurate diagnosis in very small numbers of cells on microtiter plates. This methodology should be applicable to chorionic villus samples. Mutational analysis should become more widely available for prenatal diagnosis.

Any patient shown to be responsive to thiamine should be treated accordingly. The mainstay of treatment for the majority of patients is dietary regulation. The intakes of leucine, isoleucine, and valine are maintained at levels at which the concentrations of the branched-chain amino acids in plasma are kept within normal limits. This therapy may be difficult. However, in patients in whom diagnosis is made very early a normal IQ may be achieved. Commercial products are available that are useful in management. Liver transplantation reverses the clinical and metabolic features of the disease and permits a normal diet.

Propionic acidemia and disorders of propionate metabolism

Propionic acidemia (Table 16.5) is the protypic organic acidemia. In this disorder, and in methylmalonic acidemia and multiple carboxylase deficiency, the patient presents in early infancy with life-threatening acidotic illness, characterized clinically by vomiting and dehydration and progressing to deep coma. It is characterized metabolically by massive ketosis, a low serum concentration of bicarbonate, and a low pH. There may be an elevated blood concentration of ammonia. Concentrations of glycine in blood and urine are elevated.

Recurrent episodes of metabolic acidosis are associated with the ketosis, similar to those observed in diabetic coma. Patients usually have neutropenia and thrombocytopenia, and may be anemic. Osteoporosis may be severe enough to lead to pathologic fractures. Mental retardation may occur, but this usually appears to be a consequence more of the complications of overwhelming illness in a young infant (such as shock and diminished cerebral perfusion) or of complicating hyperammonemia, than of the metabolic defect itself. However, some patients have been reported with an exclusively neurologic presentation. Such patients have had chorea and dystonia. Catastrophic acute infarction of the basal ganglia has also been reported.

Table 16.5 Disorders of Propionate Metabolism/Propionicacidemia

Discriminating features
- Deficiency of propionyl-CoA carboxylase

Consistent features
- Methylcitraturia
- Hydroxypropionaturia
- Propionicacidemia
- Recurrent episodes of ketosis and acidosis, leading to coma and potentially fatal illness
- Osteoporosis
- Vomiting
- Hypotonia
- Anorexia
- Moniliasis

Variable features
- Hyperammonemia
- Anemia
- Hyperglycinemia, hyperglycinuria
- Pathologic fractures
- Mental retardation
- Immunodeficiency
- Abnormal MRI of the basal ganglia

The diagnosis of propionicacidemia is most readily made by organic acid analysis of the urine, in which the diagnostic compound is methylcitrate. The diagnosis may be suspected by finding elevated quantities of glycine in the plasma. Other distinctive metabolites found in the urine are hydroxypropionate, tiglate, tiglylglycine, and propionylglycine.

The molecular defect is in the activity of propionyl-CoA carboxylase, an enzyme on the catabolic pathway for isoleucine, valine, threonine, and methionine, which catalyzes the conversion of propionyl CoA to methylmalonyl CoA. The enzyme has two subunits, a and b, and the genes of both have been cloned and localized to chromosomes 13 and 3, respectively. A number of mutations have been found. The enzyme may be assayed in leukocytes or cultured fibroblasts. Prenatal diagnosis has been carried out by assay of this enzyme in cultured amniocytes. However, an index of the difficulties inherent in this approach is the fact that the first pregnancy in which the prenatal diagnosis was reported was already so far advanced that termination was not feasible; a baby with propionicacidemia was born who died in infancy. This type of experience has been a stimulus for the development of more rapid methods of prenatal diagnosis. Among them has been the incorporation of [^{14}C]propionate into macromolecules, a technique that requires only two to four passages to obtain a sufficient number of amniocytes. It can be applied also to the diagnosis of methylmalonic acidemia. Propionyl-CoA carboxylase can also be assayed in chorionic villus samples. The direct chemical prenatal diagnosis of propionicacidemia can be accomplished by the demonstration of methylcitric acid in the amniotic fluid. Stable isotope dilution and selected ion monitoring gas chromatography-mass spectrometry have allowed rapid, highly sensitive prenatal diagnosis of the fetus with propionicacidemia. Patients with methylmalonic acidemia and multiple carboxylase deficiency can also be diagnosed in this way (Table 16.5).

Prenatal diagnosis permits the institution of prenatal treatment. This has been accomplished with excellent results in B_{12}–responsive methylmalonic acidemia and in biotin-responsive multiple carboxylase deficiency. Prenatal therapy of a pregnant woman carrying a fetus with methylmalonic acidemia or multiple carboxylase deficiency with pharmacologic doses of cobalamin or biotin has been highly successful. This approach permits the avoidance of the initial catabolic episode, which can occur within hours of birth and can be fatal.

Methylmalonic acidemia and multiple carboxylase deficiency also present with an identical picture of overwhelming illness that is usually fatal in the neonatal period. Infants with multiple carboxylase deficiency have, in addition, generalized erythematous cutaneous lesions and alopecia totalis. Each has a characteristic pattern of organic acid excretion. The first is characterized by the excretion of large amounts of methylmalonic acid, but 3-hydroxypropionic acid and methylcitric acid are also found in the urine. In multiple carboxylase deficiency, 3-hydroxypropionic acid and methylcitric acid are found, along with 3-methylcrotonylglycine and large amounts of 3-hydroxyisovaleric acid and lactic acid.

Patients with methylmalonic acidemia have defective activity of methylmalonyl CoA mutase. The gene for the enzyme has been localized to chromosome 6. A number of mutations have been identified. In a B_{12}–responsive subset of patients, the fundamental defect is in the conversion of hydroxocobalamin to deoxyadenosylcobalamin, the cofactor for the mutase enzyme. Similarly, patients with multiple carboxylase deficiency have abnormal activity of propionyl CoA carboxylase, 3-methylcrotonyl-CoA carboxylase, and pyruvate carboxylase, but the fundamental defect in the infantile form is in the enzyme holocarboxylase synthetase. A second form of multiple carboxylase deficiency is due to deficiency of biotinidase.

Therapy in propionicacidemia and methylmalonic acidemia requires profound restriction of the dietary intake of protein. In B_{12}-responsive methylmalonic acidemia treated with B_{12}, dietary restriction may be less severe, and in multiple carboxylase deficiency treatment with biotin, usually in doses as small as 10 mg/day, is all that is required for effective therapy.

Dietary therapy in propionicacidemia and methylmalonic acidemia requires the amounts of protein to be individually determined. For most patients, the requirements are less than 1.0 g/kg per day. Infants diagnosed early and treated with good dietary management may have normal intelligence. Episodes of intercurrent acidosis must be treated vigorously with large amounts of parenteral fluid and electrolytes containing sodium bicarbonate.

Isovalericacidemia

Isovalericacidemia is a disorder of the catabolism of leucine that is remembered as the "sweaty foot syndrome" because of the characteristic pungent odor of isovaleric acid, which does not smell at all like sweaty feet. Patients usually present with severe illness in early life, much like that of propionicacidemia; onset may occur with vomiting. Neurologic abnormalities include tremors and convulsions. The course is progressive to deep coma. Laboratory assessment reveals prominent acidosis and ketosis. Some patients have hyperammonemia. Patients with isovalericacidemia may also have leukopenia, thrombocytopenia, and anemia. Death may occur within a few days or weeks of birth.

Infants who survive the initial episode of illness are subject to recurrent attacks of vomiting, acidosis, and ataxia, progressive to coma. Such episodes may follow infections or surgery. The odor is more likely to be appreciated during an episode of acute illness, but it may be absent. Mental retardation may be the result. Some patients may have persistent ataxia, tremor, brisk deep tendon reflexes, or extrapyramidal involuntary movements.

The diagnosis is best based on the detection of isovalerylglycine in the urine. This compound is excreted in amounts up to 3 g/day. It is stable, and can also be employed to monitor the success of therapeutic measures, and especially to fine tune dietary management. 3-Hydroxyisovaleric acid is also found in the urine. Levels of glycine may be elevated. The molecular defect is in the activity of isovaleryl-CoA dehydrogenase, through which isovaleryl CoA is converted into 3-methylcrotonyl CoA. Enzyme assay is not easy and is not generally available. The gene has been sequenced and localized to chromosome 15; a number of mutations have been defined (Table 16.6).

Table 16.6 Isovalericacidemia

Discriminating features
- Isovalerylglycinuria
- Deficiency of isovaleryl-CoA dehydrogenase

Consistent features
- Episodes of acute illness
- Ketoacidosis
- Neutropenia, thrombocytopenia
- 3-Hydroxyisovaleric aciduria

Variable features
- Acrid "sweaty foot" odor
- Mental retardation
- Anemia
- Ataxia
- Convulsions

Treatment of the acute episode requires the vigorous use of parenteral fluids containing glucose and electrolytes, as outlined for the management of propionicacidemia. Hemodialysis, exchange transfusion, or peritoneal dialysis may be useful, especially in the hyperammonemic neonate. Supplemental glycine and its conjugation with isovaleric acid may be useful in acute management. Doses employed have been 250 mg/kg.

Glycine has also been employed in doses of 800 mg/day in chronic management. The mainstay of chronic treatment is restriction of dietary intake of leucine by lowering the intake of protein until the amounts of leucine ingested are those necessary for growth.

Pearls and Perils

Isovalericacidemia

- The excretion of 3-hydroxyisovalerate may engender confusion because it is a regular concomitant of this disease and of multiple carboxylase deficiency. It also occurs in any infant with ketosis. The diagnosis of isovalericacidemia requires a demonstration of the presence of isovalerylglycine.
- In the acutely hyperammonemic infant whose condition is improved by means of dialysis or exchange, resist the urge to begin protein feedings until levels of ammonia are normal and stable, and then begin with very small quantities.

Glutaric aciduria

Glutaric aciduria type I is a neurodegenerative disorder initially described in two siblings, one of whom also had a tendency to a compensated metabolic acidosis. Progressive neurologic deterioration occurs episodically following intercurrent infection. Patients have convulsions, spasticity, and involuntary movements. Among the earliest manifestations is macrocephaly. Bilateral subdural accumulations of fluid have been reported, and patients have been thought to have been victims of child abuse. Neuroimaging studies reveal marked fronto-temporal atrophy (Table 16.7).

The cardinal characteristic is the excretion of glutaric acid. This increases after lysine loading and de-

Table 16.7 Glutaric aciduria

Discriminating features
- Glutaric aciduria
- 3-Hydroxyglutaric aciduria

Consistent features
- Spasticity
- Convulsions
- Cerebral degeneration
- Involuntary movements
- Glutaconic aciduria

Variable features
- Metabolic acidosis

creases after the restriction of the dietary intake of protein. 3-Hydroxyglutaric and glutaconic acid are also found in the urine. In fact, the author has observed patients in whom 3-hydroxyglutaric acid was the only diagnostic feature of organic acid analysis. This pattern distinguishes this disease from glutaric aciduria type II, in which several organic acids are excreted in the urine, along with glutaric acid. These include a number of other dicarboxylic acids and hydroxy acids, especially ethylmalonic, adipic, suberic, and sebacic acids. Lactic acid is also present in massive amounts, and concentrations of the amino acids citrulline, lysine, ornithine, and proline may be elevated in plasma and urine.

In glutaric aciduria type I, the molecular defect is in glutaryl-CoA dehydrogenase. Glutaryl-CoA is an intermediate in the catabolism of lysine, tryptophan, and hydroxylysine. α-Ketoadipic acid is a common product of each of these three amino acids, which is decarboxylated to form glutaryl-CoA. Glutaryl-CoA dehydrogenase converts glutaryl-CoA to glutaconyl-CoA. It is a mitochondrial flavin adenine dinucleotide-dependent enzyme found in the liver and kidney. The gene is located on the short arm of chromosome 19. A splice site mutation has been identified in a population of Canadian Indians in whom glutaric aciduria is common.

Pearls and Perils

Glutaric Aciduria

- This condition raises the importance of screening for organic aciduria in a sizable population of patients with seizures and neurologic deterioration.
- The discovery of subdural effusions in a patient should suggest a search for this diagnosis in children suspected of being victims of child abuse.

Treatment of glutaric aciduria type I has been reported to be modestly effective. Treatment with a diet specifically low in tryptophan and lysine was followed by a decrease in the excretion of glutaric acid in the urine to about one-third of the usual level. A low-protein diet and treatment with riboflavin, the coenzyme for glutaryl-CoA dehydrogenase, were also followed by substantial reduction in glutaric aciduria. Clinical improvement or prevention in patients diagnosed presymptomatically has been reported. Treatment with the γ-aminobutyric acid (GABA) agonist baclofen has also been recommended. Treatment with carnitine is effective in conjugating with glutaryl CoA and removing glutarylcarnitine from the body.

The mainstay of treatment is the rapid response to intercurrent infection with the infusion of large amounts of glucose and water.

3-Hydroxy-3-methylglutaricaciduria

3-Hydroxy-3-methylglutaricaciduria differs from the other organic acidemias in that it presents as hypoketotic hypoglycemia. Thus, it must be considered in the differential diagnosis of disorders of fatty acid oxidation. However, it also presents with metabolic acidosis and hyperammonemia, so that the major problem in diagnosis is its distinction from Reye syndrome. It should always be considered in children with "recurrent" attacks of Reye syndrome. Episodes of the illness are, as usual for Reye syndrome, likely to follow an acute infectious illness.

Acute episodes of life-threatening illness occur in early infancy and may lead to coma. Persistent vomiting may be the first symptom. Apnea and death may ensue unless vigorous measures of resuscitation, including mechanical ventilation, are employed. Some patients have convulsions. Most have some hepatomegaly. One patient presented with acute pancreatitis. Chronic features may

Pearls and Perils

3-Hydroxy-3-methylglutaricaciduria

- The urine of every patient with Reye syndrome should be subjected to an organic acid analysis. In a patient who has had more than one attack, or in an infant younger than 2 years of age thought to have Reye syndrome, organic acid analysis is mandatory.
- Hypoketotic hypoglycemia is an unusual syndrome. 3-Hydroxy-3-methylglutaricaciduria is a well-defined cause of the syndrome. Look for carnitine deficiency or deficiency of carnitine palmitoyl transferase as another cause.

Table 16.8 3-Hydroxy-3-methylglutaricaciduria

Discriminating features
- 3-Hydroxy-3-methylglutaricaciduria
- 3-Hydroxy-3-methylglutaryl-CoA lyase deficiency

Consistent features
- 3-Methylglutaconicaciduria
- 3-Methylglutaricaciduria
- Hypoketotic hypoglycemia
- Acute overwhelming illness
- Metabolic acidosis
- Lethargy or coma

Variable features
- Lactic aciduria
- Lactic acidemia
- Hyperammonemia
- Hypotonia
- Hepatomegaly
- Vomiting
- Elevated liver function tests
- Convulsions
- Cerebral atrophy

include mental retardation, neurologic abnormalities, and cerebral atrophy. Death and permanent neurologic disability have been reported.

Serum concentrations of glucose may be very low. Levels less than 10 mg/dL were recorded in the first three patients. The absence of ketonuria distinguishes these patients from all others with organic acidemia. Nevertheless, a prominent metabolic acidosis and reduction in the serum bicarbonate may be present. Neonatal hyperammonemia is common. Liver function tests may be abnormal.

The organic aciduria is characteristic. The index feature is the excretion of large quantities of 3-hydroxy-3-methylglutaric acid. In addition, 3-methylglutaconic acid and 3-methylglutaric acid are found in the urine. These compounds represent successive steps in the catabolism of leucine. At times of acute illness, the urine also contains large amounts of lactic acid. The molecular defect is in 3-hydroxy-3-methylglutaryl CoA lyase, which catalyzes the conversion of 3-hydroxy-3-methylglutaryl-CoA to acetyl-CoA and acetoacetate. The activity of the lyase can be assayed in fibroblasts, leukocytes, and cultured amniocytes. The disorder is transmitted as an autosomal recessive trait. Heterozygotes may be detected by enzyme assay of leukocytes or fibroblasts (Table 16.8).

Management of the acute crisis requires large amounts of water, electrolytes, and glucose. Long-term management depends on the avoidance of fasting and attendant hypoglycemia. Parents should bring the patient in early when the oral route is compromised by vomiting or anorexia. A high-carbohydrate diet is useful, and the intake of both fat and protein should be limited. Glucose polymers and uncooked cornstarch are useful.

4-Hydroxybutyricaciduria

4-Hydroxybutyricaciduria is an inborn error of GABA metabolism that is unusual in that the compound that accumulates is of known neuropharmacologic activity. 4-Hydroxybutyric acid was once developed by the pharmaceutical industry as an intravenous anesthetic. It was designed as a GABA analog that could cross the blood–brain barrier, but it was abandoned when it was found to produce convulsions in animals. Unfortunately, the compound has been popularized as a street drug and implicated in date rape.

Affected patients have had seizures as well as mental retardation and ataxia. Ataxia has been nonprogressive. Marked hypotonia has been observed regularly. Psychomotor delay may be mild. One patient had mild ocular apraxia. Language development is usually retarded. Speech may be dysarthric. Pyramidal tract signs are not observed, and there is no sensory deficit.

The hallmark feature is the accumulation of 4-hydroxybutyric acid in urine, serum, and cerebrospinal fluid (CSF). Acidosis is characteristically absent.

The molecular defect is in the enzyme succinic semialdehyde dehydrogenase. The succinic semialdehyde that accumulates is reduced to 4-hydroxybutyric acid. The enzyme is not expressed in fibroblasts, but it is active in lymphocytes and cultured lymphoblasts, and the molecular diagnosis has been established in these cells. It is also active in chorionic villus samples. Therefore, the disease should be diagnosable prenatally by chorionic villus biopsy. Prenatal diagnosis has been accomplished by gas chromatography-mass spectometry (GC-MS) assay of 4-hydroxybutyric acid in amniotic fluid. Heterozygous carriers are detectable by assay of the enzyme in lymphocyte or lymphoblast lysates. An effective treatment regimen has not been developed.

Pearls and Perils

4-Hydroxybutyricaciduria

- This disorder presents another good reason for screening the urine for organic acids in the presence of rather nonspecific neurologic disease, such as convulsions, mental retardation, and ataxia.
- 4-Hydroxybutyric acid may be missed in some systems of organic acid analysis.

Nonketotic hyperglycinemia

Nonketotic hyperglycinemia is an inborn error of metabolism in which large amounts of glycine are found in body fluids, and there is no detectable accumulation of organic acids.

The accepted diagnostic feature is the elevated concentration of glycine in the CSF The child generally presents with severe illness within a few days of birth. Death usually occurs in the first year. Most patients develop apnea and, if admitted to a neonatal intensive care unit, usually require ventilator support. Children who survive have severe mental retardation in which there is little evidence of functional cortical activity. These infants have severe seizure disorders—many have virtually continuous seizures. Hiccuping and myoclonic seizures including infantile spasms are common.

Microcephaly, hypertonicity, and hypotonicity may be found. Deep tendon reflexes are exaggerated. Cerebral atrophy is found on CT or MRI scan. Decreased or absent myelination of the supratentorial white matter is characteristic. The EEG displays a distinctive burst suppression pattern.

Heterogeneity has also been described in this condition, and there are some patients with milder clinical pictures. Such patients may have only a modest developmental delay, but this presentation is rare. Glycine concentrations in plasma are elevated; levels usually approximate 800–1600 μm/L (6–12 mg/dL). Glycine excretion in the urine may be enormous. Concentrations in the CSF of patients with nonketotic hyperglycinemia average at least eight times the control level of 0.1 mg/dL. The ratio of the CSF concentration of glycine to that in the plasma is very useful in delineating the diagnosis. The ratio is substantially higher in patients with nonketotic hyperglycinemia than in hyperglycinemic patients with organic acidemia. Normally the ratio is only 0.02. In nonketotic hyperglycinemia the mean ratio was 0.17 ± 0.09. Patients with milder versions of the disorder than the classic phenotype tend to have lower ratios. The molecular defect is in the glycine cleavage enzyme, which catalyzes the conversion of glycine to CO_2 and hydroxymethyltetrahydrofolic acid. This is a multienzyme system, with four distinct protein components designated P, H, T, and L. Among patients with nonketotic hyperglycinemia studied definitively by assay of the enzyme system in autopsied liver or brain, individual defects have been described in the H protein, the P protein, and the T protein. The enzyme may also be assayed in transformed lymphocytes and in chorionic villus samples. The cDNA for the P protein has been cloned, and a deletion of a phenylalanine at position 756 has been identified in a Japanese patient. In Finland, where the disease is common, a substitution of leucine for serine at position 564 has been found in the gene for the P protein (Table 16.9).

Treatment is generally unsatisfactory. Heroic measures are probably not justified. Treatment with strychnine has been reported, but it is clear that it is not useful in the classic phenotype. A concerted effort to lower the CSF concentration as much as possible within the limits of the toxicity of benzoate may ameliorate seizures in a surviving patient. Dextromethorphan may aid as a glycine antagonist at the N-methyl-D-aspartate (NMDA) receptor.

Table 16.9 Nonketotic hyperglycinemia

Discriminating features
- Elevated CSF and plasma glycine ratio
- Defective glycine cleavage enzyme
- Hyperglycinemia

Consistent features
- Hyperglycinuria
- Neonatal coma and apnea
- Myoclonic seizures (infantile spasms)
- Electroencephalograph (EEG) burst suppression pattern
- Cerebral atrophy

Variable features
- Hypertonia
- Hypotonia
- Increased deep tendon reflexes
- Hiccuping

Pearls and Perils

Nonketotic Hyperglycinemia

- In the workup of an infant in metabolic coma, routine clinical laboratory tests are very helpful. First hypoglycemia must be ruled out. Metabolic acidosis and reduction of the serum bicarbonate lead one to the diagnosis of an organic acidemia. Hyperammonemia in the absence of acidosis signifies a urea cycle defect. Most other patients have nonketotic hyperglycinemia.

Homocystinuria

Homocystinuria is an inborn error of metabolism in which there is defective activity of the enzyme cystathionine synthetase. This enzyme catalyzes the conversion of homocysteine and serine to cystathionine. Homocystinuria is a disorder of connective tissue with similarities to Marfan syndrome. It is also characterized by thromboembolic disease, and therefore the resultant clinical picture is often a consequence of which vessel or vessels become involved. In homocystinuria, clinical manifestations tend to be progressive, because many of its clinical manifestations result from thrombotic complications.

A characteristic feature is subluxation of the ocular lens. In some patients, this is the only manifestation of disease. Iridodonesis may alert one to the presence of the detached lens. Myopia, cataracts, glaucoma, and other ocular manifestations may occur.

The hair is usually fair, fine, and sparse. The complexion is usually fair, and the eyes are blue. A malar flush is striking, and many patients have had livedo reticularis.

Thromboembolic phenomena are both arterial and venous, and are frequently the cause of death. Pulmonary emboli, renal artery thrombosis, and cerebral thrombosis have been common, as well as carotid or coronary thrombosis. Classic tests of clotting function are normal, but platelets from these patients show unusual adhesiveness. Furthermore, the addition of homocystine to normal blood causes the platelets to become sticky. Mental retardation is a common but by no means an invariable feature of the disease. Among retarded patients, the IQ has been 30–75. There may be acute signs of a stroke, or the insidious development of hemiplegia. Some patients have spastic paraplegia. Many have seizures, and even more have abnormalities of the EEG.

The most prominent metabolic characteristic is the excretion of homocystine in the urine. Homocysteine is an intermediate in the metabolism of methionine. Free homocysteine condenses with itself to form the disulfide homocystine, as cysteine does to form cystine. The diagnosis is made by the demonstration of homocystine in the urine or by the concentration of total homocysteine in the blood. Levels of methionine in blood and urine are usually elevated. The mixed disulfide of cysteine and homocysteine is also present in the urine.

Homocystine is unstable; therefore, testing should be performed on fresh urine. For the analysis of plasma, it is important to precipitate the protein immediately, or homocysteine will attach to the proteins and be removed before analysis. Screening of urine can be carried out by the cyanide-nitroprusside test. The enzymatic defect in the most usual form of homocystinuria is in cystathionine synthase, which catalyzes the conversion of homocysteine and serine to cystathionine. The enzyme defect can be demonstrated in biopsied liver or in cultured fibroblasts or amniotic fluid cells. The disorder is transmitted as an autosomal recessive trait, and heterozygotes have reduced cystathionine synthase activity. Defects in cobalamin metabolism may cause homocystinuria as well as methylmalonicaciduria, and defective activity of 5,10-methylene tetrahydrofolate reductase is a rare cause of homocystinuria.

The cDNA for human cystathionine b-synthase has been cloned and mapped to chromosome 21q22.3. A number of mutations have been identified. Correlations have begun to emerge between phenotype and genotype, particularly with the advent of patients uncovered by newborn screening, some of whom appear to be a different population from those uncovered by the development of symptomatology. Some genotypes, such as T353M, have been found exclusively in B_6-unresponsive patients, whereas others, such as I278T, have been found exclusively in B_6-responsive patients. Some patients respond to the administration of pyridoxine with an impressive reduction in the accumulation of homocystine. The usual doses are 100–500 mg/day, but up to 1,000 mg/day may be necessary. Those who respond are effectively managed by treatment with pyridoxine. Folate deficiency is avoided by concomitant administration of 1–15 mg/day of folate.

In patients unresponsive to pyridoxine, betaine has been used successfully to provide a methyl donor, thus reducing concentrations of homocysteine by converting it to methionine. Dietary therapy has also been recommended: methionine is restricted and supplemental cystine is provided.

Urea cycle disorders

The prototypic disorders of the urea cycle include carbamyl phosphate synthetase (CPS) deficiency, ornithine transcarbamylase (OTC) deficiency, citrullinemia, and argininosuccinic aciduria. Each presents classically with massive neonatal hyperammonemia. This picture may also be produced by transient hyperammonemia of the newborn. The classic disorder of urea cycle function is uniformly fatal in the first days of life. Transient hyperammonemia of the newborn, on the other hand—

Pearls and Perils

Urea Cycle Disorders

- Neonatal hyperammonemic coma is harmful to the brain. Most male infants with ornithine transcarbamylase (OTC) deficiency rescued with benzoate or phenylacetate treatment are retarded, and they tend to worsen with each subsequent episode. Best results are obtained in infants diagnosed prenatally who are prevented from ever having serious hyperammonemia. This may be done more easily in carbamyl phosphate synthetase (CPS) deficiency or argininosuccinicaciduria, or in the female with OTC deficiency, possibly in citrullinemia.
- Patients undergoing this type of therapy should be followed with repeated magnetic resonance imaging scans.
- Hepatic transplantation should be considered.

although lethal if untreated—resolves within 5 days with proper care, and its long-term prognosis is excellent. Most of the urea cycle disorders are autosomal recessive, but OTC deficiency, the most common single disorder of the urea cycle, is determined by a gene on the X chromosome. The disease is expressed in both males and females. Affected male infants have the classic phenotype, in which the disease is fatal in the first days of life. In affected females there is variable expression, owing probably to the variable inactivation of the X chromosome carrying the normal gene or its counterpart carrying the abnormal one.

The infant with a defect in the urea cycle is normal at birth and may do well for some time, usually until 12–48 hours after feedings begin. Refusal of feedings and lethargy develop. Some infants have convulsions. Progression is rapid to apnea and hypothermia. The appearance is that of surgical anesthesia. The patient survives only if intubated and provided with mechanical ventilation. The family history may include siblings who died very early in life.

Children with less complete deficiency of a urea cycle enzyme may present with neurologic abnormalities or mental retardation. Some have had recurrent episodes of vomiting, headaches, or ataxia. Even these patients may be at risk of death in hyperammonemic coma. Children with later-onset argininosuccinic aciduria have also had trichorrhexis nodosa, in which scalp hair is brittle and breaks off, leaving such short hair that the child may appear to be bald.

The hallmark feature in children with disorders of the urea cycle is the presence of hyperammonemia. In neonatal hyperammonemic coma, ammonia concentrations of 600–2,600 μg/dL have been observed (Table 16.10).

In hyperammonemic patients, the concentrations of glutamine and alanine, and occasionally aspartate, increase as nonspecific responses to the increased ammonemia levels. Similarly, when carbamoylphosphate accumulates, orotic acid excretion is increased. Oroticaciduria is characteristic of OTC deficiency. It also occurs in citrullinemia and argininosuccinicaciduria. Hepatomegaly and increased serum activities of serum glutamic oxaloacetic transaminase and serum glutamic pyruvate transaminase occur at times when ammonia concentration is increased and may cause diagnostic confusion with hepatic coma.

In the workup of a patient with hyperammonemia, the first step is the quantitative analysis of the amino acids of the plasma and urine. Citrulline is found in large amounts in both plasma and urine in citrullinemia; argininosuccinic acid is found in the urine in patients with argininosuccinicaciduria. In patients without elevation of an amino acid of the urea cycle, oroticaciduria is used to distinguish those with OTC deficiency from those with deficiency of CPS. To distinguish patients with transient

Table 16.10 Urea cycle disorders

Discriminating features

- Ornithine transcarbamylase (OTC) deficiency
- Carbamyl phosphate synthetase (CPS) deficiency
- Argininosuccinic synthase deficiency
- Argininosuccinase deficiency

Consistent features

- Oroticaciduria in OTC deficiency, citrullinemia and argininosuccinic aciduria
- Hyperammonemia
- Hyperglutaminemia
- Coma
- Absence of oroticaciduria in CPS deficiency
- Citrullinemia and citrullinuria in citrullinemia
- Increased concentrations of argininosuccinate in urine and cerebrospinal fluid in argininosuccinicaciduria

Variable features

- Hyperalaninemia
- Hyperaspartic acidemia
- Convulsions
- Mental retardation
- Trichorrhexis nodosa (in argininosuccinicaciduria)

hyperammonemia of the newborn from those with CPS deficiency, one looks carefully for the peaks of citrulline and arginine. They should be absent in a newborn with massive hyperammonemia because of a complete defect in CPS, whereas some of each is usually present in transient hyperammonemia of the newborn.

The molecular defect in CPS deficiency is in the first step of the urea cycle. The enzyme catalyzes the formation of carbamyl phosphate from ammonium and bicarbonate and thus provides a branch point to pyrimidine biosynthesis as well as urea synthesis. Assay of the enzyme requires liver biopsy. Biopsy is ideally postponed until the patient has been shown to be stable and able successfully to survive catabolic states such as infection. A restriction fragment length polymorphism (RFLP) for the CPS enzyme is useful in prenatal diagnosis.

Carbamyl phosphate reacts with ornithine in the presence of OTC to form citrulline. The OTC enzyme is exclusively present in the liver. Prenatal diagnosis has not been possible in the usual ways. It has been attempted by biopsy of the fetal liver and assay of the enzyme in liver tissue, but OTC activity in the liver does not develop until the second trimester. Therefore this rather heroic type of prenatal diagnosis has had to be delayed until 18–20 weeks of gestation.

The cloning of the OTC gene has permitted the early prenatal diagnosis of amniocytes and chorionic villus tissue. It also permits heterozygote detection. Deletions have been found in about 10% of affected males. A number of point mutations have been identified. In 10%, these involve mutation of a Taql restriction site. In two pregnancies at risk, a hemizygous normal male was detected in one and a heterozygous female in the other.

In citrullinemia, the molecular defect is in argininosuccinate synthase, which catalyzes the formation of argininosuccinic acid from citrulline. Argininosuccinic acid synthase has been found to be deficient in liver and in cultured fibroblasts. Heterozygotes may be detected by assay of fibroblasts, and prenatal diagnosis has been accomplished. The gene has been cloned. A number of mutations have been found in the argininosuccinate synthetase (ASS) gene, located on chromosome 9q34.1, most of which yield no immunoreactive enzyme.

Argininosuccinic acid is an intermediate in the urea cycle that is formed from citrulline and aspartic acid. It is not normally found in body fluids. In argininosuccinicaciduria, there is very efficient renal clearance of the compound, so that plasma concentrations are low and urinary concentrations very high. High concentrations of argininosuccinic acid are also found in the CSF. Argininosuccinicaciduria represents a failure in the cleavage of this compound to arginine and fumaric acid, which is catalyzed by argininosuccinase. The defective enzyme may be demonstrated in erythrocytes and cultured fibroblasts as well as in liver. The disease has been diagnosed prenatally. A number of mutations have been reported.

The treatment of disorders of the urea cycle has been altered dramatically by the advent of alternative approaches to the elimination of waste nitrogen. Thus, benzoate is given to tie up glycine as hippurate and phenylacetate or phenylbutyrate are given to tie up glutamine as phenylacetylglutamine. Both compounds are efficiently excreted in the urine. In addition arginine is provided as an essential amino acid in case of a complete block and as a source of ornithine to keep the cycle moving. This approach is especially useful in citrullinemia and argininosuccinicaciduria. In the management of the acute episode of coma, hemodialysis is more efficient than exchange transfusion or peritoneal dialysis.

Argininemia

Argininemia is a disorder of the urea cycle in which the clinical picture is very different from that of the other disorders of the cycle. The picture is that of a spastic tetraplegia first noted in the early months or years of life or convulsions in the neonatal period. Developmental delay may be the first evidence of abnormality. In the established phenotype, the patient is very spastic and opisthotonic. Muscle tone is hypertonic, and the deep tendon reflexes are accentuated. Chorea or athetosis may be present. Some patients have tremors. Drooling and dysphagia are common. The EEG shows abnormalities. Psychomotor retardation is usually severe. Ultimately, microcephaly and cerebral atrophy are observed on CT or MRI scan (Table 16.11).

Pearls and Perils

Argininemia

- The diagnosis of argininemia may be missed on the basis of a screening pattern of amino acids in the urine because the pattern may appear to be that of cystinuria. The question is readily resolved by the quantitative analysis of the amino acids of the plasma.

Concentrations of ammonia are elevated only intermittently in argininemia, and hyperammonemia, when it occurs, tends to be moderate. The diagnosis is made by the analysis of the amino acids of the blood or urine.

Plasma concentrations of arginine are four to 20 times normal. Concentrations in CSF are also markedly elevated. The concentration of arginine in the urine is elevated, but the urine also contains increased quantities of lysine, cystine, and ornithine because of competition for reabsorption by the large amounts of arginine in tubular urine. Patients with argininemia also have massive oroticaciduria. This feature of the disease is not a consequence of hyperammonemia, as it is in other urea cycle defects, but rather a consequence of the stimulation by accumulated arginine of N-acetylglutamate synthesis, which leads to increased synthesis of carbamoylphosphate. In the presence of limiting quantities of ornithine, this leads preferentially to pyrimidine biosynthesis.

The molecular defect is in the activity of arginase, which is readily measured in erythrocytes. The defect has

Table 16.11 Argininemia

Discriminating features
- Arginase deficiency
- Argininemia

Consistent features
- Spastic diplegia
- Developmental delay
- Hypertonia
- Opisthotonus
- Involuntary movements

Variable features
- Hyperammonemia
- Hepatomegaly
- Abnormal liver function tests
- Convulsions
- Electroencephalograph abnormalities

Consider Consultation When...

- A patient with apparent cerebral palsy has hyperuricemia.
- Organic acidemia, such as propionicacidemia or methylmalonic acidemia, is found; management of metabolic crisis is demanding.
- The comatose patient is found to have hyperammonemia.
- A patient presents with maple syrup urine disease.

also been demonstrated in liver, but the enzyme is not expressed in cultured fibroblasts.

The cDNA for arginase has been cloned and mapped to chromosome 6q23. A number of mutations have been identified.

Heterozygosity may be demonstrated by assay of arginase in erythrocytes. Prenatal diagnosis by enzyme assay has not been possible because the enzyme is not expressed in amniocytes. Mutational analysis is the preferred method.

Nutritional therapy designed to keep levels of arginine within normal limits has been known to lead to normal neurologic development. Sodium benzoate or phenylacetate (phenylbutyrate) may be employed not only to treat the rare hyperammonemia, but to decrease synthesis of arginine.

Annotated bibliography

Lesch-Nyhan syndrome

Bakay B, Nissinen E, Sweetman L, et al. Utilization of purine by an HPRT variant in an intelligent, nonmutilative patient with features of the Lesch-Nyhan syndrome. *Pediatr Res* 1979;13:1365–1370.
The first example of a patient with a variant enzyme whose neurologic examination was just like that of classic Lesch-Nyhan disease but who differed in that mental retardation and abnormal behavior were absent. He was shown to have an enzyme with some activity using an intact cell assay.

Christie R, Bay C, Kaufman IA, et al. Lesch-Nyhan disease: Clinical experience with nineteen patients. *Dev Med Child Neurol* 1982;24:293–306.
A compilation of the clinical phenotype in 19 patients observed as inpatients in the Clinical Research Center.

Jinnah HA, Harris JC, Nyhan WL, O'Neill JP. *The spectrum of mutations causing HPRT deficiency: An update.* Taylor & Francis, 23: 1153-1160, 2004

Lesch M, Nyhan WL. A familial disorder of uric acid metabolism and central nervous system function. *Am J Med* 1964; 36:561–570.
This is the original, classic description of the syndrome.

Nyhan WL, James TA, Teberg AJ, et al. A new disorder of purine metabolism with behavioral manifestations. *J Pediatr* 1969;74:20–27.
The initial description of a patient with a PRPP synthetase abnormality, hyperuricemia, deafness, and developmental delay.

De Gregorio L, Jinnah HA, Harris JC, et al. Lesch-Nyhan disease in a female with a clinically normal monozygotic twin. *Molec Genet Metabol* 2005;89:70–77.

Nyhan WL, Barshop BA, Ozand P. *Atlas of metabolic diseases.* London: Hodder-Arnold, 2005:431–447.
A more complete, illustrated treatment of the subject.

Purine nucleoside phosphorylase deficiency

Giblett ER, Ammann AJ, Wara DW, et al. Nucleoside phosphorylase deficiency in a child with severely defective T-cell immunity. *Lancet* 1975;1:1010–1013.
The first description of the entity.

Simmonds HA, Fairbanks LD, Timms P. Erythrocyte GPT depletion in PNP deficiency presenting with haemolytic anaemia and hypo-uricaemia. *Pediatr Res* 1985;19:776.
The first report on severe neurologic abnormalities in PNP deficiency.

Stoop JW, Zegers BJM, Hendrick GFM, et al. Purine nucleoside phosphorylase deficiency associated with selective cellular immunodeficiency. *N Engl J Med* 1977;296:651–655.
Documentation of impaired T-cell function in a patient with no tonsils. Two siblings in this family had PNP deficiency along with mild mental retardation and spastic tetraparesis.

Phenylketonuria

Burton BK, Grange DK, Milanowski A, et al. The response of patients with phenylketonuria and elevated serum phenylalanine to treatment with oral sapropterin dihydrochloride (6R-tetrahydrobiopterin): A phase II, multicentre, open-label, screening study. *J Inherit Metab Dis* 2007;30:700–707.

Jervis GA. Phenylpyruvic oligophrenia. *Assoc Res Nerv Ment Dis Proc* 1954;33:259–282.
A classic description of untreated PKU from a time before the development of treatment regimens.

Kyall P, Treacy E, Waters PJ, et al. Human phenylalanine hydroxylase mutations and hyperphenylalaninemia phenotypes: A metaanalysis of genotype-phenotype correlations. *Am J Hum Genet* 1997;61:1309.
Current analysis of the molecular biology of PKU.

Partington MW. The early symptoms of phenylketonuria. *Pediatrics* 1961;27:465–473.
A description of the earliest signs of PKU, emphasizing that vomiting is the most prominent sign.

Smith I, Beasley MG, Ades AE. Intelligence and quality of dietary treatment in phenylketonuria. *Arch Dis Child* 1990;65:472.
Best evidence for the setting of optimal levels of phenylalanine in plasma as objectives of therapy.

Woo SLC, Lidsky AS, Guttler F, et al. Prenatal diagnosis of classical phenylketonuria by gene mapping. *JAMA* 1984;251: 1998–2002.
Modern molecular biology and the cloning of the gene for phenylalanine hydroxylase permit prenatal diagnosis and heterozygote detection.

Abnormalities in the metabolism of biopterin

Bartholome K, Byrd DJ. L-Dopa and 5-hydroxytryptophan therapy in phenylketonuria with normal phenylalanine hydroxylase. *Lancet* 1975;2:1042–1043.
This paper discusses the role of biogenic amine precursors in therapy.

Danks DM, Schlesinger P, Firgaira F, et al. Malignant hyperphenylalaninemia: Clinical features, biochemical findings, and experience with administration of biopterins. *Pediatr Res* 1979;13:1150–1155.
A clinical description of the phenotype and the use of tetrahydrobiopterin in diagnosis.

Skrygan M, Bartholome B, Bonafe L, et al. A splice mutation in the GTP cyclohydrolase I gene causes dopa-responsive dystonia by exon skipping. *J Inherit Metab Dis* 2001;24:345–351.

Maple syrup urine disease

Khanna A, Hart M, Nyhan W, et al. Domino liver transplantation in maple syrup urine disease. *Liver Transplant* 2006;12: 876–882.
Not only did liver transplantation cure the crisis of metabolic in balance in the disease, but domino transplantation of the patient's liver into a recipient did not cause disease in him.

Menkes JH, Hurst PL, Craig JM. A new syndrome: Progressive familial infantile cerebral dysfunction associated with an unusual urinary substance. *Pediatrics* 1954;14:462–466.
This is the classic paper; an example of the value of careful clinical observation—and a good nose—in the definition of a new disease.

Nyhan WL, Rice-Asaro M, Acosta P. Advances in the treatment of amino acid and organic acid disorders. In: Desnick RJ, ed. *Treatment of genetic diseases.* New York: Churchill Livingstone, 1991;45–67.
Recipes for and the use of intravenous solutions for the treatment of the acute crisis in MSUD.

Nyhan WL, Rice-Kelts M, Klein J, Barshop BA. Treatment of the acute crisis in maple syrup urine disease. *Arch Pediatr Adolesc Med* 1998;152:593–598.

Scriver CR, Mackenzie S, Clow CL, Devlin E. Thiamine-responsive maple syrup urine disease. *Lancet* 1971;1:310–312.
Not many patients with MSUD respond to thiamine, but they all should be tested. If the patient is responsive, management is enormously simplified and the prognosis should be very good.

Snyderman SE. Maple syrup urine disease. In: Nyhan WL, ed. *Heritable disorders of amino acid metabolism.* New York: John Wiley & Sons, 1974;17–31.
The definitive work on the dietary management of MSUD.

Disorders of propionate metabolism

Childs B, Nyhan WL, Borden M, et al. Idiopathic hyperglycinemia and hyperglycinuria, a new disorder of amino acid metabolism. *Pediatrics* 1961;27:522–538.
This is the initial description of this order.

Naylor G, Sweetman L, Nyhan WL, et al. Isotope dilution analysis of methylcitric acid in amniotic fluid for the prenatal diagnosis of propionic and methylmalonic acidemia. *Clin Chim Acta* 1980;107:175–183.
The method for direct prenatal diagnosis by GCMS of the amniotic fluid.

Nyhan WL, Barshop BA, Ozand PT. Propionic acidemia. In: *Atlas of metabolic diseases.* London: Hodder-Arnold, 2005; 8–17.

Nyhan WL. Disorders of propionate metabolism. In: Bickel H, Wachtel U, eds. *Inherited diseases of amino acid metabolism: Recent progress in understanding, recognition and management.* Stuttgart: Georg Thieme, 1985;363–382.
This chapter summarizes the most up-to-date approach to dietary treatment of these disorders.

Nyhan WL, Gargus JJ, Boyle K, et al. Progressive neurologic disability in methylmalonic academia despite transplantation of the liver. *Eur J Pediatr* 2002;161:377–379.
These patients make the point that an absence of the acute ketoacidotic may set the stage for indolent injury to the basal ganglia.

Isovalericacidemia

Ando T, Nyhan WL, Bachmann C, et al. Isovaleric acidemia: identification of isovalerate, isovalerylglycine, and 3-hydroxyisovalerate in urine of a patient previously reported as having butyric and hexanoic academia. *J Pediatr* 1973;82: 243–248.
An index of the problems with a specific diagnosis in organic acidemia is the fact that these patients were originally described as having a different entity.

Tanaka K, Budd MA, Efron ML, Isselbacher KJ. Isovaleric acidemia: A new genetic defect of leucine metabolism. *Proc Natl Acad Sci USA* 1966;56:236–242.
This is the classic initial description of the disease.

Vockley J. Ensenauer R. Isovaleric acidemia: New aspects of genetic and phenotype heterogenicity. *Am J Med Genet C Semin Med Genet* 2006;142:95–103.

Kolker S, Garbade SF, Maier E, et al. Decline of acute encephalopathic crises in children with glutaryl-CoA dehydrogenase deficiency identified by newborn screening in Germany. *Ped Res* 2007;62:357–363.

Glutaric aciduria

Goodman SI, et al. Glutaric aciduria: A 'new' disorder of amino acid metabolism. *Biochem Med* 1975;12:386–391.
This is the classic description of the disease.

Hoffmann GF, Trefz FK, Barth PG, et al. Glutaryl-CoA dehydrogenase deficiency: A distinct encephalopathy. *Pediatrics* 1991;88:1194–1203.
The most comprehensive compendium of patient material, providing an overview of the entire spectrum of illness.

Kyllerman M, Steen G. Intermittently progressive dyskinetic syndrome in glutaric aciduria. *Neuropediatrics* 1977;8:397–404.
A good clinical description of the progressive disease.

Nyhan WL, Zschocke J, Hoffmann G, et al. Glutaryl-CoA dehydrogenase deficiency presenting as 3-hydroxyglutaric aciduria. *Mol Genet Metab* 1999;66:199–204.

3-Hydroxy-3-methylglutaricaciduria

Faull K, Bolton P, Halpern B, et al. Patient with defect in leucine metabolism. *N Engl J Med* 1976;294:1013.
This is the original description of the entity.

Gibson KM, Sweetman L, Nyhan WL, et al. 4-Hydroxy-3-methylglutaric aciduria: A new assay of 3-hydroxy-3-methylglutaryl-CoA lyase using high-performance liquid chromatography. *Clin Chim Acta* 1982;126:171–181.
This article describes the definitive enzyme assay in which the products of the reaction are isolated and quantified.

Wilson WG, Cass MB, Sovik O, et al. 3-Hydroxy-3-methylglutaryl-CoA lyase deficiency in a child with acute pancreatitis and recurrent hypoglycemia. *Eur J Pediatr* 1984;142:289–291.
This paper describes a case that presented with vomiting and abdominal pain, leading to a diagnosis of pancreatitis.

4-Hydroxybutyricaciduria

Gibson KM, Nyhan WL, Jaeken J. Inborn errors of GABA metabolism. *Bioessays* 1986;4:24–27.
A good review of the chemical and clinical features.

Gibson KM, Aramaki S, Sweetman L, et al. Stable isotope dilution analysis of 4-hydroxybutyric acid: An accurate method of quantification in physiological fluids and the prenatal diagnosis of 4-hydroxybutyric aciduria. *Biomed Environ Mass Spectrom* 1990;19:89.

Jakobs C, Bojasch M, Monch E, et al. Urinary excretion of gamma-hydroxybutyric acid in a patient with neurological abnormalities. The probability of a new inborn error of metabolism. *Clin Chim Acta* 1981;111:169–178.
The original description of the disease.

Nonketotic hyperglycinemia

Dinopoulos A, Matsubara Y, Kure S. Atypical variants of nonketotic hyperglycinemia. *Mol Gen Met* 2005;86:61–69.

Gerritsen T, Kaveggia E, Waisman HA. A new type of idiopathic hyperglycinemia with hypo-oxaluria. *Pediatrics* 1965;36:882–891.
The original description of the disease.

Hayasaka K, Tada K, Kikuchi G, et al. Nonketotic hyperglycinemia: Two patients with primary defects of P-protein and T-protein, respectively, in the glycine cleavage system. *Pediatr Res* 1983;17:967–970.
A report on the enzyme defect.

Kure S, Takayanagi M, Narisawa K, et al. Identification of a common mutation in Finnish patients with nonketotic hyperglycinemia. *J Clin Invest* 1992;90:160.

Wolff JA, Kulovich S, Yu AL, et al. The effectiveness of benzoate in the management of seizures in nonketotic hyperglycinemia. *Am J Dis Child* 1986;140:596–602.
A concerted attack on the CSF glycine level using sodium benzoate may ameliorate seizures.

Homocystinuria

Barber GW, Spaeth GE. The successful treatment of homocystinuria with pyridoxine. *J Pediatr* 1969;76:463–478.
This demonstration that some patients respond to vitamin B_6 established genetic heterogeneity in homocystinuria. It also provided a means of highly effective therapy in responsive patients.

Carson NAJ, Cusworth DC, Dent CE, et al. Homocystinuria: A new inborn error of metabolism associated with mental deficiency. *Arch Dis Child* 1963;38:425–436.
This classic description of the disease clearly lays out its clinical manifestations.

Urea cycle disorders

Ballard RA, Vinocur B, Reynolds JW, et al. Transient hyperammonemia of the preterm infant. *N Engl J Med* 1978;299:920–925.
The initial description of this syndrome.

Brusilow SW, Batshaw ML, Waber L. Neonatal hyperammonemic coma. *Adv Pediatr* 1982;29:69–103.
This paper sets out the current approaches to the management of hyperammonemia and of patients with defects of the urea cycle.

Campbell AGM, Rosenberg LE, Snodgrass PJ, Nuzum CT. Ornithine transcarbamylase deficiency: A cause of lethal neonatal hyperammonemia in males. *N Engl J Med* 1973;288:1–6.
A classic description of the lethal nature of neonatal hyperammonemic coma in urea cycle defects.

Leibowitz J, Thoene J, Spector E, Nyhan W. Citrullinemia. *Virchows Arch A* 1978;377:249–258.
Citrullinemia, too, when presenting in the neonatal period, was once uniformly fatal.

Nyhan WL, Barshop BA, Ozand PT. Introduction to hyperammonemia and disorders of the urea cycle: Ornithine transcarbamylase deficiency. In: *Atlas of metabolic diseases.* London: Hodder-Arnold, 2005;195–205.
A general overview on diagnosis and management.

Rozen R, Fox J, Fenton WA, et al. Gene deletion and restriction fragment length polymorphisms at the human ornithine transcarbamylase locus. *Nature* 2985;313:815–817.
The use of molecular biology in the assessment of OTC deficiency.

Tuchman M, Morizono H, Rajagopal BS, et al. The biochemical and molecular spectrum of ornithine transcarbamylase deficiency. *J Inherit Metab Dis* 1998;21(Suppl):40–58.

Argininemia

Terheggen HG, Schwenk A, Lowenthal A, et al. Hyperargininemia mit Arginasedetkt: Eine neue famihare Stoffwechselstorung. *Z Kinderheilkd* 1970;107:298–312.
The original description of the disease.

Terheggen HG, Lavinha F, Colombo JP, et al. Familial hyperargininemia. *J Hum Genet* 1972;20:69–84.
A description for those who do not read German.

Yoshino M, et al. Argininemia: report of a new case and mechanisms of orotic aciduria and hyperammonemia. In: Lowenthal A, Mori A, Marescau B, eds. *Urea cycle diseases.* New York: Plenum Press, 1982; 121–125.

CHAPTER 17

Neoplastic Diseases

Roger J. Packer, Tobey J. MacDonald, Brian R. Rood,

Gilbert Vezina, and Robert A. Keating

Outline

- Epidemiology
- Clinical presentation
- Staging and risk stratification
- Neuroimaging
- Neuropathology
- Molecular genetics
- General aspects of therapy
- Specific tumor types
- Common long-term sequelae of tumor/treatment

Tumors of the central nervous system (CNS) represent 16% of all malignancies that arise during childhood and adolescence. Although relatively infrequent, diagnosed in approximately 2,200 children in the United States every year, they are the leading cause of morbidity and mortality from cancer in childhood. The majority of brain tumors occurring in children will be primary CNS lesions, as metastatic tumors are considerably less frequent than in adulthood. Tumors of varying histologies occur throughout the CNS in childhood, with a relative predilection for the posterior fossa.

Although progress has been slow in the management of childhood brain tumors, for many patients long-term survival and cure is possible. Diagnosis has been simplified by the increased availability of sensitive neuroimaging techniques, especially magnetic resonance imaging (MRI). It is unclear whether earlier diagnosis has actually improved long-term survival, but MRI has undoubtedly diagnosed some forms of tumors earlier and with more precision, especially as regards extent of the neoplasm at the time of diagnosis. Therapeutic interventions are primarily surgery, radiation therapy, and chemotherapy. The latter has been increasingly employed, especially in young children with aggressive or malignant tumors. With current means of treatment, tumor- and therapy-related long-term sequelae are frequent, and "quality-of-life" for many survivors is significantly impaired.

Epidemiology

Primary CNS tumors are the second most common form of cancer in childhood and the most common form of solid tumor. The overall incidence of childhood brain tumors, in patients between 0 and 19 years of age, inclusive, is estimated to be 2.5–3.5 per 100,000 person-years (Central Brain Tumor Registry of the United States [CBTRUS] 2002). Rates are highest for neuroepithelial tumors (3.0 per 100,000 person-years), with pilocytic astrocytomas and medulloblastomas being the most common individual histologies (Figure 17.1). The incidence of pediatric brain tumors is higher among children between 0 and 4 years of age and remains relatively steady until age 7, when a 40% drop in incidence occurs. The lowest incidence occurs among children between 10 and 14. The incidence of CNS tumors varies based on histology; ependymomas and medulloblastomas in children decrease with age, and pilocytic astrocytomas peak among children between 5 and 9 years of age and then decrease over time.

Pearls and Perils

- In children with visual pathway gliomas, especially optic nerve gliomas, look carefully for stigmata of neurofibromatosis type 1.

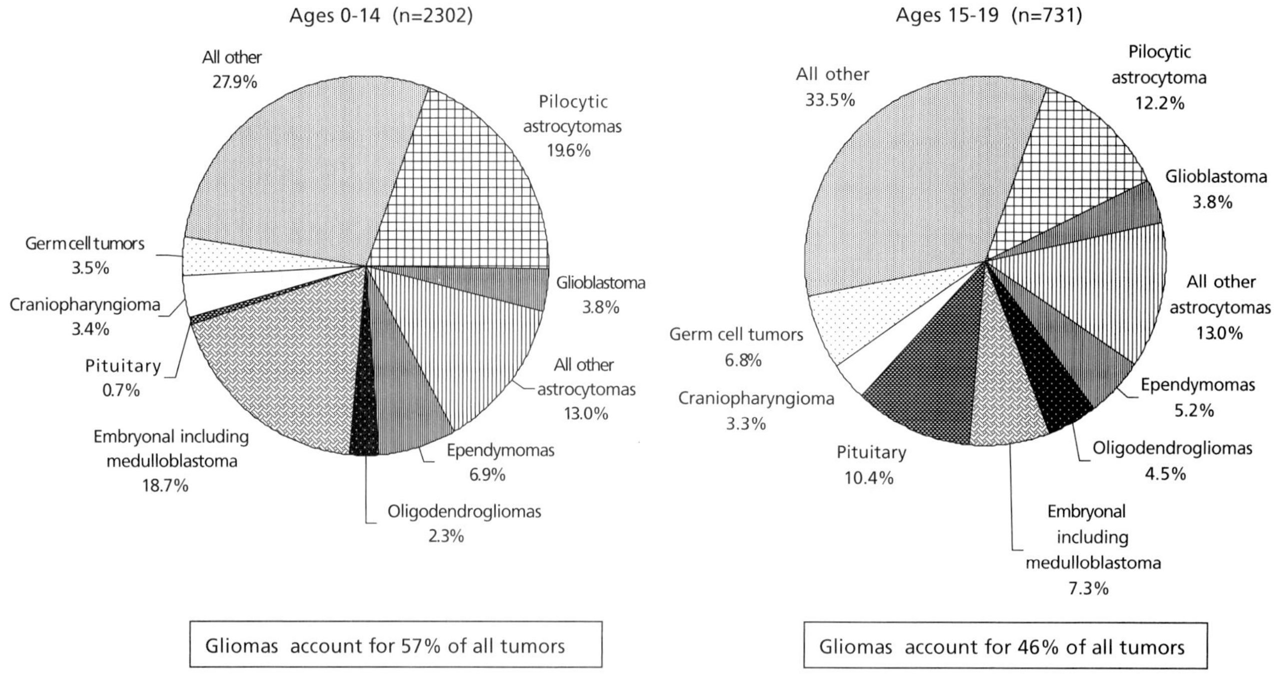

Figure 17.1 Distribution of pediatric primary brain and central nervous system tumors by histology. From the Central Brain Tumor Registry of the United States.

The reported incidence of childhood brain tumors is slightly more common in whites than in blacks. Males have a slightly higher incidence than females, with a clear male predominance for primitive neuroectodermal tumors and ependymomas.

For the majority of childhood brain tumors, no specific etiologic factors exist. Patients with neurofibromatosis type 1 (NF1) have a higher incidence of visual pathway gliomas, other glial tumors, and, to a lesser extent, other types of CNS malignancies. Patients with von Hippel Lindau syndrome and are much more likely to develop cerebellar hemangioblastomas. The Li-Fraumeni syndrome is an increasingly recognized genetic predisposition to a variety of different tumors, including gliomas. Medulloblastomas are primarily sporadic but have been linked with a variety of different genetic conditions including the autosomal dominant nevoid basal cell carcinoma syndrome (Gorlin syndrome), as well as the recessively inherited Turcott syndrome.

Regarding environmental risk factors, therapeutic doses of ionizing radiation have been linked to an increased risk of brain tumors in children (CBTRUS 2002). Inconsistent relationships have been found between the development of childhood brain tumors and other factors, such as maternal food consumption, electromagnetic waves, exposures to products containing n-nitroso compounds, pesticides, and father's occupation.

Clinical presentation

Nonspecific signs and symptoms

The signs and symptoms associated with childhood brain tumors are dependent on the location of the tumor and the age of the patient. Since brain tumors in children have a relative predilection for the posterior fossa, cerebellar or brainstem symptoms are common. Similarly, because of the predilection for the posterior fossa and other midline sites, obstruction of cerebrospinal fluid (CSF) flow occurs relatively early in many types of childhood brain tumor, resulting in nonspecific signs and symptoms of increased intracranial pressure. In some cases, the symptoms occur quite early in the disease, making diagnosis easier. However, in infiltrating midline lesions, symptoms may be insidious, nonspecific, and often nonlocalizing early in the course of illness, resulting in relatively late diagnosis (Tables 17.1 and 17.2). Some childhood brain tumors have a proclivity to disseminate throughout the nervous system early in the course of illness. This is especially true for medulloblastomas, pineoblastomas, malignant tumors in infants, and germinomas. Despite this predilection, dissemination is usually asymptomatic and overshadowed by neurologic dysfunction referable to the primary tumor site. The greatest delay in diagnosis usually occurs in infants and young children because of the relative rarity of childhood brain tumors and the tendency of such lesions to initially present with developmental

Table 17.1 Midline tumors

Discriminating features
- Craniopharyngioma
  - Pathologic examination
- Visual pathway tumor
  - Pathologic examination or characteristic CT or MRI lesion
- Tumors of the thalamus and the hypothalamus (diencephalic syndrome)
  - Pathologic examination
- Pineal region tumor
  - Pathologic examination

Consistent features
- Craniopharyngioma
  - Suprasellar mass
- Visual pathway tumor
  - Visual loss and optic atrophy
  - Asymmetric visual field loss
  - Abnormal visual evoked response
  - Nystagmus
- Tumors of the thalamus and the hypothalamus (diencephalic syndrome)
  - Failure to thrive
  - Normal intelligence
  - CT or MRI shows diencephalic mass
  - Lack of focal neurologic signs
- Pineal region tumor
  - CT or MRI shows pineal region mass
  - Lack of focal neurologic signs
  - More common in males
  - Suprasellar germinomas more often found in girls and pineal region pinealomas in boys

Variable features
- Craniopharyngioma
  - Papilledema
  - Endocrinopathies secondary to obstruction of foramen of Monro
  - Suprasellar calcification
  - Visual loss (acuity of fields)
- Visual pathway tumor
  - Headache
  - Papilledema
  - Endocrinopathies
  - Proptosis
  - Visual loss
- Tumors of the thalamus and the hypothalamus (diencephalic syndrome)
  - Visual loss
  - Nystagmus
  - Euphoria
- Pineal region tumor
  - Papilledema
  - Precocious puberty in boys
  - Elevated alpha-fetaprotein
  - Elevated chorionic gonadotropin
  - Spread throughout the cerebrospinal fluid pathways

Table 17.2 Pathology and course of midline tumors

Discriminating features
- Craniopharyngioma
  - Suprasellar location
  - Calcified cystic mass
- Visual pathway tumor
  - Tumor either intraorbital or chiasmatic
  - Pathology typically low-grade astrocytomas
- Hypothalamus
  - Usually pilocytic low-grade astrocytoma (juvenile pilocytic astrocytomas)
- Pineal region
  - Teratomas, germinomas, and pinealomas found in midline area

Consistent features
- Craniopharyngioma
  - Diabetes insipidus following surgery
  - Long-term survival is the rule
  - Must be followed and treated for panhypopituitarism
- Visual pathway tumor
  - 50% associated with neurofibromatosis
  - Long-term survival is the rule
  - Do not require treatment unless there is visual loss or evidence of progression on neuro imaging
- Hypothalamus
  - Failure to thrive seen in young child with hypothalamic tumors ("diencephalic syndrome")
  - Long tract signs seen in thalamic tumors
  - Hypothalamic tumors are more commonly associated with endocrinopathies
- Pineal region
  - Germinomas are highly radiosensitive
  - Teratomas do not respond well to radiation
  - Presence of alpha-fetoprotein or human chorionic gonadotropin suggests malignant behavior

Variable features
- Craniopharyngioma
  - Over 50% recur despite putative total removal
  - Radiation indicated in those patients who do not have total removal and in those who have a recurrence
  - Growth acceleration may occur following removal
- Visual pathway tumor
  - May be confused with spasmus nutans or congenital nystagmus
  - Long-term survivals reported regardless of form of treatment, that is, no treatment, surgery, or radiation
- Hypothalamus
  - Prognosis better in hypothalamic tumors, worse in thalamic tumors
  - Response to radiation is variable
- Pineal region
  - Prognosis predicted by histology and whether tumor seeds via CSF
  - Germinoma may resemble a primitive neuroectodermal tumor
  - Vascularity of region may limit attempts at total surgical removal

Consider Consultation When...

- The triad of morning headaches, vomiting, and lethargy requires referral to a pediatric neurologist or pediatric neurosurgeon and neuroimaging.

delay or, later in the course of illness, regression of developmental milestones. Such subtle findings are often overlooked until focal neurologic deficits become apparent.

Obstruction of CSF results in increased intracranial pressure and some of the more classic symptoms of CNS tumors, including the triad of increased intracranial pressure (ICP): morning headaches, vomiting, and lethargy (Table 17.3). Headaches are an extremely problematic issue in the diagnosis of childhood brain tumors. Although the majority of children with brain tumors will have some type of headaches by the time of diagnosis, the classical headache of increased ICP may not be apparent early in the course of illness. Headaches early in illness are often nonlocalized and, later in illness, there may be significant overlap between the types of headaches seen in childhood migraine and those caused by a CNS tumor. Headaches that wake a child from sleep or occur early in the morning suggest the possibility of increased ICP. In very young children, headache may be quite difficult to discern and may be intermittent, possibly due to the presence of open fontanels and sutures. Increased ICP may also cause other nonspecific and nonlocalizing problems such as declining academic performance, fatigue, and personality change. Headaches associated with the primary CNS tumors are usually less than 4–6 months in duration, although chronic headaches do not rule out the presence of a tumor and call for clinical evaluation in the context of focal neurologic deficits.

In patients with headaches, especially those with morning headaches associated with vomiting, funduscopic examination is critical. Although papilledema is frequently present at the time of diagnosis, it can be absent very early (in the first 1 or 2 days) of increased ICP. In longstanding increased ICP, especially due to slow growing lesions in the suprasellar region, optic pallor, rather than papilledema, may be present by the time diagnosis is made. In infants, the "setting sun" sign, manifest by impaired upgaze and a seemingly forced downward deviation of the eyes, strongly suggests either increased ICP due to CSF obstruction with third ventricular dilatation, or direct compression by the tumor of the tectal region of the midbrain.

Table 17.3 Increased intracranial pressure: Brain tumor etiology

Etiology

- Obstruction of cerebrospinal fluid (CSF) flow
- Focal mass effect (tumor and edema)
- Overproduction CSF

Signs/Symptoms

- Headache (especially morning)
- Nausea
- Vomiting
- Lethargy, obtundation
- Isolated sixth-nerve palsy
- Developmental delay; regression (infants)
- Setting sun sign (infants)

Localizing signs and symptoms: infratentorial masses

The other classical signs and symptoms of infratentorial brain tumors include deficits of balance, such as truncal unsteadiness, upper extremity coordination difficulties, and gait difficulties, with or without cranial nerve dysfunction (Table 17.4). Their presence and timing is partially dependent on tumor type. Early in the course of illness, tumors that fill the posterior fossa but do not invade the brainstem (such as medulloblastomas) may result predominantly in truncal unsteadiness. In contrast, tumors arising in the cerebellar hemisphere, such as cerebellar astrocytomas, are more likely to cause lateralizing signs early in illness, with signs and symptoms of increased ICP occurring later.

Inability to abduct one or both eyes (representing paresis of the sixth cranial nerve), may be a false localizing sign related to increased ICP rather than due to direct

Pearls and Perils

- Headaches early in the presentation of a brain tumor are usually nonlocalized or nonspecific; however, headaches that are new or have changed significantly in character raise the possibility of an intracranial lesion.

Pearls and Perils

- Crossed hemiparesis with a peripheral facial palsy on one side and hemiparesis on the other strongly suggest the possibility of an intrinsic brainstem process, especially a brainstem glioma.

Table 17.4 Posterior fossa tumors of childhood: Signs and symptoms

Tumor type	Peak age at diagnosis	Duration of symptoms prior to diagnosis	Common signs and symptoms
Medulloblastoma	3–5 years, with a second 8–12 years	1–3 months	Headaches, nausea and vomiting, truncal/gait unsteadiness
Cerebellar astrocytoma	Late first decade	2–5 months	Lateralizing cerebellar deficits, headache and vomiting (late)
Ependymoma	Mean age 5–6 years; 50% < 5 years of age	2–4 months	Ataxia, cranial nerve deficits, headaches, nausea and vomiting
Brainstem glioma (diffuse, pontine)	5–15 years of age	1–6 months	Multiple cranial nerve palsies, ataxia, long-tract signs, sensory loss, headaches, vomiting (late)
Brainstem glioma (focal)	Unclear	Variable, dependent on location	Sixth and seventh nerve palsies (focal pontine); nausea, vomiting, head tilt, unsteadiness (cervicomedullary); hydrocephalus, increased intracranial pressure (tectal)
Atypical teratoid/rhabdoid	Less than 2 years in majority	1–3 months	Vomiting, failure to thrive, development arrest/ delays, unsteadiness

brainstem dysfunction. However, inability to deviate both eyes conjugally (a gaze palsy) or the inability to adduct an eye properly on attempted lateral gaze with jerk nystagmus of the abducting other eye, implies an intrinsic brainstem disorder, the latter representing an intranuclear ophthalmoplegia. Such findings, especially when associated with other cranial nerve deficits, strongly suggest direct invasion of the brainstem and, in children, most likely the presence of a diffuse infiltrating brainstem glioma. Masses that involve the cerebellopontine angle will result in sixth, seventh, and eighth nerve dysfunction, often with associated unilateral cerebellar deficits; in children this is most commonly due to an ependymoma. Weakness of the upper and lower portions of the face, consistent with a peripheral or nuclear seventh nerve palsy, suggests an intrinsic brainstem lesion. Horner syndrome, consisting of ipsilateral ptosis and meiosis, is often overlooked and occurs in patients with hypothalamic lesions, as well as in patients with brainstem or upper cervical cord compromise.

Localizing signs and symptoms: supratentorial tumors

Symptoms and signs of supratentorial lesions in children are not particularly different than those in adults, with the exception that infants and young children with infiltrating lesions can present with delay or arrest in development (Table 17.5). After headaches, seizures are second in frequency as a presenting complaint of patients with supratentorial tumors. Approximately one-quarter of children with supratentorial tumors have seizures as their initial symptom, especially patients with tumors of the temporal or frontal region. The likelihood of an infiltrating tumor causing seizures is dependent on its histologic type, rate of growth, and location. Slow-growing cortical gliomas are most likely to result in convulsions; as many as 50% of patients with low-grade glial lesions will have such an event, in contrast to 20% of those with more aggressive lesions. With the increasing utilization of surgery to manage patients with intractable epilepsy, a significant number of children have been diagnosed with low-grade or indolent mixed neuronal glial lesions (gangliogliomas) as the cause of their uncontrollable seizures. Many of these patients have presented with complex partial seizures. In patients with epilepsy, features associated with an increased risk of a neoplasm include a change in the character of the seizure type in patients with preexisting seizures, status epilepticus at onset of seizures, prolonged postictal paralysis, resistance to medical control, focal symptoms, and associated focal deficits.

Focal neurologic findings, such as hemiparesis, hyperreflexia, and somewhat less frequently, sensory abnormalities, may also be present in the child with an underlying supratentorial malignancy. Such symptoms suggest a more aggressive tumor, but may also be found in children with lower-grade neoplasms. In neoplasms involving the so-called "silent" areas of the cortex (the frontal or parietal lobes), focal neurologic deficits may occur late in the course of illness and may be overshadowed by symptoms and signs of increased ICP. Frontal lobe lesions may also present with a long history of behavioral difficulties.

Suprasellar lesions notoriously result in delayed diagnosis, especially in very young children with brain tumors. Two major tumor types, the diencephalic glioma and the craniopharyngioma, are both relatively slow

Pearls and Perils

- An infiltrating chiasmatic mass, especially a chiasmatic glioma, more frequently results in complex visual field loss with variable loss of visual acuity than bitemporal hemianopsias.

growing tumors and may result in a slowly evolving clinical course and a delay in diagnosis. Chiasmatic gliomas and gliomas of other portions of the visual pathway may present with visual field loss or an insidious loss of visual acuity in one or both eyes, which may be difficult to diagnose in a young child. Chiasmatic tumors may also result in bitemporal hemianopsia, but more frequently result in more complex visual field loss. Chiasmatic gliomas also tend to result in unilateral or bilateral nystagmus with a head tilt and a constellation of findings that may be difficult to distinguish from more benign conditions such as strabismus, amblyopia, or spasm nutans. A relative afferent pupillary defect, the Marcus-Gunn pupil, is often an important clue in the early diagnosis of a visual pathway tumor. Craniopharyngiomas, although tending to occur in somewhat older patients than those with chiasmatic tumors, may also cause complex visual field deficits, but more classically result in a bitemporal visual field abnormality. Early signs and symptoms of craniopharyngiomas may be difficult to interpret in the presence of associated behavioral difficulties. Another syndrome of diencephalic lesions that often results in delayed diagnosis is a constellation of failure to thrive and emaciation in an otherwise seemingly "normal" child with adequate appetite and gastrointestinal function; this is known as the *diencephalic syndrome*. In retrospect, often these children are not euphoric but are rather irritable, have some component of developmental delay, and, on careful testing, may have ophthalmologic dysfunction, especially nystagmus.

Another syndrome that may become apparent in children is the Parinaud syndrome, caused by compression of the midbrain. This is primarily due to pineal region tumors, although a similar syndrome can be caused by dilatation of the third ventricle. It is manifest by poor saccadic upward gaze (with relatively preserved pursuit), slightly dilated pupils that react on accommodation but not to light, retraction or convergence nystagmus, and lid retraction.

Staging and risk stratification

Staging is a major component of the management of many forms of childhood brain tumors. The classical tumor, metastasis, nodes (TMN) staging system is generally not appropriate for childhood brain tumors, since extra-CNS spread at the time of diagnosis is very unusual and nodal involvement is not a clinical issue. However, for some tumor types that readily disseminate through the CNS at the time of diagnosis, evaluation of extent of disease at time of diagnosis is a critical part of disease planning. Tumors that have a high predilection for spread at diagnosis include medulloblastoma, pineoblastoma, germ cell tumors, and atypical teratoid tumors. Other lesions, such as cortical primitive neuroectodermal tumors, ependymomas, and high- and low-grade gliomas, may be spread at time of diagnosis, but the majority are localized to the primary site until later in disease.

Evaluation for extent of disease usually requires MRI and evaluation of CSF. To overcome the issue of postoperative artifact, MRI of the entire neuroaxis is best performed prior to surgery, if there is likelihood that the tumor is of the histologic type that may disseminate early in illness. The M-staging system is usually graded on a 0–4 basis, with M0 disease representing no evidence of metastatic spread, M1 disease denoting positive CSF cy-

Table 17.5 Supratentorial tumors of childhood: Signs and symptoms

Tumor type	Peak age at diagnosis	Duration of symptoms prior to diagnosis	Common signs and symptoms
Cortical low-grade gliomas	Variable	Month to years	Seizures, nonspecific headaches, focal deficits later
Diencephalic gliomas	More common first decade of life; Peak under age 3	Variable, often months	Visualize loss, visual field loss, diencephalic syndrome, nystagmus, hemiparesis (thalamic)
Germ cell tumors	Second decade of life; Peak 10–14 years of age	2–4 months pineal; ? longer suprasellar	Headaches, vomiting, Parinaud syndrome (pineal), precocious or delayed puberty (suprasellar)
Ependymoma	Peak in infancy	Variable; usually brief	Seizures, focal deficits, headache
Craniopharyngioma	Any time, median age 8 years	Often prolonged, > 6 months	Headache, visual field loss, change in personality, falling school performance

Pearls and Perils

- Evaluation for tumor dissemination requires both magnetic resonance imaging (MRI) and cerebrospinal fluid (CSF) analysis; MRI of the entire neuroaxis is best performed prior to surgery.

Consider Consultation When...

- Consider consultation with a neuroradiologist when a brain tumor is believed likely to determine the optimum imaging that should be undertaken, including the potential utility of magnetic resonance spectroscopy (MRS) and functional magnetic resonance imaging (fMRI).

tology, and M2–M3 disease denoting spread of disease visible on neuroimaging to the spinal leptomeninges or other regions of brain. Spread outside the CNS at the time of diagnosis (M4 disease) is quite infrequent and occurs primarily in young infants.

When staging was initially introduced into the management of childhood brain tumors, the T-stage, or tumor size, was often assessed on the combination of preoperative imaging and the impressions of the surgeon at the time of surgery. This type of T-staging has essentially been supplanted by postoperative imaging. In an attempt to avoid confusion between residual tumor and postsurgical changes, such postoperative imaging is usually performed within 48 hours after surgery.

Age at the time of diagnosis, although not a true staging parameter, is also utilized to stratify patients, as a very young age at the time of diagnosis (less than 3 years of age for children with medulloblastoma) has been related to a poorer outcome for children with medulloblastoma. It is unclear whether this is related to an age-dependent biologic difference between tumors and/or because treatment utilized for younger children differs from that given to older patients.

The results of staging studies are utilized for treatment planning and stratification of tumors into risk groups. It is likely that current disease stratification schemas will dramatically change with the incorporation of molecular genetic tumor findings.

Neuroimaging

Magnetic resonance imaging is clearly the imaging modality of choice for assessment of brain tumors, offering improved sensitivity over computed tomography (CT). The speed and availability of CT, however, often results in it being used as first line imaging for children with suspected intracranial pathology. CT can also provide complementary information to MRI. Intratumoral calcifications, for example in craniopharyngioma, and bony erosion or remodeling, are better detected by CT. Further, CT can provide useful information on hemorrhage and tumor cellularity.

The superior image contrast of MRI allows early detection of changes in tissue composition, while its multiplanar capabilities offers improved tumor localization. MRI makes it possible for a tumor to be accurately located within either the intra- or extra-axial space or the ventricular system, an important distinction for subsequent differential diagnosis. High-resolution 3D imaging provides even more detailed anatomy, an important adjunct for surgical or radiotherapy planning. Functional MRI (fMRI) can prove to be a useful adjunct to surgical planning of brain tumors, providing valuable data on the tumor location with respect to important structures, such as the sensorimotor cortex.

MRI offers more than simple detection and localization of a tumor, it also provides the means to assess tumor composition, thus help determine pathologic type. A multitude of MR sequences are available to offer improved tissue characterization.

Post-gadolinium T1-weighted sequences also provide a sensitive means for detecting leptomeningeal or subependymal metastases, although there is some indication that post-gadolinium fluid attenuated inversion recovery (FLAIR) images may be even more sensitive in some tumors. In tumors in which metastatic involvement of the spine is common, it is preferable to undertake full staging prior to surgery, as postoperative findings can cause false-positive findings.

MR spectroscopy (MRS), diffusion, and perfusion imaging offer a further means of improving imaging specificity by supplementing anatomic findings with functional data. MRS can be performed with single-voxel or multi-voxel techniques. Single-voxel studies have faster acquisition times and better spectral resolution, and require a fairly large voxel size (6–8 cm^3); tissue composition within the voxel must be homogeneous, otherwise partial volume averaging of tissue of various compositions occurs. Spectroscopic analysis of a large volume of cerebral tissue with multiple small voxels (1 cm^3) is feasible with multi-voxel studies (or MRS imaging, MRSI). MRS can differentiate normal from tumor tissue, as tumor tissue in general shows elevation of choline and decrease in N-acetyl-aspartate (NAA).

Signal on diffusion images can reflect cellular density and microarchitecture. The apparent diffusion coefficient (ADC), a measure of the ability of tissue to restrict water diffusion, decreases with increasing cellularity and tumor grade.

Perfusion imaging can be performed with techniques based on dynamic susceptibility contrast (DSC) or based on vascular permeability. Regional blood volume (rCBV) can be estimated from either technique; rCBV can reflect the neovascularization associated with tumor growth (tumor angiogenesis); in nonpilocytic glial tumors, angiogenesis is highly correlated to tumor grade.

Neuropathology

Primary brain tumors constitute a remarkably diverse group of lesions, derived from any of the many normal cellular constituents, with all possible degrees of differentiation. They have a wide variety of macroscopic and histologic appearances; therefore, it is not surprising that many attempts have been made to produce a classification that would be universally accepted. The first attempt is nearly 150 years old; the last one—only a few years old—has become the official World Health Organization (WHO) classification.

The revised WHO classification has adopted the basic principle of histologic typing, in which tumors are defined primarily by morphologic appearances, including constituent cell type and tissue pattern. The overall aim is to classify the neoplasms, whenever possible, according to their histogenesis. From this point of view, modern investigative techniques, such as those of genetics and immunohistochemistry, are of great help.

Molecular genetics

To date, only a small number of genetic alterations have been identified for childhood brain tumors; most have been described in medulloblastoma. However, with the advent of technology that allows for high-throughput genetic screening, a broader range of gene expression patterns in various childhood brain tumors is beginning to emerge, and their molecular pathogenesis is becoming more clearly defined.

Medulloblastoma and supratentorial primitive neuroectodermal tumors

Isochromosome 17q is the most common cytogenetic alteration in medulloblastoma, occurring in up to 50% of tumors; however, a clear association between 17p loss and clinical outcome has not been found. Supratentorial primitive neuroectodermal tumors (PNETs), which have an identical histologic appearance, do not have isochromosome 17q, suggesting that these tumors are molecularly distinct.

The neurotrophin-3 receptor TRKC was the first molecular alteration that was shown to be an independent predictor of medulloblastoma outcome (Grotzer et al. 2002) Tumor expression of TRKC directly correlates with good outcome, presumably by acting to promote the differentiation of primitive medulloblastoma cells. Expression of ErbB2, a member of the epidermal growth factor receptor (EGFR) family, and the *MYCC* oncogene independently correlates with adverse outcome in medulloblastoma. ErbB2 protein has been detected in up to 85% of medulloblastomas. *MYCC* amplification is seen in only 5% of medulloblastomas, but its presence is associated with the aggressive large-cell anaplastic medulloblastoma variant, which is uniformly fatal.

Medulloblastomas arise in patients with nevoid basal cell carcinoma syndrome (Gorlin syndrome), a condition caused by a somatic mutation of the patched (PTCH) gene on chromosome 9q22. *PTCH* is an important regulator of the sonic hedgehog (Shh) pro-mitogenic signaling pathway. Gorlin syndrome accounts for 1–2% of all medulloblastomas, most commonly of the desmoplastic subtype. Mutations in this pathway have also been identified in 2–10% of sporadically occurring medulloblastomas. Metastatic medulloblastoma, in comparison to nonmetastatic medulloblastoma, is associated with significant overexpression of the platelet-derived growth factor (PDGF) receptor and the downstream RAS oncogenic pathway (MacDonald et al. 2001).

Glioma

In comparison to adult gliomas, the molecular changes associated with childhood gliomas are less well defined. Low-grade gliomas, usually of the optic nerves and chiasm, occur in about 15% of children with NF1, and more than half of all patients diagnosed with optic pathway gliomas will have underlying NF1.

More recent evidence shows that childhood and adult gliomas differ in the incidence of EGFR gene amplification and mutations of the TP53 and PTEN tumor suppressor genes. Overexpression of EGFR is seen in 60–80% of high-grade gliomas in children and adults, but amplification of the EGFR gene, found in 40% of adult high-grade tumors, is rarely seen in childhood gliomas. *PTEN* mutations occur in only 8% of high-grade lesions in children, compared to 30% of adult high-grade tumors; however, *PTEN* mutations are associated with decreased survival among children with high-grade gliomas.

Atypical teratoid/rhabdoid tumors

One of the most important molecular genetic alterations in childhood brain tumors is the discovery of hSNF5/INI1 gene mutations in association with atypical teratoid/rhabdoid tumors (AT/RT). AT/RT has sometimes been confused with medulloblastoma and PNET, but now screening for hSNF5/INI1 mutations can confirm the molecular diagnosis of AT/RT, which has important prognostic and therapeutic implications.

General aspects of therapy

Surgery

Considerable changes occurring over the past decade have facilitated increased success in obtaining meaningful tumor resections while concomitantly decreasing perioperative surgical morbidity and mortality. A number of studies have demonstrated the effectiveness of total or "near-total" resections in improving long-term survival of children with malignant brain tumors. Surgical techniques have improved because of better preoperative planning, minimal exposure, safer intraoperative methods of tumor resection, and the increasing utilization of real-time visualization of tumor location.

In the operating room, current technology permits real-time localization of tumor and surrounding brain when coupled with preoperative CT, MRI, and angiographic studies. The wider availability of intraoperative MRI has led to improved capabilities of assessing the degree of surgical resection in the operating room and, consequently, a more exact intraoperative assessment of the extent of surgical removal of tumor. These advances have been critical in allowing minimalization of the surgical arena, which allows localization of tumors with a 1–2 mm degree of accuracy, and offers the surgeon the opportunity to plan surgical trajectories while avoiding adjacent critical structures. Current systems utilizing a fixed-pin rigid immobilization of the patient's head are being improved to permit surface mapping of the patient's head and face, which will bring this advance to the previously excluded group of infants. In the push for minimizing surgical exposure and risk to surrounding brain, endoscopic techniques continue to evolve. Intraventricular tumors are particularly amenable to this approach and may be successfully biopsied through a burr hole and removed by the endoscope. This is particularly valuable for pineal tumors with extension into the third ventricle, colloid cysts, and other intraventricular lesions. Tumor resection techniques have also improved, offering the surgeon a number of different methods for safer removal. Laser (YAG, CO_2), ultrasonic aspiration, and electromechanical disruption now offer the surgeon the ability to safely remove lesions in previously inaccessible locations while minimizing direct trauma to surrounding tissues.

Radiotherapy

Radiotherapy is a component of management of all malignant and many benign brain tumors of childhood. Children are a special challenge to radiation oncologists, and sedation or anesthesia is usually necessary for younger patients to allow for the precision required. Pre- and post-treatment MRI and CT are often co-registered to most exactly define the target volume. A variety of newer treatment planning systems allow optimization of dose distribution in three dimensions. These techniques have different names, but all are a variation of conformal therapy utilizing multiple beams, with individual beams shaping the radiation portal. The primary form of radiotherapy used is photons. Electrons have also been used to treat the spinal axis and, more recently, proton beam irradiation has been utilized at a few select centers to spare radiation exposure to the noninvolved brain and other surrounding organs.

The choice of the total dose and volume of radiotherapy is not only dependent on the type of tumor present but, in great part, on the tolerance of the normal surrounding brain. The latter is related to the age of the child, the volume of radiotherapy needed, and other poorly understood host factors. Conventionally, daily fractions of 1.8 cGy of radiation therapy are utilized. Total doses of local radiotherapy range between 4,500 and 5,580 cGy, with children harboring aggressive lesions requiring the higher doses of radiotherapy. For many pediatric tumors, including medulloblastoma, pineoblastoma, and germ cell tumors, treatment is initiated with craniospinal radiotherapy because of the high likelihood of spread or disease recurrence outside the primary site, with additional local boost radiotherapy given to control primary site disease. Doses of craniospinal radiotherapy are also, in part, age-dependent. A dose of 3,600 cGy of craniospinal radiation therapy has been conventionally utilized for aggressive CNS tumors. The neurocognitive and endocrinologic sequelae associated with such treatment have resulted in a reduction of radiation dose in craniospinal radiation therapy by one-third (to 2,400 cGy) or greater to decrease long-term sequelae. Similarly, for younger children, craniospinal radiation therapy is often reduced or delayed, in an attempt to diminish permanent damage.

Alterations in the dose fractionation schedule of radiotherapy, such as utilizing radiotherapy in smaller doses multiple times per day instead of larger doses once per day, have theoretical advantages; however, such approaches have yet to show improved survival or decreased sequelae.

Local treatment failure remains the predominant form of disease relapse; thus, there has been significant interest in using other types of radiotherapy to improve local disease control. These include techniques such as brachytherapy, stereotactic irradiation (including boost radiotherapy), and the use of radioactive colloidal solutions. Stereotactic radiation therapy includes an increasing array of options such as the cobalt-60 beam system (the knife) or other focused radiotherapy techniques. Because of the types of tumors occurring in children and the risk of at least transient increased swelling with these techniques, they are appropriate for only a minority of patients. Stereotactic radiation may also be utilized to deliver fractionated treatment, which may result in a reduced exposure of the surrounding brain, with fewer short-term sequelae. Radiocolloid solutions have been predominantly utilized to treat cysts, especially in patients with craniopharyngiomas. Brachytherapy, although having significant theoretic advantages, has not been widely utilized in pediatrics. Attempts are being made to increase cellular radiosensitivity using specific hypoxic cell sensitizers and chemotherapeutic agents that possess radiosensitizing properties (such as the platinum derivatives).

Chemotherapy

Within the last decade, chemotherapy has had an expanded role in the treatment of childhood brain tumors, largely because of efforts to avoid or delay the need for radiotherapy, particularly in infants and young children in whom the risk of radiation-induced neurotoxicity is greatest. Yet, the success of chemotherapy has remained somewhat limited. Two major reasons for this limitation are impediment to drug delivery across the blood–brain barrier (BBB) and chemotherapy resistance. Newer therapeutic strategies have thus been designed to (a) overcome the BBB, (b) decrease resistance to chemotherapy, or (c) utilize drugs that specifically target tumor biology.

The goal of high-dose chemotherapy (HDCT) is to effectively increase the delivery of cytotoxic agents to the tumor by overcoming the limited permeability of the BBB. Several trials have been conducted in children with primary and refractory malignant brain tumors utilizing myeloablative or myelosuppressive HDCT, with either autologous bone marrow transplant (ABMT) or peripheral blood stem cell (PBSC) support. Classic lipid-soluble alkylating agents, which have non-overlapping hematologic toxicities and show little cross-resistance, have been predominantly investigated. The most impressive responses have been noted in medulloblastoma and possibly malignant tumors arising in children younger than 3 years of age. Despite the promising responses observed, the toxicity associated with these regimens was high (5–15% death rate). In an effort to reduce this toxicity, more recent investigations have used multiple cycles of somewhat lower doses of chemotherapy followed by PBSC support.

Consider Consultation When…

- Early in the course of treatment a pediatric oncologist or neuro-oncologist should be involved to determine the potential benefit of adjuvant chemotherapy.

Intrathecal or intraventricular administration of cytotoxic agents is an alternative method to increase tumor exposure to chemotherapy, as well as to control leptomeningeal tumor dissemination. To date, these methods have been limited by the lack of available active agents that can be given by this route of administration. Convection-enhanced intracavitary and intratumoral delivery of radionuclide- and immunotoxin-conjugated antibodies is the most recent regional strategy that has the added advantage of directed tumor targeting, but these agents have yet to demonstrate improved survival.

The BBB is disrupted and leaky at various sites within the tumor vasculature and is one reason why water-soluble alkylators and platinum compounds have shown activity against pediatric brain tumors. For these reasons, agents that further disrupt the BBB, such as synthetic bradykinin agonists, have been developed to take advantage of the physiologic response to active hydrophilic compounds, but they have yet to show clear-cut benefit. Other means to disrupt the BBB by using compounds such as mannitol prior to chemotherapeutic drug infusion have been used with some evidence of increased efficacy.

Strategies to overcome tumor resistance to drug therapy have been employed with some success. A key example of this has been with the alkylator, temozolomide, which has shown activity against malignant gliomas in adults. A major resistance mechanism against this drug is DNA alkylation repair via the enzyme AGT. The drug 0-6-benzylguanine depletes tumor AGT levels thus rendering the tumor more sensitive to temozolomide.

Biologic therapy

Therapy that specifically targets tumor biology has gained recent attention. In contrast to traditional chemotherapy, biologic therapy can be cytostatic rather than cytotoxic. Examples of this include differentiation therapy with retinoid derivatives, gene therapy with thymidine kinase and ganciclovir treatment, angiogenesis inhibitors, receptor tyrosine kinase inhibitors such as anti-EGFR small molecules, and farnesyl transferase inhibitors that block Ras oncogene activation. All of these approaches are in active study.

Specific tumor types

Medulloblastoma

Medulloblastoma is the most common malignant primary CNS tumor of childhood, accounting for 40% of all posterior fossa tumors and 15–20% of all brain tumors (Packer et al. 1994) (Table 17.6). The tumor has a bimodal peak in incidence, arising most commonly in children between 3 and 5 years of age and then again peaking at the end of the first decade of life. Medulloblastomas

Table 17.6 Posterior fossa tumors

Discriminating features
- Cerebellar astrocytoma
  - Pathologic examination
- Medulloblastoma
  - Pathologic examination
- Brainstem tumor
  - Fusiform swelling of brainstem on MRI or computed tomography (CT)
- Ependymoma
  - Pathologic examination

Consistent features
- Cerebellar astrocytoma
  - Ataxia (usually appendicular, may be truncal)
  - Papilledema
  - CT or MRI shows cystic lesion with mural nodule in cerebellum
- Medulloblastoma
  - Truncal ataxia
  - Short course
  - Papilledema
  - Neuroimaging shows noncystic midline cerebellar lesion
- Brainstem tumor
  - Ataxia
  - Long tract signs
  - Cranial nerve signs
  - Short course
- Ependymoma
  - Ataxia
  - Obliteration of fourth ventricle on CT or MRI
  - Papilledema

Variable features
- Brainstem tumor
  - Feeding and swallowing abnormalities
  - Symptoms and signs of intracranial pressure (late)
- Ependymoma
  - Symptoms and signs of increased intracranial pressure
  - Neck pain and stiffness

are more common in males, with a 2:1 male-to-female ratio.

In children, medulloblastomas most commonly arise in the midline, seeming to arise from the cerebellum in the region of the roof of the fourth ventricle, causing early symptoms and signs of increased ICP, as the tumor fills the fourth ventricle and causes obstruction of CSF flow. Although up to one-third of patients with medulloblastoma will have disseminated disease at the time of diagnosis, usually this dissemination is subclinical, and back pain and leg weakness secondary to spinal cord involvement is uncommon at presentation (Table 17.7).

In young children, clinical presentation may be subtle, as cerebellar deficits are often overlooked early in the

Table 17.7 Pathology and course of posterior fossa tumors

Discriminating features
- Cerebellar astrocytoma
  - Cerebellar hemisphere or midline
  - Cystic with mural nodule
  - Less frequently diffuse
  - Seldom spreads
- Medulloblastoma
  - Mostly midline of cerebellum
  - Seeds subarachnoid space early in course
- Brainstem tumor
  - Triad of ataxia, cranial neuropathies, and long tract signs suggests brainstem pathology
- Ependymoma
  - In ventricle
  - May invade brainstem

Consistent features
- Cerebellar astrocytoma
  - Papilledema secondary to obstructive hydrocephalus
  - Greater than 95% survival rate for cystic type, somewhat less for diffuse
  - Cured with surgery alone if mural nodule removed
- Medulloblastoma
  - Respond to radiotherapy
  - Midline mass without cyst on CT
  - Rapidly progressive with short course of symptoms
- Brainstem tumor
  - Astrocytomas most common pathology
  - Hypodense lesion on CT suggests malignant course
  - Rapid course to death
- Ependymoma
  - Require adjuvant therapy following surgery
  - Homogeneous fourth-ventricle mass on CT

Variable features
- Cerebellar astrocytoma
  - On recurrence may require radiotherapy
  - Malignant glioma unusual
- Medulloblastoma
  - Survival rate of 50% to 70%, depending on age, location, and degree of removal at surgery
  - Certain subsets respond to chemotherapy
- Brainstem tumor
  - Response to therapy limited
  - Survival rate of 15% to 30 five-year
  - A small subset may be long-term survivors
  - Surgery may be effective in patients with cervical/medullary or exophytic tumors
- Ependymoma
  - May metastasize to CSF
  - Clinical course and response to radiotherapy and chemotherapy variable
  - Survival varies with age, location, degree of surgical removal, and presence of CSF seeding

course of illness and there may be macrocephaly, intermittent lethargy, a bulging fontanel, and the setting-sun sign. Patients with medulloblastoma may also present in extremis with abrupt onset or change in mental status, severe headaches, and obtundation. Although this may be due to acute obstruction of CSF flow, it may also be due to hemorrhage within the tumor and sudden expansion of the lesion.

Neuroimaging

In young children, medulloblastoma commonly occurs as a midline posterior fossa mass, originating in the inferior medullary velum and expanding to fill the fourth ventricle. (Figure 17.2). In approximately a third of cases, medulloblastoma invades the posterior aspect of the brainstem. In older children and adolescents, medulloblastoma often arises laterally near the cerebellopontine angle or in the cerebellar hemisphere. Mild to moderate surrounding edema may be evident, and obstructive hydrocephalus commonly occurs. The tumor's dense cellularity results in hyperdensity on CT, isointense signal on FLAIR T2-weighted images, and bright signal on diffusion images. Following contrast, the tumor shows moderate to brisk enhancement in about 75% of cases, and little or no enhancement in 25%. The tumor is usually homogeneous in appearance; however, the presence of foci of calcification or necrosis may cause a more heterogeneous pattern. Metastatic disease, when present, is commonly seen in the posterior fossa cisterns, the anterior third ventricle, the sylvian fissures, the spinal subarachnoid space and, rarely, within brain parenchyma.

Microscopy

The classic medulloblastoma is composed of densely packed cells with hyperchromatic, round to oval or carrot-shaped nuclei and indiscernible cytoplasm (Figure 17.3).

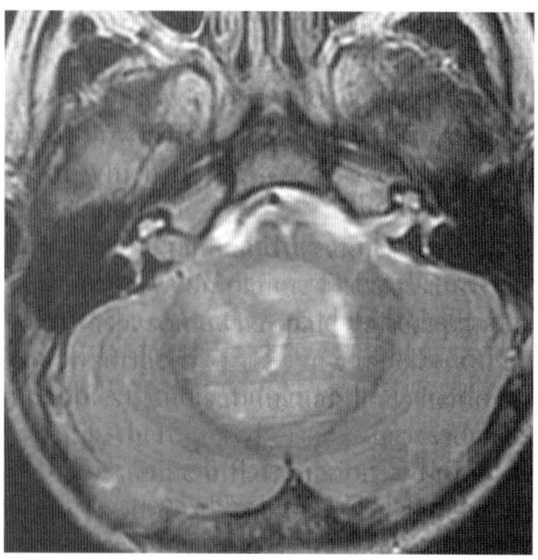

Figure 17.2 Axial T2-weighted image of the posterior fossa shows a characteristically isointense medulloblastoma filling the fourth ventricle and involving the right internal auditory canal.

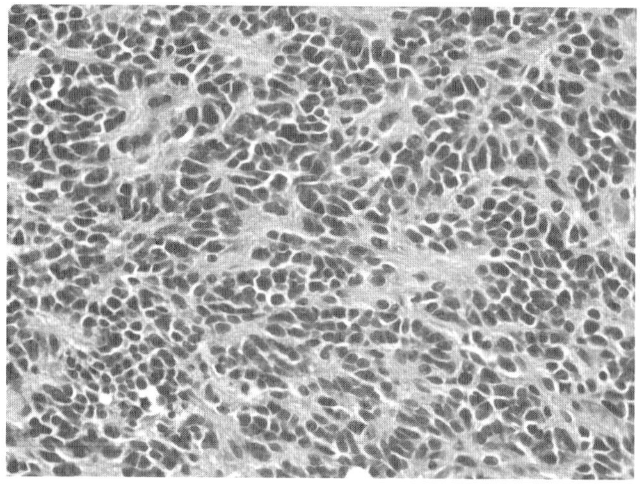

Figure 17.3 Classical medulloblastoma is characterized by Homer-Wright rosettes, histologic expression of neuroblastic differentiation (hemolysin and eosin stain).

Homer Wright rosettes, which consist of tumor cell nuclei disposed in a circular fashion around tangled cytoplasm processes, are a histologic hallmark of medulloblastomas but are observed in only 40% of cases. Mitoses are usually numerous and the growth fraction, as determined by the antibodies Ki-67/MIB-1, has been reported to vary greatly, with values up to 40%. These tumors may be strongly immunoreactive for vimentin and at least focally for synaptophysin. The desmoplastic variant is characterized by a dense intercellular network of reticulin fibers with lucent, reticulin-free nodular zone or "pale island." The large cell/anaplastic medulloblastoma is an uncommon, highly malignant variant, histologically characterized by monotonously large cells with vesicular nuclei, prominent nucleoli and more abundant cytoplasm.

Management and outcome

Of all primary CNS tumors of childhood, staging is most integral to the management of medulloblastoma (Table 17.8). Depending on age, 10–30% of children with medulloblastoma will have evidence of dissemination, as confirmed by pre- or post-MRI of the entire neuroaxis and lumbar CSF cytological examination. Determination of neuroaxis dissemination can be quite difficult in patients

Table 17.8 Stratification: Medulloblastoma

	High risk (any factor)	Average risk
Age	<3 years	≥3 years
Resection	Subtotal; biopsy	Total; Near-total
Extent	Disseminated	Localized
Histology	Anaplastic	Desmoplastic
Biologic parameters	↑ Erbb2, ↑ nMyc	↑ TrKC

Key Clinical Questions

Prior to initiation of therapy, clinical information which must be addressed for children with medulloblastoma include:

- What is the extent of disease at the time of diagnosis, as assessed by neuroimaging of the entire neuroaxis and cerebrospinal fluid cytologic examination?
- What is the degree of surgical resection necessary, as assessed by postoperative neuroimaging?

Other important factors may include the histopathologic appearance of the tumor and specific molecular genetic tumor characteristics.

with nonenhancing lesions. In multicentered studies, central neuroradiographic review disclosed incorrectly interpreted studies in nearly 10% of patients and suboptimally obtained images in another 10–15% (Packer et al. 2006). Dissemination within the neuroaxis is most common in infants, and occurs in approximately 10% of adolescents and teenagers. Based on the amount of disease left after surgery, the extent of neuroaxial spread at the time of diagnosis, histologic features, and the age of the patients, children with medulloblastoma have been separated into so-called "average-risk" or "high-risk" disease.

Extraneural spread can occur in patients with medulloblastoma, but probably is present at the time of diagnosis in less than 1% of patients. Infants are at somewhat higher risk of having extraneural spread, but staging for disease outside the nervous system, with techniques such as bone scans and bone marrows, are infrequently informative. Molecular genetic findings are likely to significantly alter the way medulloblastoma patients are stratified. Tumor overexpression or upregulation of a variety of different genes have been related to prognosis, but these molecular markers have not yet been fully incorporated into stratification schemas (Pomeroy et al. 2002).

Multiple studies have demonstrated that the extent of resection is related to outcome, as patients who undergo a "complete" resection have a better prognosis. Extent of surgical resection has never been shown to be predictive of outcome in patients with disseminated disease at the time of diagnosis. Furthermore, no clear evidence suggests that patients who undergo a significant tumor resection (a near-total resection) have a different prognosis than patients who have had a "total" resection. Surgical resection has been associated with morbidity. Between 10% and 25% of patients with medulloblastoma will develop the "posterior-fossa mutism syndrome" following surgery (Robertson et al. 2006). This is an ill-defined constellation of findings, which includes the delayed onset mutism, cranial nerve dysfunction (suprabulbar dysfunction), hypotonia, cerebellar deficits, and severe emotional lability (Table 17.9). This syndrome results in significant long-term sequelae in nearly 50% of affected patients. The etiology of the posterior fossa mutism syndrome is not fully understood, and it has not been clearly related to surgical technique. Damage to the cerebellar vermis, with resultant disruption of critical neural pathways, has been implicated as the most likely cause of the syndrome.

Table 17.9 Posterior fossa mutism syndrome

- Can occur post-op in any posterior-fossa tumor; primarily medulloblastoma
- Delayed onset (? 24 hours) mutism
- Other symptoms
  - Hypotonia
  - Ataxia
  - Supranuclear cranial nerve palsies
  - Agitation
  - Emotional liability
- Visual loss

Standard postoperative treatment for children with medulloblastoma over 3 years of age includes the use of craniospinal radiotherapy coupled with adjuvant chemotherapy. Although chemotherapy has never been demonstrated in a prospective randomized trial to improve survival over treatment with radiotherapy alone, it has become a basic component of treatment for all children with medulloblastoma, based primarily on the results of single-armed studies. Chemotherapy given prior to radiotherapy has been shown, in some studies, to result in decreased overall survival, as compared to treatment with immediate postoperative radiotherapy and chemotherapy during and after radiotherapy. Radiotherapy has conventionally been given to the entire neuroaxis at the time of diagnosis, as treatment with local radiotherapy alone results in long-term disease control in probably less than 10% of patients. The dose of craniospinal radiation therapy can safely be reduced to 2,400 cGy in patients with localized disease at the time of diagnosis. The dose to the primary site has remained at 5,400–5,580 cGy, and studies are presently underway to determine if the volume of local site irradiation can be safely decreased, with conformal techniques, to the tumor site alone, instead of the entire posterior fossa. This is being performed primarily in attempts to avoid cochlear irradiation and decrease ototoxicity.

For patients with poor-risk disease (see Table 17.4), treatment with radiotherapy alone (3,600 cGy of craniospinal radiotherapy and 5,580 cGy of local radiotherapy) usually results in a 40% or less likelihood of long-term survival. The addition of chemotherapy probably increases the likelihood of disease control by another

20% (Gajjar et al. 2006). Attempts are presently under way to improve survival by altering the timing or type of chemotherapy utilized. High-dose chemotherapy, supported by peripheral stem cell rescue, is one approach under evaluation. Another therapeutic intervention being explored is the use of chemotherapy or other agents during radiotherapy in attempts to enhance the efficacy of the radiotherapy delivered.

The management of infants with medulloblastoma remains problematic. The use of radiotherapy in infants and very young children carries with it a high risk of severe, long-term neurocognitive and endocrinologic sequelae. Present management of infants and young children include the use of chemotherapy with agents such as cisplatinum, cyclophosphamide, vincristine, and VP-16. Investigations are under way to intensify the use of chemotherapy, especially with the use of peripheral stem cell support, and incorporate newer chemotherapeutic agents or chemotherapy delivered intrathecally (methotrexate), in an attempt to prevent leptomeningeal disease progression or relapse. Preliminary evidence suggests that these high-dose regimens may be more effective. In some subsets of infants with medulloblastoma, primarily in those with desmoplastic tumors, chemotherapy alone has resulted in a 70% or higher likelihood of long-term control. There is also the consideration of utilizing local radiotherapy after chemotherapy in those children with localized disease, although this approach carries with it the likelihood of increased neurologic sequelae.

Ependymoma

Ependymomas most frequently occur in young children, with more than half of the cases diagnosed before 5 years of age (Horn et al. 1999). These tumors typically present with nonspecific and nonlocalizing signs and symptoms related to increased ICP. Infratentorial tumors often display cerebellar dysfunction and multiple lower cranial nerve findings, especially VI, VII, VIII, IX, and X. Supratentorial tumors may present with seizures and focal cerebral deficits.

Neuroimaging

The majority of posterior fossa ependymomas arise within the fourth ventricle; however, occasionally they may arise from ependymal rests located within the cerebral hemispheres (Figure 17.4). Insinuation of a fourth ventricular tumor inferiorly into the foramen of Magendie, or laterally in the foramen of Luschka, provides supportive evidence for an ependymoma, over other posterior fossa tumors. Tumors commonly cause obstructive hydrocephalus. Supratentorial tumors are commonly large at presentation, most often presenting as a cortical mass; lesions often comprise large cysts, with significant surrounding mass effect.

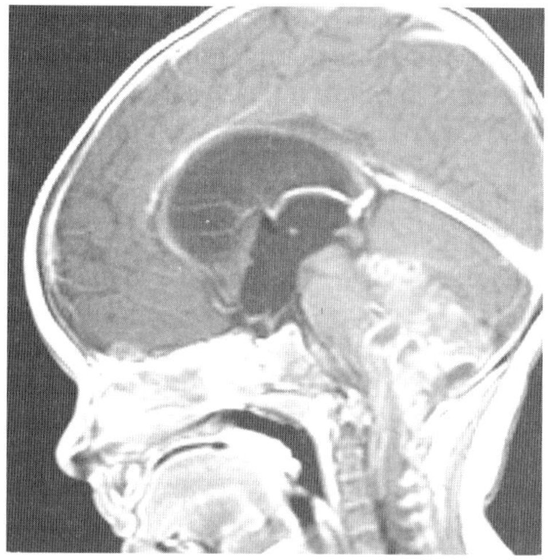

Figure 17.4 Sagittal post-gadolinium T1-weighted image of the brain shows an enhancing ependymoma filling the fourth ventricle, extending into the upper cervical spinal canal, in front of and behind the spinal cord.

Posterior fossa ependymomas have calcification in about 50% of cases, occasional small cysts, and hemorrhage; thus, they have a more heterogeneous imaging appearance than medulloblastoma. Imaging characteristics are therefore variable; however, solid tumor components are often iso- or hyperdense on CT and isointense to gray matter on T2-weighted imaging. As would be expected, contrast enhancement is heterogeneous. Subarachnoid spread is far less common than with medulloblastoma.

Microscopy

The classical variant of this tumor is characterized by a peculiar cellular pattern. The WHO classification distinguishes four subtypes: cellular, papillary, clear cell, and tanycytic. The cellular type is composed of densely packed cells with little tendency to form pseudorosettes and rosettes. Papillary ependymoma resembles choroid plexus papilloma without assuming the frond-like, overtly papillary characteristics of the latter. The clear-cell tumors are composed of cells with well-demarcated, clear cytoplasm and need to be distinguished from oligodendrogliomas. Finally, the tanycytic variant is characterized by markedly elongated cells with highly fibrillary processes.

Management and outcome

Therapeutic intervention begins with an accurate histologic diagnosis, as well as reasonable attempt at total tumor resection. The single greatest factor in determining long-term survival is the degree of tumor resection for both supratentorial and infratentorial tumors (Horn et al. 1999). Surgical considerations will vary by tumor location. Resection of midline posterior fossa ependymomas often involves dissection of the floor of the fourth ventricle with an expected high level of morbidity, whereas

Pearls and Perils

- The most important determinant of outcome for patients with ependymomas is the degree of surgical resection.

more lateral lesions originating in the cerebellopontine angle often manifest complications related to cranial nerve manipulation or ischemic changes due to vascular insufficiency after spasm or direct vessel injury. Due to the tumor or its resection, multiple lower cranial nerve palsies and long-term neurologic impairment may occur. In addition, the 20–40% progression rate for patients without residual disease on postoperative imaging suggests that a significant number of tumors have extensive microscopic residual disease. Progression in almost all cases is local, with distant relapse occurring in less than 10% of cases. The positive role of complete resection and the predominance for local recurrence has led to the concept of second-look surgery for tumors that have been incompletely resected.

Conformal radiotherapy to 50–55 Gy for supratentorial tumors and 55–59 Gy for infratentorial tumors is the standard postoperative treatment of nondisseminated ependymomas. Five-year survival is best for patients who have been totally resected and receive postoperative local radiotherapy, ranging in the 60% to as high as 75% range rate in some series (Merchant et al. 2005). Studies are presently under way assessing the feasibility of omitting radiation, until the time of progression, for patients with "totally" resected "benign," supratentorial tumors.

Despite several trials demonstrating measurable disease responses, the role of chemotherapy in the treatment of ependymoma has not been established (Robertson et al. 1998). In single-agent trials, platinum compounds have been the most active, and increasing evidence suggests that ependymomas are somewhat chemosensitive.

Preliminary studies support the potential use of chemotherapy in infants in an effort to delay radiation therapy or in children with incompletely resected tumors as an adjunct to second-look surgery prior to radiation therapy. Objective response may be seen in nearly 50% of patients, and chemotherapy-only regimens have controlled disease in up to 40% of infants (Grundy et al. 2007).

Cerebellar Astrocytoma

Infratentorial astrocytomas account for 12–18% of all pediatric brain tumors. The majority of childhood cerebellar astrocytomas are low-grade, primarily pilocytic astrocytomas.

Patients with cerebellar astrocytomas may present with increased ICP or with focal findings secondary to direct compression of adjacent neural structures (e.g., tectum, cranial nerves, etc.). Compression of the aqueduct of Sylvius or the fourth ventricular outflow may lead to the development of hydrocephalus with the attendant pressure-related symptoms. More direct involvement of cranial nerves and cerebellar nuclei may manifest with variable cranial neuropathies, dysconjugate gaze, tinnitus, vertigo, or dysmetria.

Neuroimaging

The cerebellar astrocytoma arises more commonly from the vermis than the hemisphere. Rarely, it may arise solely within a cerebellar hemisphere (Figure 17.5). Surrounding mass effect is common, leading to obstructive hydrocephalus at the fourth ventricle.

The typical appearance of the tumor is that of a predominantly cystic lesion with a mural nodule. The tumor nodule is either rounded or plaque-like; the cyst can be round or ovoid and is usually unilocular. The walls of the cyst are usually thin and do not enhance. Other tumors will be solid (20%) or present mixed solid and microcystic components. Ten to 20% are calcified on CT. The solid portions are commonly iso- to hypodense on CT, hypointense on T1-weighted imaging and hyperintense on T2-weighted imaging. At least some part of the tumor shows evidence of strong enhancement, commonly the mural nodule, or the more solid part of a necrotic tumor.

Microscopy

The typical tumor demonstrates a biphasic pattern in which highly fibrillated, pilocytic areas are intermingled

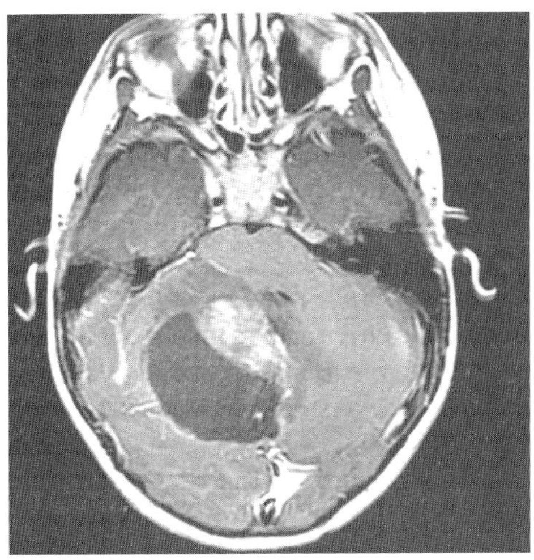

Figure 17.5 Axial post-gadolinium T1-weighted image of the posterior fossa reveals a cystic mass with a large enhancing tumor nodule within the deep cerebellum. Surrounding low-T1 signal edema is evident. The fourth ventricle is compressed, indicating a tumor originating outside the ventricular system.

with loosely structured, microcystic tumor tissue in a mucinous background. In areas of mucoid degeneration and microcyst formation the cells become round or stellate with plump or indiscernible processes. Rosenthal fibers are characteristic of pilocytic, fibrillated areas. They appear as bright eosinophil bodies with a shape resembling a sausage, corkscrew, or carrot, and their numbers vary considerably.

Pilocytic astrocytomas are slowly growing neoplasms with absent or rare mitoses but show focal proliferative activity with a Ki-67/MIB-1 labeling index up to 4%. Necrosis is rare, without pseudopalisading, but vascular proliferation may be extensive, especially along the walls of the tumor cysts.

Management and outcome

Management of infratentorial gliomas relies predominantly upon surgical excision. In addition to obtaining tissue for pathologic confirmation, the surgical objective is a total resection of the tumor, achievable in up to 90% of astrocytomas (Schneider et al. 1992). Whereas preexisting hydrocephalus can be addressed with placement of a ventricular drain prior to or at the start of surgery, an attempt to defer shunt placement is often made. In the patient eventually requiring CSF diversion, an endoscopic third ventriculostomy may avoid the need for long-term hardware. It is imperative to remove the solid tumor nodule but removal of the gliotic cyst wall is not required. Cerebellar mutism (posterior-fossa mutism syndrome) has been reported in some patients following surgery, but is less common than after surgery for medulloblastoma.

Although some tumors characterized by increased MIB-1 labeling have a higher likelihood of relapse, low-grade tumors (juvenile pilocytic astrocytomas) have a 95–100% survival rate after gross total resection.

Brainstem gliomas

Brainstem gliomas comprise between 10% and 15% of all childhood primary CNS tumors. They arise at a median age of 5–9 years and occur equally in males and females. The majority of brainstem gliomas are diffuse infiltrating lesions involving the pons, but may also involve the midbrain, medulla, and other contiguous sites. They often present with multiple cranial nerve palsies, most commonly sixth and seventh nerve palsies, associated with long tract signs and cerebellar deficits. The majority of patients will be diagnosed within 3 months of onset of symptoms. Increased ICP is present in approximately one-third of patients at the time of diagnosis. Twenty percent of brainstem gliomas will be more focal.

Tectal tumors present with hydrocephalus and few, if any, localizing deficits. Tumors usually take an indolent course with no further progression for years following CSF diversion. Cervicomedullary brainstem gliomas tend to be dorsally exophytic and are often low grade. Such lesions may present with headache and unsteadiness, but may also cause intermittent nausea and vomiting for weeks to months before causing any other symptoms.

> **Key Clinical Questions**
>
> In the management of brainstem gliomas, key questions include:
>
> - Is surgery required for diagnosis?
> - Does surgical intervention improve the likelihood of long-term survival?

> **Pearls and Perils**
>
> - Not all childhood brainstem gliomas carry a poor prognosis; 20% will be more focal lesions either emanating from the cervicomedullary junction or arising in the tectum.

Neuroimaging

Diffuse, infiltrative brainstem gliomas almost always arise in the pons. Anteriorly, the tumor commonly engulfs the basilar artery; posteriorly, it may extend into the cerebellar peduncles; superiorly, it may extend into the midbrain and cerebral peduncles and beyond; inferior extension into the spinal cord is uncommon (Figure 17.6). Although gliomas may cause posterior displacement of the fourth ventricle, hydrocephalus is relatively uncommon. This tumor shows hypodensity on CT and homogeneous signal increase on T2-weighted imaging. Enhancement is rare at presentation, although may occur following radiation.

By comparison, focal brainstem gliomas are more common in the midbrain or medulla. In the midbrain, the tectum is the most common site; tectal gliomas often do not enhance, show isointense T1 signal and mild increased T2 signal, and little or no enhancement; they almost universally present with aqueductal obstruction and hydrocephalus. Focal dorsal exophytic medullary tumors often originate in the upper cervical cord; the lesion takes a dorsal exophytic turn within the medulla as the tumor cells encounter the pyramidal decussation. These tumors are often low grade, may contain cysts, and show bright T2 signal and enhancement of the solid portions on MR images following gadolinium injection.

Management and outcome

Treatment of diffuse intrinsic brainstem gliomas has not been effectively improved over the past decades (Packer et

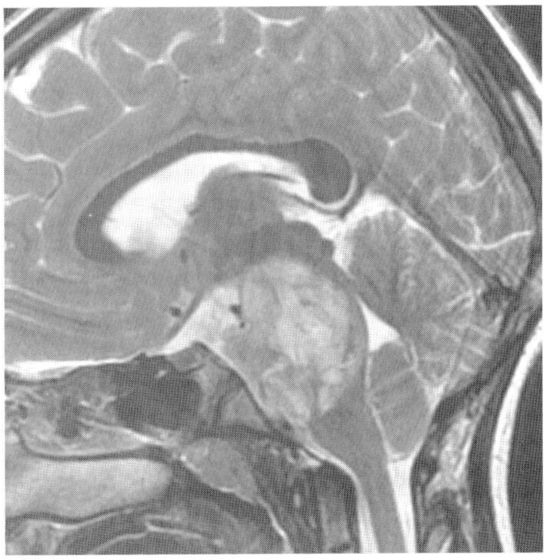

Figure 17.6 Sagittal T2-weighted image demonstrates the diffuse homogeneous T2 hyperintense tumor, with an anterior exophytic component. The lesion extends into the lower midbrain and spares the medulla.

al. 1990). Although biopsy and partial resections can be undertaken, they have not been shown to affect the natural history of the disease, and the information obtained at the time of biopsy usually does not change management. Radiotherapy remains the only proven treatment for brainstem gliomas, resulting in disease stabilization or clinical improvement in approximately 90% of patients. Doses of local radiotherapy, ranging between 5,400 and 6,000 cGy, will result in tumor shrinkage in approximately one-half of patients, but 90% of patients will progress and die of disease within 18 months of diagnosis.

Alterations in radiation schedule and dose, as well as the addition of chemotherapy, either prior to, during, or after radiotherapy, have not improved survival. Studies are presently under way attempting to improve the efficacy of radiation therapy by the concomitant use of radiosensitizing chemotherapeutic or biologic agents. Due to the severe neurologic compromise of patients with brainstem gliomas at the time of diagnosis and during their disease, corticosteroids are often utilized in an attempt to improve neurologic function. Although corticosteroids may improve neurologic function temporarily, they have no long-term benefit and their chronic use is associated with significant side effects including hypertension, hyperglycemia, gastrointestinal irritation, cushingoid appearance, and uncontrollable appetite. These symptoms result in increased morbidity; corticosteroids should be tapered and, if possible, discontinued early in the course of treatment.

The management of more focal lesions within the pons remains relatively empiric. Focal lesions within the pons, especially cystic ones presenting with isolated cranial nerve palsies, are often pilocytic astrocytomas. Biopsy and cyst drainage followed by focal radiotherapy can result in prolonged disease control for many patients. Patients with tectal tumors may require no treatment other than CSF diversion for many years after diagnosis. Biopsy is usually not required for diagnosis in these patients, and if there is progression, treatment with either chemotherapy (in very young children) or focal radiotherapy is usually effective. In contrast, dorsally exophytic cervicomedullary lesions are usually treated with surgery and are usually found to be pilocytic astrocytomas. Although extensive resections are possible, such resections may cause significant neurologic morbidity. Therefore, patients with cervicomedullary gliomas are successfully treated with partial surgical resection followed by either local radiotherapy or chemotherapy.

Diencephalic gliomas/visual pathway gliomas

Gliomas of the visual pathway, including the optic nerves, chiasm, and optic tracts, constitute approximately 5% of all primary CNS tumors. More than 75% of isolated optic nerve gliomas occur in the first decade of life. Neurofibromatosis type-1 is present in 50–80% of patients with isolated optic nerve tumors, and in approximately 15–20% of those with chiasmatic or tumors that diffusely infiltrate the visual pathway.

Children younger than 3 years of age are often brought to medical attention because of strabismus, proptosis, or nystagmus. Infants may display the triad of head tilt, head bobbing, and monocular or disassociated asymmetric nystagmus. Similar symptoms can be found in children with spasms nutans, and clinical differentiation is difficult.

At the time of diagnosis, patients with isolated optic nerve tumors usually have some decreased visual acuity in the involved eye; however, vision may be remarkably maintained, especially in patients with NF1. Funduscopic examination usually discloses optic pallor and atrophy in the involved eye, rather than papilledema. In patients with chiasmatic involvement, decreased visual acuity is usually associated with some type of visual field abnormality. Patients may have fine, rapid unilateral or bilateral nystagmus, which may or may not be associated with decreased visual acuity. Growth and endocrine disturbance may be present, especially in patients with extensive hypothalamic involvement. The diencephalic syndrome (as described earlier) is a classical presentation for patients with hypothalamic gliomas.

Neuroimaging

Optic pathway gliomas can variably involve one or both optic nerves, the chiasm, and the optic tracts. Chiasmatic tumors can infiltrate superiorly into the hypothalamus, septum pellucidum, and the third ventricle; optic tract disease can extend superiorly into the internal capsules and inferiorly into the cerebral peduncles and beyond. Tumors extending into the third ventricle may cause obstructive hydrocephalus at the foramen of Monro. Small tumors are generally homogeneously hypodense on CT, isointense on T1-weighted imaging, and hyperintense on T2-weighted imaging. Larger tumors in the chiasm may harbor cystic elements, especially in children without neurofibromatosis, and usually enhance. Infiltration within the optic tracts and cerebral parenchyma is accompanied by bright T2 FLAIR signal; the majority of the abnormal T2 signal often does not enhance (Figure 17.7).

Management and outcome

For patients with isolated optic nerve gliomas, management is dependent on the degree of proptosis and associated cosmetic abnormalities and visual acuity. In patients with significant proptosis and a blind eye, resection is usually undertaken to remove as much of the optic nerve as possible. However, there remains little evidence that the majority of patients with isolated optic nerve tumors will develop tumor deeper into the visual pathway, even if the tumor is left alone.

In patients with maintained vision, radiotherapy may result in shrinkage of the optic nerve and maintenance of vision. However, radiotherapy may also have long-term cosmetic sequelae because of involvement of the overlying bone, and secondary mutagenesis is an important issue, especially in children with NF1.

For patients with chiasmatic, hypothalamic, or more extensive visual pathway infiltration, the role of surgery is more limited. Patients with NF1 do not require biopsy to confirm the presence of a glioma. In non-NF1 patients with chiasmatic or hypothalamic disease, biopsy may distinguish the rare patients with a higher-grade infiltrating glioma. Patients with extensive visual pathway gliomas are not amenable to gross total resection. Partial resection may relieve obstructive hydrocephalus and, in selected patients, may result in disease stabilization and delay the need for more definitive therapy.

Radiotherapy results in visual stabilization in the majority of patients with visual pathway gliomas. Visual improvement has been reported after radiotherapy in a variable proportion of patients ranging between 9% and 44%. Irradiation of large chiasmatic/hypothalamic lesions results in disease stabilization in the majority of patients and 5- and 10-year progression-free survival rates ranging between 70% and 90%. The doses of radiotherapy required (4,500–5,500 cGy) will result in significant endocrinologic deficits in the majority of patients. The latter long-term effects may include the development of vascular malformations (which may be life-threatening) and significant neurocognitive sequelae, especially in very young children.

To delay, if not obviate, the need for radiotherapy, chemotherapy has been used in children with progressive visual pathway gliomas (Packer et al. 1997). The combination of carboplatin and vincristine has been shown to result in disease stabilization in over 90% of patients with progressive lesions and radiographic shrinkage in 60%. Other drug regimens such as carboplatin alone, or more aggressive regimens, may result in disease control. It is unclear whether these more aggressive regimens are needed to halt disease progression.

For children with NF1 and visual pathway gliomas, interventions must be undertaken cautiously (Listernick et al. 1995). The natural history of tumors of the optic nerve or visual pathway is extremely erratic in patients with NF1. The majority of children diagnosed on screening examinations, who are not clearly symptomatic or progressive, will require no immediate treatment. Management includes careful neurologic, visual, endocrinologic, and neuroradiographic follow-up and treatment only if there is clear-cut progression. Because of the potential risks of radiotherapy, patients with progressive disease are often initially treated with chemotherapy.

Cortical Gliomas

Up to one-half of cortical gliomas are located in the cerebral hemispheres. The remainder occur in the deep midline structures of the diencephalon and basal ganglia. Children may often have mixed neuronal-glial tumors (Table 17.10) The major clinical signs at diagnosis are nonspecific and nonlocalizing features related to in-

Key Clinical Questions

Before treatment of childhood visual pathway gliomas ask:

- What part of the visual pathway is involved?
- Does the child have neurofibromatosis type 1?
- Is there evidence for clear-cut tumor progression at time of diagnosis?
- What would be the potential detrimental effects of treatment?

Table 17.10 Rarer cortical childhood glial, neuronal, and mixed neuronal/glial tumors

Neuronal/Mixed
- Gangliogliomas/gangliocytomas
- Desmoplastic infantile astrocytoma and ganglioglioma
- Dysembryoplastic neuroepithelial tumor
- Central neurocytoma
- ? Giant-cell

Astrocytic
- Pleomorphic xanthoastrocytoma
- Oligodendroglioma
- Oligoastrocytoma

Pearls and Perils

- Cortical gliomas, especially in infants, may be quite complex and be extremely large at the time of diagnosis, but they have a relatively favorable prognosis.

creased ICP (headache, morning emesis, lethargy) occurring in up to 75% of patients, regardless of tumor histology and location. Seizures, most frequently grand mal, are present at diagnosis in at least 25% of patients. The frequency of seizures is higher in the more slowly evolving low-grade tumors, where they may precede diagnosis by months to years, particularly for ganglioglioma and oligodendroglioma.

Neuroimaging

Cortical tumors have a wide variety of appearances, reflecting their different histologies, but all involve the cortical gray matter. The ganglioglioma and dysembryoplastic neuroepithelial tumor (DNET) are well-defined tumors, commonly found in the frontal and temporal lobe; both can have a "soap bubble" appearance on CT and MRI that can be confused with cystic encephalomalacia. The ganglioglioma is generally of a mixed solid-cystic composition, showing hypodensity on CT, hypointensity on T1-weighted imaging, hyperintensity on T2-weighted imaging, and variable enhancement. The DNET may present as an enlarged gyrus, showing a lobulated contour. Again hypodense on CT and hyperintense on T2-WI, approximately one-third of cases show calcification or enhancement. Both tumors can remodel the inner table of the skull and show little or no surrounding edema. The desmoplastic infantile ganglioglioma presents as a very large hemispheric mass with both cystic and solid components. The solid regions tend to be located more peripherally and show a slight increase in density on CT and isointensity on T2-weighted imaging. They strongly enhance, the result of an intense desmoplastic reaction. The pleomorphic xanthoastrocytoma (PXA) commonly presents as a mixed solid-cystic mass, with a superficial mural nodule and adjacent to the leptomeningeal infiltration. It is hypodense on CT, hypointense on T1-weighted MRI, and iso- to hyperintense on T2-weighted imaging. The mural nodule commonly enhances.

Microscopy

Diffuse, fibrillary astrocytomas (WHO grade II) are composed of infiltrating, neoplastic astrocytes with scant cytoplasm and nuclear atypia, but without mitoses, and higher-grade tumors such as anaplastic astrocytomas (WHO grade III) demonstrate increased cellularity, cellular pleomorphism, nuclear hyperchromasia, and mitotic activity. The highest grade of astrocytic tumor, glioblastoma multiforme (WHO grade IV), rare in children, demonstrates higher cellularity, greater pleomorphism with possible giant cells, pseudopalisading necrosis, exuberant microvascular proliferation, and numerous mitoses.

Oligodendroglioma (WHO grade II) are composed of cells with uniform round to ovoid nuclei and empty-looking cytoplasm (fried egg artifact), bounded by a distinct cell membrane producing a classical, low-power, "honeycomb" appearance.

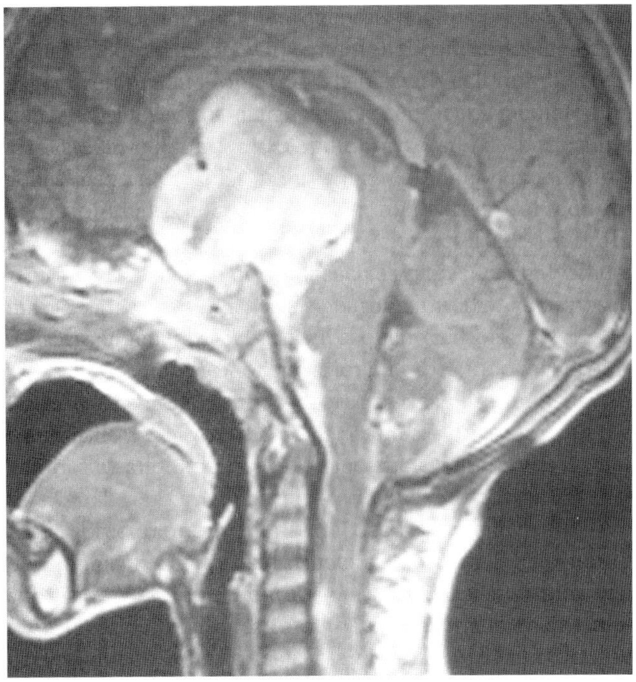

Figure 17.7 Sagittal post-gadolinium T1-weighted image of the brain reveals a very large suprasellar tumor extending superiorly into the hypothalamus and anterior third ventricle and posteriorly, resulting in mass effect on the brainstem. There is diffuse enhancement within the subarachnoid spaces surrounding the brainstem and upper cervical cord, as well as in the cisterna magna.

High-grade glioma: management and outcome

Radical (>90%) surgical resection is the most powerful predictor of favorable outcome in high-grade glioma (HGG) when followed by irradiation. However, only 49% of tumors in the superficial hemisphere and 8% of tumors in the midline or deep cerebrum are amenable to radical resection. In addition, training of the neurosurgeon (pediatric versus adult neurosurgery) has a significant impact on the extent of surgical resection. Local (2- to 4-cm margin around the area of edema defined by imaging) or wide-field irradiation to 5,000–6,000 cGy is the mainstay of therapy.

The addition of radiation therapy has improved 5-year survival rates (10–30%) compared to surgery alone

(0%). All patients are thus considered candidates for radiotherapy following surgery, with the exception of very young children, in whom attempts have been made to eliminate or delay the use of radiotherapy because of concern regarding neurodevelopmental morbidity. Newer techniques, such as conformal radiation and stereotactic radiosurgery (γ-knife), which allow for higher doses of radiation delivered to the tumor bed while minimizing exposure to adjacent normal tissue, are currently under investigation. To date, no large randomized prospective clinical trial has clearly demonstrated a benefit of adjuvant chemotherapy.

The outcome of children with high-grade cortical gliomas remains poor. The 5-year survival rate ranges from 16% to 46% with the use of postoperative radiotherapy and chemotherapy.

Low-grade gliomas: management and outcome

Complete surgical resection is curative for most low-grade gliomas (LGG), and even with incomplete excision, long-term progression-free survival is common. If subsequent progression occurs then re-resection is generally first undertaken. Surgical morbidity depends largely on tumor location and is highest in diencephalic tumors, in which the incidence of hemiparesis or visual field deficits may be 10–20%. Gross total excisions are possible in up to 90% of hemispheric tumors (Tables 17.11 and 17.12). For patients with progressive disease not amenable to resection, local conformal irradiation to 5,000–5,500 cGy to the area of the tumor plus a 2-cm margin is warranted. The use of chemotherapy as initial treatment in newly diagnosed LGG involving the optic chiasm and hypothalamus has become a standard approach only among very young children and infants, in whom the goal is to avoid radiation neurotoxicity. The use of such therapy in older patients is questionable since outcome is generally good with surgery and irradiation. Overall 5-year survival for low-grade cortical glioma is 95%, while progression-free survival is 88%.

Table 17.11 Hemispheric tumors

Discriminating features
- Low-grade astrocytoma
  - Pathologic examination
- High-grade astrocytoma
  - Pathologic examination
- Primitive neuroectodermal tumors
  - Pathologic examination
- Oligodendroglioma
  - Pathologic examination

Consistent features
- Low-grade astrocytoma
  - Lateralizing signs
  - Slow progression
  - Long duration of symptoms
- High-grade astrocytoma
  - Rapid progression
  - Short duration of symptoms
  - Enhancing mass on CT and MRI
  - Lateralizing signs
- Primitive neuroectodermal tumors
  - Large mass on CT or MRI
  - Papilledema
  - Subtle signs
- Oligodendroglioma
  - Long duration of symptoms

Variable features
- Low-grade astrocytoma
  - Seizures
  - Nonenhancing CT, MRI
  - Symptoms and signs of increased intracranial pressure
- High-grade astrocytoma
  - Symptoms and signs of increased intracranial pressure
  - Seizures
  - Subarachnoid spread
- Primitive neuroectodermal tumors
  - Calcification
  - Cranial neuropathy associated with subarachnoid seeding
  - Seizures
- Oligodendroglioma
  - Seizures
  - Lateralizing signs

Craniopharyngiomas

Despite over 70 years of experience in the neurosurgical arena, successful treatment of craniopharyngiomas remains open to controversy (Scott et al. 1994). They account for 5–10% of all childhood brain tumors. Although these tumors are benign and represent embryonic remnants of Rathke's pouch in the region of the sella, their location in proximity to the hypothalamus, optic pathways, and carotid vessels and their propensity to grow to large sizes, as well as develop calcification, make their safe and total removal exceedingly difficult. A bimodal incidence is seen with children between the ages of 6 and 10 years, as well as at 11–15 years, and gender predilection appears to be equal, although some studies support a slightly greater male incidence. Clinical presentation may be variable and may include symptoms secondary to increased intracranial hypertension due to hydrocephalus or from direct tumor/cyst extension. Headaches, nausea, vomiting, visual changes, hormonal insufficiency, memory deficits, and seizures are commonly seen in the setting of craniopharyngioma. Visual symptoms are noted in approximately 50% of affected individuals, and compression of the optic chiasm constitutes an emergent clinical situation to preserve vision. Hormonal insufficiency is common (>70%) and may include failure of growth, delayed sexual maturation, excessive weight gain and, in 10–20% of children, diabetes insipidus.

Table 17.12 Pathology and course of hemispheric tumors

Discriminating features

- Low-grade astrocytoma
  - Supratentorial hemispheric mass with pilocytic, fibrillary, or gemistocytic appearance
- High-grade astrocytoma
  - Supratentorial hemispheric mass with mitoses, necrosis, hemorrhage, endothelial proliferation, and multinucleated giant cells
- Primitive neuroectodermal tumors
  - 90% to 95% undifferentiated, mitoses, necrosis, endothelial hyperplasia
  - Focal areas of differentiation (possibly)
- Oligodendroglioma
  - Honeycomb appearance, microcalcification

Consistent features

- Low-grade astrocytoma
  - Slow progression
  - Long duration of symptoms
  - Up to 70% five-year survival
- High-grade astrocytoma
  - Ring enhancement, mass effect, edema on CT or MRI
  - Rapid progression
  - Short-duration symptoms
  - Increased intracranial pressure
  - Focal signs
  - Rapid downhill course, limited survival
- Primitive neuroectodermal tumors
  - Increased intracranial pressure, mass effect, focal signs
  - Cysts, hemorrhage, and enhancement on CT or MRI
  - Rapid downhill course
- Oligodendroglioma
  - Calcification, decreased density, mass lesions
  - Slow wave focus on EEG
  - May be cured with surgery, with or without radiation

Variable features

- Low-grade astrocytoma
  - Contrast enhancement variable
  - Slow wave focus on EEG
  - Seizures, headache, focal motor/sensory signs, visual field abnormalities
- High-grade astrocytoma
  - Seizures, subarachnoid spread, extraneural metastases
- Primitive neuroectodermal tumors
  - Seizures, personality change, subarachnoid metastases, extraneural metastases
- Oligodendroglioma
  - Subarachnoid metastases (uncommon), seizures, common focal motor signs
  - Infrequently hemorrhage

Pearls and Perils

- Although long-term survival is common in children with craniopharyngiomas, quality of life can be greatly impaired in long-term survivors. Sequelae include severe emotional difficulties, obesity, and visual impairment.

Neuroimaging

The adamantinomatous craniopharyngioma, most common in children, presents as a well-defined, lobulated, heterogeneous mass. The tumor almost always contains cystic components, which are T2 hyperintense and commonly quite hyperintense on T1-weighted imaging due to high cholesterol content. After contrast administration, the solid components, as well as the cyst walls, enhance intensely, but not the cyst contents. Calcification is almost universal, occurring either as a thin rim around a cyst or larger internal foci.

Management and outcome

Therapeutic direction must take into account numerous factors, which not only include surgical consideration of tumor size and location but also reflect whether the tumor is primary or recurrent, as well as preoperative visual and endocrinologic status. Preoperative evaluation should include formal visual field testing as well as extensive endocrine and metabolic evaluation. Not uncommonly, patients with craniopharyngiomas may demonstrate endocrine dysfunction without overt symptoms.

The surgical goal remains total extirpation, if possible. Due to the proximity of the carotid vessels, optic chiasm, and hypothalamus, tumors with significant adherent calcification may prevent total excision in a safe fashion. Although this has been a contentious issue for many clinicians up until recently, recent studies appear to support the role for limited resection of craniopharyngiomas when vital structures are at risk. Residual tumor may be subsequently treated with stereotactic radiosurgery, intracavitary brachytherapy utilizing ^{32}P or ^{90}Y, and cyst aspiration, as well as intracavitary bleomycin. Indications for type of treatment as well as long-term outcome are still in evolution, although irradiation has been demonstrated to offer 50–90% 5- and 10-year disease-free survival. Primary tumors presenting within the sella occur 3–15% of the time and may be removed successfully via a transsphenoidal approach, with an attendant reduction in overall risk to the patient. Whereas peril to the chiasm and carotid vessels is diminished, endocrine disturbances are expected if the pituitary stalk is not preserved.

Total resection, confirmed by postoperative radiographs, is now possible in 80–90% of individuals, whereas mortality has decreased to 0–2% over the past decade. Hormonal replacement is necessary in approximately 80% of children and most frequently involves diabetes insipidus, requiring DDAVP therapy in 75% of children, as well as thyroid and cortisol supplementation. Visual deterioration is seen in nearly 20% of patients, whereas 50–60% will show improvement. Neuropsychological impact remains controversial, and is dependent upon baseline memory and intelligence. Recent studies, however, have demonstrated normal psychosocial integration as well as academic performance in 70–87% of children treated by experienced surgeons and centers.

Germ cell tumors

Germ cell tumors may arise throughout the neuroaxis, with a propensity to occur in a suprasellar location and more commonly in the pineal region (Packer et al. 2000). Confirmed tissue histology prior to the advent of adjuvant therapy remains a cornerstone of pineal/suprasellar tumor therapy, except for those tumors that can be diagnosed by measurement of CSF markers.

Because germ cell tumors generally arise in the midline pineal area, the dominant signs and symptoms of these tumors are typically the nonspecific and nonlocalizing features of increased ICP secondary to tumor extension and compression of the third ventricle. Other findings depend on the location and extent of tumor spread. Tumors extending to the midbrain (tectum) may cause varying degrees of vertical gaze palsy characteristic of Parinaud syndrome. Tumors that infiltrate the thalamus may cause hemiparesis, incoordination, visual deficits, or movement disorders. The suprasellar region also frequently harbors germ cell tumors that may produce pituitary and hypothalamic dysfunction, including diabetes insipidus, hypothyroidism, precocious puberty, and emotional as well as thermoregulatory dysfunction. Somewhat surprisingly, although malignant tumors, a delayed diagnosis due to subtle initial symptoms is not uncommon (Crawford et al. 2007).

Neuroimaging

Germinomas can present as well-defined, homogenous masses located either in the pineal region or, less commonly, in the third ventricle; when large they may show internal heterogeneity. Germinomas commonly show strong uniform enhancement. Metastatic spread throughout the CSF is common as the tumors are not encapsulated. By comparison, the teratoma is extremely heterogeneous, with evidence of fat, calcification, and soft tissue within the tumor. This gives a very varied appearance on CT and MR. Enhancement is unusual unless there has been malignant degeneration. Embryonal cell carcinoma and endodermal sinus tumors have few individual defining imaging features. Choriocarcinoma may undergo hemorrhage and should be considered when a hemorrhagic pineal mass is present.

> **Pearls and Perils**
>
> - Germinomas, although often aggressive lesions that frequently disseminate the neuroaxis, may present insidiously; a delay of 6 months or more from onset of symptoms and diagnosis is not infrequent.

Microscopy

Germinomas are the most frequently occurring intracranial germ cell tumors and are composed of sheets or lobules of large cells with abundant clear cytoplasm, round vesicular nuclei, and prominent nucleoli. Often the tumor cells are intermixed with small T-lymphocytes along fibrovascular septa. Teratomas recapitulate, albeit in disorganized fashion, the somatic differentiation by the embryonic ectoderm, endoderm, and mesoderm. These tumors may be mature, if composed of fully differentiated, "adult-type" tissue elements, or immature, if composed of incompletely differentiated elements resembling fetal tissue. Mixed germ cell tumors demonstrate any combination of germinomas and/or teratomas with other malignant component such as embryonal carcinomas, endodermal sinus tumors, and choriocarcinomas.

Management and outcome

Cerebrospinal fluid including α-fetoprotein (AFP), β-human chorionic gonadotrophin (β-HCG), and placental alkaline phosphatase (PLAP) levels should be measured on ventricular and, if safe, lumbar fluid and compared to serum counterparts. In addition, CSF is assayed for cytology, as part of a preoperative attempt at diagnosis. Elevated levels of AFP and β-HCG confirm the presence of mixed germ cell tumors, whereas highly elevated β-HCG is diagnostic of a choriocarcinoma. Mildly elevated β-HCG suggests the syncytiotrophoblastic form of germinoma. In suspected cases of nonsecreting germinomas or non–germ cell pineal region tumor, stereotactic or endoscopic methods of obtaining tissue remain a viable approach to limit perioperative morbidity.

Individuals presenting with hydrocephalus may subsequently be good candidates for endoscopic biopsy of pineal region lesions that project into the posterior third ventricle. In addition to relatively minimal morbidity, it is often possible to perform an endoscopic third ventriculostomy at the same time.

Patients with radiographic features of benign disease, or whose biopsy demonstrates tumor histology insensitive to adjuvant therapy, are best served by an attempt at total tumor resection for long-term control of disease. This may be accomplished via an infratentorial approach using a supracerebellar exposure or through a supratentorial avenue via a posterior corpus callosum dissection. In individuals with large lesions extending into both the supra- and infratentorial compartments, a combined approach of splitting the tentorium may offer excellent visualization of the tumor and surrounding vascular structures. Despite decreasing morbidity over the past decade with improvements in surgical technique and postoperative care, such surgical avenues, while offering the possibility of total tumor resection, still carry significant risks of perioperative morbidity and mortality.

Craniospinal irradiation (36 Gy for nongerminomatous and 24 Gy for germinomas) supplemented with radiation to the primary tumor site, has been the standard treatment for all germ cell tumors. However, given the chemosensitive nature of these tumors, an alternative approach is to use chemotherapy prior to radiotherapy as a means to eliminate, or reduce, the dose of irradiation needed in patients without metastatic spread. Some investigators have recommended that only cranial or whole ventricular irradiation be used in nondisseminated patients. Metastatic tumors still require craniospinal irradiation with boost to the sites of bulk disease. The specific chemotherapeutic regimens vary according to the histology and response to initial treatment; however, most contain regimens with an alkylating agent (ifosfamide or cyclophosphamide), platinum agents (carboplatin or cisplatin), and etoposide.

The most important predictive feature of outcome for germ cell tumors is histologic subtype. Pure germinomas, which have negative serum and CSF markers for malignant germ cell elements (negative AFP and negative to low β-HCG), are sensitive to irradiation, and as such, have a greater than 95% survival rate. Attempts to treat these tumors with chemotherapy alone have shown radiographic response rates of 78%, but only 60–70% chance of disease-free survival. Patients with mixed germ cell tumors have a much worse prognosis. The best results have been obtained with platinum-based chemotherapy and full-dose craniospinal irradiation, although 5-year survival remains 40–50%. Pure teratomas are typically unresponsive to chemotherapy or radiotherapy and surgery is the only proven treatment.

Choroid plexus tumors

Although choroid plexus tumors are uncommon entities and constitute only 1–5% of all pediatric tumors, they nevertheless represent a greater percentage (4–12%) of tumors in patients younger than 1 year of age. Due to their intraventricular location, they frequently present with hydrocephalus secondary to CSF overproduction as well as obstruction of intraventricular pathways. Not infrequently, infants are born with large lesions within the ventricles in association with hydrocephalus, and these may even be identified during prenatal evaluation via ultrasound. In addition to presenting with increased ICP (macrocephaly, full fontanelle, split sutures, Parinaud phenomenon, vomiting, irritability, etc.), patients may also present with seizures, intraventricular hemorrhage, or focal neurologic findings. Tumors may arise from any of the ventricles with 75% occurring in the lateral ventricle, in particular the atrium. Although choroid plexus lesions occur most commonly in the fourth ventricle in adults, this location is infrequently seen in children. Extraventricular locations have also been observed, in addition to multiple locations, including metastasis, throughout the neuroaxis.

Neuroimaging

The papilloma presents as a well-defined, lobulated mass that replicates the appearance of an enlarged choroid plexus. On CT, it is commonly iso- or hyperdense, occasionally showing punctate calcifications or hemorrhage. MRI reveals T1 isointensity and relative T2 hypointensity (Figure 17.8). The tumor shows strong homogeneous enhancement. Choroid plexus carcinoma shows a more aggressive appearance, with an irregular contour and invasion of adjacent brain, where it induces vasogenic edema; it displays marked heterogeneity with evidence of necrosis, mixed densities and signal intensities, and prominent enhancement.

Microscopy

Choroid plexus tumors manifest pathologic features that range from benign, well-delineated papillomas to invasive,

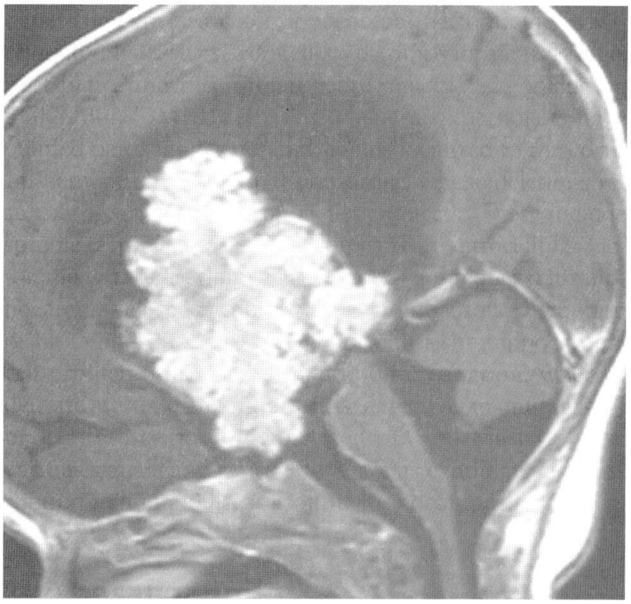

Figure 17.8 Sagittal post-gadolinium T1-weighted image of the brain reveals an extremely large lobulated mass within the third ventricle, showing strong contrast enhancement.

poorly differentiated carcinomas. The choroid plexus papilloma has a distinct papillary pattern with a well-vascularized connective tissue core, surmounted by a single layer of cuboidal or columnar epithelium. The tumor is well-circumscribed, without invasion of brain and with low mitotic activity. The malignant counterpart, carcinoma, is characterized by loss of papillary architecture, with the neoplastic cells forming large solid sheets. Anaplastic features include increased mitotic activity, nuclear atypia, necrosis, and frank invasion of adjacent neuronal tissue.

Management and outcome: choroid plexus papillomas

Therapeutic considerations predominantly involve surgical extirpation, with complete excision of tumor if possible. In many instances, the need for permanent CSF diversion may not be necessary after the removal of a hypersecreting tumor. Choice of surgical approach takes into consideration the vascular supply of the tumor. Lesions in the lateral ventricle not uncommonly have blood supply from both the anterior and lateral posterior choroidal arteries, whereas third ventricle tumors are supplied from the medial posterior choroidal artery. Tumors arising in the fourth ventricle are vascularized by branches from posterior inferior cerebellar or superior cerebellar arteries. Larger tumors often require piecemeal resection to eventually reach their blood supply, and may manifest considerable bleeding before vascular control is undertaken. Consequently, removal of large atrial lesions in the newborn carries considerable risk of life-threatening hemorrhage and should be deferred to a later age if possible. Preoperative embolization may also be considered as an adjunct to reducing intraoperative bleeding, but is usually reserved for the older patient with sufficiently larger vessels. Continued advances in surgery have led to decreasing surgical morbidity and mortality; however, mortality is still reported to be as high as 24% in some series. Long-term outcome will be dependent upon the degree of tumor resection as well as the histopathology. Benign papillomas with complete resection understandably carry an excellent prognosis.

Management and outcome: choroid plexus carcinomas

Surgical resection is also the cornerstone of treatment of choroid plexus carcinoma. The surgical approach chosen depends on the location and vascularization of the tumor. Resection of ventricular tumors can be complicated by hemorrhage from arterial feeding vessels or deep venous drainage vessels, and appropriate care must be taken to isolate and ligate these vessels. Preoperative embolization has been used to help mitigate the risk of hemorrhagic complications.

Successful gross total resection (GTR) is the most important predictor of successful therapy for CPC. In 277 patients with CPC, 2-year survival rates were 72% versus 34% for those with GTR or subtotal resection, respectively. When not initially possible, a GTR may be possible following adjuvant therapy.

Irradiation may be of benefit for those patients who have had a subtotal resection. Adjuvant therapy has been purported to be necessary in the treatment of subtotally resected CPC. Chemotherapy has also been used as adjuvant therapy in young children as well as in combination with radiation. Chemotherapeutic regimens employed usually include cyclophosphamide, etoposide, and a platinum agent. Although responses have been noted, a positive impact on long-term survival has been difficult to gauge owing to the small number of patients in each report and the heterogeneity of chemotherapy regimens.

> **Pearls and Perils**
>
> ▸ Despite their aggressive histology, choroid plexus carcinomas may require only complete resection for long-term control.

Atypical teratoid/rhabdoid tumors

The atypical teratoid/rhabdoid tumor was first clearly described in 1987 (Rorke et al. 1996). This tumor, diagnosed by light microscopy and immunohistochemical findings, comprises approximately 10–15% of all embryonal tumors occurring in children younger than 3 years of age. Although its exact incidence is unknown, the ratio of atypical teratoid/rhabdoid tumors to primitive neuroectodermal tumors is approximately 1:4 in children younger than 3 years of age. More recently, atypical/rhabdoid tumors have been diagnosed in older patients.

Approximately one-half of all atypical teratoid/rhabdoid tumors will arise in the posterior fossa. The tumor has also been found throughout the nervous system, including the suprasellar region, pineal region, spinal cord, and extramedullary sites. When arising in the posterior fossa, atypical teratoid/rhabdoid tumors present similarly to medulloblastomas. However, there seems to be a predilection for the cerebellopontine angle, with children often presenting with sixth and seventh nerve palsies. Supratentorial lesions tend to be quite large at the time of diagnosis, resulting in focal neurologic deficits, as well as symptoms of increased ICP. Cerebrospinal fluid dissemination occurs at the time of diagnosis in one-third to one-half of patients.

Neuroimaging

These tumors are often large by the time of presentation and commonly show a heterogeneous appearance, due to presence of calcifications, hemorrhage, cysts, and necrosis. Solid tumor components often show similar imaging characteristics to medulloblastoma or PNET, namely CT hyperdensity, T1 hypointensity, and T2 isointensity, as well as contrast enhancement. Surrounding edema is common. In the posterior fossa, there is a predilection for the cerebellopontine angle; this location, and the marked heterogeneity, often differentiates the atypical teratoid/rhabdoid tumor from a medulloblastoma an infant or young child.

Microscopy

The typical rhabdoid cell is medium-sized, round to oval with distinct borders, eccentric nucleus, and commonly prominent nucleolus (Figure 17.9). Cytoplasm has a fine granular character or may contain a poorly defined pink "body" resembling an inclusion. Mitoses are abundant and field necrosis is common. The immunophenotype is broad, as the large rhabdoid cells display a range of immunoreactivity with clusters of cells almost always positive for epithelial membrane antigen (EMA) and vimentin. Also frequent is reactivity for glial fibrillary acidic protein (GFAP) and cytokeratin and less frequent for smooth muscle actin (SMA) and neurofilament protein. The rhabdoid cells are negative for desmin and any of the markers for germ cell tumors.

Management and outcome

The management of atypical teratoid/rhabdoid tumors remains suboptimal. In the majority of patients younger than 2 years of age, treatment with chemotherapy alone or chemotherapy plus local radiotherapy will result in a long-term disease control rate of less than 10%, although recent studies suggest somewhat better outcomes after the use of "sarcoma" drug regimens. Treatment with chemotherapy followed by early craniospinal and local boost radiotherapy or initial radiotherapy supplemented by high-dose chemotherapy has been shown to result in a better outcome in older patients. The management approaches utilized for patients with poor-risk medulloblastoma are often utilized for children with atypical teratoid/rhabdoid tumors; however, recent studies have suggested that therapy will need to be intensified to improve disease control.

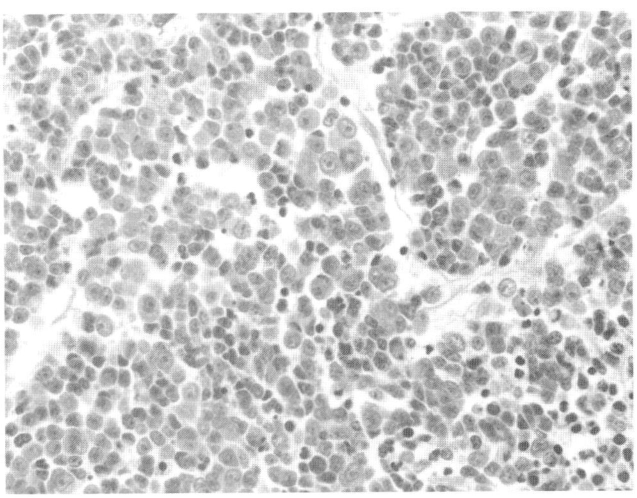

Figure 17.9 The cells forming trabeculae have abundant cytoplasm with eosinophilic inclusions, large nuclei and prominent nucleoli (hemolysin and eosin stain).

Spinal cord tumors

Spinal cord tumors are relatively rare entities accounting for only 4–10% of all CNS neoplasms. A variety of tumors may arise in the spinal cord as primary lesions or as metastatic secondary masses. The most common primary lesions include astrocytomas, ependymomas, schwannomas, and lipomas, as well as inclusion cysts (i.e., dermoid, epidermoid). Less common lesions may include ganglioglioma, ganglioneurocytoma, teratoma, hemangioblastoma, and germinoma, in addition to leptomeningeal metastases from PNET, pineal tumors, ependymomas, and malignant astrocytomas.

Spinal cord tumors may present as intrinsic, intramedullary lesions or as extramedullary masses with extrinsic compression of the cord and adjacent nerve roots. Approximately one-third of pediatric spinal cord tumors are intramedullary, with the vast majority of lesions being astrocytomas in the younger patient and ependymomas in the older child. Primary intramedullary tumors (astrocytomas, ependymomas, gangliogliomas) clinically present with intrinsic cord compression and may manifest by weakness, sensory changes including paresthesias, pain, gait changes, scoliosis, and bowel or bladder difficulties. Extrinsic tumors, which may include schwannomas, metastases, dermoid/epidermoid, lipomas, and others, frequently present with a combination of myelopathic changes as well as peripheral nerve findings. Peripheral nerve involvement may include back or radicular pain, motor or sensory disturbances, and spasticity, as well as bowel and bladder changes.

Diagnostic evaluation predominantly involves radiological investigation. Electromyographic (EMG)/nerve conduction velocities (NCV) tests are infrequent adjuncts in today's workup of spinal cord tumors. Somatosensory evoked potentials remain a valuable preoperative as well as intraoperative method of assessing neurophysiological function and integrity of the spinal cord during the course of surgery, alerting the surgeon in the event that manipulation of the cord is causing dysfunction. In addition, urodynamic testing may demonstrate early evidence for neurogenic bladder and may also provide a relative baseline for long-term surveillance.

Neuroimaging

MRI commonly reveals an enlarged, T2 hyperintense cord, although subjects may present with a thin syrinx (Figure 17.10). Ependymomas may show areas of hemorrhage,

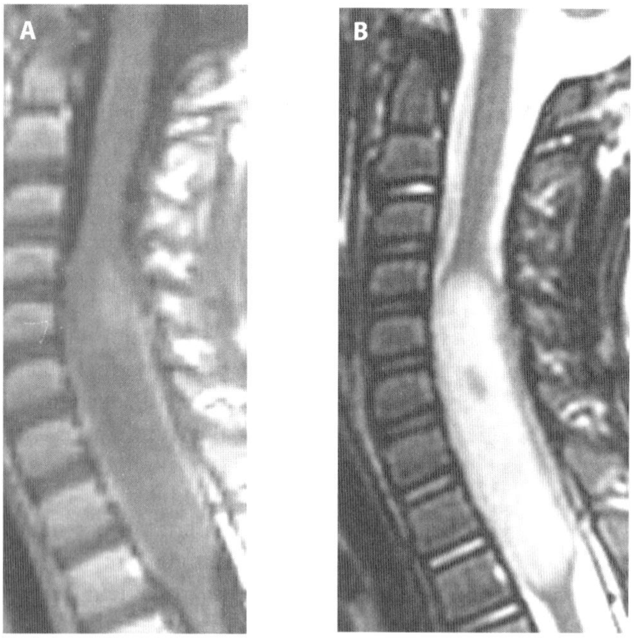

Figure 17.10 (A) Sagittal T1 (*left*) and (B) T2 (*right*) images of the cervical spine reveal cord expansion and diffuse T2 hyperintensity extending from C2 through T2 levels. Faint enhancement is evident at the periphery and superiorly.

detectable as T2 hypointensity surrounding the tumor. Analysis of T2 and postcontrast T1 signal behavior is required to distinguish tumor from surrounding edema or intra- or peritumoral cyst formation, common findings in intramedullary spinal tumors. Most spinal cord tumors enhance, although some glial low-grade infiltrative tumors do not. Ependymomas tend to be more sharply circumscribed following gadolinium enhancement, however the rarer germinomas and gangliogliomas also show this finding. By comparison, astrocytomas show a more infiltrative pattern, and tumor cells may extend beyond the area of enhancement.

Management and outcome

Current management of spinal cord tumors consists of surgical extirpation in the setting of a majority of benign tumors. Most lesions are low-grade or benign, with the greatest challenge resting with defining a surgical plane between normal cord and tumor.

A number of technological advances have played a role in decreasing surgical morbidity over the past decade. The operating microscope in conjunction with intraoperative electrophysiological monitoring as well as the CO_2 or YAG laser, real-time ultrasound, and ultrasonic aspiration have all contributed significantly to improve the outcome of these operations. Astrocytomas are often low-grade lesions, yet their failure to manifest a clear tumor/cord plane often makes a complete excision impossible to perform and commonly results in recurrent disease. Benign ependymomas often present with a discernible tissue plane that simplifies a possible total removal, whereas more aggressive ependymomas will have a less defined tumor interface and, subsequently, more often result in incomplete resection. Other cord lesions, in particular extramedullary lesions such as inclusion cysts (dermoid, epidermoid) and neurofibromas, may be removed in their entirety, with the exception of the congenital lipoma. Postoperative courses may be complicated by neurologic deficits (new and/or increased) in addition to infection, CSF leak, and kyphoscoliosis. Patients with significant neurologic compromise prior to the start of surgery are at considerable risk for increased deficits after surgery. Individuals with extensive laminectomies for tumor removal will be at risk of developing progressive kyphoscoliosis over time.

Outcomes are generally excellent for benign or low-grade lesions. Benign lesions undergoing total excision fare the best, with low-grade astrocytomas often enjoying long-term, progression-free survival without adjuvant therapy. Subtotal resection of high-grade lesions such as malignant ependymomas as well as glioblastoma, is followed by radiation therapy as an adjunct therapy. Although patients (especially those younger than 5 years of age) are at risk for developing radiation myelitis as well as secondary malignancies at a later date, they are felt to benefit from radiotherapy. Chemotherapeutic approaches have become more commonly employed, with variable success to date. Additional protocols are in evolution and may benefit from greater molecular understanding of these tumors.

Common long-term sequelae of tumor/treatment

As has been noted in the various general and specific sections in this chapter, childhood brain tumors and their treatment are associated with significant long-term sequelae (Table 17.13). The etiology of the sequelae are often multiple and include factors such as the size of the tumors and its location, the degree of spread of tumor at the time of diagnosis, the presence and degree of hydrocephalus at diagnosis, surgical complications, and short- and long-term effects of radiotherapy and chemotherapy.

Residual neurologic and neurosensory abnormalities have been poorly characterized. In a recent study of over 1,800 long-term survivors of childhood brain tumors, it was noted that a significant proportion of patients had permanent focal neurologic deficits, including residual hemiparesis and cerebellar deficits (Packer et al. 2003). In addition, children with both infratentorial and supratentorial lesions had seizures. Psychological difficulties were common, as were difficulties re-entering into society, holding jobs, and having families.

Table 17.13 Common long-term sequelae of tumor/treatment

- Neurocognitive dysfunction
  May be related to tumor, hydrocephalus, postoperative complications, delayed effect (progressive) of cranial radiation
- Endocrinologic dysfunction
  May be related to hypothalamic/pituitary tumor, late effect of suprasellar/whole brain radiotherapy
- Hearing loss
  May be related to cerebellopontine tumors/resection, long-term effect of radiotherapy, cisplatinum use
- Secondary tumors
  May be secondary to radiotherapy, ? chemotherapy, genetic predisposition
- Psychologic/behavioral dysfunction
  May be secondary to tumor (? cortical, frontal), sequelae of treatment

Much of the focus of long-term sequelae research has been centered on the potential detrimental affects of radiotherapy. Radiotherapy tends to induce transient, acute neurologic difficulties due to tumor-related swelling; however, the most common difficulties encountered are late effects. These delayed sequelae include neurocognitive deficits and endocrinologic sequelae. Whole-brain radiotherapy and extensive cortical radiotherapy has been shown to result in overall declines in intelligence, primarily in younger children (especially those younger than 7 years of age), and results in significant, albeit more subtle deficits in learning in older children (Ris et al. 1999). Specific forms of cognitive difficulties may be present, including executive function disabilities and attentional deficits. These are targets for intensive educational interventions and possibly pharmacologic therapies. The detrimental effects on cognition of more focal radiotherapy, especially radiotherapy given to the posterior fossa, are less clear.

Radiotherapy to the suprasellar region and whole-brain radiotherapy has been related to a host of endocrinologic sequelae, most commonly growth hormone and thyroid deficiency. The impact of growth hormone deficiency is often exacerbated by poor vertebral growth

Pearls and Perils

- Children surviving brain tumors are at risk for significant neurologic, neurocognitive, psychological, and endocrinologic sequelae. The success of treatment cannot only be assessed on the basis of survival, but also on quality of life.

Pearls and Perils

- Years after successful treatment, secondary brain tumors may occur, especially when radiotherapy was used in initial management.

secondary to spinal radiation therapy, required for tumors with a proclivity to disseminate to the nervous system. Growth hormone replacement therapy has been shown to be relatively safe and partially ameliorates growth retardation. Other endocrinologic sequelae also may occur, and the issue of gonadal deficiency and fertility is a complex and understudied complication.

Secondary tumors, including primary CNS tumors and systemic cancers, are a devastating late occurrence in children with brain tumors. Their exact incidence is not known, but secondary tumors may occur in as many as 1–2% of long-term survivors. The development of this complication is multifactorial and probably relates to genetic predisposition, as well as to the long-term effects of both radiotherapy and chemotherapy. Primary CNS tumors that occur most frequently following successful treatment of a brain tumor include high-grade gliomas, which may occur as early as 4 years after treatment and have been extremely resistant to any form of subsequent therapy, and meningiomas, which occur at increasing frequency many years (7–10 plus) after radiotherapy.

Chemotherapy has been employed in an attempt to improve survival and to delay, if not obviate, the need for radiotherapy, but chemotherapy also may result in significant long-term sequelae. Because of the additive neurotoxicity of methotrexate, this drug has not been recently utilized in most chemotherapeutic regimens for children with brain tumors, but is being reintroduced in some protocols. Methotrexate may result in significant neurologic impairment, including leukoencephalopathy, myelopathy, and, if given intrathecally, significant spinal cord dysfunction and radiculopathy.

Cis-platinum, which is an active agent in childhood primitive tumors, especially medulloblastoma, often results in significant hearing loss, which may be additive to the effects of radiotherapy delivered to the cochlear region. Vincristine, another commonly used chemotherapeutic agent, often results in some degree of peripheral neuropathy, which may be permanent if this complication is not appreciated early in treatment. The wider use of high-dose chemotherapy carries with it other risks, and the use of intensive drug regimens supported by bone marrow transplant or peripheral stem cell rescue may result in significant permanent neurologic difficulties, including seizures. Some chemotherapeutic agents, as stated previously, also may increase the risk of mutagenesis.

Annotated bibliography

Central Brain Tumor Registry of the United States (CBTRUS). Statistical Report: Primary Brain Tumors in the United States, 1995–1999. Central Brain Tumor Registry of the United States, 2002.
A study of the epidemiology of childhood and adult brain tumors.

Crawford J, Vezina LG, Packer RJ. Central nervous system germ cell tumors of childhood, presentation and delay in diagnosis. *Neurology* 2007;68:1668–1673.
A retrospective review demonstrating frequent reasons for delay in diagnosis of germ-cell tumors.

Duffner PK, Horowitz MD, Krischer JP, et al. Postoperative chemotherapy and delayed radiation in children less than three years of age with malignant brain tumors. *N Engl J Med* 1993;328:1725–1731.
A large series of infants and children under age 3 treated with chemotherapy and delayed radiotherapy for predominantly high-grade tumors.

Evans AE, Jenkin RD, Sposto R, et al. The treatment of medulloblastoma: Results of a prospective randomized trial of radiation therapy with and without CCNU, vincristine, and prednisone. *J Neurosurg* 1990;72:572–582.
The first study demonstrating the benefits of adjuvant chemotherapy for some children with newly diagnosed medulloblastoma.

Gajjar A, Chintagumpala M, Ashley D, et al. Risk-adapted craniospinal radiotherapy followed by high-dose chemotherapy and stem-cell rescue in children with newly diagnosed medulloblastoma (St. Jude Medulloblastoma-96): Long-term results from a prospective, multicentre trial. *Lancet* 2006;7:813–820.
The preliminary results of a single-arm study using post-radiotherapy high-dose chemotherapy and peripheral stem cell support.

Gajjar A, Hernan R, Kocak M, et al. Clinical, histopathologic, and molecular markers of prognosis: Toward a new disease risk stratification system for medulloblastoma. *J Clin Oncol* 2004;15;22(6):984–993.
A paper discussing the addition of molecular genetic tests into the stratification schema of medulloblastoma.

Geyer JR, Jennings M, Sposo R, et al. Multiagent chemotherapy and deferred radiotherapy in infants with malignant brain tumors: A report from the Children's Cancer Group. *J Clin Oncol* 2005;23:7621–7631.
A multi-institutional prospective study of the efficacy of chemotherapy for infants with malignant brain tumors.

Grotzer MA, Janss AJ, Fung K, et al. TrkC expression predicts good clinical outcome in primitive neuroectodermal brain tumors. *J Clin Oncol* 2000;18:1027–1035.
A series demonstrating that molecular genetic findings are predictive of outcome in children with medulloblastoma.

Horn B, Heideman R, Geyer R, et al. A multi-institutional retrospective study of intracranial ependymoma in children: Identification of risk factors. *J Pediatr Hematol Oncol* 1999;21:203–211.
A large multi-institutional retrospective series of intracranial ependymomas.

Listernick R, Darling C, Greenwald M, et al. Optic pathway tumors in children: The effect of neurofibromatosis type 1 on clinical manifestations and natural history. *J Pediatr* 1995;127:718–722.
A study of the natural history of optic nerve tumors in children with neurofibromatosis type 1.

MacDonald TJ, Brown KM, LaFleur B, et al. Expression profiling of medulloblastoma: PDGFRA and RAS/MAPK pathway as therapeutic targets for metastatic disease. *Nat Genet* 2001;29:143–152.
An article demonstrating that genomics can be used to predict outcome and possibly lead to new and better understanding of ways to treat childhood medulloblastoma.

Merchant TE, Mulhern RK, Krasin MJ, et al. Preliminary results from a phase II trial of conformal radiation therapy and evaluation of radiation-related CNS effects for pediatric patients with localized ependymoma. *J Clin Oncol* 2004;22:3156–3162.
A study demonstrating improved disease control in children with ependymoma.

Neglia JP, Robison LL, Stovall M, et al. New primary neoplasms of the CNS in survivors of childhood cancer: A report from the childhood Cancer Survivor Study. *J Natl Cancer Institute* 2006;98:1528–1537.
Incidence of second malignancies after treatment of childhood cancer.

Packer RJ, Allen JC, Goldwein JL, et al. Hyperfractionated radiotherapy for children with brainstem gliomas: A pilot study using 7,200 cGy. *Ann Neurol* 1990;27:167–173.
An article describing outcome of children with brainstem gliomas and the transient ability of radiation to control disease.

Packer RJ, Ater J, Allen J, et al. Carboplatin and vincristine chemotherapy for children with newly diagnosed progressive low-grade gliomas. *J Neurosurg* 1997;86:747–754.
A large series documenting the potential efficacy of chemotherapy for low-grade gliomas.

Packer RJ, Cohen BH, Cooney K. Intracranial germ cell tumors. *Oncologist* 2000;5:312–320.
A review of therapy of germ cell tumors.

Packer RJ, Gajjar A, Vezina G, et al. Phase III prospective randomized study of craniospinal radiation therapy followed by one of two adjuvant chemotherapy regimens for newly-diagnosed average risk medulloblastoma. *J Clin Oncol* 2006; 24:4202–4208.
Results of a randomized trial demonstrating an 80% event-free survival rate for children with medulloblastoma.

Packer RJ, Gurney JG, Pynyko JA, et al. Longterm neurologic and neurosensory sequelae in adult survivors of a childhood brain tumor: Childhood Cancer Survivor Study. *J Clin Oncol* 2003;21:3255–3261.

Pomeroy SL, Tamayo P, Gaasenbeck M, et al. Prediction of CNS embryonal tumour outcome based on gene expression. *Nature* 2002;415:436–442.
An article describing the potential power of genomics to increase understanding and change therapeutic approach to pediatric embryonal tumors.

Ris MD, Packer R, Goldwein J, et al. Intellectual outcome after reduced-dose radiation therapy plus adjuvant chemotherapy for medulloblastoma: A Children's Cancer Group study. *J Clin Oncol* 2001;19:3470–3476.
The results of assessment of neurocognitive in children with medulloblastoma treated with radiotherapy and chemotherapy.

Rutkowski S, Bode U, Deinlein F, et al. Treatment of early childhood medulloblastoma by postoperative chemotherapy alone. *N Engl J Med* 2005;352(10):978–986.

A study demonstrating long-term control in infants with medulloblastoma treated with chemotherapy alone, including intrathecal methotrexate.

Robertson PL, Muraszko KM, Holmes EJ, et al. Incidence and severity of postoperative cerebellar mutism syndrome in children with medulloblastoma: A prospective study by the Children's Oncology Group. *J Neurosurg* 2006;105(S6 Pediatrics): 444–451.

A study of the incidence of the posterior fossa mutism syndrome in children with medulloblastoma treated in two prospective North American clinical trials.

Robertson PL, Zeltzer PM, Boyett JM, et al. Survival and prognostic factors following radiation and chemotherapy for ependymomas in children: A report of the Children's Cancer Group. *J Neurosurg* 1998;88:685–694.

A series demonstrating the lack of efficacy of chemotherapy for ependymomas.

Rorke LB, Packer RJ, Biegel JA. Central nervous system atypical teratoid/rhabdoid tumors of infancy and childhood: definition of an entity. *J Neurosurg* 1996;85:56–65.

The first comprehensive description of childhood atypical teratoid/rhabdoid tumors.

Schneider JM, Raffel C, McComb JG. Benign cerebellar astrocytomas of childhood. *Neurosurgery* 1992;30:58–62.

A review of outcome in children with cerebellar astrocytoma.

Scott RM, Hetelekidis S, Barnes PD et al. Surgery, radiation, and combination therapy in the treatment of childhood craniopharyngioma: A 20-year experience. *Pediatr Neurosurg* 1994;21:75–81.

A balanced review of approaches of management of craniopharyngiomas in childhood.

Smith MA, Freidlin B, Glocker-Ries LA, Simon R. Trends in reported incidence of primary malignant brain tumors in children in the United States. *J Nat Cancer Instit* 1998;90: 1269–1277.

A discussion of the incidence of childhood brain tumors and reasons for an apparent increase in incidence.

CHAPTER 18

Neuromuscular Disease in Children

John T. Sladky

Outline

- Neuromuscular disorders presenting at birth
- Neuromuscular disorders presenting in the infant/toddler
- Evaluation of the preadolescent with neuromuscular disease
- Differential diagnosis of neuromuscular disease in the newborn

The traditional approach to the topic of neuromuscular disease is to highlight constituents of the lower motor unit and discuss pathologic processes that affect particular components, such as anterior horn cells, peripheral nerves, neuromuscular junctions, and muscle. Although this has proven to be a useful pedagogical strategy, it is not economical, practically or intellectually, when dealing with children with neuromuscular disorders. An alternative approach is to take advantage of the fact that certain diseases present stereotypically in terms of the clinical features and the age at which they become manifest. Unlike adults, in whom the age of onset of symptoms may be of little help in suggesting their etiology, in children the age of presentation and incidence of particular disease entities can be used to structure a differential diagnosis.

Neuromuscular disorders presenting at birth

Common neuromuscular disorders that present at birth are listed in Table 18.1.

Congenital myopathies

Congenital myotonic dystrophy (DM-1) is probably the single most common neuromuscular disorder presenting at birth. Children with congenital myotonic dystrophy are almost exclusively born to mothers with myotonic dystrophy. Because of the marked variability in gene

Pearls and Perils

Congenital Myopathies

- Several somatic features are common to congenital myopathies of diverse etiologies. Hypomotility of the extremities in utero may result in arthrogryposis multiplex congenita. Although lower extremities typically are more involved, it is rare in the face of hip, knee, and ankle joint involvement not to find restricted range of motion at elbow and shoulder joints.
- Bulbar weakness with diminished swallowing in utero results in polyhydramnios. During embryogenesis, the palate develops from a narrow and highly arched configuration. The upward pressure from the tongue during the process of swallowing during gestation flattens the palate, resulting in horizontal expansion of the midface and transverse orientation of the lips.
- Infants with centronuclear myopathy, like other congenital myopathies, may present with arthrogryposis multiplex congenita. By virtue of the multiple joint contractures, one assumes that joint movement must have been markedly limited during early gestation. Although joint range of motion is restricted, muscle strength may be, paradoxically, only mildly diminished.

Table 18.1 Neuromuscular disorders presenting at birth

Discriminating features
- Hypotonia at rest
- No improvement in muscle tone with stimulation
- Weakness of appendicular muscles:
  - Diminished grasp (palmar and plantar)
  - Inability to raise limbs against gravity (or resistance)
- Weakness of axial muscles:
  - Inability to raise head to neutral in Landau posture
  - Diaphragmatic breathing
  - Respiratory compromise
- Weakness of facial and bulbar muscles
  - Facial diplegia
  - Ptosis
  - External ophthalmoplegia
  - Swallowing difficulty
  - Tongue fasciculation
- Diminished or absent reflexes

Associated clinical features
- Long, narrow facial features
- Tented upper lip
- High, arched palate
- Polyhydramnios
- Arthrogryposis

Associated laboratory features
- Elevated creatine phosphokinase
- Abnormal nerve conduction/electromyography testing
- Bell-shaped thorax on x-ray

Most common neuromuscular disorders presenting at birth
- Congenital myotonic dystrophy
- Congenital myopathy
- Brachial plexopathy
- Mononeuropathy
- Neonatal myasthenia gravis
- Motor neuron disease (usually not spinal muscular atrophy)

penetrance, the mother may be unaware of her disorder. Thus, myotonic dystrophy is a dominantly inherited disorder in which about half of infants of mothers with DM-1 are symptomatic at birth with gradual improvement in the severity of weakness with maturation. The genetic substrate for the disease is an expansion of a CTG repeat sequence within the 3' untranslated portion of the DM protein kinase gene (DMPK) on chromosome 19. In normal individuals, the CTG repeat may range from 5 to 37 repeats. Individuals affected with DM-1 show greater than 50 repeats and up to 6,000. The greater the number of repeats, the earlier and more severe the clinical presentation. The CTG sequence is unstable and, with succeeding generations, undergoes progressive expansion thus providing the molecular explanation for the clinical phenomenon of *genetic anticipation*, or the observation that offspring of affected individuals frequently have an earlier presentation and more severe disease. Why a congenital disorder, which is inherited through a dominant mode, is transmitted almost exclusively via affected mothers is incompletely understood. One hypothesis contends that the size of the repeat expansion confers a burden on the spermatozoa, resulting in impaired migration or fertilization, such that the sperm carrying the unaffected allele is far more likely to fulfill its procreative destiny. This explanation may be an oversimplification, and other factors may also play a role in this phenomenon.

Other congenital myopathies may present with a similar clinical picture. A host of myopathic disorders present in infancy, some of which have specific and unique gene defects, whereas others are genetically heterogeneous (Table 18.2). These disorders are classified on the basis of abnormalities of myofibrillar structure on histochemical studies and on electron microscopy. Some congenital myopathies are identified based on abnormal inclusions, such as nemaline or rod-body myopathy or fingerprint body myopathy, whereas others have myofibrillar abnormalities like central core disease or mini-core disease. Myotubular myopathy, also known as centronuclear myopathy, is characterized by myofibers that are similar to developing muscle in early gestation, in which myofibers have a tubular appearance with centrally located nuclei. Centronuclear or myotubular myopathy derives its name from the similarity in appearance of the muscle histology at term in these infants to a much earlier stage in muscle development. Early in gestation, myocytes are multinucleate tubular structures with centrally located nuclei. The metabolic differentiation of myofibers into different fiber types is also rudimentary at that stage. With maturation, myofibers expand in caliber, with peripheral migration of myonuclei and metabolic differentiation into a normal distribution of types I and II myofibers. Histochemical examination of muscle biopsies from infants with centronuclear myopathy confirms an immature appearance of myofibers with normal biochemical fiber type differentiation. These observations have engendered the hypothesis that centronuclear myopathy, in part, represents a process of delayed myofibrillar maturation, with profound weakness early in embryogenesis resulting in restricted joint movement and contracture formation. Muscle strength is thought to improve later in gestation in some infants, resulting in only minimal weakness at term.

Molecular techniques are rapidly expanding our ability to offer genotypically specific diagnoses in this group of diseases. The prognosis in these disorders is highly variable as there are, in many cases, multiple genotypes with similar phenotypical expressions. Many severely affected children at birth, even those requiring

Table 18.2 Congenital myopathies

Discriminating features
- Central core disease
  - Presence of central cores on biopsy
- Nemaline (rod body) myopathy
  - Rod bodies originating from Z bands
- Centronuclear (myotubular myopathy)
  - Chains of central nuclei
- Congenital fiber-type disproportion
  - A combination of clinical features and type I fiber predominance
- Congenital muscular dystrophy
  - A combination of clinical features and myopathic muscle biopsy

Consistent features
- Central core disease
  - Autosomal dominant
  - Benign course
  - Type I fiber predominance
- Nemaline (rod body) myopathy
  - Autosomal dominant
  - Type I fiber predominance
  - Moderate atrophy
- Centronuclear (myotubular myopathy)
  - Type I fiber predominance
  - CK elevation
  - Absent reflexes
- Congenital fiber-type disproportion
  - Autosomal dominant
  - Contractures and skeletal deformities
  - Short stature
- Congenital muscular dystrophy
  - Autosomal recessive
  - Elevated CK
  - Contractures and skeletal deformities

Variable features
- Central core disease
  - Skeletal deformities
- Nemaline (rod body) myopathy
  - Skeletal deformities
  - Bulbar weakness
- Centronuclear (myotubular myopathy)
  - Autosomal recessive
  - Extraocular muscle movement
- Congenital fiber-type disproportion
  - Myopathic EMG
- Congenital muscular dystrophy
  - Benign and severe forms

mechanical ventilatory support, may improve over time and survive into adulthood. Although scientifically unsatisfying, an augury of the prognosis may be observed over the first few months. Those infants who improve will, in general, continue to do so. Those who deteriorate progressively worsen, and those with a static course have an indeterminate prognosis, although the outcome is more likely to be unfavorable.

Congenital muscular dystrophy

The primary distinction between congenital myopathies and congenital muscular dystrophies (CMD) is based on the presence of myofibrillar necrosis and regeneration, along with endomysial fibrosis and deposition of fat on histopathologic examination of muscle biopsy in the dystrophic disorders. In addition to weakness and hyporeflexia (usually areflexia), these children may have elevated creatine phosphokinase measurements of several times the upper limit of normal. Most of these disorders are inherited in an autosomal recessive fashion. The initial step in classifying these diseases is based on the presence or absence of merosin (α-2 chain of laminin 2) on immunocytochemical studies of muscle biopsies or Western blots. Absence of the protein can be a primary or secondary phenomenon. Congenital muscular dystrophies, therefore, are described as those which are merosin-deficient or are merosin-positive, the latter of which accounts for about half of CMDs. Some of the CMDs are associated with central nervous system (CNS) abnormalities, including structural abnormalities on magnetic resonance imaging (MRI) and mental retardation. In Japan, the Fukayama type of CMD is the most common form. This disorder is inherited in a recessive mode from a defect in the gene that codes for the protein fukutin. The DNA coding for fukutin occupies a 100-kb genomic sequence consisting of 10 exons and 9 introns localized to 9q31.

Pearls and Perils

Congenital Muscular Dystrophy (CMD)

- The clinical course in CMDs is heterogeneous. Some children eventually walk while others grow progressively weaker and die from respiratory failure. Measures of serum creatine phosphokinase levels and pathological features on routine histochemical studies of muscle biopsy specimens are of limited value in discussing prognosis with families.
- As a rule, merosin positive CMDs are more likely to have normal cognitive development, normal cerebral magnetic resonance imaging studies, and overall a less severe course.
- Severe cognitive impairment along with abnormalities in brain imaging studies is commonly associated with both primary and secondary merosin deficiency.

Moderate to severe mental retardation typically occurs, with variable structural brain abnormalities including pachygyria/microgyria, and high signal intensity changes in white matter on T2 MRI sequences. Other examples of congenital muscular dystrophy associated with CNS abnormalities include Walker-Warburg syndrome and muscle-eye-brain disease. These are closely related disorders due to defects in glycosylation of α-dystroglycan, resulting in impaired binding to the extracellular matrix. Diminished expression of laminin 2 is thought to be a secondary phenomenon in this disorder.

Congenital myasthenic syndromes

Congenital myasthenia gravis may result in transient weakness in the newborn. This syndrome occurs in infants of mothers with active autoimmune myasthenia. Maternal IgG directed against epitopes associated with the postsynaptic acetylcholine receptor is passively transferred across the placenta in late gestation, resulting in receptor blockade with concomitant transient bulbar and somatic weakness. In a poorly controlled myasthenic mother who produces antibodies that cross-react with the fetal acetylcholine receptors (AChRs), transplacental diffusion of the IgG may result in diminished fetal movement, resulting in arthrogryposis. As AChRs mature, they are no longer primarily targeted by the antibody. Other congenital myasthenic syndromes may also present in the newborn period. These are typically inherited disorders with either autosomal dominant or recessive modes of transmission. The electrochemical defect can be presynaptic, postsynaptic, or at the end-plate itself. A primary AChR deficiency accounts for most of the nonautoimmune congenital myasthenic syndromes.

Focal nerve injuries

Peripheral nerve injuries are reasonably common including intrauterine, intrapartum, and postpartum events occurring in the nursery. Although the incidence of this collective category is not known, the most frequently encountered of these is brachial plexus injury, which has been variously estimated to occur in between 0.4 and 2.3 per 1,000 live births. Although most of these injuries are associated with macrosomic infants and often attributed to traction injury during delivery, there are reports of infants with brachial plexopathy after cesarean section or atraumatic vaginal delivery, reinforcing the hypothesis it may be due to the forces of intrauterine contraction alone. Thus, injury during delivery should not be assumed to be the cause of neonatal brachial plexopathy in all cases. The prognosis for recovery in these infants, particularly those with partial plexus involvement involving more proximal myotomes, is usually favorable. Compression neuropathies, especially involving radial and peroneal nerves, can be present at delivery, probably related to intrauterine position. They may develop postnatally in the neonatal intensive care unit (NICU), probably due to focal nerve compression.

Disorders of motor neurons

Disorders affecting motor neurons may present in the newborn period. Interestingly, it is rare for spinal muscular atrophy to be diagnosed in the neonatal nursery. For the most part, anterior horn cell diseases that are symptomatic at birth are related to hypoplasia of spinal motor neurons, or to intrauterine injury. Occasionally there is a history of maternal viral-like illness during gestation; however, causality can only be assumed and generally these disorders are considered to be of undetermined etiology. There may be associated arthrogryposis. This group of disorders tends to be nonprogressive, and affected infants may demonstrate improvement in motor function over time.

Evaluation of the newborn with suspected neuromuscular disease

The essential question to be addressed by the neurologist in the NICU is whether the infant has central hypotonia or neuromuscular disease. The findings of weakness and areflexia are probably the two most definitive discriminators between the two categories. Although encephalopathy and seizures point to a central cause, a congenital neuromuscular disease does not indemnify the infant against perinatal hypoxia–ischemia. Microcephaly and other congenital anomalies push the clinician to think along the lines of a global disorder affecting the ontogeny of multiple organ systems, with cerebral dysgenesis the likely cause for hypotonia. The bedside clinical examination may be sufficient to make the distinction. Ancillary laboratory studies can be useful screening tools:

- Brain imaging if hypotonia is thought to be on a central basis. Consider performing an electroencephalogram (EEG) to assess physiologic maturity/activity.
- Nerve conduction studies and electromyography (EMG) are extremely helpful in confirming that hypotonia and weakness are due to a neuromuscular disorder and to identify the nature of the disease (e.g., peripheral neuropathy, anterior horn cell disease, etc.).
- If the nerve conduction studies are normal but EMG demonstrates widespread denervation, causes of motor neuron disease should be explored. A blood test to evaluate possible mutations in the survival motor neuron gene will detect the majority of cases of spinal muscular atrophy (Werdnig-Hoffman disease) in this age group.

- If the study suggests a myopathic process, careful examination of the parents, especially the mother is essential. Myotonic dystrophy is the commonest inherited neuromuscular disease in the population and often is not recognized in affected adults. Clinical examination of the mother will often be consistent with the diagnosis of DM-1. The diagnosis can be confirmed with genetic testing.
- If the parents are normal, a muscle biopsy is often the next step in evaluating a patient with congenital myopathy. A caveat that must be confronted, and explained to family members, is that many disorders classified under the broad category of congenital myopathy have nonspecific morphologic changes on muscle biopsy, in which case, the biopsy may not lead to more specific understanding of the disorder.

Neuromuscular disorders presenting in the infant/toddler

Typically, in this age group, medical attention is sought because of failure to attain motor developmental milestones. Once again, the evaluation requires making a distinction between central hypotonia and neuromuscular disease. Fortunately, this task becomes less difficult as children grow older. It is useful to inquire of the parents, "When the child is very angry or upset, does his strength improve?" This phenomenon is quite typical of children with central hypotonia. It is often necessary to examine the child when they are very annoyed to confirm the parents' observation. Common neuromuscular disorders of the infant/toddler years are listed in Table 18.3.

Table 18.3 Neuromuscular disorders presenting in the infant/toddler

Clinical features

- Failure to achieve motor milestones
- Hypotonia
- Weakness, generalized or of selected muscle groups:
  - Appendicular muscles
  - Difficulty reaching for and grasping objects
  - Inability to bear weight on lower extremities
  - Axial muscles
  - Immature Landau posture
  - Inability to sit up
  - Poor head control
  - Diaphragmatic breathing
  - Respiratory compromise
  - Bulbar muscles
  - Facial weakness
  - Impaired suck/swallow
  - Nasal regurgitation
  - Ptosis
  - External ophthalmoparesis
  - Tongue fasciculations
- Diminished or absent tendon reflexes

Evaluation of the infant/toddler with neuromuscular disease

The clinical picture is usually clearer in this age group than in the newborn, in whom the potential explanation for the child's illness is often multifactorial. Two typical scenarios arise when evaluating children in this age group. The first is that of delayed or completely stagnant motor development dating back to birth. The second is that of normal early development with the subacute evolution of neuromuscular symptoms.

Group I: chronic delay, no clear onset of weakness

The symptoms in this group may be relatively static or indolently progressive; often it is difficult to be certain. Assuming that cognitive development is normal:

- Nerve conduction velocity tests and EMG are reliable screens for neuromuscular disorders with this type of presentation.
- Spinal muscular atrophy is probably the most common single entity that shows up in this context. The nerve conduction velocity tests and EMG should localize the disease process to the anterior horn cell. Genetic screening for a mutation in the survival motor neuron (SMN) loci should confirm the diagnosis in over 95% of children.
- Screening for creatine phosphokinase and aldolase will help to identify myopathic disorders with defective cytoskeletal proteins (dystrophin, sarcoglycan, merosin, etc.) or other disorders with significant myonecrosis (inflammatory myopathies). With the exception of dystrophinopathies, a biopsy may be required for diagnosis.
- Demyelinating/hypomyelinating neuropathies can present in this age group. Some of those, which are genetically determined, may be identified with DNA analysis for associated gene mutations. When these studies are unrevealing, nerve biopsy may be required to more accurately characterize the nature of the disorder.

Table 18.4 Common neuromuscular disorders presenting in the infant/toddler: Group I

- Spinal muscular atrophy
- Congenital myopathies
- Congenital muscular dystrophy
- Genetically determined neuropathy

Common neuromuscular disorders presenting in the infant/toddler: Group I

Table 18.4 presents the common neuromuscular disorders of Group I that present in infants and toddlers.

Spinal muscular atrophies

Spinal muscular atrophy (SMA) types I and II, also known as Werdnig-Hoffman disease, are typically diagnosed postnatally when a failure to attain motor milestones is recognized by parents and physicians. Clinical findings are generalized hypotonia, weakness of axial and appendicular muscles with relative sparing of facial and bulbar muscles (early on), and areflexia. Electrodiagnostic testing will document normal sensory nerve conduction with widespread denervation on EMG localizing the disorder to a process at the level of motor neurons.

The disease is caused by a homozygous deletion involving exons 7 and 8 in the survival motor neuron gene (SMN1) and modified by the expression of a second duplicate homologous gene (SMN2). Both are located on chromosome 5q and closely linked, with SMN1 located on the telomeric side of the duplication. Children with severe early-onset SMA have typical deletions in SMN1 genes with only one or two residual copies of the SMN2 genes. Those with milder phenotypes have the SMN1 deletions but also possess three or more copies of SMN2. Deletion of both SMN1 and SMN2 genes is probably a lethal permutation since this genotype has not been described in affected humans.

> **Pearls and Perils**
>
> **Spinal Muscular Atrophy**
>
> - The spinal muscular atrophies, particularly in children with onset under 1 year of age, are often associated with a defect in Ω-fatty acid oxidation. During periods of metabolic stress or fasting, which often occur with intercurrent infection, dicarboxylic aciduria may be present as a manifestation of the metabolic defect. In this setting, the child's weakness may precipitously worsen.
> - Children admitted because of clinical deterioration with evidence of metabolic decompensation and increasing weakness will often benefit from infusions of high levels of glucose. This approach can help to mitigate the effects of systemic stress, normalize metabolic defects, and increase strength. Even modest increases in respiratory muscle strength may be very helpful in the face of impending or frank respiratory failure.

Chronic symmetrical peripheral neuropathies

Most of the peripheral neuropathies presenting early in life are associated with slowing of sensory and motor nerve conduction velocities and absent or diminished amplitude of sensory nerve, and compound motor action potentials (Table 18.5). They are incorporated under the rubric of *demyelinating neuropathies*, often, more accurately, *hypomyelinating neuropathies*, since there is rarely evidence of formation of normal myelin sheaths on large caliber axons. Congenital hypomyelinating neuropathy may be evident at birth; however, more commonly, it is diagnosed at a later date. Since respiratory muscles and bulbar muscles are usually spared, at least in infancy, in these disorders, normal feeding and respiratory patterns reinforce the perception of normal infant behavior. When examined, these children are typically hypotonic with generalized weakness and absent reflexes. Motor nerve conduction velocities are diminished and may be as slow as 2 m/sec. Only limited correlation exists between the magnitude of conduction velocity slowing and the severity of the clinical syndrome. In one series, it was reported that the presence of arthrogryposis multiplex congenita and the absence of onion bulb formations within the endoneurium were histopathologic markers associated with a poor prognosis. This category of peripheral neuropathy has been referred to as *Dejerine-Sottas syndrome*. The term brings with it little specificity, since the diagnosis includes children with substantial variability in terms of both genotype and phenotype. In fact, the limitations in nosology closely reflect the reality of the situation; homologous gene defects result in different phenotypes, and diverse gene mutations produce similar clinical presentations.

Group II: normal early development, subacute onset of symptoms

These children have a history of normal perinatal events and early acquisition of motor skills with a clearly identifiable time of onset of disability. In my experience, the majority of children in this group have disorders of neuromuscular transmission. These children present with bulbar symptoms along with axial and appendicular weakness. In young infants (1–5 months of age) the etiology is usually infant botulism. In older infants/toddlers (12–24 months of age) the cause is often myasthenia gravis. Other acquired, immune-mediated disorders can present in this age although are more common in older

Table 18.5 Peripheral neuropathies

Discriminating features

- Charcot-Marie-Tooth neuropathy, hereditary motor and sensory neuropathy (HMSN)-1
  - Demyelinating neuropathy and dominant inheritance
  - C17p11.2 duplication
- HMSN-2
  - Axonal neuropathy
- Déjérine-Sottas neuropathy HMSN-3
  - A combination of clinical features and pattern of inheritance
  - C17p11.2 duplication or point mutation
- Guillain-Barré syndrome
  - Albuminocytologic dissociation in cerebrospinal fluid (cerebrospinal fluid protein elevation without pleocytosis)

Consistent features

- Charcot-Marie-Tooth neuropathy HMSN-1
  - Onion bulb formation
  - Hypertrophic nerves
  - Pes cavus and hammertoes
  - Linkage to Duffy locus
  - Slow conduction velocities
- HMSN-2
  - Nerves are not palpable
  - Pes cavus and hammertoes
  - Axonal degeneration
- Déjérine-Sottas neuropathy HMSN-3
  - Infantile onset
  - Hypertrophic nerves
  - Autosomal dominant
  - Demyelinating and axonal neuropathy
  - Marked onion bulb formation
  - Severe hypotonia
  - Elevated cerebrospinal fluid protein
- Guillain-Barré syndrome
  - Demyelination
  - Early muscle pains
  - Facial weakness
  - Depressed reflexes
  - Slow conduction velocities with blocks

Variable features

- Charcot-Marie-Tooth neuropathy HMSN-1
  - Degree of weakness
- HMSN-2
  - Degree of weakness
- Déjérine-Sottas neuropathy HMSN-3
  - Degree of weakness
- Guillain-Barré syndrome
  - Axonal degeneration
  - Respiratory involvement

children. Metabolic disorders, mitochondrial cytopathies in particular, may present with loss of motor skills, often acutely and related to intercurrent infection.

- Electrodiagnostic testing is highly reliable in confirming the diagnosis of infant botulism long before tests for the organism or toxin are available.
- Confirming a postsynaptic defect in neuromuscular transmission in this age group can be difficult. When a myasthenic syndrome is suspected, a trial of Mestinon may help to clarify the diagnosis.
- Metabolic screening for lactic acidosis, especially during an acute episode, along with analysis of urine organic acids and serum amino acids may identify those children with disorders of oxidative phosphorylation. MRI spectroscopy can noninvasively document elevation in intracerebral lactate in children with phenotypical features suggesting a disorder of oxidative phosphorylation. A number of mitochondrial cytopathies can be confirmed by identification of mutations in the mitochondrial genome. The majority of mitochondrial disorders, however, are related to mutations in nuclear genes.

Common neuromuscular disorders in the infant/toddler: Group II

The commonly presenting neuromuscular disorders of Group II in infants and toddlers are listed in Table 18.6.

Infant botulism

This disease results when botulinum spores are ingested, germinate in the gastrointestinal tract, and slowly elaborate botulinum toxin, which is absorbed and disseminated through systemic circulation, ultimately interrupting neuromuscular transmission. Germination of botulinum spores only occurs in infancy due the lower acidity of the immature stomach, which doesn't destroy the ingested spores. The toxin binds at a presynaptic site on the neuronal membrane. It then traverses the neurolemma, probably by endocytotic mechanisms, and enters the cytoplasm where it binds to acetylcholine release sites and prevents synaptic release of acetylcholine vesicles. Once the toxin

Table 18.6 Common neuromuscular disorders in the infant/toddler: Group II

- Infant botulism
- Myasthenia gravis
- Metabolic myopathies
- Inflammatory myopathies

> **Pearls and Perils**
>
> **Infant Botulism**
>
> - The time course and severity of infant botulism caused by type A toxin tends to be shorter and less severe than type B.
> - A hallmark feature in Eastern, or type B, infant botulism is the presence of internal and external ophthalmoparesis. Observers in Rocky Mountain states and West describe this phenomenon in a minority of cases related to the type A toxin.
> - Some authors have suggested that the typical (virtually diagnostic) electrophysiologic findings on repetitive motor nerve stimulation in infants with botulism are often absent or inconclusive. This may be related to the nature and number of muscles tested. Ideally, repetitive stimulation should be performed on a muscle in which the compound motor action potential amplitude is only mildly to moderately diminished. One may be unable to demonstrate a meaningful increment or decrement in a severely affected muscle in which the majority of neuromuscular junctions are inactivated.

is internalized, it irreversibly blocks acetylcholine release. The latter steps in this process, internalization of the toxin and blockade of vesicle release, are both temperature- and activity-dependent. One would, therefore, predict that those neuromuscular junctions that are warmer and more active would be the earliest to be affected. In fact, among the earliest manifestations of infant botulism are constipation, external ophthalmoparesis, and feeding difficulty. The clinical severity of the disorder in these infants typically progresses after initial presentation, usually over a relatively short period of time. Many of these patients will require mechanical ventilatory support. Autonomic dysfunction may accompany weakness, especially in the more severely affected infants.

The disease can be caused by several *Clostridium botulinum* species, types A through G, which are subclassified based on the characteristics of the elaborated toxin. The vast majority of cases of infant botulism are caused by types A and B. The spores of *C. botulinum* are essentially ubiquitously distributed and typically present in soil. The often-described exposure to honey is overemphasized, and colonization from honey containing spores accounts for a small fraction of cases. Types A and B *C. botulinum* have a geographically distinct distribution, with type A predominantly found in states from the Rocky Mountains and west, whereas type B is located in regions east of the mountain range. Diagnosis of the disease can be based on typical clinical findings in the context of the subacute evolution of symptoms in a previously healthy infant including the external ophthalmoparesis, bulbar dysfunction, generalized weakness, and, commonly, areflexia. A firm diagnosis can also be based on the electrophysiologic characteristics from nerve conduction studies and EMG. The nature and presynaptic localization of neuromuscular blockade in these infants results in a reproducible constellation of findings. The hallmark features of electrodiagnostic testing are the presence of a decremental response in the compound muscle action potential (CMAP) amplitude with low-frequency repetitive motor nerve stimulation (2–3 Hz) and a marked increment with higher rates of stimulation (10–50 Hz). Electromyography reveals mixed features, including widespread fibrillation potentials due to chemical denervation of myofibers along with abundant small-amplitude, short-duration, myopathic-appearing motor unit potentials. This latter finding is related to the electrochemical inexcitability of myofibers scattered within the motor unit, resulting in motor unit potentials with reduced amplitude and a polyphasic morphology.

Despite the severity of the clinical syndrome, with adequate supportive care, the vast majority of these infants recover fully. The mechanism of recovery from the disease is probably multifactorial. The first step is likely recognition of the toxin by the immune system and elaboration of an antibody response to the toxin. During, and in some cases, after recovery, toxin can still be recovered from the gastrointestinal tract. If there is sufficient binding and internalization of toxin at a particular neuromuscular junction, transmission at that junction is permanently blocked, with subsequent degeneration of that nerve terminal. Neuromuscular transmission to that myofiber is reestablished by sprouting of a new axon from the distal nerve fiber and the generation of a new neuromuscular junction. The pace of recovery can be enhanced by the early administration of an antibody directed toward botulinum toxin.

Myasthenia gravis

Myasthenia gravis (MG) is an autoimmune disorder characterized by a deficiency of AChRs on postsynaptic nerve terminals at neuromuscular junctions. The salient clinical manifestation of this disorder is weakness. The most common expression of MG is ptosis with variable involvement of other muscles. Conventionally, MG has been said to comprise three clinical syndromes: ocular, bulbar, and generalized myasthenia. Pure ocular MG accounts for about 15–25% of autoimmune myasthenia in children, depending on the age group and ethnic background. It is often the herald symptom, antedating the appearance of weakness in other muscle groups. Among those children who present with symptoms of ocular MG, roughly 75% will progress to involve bulbar muscles or develop generalized MG. Ptosis with variable degrees of external ophthalmoparesis can develop at any age, including children and adults, and evolve to include nearly any combination of striate muscles. Most children who present with ocular symptoms that later generalize do so within the first year. The symptoms typically wax and wane, and may be exacerbated by intercurrent infection that up-regulates activity of the immune system. Typically, fluctuation also occurs in the severity of symptoms in proportion to the degree of exertion, hence the frequently heard complaint that ptosis and other weakness increases during the course of the day. Myasthenia gravis may take a heavy toll on the patient's psychological well-being, especially in older age groups. This is engendered because of the marked, unpredictable fluctuations in strength and functionality in some myasthenic patients.

Myasthenia gravis is an immune-mediated disorder with predominantly IgG class of antibodies directed toward various epitopes of the postsynaptic AChR. These antibodies are detectable in 50–75% of children with generalized MG. Although the disease is thought to be mediated predominantly via anti-AChR antibodies, evidence suggests that cellular immune mechanisms also play a role in orchestrating the elimination of postsynaptic receptors. Roughly 25–50% of children, especially in younger age groups, will be found to be seronegative. It is difficult to quantitate precisely, but a proportion of these seronegative patients, influenced again by age and ethnic background, have pathogenic autoantibodies to muscle specific tyrosine kinase (MuSK). MuSK is localized on the sarcolemmal surface of the neuromuscular junction. This kinase participates in the agrin-induced clustering of AChRs on the postsynaptic nerve terminal during the ontogenesis of the neuromuscular junction. The role this molecule plays in the mature neuromuscular junction is not precisely understood. It is thought, however, that immune-mediated reduction in MuSK results in diminished numbers or inappropriate distribution of AChRs at the postsynaptic nerve terminal. Anti-AChR antibodies and anti-MuSK antibodies appear to be mutually exclusive, in that these two antibody species do not coexist in individual patients with myasthenia. The autoimmune-mediated attack directed at epitopes from either of these entities results in similar clinical manifestations.

The first line of therapy in MG is usually pyridostigmine. It is most useful in patients with pure ocular involvement, in whom immunosuppression may not be warranted. There is little data on which to base recommendations for an optimal therapeutic algorithm. Corticosteroids are almost always efficacious; however, side effects may become unacceptable when prolonged, high-dose treatment is necessary.

Incorporation of both plasmapheresis and intravenous immunoglobulin (IVIg) administration should be considered as steroid-sparing strategies. The latter usually is accompanied by fewer logistical impediments; however, it may have a longer latency between treatment initiation and therapeutic response. Cyclosporine A is a particularly useful adjunct therapeutic agent. Because toxicities are, for the most part, dose-dependent, the ability to monitor drug levels provides a mechanism to adjust dosage to achieve blood concentrations of the drug within the desired range, and to avoid toxic levels with anticipated side effects. Mycophenolate is also effective and generally well tolerated.

The relationship of thymoma and myasthenia gravis is well established and occurs in roughly 30 % of adults with the disease. By contrast, thymic hyperplasia is the predominant finding in children, with thymoma being exceedingly rare. Conventional wisdom holds that thymectomy confers an increased likelihood of achieving remission and that the procedure is more likely effective in achieving this objective when performed within 1 year of the onset of symptoms. On review, available data support this contention; however, the design of many of the studies is less than rigorous. There is a long history of vigorous debate regarding the optimal surgical approach for thymectomy including transsternal, supraclavicular, and, more recently, endoscopic techniques. The fundamental contention relates to the ability to detect ectopic thymic tissue. The data in this arena are even more difficult to sort out; however, contemporary practitioners assert that the endoscopic exploration of the thoracic cavity is equally thorough compared to open exposures and is less invasive, with less morbidity and earlier recovery. The ultimate criteria for endorsement of any of these procedures is the long-term outcome of the disease, and that question awaits a definitive answer. It is generally accepted that thymectomy does not have a role in cases of myasthenia with anti-MuSK antibodies.

Metabolic myopathies

The topic of metabolic disorders affecting muscle is a broad one that precludes detailed elucidation in the context of this chapter. The majority of metabolic myopathies can be classified into three broad categories: glycogen storage disorders, defects in fatty acid oxidation, and mitochondrial cytopathies (Table 18.7). It is axiomatic that these metabolic disturbances often affect other organ systems, and weakness may not be the predominant factor that precipitates seeking medical attention.

A common clinical theme with many of the glycogenoses is the presence of exercise intolerance and muscle cramps. Many of the disorders that present in this fashion may also be associated with episodic myoglobinuria. Four of the more well recognized glycogen storage disorders are myophosphorylase deficiency (glycogenosis type V or McArdle disease), phosfructokinase deficiency (glycogenosis type VII or Tauri disease), α-glycosidase deficiency (glycogenosis type II or Pompe disease), and debrancher enzyme deficiency (glycogenosis type III or Forbes disease). The first two of these disorders may have

Pearls and Perils

Metabolic Myopathy

- The symptoms of exercise intolerance, myalgias, and episodic rhabdomyolysis are shared by all three categories of metabolic defects described. An optimal sequence of diagnostic investigations is difficult to codify. Measurement of serum lactate, pyruvate, and quantitative amino acids, along with determination of quantitative organic acid concentrations in urine are effective screening tools.
- Some children will require skin biopsy and isolation of cultured fibroblasts for studies of lipid metabolism. In selected patients, muscle biopsy may be necessary for enzyme determination, oxidative phosphorylation studies, mitochondrial DNA analysis, routine histochemistry, and ultrastructural studies of muscle.
- Careful electrodiagnostic studies may help to identify those children in whom mitochondrial disease is more likely. Evidence of peripheral neuropathy on nerve conduction studies is often present in mitochondrial cytopathies, often with features of demyelination, even if clinically not apparent. Mild myopathic characteristics seen in proximal muscles in these patients may be obscured by changes due to denervation in distal muscles. This combination (peripheral neuropathy with mild myopathic changes in proximal muscles) is typical of mitochondrial disorders but may be overlooked unless specifically sought.

similar clinical manifestations, often presenting with exercise intolerance and muscle cramps as the herald symptoms. Either disease can present at almost any age; however, they are more likely to present in mid-childhood or later, at a time when strenuous physical exertion is more likely to occur. Prolonged exercise may result in rhabdomyolysis and pigmenturia. In severe cases, this can result in predominantly transient renal failure. In a similar vein, α-glucosidase deficiency and debrancher deficiency may present in children or adults, but both may cause hypotonia and weakness in infancy or early childhood. These latter disorders are not typically associated with episodes of rhabdomyolysis. In addition to involvement of striatal muscle, both of these diseases may involve other organ systems, with progressive encephalopathy in Pompe disease and cardiomyopathy a prominent feature in both.

Carnitine palmitoyltransferase II (CPT II) deficiency is arguably the most often identified disorder of fatty acid oxidation. Like many enzyme deficiency diseases, it is genetically determined and has an autosomal recessive mode of inheritance. The salient clinical feature of the disorder

Table 18.7 Metabolic myopathies

Discriminating features

- Glycogen metabolism disorders
  - Glycogen storage disease types 5, 7, 9, and 10
    - Assays for specific enzyme deficiencies
  - Acid maltase deficiency
    - Absent specific enzyme activity in all forms
- Lipid metabolism disorders
  - Carnitine palmitoyltransferase (CPT) deficiency
    - Low CPT activity in muscles
- Mitochondrial disorders
  - Mitochondrial myopathies
    - Respiratory chain component assays or DNA analysis

Consistent features

- Glycogen metabolism disorders
  - Glycogen storage disease types 5, 7, 9, and 10
    - Exercise intolerance
    - Positive forearm ischemic exercise test
    - Autosomal recessive
    - Myoglobinuria
    - Muscle pain and cramps
    - Fatigue
  - Acid maltase deficiency
    - Severe myopathy in the infantile form with organomegaly and cardiomyopathy
    - Autosomal recessive
    - Vacuolar myopathy
    - Creatine kinase K elevation
- Lipid metabolism disorders
  - CPT deficiency
    - Exercise intolerance
    - Muscle pain and tenderness
    - No weakness
    - Increased lipid in muscles
    - Normal electromyelogram (EMG)
    - Precipitated by fasting
    - Myoglobinuria
- Mitochondrial disorders
  - Mitochondrial myopathies
    - Exercise intolerance
    - Lactic acidosis
    - Ragged red fibers

Variable features

- Glycogen metabolism disorders
  - Glycogen storage disease types 5, 7, 9, and 10
    - Permanent weakness
    - Myopathic EMG and muscle biopsy
  - Acid maltase deficiency
    - Slower rate of progression in the mild form with variable organomegaly
- Lipid metabolism disorders
  - CPT deficiency
    - Cramps and contractures
- Mitochondrial disorders
  - Mitochondrial myopathies
    - Variable degrees of myopathy
    - Deafness
    - Ophthalmoplegia
    - Cardiomyopathy
    - Pigmentary retinal degeneration

is recurrent rhabdomyolysis. Unlike the glycogenoses, there is usually no exercise intolerance in CPT II deficiency. Affected individuals will generally not experience muscle pain or cramping during vigorous exertion. Rather, after an episode of prolonged exercise, they will develop muscle pain followed by pigmenturia. Often, similar bouts will occur spontaneously or in association with intercurrent infection. Between bouts of rhabdomyolysis, these individuals appear normal and very rarely develop weakness. The most important risk from CPT II deficiency is renal failure induced by myoglobinuria. For unclear reasons, the frequency and severity of episodes of rhabdomyolysis seem to improve with maturation.

Another well-recognized category of fatty oxidation disorders includes the various species of acyl-CoA dehydrogenase deficiency or CAD. The acyl-CoA dehydrogenases participate in the process of mitochondrial B-oxidation and are specific for the length of the associated fatty acid, short-chain (4 carbon; SCAD), medium-chain (8 carbon; MCAD), and long-chain (up to 18 carbon; LCAD) acyl-CoA dehydrogenase. Again, at the risk of oversimplification, children with these disorders most commonly present with an acute encephalopathy, nonketotic hypoglycemia, and features similar to Reye syndrome. These episodes may be associated with rhabdomyolysis, however, this is usually a less dramatic feature of the diseases. The episodes are often precipitated by prolonged fasting. This often occurs in the setting of intercurrent infection. Over time, slowly progressive weakness may evolve, particularly in SCAD and LCAD.

In recent years, there has been increasing recognition and understanding of disorders of oxidative phosphorylation. This group of disorders is multifaceted in molecular etiology and protean in clinical manifestations. The prototypical mitochondrial disorder is the Kearns-Sayre syndrome. The clinical characteristics of this disorder include short stature, external ophthalmoparesis, myopathy, pigmentary retinopathy, and cardiac conduction defects. When followed over the long term, the majority of these patients will develop cardiomyopathy, progressive encephalopathy, and blindness. Like many of the classic, phenotypically characterized mitochondrial disorders, such as myopathy, encephalopathy, and ragged red fibers (MERRF); mitochondrial encephalopathy, lactic acidosis, and stroke-like episodes (MELAS); or Leigh syndrome, Kearns-Sayre syndrome is inherited via the maternal transmission of the defective mitochondrial gene. In addition to the clinical features just enumerated, multiorgan involvement is typical in oxidation/phosphorylation (OX/PHOS) disorders where symptoms may include ataxia, deafness, anemia, liver or kidney failure, gastrointestinal hypomotility, autonomic failure, and peripheral neuropathy.

Considerable variability may occur in the severity of the expression of homologous gene defects in members of the same kinship. The variable phenotypic manifestations of the disease in different individuals and different organ systems is thought to be attributable to at least two independent factors. The first is determined by the basal metabolic requirements of particular cell and tissue types. Those organ systems with the highest energy substrate requirements are likely to be preferentially susceptible to injury due to defective production of high-energy phosphate intermediates. Inheritance of mitochondrial DNA occurs through the maternal lineage, in which the gene may be heterogeneous for mutations, with each cell containing both mutated and normal mitochondrial DNA within the cell cytoplasm. This results, during the earliest phases of embryonal development, in primordial stem cells with variable ratios of abnormal to normal mitochondria. This heterogeneous group of embryonic cells is segregated into progenitor cell lines, which develop into tissues with variable burdens of dysfunctional mitochondria. These factors result in a mismatch between the level of basal energy substrate requirements in a particular tissue and the ability of that tissue to generate the required amount of energy. Hence, different thresholds for energy failure among different organ systems and individual patients.

Only a minority of mitochondrial disorders are maternally inherited due to mutations of the mitochondrial genome. The majority of these diseases are related to mutations of nuclear-encoded genes or their processing. A prototypical disease in this category is Friedreich ataxia. Friedreich ataxia is inherited in a recessive mode due to an expanded GAA repeat sequence on chromosome 9q resulting in defective expression of the protein frataxin. This protein is thought to regulate iron content within mitochondria, with diminished amounts of frataxin resulting in increased iron concentrations within mitochondria, resulting in diminished thresholds for oxidative stress, and consequent cell injury. Analogous to other mitochondrial diseases, Friedreich ataxia exhibits multiorgan involvement, with cardiac muscle, motor neurons, and subpopulations of sensory neurons within dorsal root ganglia being preferentially affected.

Evaluation of the preadolescent with neuromuscular disease

The chief complaint, by the parents and family members, with the onset of neuromuscular disease in this age group (roughly 3–10 years of age), is commonly clumsiness or loss of balance. In children with myopathic processes, this perception is due to the inability of these children to right themselves when their center of gravity is displaced from its point of equilibrium due to weakness of proximal hip girdle muscles. In peripheral neuropathies, the weakness of foot dorsiflexors results in "tripping" when the child encounters trivial environmental obstacles. In both cases, the family will complain that the child is falling down. Generally, by the time these phenomena are apparent, muscle weakness is quite evident on examination. A more subtle manifestation is loss of endurance. A careful history will often reveal that inability to keep up with peers and diminished endurance antedated the onset of falling down. In cases of very mild weakness, early fatigueability may be the only historical feature, and examination may be normal or nearly so. In patients with peripheral neuropathies, in addition to a history of weakness or foot drop, it is necessary to inquire about "weak ankles," high arches, and hammertoes in family members, in order to confirm the hereditary nature of the disease. The most common chronic neuromuscular disorders to present in this age group are genetically determined: Duchenne and Becker muscular dystrophies and Charcot-Marie-Tooth disease or the hereditary sensory-motor neuropathies.

The clinical features of preadolescent neuromuscular diseases are listed in Table 18.8.

Table 18.8 Preadolescent neuromuscular disease

Clinical features

- Loss of motor skills, apparent loss of balance
- Decreased endurance
- Weakness, generalized or of selected muscle groups
  - Appendicular muscles
  - Diminished grasp
  - Gower maneuver
  - Foot drop
  - Axial muscles
  - Inability to do a sit-up
  - Poor head control
  - Bulbar muscles
  - Facial weakness
  - Nasal regurgitation
  - Ptosis
  - External ophthalmoparesis
  - Tongue fasciculations
- Diminished or absent tendon reflexes

Associated clinical features

- Exaggerated lumbar lordosis
- Muscle pseudohypertrophy
- Pes cavus deformities
- Hammertoes
- Cutaneous nodules
- Toe walking
- Muscle wasting
- Pes planus deformities
- Heliotrope malar rash

Common neuromuscular disorders presenting in the preadolescent period

- Duchenne/Becker muscular dystrophy
- Hereditary sensory and motor neuropathies
- Myasthenia gravis
- Inflammatory myopathies
- Guillain-Barré syndrome
- Chronic inflammatory demyelinating neuropathy

Duchenne/Becker muscular dystrophy

These disorders are probably the commonest, and also most clinically stereotypical, among diseases affecting males in this age group. The Duchenne variety generally presents early in the first decade of life, whereas the Becker phenotype may not become clinically evident until late adolescence. These boys exhibit proximal weakness and muscle pseudohypertrophy, and most will have a mutation in the dystrophin gene. The Duchenne variety occurs when a nonsense mutation occurs in the gene, typically an out-of-frame deletion or a stop codon resulting in complete failure of transcription. Becker dystrophy is caused by a missense mutation, usually an in-frame deletion, resulting in a truncated protein that has the capacity to moderate disease severity. Dystrophin is a cytoskeletal protein which, among others, is critical in stabilizing the link between the intracellular contractile apparatus, the sarcolemmal membrane, and the extracellular matrix. In the absence of the protein, the sarcolemmal membrane is fragile and susceptible to fenestration during myofibrillar contraction and relaxation. Defects in the sarcolemma result in permeability to extracellular ions and subsequent accumulation of intracellular calcium, which initiates several pathways and ultimately results in cell death.

Although the clinical features of the disorder are quite stereotypical, several laboratory studies can reinforce the diagnostic impression. A markedly elevated level

Pearls and Perils

Muscular Dystrophy

- Conventional wisdom is that children with Duchenne type muscular dystrophy (DMD) present at between 3 and 5 years of age with a complaint of weakness. In fact, parents often notice symptoms at a much earlier stage and may have brought their concerns to the child's pediatrician but were reassured that all was well.
- Parents frequently state the reason for bringing their child with muscular dystrophy for evaluation is clumsiness or impaired balance.
- Pseudohypertrophy in DMD is not restricted to calves, but may also involve proximal leg and shoulder girdle muscles.

of creatine phosphokinase in serum is often present. DNA analysis from peripheral blood samples can be diagnostic with a deletion at Xp21, which can be demonstrated in about two-thirds of these boys using traditional polymerase chain reaction (PCR) techniques. Full-length screening of the coding sequences of the dystrophin gene will define a mutation in an additional segment of the boys in whom there is no detectable deletion. As noted, a serum creatine phosphokinase level that is elevated 50- to 100-fold is nearly pathognomic for dystrophinopathy in this age group, although other defects in cytoskeletal proteins can mimic dystrophin deficient muscular dystrophy (e.g., sarcoglycan deficiency or severe childhood autosomal recessive muscular dystrophy [SCARMD]) along with other limb-girdle muscular dystrophies. These are most often inherited in an autosomal recessive fashion and, therefore may affect either sex.

As noted earlier, DNA analysis is a readily available tool and will identify a mutation in the majority of boys with Duchenne/Becker muscular dystrophies. The accuracy with which the molecular geneticist can predict the disease phenotype (Becker or Duchenne) varies considerably from lab to lab and with the nature of the mutation. When no family history suggests the likely rate of progression of the myopathy, a muscle sample for immunocytochemical staining or Western blot analysis of the dystrophin protein will distinguish between the Duchenne and Becker variants.

Despite the widespread enthusiasm for the use of corticosteroids in the treatment of boys with muscular dystrophy, these drugs are, realistically, symptomatic and not curative. Two agents, prednisone and deflazacort, have been shown in randomized controlled trials to improve muscle strength along with motor function. These drugs retard the rate of progression of the disease which, however, is inexorable. Management of the side effects of long-term corticosteroid therapy are an ongoing challenge. These may include weight gain, behavioral changes, hypertension, hyperglycemia, growth retardation, osteopenia, cataracts, and immunosuppression. All require judicious monitoring and alteration of the corticosteroid regimen as necessary. (Although not established in controlled trials, patients with Becker muscular dystrophy may respond well to treatment with corticosteroids, often at a low dose of <0.5 mg/kg/day).

A linch-pin in the management of muscular dystrophy is anticipatory, supportive therapy. Physical therapy should be instituted early in the course of the illness. Because boys with a Duchenne pattern of proximal lower extremity weakness become obligate toe walkers, Achilles contractures are nearly inevitable. Initiating an aggressive stretching program can usually forestall functionally disabling contractures in ambulatory boys. When the contractures progress despite rigorous physical therapy, with compliant participation of the family, introduction of night splints may be helpful to maintain the foot and ankle in a physiologic position during sleep. Some boys will benefit from orthotics during ambulation, while others find them an impediment. The increasing exaggeration of the lumbar lordosis, which evolves along with progression of hip girdle weakness, is an unavoidable anatomic consequence of compensatory alterations in gait to maintain ambulation.

Cardiomyopathy is a ubiquitous feature of the disease. In most boys, it is asymptomatic until the end stage of the illness. It is prudent to obtain a cardiologic evaluation relatively early in the course. Evidence suggests that treatment with angiotensin-converting enzyme inhibitors may retard the progression of cardiomyopathy.

Scoliosis is generally a complication that evolves after loss of ambulation and should be evaluated radiographically on a regular basis. Early surgical intervention will stabilize the curve and prevent the additional burden that spinal and chest wall deformities add to the restrictive lung disease due to progressive weakness of respiratory muscles. Interval pulmonary function studies are helpful in following the pace of the progression of respiratory muscle weakness and provide insights regarding the timing for introduction of additional therapeutic strategies, such as assistive cough devices, nocturnal oxygen supplementation, or ventilatory assistance.

A segment of nearly every visit to the clinic will be spent discussing the progress of research for a cure for the disease. Over the past few years, several therapeutic strategies have emerged that appear to be promising. The longest standing of these approaches is viral vector–mediated introduction of functional dystrophin genes into muscle. This approach is currently undergoing clinical trials in humans. Other pathways include pharmacologically induced read-through of stop codons, oligonucleotide-mediated gene editing, and stem cell transplantation. Comprehensive review of this research is outside the scope of this discussion; however, assurance that progress is ongoing in this enterprise is often helpful to patients and their families coping with DMD.

Inflammatory myopathy

Inflammatory myopathies, although relatively rare, are more commonly seen in childhood. These disorders are conventionally divided into three broad categories: infectious myositis, autoimmune polymyositis, and dermatomyositis (Table 18.9). A host of viruses with myotrophic properties can produce focal or generalized muscle inflammation and injury. A not unusual scenario is a child in the mid-first decade of life who, rather acutely, complains of calf pain and is reluctant or unable to walk. In general, there will be tenderness to palpation in affected muscles. Serum creatine phosphokinase and muscle transaminases may be elevated. These symptoms usually resolve over several days and further evaluation is rarely necessary.

Table 18.9 Inflammatory myopathies (dermatomyositis)

Discriminating features
- A combination of the characteristic rash and typical muscle biopsy

Consistent features
- Violaccous rash
- Proximal weakness
- Perifascicular atrophy on muscle biopsy
- Elevated CK
- Inconsolable child

Variable features
- Bulbar and respiratory weakness
- Gastrointestinal symptoms
- Myocarditis and pericarditis
- Arthralgias

Autoimmune inflammatory myopathies, for the most part, fall into the category of polymyositis or dermatomyositis. Many children with polymyositis present with complaints of fatigue or weakness with or without muscle swelling or tenderness. Electrodiagnostic testing will confirm a myopathic disorder, frequently without "irritable" features typically associated with muscle inflammation. The serum creatine phosphokinase level may be mildly or massively elevated, with variable elevations in the erythrocyte sedimentation rate and other satellite markers for inflammation or other autoimmune disorders. Magnetic resonance imaging of muscle may demonstrate multifocal areas of increased signal intensity on T2 spin echo sequences representing regions of edema. Muscle biopsy may be normal because of the multifocal nature of inflammation. When an active area of inflammation is sampled, typical features include myofibrillar degeneration and regeneration with primary endomysial inflammation and occasionally perivascular collections of inflammatory cells, without evidence of vasonecrosis.

Dermatomyositis is one of few disorders in clinical neurology in which the nosology accurately reflects the pathology of the disease. Children with this disease may present with muscle pain and weakness or with a painful rash as their primary complaint. The classic syndrome features a malar rash, somewhat pale, raised, papular lesions over extensor surfaces of the fingers, elbows, and knees (Gottron papules), and subungual flame hemorrhages. As in polymyositis, there may be serologic evidence of muscle injury and systemic inflammation. Testing in the electrophysiology laboratory may be similar to polymyositis as well, and muscle MRI may demonstrate evidence of multifocal myoedema. Dermatomyositis is a vasculitic myopathy so that, in addition to the biopsy features seen in polymyositis, there is evidence of frank vasonecrosis indicative of active vasculitis. A hallmark histopathologic feature of dermatomyositis is perifascicular myofibrillar atrophy. This is due to the distribution of endomysial blood flow, with areas of ischemia most commonly affecting the periphery of the fascicle.

Unlike the situation in adults, in whom dermatomyositis is commonly a paraneoplastic disease, often associated with small-cell carcinoma of the lung, neoplasia is almost never a feature of the disease in children. Therapy in dermatomyositis and polymyositis consists of immunosuppression. Corticosteroids are probably the first-line therapeutic agents. IVIg and methotrexate can be quite helpful in avoiding or reducing chronic steroid side effects.

Rare myopathies associated with other connective tissue disorders, systemic vasculitides, or paraneoplastic syndromes will not be addressed in this chapter.

Hereditary motor and sensory neuropathy

The peroneal muscular atrophy syndrome was originally described in 1886 by Howard Henry Tooth, an English medical student. Later that year, a more detailed description of the disorder was published by the French neurologists Charcot and his pupil Marie. The clinical features of the disease are progressive loss of strength in a fiber length–dependent distribution and, usually to a lesser degree, diminished sensation, predominantly involving those modalities related to large-caliber myelinated axons. Myotactic reflexes are diminished or absent at early stages of the disease.

The initial subclassification of these disorders, for most of the 20th century referred to as Charcot-Marie-Tooth disease, resulted from work by Dyck and Lambert. Electrophysiologic testing permitted distinction between kinships with autosomal dominantly inherited neuropathies based on motor nerve conduction velocities in the forearm. Patients with nerve conduction velocity below 40 m/sec were classified as having the demyelinating form of the disease (type I), whereas those with motor conduction velocity of greater than 40 m/sec were classified as the axonal form (type II). This classification schema was validated by histopathologic features on sural nerve biopsies wherein the predominant pathologic features were either of axons showing evidence of demyelination and remyelination or features of axonal degeneration and regeneration. Genetic analysis is available to confirm the diagnosis in many hereditary motor and sensory neuropathy (HMSN) subtypes. The initial mutations identified in autosomal dominantly inherited demyelinating neuropathies were in genes encoding peripheral myelin protein 22 (PMP22) and myelin protein 0 (MPZ). Mutations in the Connexin 32 gene (Cx32) were shown to be responsible for an X-linked pattern of inherited demyelinating neuropathy. Since then, numerous genes have been identified to be associated with both axonal and demyelinating subtypes of HMSN.

Pearls and Perils

Hereditary Motor and Sensory Neuropathy (HMSN)

- The demyelinating forms of HMSN have, in the past, been referred to as hypertrophic demyelinating neuropathies because of nerve enlargement due to endoneurial Schwann cell proliferation and collagen deposition. This is manifested by peripheral nerve enlargement that permits distinction between HMSN I and HMSN II phenotypes at the bedside based on the presence of palpably enlarged peripheral nerves.
- Peripheral nerve enlargement can be appreciated in the ulnar nerve at the elbow or the peroneal nerve at the fibular head. After extension and rotation of the fibular head, enlargement of the posterior auricular nerve can be seen and palpated over the posterior-lateral neck.
- When pursuing a family history of genetically determined neuropathy, it is often necessary to inquire about symptoms and signs in family members rather than asking whether peripheral neuropathy is present in the kinship. Useful examples are pes cavus and hammertoes in the family, frequent ankle sprains in childhood and adolescence, or inability to roller skate or ice skate.

As noted earlier, the patterns of inheritance are variable, and kinships with autosomal dominant, recessive, and sex-linked modes of transmission are reported. There also appear to be instances of spontaneous mutation, although this phenomenon is probably quite rare. To make matters more difficult, mutations in the same gene in different kinships can result in divergent phenotypes, with features of either axonal or demyelinating neuropathy. This phenomenon is most likely related to the effect of specific mutations at different sites within the gene resulting in altered protein products with differing pathologic effects on the functional integrity of Schwann cell–axonal relationships.

Guillain-Barré syndrome

In nations with widespread immunization programs, Guillain-Barré syndrome (GBS) is the single commonest cause of acute flaccid paralysis in children and adults. The incidence of the disease has been variously estimated to be between 0.5 and 1.5/million in children younger than 18 years of age. In most series, there is male predominance with a male-to-female ratio of approximately 1.2:1. A typical patient might describe ascending weakness beginning in the legs and advancing to involve the arms, associated with moderate to severe back and leg pain. The accepted diagnostic criteria are purely clinical, consisting of the subacute or acute onset of progressive weakness involving more than one extremity along with diminished or absent stretch reflexes. Laboratory investigations can serve to reinforce the accuracy of the diagnosis, including the presence of albumino-cytologic dissociation on spinal fluid examination and electrodiagnostic testing.

Pearls and Perils

Guillain-Barré Syndrome (GBS)

- Guillain-Barré syndrome can occur in any age group including neonates. Passively transferred antibodies have even produced the disorder in utero with clinical findings evident at birth.
- Pain is often the presenting complaint and, in children, may obscure weakness in the early stages of the disease. These painful symptoms are commonly attributed to arthralgia, and the neurologist may be the second or third specialist consulted, after orthopedics and rheumatology.
- Pain is a component of the morbidity in GBS in the majority of cases. In children with severe disease, those requiring mechanical ventilation in particular, it is nearly ubiquitous and is, in some cases, excruciating. Pain should be treated aggressively, and the clinician should not hesitate to incorporate narcotic analgesics into the therapeutic armamentarium.
- It is likely that in GBS the majority of peripheral nerve injury occurs at the outset, within the first few days of symptoms. Unless underlying chronic inflammatory demyelinating neuropathy (CIDP) is suspected, repeat treatment episodes with plasmapheresis or intravenous immunoglobulin (IVIg) are unlikely to alter the clinical course.
- Guillain-Barré syndrome is a disease in which rehabilitation needs to begin in the intensive care unit. Early, proactive attention to potential contractures and other complications from prolonged immobility will enhance long-term outcomes.

Roughly two-thirds of GBS patients will identify an antecedent event in the 30–60 days prior to the onset of symptoms. These events are diverse in character and dissociate in nature, ranging from infections, immunizations, trauma, surgery, and parturition to animal exposures and insect bites. When a query regarding the list of antecedent events is narrowed, upper respiratory infection is the most commonly identified. Over the past few years, it has come to be appreciated that *Campylobacter* enteritis may be the commonest antecedent infection to instigate an immune response resulting in GBS. This is particularly true in developing countries and in areas where the water supply may be contaminated.

The clinical course of GBS conforms to a triphasic model. An initial progressive phase includes the interval from the first appearance of symptoms until the point of maximal clinical severity. This is followed by a plateau phase, which lasts until the beginning of recovery. Finally, there is a recovery phase, which is typically considerably more prolonged than the progressive phase. Review of several series describing the natural history of GBS in adults and children reveals remarkable consistency, with the mean duration of the progressive and plateau phases each lasting approximately 10–11 days. The recovery phases were much more variable among the different series.

The clinical severity at the nadir of the disease in children hospitalized for GBS was also fairly consistent. Approximately 25% of patients retained the ability to ambulate 5 m without assistance. Roughly 20% of children could ambulate 5 m with assistance or a walker. Forty percent of children were bed- or wheelchair-bound, with the balance requiring mechanical ventilatory support. The prognosis for recovery is, in general, excellent. A large series from western Europe with consistent follow-up reported that after 6 months all children were ambulatory and, at worst, had minimal functional deficits. In tertiary care centers with sophisticated life support facilities, where most of the more severely affected patients are treated, the mortality in childhood GBS is virtually zero.

The pathobiology of GBS remains incompletely understood, and a comprehensive discussion of this topic is outside the scope of this chapter. It is reasonable to conceptualize the pathogenesis as reflecting a series of discrete processes that ultimately orchestrate an immune-mediated attack on the peripheral nervous system. Whether identifiable or not, there must be an event that initiated an autoimmune process. This then is followed by breakdown of immune tolerance. The immune system then targets specific epitopes on Schwann cells or axons, or both, within peripheral nerves. Specific immune components, including immunoglobulin, T cells, macrophages, and proinflammatory cytokines, must traverse the blood–nerve barrier. This cascade of events ultimately results in a T-cell and immunoglobulin orchestrated, macrophage-mediated attack on endoneurial contents.

The specific endoneurial components that are targeted and injured in this autoimmune process determine the electrophysiologic, histopathologic, and clinical phenotype in the affected child. These criteria have been employed to subclassify GBS into several distinct syndromes. The most common manifestation of GBS in North America and western Europe is acute, inflammatory, demyelinating polyradiculoneuropathy (AIDP). This disorder accounts for more than 90% of cases of GBS in these regions. These children present with typical ascending paralysis with electrophysiologic and histopathologic evidence of multifocal demyelination. A second, much less frequent GBS subtype is acute motor and sensory axonal neuropathy or AMSAN. In this syndrome, the electrophysiology and histopathology are indicative of axonal degeneration rather than demyelination, affecting both sensory and motor axonal populations. Fisher syndrome is a clinical diagnosis based on the triad of external ophthalmoplegia, ataxia, and areflexia. Often children presenting with this clinical triad will develop evidence of more widespread involvement within the peripheral nervous system. This syndrome has been estimated to account for approximately 2% of cases of childhood GBS. A fascinating syndrome, which is extremely rare in North America and western Europe, is acute motor axonal neuropathy (AMAN). Electrodiagnostic testing in this syndrome reveals normal motor and sensory nerve conduction velocities with preservation of sensory nerve action potential amplitudes. Histopathologic studies have demonstrated sparing of sensory axons, with axonal degeneration discretely limited to the motor axonal population. Although rare in the United States, this disorder may account for up to 70% of cases of GBS in China, South America, and elsewhere. A significant correlation exists with *Campylobacter* infection and the absence of water treatment facilities.

There is no scientific rationale on which to base a decision regarding optimal treatment of children with GBS. There are numerous case series in the literature, some employing historical controls, examining the efficacy of both plasmapheresis and human IVIg in the treatment of children with GBS. Many of these series describe a more rapid recovery in children treated with either modality. There have been no randomized controlled trials of treatment for GBS in children. Data are available for several large randomized trials in adults with GBS using plasmapheresis or IVIg. These treatments have been found to be equivalent in reducing morbidity in GBS. The individual treatments of plasmapheresis and IVIg have also been compared to a combination of both and each of the three arms of this randomized controlled trial showed equivalent paces of recovery. Several trials have documented an increased incidence of adverse events in the plasmapheresis-treated cohorts compared to the patients treated with IVIg, attributable to the need for large-caliber venous access for the duration of the plasmapheresis, heparinization of the patient, and a need to "prime the pump" with blood products. In the absence of evidence of the superiority of plasmapheresis, many neurologists believe that IVIg is the treatment of choice in children.

Chronic inflammatory demyelinating neuropathy

Chronic inflammatory demyelinating neuropathy (CIDP) is reasonably easily identified when it presents acutely, mimicking GBS followed by sequential relapses, or the symptoms of the disorder evolve subacutely in the context of a previously well child. In some cases, however, the onset is indolent with slow progression. In this setting CIDP can mimic virtually any inherited neuropathy and should always be kept in mind in a child with neuropathy

> **Pearls and Perils**
>
> **Chronic Inflammatory Demyelinating Neuropathy (CIDP)**
>
> - Clinical manifestations of CIDP may be protean. Any sensory-motor modality that relies on peripheral nerve for executive or reporter functions may be affected.
> - Despite obvious sensory ataxia, careful examination may document little or no impairment of proprioception. Vibratory sensation, in this scenario, will commonly be more obviously diminished. Bulbar involvement, which is more frequent in acute, inflammatory, demyelinating polyradiculoneuropathy (AIDP), may be present in CIDP. Cranial neuropathies including optic nerve involvement with papilledema have been reported.
> - Peripheral neuropathy associated with mitochondrial diseases can replicate the clinical, electrophysiological, and histopathologic characteristics of CIDP.

when no other evidence of disease can be confirmed in the kinship. Because many of the inherited neuropathies are transmitted in a dominant mode, careful family history, and, when practical, examination of available family members, may establish a presumptive genetic cause for the neuropathy. On occasion, electrodiagnostic testing will distinguish hereditary from acquired neuropathies; however, asymmetrical slowing of nerve conduction velocities, conduction block, and other features suggestive of an acquired demyelinating neuropathy may not be evident. To further muddy the waters, electrodiagnostic features may be indicative of an axonal neuropathy. DNA analysis for common mutations associated with hereditary neuropathies may clarify the issue if a mutation is detected that appears consonant with the clinical picture. In the absence of a detectible mutation, however, it may be necessary to perform a nerve biopsy or undertake a trial of an immunosuppressant to sort these issues out.

Several immunosuppressant agents have been shown to be effective in the treatment of CIDP. The choice of treatment in this disorder is individual and idiosyncratic. Corticosteroids are often a first-line therapy because they are relatively inexpensive, and the majority of children with CIDP initially respond well to this treatment. If there is an inadequate response or if cumulative side effects occur because of an ongoing high dosage requirement, additional steroid-sparing strategies can be employed. Plasmapheresis, IVIg, cyclosporine, azathioprine, and cyclophosphamide all have been used with variable success.

Differential diagnoses

Tables 18.10 through 18.12 present differential diagnoses for various neuromuscular diseases of children.

Table 18.10 Differential diagnosis of neuromuscular disease in the newborn

Anterior horn cell disease
- Intrauterine infection
- Hypoxic–ischemic injury
- Genetic disease; spinal muscular atrophy

Peripheral neuropathies
- Congenital hypomyelinating neuropathy
- Congenital axonal neuropathy
- Immune-mediated demyelinating neuropathy
- Guillain-Barré syndrome/chronic inflammatory demyelinating neuropathy

Disorders of the neuromuscular junction
- Myasthenia gravis (passive transfer of maternal antibody)
- Congenital myasthenic syndromes
- Hypermagnesemia

Diseases affecting muscle
- Congenital myopathy
  - Congenital myotonic dystrophy
  - Congenital myopathies with specific cytoarchitectural characteristics
  - Myotubular myopathy
  - Centronuclear myopathy
  - Nemaline myopathy
  - Central core disease
  - Congenital fiber type disproportion
- Congenital muscular dystrophy
  - Dystrophin deficiency
  - Fukayama-type dystrophy
  - Dystrophin-associated glycoprotein deficiencies
  - With dystrophic cerebral white matter
  - Without CNS involvement
  - Inflammatory myopathy

Table 18.11 Differential diagnosis of neuromuscular diseases presenting in the infant/toddler

Anterior horn cell disorders
- Infection (polio, enteroviruses, rabies)
- Genetic (spinal muscular atrophies)

Peripheral neuropathies
- Genetically determined neuropathy
- Hereditary sensory-motor neuropathies (HMSN types Ia, Ib, Ix, II)
- Guillain-Barré syndrome
- Chronic inflammatory demyelinating neuropathy

Disorders affecting the neuromuscular junction
- Myasthenia gravis
- Congenital myasthenic syndromes
- Infant botulism

Disorders affecting muscle
- Congenital myopathy
- (Not myotonic dystrophy in infants)
- Congenital muscular dystrophy
- Inflammatory myopathy
- Metabolic disorders
- Hypokalemia
- Periodic paralysis
- Metabolic myopathies
- Pompe disease
- Phosfructokinase deficiency
- Debrancher deficiency
- Phosphoglycerokinase deficiency
- Methylglutaconic aciduria
- Acyl-CoA-dehydrogenase deficiency (multiple variants)
- Mitochondrial disorders

Key Clinical Questions

- Is the infant's diminished spontaneous movement due to a neuromuscular disorder or a systemic disease?
- Is the hypotonia due to a central or peripheral process?
- Does hypotonia improve with stimulation?
- Are reflexes normal or diminished?
- Is motor development improving, static, or worsening?
- Is the pattern of weakness predominantly proximal or distal?
- Is there evidence of associated sensory loss?
- Does weakness and sensory loss conform to a length dependent pattern of severity?
- Is diminished sensation predominantly related to dysfunction of myelinated or unmyelinated axons?
- Is motor dysfunction due to weakness or pain?
- Is internal or external ophthalmoplegia present?
- Do symptoms fluctuate in the course of the day, during the week, over several months, or at all?
- Is ataxia sensory or cerebellar?

Table 18.12 Differential diagnosis of neuromuscular disorders presenting in the preadolescent

Anterior horn cell disorders
- Infection (polio, enteroviruses, rabies)
- Genetic (spinal muscular atrophies)

Peripheral neuropathies
- Genetically determined neuropathies
- Hereditary motor and sensory neuropathy (HMSN types Ia, Ib, Ix, II)
- Guillain-Barré syndrome
- Chronic inflammatory demyelinating neuropathy

Disorders affecting neuromuscular transmission
- Myasthenia gravis
- Congenital myasthenic syndromes
- Botulism (food-borne or wound)

Disorders affecting muscle
- Duchenne/Becker muscular dystrophy
- Severe childhood autosomal recessive muscular dystrophy and other limb-girdle muscular dystrophies
- Myotonic dystrophy
- Congenital myopathy
- Inflammatory myopathy
- Metabolic disorders
- Hypokalemia
- Periodic paralysis
- Metabolic myopathies

Annotated bibliography

Brooke MH. *A clinician's view of neuromuscular diseases*. Baltimore: Williams & Wilkins, 1986.

At more than 20 years, this edition is dated, particularly with respect to molecular genetics. This single-author text, however, remains among the most readable and lucid monographs describing the clinical features of neuromuscular disorders.

Jones HR, DeVivo DC, Darras BT. *Neuromuscular disorders of infancy, childhood, and adolescence: A clinician's approach*. Philadelphia: Butterworth Heinemann, 2003.

A substantial text devoted to pediatric neuromuscular disease. Currently, this is the definitive work in the field.

Engel AG. *Myology*, 3rd ed. New York: McGraw-Hill, 2004.

The two-volume text is a comprehensive reference source regarding muscle and disorders of that tissue.

Dyck PJ, Thomas PK. *Peripheral neuropathy*, 4th ed. Philadelphia: Saunders, 2005.

Definitive text regarding the neurobiology of peripheral nerve and peripheral neuropathies.

CHAPTER 19

Order of Nervous System Development

Emanuel DiCicco-Bloom

Outline

- The neural plate and neurulation
- The ventricular and subventricular proliferative zones
- Radial and tangential patterns of neurogenesis and migration
- Specific inductive signals and patterning genes in development
- The spinal cord
- The cerebral cortex
- The hippocampus
- The basal ganglia
- Neuronal specification
- Regulation of neurogenesis by extracellular factors
- Cell migration
- Differentiation and neuronal process outgrowth

Nervous system development is generally conceived of as a sequence of processes including precursor proliferation and cell cycle withdrawal, cell migration, axon and dendrite formation, neurotransmitter system expression, axonal growth to targets, synapse elaboration, and selective neuron survival based on appropriate target innervation. Although it is convenient to separate these events into discrete processes, many of them occur simultaneously within brain regions and even in the same cell. This is important to recognize, since it alters the conceptual models we construct regarding the possible effects of changing one process, and how it may alter several concurrent processes. For example, the presence of neurotransmitter receptors on very early precursors, those engaged in cell proliferation, allows neurotransmitters themselves, and therapeutic drugs we administer, to directly affect neuron production during development. Thus, following a general overview of development, we examine several of these processes and describe the important roles in development and disease pathogenesis of neural patterning genes, extracellular signals regulating neurogenesis, and molecular mechanisms of cell migration and process outgrowth.

Several principles guide our understanding of brain development. First, different brain regions and neuron populations are generated at distinct times and exhibit specific temporal schedules. Second, the sequence of cellular processes comprising ontogeny predicts that abnormalities in early events necessarily lead to differences in subsequent stages. Third, specific molecular signals, such as extracellular growth factors, play roles at multiple developmental stages of the cell. Thus, changes in expression or regulation of a ligand or its receptor, by environmental insults or genetic mechanisms, will have effects on multiple developmental and maturational processes.

The neural plate and neurulation

The human nervous system first appears between 2.5 and 4 weeks of gestation. During development, emergence of new cell types, including neurons, results from interactions between neighboring layers of cells. On gestational day 13, the embryo consists of a sheet of cells. Following gastrulation (day 14–15), which forms a two-cell layered embryo consisting of ectoderm and endoderm, the neural plate region of the ectoderm is delineated by the underlying mesoderm, which appears on day 16. The mesoderm forms by cells entering a midline cleft in the ectoderm, called the *primitive streak*. After migration, the mesodermal layer lies between ectoderm and endoderm and induces overlying ectoderm to become neural plate. Induction usually involves release of soluble growth factors from one group of cells, which in turn bind receptors on neighboring cells, eliciting changes in nuclear

Key Clinical Questions

All Disorders of Brain Development

- *Were there any prenatal maternal infections?*
  A history of prenatal infections raises the possibility of an environmental, rather than a genetic cause, for brain malformations. Cytomegalovirus can result in polymicrogyria, rubella can cause microcephaly, and toxoplasmosis often leads to scattered calcifications.
- *Is there a history of clotting disorders?*
  Clotting disorders can cause cerebral infarctions. Early prenatal infarctions may result in porencephaly, which is distinguished from schizencephaly by the gray matter that lines the cleft of a schizencephalic defect. Complete occlusion of both internal carotid arteries results in hydrencephaly, which is distinguished from aprosencephaly by the membranous covering that overlies a hydrencephalic defect.
- *Is there a family history of developmental delays, learning disabilities, or seizures?*
  Some disorders of brain formation have widely variable clinical phenotypes ranging from mild learning disabilities to severe mental retardation, spastic quadriparesis, and epilepsy. Periventricular nodular heterotopia, for instance, is clinically silent in as many as 25% of affected patients. The mother of an affected patient may herself have the disorder without knowledge of it. A history of mild learning disabilities may be the only sign of maternal involvement.
- *How is the child doing developmentally?*
  Developmental concerns are common among all disorders of brain formation and are often the presenting sign of the disorder. It is therefore important to review developmental progress and initiate any therapies that are needed.
- *Have there been any seizures?*
  Seizures are also common among all disorders of brain formation. Infantile spasms are particularly prevalent in lissencephaly and tuberous sclerosis and should always be considered in infants with these conditions.
- *Are the parents planning more children in the future?*
  Family planning is among the most important considerations for parents of an affected child. It is therefore necessary to pursue genetic testing and provide genetic counseling, particularly for families planning to expand.

transcription factors that control downstream gene expression. In some cases, cell–cell contact-mediated mechanisms are involved.

The neural plate, whose induction is complete by 18 days, is a sheet of columnar epithelium, surrounded by ectodermal epithelium. After formation, the edges of the neural plate elevate, forming the neural ridges. Subsequently, changes in intracellular cytoskeleton and cell–extracellular matrix attachment cause the ridges to merge in the midline and fuse, a process termed neurulation, forming the neural tube, with a central cavity presaging the ventricular system. Fusion begins in the cervical region at the hindbrain level (medulla and pons) and continues rostrally and caudally. Neurulation occurs at 3–4 week of gestation in humans, and its failure results in anencephaly rostrally and spina bifida caudally. Neurulation defects are well known following exposure to retinoic acid in dermatologic preparations, anticonvulsants, especially valproic acid, and diets deficient in folic acid.

Another product of neurulation is the neural crest, whose cells derive from the edges of the neural plate and dorsal neural tube. Neural crest cells migrate dorsolaterally, under the skin to form melanocytes, and ventromedially to form dorsal root sensory ganglia and sympathetic chains of the peripheral nervous system and ganglia of the enteric nervous system. The neural crest also gives rise to diverse tissues including neuroendocrine, cardiac, mesenchymal, and skeletal systems, forming the basis of many congenital syndromes involving the brain and other organs. Neural crest abnormalities underlie the neurocutaneous disorders, including tuberous sclerosis and neurofibromatosis. Another structure of mesodermal origin found on the ventral side of the neural tube, the notochord, plays a critical role during neural tube differentiation, since it is a source of soluble growth factors, especially sonic hedgehog (Shh), which impact gene patterning and cell determination of the ventral spinal cord and hindbrain.

After closure, the neural tube expands differentially to form major morphologic subdivisions that precede the major functional divisions of the brain. These subdivisions are important developmentally since different regions are generated according to specific schedules of proliferation and subsequent migration and differentiation. The neural tube can be described in three dimensions: longitudinal, circumferential, and radial. The longitudinal dimension reflects the rostrocaudal (anterior-posterior) organization, which most simply consists of the brain and spinal cord. The circumferential organization represents two major axes: in the dorsoventral axis cell groups are uniquely positioned from top to bottom. In the medial to lateral axis there is mirror image symmetry. The radial dimension extends from the innermost cell layer adjacent to the ventricles to the outermost surface, and exhibits region-specific cell layering. At 4 weeks, the human brain is divided longitudinally into prosencephalon (forebrain), mesencephalon (midbrain), and rhombencephalon (hindbrain). These three "vesicles" divide further into five divisions by 5 weeks, with the prosencephalon forming telencephalon (including cortex, hippocampus, and basal ganglia) and diencephalon (thalamus and hypothalamus), the mesencephalon (midbrain), and the rhombencephalon forming metencephalon (pons and cerebellum) and myelencephalon (medulla). Morphologic transformation into five vesicles depends on region-specific proliferation of precursor cells adjacent to the ventricles, the so-called ventricular zones (VZ). Proliferation depends on soluble growth factors made by proliferating cells themselves or released from regional signaling centers. In turn, growth factor production and cognate receptor expression also depend on region-specific patterning genes. We now know that VZ precursors, which appear morphologically homogeneous, express a checkerboard array of molecular genetic determinants that control the generation of specific types of neurons in specific regions. Although an individual gene may be expressed over an extensive range, such as the rostral cerebral cortex, a specific combination of partially overlapping genes may define a distinct domain, such as the medial aspect of the superior frontal cortex.

Circumferentially, organization begins very early and extends over many rostrocaudal subdivisions. In the spinal cord, the majority of tissue comprises the lateral plates, which later divide into dorsal or alar plates, consisting of sensory interneurons, and motor or basal plates, consisting of ventral motor neurons. Two other diminutive plates, termed roof plate and floor plate, are virtually absent in maturity, but play critical regulatory roles as growth factor signaling centers in the embryo. Indeed, the floor plate, in response to the growth factor, Shh, from the notochord, produces its own Shh, which in turn induces neighboring cells in the ventral spinal cord and brainstem to express region-specific transcription factors that specify cell phenotype and function. For example, floor plate Shh induces midbrain precursors to differentiate into dopamine-secreting neurons of the substantia nigra. Similarly, the roof plate secretes bone morphogenetic proteins (BMPs), which induce dorsal neuron cell fate in spinal cord. In the absence of the roof plate, dorsal structures, such as cerebellum, and midline hippocampal structures, fail to form. In the radial dimension, the organization of layers is subdivision-specific and is produced by differential proliferation of VZ precursors and selective patterns of neuronal cell migration.

The ventricular and subventricular proliferative zones

The distinct patterns of precursor proliferation and migration in different regions generate radial nervous system organization. In each subdivision, control of neurogenesis matches production to the final size of a region. Although many cells produced during development undergo genetically programmed cell death (up to 10–40%), initial cell generation roughly matches regional size requirements, indicating that neurogenesis itself is precisely controlled. This contrasts with traditional concepts suggesting excess cell production everywhere, with cell number regulation achieved through selective cell death mediated by target-derived survival (trophic) factors. The patterning genes play major roles in directing regional precursor proliferation that is coordinated with final structural requirements. Consequently, in diseases characterized by brain regions smaller than normal, such as schizencephaly, there may be a failure to generate neurons initially, as opposed to normal generation with subsequent cell loss.

The generation of specific cell types involves proliferation of undifferentiated precursor cells (or progenitors), followed by cessation of proliferation (exit from the cell cycle) and expression of specific phenotypic characters, such as neurofilaments and neurotransmitter systems. Precursor proliferation occurs primarily in two densely packed regions during development. The primary site is the VZ lining the walls of the entire ventricular system, which contributes to all brain regions in the rostrocaudal dimension. For select regions, however, including the cerebral cortex, hippocampus, and cerebellar cortex, precursors from the VZ migrate out to secondary zones where they generate a more restricted range of cell types.

In the early embryo, neural tube VZ progenitors are arranged as a one-cell-layer–thick, pseudostratified neuroepithelium. Ventricular zone precursors have cytoplasmic processes that span from the ventricular to the pial surface. During the cell cycle, the VZ appears multilayered, or stratified, because cell nuclei undergo movements, called *interkinetic nuclear migration*. The cell cycle that produces new cells comprises four stages: mitosis (M), when nuclei and cells divide; G1, when cells grow in size before dividing; S phase, when cells synthesize DNA and replicate chromosomes; and G2, a brief delay followed by M phase. Precursor cell division occurs at the ventricular margin, producing two new cells. The progeny then re-enter G1 as they move outward within the VZ. Under the influence of extracellular signals, cells become committed to another round of division, marked by entry into S phase, which occurs near the upper VZ margin. After DNA replication, during G2, nuclei move down to the ventricular surface, where they undergo mitosis and divide. Although the role of nuclear migration is not known, several human genetic mutations interfere with interkinetic nuclear movement and cell migration, producing heterotopic neurons and epilepsy syndromes as well as "smooth brain" or lissencephalies.

At early stages, VZ cells divide to increase the pool of progenitors. Then, during neurogenesis, each cell cycle division gives rise to both a postmitotic neuron and another dividing precursor. At the end of neurogenesis, precursor division gives rise to two postmitotic neurons only, greatly increasing neuron production and depleting the precursor pool. Newly born neurons migrate out of the

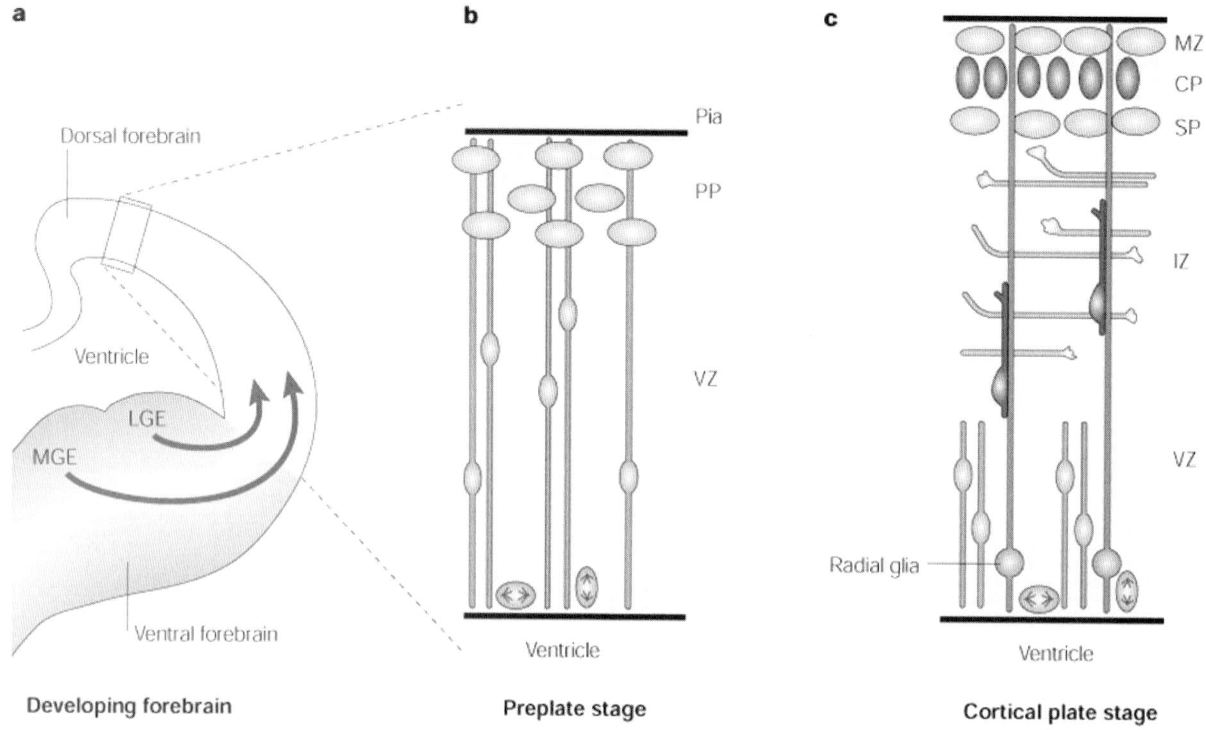

Figure 19.1 Schematic drawing of radial and tangential migration during cerebral cortex development. (A) A coronal section of one-half of the developing rat forebrain. The dorsal forebrain gives rise to the cerebral cortex. The medial and lateral ganglionic eminences (MGE and LGE) of the ventral forebrain generate neurons of the basal ganglia and the cortical interneurons. The arrows indicate the tangential migration route for γ-aminobutyric acid (GABA) interneurons to the cortex. The boxed area (enlarged in B and C) shows the developing cortex at early and late stages. (B) In the dorsal forebrain, the first cohort of postmitotic neurons migrate out from the ventricular zone (VZ) and create a preplate below the pial surface. (C) Subsequent postmitotic neurons will migrate along radial glia through the intermediate zone (IZ) and take position in the middle of the preplate, creating a cortical plate (CP) between the outer marginal zone (MZ) and inner subplate (SP). Ultimately the CP will be composed of six layers that are born sequentially, migrating in an inside-to-outside pattern. Horizontal processes in the IZ represent axon terminals of thalamic afferents. (From Nadarajah & Parnavelas, 2002.)

VZ to their final destinations, such as the cerebral cortical plate, traveling along the processes of radial glial cells (Figure 19.1C). A recent discovery is that the radial glia that have one process associated with the ventricular surface and the other reaching the pial surface, are, in fact, the dividing VZ precursors (Noctor et al. 2001; Noctor et al. 2002). The association between newborn neurons and radial glial process allows cells generated within localized VZ domains, known to express distinct patterning genes, to migrate to specific cortical functional areas. This suggests that VZ precursors already have their phenotypic fate specified at the genetic level, prior to ceasing cell division and beginning migration. However, there is active debate about the relative roles of early expressed VZ genes versus the thalamic afferents that synapse on cortical neurons in determining neuronal cell fate and function. Unlike rodents, in which neurons are generated prior to birth and glia are produced after, in the human brain neuron production largely occurs during the first 4 months of gestation. From 16 weeks to birth neurons undergo migration and glial precursors proliferate, migrate, and produce myelin.

Supplementing this general plan of neurogenesis, there are distinct regions where other cells are produced in secondary proliferative zones. For example, in the cerebral cortex and thalamus, the subventricular zone (SVZ) produces astroglial cells, although debate continues as to whether it also produces oligodendrocytes and neurons. In the hippocampus, the hilus and later the subgranular zone produce dentate gyrus granule neurons, a lifelong process of neurogenesis. In newborn cerebellum, the overlying external germinal layer (EGL) generates granule neurons for several weeks in rodents and for 7–20 months in humans (a population of cells likely affected by therapeutics administered in the neonatal intensive care unit, such as neurodevelopmental effects of perinatal steroids). Unlike VZ, secondary zone cells do not exhibit nuclear movements, suggesting distinct regulatory mechanisms. After neurogenesis, the VZ differentiates into ciliated ependymal cell lining. Underlying the ependyma, undifferentiated cells of the SVZ, referred to as subependyma, have been identified as a neural stem cell population, capable of generating neurons and glia throughout life, a potential source for repair and neoplasia. This represents a major change in concept that mammalian neurogenesis is restricted to gestation.

Radial and tangential patterns of neurogenesis and migration

Three well-recognized spatio-temporal patterns of neurogenesis underlie regional brain formation, including two patterns of radial migration and a third, termed *tangential migration*. The two radial patterns of migration from the VZ utilize radial glial processes and are termed *inside-to-outside* and *outside-to-inside*. The different radial patterns reflect whether a structure is phylogenetically older, such as spinal cord, tectum, and hippocampal dentate gyrus, or more recently evolved, like cerebral cortex. In more primitive structures, early generated cells are positioned outside, with later-born cells residing inside, closer to the VZ. This pattern suggests that more recently generated cells passively move earlier-born cells farther away. In the second pattern relevant to cerebral cortex, early-born cells are located inside, with later-born cells migrating past earlier ones to take up position outside. This inside-to-outside gradient requires a more complex mechanism, and cannot rely solely on passive cell movement. We now know that radial glial cell function is required for both types of migration. Finally, cells originating from distant or secondary proliferative zones may enter into a region by nonradial, tangential migration, relevant to γ-aminobutyric acid (GABA) interneurons in the cortex and hippocampus, or granule neurons in the cerebellum, hippocampal dentate gyrus, and olfactory bulb.

The cerebral cortex is the paradigmatic model of inside-to-outside neurogenesis. Derived from the embryonic telencephalic vesicles, its six cell layers represent a common cytoarchitectural and physiologic basis for neocortical function. Within each layer, neurons exhibit related axodendritic morphologies, use common neurotransmitters, and establish similar afferent and efferent connections. In general, pyramidal neurons in layer 3 establish synapses within and between cortical hemispheres, whereas deeper-layer 5/6 neurons project primarily to subcortical nuclei, including the thalamus, brainstem, and spinal cord. The majority of cortical neurons originate from the forebrain VZ and secrete the excitatory transmitter glutamate. At the earliest stages, the first postmitotic cells migrate from the VZ to establish a superficial layer termed the *preplate*, which consists of Cajal-Retzius cells that form outermost layer 1 or marginal zone, and subplate neurons that lie beneath future layer 6 and serve a temporary role. These distinct regions form when later-born cortical plate neurons migrate within and divide the preplate in two (Figure 19.1). Cajal-Retzius cells produce the extracellular glycoprotein reelin, an important signal for neuronal migration. When reelin gene is genetically deleted in mice, cortical neuron migration is inverted, yielding an outside-to-inside pattern. Thus, early-born neurons now aberrantly appear farthermost from the VZ, and latest-born cells remain closest to the ventricles. Abnormal levels of reelin protein and mRNA have been found in bipolar depression and schizophrenia, and human reelin mutation is associated with autism as well as lissencephaly (smooth brain), a malformation with loss of forebrain gyri and sulci, abnormalities in the cerebellum, seizures, and mental retardation.

After preplate formation, the cortical VZ generates in inside-to-outside fashion first-layer 5/6 neurons, and then more superficial layers in temporal sequence. Thus, the day on which a VZ precursor exits the cell cycle, its birthday, determines the kind and localization of the generated neuron, predicting that insults on specific days of gestation will produce layer-specific defects. Currently, molecular mechanisms mediating this correlation are being defined, including specific stimulatory and inhibitory proliferative signals, as well as intrinsic patterning gene expression.

Unlike excitatory pyramidal neurons, inhibitory GABA-secreting interneurons originate from mitotic precursors of the ganglionic eminences that generate neurons of the basal ganglia. Subsets of interneurons also secrete neuropeptides, such as neuropeptide Y (NPY) and somatostatin, and express nitrous oxide generating enzyme, nitrous oxide synthetase (NOS), and the calcium-binding proteins, calretinin, calbindin, and parvalbumin. Not associated with radial glia, GABA interneurons reach the cortical plate by migrating tangentially, in the superficial marginal zone or in the subplate region where thalamic afferents are also growing. Thus, cortical development represents convergence of two principal patterns of neurogenesis: radial and nonradial migration of neurons.

The phylogenetically older regions of the nervous system, such as the hypothalamus, spinal cord, and hippocampal dentate gyrus, exhibit the reverse order of cell generation. First-formed postmitotic neurons lie superficially and last-generated cells localize toward the center, with migration depending also on radial glia and specific migration signaling molecules. Cells do not always lie in direct extension from their locus of VZ generation, with some migrating to specific locations, like the inferior olivary nuclei.

Hippocampal development depends on both radial and nonradial patterns of neurogenesis. The pyramidal cell layer, Ammon horn CA 1–3 neurons, is generated in a typical outside-to-inside fashion from 7 to 15 weeks of gestation. However, the other major population, dentate gyrus granule neurons, starts appearing at 18 weeks and exhibits prolonged outside-to-inside postnatal neurogenesis, originating from several migrating secondary proliferative zones. In rat, granule neurogenesis starts at embryonic day (E)16 with proliferative precursors in the forebrain VZ, which then migrate into the dentate gyrus, and after residing in the dentate hilus for 1 month, ultimately localize just beneath the granule cell layer. These subgranular zone (SGZ) precursors produce neurons throughout life in adult rats, primates, and humans and proliferate in response to cerebral ischemia, tissue injury, and seizures, as well as growth factors, thus identifying potential sources for brain response to damage.

A different combination of radial and nonradial migration occurs in cerebellum, a region recently recognized to play important functions in nonmotor tasks. Except for granule cells, the other major neurons, including Purkinje and deep nuclei, originate from the primary VZ of the fourth ventricle at E13–15 in rat and 5–7 weeks in humans, coincident with other brainstem neurons. The granule neurons originate in the secondary proliferative zone, the external germinal layer (EGL), which is fate-restricted to these neurons and covers newborn cerebellum at birth. The rat EGL proliferates for 3 weeks, whereas in humans EGL precursors exist for at least 7 weeks and up to 2 years. When an EGL precursor stops proliferating, the cell body sinks below the surface, grows bilateral processes that extend transversely in the molecular layer, and then the soma migrates farther down along radial Bergmann glial processes into the internal granule layer, the IGL. Clinically, this postnatal population of neurons, which is the origin of medulloblastomas, makes cerebellar neurogenesis vulnerable to infectious and other insults of early childhood, and an unintended target of therapeutic drugs, such as anticonvulsants and steroids, well known to inhibit cell proliferation.

Specific inductive signals and patterning genes in development

Central nervous system (CNS) induction begins at the neural plate stage when the notochord, underlying mesenchyme, and surrounding epidermis produce signaling molecules that affect the identity of neighboring cells. The ectoderm produces BMPs that promote and maintain epidermal differentiation. Significantly, in the absence of BMPs, neural differentiation occurs because it is a default state. Thus, control of neural induction is regulated through BMP-inhibiting proteins, such as noggin, follistatin, and chordin, that are secreted by the Hensen node, a signaling center at the rostral end of the primitive streak. After neural tube closure, the roof and floor plates become new signaling centers, organizing dorsal and ventral neural tube respectively. As a principle stated earlier, the same ligand/receptor system is used sequentially for multiple functions during development. BMPs are a case in point, since they prevent neural development at neural plate stage, whereas after neurulation, the factors are produced by the dorsal neural tube itself to induce sensory neuron fates. Consequently, interfering with this single signal will have complex developmental effects, such as cyclopia.

The spinal cord

The synthesis, release, and diffusion of inductive signals from signaling sources produce concentration gradients that impose distinct neural fates in the spinal cord. The notochord and floor plate secrete Shh, which induces motor neurons and interneurons ventrally, while epidermal ectoderm and roof plate release BMPs that impart neural crest and sensory interneuron fates dorsally. Growth factor inductive signals initiate discrete regions of transcription factor gene expression. For instance, Shh induces the winged helix transcription factor Hnf3β gene in floor plate cells and Nkx6.1and Nkx2.2 in ventral neural tube, while more dorsal genes, Pax6, Dbx1, Dbx2, Irx3, and Pax7, are repressed. In response to Shh, ventral motor neurons express transcription factor gene Isl1, which is essential for neuron differentiation. In contrast, BMPs and Wnt proteins from the dorsal cord and roof plate induce a distinct cascade of patterning genes to elicit sensory interneuron differentiation. In aggregate, the coordinated actions of Shh and BMPs induce the dorsoventral dimension of the spinal cord. Neuropathologically, a Shh-regulated patterning gene of the Pax family interacts with platelet-derived growth factor (PDGF) receptor and folic acid metabolism in spina bifida causation.

Similar to the dorsoventral dimension, the rostrocaudal organization of the CNS depends on inductive signals; retinoic acid anteriorly, an upstream regulator of Hox patterning genes, and the FGFs posteriorly. The overlapping and unique expression of the many Hox gene family members is important for establishing the segmental pattern in the anterior–posterior axis of the hindbrain and spinal cord. The patterning gene, ZIC2 transcription factor, is associated with hindbrain deformity, Dandy-Walker syndrome, and holoprosencephaly (HPE), whereas ENGRAILED 2 is associated with autism spectrum disorders (Benyaol et al.; DiCicco-Bloom et al.; Gharani et al.).

The cerebral cortex

Based on embryonic studies, the forebrain can be divided into a checkerboard-like grid pattern of domains generated by intersecting longitudinal columns and transverse segments of gene expression. The columns and segments (prosomeres) exhibit restricted expression of patterning genes, allowing for unique combinations of factors within each embryonic subdivision. Many of these genes, including Hnf3β, Emx2, Pax6, and Dlx2, are first expressed even before neurulation in the neural plate and are then maintained, providing molecular determinants of the proliferative VZ. As in spinal cord, initial forebrain gene expression is influenced by soluble factors arising from signaling centers, such as Shh, BMP, and retinoic acid. In the dorsal midline, signaling initiates from the anterior neural ridge, an anterior cranial mesenchyme secreting FGF8, the roof plate, and the cortical hem (Figure 19.2), while other factors originate laterally from the dorsal-ventral forebrain junction. Initial forebrain development starts with formation of two telencephalic vesicles from the rostral-most neural tube, the prosencephalon, influenced by anterior neural ridge–secreted signals, including FGF8 and Shh.

Genetic studies have begun to provide insight into the mechanisms producing the diversity of cerebral cortical regions. After telencephalic vesicles form, opposing gradients of patterning genes are critical in specifying the rostrocaudal area characteristics of the cortex: rostral/lateral cortex expresses high levels of homeodomain gene Pax6, whereas caudal/medial cortex exhibits Emx2, Lhx2, and Lhx5 (Figure 19.2). A prediction would be that altering gene expression should cause a change in cortical areas. Indeed, in mice mutant for Pax6, the motor cortex is markedly diminished, accompanied by a proportionate increase in caudal sensory cortex. Moreover, there is also change in the dorsoventral dimension: Genes usually restricted to the ventral striatum and pallidum, namely Gsh and Dlx, are expressed ectopically in dorsal territory. These observations indicate that patterning genes exert reciprocal inhibitory functions in several dimensions, a mechanism for establishing developmental boundaries between areas. The influence of signaling molecules on the patterning genes has also been demonstrated: Overexpression of FGF8 in the anterior neural ridge causes a posterior shift of cortical areas, whereas overexpressing a FGF8 receptor inhibitor shifts borders anteriorly, suggesting that FGF8 (and other soluble signals) alters the ratios of Pax6 and Emx2 levels in the cortical neuroepithelium. Downstream molecular targets of patterning genes are proteins that mediate cell–cell interactions, such as adhesive cadherins, membrane-bound ephrins and their Eph receptors, and members of the immunoglobulin superfamily, which play roles in cell differentiation, cell migration, and neuronal process outgrowth.

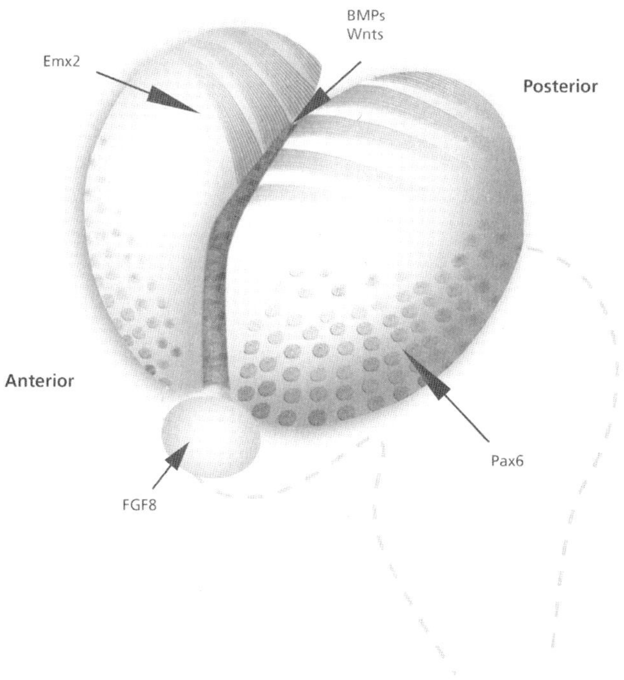

Figure 19.2 Patterning genes and signaling centers in the developing cerebral cortex. This schematic diagram shows a lateral-superior view of the two cerebral hemispheres of the embryonic mouse, sitting above the midbrain and hindbrain (broken lines). The anterior-lateral extent of Pax6 gene expression is indicated by circles. The posterior-medial domain of Emx2 expression is indicated by stripes. The genes exhibit continuous gradients of expression that decrease as they extend to the opposite poles. The signaling factor FGF8 is produced by and released from mesenchymal tissue in the anterior neural ridge, which regulates Pax6 and Emx2 expression. In the midline, bone morphogenetic proteins (BMPs) and Wnts are secreted from other signaling centers, including the roof plate and cortical hems. (Designed by E. DiCicco-Bloom, MD, and drawn by Karen Forgash.)

The hippocampus

As a region of major importance in learning and memory, epilepsy, autism, depression, and schizophrenia, identifying mechanisms regulating hippocampal formation may provide clues to the developmental bases of these disorders. The expression of hippocampal patterning genes is regulated by factors secreted by the anterior neural ridge, roof plate, and the cortical hem (Figure 19.2), including FGF8, Shh, BMPs, and Wnts. Genetic experiments have defined patterning genes and signals localized to the cortical hem and hippocampal primordia, whose deletions result in a variety of morphogenetic defects. These include soluble factor Wnt3a and its downstream intracellular factor, the Lef1 gene, thus suggesting they are required for hippocampal cell specification and/or proliferation. Disruption of Lhx5 and Lhx2 produce abnormalities in hippocampal cell proliferation, migration, and differentiation, whereas dentate gyrus differentiation is defective in mutants of bHLH transcription factors NeuroD and Mash1. These various signals and genes now serve as candidates for disruption in human diseases of the hippocampus.

The basal ganglia

In addition to motor and cognitive functions, the basal ganglia take on new importance in neocortical function, since they are the embryonic origin of all adult GABA interneurons, reaching the neocortex through tangential migration (Figure 19.1). As in dorsal cortex, transcription factor expression establishes boundaries between different precursor zones in the ventral forebrain VZ, acting through mutual repression. As a simplified model, the medial ganglionic eminence (MGE) expresses Nkx2.1 and produces most GABA interneurons of the cortex and hippocampus, whereas the lateral ganglionic eminence (LGE) expresses Gsh2 and generates GABA interneurons of the SVZ and olfactory bulb. When Nkx2.1 is deleted, LGE transcription factor expression spreads ventrally into the MGE territory, and a 50% reduction occurs in neocortical and striatal GABA interneurons. In contrast, Gsh2 deletion leads to ventral expansion cortical markers and decreases in olfactory interneurons. The final phenotypes are complex, because factors exhibit unique and overlapping expression and interact to control cell fate.

Neuronal specification

Throughout the nervous system, transcription factors participate in decisions at multiple levels, including determining the generic neural cell, such as neuron or glial cell, as well as neuron subtypes. In basal ganglia, transcription factors regulate both the timing of differentiation and specification of interneuron subtype. Early-born cells express Mash1, which is followed in maturing neurons by bHLH family members Dlx1/Dlx2 that then target Dlx5/Dlx6. In fact, Mash1 regulates Dlx expression, whereas Dlx2 induces expression of GABA synthetic enzyme, glutamic acid decarboxylase (GAD) 67. We may predict then that genetic mutants may exhibit similar defects. Deletion of Mash1 results in reduced cortical GABA interneurons and striatal cholinergic interneurons. In Dlx1/Dlx2 double-knockout mice, interneurons are reduced 75% in neocortex and absent in hippocampus, whereas olfactory neurons are preserved. Similarly, Nkx2.1 deletion leads to complete loss of cortical interneurons expressing NPY, somatostatin, and NOS. These studies suggest that transcription factors play roles at multiple stages in neuronal production, including generic neuronal fate specification, as well as neuron subtype determination. Furthermore, transcription factors demonstrate region/cell type–specific actions: bHLH factor Olig1/2 promotes oligodendrocyte development in the forebrain, whereas it promotes motor neuron differentiation in the spinal cord, indicating that the variety of factors expressed in a specific cell leads to combinatorial effects, thus diverse outcomes for cell differentiation. Other examples include bHLH inhibitory factor Id in sensorimotor cortex specification, NeuroD and Math1 in dentate gyrus granule neuron fate, and Tbr1, Otx1, and Pax6 in cerebral cortical layer specification.

Regulation of neurogenesis by extracellular factors

The interaction of extracellular factors with intrinsic genetic determinants controlling region-specific neurogenesis includes signals that regulate cell proliferation. Patterning genes control the expression of growth factor receptors and cell cycle machinery. Extracellular factors originate from the cells themselves (autocrine), neighboring cells (paracrine), or the general circulation (endocrine). Mitogenic growth factors are well-characterized in vivo, including those stimulating proliferation, such as basic fibroblast growth factor (bFGF), EGF, IGF-I, Shh, and signals inhibiting cell division, such as pituitary adenylate cyclase-activating polypeptide (PACAP), GABA and glutamate, and members of the transcribing growth factor (TGF)-β superfamily. In addition to stimulating reentry into the cell cycle, a mitogenic effect, extracellular signals also enhance proliferation by promoting survival of the mitotic population, a trophic action. Several of the neurotrophins, especially BDNF and neurotrophin-3 (NT3), promote survival of mitotic precursors, as well as of the newly generated progeny.

The developmental significance of extracellular mitogens is demonstrated by factor and receptor expression in regions of neurogenesis, and the profound and permanent consequences of altering their activities during development. Changes in proliferation in prenatal cortical VZ, and postnatal cerebellar EGL and hippocampal dentate gyrus produce lifelong modifications in brain region population size and cell composition, potentially relevant to structural differences observed in autism, depression, and schizophrenia. In the cerebral cortex VZ of the embryonic rat, proliferation is controlled by promitogenic bFGF and antimitogenic PACAP, which are expressed as autocrine/paracrine signals. Positive and negative effects were shown in living embryos in utero by performing intracerebroventricular (ICV) factor injections. bFGF produced a larger adult cortex composed of 87% more glutamate neurons, thus increasing the ratio of excitatory pyramidal-to-GABA inhibitory neurons, which were unchanged. Conversely, embryonic PACAP injection inhibited proliferation of precursors by 26%, reducing the number of labeled cortical neurons by 40% (Figure 19.3A). A similar reduction was accomplished by genetically deleting promitogenic bFGF, diminishing cortical size. Furthermore, effects of mitogenic signals depended critically on the stage-specific program of regional development, since bFGF injection at later ages when gliogenesis predominates, affected glial numbers selectively. Thus, developmental dysregulation of mitogenic pathways due to genetic or environmental factors (hypoxia, maternal/fetal infection, drug or toxin exposure) may produce subtle changes in the size and composition of the developing cortex.

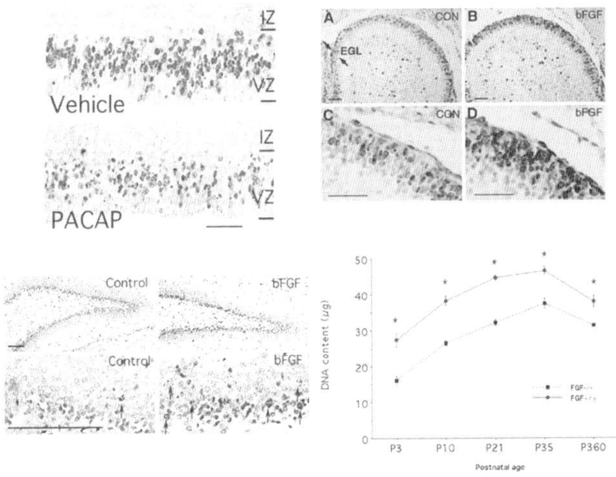

Figure 19.3 Extracellular growth factors stimulate or inhibit neuronal precursor proliferation during brain development. (A) Intracerebroventricular injection of antimitogenic peptide *pituitary* adenylate cyclase activating polypeptide (PACAP) into the rat embryo in utero inhibits mitosis in ventricular zone (VZ) precursors of the cerebral cortex. Fewer VZ precursors exhibit nuclear labeling with DNA syntheses marker, BrdU, in embryos exposed to PACAP, indicating that the cells were prevented from entering S phase of the mitotic cell cycle. Three and 5 days later, there were ~40% fewer mitotically labeled neurons in the cortical plate. BrdU-positive cells appear brown, and toluidine counterstain appears blue. Scale bar = 50 µm. (Suh et al. 2002). (B) Eight hours after subcutaneous injection of bFGF in newborn rat pups, 30% more cerebellar EGL precursors are in mitotic S phase, as indicated by brown nuclear staining compared to the saline-injected littermate. Thus, peripherally injected factors rapidly alter ongoing neurogenesis in the developing brain. Parts A and B show low magnification of a single cerebellar folium, parts C and D show high magnification. CON, control saline injection (A and C); bFGF, growth factor injected (B and D). Nuclear BrdU stain appears brown, and basic fuschsin counterstain appears pink. Scale bar = 100 µm. (Tao et al 1996). (C) Three weeks after bFGF injection at birth, there are many more mitotically labeled (*arrows*) dentate gyrus granule neurons in the hippocampal formation. BrdU-positive nuclei indicated by arrows in control, factor-treated animals appear brown, and thionin counterstain appears blue. There were 33% more granule neurons quantified by stereologic counting, an increase that was maintained throughout life. The postnatal day 21 dentate gyrus is pictured at low (*top*) and high magnification (*bottom*). Scale bar = 100 um. (Cheng et al. 2002). (D) Mice with genetic deletion of bFGF exhibit a lifelong reduction in total cells in the hippocampal formation, reflected by diminished total DNA in microgram per hippocampus. Absolute cell counting revealed 30% decreases in the number of dentate gyrus granule layer neurons, as well as astrocytes at 3 weeks of age. (Cheng et al. 2002).

Later-generated populations, such as granule neurons of cerebellum and hippocampal dentate gyrus, are also sensitive to growth factor manipulation, especially relevant to therapies administered intravenously to premature and newborn infants in the neonatal nursery. In the rat, cerebellar granule neurons are produced postnatally for only 3 weeks; however, dentate gyrus neurons are produced throughout life, as in humans. Remarkably, a single peripheral injection of bFGF into newborn rat pups rapidly crossed into the cerebrospinal fluid and stimulated proliferation in the cerebellar EGL by 30%, as well as hippocampal dentate gyrus by 100%, consistent with an endocrine mechanism of action (Figure 19.3B). The consequences of bFGF stimulation in cerebellum were a 33% increase in granule neurons and a 22% larger cerebellum. In the hippocampus, the mitotic dentate gyrus granule neuron number increased by 33%, producing a 25% larger hippocampus containing more neurons and astrocytes, a change that persisted lifelong. Conversely, genetic deletion of bFGF resulted in smaller cerebellum and hippocampus at birth and throughout life, indicating that levels of the growth factor were critical for normal brain region formation (Figure 19.3D).

There are clinical implications of growth factor effects observed in fetuses and newborns. It is necessary to investigate possible neurogenetic effects of therapeutic agents administered during pregnancy and in the newborn nursery for long-term consequences. For example, steroids, which inhibit neurogenesis, are frequently used during the perinatal period to promote lung maturation and treat infections and trauma. At least in very-low-birth-weight premature infants (<1,000 g), postnatal steroid use is associated with worse neurodevelopmental outcome, supporting recent cautions about their use in this population. Further, neurodevelopment delay is well known in children experiencing serious systemic illness; to what degree this reflects interference with neurogenesis and concomitant processes, potentially producing long-term sequelae, is an important area for investigation.

Cell migration

Throughout the nervous system, newly generated neurons normally migrate away from proliferative zones to achieve their final destinations. If disrupted, abnormal cell localization occurs, resulting in abnormal function. As described earlier, three well-described patterns of neurogenesis and migration exist, including two forms of radial migration and tangential migration. Neurons migrate from proliferative zones along radial glial processes in inside-to-outside (e.g., hippocampus, tectum, spinal cord) and outside-to-inside (cerebral cortex) fashion. Alternatively, cells migrate tangentially from basal ganglia to provide GABA interneurons. The most commonly recognized disorders of human neuronal migration are the extensive lissencephalies (described later), although incomplete migration of more restricted neuron aggregates (heterotopias) frequently underlies focal seizure disorders.

In man, more than 25 syndromes with disturbed neuronal migration have been described, most of which produce various levels of mental retardation and epilepsy. Animal models have been essential in defining molecular pathways. Cell movement requires signals to start and stop migration, adhesion molecules to guide migration, and functional cytoskeleton to mediate cell translocation. The best characterized mouse model of aberrant migration is reeler, in which cortical neuron laminar position is inverted, being generated in outside-to-inside fashion. Reelin is a large, secreted, extracellular glycoprotein produced embryonically by the earliest neurons in the cortical preplate, Cajal Retzius cells, and also in the hippocampus and cerebellum. Reelin signals through at least two receptors, the very-low-density lipoprotein receptor (VLDLR) and the apoprotein E receptor 2 (ApoER2), and the intracellular adapter protein, disabled 1 (Dab1), identified in the scrambler mutant, which is a reelin phenocopy. The reelin system is considered as one mediator of radial glial-guided neuronal migration. The roles of VLDL and ApoE2 receptors are intriguing given their contributions to Alzheimer disease risk. Human reelin gene (*RELN*) mutations are associated with autosomal recessive lissencephaly and perhaps autism.

Cell migration also depends on molecules mediating cell adhesion, or inducing attraction or repulsion. Astrotactin is a major glial protein involved in neuronal migration on radial glial processes, whereas neuregulins and their receptors, ErbB2–4, play roles in neuronal–glial migratory interactions, interesting because neuregulin polymorphisms are highly associated with schizophrenia. In addition to adhesion signals, early appearing neurotransmitters, GABA and glutamate, and PDGF appear to regulate migration speed. In contrast to radial migration, GABA interneurons generated in ganglionic eminences migrate from ventral forebrain tangentially into cerebral cortex, guided by Slit protein and Robo receptor, the semaphorins and their neuropilin receptors, and hepatocyte growth factor and its c-Met receptor, all of which appear to repel GABA interneurons, promoting their tangential migration (Figure 19.1). Several forms of congenital muscular dystrophy with severe brain and eye migration defects result from gene mutations in enzymes that transfer mannose sugars to serine/threonine –OH groups in glycoproteins, interrupting interactions with several extracellular matrix molecules, producing type II cobblestone lissencephalies (discussed in Chapter 20).

Differentiation and neuronal process outgrowth

After newly produced neurons and glial cells reach their final destinations, they differentiate into mature cells. For neurons, this involves outgrowth of dendrites and extension of axonal processes, formation of synapses, and production of neurotransmitter systems, including receptors and selective reuptake sites. Most axons will become insulated by myelin sheaths produced by oligodendroglial cells. Many of these events occur with a peak period from 5 months of gestation onward. During the first several years of life, many neuronal systems exhibit exuberant process growth and branching, which is later decreased by selective "pruning" of axons and synapses dependent on experience. In contrast, myelination continues for several years after birth and into adulthood.

Although there is tremendous synapse plasticity in adult brain, a fundamental feature of the nervous system is the point-to-point, or topographic, mapping of one neuron population to another. During development, neurons in various brain regions extend axons to innervate diverse distant targets, such as cortex and spinal cord. The structure that recognizes and responds to cues in the environment is the growth cone, located at the axon tip. The growth cone has rod-like extensions called *filopodia* that bear receptors for specific guidance cues, which are present on cell surfaces and in the extracellular matrix. Interactions between filopodial receptors and environmental cues cause growth cones to move forward, turn, or retract. The region-specific expression of extracellular guidance molecules, such as cadherins regulated by patterning genes Pax6 and Emx2, results in highly directed outgrowth of axons, termed *axonal pathfinding*. These molecules affect the direction, speed, and fasciculation of axons, acting through either positive or negative regulation. Guidance molecules may be soluble extracellular factors, or alternatively, may be bound to extracellular matrix or cell membranes. In the latter class of signal is the newly discovered family of transmembrane proteins, the ephrins. Ephrins play major roles in topographic mapping between neuron populations and their targets, and act via the largest known family of tyrosine kinase receptors in brain, Eph receptors. Ephrins frequently serve as chemorepellent cues, negatively regulating growth by preventing developing axons from entering incorrect target fields. For example, the optic tectum expresses ephrins A2 and A5 in a gradient that decreases along the posterior to anterior axis, whereas innervating retinal ganglion cells express a gradient of Eph receptors. Ganglion cell axons from the posterior retina, which possess high Eph A3 receptor levels, will preferentially innervate the anterior tectum, since low-level ephrin expression will not activate the Eph kinase that causes growth cone retraction. In the category of soluble molecules, netrins serve primarily as chemoattractant proteins secreted, for instance, by the spinal cord floor plate to stimulate spinothalamic sensory interneurons to grow into the anterior commissure, whereas Slit is a secreted chemorepulsive factor which, through its roundabout (Robo) receptor, regulates midline crossing and axonal fasciculation and pathfinding.

In the neocortex, layer 5 and 6 axons exit the hemisphere laterally via the internal capsule to reach subcortical destinations, whereas layer 3 axons extend medially through corpus callosum to innervate the opposite hemisphere. The internal capsule carries bidirectional axons, from cortex to thalamus and beyond, as well as thalamocortical processes, exhibiting precise connections between individual thalamic nuclei and distinct cortical domains. During development, thalamic axons must travel a complex route, passing through lateral ventral thalamus, turning to enter the internal capsule, and turning dorsally to reach cortical targets. However, thalamic axons reach the developing neocortex before target neurons have completed their migration to appropriate layers. Instead, the early-generated subplate neurons projecting to the internal capsule may function as guidepost cells, serving as temporary targets for thalamic axons. The subplate neurons express two guidance systems, including the chemoattractant netrin 1, and chemorepellant cell surface molecule, ephrin-A5, which is complemented by Eph receptor expression by thalamic axon growth cones. After cortical neurons complete laminar migration, thalamic axons leave subplate neurons, which apparently undergo degeneration, and extend into proper cortical layers guided by a number of cues, including chondroitin sulfate proteoglycans, ephrins, and cadherins under patterning gene regulation. In similar fashion, thalamic afferents to limbic cortex, which express Eph A5 receptor, may be repelled from the sensorimotor cortex by ephrin A5. Numerous experiments demonstrate misrouted axon terminals in developing brain when ephrin/Eph expression is altered. Thus, changes in ephrin/Eph signaling during brain development may cause abnormal cell migration and/or axonal process termination. Such abnormalities may contribute to cognitive and/or motor dysfunction of genetic or environmental origin.

Annotated bibliography

Benayed R, Gharani N, Rossman I, et al. Support for the homeobox transcription factor, ENGRAILED 2, as an autism spectrum disorder (ASD) susceptibility locus. *Am J Hum Genet* 2005;77:851–868.

DiCicco-Bloom E, Lord C, Zwaigenbaum L, et al. The developmental neurobiology of autism spectrum disorder. *J Neurosci* 2006;26:6897.

Englund C, Fink A, Lau C, et al. Pax6, Tbr2, and Tbr1 are expressed sequentially by radial glia, intermediate progenitor cells, and postmitotic neurons in developing neocortex. *J Neurosci* 2005;25(1):247–251.

Gharani N, Benayed R, Mancuso V, et al. Association of the homeobox transcription factor, ENGRAILED 2, 3, with autism spectrum disorder. *Mol Psychiatry* 2004;9:474–484.

Noctor SC, Flint AC, Weissman TA, et al. Neurons derived from radial glial cells establish radial units in neocortex. *Nature* 2001;409(6821):714–720.

Noctor SC, Flint AC, Weissman TA, et al. Dividing precursor cells of the embryonic cortical ventricular zone have morphological and molecular characteristics of radial glia. *J Neurosci* 2002;22(8):3161–3173.

CHAPTER 20

Disorders of Nervous System Development: Cellular and Molecular Mechanisms

John N. Gaitanis and David E. Mandelbaum

Outline

Many neurologic conditions represent the consequences of altered nervous system development. These include epilepsy syndromes, attentional and cognitive deficits, autism spectrum disorders, neurocutaneous syndromes, primitive neuroectodermal tumors (PNET), medulloblastomas, and congenital malformations. Evidence indicates that psychiatric diseases, including schizophrenia and bipolar depression, are also secondary to abnormal brain development. Thus, knowledge of current principles of developmental neuroscience may provide insights into disease causation as well as a basis for therapeutic interventions. In Chapter 19, normal brain development was reviewed, with a focus on cellular and molecular mechanisms. In this chapter, syndromes known or thought to result from disorders of nervous system development are discussed.

The symptoms of disorders of brain development will depend on which phase of brain development is disrupted and to what degree. In some disorders, this occurs very early in fetal development, resulting in a devastating abnormality. In the case of some of the neurocutaneous disorders, symptoms may occur after birth, resulting in very mild symptoms or *forme fruste* that is not even detected until a family member presents with more severe manifestations. Despite this wide range of presentations, all these conditions represent disorders of brain development, often genetically mediated, and thus warrant being discussed as a group.

Classification

Early classification schemes of brain malformations relied on pathology and radiographic findings. More recent classifications have taken genetics into account. Clinicians, radiologists, pathologists, embryologists, and geneticists have different areas of focus and each discipline is inclined to align a classification scheme according to its primary area of interest. The fact that a given gene defect can cause different phenotypic expressions and that a single phenotype may have multiple gene abnormalities associated with it illustrates the complexity in attempts at classification.

This chapter arranges cortical malformations according to the earliest embryologic stage in which the abnormality has its origin (Barkovich et al. 2001). Yet, this too is an artificial distinction since the stages of cortical development overlap in time and lack discrete boundaries. Moreover, some gene defects exert influence in more than one developmental stage. Thus, the classification system presented here will undoubtedly be modified as understanding of these conditions increases.

Overview of embryology

As discussed in great detail in Chapter 19, the brain and spinal cord form from the dorsal aspect of the embryo through neurulation, the process of neural tube formation occurring in the third and fourth weeks of gestation. In the fifth and sixth weeks, prosencephalic development, the process by which the brain takes shape, begins. Cortical formation in humans spans weeks 8–24 of gestation (Crino & Eberwine 1997a,b) and can be divided into stages of cell proliferation (both neural and glial precursor cells are generated), neuronal migration (cells travel from the proliferative zone to their designated destination), and cortical organization (cell networks are determined) (Barkovich et al. 1996, 2001). Myelination is the final step of brain development and continues well beyond birth (Brody et al. 1987). As noted earlier, assigning strict temporal divisions is misleading, since different stages take place concurrently. It is nevertheless helpful to define stages for the purpose of classification of the disorders.

Disorders of neurulation

Fusion of the neural tube begins at the level of the hindbrain (medulla and pons) and proceeds rostrally and caudally. Failure of rostral fusion results in dysraphic states of the brain (anencephaly, encephalocele; Table 20.1) and incomplete caudal fusion causes spinal dysraphism (myelomeningocele). The anterior end of the neural tube closes by 24 days, and posterior closure, to the level of the lumbar sacral region, happens by day 26 (lower sacral and coccygeal closure occurs by a separate process termed secondary neurulation, which is not complete until after birth). Disorders of neurulation differ in severity depending on the timing of the disruption. The most severe disorder, craniorachischisis totalis, in which the brain and spinal cord fail to develop because of a complete absence of neurulation, occurs no later than 20–22 days of gestation. Anencephaly, a complete failure of anterior neural tube closure resulting in an absence of brain formation, occurs no later than 24 days. Encephalocele, a restricted failure of anterior neural tube closure, happens around day 26. Likewise, myelomeningocele, a restricted failure of posterior neural tube closure, also occurs by day 26.

Myelomeningocele is the most clinically important disorder of neurulation since patients with it usually survive. Its incidence in the United States is approximately 0.2–0.4 per 1,000 live births (Yen et al. 1992). The neurologic features of myelomeningocele relate to the level of involvement, presence of hydrocephalus, and other associated malformations (Table 20.2).

Table 20.1 Encephalocele

Discriminating features
- Meningeal extrusion through bony defect
- Abnormal cortical tissue extending through defect

Consistent features
- Midline skull defects

Variable features
- Location
- Other central nervous system structural abnormalities
- Cognitive function
- Anomalies of other systems

Table 20.2 Myelomeningocele/spina bifida

Discriminating features
- Absence of overlying skin
- Absence of meninges
- Malformed spinal cord

Consistent features
- Failure of vertebral arch fusion
- Arnold-Chiari malformation

Variable features
- Extent and levels of cord malformation
- Number of vertebral arches involved
- Extent of skin defect
- Other central nervous system abnormalities
- Cognitive function
- Presence of seizure disorder
- Tethered cord below lesion

Impairment of motor, sensory, and sphincter function relate directly to the level of involvement. Ambulation is one of the most important clinical concerns, and retained strength of the iliopsoas and quadriceps muscles are required for walking. Lesions at or below S1 rarely affect ambulation, whereas higher defects, above L2, almost always do. Among patients with intermediate lesions (L3, L4, L5), approximately half will walk, but braces or other assistive devices may be required. A clinical adage, while a bit simplistic, summarizes it as follows: "If they can move their hips they can walk and if they can move their knees they can run."

Hydrocephalus is seen in approximately 90% of patients with lumbar lesions. The usual signs of increased intracranial pressure (lethargy, irritability, limited upward gaze, rapidly expanding head circumference) are not essential for diagnosis and are present in only 15% of newborns with myelomeningocele. If clinical signs are present, they usually develop 2–3 weeks after birth and are almost certain to be present by 6 weeks. Their frequent absence necessitates serial neuroimaging for the prompt diagnosis of hydrocephalus. Infants demonstrating hydrocephalus at birth require shunt placement immediately following myelomeningocele closure (usually within a single sedation). The closure stops cerebral spinal fluid leakage, and can therefore worsen hydrocephalus if a shunt is not placed.

When myelomeningocele and hydrocephalus are combined with inferior displacement of the medulla and lower cerebellum through the foramen magnum, it is termed the *Arnold-Chiari malformation* (Chiari type II).

Other features of this disorder include elongation and thinning of the upper medulla and pons and bony defects of the foramen magnum, occiput, and upper cervical vertebrae. Brainstem and cortical malformations are common. Resulting brainstem dysfunction is a significant cause of morbidity and mortality. It may result in apnea, stridor, cyanotic spells, and dysphagia. The overall mortality rate in patients with brainstem dysfunction is 21%, but when all four symptoms are present, the mortality rate is as high as 60%. Cortical malformations are an important cause of morbidity such as intellectual disability and epilepsy. They are also very common in patients with Arnold-Chiari malformations, being present in as many as 92% (Table 20.3).

Treatment of myelomeningocele and Arnold-Chiari malformation begins prior to birth. Delivery by cesarean section before the onset of labor is necessary to preserve motor function. Animal models of myelomeningocele have shown that intrauterine repair results in improved outcome. This suggests that the exposed spinal cord undergoes progressive in utero damage (Walsh et al. 2001). Whether this is relevant to human forms of myelomeningocele, and whether intrauterine repair would be beneficial is, as yet, unknown. Following delivery, early closure of the myelomeningocele prevents infection. Closure typically takes place within the first week, often in the first 48 hours. Early diagnosis and treatment of hydrocephalus is necessary, and placement of a ventriculoperitoneal shunt, if needed, should take place early into the infant's course. Evidence suggests that shunt placement at the time of myelomeningocele closure can reduce back wound morbidity without increasing shunt complications (Miller et al. 1996).

Brainstem dysfunction is less easily managed. Decompressive upper cervical laminectomy has been used and is best performed within the first weeks after birth. Otherwise, treatment is largely symptomatic and focuses on maintaining a patent airway and preventing aspiration.

Table 20.3 Arnold-Chiari malformation

Discriminating features
- Myelomeningocele combined with inferior displacement of medulla and lower brainstem

Consistent features
- Elongation of cerebellar tonsils through foramen magnum
- Elongation and thinning of upper medulla and pons
- Bony defects of the foramen magnum, occiput, or upper cervical vertebra

Variable features
- Progressive hydrocephalus
- Presence and degree of brainstem dysfunction
- Presence of cortical malformations
- Presence and degree of cognitive impairment
- Presence of seizure disorder

Avoiding urinary tract complications begins with urodynamic evaluation. Daily catheterization is often required to prevent urinary tract infections in patients with incoordination of the detrusor muscle and external urethral sphincter. For patients who are nonambulatory, close orthopedic follow-up is needed for prevention and management of scoliosis and contractures. Given the wide range of systems affected in myelomeningocele, multidisciplinary clinics are helpful for coordinating care.

Disorders of prosencephalic development

Prosencephalic development is the process in which the forebrain (telencephalon and diencephalon) takes shape. It begins during the fifth week and continues through the second and third months of gestation. Prosencephalic development also influences formation of the face, and a severe disruption at this stage will result in characteristic facial anomalies. Development of the forebrain can be divided into three stages: formation, cleavage, and midline development. The resulting disorders depend on the stage affected. Disruption of prosencephalic formation results in the most severe anomalies, including aprosencephaly (complete absence of the telencephalon and diencephalons) or atelencephaly (with preservation of the diencephalon). Maintenance of the skull and dermal covering readily distinguish these from anencephaly. Because disorders of prosencephalic formation are not compatible with life, they bear little clinical relevance in comparison to disruption of prosencephalic cleavage or midline development.

Holoprosencephaly

Included among disorders of prosencephalic cleavage is holoprosencephaly (HPE), in which disruption of the roof plate and absence of hemispheric separation result in a single, large, forebrain ventricle. In its most severe form, alobar HPE, the brain is a single spherical structure with a common ventricle and a malformed cortical mantle. The optic nerves are dysplastic and the olfactory bulbs and tracts may be absent. The hypothalamus does not separate normally into two halves. Facial anomalies, ranging from cyclopia to a single central incisor, are observed. Less severe forms, semilobar and lobar HPE, have lesser degrees of the same anomalies. For instance, in semilobar HPE, the frontal and parietal lobes remain fused and the interhemispheric fissure is only present posteriorly. In contrast, in lobar HPE most of the left and right hemispheres and lateral ventricles are separated and fusion is seen only at the most ventral aspect of the frontal lobes. Clinical severity relates directly to the degree of structural change. Neurologic dysfunction inversely correlates with the degree of hemispheric separation, with less separation

Pearls and Perils

Holoprosencephaly (HPE)

- Craniofacial anomalies accompany HPE in about 80% of patients, but patients with all types of holoprosencephaly can have relatively normal facial appearances. A correlation often exists between the facial anomalies and the subtype of holoprosencephaly.
- Ventricular enlargement of the occipital horns, termed *colpocephaly*, is a common finding in holoprosencephaly and does not reflect progressive hydrocephalus.
- Clinically, infants with septo-optic dysplasia have impaired vision (often presenting with nystagmus) and endocrine dysfunction (hyponatremia, hypoglycemia, and impaired growth).
- Agenesis of the corpus callosum in combination with chorioretinal lacunas, mental retardation, and infantile spasms constitutes Aicardi syndrome.

resulting in greater impairment. Endocrinopathies correlate with the severity of hypothalamic separation. Associated cortical malformations frequently cause epilepsy, which is often refractory. Careful attention to the neuroimaging features is necessary in providing an accurate prognosis (Plawner et al. 2002) (Table 20.4).

Holoprosencephaly is a heterogeneous condition, with both genetic and environmental causes. The most common environmental cause is maternal diabetes, which carries a 1% risk of HPE (200 times greater than in the normal population). Cytogenetic abnormalities account for approximately 25–50% of holoprosencephaly cases, with trisomy 13 and 18 being the most common. Single gene mutations are found in roughly 25% of patients. Several genes are known to be causative. The first gene discovered, the sonic hedgehog gene (Shh) at 7q36, appears to be the most common. Shh plays an important role in dorsal-ventral patterning—the process by which the dorsal and ventral regions of the nervous system acquire their anatomical and functional properties (Thakur et al. 2004). Genetic testing is currently available for seven different single gene mutations, and many more may exist. Holoprosencephaly is also seen in cases of Smith-Lemli-Opitz syndrome, in which a defect in the biosynthesis of cholesterol leads to reduced Shh activity. Assuming a clear environmental cause is not found, the evaluation typically begins with a karyotype followed by molecular genetic testing if the karyotype is unremarkable. Genetic counseling is important given the heterogeneity of these disorders.

Table 20.4 Holoprosencephaly

Discriminating features
- Impaired forebrain cleavage

Consistent features
- Incomplete separation of forebrain

Variable features
- Degree of cleavage defect (alobar, semilobar, lobar)
- Endocrinopathies
- Associated cortical malformations
- Cognitive impairment
- Optic nerve dysplasia
- Presence of seizure disorder

Abnormalities of midline prosencephalic development are typically less severe than HPE. They include agenesis of the corpus callosum and septo-optic dysplasia (SOD). Agenesis of the corpus callosum can be either partial or complete. With partial agenesis, the posterior portion is more affected. It is commonly associated with other brain anomalies including Arnold-Chiari II malformations and neuronal migration disorders. Septo-optic dysplasia, on the other hand, is characterized by optic nerve hypoplasia in combination with absence of the septum pellucidum and pituitary dysfunction. Clinically, it may present with visual impairment (which may be recognized because of congenital nystagmus), endocrinopathies, or both. The causes are heterogeneous, including both environmental and genetic etiologies. One gene associated with SOD is *HESX1*, a homeobox gene essential for pituitary and forebrain development.

Disorders of neuronal proliferation

Neuronal proliferation takes place between the second and fourth months of gestation (Volpe 2001). Radial glial cells, which play a critical role in neuronal migration, are also formed at this time. Neurons and glia have their origin in the ventricular and subventricular zones. In the earliest phases of neuronal proliferation, neuronal-glial stem cells divide to form further stem cells (Rakic 1988, 1995). Later, stem cell division becomes asymmetric so that one daughter cell is postmitotic while the other remains a stem cell. Eventually, fewer and fewer stem cells are produced, and all of the neurons within the proliferative unit are postmitotic (Kornack 1998). Abnormal neuronal proliferation may result in conditions characterized by too many or too few neurons. Incomplete differentiation of postmitotic neurons is included within this category.

Decreased proliferation

Microcephaly/microlissencephaly

Primary microcephaly (microcephaly vera) is diagnosed when the head circumference at birth is three or more standard deviations below normal (Table 20.5). Primary

Table 20.5 Primary microcephaly

Discriminating features
- Head circumference >3 standard deviations below normal at birth

Consistent features
- Developmental delay (cognitive and/or motor impairment)

Variable features
- Etiology (destructive versus genetically determined)
- Degree of gyral simplification

microcephaly is a heterogeneous condition and can be caused by destructive processes (hypoxia–ischemia, intrauterine infections) or from a genetically determined reduction in neuronal proliferation. Most genetic forms are recessively inherited. The most common of these conditions may be microcephaly 5 (MCPH5), caused by mutations in the abnormal spindle-like microcephaly associated gene (*ASPM*) (Bond 2003). *ASPM* may be essential for normal mitotic spindle activity in neuronal progenitor cells, and its disruption therefore affects neuronal proliferation (Bond 2002). Mental retardation and a generalized simplification of the gyral pattern are common, but more severe gyral abnormalities have not been described.

Microcephaly is sometimes associated with a more simplified gyral pattern or, in severe cases, with a smooth cortex, termed *microlissencephaly* (Barkovich et al. 1998; Dobyns & Truwit 1995). These cases can be associated with cerebellar and callosal abnormalities (Barth 1982) in addition to extracranial dysmorphism (McComb 1991). Seizures and global developmental delays are uniformly present (Kroon 1996). Microlissencephaly is thought to be distinct from the syndrome of microcephaly with simplified gyral pattern (Dobyns 1999).

Disordered proliferation

Hemimegalencephaly

When there is enlargement of just one cerebral hemisphere, it is termed *hemimegalencephaly*. It probably results when a disturbance of cellular differentiation and proliferation interacts with the genetic expression of body symmetry (Flores-Sarnat 2002) (Figure 20.1). In addition to increased size of the affected hemisphere, neuroimaging may reveal abnormal gyration, ventriculomegaly, and increased T2 signal of the white matter (Flores-Sarnat 2002; Sasaki 2000). Histology reveals disorganized cortical lamination, subcortical heterotopia, and large, dysmorphic neurons, termed *balloon neurons* (Crino 1997a; DeRosa 1992; Woo 2001). The opposite hemisphere may be normal or have mild dysplasia and heterotopia (Crino 1997b). Hemimegalencephaly can be associated with tuberous sclerosis complex (Galluzzi 2002), hypomelanosis of Ito (Woo 2001), and linear nevus sebaceous syndrome (Herman 2001). All patients have epilepsy; hemispherectomy is often required for intractable cases (Devlin 2003; Flores-Sarnat 2002).

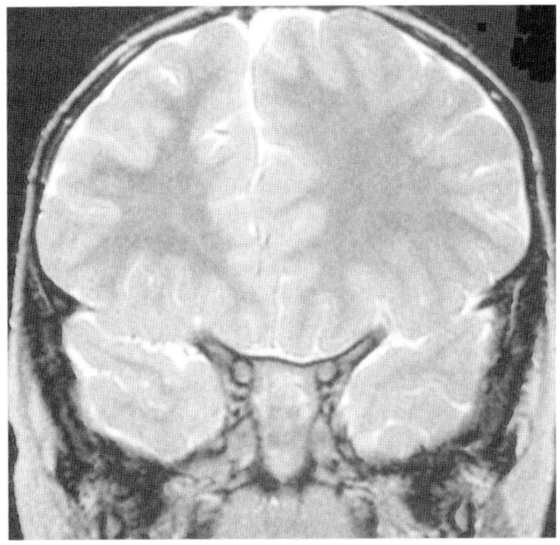

Figure 20.1 When unilateral enlargement of just one cerebral hemisphere exists, it is termed hemimegalencephaly. It probably results when a disturbance of cellular differentiation and proliferation interacts with the genetic expression of body symmetry.

Abnormal neuronal differentiation/maturation

In abnormalities of maturation or differentiation, neurons exhibit immature or glial features. The large, dysplastic neurons of cortical dysplasia possess markers of neuronal immaturity, such as microtubule associated protein 2c (MAP2c), MAP1B, and nestin (Crino 1997a; Yamanouchi 1996). Balloon neurons contain abnormally large amounts of cytoplasm and stain for both neuronal and glial markers (Barkovich et al. 2001), indicating a failure to commit to a specific cell lineage (Robain 1996). Balloon and dysplastic neurons are seen in cortical dysplasia and in the cortical hamartomas of tuberous sclerosis complex (Cravioto 1960; Crome 1957). Evidence of disrupted neuronal migration, including disorganized or absent lamination, malpositioned neurons, and heterotopic neurons within the white matter (Crino 1997b) are also present in these disorders. Such conditions must, therefore, involve abnormalities of both maturation and migration, indicating that dysplastic and balloon neurons lack the cellular machinery to migrate properly through the cortical plate (Crino 1997b).

Tuberous sclerosis complex

Tuberous sclerosis complex (TSC) is a multisystem, dominantly inherited condition. It has a high rate of spontaneous mutations and approximately half of all patients do not have an affected parent. Two genes have been

Pearls and Perils

Tuberous Sclerosis Complex

- About 25% of children with infantile spasms have tuberous sclerosis.
- Vigabatrin may be preferable to adrenocorticotropic hormone (ACTH) for the treatment of infantile spasms in patients with tuberous sclerosis
- Cranial imaging, abdominal (renal) ultrasound study, and echocardiograms should be considered in screening parents of patients with tuberous sclerosis for manifestations of the disease.
- Surgical decompression, possibly percutaneous, may ameliorate clinical symptoms of renal cysts.
- Retinal hamartomas are not symptomatic and do not change significantly with age.
- Pulmonary lymphangiomyomatosis, although very rarely seen in tuberous sclerosis, is pathognomonic for the disorder.
- The fat content of hepatic angiomyolipomas is diagnostic on ultrasound or computed tomography.
- Dental enamel pitting can be easily demonstrated with plaque-disclosing solution and dye. The diffuse small pits have been seen in 75–100% of adults with tuberous sclerosis.

cloned for TSC. Both result in similar clinical features. *TSC1*, located on chromosome 9q34, codes for a novel protein called hamartin, which indirectly links the cell membrane to the cytoskeleton (Narayanan 2003). *TSC2*, located at chromosome 16p13.3 encodes for the protein tuberin, which may function in cellular signaling pathways (Narayanan 2003). Hamartin and tuberin interact together as part of a larger protein complex (Narayanan 2003), which functions to negatively regulate mTOR (Gao 2002; Potter 2001). When tuberin or hamartin are nonfunctional, mTOR is active, resulting in increased cell growth and proliferation (Inoki 2005). Rapamycin acts as an mTOR inhibitor and has shown efficacy in the treatment of subependymal giant cell astrocytomas in patients with TSC (Franz 2006).

The clinical diagnosis of TSC is divided into three subheadings: definite, probable, and suspect, based on the type and number of abnormalities (Roach 1992). The clinical expression of TSC is based on the location and severity of organ involvement. The primary targets are the skin, kidneys, heart, and central nervous system. Hypopigmented macules (Figure 20.2) are the most common skin lesions and are present in as many as 90% of affected patients. Adenoma sebaceum, an angiofibromatous lesion occurring in a butterfly distribution about the nose and cheeks, is seen in 50% (Figure 20.3). Other skin lesions

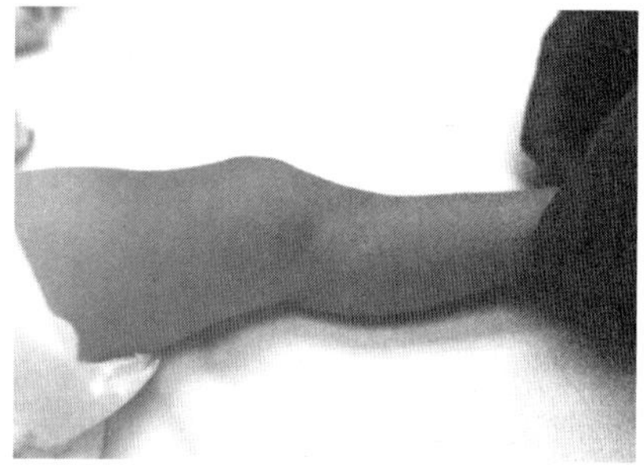

Figure 20.2 Hypopigmented macules (ash-leaf) spots are the most common skin lesions in tuberous sclerosis and are present in as many as 90% of affected patients.

include the shagreen patch (over the lumbosacral or gluteal region), café-au-lait spots, and subungual fibromas. Tumors are common and are seen in multiple organs, such as renal angiomyolipomas, cardiac rhabdomyomas, and retinal hamartomas (Table 20.6).

In the brain, the characteristic features include cortical hamartomas (cortical tubers), subependymal hamartomas (subependymal nodules), and giant-cell astrocytomas. Cortical tubers are firm and nodular, with a consistency resembling the potato tubers for which they are named. On magnetic resonance imaging (MRI) cortical tubers appear as enlarged, atypically shaped gyri with abnormal signal intensity in the subcortical white matter (Barkovich et al. 1995). Microscopically, they resemble focal cortical dysplasia (Taylor 1971) with disorganized lamination and balloon neurons (Crino 1997b). Beneath the cortex, subependymal nodules are at risk of trans-

Table 20.6 Tuberous sclerosis complex

Discriminating features
- Cortical and retinal hamartomas (tubers)
- Dermal angiofibromas
- Multiple renal angiomyolipomas

Consistent features
- Hypomelanotic macules

Variable features
- Epilepsy, including infantile spasms
- Mental retardation
- Cardiac rhabdomyomas
- Thyroid adenoma
- Gingival fibromas
- Shagreen patch
- Subungual fibromas
- Adenoma sebaceum
- Subependymal nodules
- Subependymal giant cell astrocytoma

From Roach ES, Smith M, Huttenlocher P, et al. Diagnostic criteria: tuberous sclerosis complex. Report of the Diagnostic Criteria Committee of the National Tuberous Sclerosis Association. *J Child Neurol* 1992;7:221–224.

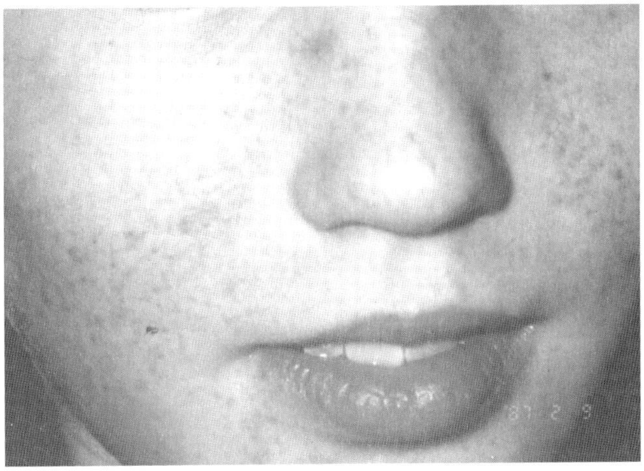

Figure 20.3 Adenoma sebaceum, an angiofibromatous lesion occurring in a butterfly distribution about the nose and cheeks, is seen in 50% of patients with tuberous sclerosis and typically develops in adolescence.

forming into subependymal giant cell astrocytomas (Kwiatkowski et al. 2002).

Cortical tubers often result in epilepsy. Under 1 year of age, infantile spasms predominate. Vigabatrin is a particularly effective treatment for infantile spasms in TSC patients (Elterman 2001) and is widely considered to be first line therapy in this setting (Chiron 1997; Hancock 1999). Later in life, generalized tonic–clonic seizures predominate, but simple and complex-partial seizures are also common. Refractory epilepsy is a common problem in TSC; surgical resection of an epileptogenic cortical tuber is possible, and is most successful when a single epileptogenic area is identified (Guerreiro 1998).

The presence of epilepsy is a predictor of cognitive impairment—this is particularly true when seizures develop under 2 years of age or when infantile spasms occur. Cognitive impairment can also be predicted by the burden of cortical tubers, with more tubers correlating with greater impairment (O'Callaghan et al. 2004). Autism is common in patients with TSC. It is more likely to develop in those with temporal tubers, seizure onset before age 3, or a history of infantile spasms (Bolton et al. 2002). Attention, language, and behavioral problems are also seen. Most of these patients have epilepsy as well. In general, only those TSC patients who are cognitively normal are seizure-free, and vice versa.

Nodular, periventricular collections of small cells resembling candle drippings are termed *subependymal nodules*. In some instances, they will transform over time into subependymal giant-cell astrocytomas (SEGAs); SEGAs typically develop in the region of the foramen of Monro and can obstruct cerebral spinal fluid flow, resulting in hydrocephalus. Presenting symptoms include headache, vomiting, obtundation, or focal neurologic deficits. Early recognition is important. Incompletely calcified periventricular nodules greater than 5 mm, and nodules demonstrating gadolinium enhancement are at greater risk of transformation. Yet, the most important criterion for recognizing SEGAs is progressive enlargement of the lesion. Neuroimaging is recommended prior to 2 years to screen for such lesions, and yearly follow-up may be necessary if suspicious periventricular nodules are discovered (Nabbout 2001).

Focal cortical dysplasia

Focal cortical dysplasia (FCD) strongly resembles the cortical tubers of TSC. Macroscopically, the lesions display wider than normal gyri and blurring of the gray–white junction (Cotter et al. 1999). Microscopic findings include disordered cortical lamination with dysplastic, cytomegalic-appearing neurons and balloon cells. The underlying white matter is hypomyelinated and contains radially oriented balloon cells (Urbach et al. 2002). The histology of FCD resembles tuberous sclerosis to such an extent that they have been postulated to be the same entity, with FCD representing a *forme fruste* of TSC. Although patients with FCD do not demonstrate the cutaneous or other systemic manifestations of TSC, they have the same genetic alterations as TSC, an increase in *TSC1* polymorphisms and loss of heterozygosity at the *TSC1* locus (Becker et al. 2002), suggesting a common pathway in these two disorders. On MRI, FCD are slightly hyperintense on T2-weighted sequences. The hyperintense regions have a funnel-shaped appearance, with the base of the funnel oriented toward the pial surface and the tip extending to the white matter (Urbach et al. 2002). Seizures resulting from FCD are commonly refractory to pharmacotherapy, and surgical resection is often required to control them (Urbach et al. 2002).

Hypomelanosis of Ito

The brain malformations of hypomelanosis of Ito (HI) include abnormalities of neuronal differentiation such as cortical dysplasia and hemimegalencephaly. Malformations characteristic of later stages of brain development (heterotopia, polymicrogyria) are also seen, suggesting heterogeneity within the disorder. The skin lesions of HI consist of whorls and streaks of decreased pigmentation, which follow the lines of Blaschko. There are no preceding inflammatory or vesicular eruptions as in incontintia pigmenti (see later discussion), and the palms, soles, and mucous membranes are spared. The skin lesions are more prominent over the ventral surface of the torso and on the flexor surface of the extremities. They may be unilateral, in which case they exhibit a midline cutoff. In patients with HI and hemimegalencephaly, the skin lesions are contralateral to the brain abnormality. Hypohidrosis is present over the hypopigmented areas and can be diagnosed by applying iodine and starch on the skin, fol-

Pearls and Perils

Hypomelanosis of Ito

- Genetic mosaicism has been discovered in children with the disorder. Circulating lymphocytes do not demonstrate the chromosomal variations; skin fibroblasts are needed.
- If a clear family history is present, the possibility of the wrong diagnosis exists. Patients with incontinentia pigmenti may have similar appearing skin signs, which are distinguishable by biopsy.
- Although half the children with hypomelanosis of Ito have clear, hard neurologic abnormalities, the prevalence of less severe problems (such as migraine, attention deficit, or learning disabilities) may be higher than expected in the other half of the population.

Pearls and Perils

Schizencephaly

- The walls of the schizencephalic cleft are lined by polymicrogyria. Without the adjacent gray matter, the defect is more likely to be a porencephalic cleft.
- The septum pellucidum is absent in 80–90% of patients with schizencephaly. Septo-optic dysplasia has also been described.
- Intractable seizures are common in schizencephaly. Several different seizure types (including generalized tonic–clonic, simple partial, complex partial, and infantile spasms) can exist. The severity and subtype of schizencephaly do not correlate with the presence of or type of epilepsy.

lowed by subcutaneous injection of pilocarpine hydrochloride. Systemic manifestations include ophthalmologic, cardiac, musculoskeletal, and genital anomalies (Table 20.7).

The neurologic manifestations include epilepsy and mental retardation. Generalized tonic–clonic seizures are the most common, but infantile spasms, focal, and myoclonic seizures are also observed. Autistic behaviors are sometimes seen and are usually present in children with epilepsy. Pathology may reveal polymicrogyria, heterotopia, cortical dysplasia, or hemimegalencephaly. The etiology of HI is likely to be heterogeneous; several different chromosomal abnormalities have been associated with it, and most patients are chromosomal mosaics.

Schizencephaly

The term schizencephaly refers to a cleft extending between the pial and lateral ventricular surfaces. Lining the cleft on both sides are abnormally small gyri, termed *polymicrogyria*. The presence of polymicrogyria helps distinguish this malformative lesion from destructive disorders (i.e., porencephaly) with a similar appearance (Yakolev et al. 1946). Schizencephaly is heterogeneous in appearance. Lesions vary in size from small closed-lip to large open-lip schizencephaly, and they may occur in one or both hemispheres. Possible etiologies are similarly heterogeneous. Environmental causes, such as fetal hypotension, exposure to organic solvents, and viral infections, may be causative (Denis et al. 2000). Vascular anomalies have also been reported in association with schizencephaly (Denis et al. 2000). Familial cases exist, indicating a genetic mechanism in some instances. In 1996, Brunelli and colleagues reported heterozygous mutations in the homeobox gene *EMX2* in seven sporadic cases (Brunelli et al. 1996). The same group later reported two brothers with the same *EMX2* deletion and different degrees of schizencephaly (Granata et al. 1997). The authors postulate that although the gene mutation is

Table 20.7 Hypomelanosis of Ito

Discriminating features
- Characteristic hypomelanotic skin lesion or lesions (prominent over the ventral surface of the torso and on the flexor surface of the extremities)

Consistent features
- Characteristic hypomelanotic lesion

Variable features
- Mental retardation
- Epilepsy
- Central nervous system migration defects (heterotopia, polymicrogyria)
- Hemihypertrophy
- Syndactyly

Table 20.8 Schizencephaly

Discriminating features
- Cleft extending between the pial and lateral ventricular surfaces

Consistent features
- Polymicrogyria lining the cleft

Variable features
- Size of cleft (open or closed lip)
- Unilateral or bilateral clefts
- Epilepsy
- Motor impairment
- Cognitive impairment
- Etiology (environmental versus genetic)

causative, environmental factors may impact on severity (Table 20.8). In 2007, Tietjen sequenced *EMX2* in a cohort of 84 patients with schizencephaly and found no pathologic mutations, indicating that *EMX2* is an uncommon etiology (Tietjen 2007).

The clinical severity relates to the degree of structural involvement. Unilateral clefts commonly present with hemiparesis and mild, if any, cognitive delay. Bilateral clefts, on the other hand, are associated with quadriparesis and significant cognitive impairment (Denis et al. 2000). Likewise, the size of the lesion is an important determinant of outcome. For example, patients with large or medium open-lip schizencephaly display significantly worse motor and intellectual function than do patients with close-lip or small open-lip lesions (Barkovich & Kjos 1992b). The severity of epilepsy, however, is generally unrelated to the structural findings (Packard et al. 1997).

Disorders of neuronal migration

Migration takes place between the third and fifth months of gestation (Volpe 2001). During migration, postmitotic neurons move from the ventricular and subventricular layers to their final sites within the cerebral cortex. Migration occurs in radial (perpendicular to the pial surface) and tangential (parallel to the pial surface) fashions.

Heterotopia

Heterotopia are collections of ectopic neurons located outside of the cortex (Barkovich et al. 2000). Unlike cortical dysplasia, the neurons within heterotopia are normal. Thus, on imaging, heterotopia are isointense with normal gray matter, lacking the abnormal signal intensity seen in dysplasia. The cortex overlying heterotopia may be abnormally thin with shallow sulci (Barkovich et al. 2000).

Familial periventricular heterotopia (PH) are characterized by periventricular nodules of neurons resting beneath an otherwise normal-appearing cortex (Dobyns et al. 1996). The nodules are rounded, irregular, and separated from each other by myelinated fibers (Figure 20.4).

Table 20.9 Periventricular (nodular) heterotopia

Discriminating features
- Nodular collections of neurons within the subependymal region

Consistent features
- Rounded nodules of neurons resting beneath an otherwise normal-appearing cortex

Variable features
- Cognitive impairment
- Epilepsy

Pearls and Perils

Familial Periventricular Heterotopia

- Nearly 25% of patients are reported to be asymptomatic, but some of these patients may actually have undiagnosed learning disabilities or other subtle deficits.
- Male patients have been described and may represent a distinct genetic cause from *FLNA*.

In PH, some neurons migrate fully to form a normal-appearing six-layer cortex, whereas others have a complete failure of migration and remain in nodular collections within the subependymal region. The cortex functions surprisingly well, and most patients have normal intelligence. Epilepsy is common and generally develops in the mid teenage years (Fox & Walsh 1999) (Table 20.9).

Familial PH commonly displays X-linked dominant inheritance and is lethal in hemizygous male embryos (Eksioglu et al. 1996). Approximately half of patients have a de novo mutation. Because epilepsy is mild or absent in approximately one-quarter of all patients, a family history is not always confirmed until neuroimaging of a patient's mother is performed. Periventricular heterotopia most often results from a mutation of the Filamin A (*FLNA*) gene on chromosome Xq28, which encodes a large actin-binding protein involved in structuring actin

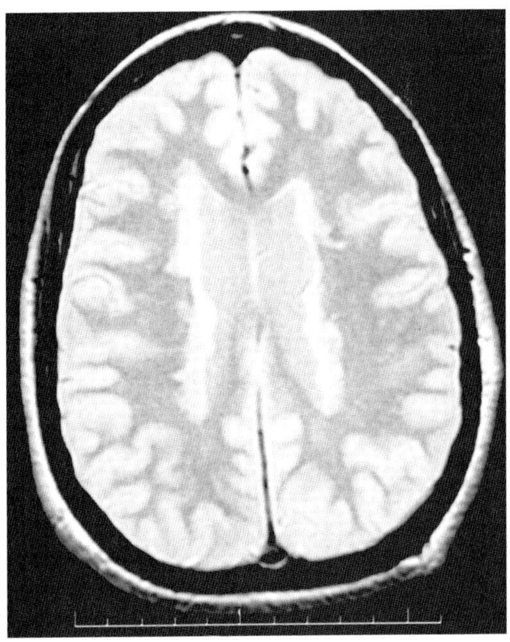

Figure 20.4 Periventricular heterotopia (PH) are characterized by periventricular nodules of neurons resting beneath an otherwise normal-appearing cortex. The nodules are rounded, irregular, and separated from each other by myelinated fibers.

networks at the leading edge of motile cells, thus necessary for migration (Fox et al. 1998; Fox & Walsh 1999).

Lissencephaly

Lissencephaly refers to a paucity of normal gyri and sulci resulting in a "smooth brain." It is a heterogeneous condition, which is traditionally divided into two pathologic subtypes: classical (type I) and cobblestone (type II). Radiographically, the cortex appears smooth in both types, but beyond that, few similarities exist. Classical lissencephaly results from an arrest of neuronal migration, whereas cobblestone lissencephaly results from overmigration. In both cases, lissencephaly is associated with epilepsy and severe developmental delay.

Classical lissencephaly (agyria–pachygyria complex)

Most patients with classical (type I) lissencephaly have a combination of agyria (a total absence of gyri) and pachygyria (a reduced number of abnormally large gyri). Radiographically, the surface of the brain appears smooth in agyria, with diminished white matter and shallow sylvian fissures (Barkovich et al. 2000). In pachygyria, gyri are reduced in number and abnormally broad and flat (Barkovich et al. 2000). Microscopically, agyria has a disorganized outer cortical layer and a thick layer of ectopic neurons in the periventricular region; pachygyria displays better cortical organization (Table 20.10). Clinical severity is largely related to the degree of structural abnormality, with greater gyral simplification resulting in greater clinical impairment. In cases of agyria, epilepsy is universal and infantile spasms are a particularly common seizure type. Electroencephalography reveals characteristic, high-voltage activity (Liang et al. 2002). Neurodevelopmental disabilities are severe; many patients have mental retardation, spastic quadriparesis, and microcephaly. In patients with pachygyria, particularly when focal and unilateral, epilepsy and developmental delays remain common but are less severe (Çakmakçi et al. 2004).

Table 20.10 Classical (type I) lissencephaly

Discriminating features
- Smooth cerebral cortex (agyria and pachygyria)

Consistent features
- Abnormally thick cortex
- Disorganized cortical lamination
- Cognitive and motor impairment
- Epilepsy

Variable features
- Degree of motor and cognitive impairment
- Severity of epilepsy
- Etiology (*LIS1* versus *DCX* mutations)
- Craniofacial or systemic malformations

Pearls and Perils

Classical (Type I) Lissencephaly

- Facial anomalies can be associated with isolated lissencephaly sequence and offer clues as to the underlying genetic defect. In Miller-Dieker syndrome (associated with *LIS1* defects), a prominent forehead, low nasal bridge, or short nose can be seen. These facial changes may become less prominent with age. In X-linked lissencephaly (*XLIS*), a low nasal bridge, prominent epicanthal folds, and flat midface can be seen.
- The pattern of gyral abnormality also differs between *LIS1* and *XLIS*. Mutations of *LIS1* generally have a posterior-to-anterior gradient, with agyria being most prominent posteriorly and increasing pachygyria anteriorly. Mutations of *XLIS*, on the other hand, are associated with an anterior-to-posterior gradient of lissencephaly.
- Cerebellar hypoplasia is more common in *XLIS* than *LIS1* mutations and is also seen in abnormalities of *RELN*.
- If the birth head circumference is less than three standard deviations below normal, microlissencephaly (which is genetically distinct from *LIS1* and *XLIS*) is the likely diagnosis.

Classical lissencephaly is most commonly caused by a disruption of the platelet-activating factor acetylhydrolase gene (*PAFAH1B1*; also known as *LIS1*) located on chromosome 17p13.3 (Reiner et al. 1993). The *LIS1* gene product interacts with microtubules, and related motor components, dynein and dynactin, as well as doublecortin, a protein that may regulate microtubule stability. Almost all patients have spontaneous, heterozygous deletions of *LIS1*, which are not present in the parents. The risk of having a second affected child is therefore low. When a large deletion occurs, other congenital anomalies (craniofacial, renal, cardiac, or gastrointestinal malformations) can result and together are termed the Miller-Dieker syndrome (Dobyns et al. 1993).

Abnormalities of the doublecortin (*DCX* or *XLIS*) gene, located on the X chromosome, are also known to cause classical lissencephaly (Gleeson et al. 1998). In hemizygous males, the phenotype is nearly indistinguishable from *LIS1*. Yet, in heterozygous females, a disorder termed double cortex (DC), also known as subcortical band heterotopia, results. In DC, the outer cortex displays normal six-layered architecture, but an inappropriate accumulation of neurons exists in the subcortical white matter (Figure 20.5). Random inactivation of an X chromosome accounts for this pattern. Half of the neurons express a normal copy of the doublecortin gene and

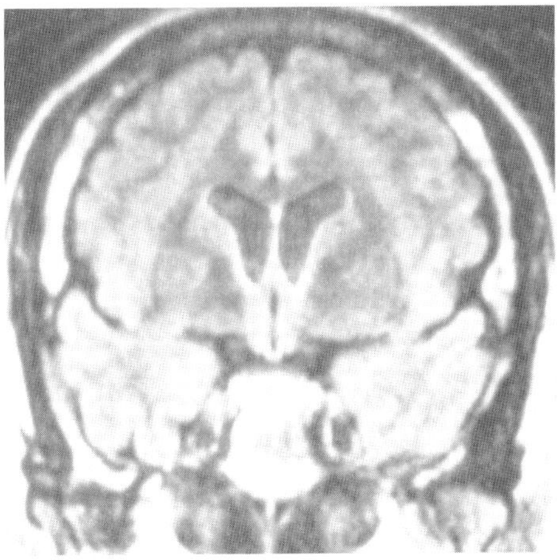

Figure 20.5 In double cortex (DC), females heterozygous for a doublecortin gene mutation display two discrete areas of cerebral cortex. The outer layer may appear normal and has an appropriate six-layered architecture, but an inappropriate accumulation of neurons also exists in the subcortical white matter. X-inactivation likely accounts for this divergent pattern of neuronal migration. In males, only one X chromosome exists, so the mutation affects all neurons and the more severe phenotype of classical lissencephaly occurs.

undergo normal migration, whereas the other half express the mutant copy and remain arrested in the subcortical white matter. In males, only one X chromosome exists, so the mutation affects all neurons. Hence, the more severe phenotype of classical lissencephaly occurs in males. Females with DC display mild to moderate mental retardation, and their epilepsy is generally less severe than in males with lissencephaly (Berg et al. 1998).

Cobblestone (type II) lissencephaly

Cobblestone lissencephaly develops from an overmigration of neurons beyond the pial surface and onto the overlying subarachnoid tissue. Cobblestone lissencephaly is sometimes associated with congenital muscular dystrophy and eye abnormalities, such as Fukuyama congenital muscular dystrophy (FCMD), Walker-Warburg syndrome (WWS), and muscle-eye-brain disease (MEB). These disorders are believed to result from an impairment of glycosylation (Grewal et al. 2003). More specifically, they affect O-mannosylation, which is important to brain, nerve, and skeletal muscle, explaining the distribution of involved tissues in these disorders (Endo et al. 1999).

Of all three disorders, WWS has the most severe phenotype and is often fatal in the first year of life (Dobyns et al. 1989). In addition to cobblestone lissencephaly, patients with WWS sometimes display agenesis of the corpus callosum, cerebellar hypoplasia, hydrocephaly, and encephalocele. Neuroimaging reveals a thickened cortex with few, abnormally shallow sulci. The gray–white matter junction is irregular due to disorganized collections of neurons misplaced in the white matter. Hypomyelination is common (Barkovich et al. 2000). Ocular anomalies include microphthalmos and congenital glaucoma (Barkovich et al. 2000). Genetically, WWS is recessively inherited. The syndrome results from mutations in the O-mannosyltransferase 1 (*POMT1*) gene (Beltrán-Valero de Bernabé et al. 2002), implicating a failure of glycosylation as the primary defect (Table 20.11).

Muscle-eye-brain disease is also an autosomal recessive condition and is most prevalent in Finland. The clinical severity is intermediate to WWS and FCMD (Santavuori et al. 1989), as is the radiographic appearance (Barkovich et al. 2000). Muscle-eye-brain disease results from loss of function mutations in the gene encoding protein O-linked mannose 1,2-N-acetylglucosaminyltransferase 1 (*POMGnT1*) (Yoshida et al. 2001). A genotype–phenotype correlation exists in MEB patients with mutations close to the 5' terminus of the *POMGnT1* gene, resulting in a severe clinical picture and mutations at the 3' terminus leading to milder impairments (Taniguchi et al. 2003).

Pearls and Perils

Cobblestone (Type II) Lissencephaly

- Fukuyama congenital muscular dystrophy, muscle-eye-brain disease of the Finnish type (MEB), and Walker-Warburg syndrome present in infancy with hypotonia, severe weakness, and a poor suck and cry. Walker-Warburg is the most severe form and Fukuyama congenital muscular dystrophy is the mildest of the three, but considerable overlap exists, and the three disorders are sometimes difficult to distinguish on clinical grounds only.

Table 20.11 Cobblestone (type II) lissencephaly

Discriminating features
- Excessive number of abnormally small cortical gyri (polymicrogyria)

Consistent features
- Thickened cortex with few, abnormally shallow sulci
- Cognitive and motor impairment

Variable features
- Ocular abnormalities
- Muscle abnormalities
- Epilepsy
- Degree of cognitive and motor impairment

Fukuyama congenital muscular dystrophy is the mildest of the three disorders. It presents with hypotonia and global developmental delays. Seizures develop in the first year of life in half of patients (Toda et al. 2000). Fukuyama congenital muscular dystrophy is associated with mutations of the gene fukutin on chromosome 9q31 (Toda et al. 1993). The exact function of fukutin is unknown, but its structure predicts it to be an enzyme involved in the modification of surface glycoproteins or glycolipids (Aravind & Koonin 1999).

Fukuyama congenital muscular dystrophy is seen primarily in Japan, where 94% of the affected individuals share a common haplotype, indicating a single founder in the Japanese population (Kobayashi et al. 1998). Patients who are homozygous for the founder mutation have a higher residual activity of fukutin and a milder phenotype than do patients with a spontaneous point mutation on the second allele (compound heterozygotes) (Toda et al. 2000). It is difficult to distinguish severely affected FCMD cases from WWS patients. Two Turkish individuals with mutations of fukutin were reported as displaying a WWS phenotype (Beltrán-Valero de Bernabé 2003; Silan 2003). Such overlap implies a shared pathway in the pathophysiology of these disorders.

Symmetric polymicrogyria

Polymicrogyria is thought to develop at the latest stages of neuronal migration or the earliest phases of cortical organization (Barkovich et al. 2001). It often results from external causes such as intrauterine cytomegalovirus infection (Barkovich et al. 1994) or placental perfusion failure (Baker et al. 1996). Yet, genetic causes do exist and tend to result in focal but symmetrical lesions. Syndromes affecting every conceivable region—frontoparietal, perisylvian, parieto-occipital—have been observed. Epilepsy and cognitive delays are common among all of the syndromes; additional symptoms depend upon the specific region(s) affected.

Bilateral frontoparietal polymicrogyria (BFPP) is characterized by bilateral, symmetric polymicrogyria in the frontoparietal regions (Chang et al. 2003). There is a decreasing gradient of severity from the anterior to posterior direction. The white matter is thin, with areas of T2 prolongation, the ventricles are enlarged, and the pons and cerebellar vermis are abnormally small (Chang 2003). The clinical manifestations are consistent: motor abnormalities, seizures, and global developmental delay are universal (Guerrini 2000; Chang et al. 2003). Cerebellar abnormalities and dysconjugate gaze are also common (Chang et al. 2003). The disorder has been mapped to chromosome 16q12.2–21 (Chang et al. 2003; Piao 2002). Bilateral frontoparietal polymicrogyria patients are characteristically from the Middle East or Indian subcontinent, and many share a single haplotype, indicating a common founder mutation (Chang et al. 2003; Piao et al. 2002).

Bilateral perisylvian polymicrogyria (BPP) results in a clinical syndrome manifested by mild mental retardation, epilepsy, and pseudobulbar palsy (Kuzniecky et al. 1993). The pseudobulbar palsy specifically affects expressive speech and feeding. Bilateral perisylvian polymicrogyria is often a sporadic condition. It has been described in association with unrelated disorders including neurofibromatosis type I (Balestri et al. 2003) and Kabuki syndrome (Powell 2003). Bilateral perisylvian polymicrogyria is therefore likely to be heterogeneous. In some pedigrees, BPP follows an X-linked inheritance pattern, and linkage analysis places the critical region at Xq28 (Villard et al. 2002). Sixty-six genes are known to exist in that interval, including the Filamin A gene. *SRPX2* is also on Xq28 and was found to carry a mutation in a boy with BPP and Rolandic seizures. The gene is therefore likely to play an important role in peri-sylvian development (Roll 2006).

Disorders of myelination and cortical organization

Cortical organization and myelination are the final steps of brain development and continue well after birth. Abnormalities at these stages may be less obvious on neuroimaging than earlier malformations, but they nonetheless can have profound effects. Cognitive and motor impairments are commonly associated with both abnormalities; spasticity is more specific to problems with myelination, whereas hypotonia is frequently seen in disorders of cortical organization.

Cortical organization begins in the fifth month of gestation and continues through the first several years of life. Abnormalities of cortical organization are commonly associated with mental retardation. The most consistent anatomic correlates of mental retardation are dendritic anomalies, such as deficient branching. Such abnormalities cannot be detected by neuroimaging, explaining why many patients with mental retardation have normal MRIs.

Myelination begins in the second trimester of pregnancy and continues into adulthood. Normal myelination is impaired when oligodendrocytes are deficient in number (either from injury or failure to proliferate) or are unable to deposit myelin around axons. Insufficient oligodendrocytes are observed in periventricular leukomalacia, in which differentiating oligodendroglia are injured and therefore unable to produce myelin. Other disorders, such as hypothyroidism, malnutrition, amino and organic acidopathies (maple syrup urine disease, homocystinuria), cause functional impairment of myelination. Primary disturbances of myelination are distinguished from leukodystrophies in that leukodystrophies result from injury to previously myelinated axons.

Neurofibromatosis type I

The primary disorder in neurofibromatosis (NF) relates to oncogene regulation and tumor formation, but the white matter abnormalities seen in NF can be categorized as a disorder of myelination. Additionally, a study showing increased volume of gray and white matter in children with NF type 1 (NF1) suggests that brain overgrowth is an intrinsic component of this disease (Greenwood et al. 2004).

Neurofibromatosis type 1, also known as *peripheral neurofibromatosis*, is an autosomal dominant, single-gene defect affecting multiple organ systems. The NF1 gene localizes to chromosome 17q11.2 and encodes the protein product neurofibromin. The incidence of NF1 ranges between 1 in 3,000 to 1 in 4,000. Approximately 50% of patients with NF1 lack a family history and likely represent new mutations (Lynch 2002). The diagnosis is based on National Institutes of Health (NIH) consensus criteria and requires two or more of the following: six or more café-au-lait spots (0.5 mm or larger in prepubertal and 1.5 mm or larger in post pubertal individuals), two or more neurofibromas of any type or one plexiform neurofibroma, axillary or groin freckling, two or more Lisch nodules, optic nerve glioma, dysplasia of the sphenoid bone or long bone cortex, or a first-degree relative with NF1 (Table 20.12). Of these features, café-au-lait spots are the most easily recognized and are often the presenting feature of the disease (Figure 20.6). They are evenly pigmented macules, which increase in size and number with age. They may be the only sign present in infancy, making a definitive diagnosis difficult to establish until later in life.

Pearls and Perils

Neurofibromatosis Type I (NF1)

- Hyperpigmented patches over the midline of the back indicate an underlying neurofibroma involving the spinal cord or adjacent roots.
- The characteristic bony lesions, sphenoid wing hypoplasia, and tibial and radial pseudoarthroses should be considered diagnostic for neurofibromatosis in children
- Probably the most common false-positive diagnostic sign is multiple café-au-lait spots. Very few patients with neurofibromatosis have these features as the only markers of the disorder.
- The subcutaneous nerves in the neck are easily seen on clinical examination. They are often the nerves first recognized as involved by neurofibromatosis.
- Slit-lamp ophthalmologic examination of parents is a rapid, accurate screen for the presence of the gene.
- Pigmentary skin features are more useful in prepubertal siblings.
- Genetic testing is of limited sensitivity and a negative study does not exclude the disorder.

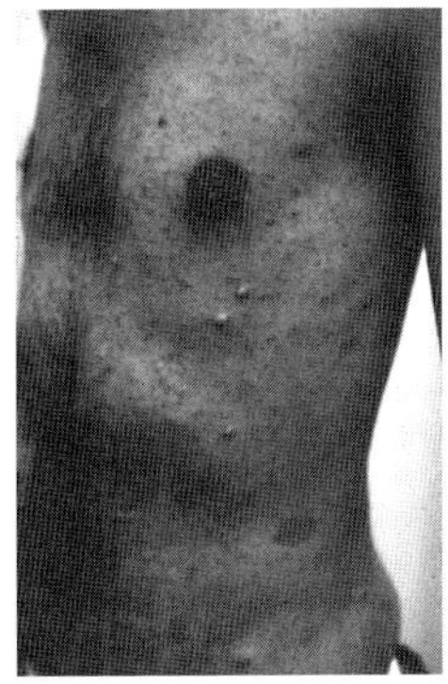

Figure 20.6 This patient with neurofibromatosis type I demonstrates multiple cutaneous neurofibromas and cafe-au-lait spots.

In childhood, the most common complication of NF1 is cognitive impairment. A broad range of effects are seen including low IQ, behavioral problems, and learning disabilities. IQ scores in NF1 patients have a bimodal distribution; some children have intellectual impairment whereas others do not. This separation may have its basis in the white matter T2 hyperintensities, also known as unidentified bright objects (UBOs), common to NF1 patients. They represent dysplastic glial proliferation and aberrant myelination in the underdeveloped brain. When compared to children without T2 hyperintensities, those with the lesions have significantly lower mean values for IQ and language scores and significantly impaired visuo-

Table 20.12 Neurofibromatosis type I (NF1)

Discriminating features
- Plexiform neurofibromas
- Optic nerve glioma

Consistent features
- Multiple café-au-lait spots
- Lisch nodules
- Autosomal dominant inheritance

Variable features
- Neurofibromas
- Pilocytic astrocytoma
- Axillary or groin freckling
- White matter T2 hyperintensities (unidentified bright objects)
- Macrocephaly
- Cognitive impairment
- Epilepsy

motor integration and coordination (North 1995). T2-hyperintensities in childhood are also a predictor of cognitive dysfunction in adulthood (Hyman 2003). Denckla and colleagues (1996) found that children with NF1 had a lowering of their IQ score as a function of the distribution of UBOs, rather than the number of lesions. A study showing a correlation between increased white matter volume and visual-perceptual deficits suggests that brain overgrowth may be a factor in the associated cognitive deficits (Greenwood et al. 2004).

Tumors and malignancies are common in NF1, and are a major cause of morbidity. Neurofibromas, the tumors for which the disorder takes its name, are peripheral nerve sheath tumors with unpredictable growth patterns. They are benign tumors without risk of malignant transformation, and typically develop in adolescence. Although they are unlikely to cause neurologic deficit, spinal neurofibromas arising from the dorsal nerve roots can lead to severe pain. Plexiform neurofibromas, on the other hand, are more likely to be present at birth. They can be found anywhere within the body and cause a variety of presenting symptoms depending on their location. Serious complications include pain, spinal cord compression, and spread to the orbit with resulting sphenoid wing dysplasia and pulsating exophthalmos. Plexiform neurofibromas can undergo transformation to malignant peripheral nerve sheath tumors.

Optic nerve gliomas are pilocytic astrocytomas involving the optic nerve, chiasm, or tract. They usually develop prior to age 7 and can be insidious in their onset. Yearly ophthalmologic assessments are therefore important for early diagnosis and management of these tumors. Abnormalities on the ophthalmologic examination necessitate an MRI. Treatment should be withheld for stable, nonprogressive tumors, since it adds to neurologic, endocrine, or visual morbidity (Tow 2003). Progressive tumors, however, do require treatment. Intraorbital tumors are best managed with resection, whereas posterior (chiasmatic or optic tract) tumors are treated with radiotherapy. Given the young age of most of these children, endocrinopathies and cognitive impairment from radiotherapy are major concerns. Chemotherapy has been tried as a means of either avoiding or delaying radiotherapy; initial results suggest that this approach spares the intellectual impairments common to radiotherapy (Lacaze 2003). Further study is needed to determine what the role of chemotherapy should be in these patients.

Other malignancies observed in NF1 include CNS tumors (particularly astrocytomas), pheochromocytomas, and leukemia. Given the prevalence of tumors in NF1, it should come as no surprise that an oncogene is responsible for the condition; neurofibromin functions as a tumor suppressor protein, the loss of which promotes tumor formation.

The workup for NF1 is aimed at the early identification of potential complications, with tumor formation being the main concern. The American Academy of Pediatrics Committee on Genetics recommends yearly physical examinations and ophthalmologic assessments. The physical examination focuses on the organ systems involved. The skin is screened for new neurofibromas or plexiform neurofibromas. Blood pressure is followed to assess for renal (renal artery stenosis) or endocrine (pheochromocytomas and adrenal tumors) abnormalities. A skeletal examination looks for pseudoarthrosis of the tibia, bowing of the long bones, scoliosis, and orbital defects. The neurologic examination may reveal macrocephaly, learning disabilities, or cognitive impairment. The ophthalmologic evaluation helps exclude optic nerve gliomas, choroidal hamartomas, and Lisch nodules.

Laboratory investigations confirm the diagnosis and explore any abnormalities disclosed on the physical examination. Molecular genetic testing is available for NF1, but the size and complexity of the gene, combined with the genetic heterogeneity of the disorder, have been obstacles to routine DNA testing. Gene testing is nonetheless helpful for genetic counseling and even makes preimplantation diagnosis possible (Verlinsky 2002). Because tumors are the most serious consequence of NF1, neuroimaging, preferably with MRI, is an important tool for the management of this condition. Imaging is required whenever the history or physical examination raise a question of tumor development.

Neurofibromatosis type II

Like NF1, NF type II (NF2) is an autosomal dominant, single gene deficit, which, in NF2, localizes to chromosome 22. The gene product, merlin, also has tumor suppressor function. Tumors and malignancies are, therefore, common in both conditions. Beyond that, few similarities exist. Café-au-lait spots are rarely seen in NF2, and neurofibromas are surprisingly uncommon considering that the disorder takes its name from this tumor type. NF2 is seen much less commonly than NF1, with an incidence of only 1:30,000 to 1:40,000.

Pearls and Perils

Neurofibromatosis Type II (NF2)

- A careful family history should be obtained from all patients with acoustic neuromas. The younger the patient, the more likely the diagnosis of NF2.
- The tumors of NF2 do not seem to respond to hormonal changes as do those of NF1.

Table 20.13 Neurofibromatosis type II

Discriminating features
▶ Bilateral acoustic neuromas
▶ Multiple schwannomas
▶ Multiple meningiomas
Consistent features
▶ Bilateral deafness
▶ Fewer than five café-au-lait spots
▶ Autosomal dominant inheritance
Variable features
▶ Tinnitus
▶ Headaches
▶ Cranial nerve palsy
▶ Retinal hamartomas

Common tumors in NF2 include schwannomas (which are usually multiple), meningiomas, ependymomas, and gliomas. Vestibulo-cochlear schwannomas are particularly common and sometimes bilateral (in which case, a diagnosis of NF2 is certain). Roughly half of NF2 patients present because of hearing loss, tinnitus, and vertigo resulting from a vestibulo-cochlear schwannoma. The peak age of diagnosis is the third decade. In children, ocular abnormalities (diplopia, vision loss) are the most common presenting symptoms (MacCollin et al. 1998). These are caused by hamartomas of the retina, optic nerve sheath meningiomas, or juvenile posterior subcapsular lenticular opacities (a specific type of cataract). Meningiomas at a young age should also raise a suspicion of NF2; both intracranial and spinal meningiomas occur. Schwannomas and ependymomas may develop in the spine, in which case, back pain and paraplegia may result (Table 20.13).

Disorders of vascular supply of brain tissue (known or postulated)

The following disorders result from vascular abnormalities, and are therefore difficult to organize within the embryologic classification presented earlier. However, each results in developmental abnormalities of the brain, justifying inclusion in this discussion.

Bilateral parasagittal parieto-occipital polymicrogyria

Unlike the other symmetrical polymicrogyria syndromes, bilateral parasagittal parieto-occipital polymicrogyria is unlikely to have a genetic basis. Of nine patients described, none had a familial distribution. Given that the lesion occurs in a vascular watershed region, perfusion failure is postulated to be the cause. All patients develop seizures and cognitive abilities range from normal to mild retardation (Guerrini 1997) (Figure 20.7).

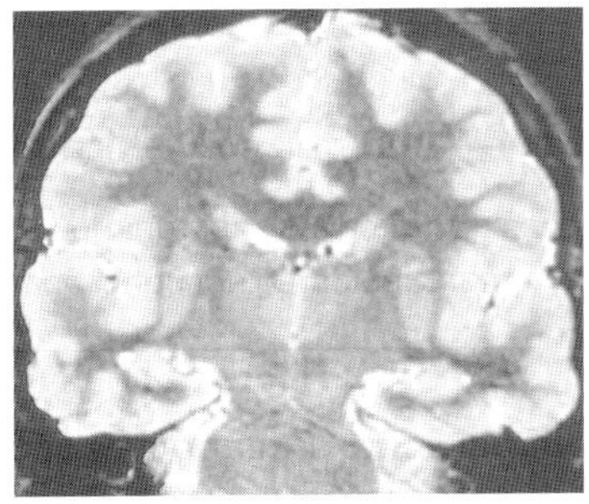

Figure 20.7 Bilateral perisylvian polymicrogyria (BPP) results in a clinical syndrome manifested by mild mental retardation, epilepsy, and pseudobulbar palsy. The pseudobulbar palsy specifically affects expressive speech and feeding, as would be predicted by the motor homunculus.

Incontinentia pigmenti

Incontinentia pigmenti (IP) is a rare, X-linked, dominant, neurocutaneous disorder with the onset of skin changes in the first 6 weeks of life. The cutaneous disorder follows a characteristic evolution from vesicular to verrucous to hyperpigmented and finally atrophic changes. The vesicles and bullae from the original eruption in infancy later give rise to the characteristic swirling pattern of hyperpigmentation. Hair, nail, dental, and ophthalmologic abnormalities are also observed. Neurologically, these infants may develop epilepsy, mental retardation, microcephaly, spasticity, or ataxia. A recent case report demonstrating periventricular hemorrhagic infarctions in infancy strongly suggests microangiopathy as the cause of the neurologic changes (Hennel 2003). The gene for incontinentia pigmenti is *NEMO* (NF-κB essential modulator)/IKK (I B kinase-γ) and is located on Xq28. *NEMO* is 200

Pearls and Perils

Incontinentia Pigmenti

- Boys with the disorder have been diagnosed (14 out of 255 cases). Some have had polyploidy of the X chromosome, notably Klinefelter syndrome.
- Children with incontinentia pigmenti are small-for-gestational-age infants more frequently than predicted in the general population.
- Retrolental fibroplasias in an infant not exposed to a high concentration of oxygen should suggest the diagnosis of incontinentia pigmenti

Table 20.14 Incontinentia Pigmenti

Discriminating features
- Characteristic swirled hyperpigmented lesions

Consistent features
- Female sex

Variable features
- Mental retardation
- Epilepsy
- Hemihypertrophy

kilobases proximal to the factor VIII locus and is important for immune, inflammatory, and apoptotic pathways (Smahi 2000). The disorder is lethal in most males, accounting for its 20:1 female to male predominance (Table 20.14). Males with IP have been described, but commonly have features of IP in only a limited distribution. Somatic mosaicism is a likely mechanism in such cases (Pacheco 2006).

Sturge-Weber syndrome

Sturge-Weber syndrome is characterized by angiomata of the leptomeninges and skin (Figure 20.8). The cutaneous lesion, also known as a port-wine stain, typically involves the ophthalmic and maxillary distributions of the trigeminal nerve. The leptomeningeal angiomata may be either unilateral or bilateral, but unilateral lesions are more common. The specific neurologic effects are dependent on the location of the lesion, which is most commonly parietal or occipital. Neurologic impairment results in large part from stasis and a vascular steal phenomenon. Laminar cortical necrosis with neuronal loss, gliosis, cerebral atrophy, and calcifications are seen histologically. The calcifications take on a classic train-track appearance on plain films and computed tomography (CT). MRI, if

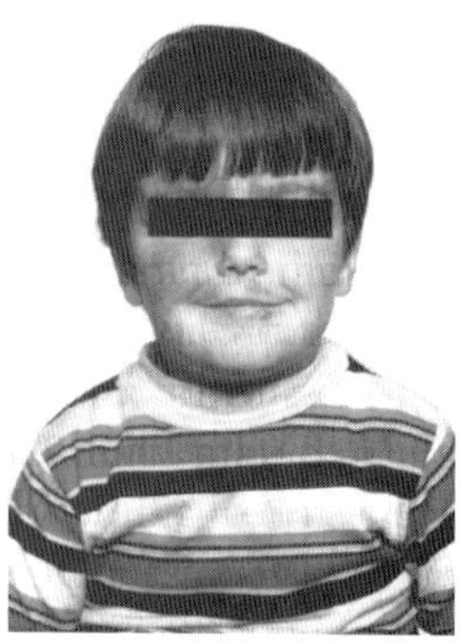

Figure 20.8 This patient with Sturge-Weber syndrome demonstrates the typical leptomeningeal angiomata (port-wine stain) of the ophthalmic and maxillary distributions of the trigeminal nerve. Leptomeningeal angiomata may be either unilateral or bilateral, but unilateral lesions are more common.

Pearls and Perils

Sturge-Weber Syndrome

- Hemihypertrophy, seen in the disorder, is usually associated with a vascular malformation of the affected limb or limbs. A similar enlargement is seen in the skull ipsilateral to the port-wine stain.
- Migraine is more common in Sturge-Weber patients than in the general population, and it is more likely to occur at younger ages and be associated with neurologic deficits.

done, should be performed with gadolinium to allow for appreciation of the angiomata. The clinical manifestations include hemiparesis, stroke-like episodes, mental retardation, epilepsy, and headaches. Epilepsy is present in 75–90% of patients, and the seizures are typically focal. Many patients have refractory epilepsy, in which case cortical resection and possibly hemispherectomy are considered. An important non-neurologic effect is glaucoma, which can occur at any age (Table 20.15).

Ataxia-telangiectasia

The reader is referred to Chapter 12 on Movement Disorders for a discussion of this condition.

Clinical aspects of nervous system malformations

Clinical–radiographic correlation

Structure predicts function. Hence, most cerebral malformations display a clinical–radiographic correlation. Diffuse lesions, such as classical lissencephaly, are associated with severe global developmental delay. Bilateral,

Table 20.15 Sturge-Weber syndrome

Discriminating features
- Port-wine stain (nevus flammeus) in trigeminal distribution
- Ipsilateral meningocortical venous malformation

Consistent features
- Progressive cortical deficits
- Epilepsy (focal)
- Glaucoma

Variable features
- Cutaneous vascular malformations on trunk or limbs
- Mental retardation
- Hemihypertrophy/hemiatrophy

focal lesions may result in bilateral motor dysfunction and moderate to severe developmental impairment (Barkovich & Kjos 1992a). Unilateral lesions can be associated with contralateral hemiplegia and mild, if any, cognitive delay. The size of focal lesions is an important determinant of outcome. For example, patients with large or medium open-lip schizencephaly display significantly worse motor and intellectual function than patients with close-lip or small open-lip lesions (Barkovich & Kjos 1992b). Location is also relevant; frontal dysplasia and polymicrogyria are strongly associated with motor impairment (Barkovich & Kjos 1992b; Guerrini et al. 2000).

Clinical–genetic correlation

Genetic heterogeneity makes it difficult to predict the clinical phenotype solely from knowing the gene involved. Nonetheless, occasionally, knowledge of the details of the mutation aid in determining the prognosis. In general, the degree of residual protein function correlates with severity. Function can range from complete absence of protein production, as is seen in large deletions, to normal production with reduced activity, which may occur with certain point mutations. Such is the case with lissencephaly/subcortical band heterotopia from *DCX* mutations. Familial cases, most of which possess missense mutations, have a milder phenotype than sporadic cases in which protein truncation mutations are more common (Matsumoto et al. 2001). For X-linked disorders, X inactivation is tremendously important in determining the phenotype, but is nearly impossible to study since brain tissue, which is optimal for looking at this question, is difficult to obtain. Cultured fibroblasts or lymphocytes can be used as a substitute, but the results from these tissues are less conclusive. In deletions, it is important to consider the impact of contiguous genes, since their involvement can alter the clinical phenotype. Such is the case in Miller-Dieker syndrome, where impairment of genes contiguous to *LIS1* accounts for a more severe degree of lissencephaly and other systemic anomalies (Cardoso et al. 2003). Gene–gene interactions are also relevant. In PH, only some of the neurons demonstrate a failure of migration whereas others go on to form a normal six-layered cortex. Traditionally, this was attributed to genetic mosaicism from random X-inactivation. Yet, males with PH from *FLNA* mutations have been described (Sheen et al. 2001), arguing against X-inactivation as the basis for the divergent behavior of neurons in PH. The highly homologous protein, Filamin B (*FLNB*), may help compensate for the loss of *FLNA* function and allow for proper neuronal migration of some neurons (Sheen et al. 2002).

As a result of genetic heterogeneity, abnormalities of a given gene can result in a wide spectrum of different phenotypes. Conversely, a single phenotype may be caused by different genes. An important issue for the clinician to

Consider Consultation When...

Endocrinology

- Consider an endocrinology consultation for patients with holoprosencephaly, septo-optic dysplasia, or other abnormalities of prosencephalic development. Consultation with an endocrinologist is essential if hypoglycemia, diabetes insipidus, growth hormone deficiency, or other signs of hypothalamic-pituitary dysfunction are present.
- Also consider an endocrine consultation for patients with catamenial epilepsy who are refractory to traditional antiepileptic agents.

Ophthalmology

- Patients with septo-optic dysplasia or other abnormalities of prosencephalic development are at risk of optic nerve atrophy. Patients with severe cortical malformations, such as lissencephaly, are more likely to have cortical visual impairment. Walker-Warburg, muscle-eye-brain, and Fukuyama congenital muscular dystrophy patients may exhibit myopia, strabismus, congenital glaucoma, retinal folds, and retinal and optic nerve hypoplasia.

Orthopedics

- Axial hypotonia with spasticity of the extremities is common in many cortical malformations such as lissencephaly. Such patients often require bracing, botulinum toxin, or surgery to reduce spasticity and contractures. In disorders with accompanying muscle disease, such as Fukuyama congenital muscular dystrophy, severe hypotonia, and weakness place patients at risk of developing scoliosis.

Cardiology

- For patients with Miller-Dieker syndrome, consideration should be given to performing an echocardiogram, since congenital heart disease can associated with the disorder.
- Cardiac rhabdomyomas may be found in children with tuberous sclerosis. They are generally clinically insignificant and usually regress over time, but they may cause mechanical obstruction, heart failure, or arrhythmias.

Pulmonary/Gastroenterology

- Patients with severe motor impairment from their cortical malformations are at risk of developing aspiration pneumonia. A swallow study should be considered if coughing or gagging develop with feeds. G-tube placement and cessation of oral feeds may be required in patients with aspiration.

Genetics

- Family planning is one of the most important social issues related to brain malformations. Consultation with a geneticist and genetics counselor is strongly advised, particularly for parents who are considering having more children.

recognize is that the initial description of genetic conditions is biased toward more severe phenotypes. Over time, as more patients are evaluated for a given genetic condition, the known phenotypes broaden to include more subtle cases.

Conclusion

For children with disorders of nervous system development few specific therapeutic interventions are available beyond physical, occupational, and speech therapy and remedial education. Epilepsy resulting from brain malformations is often refractory to pharmacotherapy but surgical resection of epileptogenic cortical malformations may be an option for some of these children. A crucial role for the treating physician is to provide counseling and guidance. This is particularly important in newly diagnosed children whose parents are burdened by uncertainty. A thoughtful, compassionate approach to the radiographic and genetic assessment can offer the parents insight to their child's condition, even given the limitations in predicting outcome. The genetic evaluation is particularly important for purposes of family planning.

Annotated bibliography

Barkovich AJ, Kuzniecky RI, Dobyns WB, et al. A classification scheme for malformations of cortical development. *Neuropediatrics* 1996;27:59–63.

Barkovich AJ, Kuzniecky RI, Jackson GD, et al. Classification system for malformations of cortical development. *Neurology* 2001;57:2168–2178.

In these papers, Barkovich et al. identify a classification scheme for disorders of cortical development, arranging them based on the earliest embryologic stage in which the malformation has its origin. The more recent paper serves as an update to the original.

Taylor DC, Falconer MA, Bruton CJ, Corsellis JAN. Focal dysplasia of the cerebral cortex in epilepsy. *J Neurol Neurosurg Psych* 1971;34:369–387.

Taylor describes the neuropathology of focal cortical dysplasia. This description includes features such as giant dysmorphic neurons and balloon cells. Focal cortical dysplasia with these features is now referred to as Taylor-type dysplasia.

Tassi L, Colombo N, Garbelli R, et al. Focal cortical dysplasia: Neuropathological subtypes, EEG, neuroimaging and surgical outcome. *Brain* 2002;125:1719–1732.

In this paper, three subtypes of focal cortical dysplasia, along with their clinical and radiographic correlates, are described. Patients with Taylor-type cortical dysplasia have readily identifiable lesions on imaging and the best surgical outcome postoperatively, with 75% being seizure-free after 1 year of follow-up. This study highlights the relationship of pathology to the clinical phenotype.

Barkovich AJ, Kjos BO. Nonlissencephalic cortical dysplasias: Correlation of imaging findings with clinical deficits. *AJNR* 1992a;13:104–106.

Barkovich AJ, Kjos BO. Schizencephaly: Correlation of clinical findings with MR characteristics. *AJNR* 1992b;13:104–106.

Both of these papers highlight the clinical–radiographic correlation of brain malformations. The first focuses on cortical dysplasias and the second on schizencephaly. In both cases, the anatomy of the lesion, as identified based on neuroimaging, is shown to correlate with the clinical outcome.

Cardoso C, Leventer RJ, Ward HL et al. Refinement of a 400-kb critical region allows genotypic differentiation between isolated lissencephaly, Miller–Dieker syndrome, and other phenotypes secondary to deletions of 17p13.3. *Am J Hum Genet* 2003;72:918–30.

Toda T, Kobayashi K, Kondo-Iida E, et al. The Fukuyama congenital muscular dystrophy story. *Neuromusc Dis* 2000;10: 153–159.

Both of these papers demonstrate genotype–phenotype correlations. The first demonstrates how deletions of contiguous genes in the 17p13.3 locus can result in varied clinical phenotypes, ranging from isolated lissencephaly to the Miller-Dieker syndrome. In the second, Fukuyama congenital muscular dystrophy patients homozygous for the founder mutation of fukutin are demonstrated to have a milder phenotype of the disorder than those with a spontaneous point mutation on the second allele.

CHAPTER 21

Disorders of Motor Execution I: Cerebral Palsy

Barry S. Russman

Outline

In a series of lectures entitled "Deformities of the Human Frame," in 1843, William Little is given the credit for first defining cerebral palsy (CP) as a motor deficit resulting from damage to the brain during infancy and, more specifically, secondary to a preterm birth or to perinatal asphyxia. He also noted that associated problems could occur in children with CP, including behavior problems and epilepsy. In 1889 Osler wrote a paper entitled "The Cerebral Palsies of Children." He was the first to develop a classification system based on the anatomic findings of the physical examination, describing infantile hemiplegia, bilateral hemiplegia and spastic paraplegia. Freud, in 1893, emphasized that the etiology was more related to prenatal or postnatal causes and not necessarily secondary to "birth trauma." From 1900 to 1950, the CP literature emphasized the treatment of CP, including physical therapy, bracing, and surgical intervention (Weiss & Betts 1967).

The American Academy of CP (to become the American Academy of CP and Developmental Medicine, AACPDM) was formally organized in 1946. Following the compilation of the answers to a questionnaire, the Academy adopted the definition of CP as any "symptom complex" arising from a nonprogressive brain lesion(s), leading to a motor impairment (Minear 1956).

In 1964, Bax was the senior author of a paper that emphasized as part of the definition that the nonprogressive lesion had to occur in the immature brain (Bax 1964). The definition of immature was not further defined. Mutch was the senior author of another consensus document defining CP as "an umbrella term" for a group of nonprogressive but often changing motor impairment syndromes secondary to a lesion or anomaly of the brain that occurred in the early stages of development (Mutch et al. 1992). That the motor impairment, and specifically the muscle tone, could change in spite of the fact that the lesion to the central nervous system (CNS) remained the same became part of the definition of CP for the first time.

A consensus conference held in 2005 to review the definition and classification of CP resulted in the publication of a supplement to the journal *Developmental Medicine and Child Neurology* (Rosenbaum et al. 2007). Currently defined, CP is a group of permanent disorders of (a) movement and posture, (b) causing activity limitation, (c) which are attributed to nonprogressive disturbances that occur in the developing fetal or infant brain. (d) The motor disorders of CP are often accompanied by disturbances of sensation, perception, cognition, communication, behavior difficulties, and epilepsy. (e) Secondary musculoskeletal problems may develop.

Classification

The classification system is a clinical one based on the physiology of the motor dysfunction, the number of limbs involved, and the functional status of the child. The sys-

Key Clinical Questions

- The diagnosis of CP is established by:
  - The finding of an abnormal MRI scan of the brain
  - A history of hypoxic ischemic encephalopathy in the neonatal period
  - A history of a motor deficit that is not worsening and examination indicating that an abnormality of the brain is responsible for the motor deficit.
  - The presence of spasticity or dystonia on examination
  - All the above

A history of a motor deficit that is not worsening and examination indicating that an abnormality of the brain is responsible for the motor deficit.

- The evaluation of a child who has been diagnosed with CP and whose cause is not obvious from the past history such as IVH, encephalitis, and meningitis should consist of:
  - Magnetic resonance imaging (MRI)
  - Coagulation evaluation if the child has hemiplegia
  - Metabolic testing including urine for organic acids
  - Electroencephalogram (EEG)
  - All of the above

An MRI is the best diagnostic tool in determining the presence of CP.

- The use of botulinum toxin A medication is indicated for those children who have:
  - Spasticity
  - Dystonia
  - Hemiballismus
  - All of the above
  - None of the above

Botulinum toxin A is indicated for those children with any of the listed disorders.

- Surgical intervention in children with CP should take place when:
  - As soon as fixed contractures develop
  - Only when the child reaches adolescence
  - Only when the contractures cause a dysfunction
  - Preferably after the age of six
  - None of the above

Surgical interventions should be delayed until after the child is 6 years of age.

- Which of the problems occur in children with CP as frequently as able-bodied children?
  - Strabismus
  - Seizures
  - Urinary tract infections
  - Severe learning deficits

Urinary tract infections have an equal incidence of occurrence in both children with CP and able-bodied children.

Pearls and Perils

Classification

- The original classification system for cerebral palsy (CP) is a descriptive one, based on anatomy and physiology of the impairment. This system affords a shorthand way of communicating the patient's deficits. It does not afford a prognosis or a treatment program.
- A recently validated system classifies patients by gross and fine motor *functions*. This affords a shorthand way of communicating the patient's functional deficits. A correlation exists between the function class and associated problems.

tem establishes an orderly approach to describing a patient's disability but does not afford insight into the etiology or pathology.

Physiologic (Motor) Grouping

Table 21.1 summarizes the physiologic and anatomic groupings. *Spasticity* is defined as velocity-dependent increased muscle tone, determined by passively flexing and extending muscle groups across a joint (Lance 1980). A satisfactory, reproducible system of grading muscle tone has never been developed, although the Ashworth and Tardieu scales are commonly used in research (Boyd & Graham 1999). Most physicians describe the tone as being normal, increased, or decreased. Associated with spasticity are enhanced deep tendon reflexes, usually associated with clonus and extensor plantar responses. However, the latter are sometimes difficult to elicit in the infant and even in the older child with spastic CP.

Dyskinesia is defined as abnormal motor movements that become obvious when the patient initiates a movement. When the patient is totally relaxed, usually in the supine position, a full range of motion and decreased muscle tone may be found. Dyskinetic patients are subdivided into two subgroups. The hyperkinetic or *choreoa-*

Table 21.1 Classification of cerebral palsy by physiology and anatomy

Physiology	Anatomy
Spasticity	Diplegia
Dyskinesia	Hemiplegia
Choreoathetosis	
Dystonia	
Ataxia	Quadriplegia
Mixed	Double hemiplegia

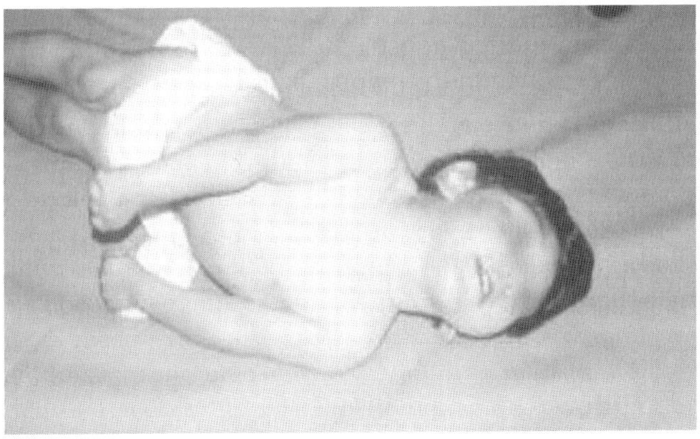

Figure 21.1 This patient's arms and legs are extended and some twisting of the upper extremities is quite noticeable; an excellent example of dystonia.

thetoid children show purposeless, often massive involuntary movements with motor overflow; that is, the initiation of a movement of one extremity leads to movement of other muscle groups. The *dystonic* group manifest abnormal shifts of general muscle tone induced by movement. Typically, these children assume and retain abnormal and distorted postures in a stereotyped pattern (Figure 21.1). Both types of dyskinesia may occur in the same patient. Simply stated, spasticity you feel; dystonia you see (Sanger et al. 2003).

Patients with ataxias have a disturbance of the coordination of voluntary movements due to muscle dyssynergia. These patients may be *hypotonic* during the first 2 or 3 years of life. They commonly walk with a wide-based gait and have a mild intention tremor (dysmetria). A rare subgroup in the ataxia category is called the *disequilibrium syndrome* (Sanner & Hagberg 1974). These patients not only have dysmetria but also have a pronounced difficulty in maintaining posture and equilibrium. They tend to be hypotonic for the first several years of life, prior to the development of useful function. Mental retardation is almost invariable in this group. Until further studies are published, patients placed in this category should be considered to have a genetic disease.

The fourth category that is commonly used in the physiologic classification is the *mixed group*. Patients in this category commonly have mild spasticity, dystonia, and/or athetoid movements. Ataxia may also be a component of the motoric dysfunction in patients placed in this group.

Anatomic Grouping

Diplegia refers to involvement predominantly of the legs. *Quadriplegia* refers to dysfunction of all four extremities; in some children one upper extremity might be less involved and the term *triplegia* then would be substituted. *Hemiplegia* refers to individuals with unilateral motor dysfunction; and in most children, the upper extremity is more severely involved than the lower. Finally, an unusual situation may occur where the upper extremities are much more involved than the lower; the term *double hemiplegia* is applied to this group of patients.

Functional Classification

A functional classification for gross motor skills, now in general use, was first described in 1997 (Palisano et al. 1997) (Table 21.2A–C). The following is a brief synopsis of the Gross Motor Functional Classification System (GMFCS) scale. Level 1 refers to a child who is basically clumsy but otherwise has full mobility. The child in level 2 walks without assistive devices but has limitations walking outdoors and in the community. The level 3 patient walks with assisted mobility devices and does have some limitations in walking outdoors. Level 4 children have self-mobility that is severely limited even with the use of assistive technology. Level 5 children have no self-mobility even with assistive technology. Subsequent studies have found that this classification system also correlates with some CP-associated problems (Beckung & Hagberg 2000). For example, the level 4 and 5 children have a significantly increased incidence of cognitive disabilities and epilepsy.

Classifying children who use several types of assistive devices and wheelchairs can be difficult using the GMFCS alone. The Functional Mobility Scale (FMS) addresses some of these issues by classifying the level of support required in the home, school, and community settings (Graham et al. 2004). The Manuel Ability Classification system (MACS) was recently developed (Eliasson et al. 2006). It is similar to the GMFCS; namely, it is based on 5 levels of function: A level 1 refers to a child who can handle objects easily and successfully; level 5 refers to a patient who does not handle objects and has severely limited ability to perform even simple actions. Functional scales for oromotor deficits have not been developed.

Epidemiology

All definitions of CP contain three common criteria: (a) a disorder of movement or posture, (b) which occurs as a result of a static abnormality of the brain, and (c) is acquired early in life. Several problems with this definition make epidemiologic studies problematic. The severity of the movement abnormality is not further defined (Blair & Watson 2006). For example, should children with a coordination motor disorder (developmental dyspraxia) be considered under the rubric of CP? Also, the words "immature brain" have not been further defined. What happens if the abnormality or the injury to the brain occurs at age 3? Should children with a motor abnormality

Table 21.2A Gross motor functional classification system (GMFCS)

- Level 1: Clumsy child; no assistive devices
- Level 2: Walks independently but limited in outdoor activities
- Level 3: Walks with assistive mobility devices
- Level 4: Self-mobility severely limited even with assistive devices
- Level 5: No self-mobility even with assistive devices

From Palisano R, Rosenbaum P, Walter S, et al. Development and reliability of a system to classify gross motor function in children with cerebral palsy. *Dev Med Child Neurol* 1997;39:214–223.

Table 21.2B Functional mobility system

- Uses wheelchair, stroller, or buggy: May stand for transfers and may do some stepping supported by another person or using a walker/frame
- Uses K-Walker or other walking frame: Without help from another person
- Uses two crutches: Without help from another person
- Uses one crutch or two sticks: Without help from another person
- Independent on level surfaces: Does not use walking aids or need help from another person. If uses furniture, walls, fences, shop fronts for support, please use 4 as the appropriate description
- Independent on all surfaces: Does not use any walking aids or need any help from another person when walking, running, climbing, and climbing stairs.

From Graham HK, Harvey A, Rodda J, et al. The Functional Mobility Scale (FMS). *J Pediatr Orthoped* 2004;24(5):514–520.

Table 21.2C Manual ability classification system

- Handles objects easily and successfully
- Handles most objects, but with a reduces quality and/or speed of achievement
- Handles objects with difficulty and needs help to prepare and/or modify activities
- Handles a limited selection of easily managed objects in adapted situations
- Does not handle objects

From Eliasson AC, Krumlinde-Sundholm L, Rosblad B, et al. The Manual Ability Classification System (MACS) for children with cerebral palsy: Scale development and evidence of validity and reliability. [see comment.] *Dev Med Child Neurol* 2006;48(7):549–554.

secondary to a problem occurring at age 3 (for example, a stroke) be considered in the epidemiology of CP? Should a child who dies at age 4 months and who has not yet shown the signs of CP but in fact has a brain lesion (such as periventricular leukomalacia [PVL], which is associated with CP) be included in the incidence of CP? In addition to these issues, the causes of CP in the developing

Pearls and Perils

Epidemiology

- CP as an outcome of difficult labor has not been clearly established.
- Most children who had low birth weight, breech presentation, or clinical depression at birth were perfectly normal 7 years later.
- Risk factors or causation are established in only 50% of patients with CP.
- A diagnosis of CP is based on history and physical examination, not on the presence or absence of risk factors. The lack of a history of prematurity or "birth trauma" neither precludes nor implies the diagnosis of CP.

countries are much different from the causes in developed countries. Taking these issues into consideration, Blair and Watson argue that it is "more informative to estimate trends and frequency by the major risk factors, namely gestational duration, plurality and uterine infections and, for service implications, by severity of impairments" (Blair & Watson 2006).

Recognizing these issues, the epidemiology data most quoted is as follows. The worldwide incidence of CP is approximately 2–2.5 per 1,000 live births (Hagberg et al. 2001). Each year, about 10,000 babies born in the United States develop CP (Boyle et al. 1996). The ninth report from the western Swedish study of the prevalence and origin of cerebral palsy was published in 2005 (Himmelmann et al. 2005). Of 88,371 live births, 170 children were diagnosed with CP (i.e., a prevalence of 1.92 per 1,000 live births; Table 21.3). The clinical types of CP are presented in Table 21.3C, and the origin of CP is noted in Table 21.3D. Hemiplegia was the most predominant form of CP, presumably due to the decline in preterm diplegia. Further, an increase in full-term dyskinetic cerebral palsy was noted. The origin of cerebral palsy in children born at term was considered to be prenatal in 38%, perinatal in 35%, and unclassifiable in 27%, whereas in children born preterm it was 17%, 49%, and 33%, respectively.

Pathogenesis

The diagnosis of CP is established by a history and physical examination (Table 21.4). An attempt to establish an etiology is necessary for many reasons including genetic counseling and for concluding that "birth trauma" was not the cause (Fisher & Russman 1974; Hughes & Newton 1992). However, most of the time, only risk factors can be identified. Although several risk factors for the de-

Table 21.3A Epidemiology of cerebral palsy

Weight	Number	Percent
<1,000 g	86	35.5
1,000–1,555 g	60	24.8
1,501–2,500 g	6	2.4
Hemiplegic		33
Diplegic		44
Quadriplegic		12
Ataxic		4

From Hagberg B, Hagberg G, Beckung E, Uvebrant P. Changing panorama of cerebral palsy in Sweden. VIII. Prevalence and origin in the birth year period 1991–94. *Acta Paediatr* 2001;90(3):271–277.

Table 21.3B Birth prevalence of cerebral palsy among babies of different gestational ages

Gestational age (weeks)	Prevalence/ 1,000 live births	Birthweight	Prevalence/ 1,000 live births
< 28	76.6	<1,000	82
28–31	40.4	1,000–1,499	54
32–36	6.7	1,500–2,500	6.7
>36	1.11	>2,500	1.2

From Himmelmann K, Hagberg G, Beckung E, et al. The changing panorama of cerebral palsy in Sweden. IX. Prevalence and origin in the birth-year period 1995–1998. *Acta Paediatrica* 2005;94(3):287–294.

Table 21.3C Clinical types of cerebral palsy

Type of cerebral palsy	Percent
Spastic hemiplegia	38
Spastic diplegia	35
Spastic quadriplegia	6
Dyskinetic	15
Ataxic	6

Table 21.3D Origin of cerebral palsy by gestational age

	Preterm	Term
Prenatal	17	38
Perinatal	49	35
Unclassifiable	33	27

Table 21.4 Cerebral palsy etiologic groups

- Obvious prenatal
  - Simple inheritance
  - Defined prenatal syndromes
  - Unequivocal prenatal syndromes
  - Cerebral malformations
- Potential prenatal or prenatal
  - Presence of one or more risk factors
- Obvious postnatal
- Unknown: None of the above

velopment of CP have been clearly identified, the majority of children born with known risk factors will *not* develop CP.

Neuroimaging not only can establish the lesion responsible for the motor dysfunction of CP but also can determine when the abnormality occurred during the pregnancy. The finding of a congenital malformation by MRI is usually indicative of an injury during the first half of the pregnancy (Barkovich et al. 2001). Primary white matter damage, such as PVL or periventricular hemorrhagic infarction (PVH), represents residual from insults operating between 24 and 34 gestational weeks (Back 2001). When found in a neonate born at term, PVL should be considered as having occurred in utero. When the brain reaches a maturity close to term, gray matter is more sensitive to injury than white matter. Focal cortical damage, most often in the territory of the middle cerebral artery is, on the other hand, thought to be related to hereditary or acquired thrombophilias and environmental factors (Nelson & Lynch 2004; Truwit et al. 1992). Unfortunately, a "stroke" in utero that might be associated with a known genetic finding in the mother, such as the presence of a factor Leyden abnormality, cannot necessarily be prevented and does not suggest that future pregnancies might be at risk for in utero strokes. Further, the finding of a stroke in a newborn does not imply the need for anticoagulation (Nelson & Lynch 2004).

Risk Factors Correlated with Prenatal and Perinatal Events

A univariate analysis of risks associated with the future development of CP identified separate *maternal*, *pregnancy*, *labor*, and *delivery* characteristics (Table 21.5) (Nelson & Ellenberg 1985). *Maternal* factors, such as level of maternal education, marital status, parity, paternal age, pregnancy spacing, smoking history, and intercourse frequency were not associated with an increased risk of the child developing CP. Unexpectedly, a history of maternal diabetes and the length of time to become pregnant also were *not* predictive of future CP. On the other

Table 21.5 Cerebral palsy risk factors

Prenatal

- Two or more previous abortions
- Maternal mental retardation
- Bleeding during pregnancy in births at term
- Preeclamptic signs
- Small-for-gestational-age baby
- Placental infection
- Multiple births
- Maternal hypothyroidism

Perinatal

- Asphyxia producing clinical encephalopathy
- Cerebral hemorrhage
- Placental ablation
- Hypoxia
- Hyperbilirubinemia
- Central nervous system infection

hand, maternal mental retardation, epilepsy, and hypothyroidism prior to the pregnancy were significantly associated with the development of CP in the child.

Pregnancy problems, which were identified as relative risk factors associated with future CP, included severe toxemia and incompetent cervix, when associated with premature birth. Third-trimester bleeding, but not first- or second-trimester bleeding was also a significant factor. Kidney and bladder infections, radiation exposure, and hyperemesis gravidarum were not associated with increased risk. Finally, a high prevalence of CP in twins compared to singletons has been noted (Grether et al. 1992). Risk factors identified during the *labor* and *delivery* periods include vaginal bleeding at the time of admission, and placental complications such as abruptio, premature rupture of the membranes, chorionitis, and breech presentation. However, many of these risk factors were significant only if a baby weighed less than 2,500 g at birth. In addition, some of the risk factors, such as oxytocin augmentation, cord prolapse, or breech delivery, were relevant only if they were associated with low Apgar scores.

Finally, children born after in vitro fertilization (IVF) have an increased risk of CP, primarily because of preterm delivery and increased possibility of twin pregnancy (Hvidtjorn et al. 2006).

Risk Factors Associated with Type of Cerebral Palsy

The Swedish studies also correlated the anatomic and physiologic findings with prenatal and perinatal risk factors. Children with spastic diplegia were almost universally appropriate for gestational age; 55% were born preterm. Furthermore, there was a lower proportion of prenatal risk factors among this group of infants. The diplegic children born at term had a much more complex situation, having both prenatal and perinatal risk factors in a much higher frequency. These included toxemia, placental infarction, and evidence of intrauterine asphyxia, including meconium staining.

The dyskinetic syndromes are most likely to occur with perinatal risk factors, such as asphyxia and hyperbilirubinemia. Of these patients, 37%, in addition to having perinatal risk factors, also had prenatal risk factors present such as fetal deprivation (Brun & Kyllerman 1979; Kyllerman et al. 1982; Kyllerman 1982). Rosenbloom has suggested that a pattern of perinatal events in term babies may lead to dyskinetic CP, a pattern that differs from that leading to spastic quadriplegia (Rosenbloom 1994). Based on an analysis of 17 patients with dyskinetic CP, 10 experienced severe fetal distress occurring late in labor; the birth asphyxia was severe but short-lived and the hypoxic–ischemic encephalopathy was only mild or moderate.

Diagnosis

The diagnosis of CP is established by a history that the child is "delayed" in motor development, is not losing skills, and the examination suggests that an abnormality of the brain is responsible (increased deep tendon reflexes, ankle clonus, etc.). The child who is not developing normally and who has normal or decreased muscle tone presents a common diagnostic problem. Persistent primitive reflexes or the lack of development of the protective reflexes at the expected time are important findings on the neurologic examination, suggesting corticospinal tract impairment (O'Shea et al. 1992). Moro reflex should be un-

Pearls and Perils

Diagnosis

- Handedness should not develop before 18–24 months of age; look for dysfunction on the less-used side.
- Poor head control, present at 3 months of age, should make one suspicious of CP. The presence of risk factors should heighten the diagnostic concern.
- The most common diagnosis for the floppy baby is CP. It is not uncommon for a floppy baby to develop a dyskinesia by or even after age 2 years.
- CP does not mean mental retardation. It is important to highlight this issue when discussing the diagnosis with the parents.

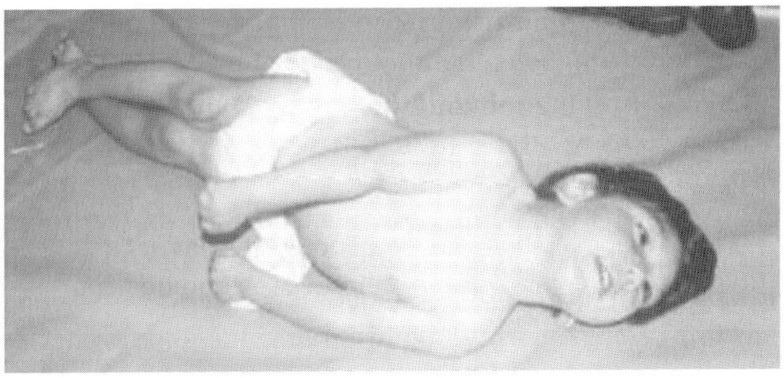

Figure 21.2 With a movement of any body part (e.g. neck movement) twisting and repetitive movements or abnormal postures or positions are noted.

obtainable after 6 months of age (Figure 21.2). The asymmetric tonic neck response should never be obligatory when the patient is placed in the appropriate position; that is, the infant should "break" the tonic neck posture spontaneously after 15–30 seconds, and it should be unobtainable after 6 months of age (Figure 21.3). The side protective reflexes should be evident after 5 months of age, and the parachute reflex is typically obtained after 10 months of age (Figures 21.4 and 21.5). Another important observation is the finding of hand preference. A child should not cross the midline when reaching for an object until after 1 year of age and should not show clear hand preference on examination until 18–24 months of age. The development of handedness prior to this time suggests a hemiplegia (Figure 21.6) or a brachial plexus injury.

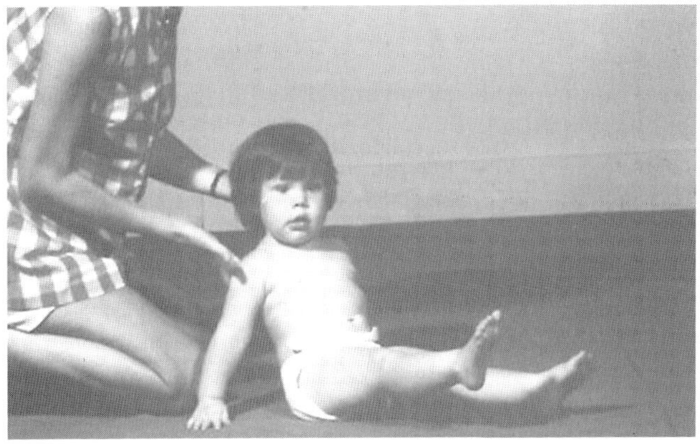

Figure 21.4 The side prop is a protective reflex that develops prior to when the child is able to sit independently when placed. Place the child in the sitting position and gently push from one side; the opposite arm should extend.

Evaluation of the patient with cerebral palsy

Role of Imaging

Once the diagnosis is established (which may require two visits a few months apart), it is necessary to establish an etiology. The evaluation of the child with CP should start with an imaging study (Ashwal 2004), assuming that an obvious brain lesion had not been established during the neonatal period (Ment et al. 2002). Magnetic resonance imaging (MRI) is the preferred study; 75% of children

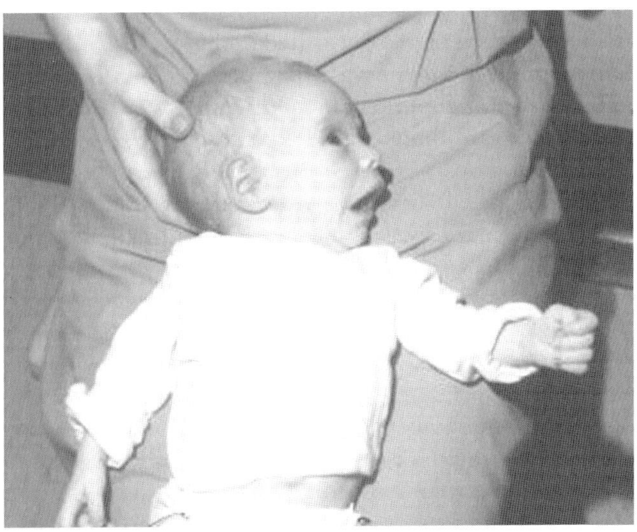

Figure 21.3 The tonic neck reflex, asymmetric tonic neck reflex or 'fencing posture': When the child's head is turned to the side, the arm on that side will straighten and the opposite arm will bend (sometimes the motion will be very subtle or slight).

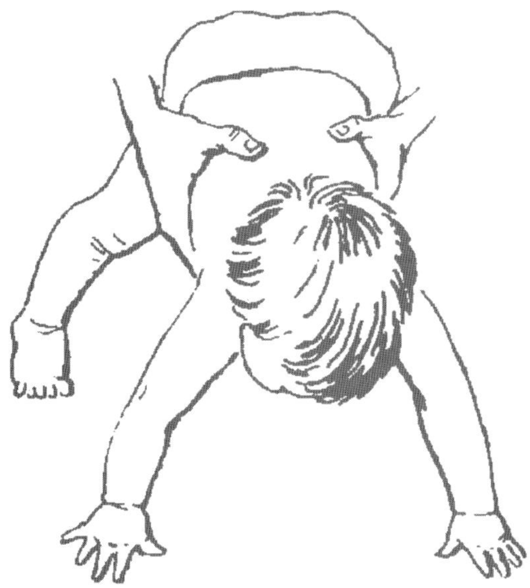

Figure 21.5 The parachute reflex is also a protective reflex and should develop prior to walking. Holding the child at the waist, gently drop the head towards the examining table; the arms should extend, 'breaking the fall.'

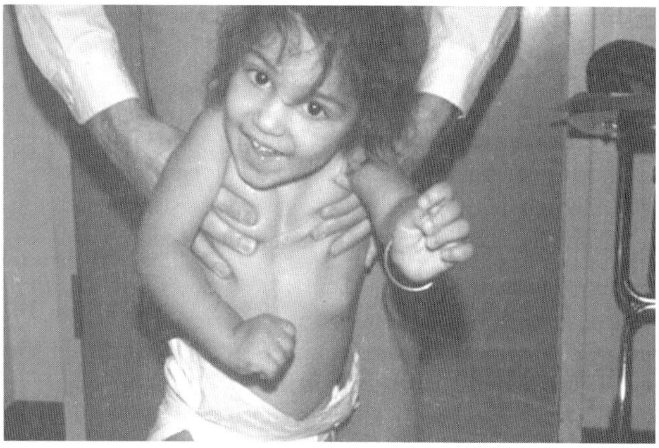

Figure 21.6 When reaching for an object, the hand should not twist; further the child should not develop hand preference prior to 18–24 months.

with CP have an abnormal computed tomography (CT) scan (Table 21.6); more than 85% of MRIs are abnormal (range 68–100%) (Table 21.7). The abnormal findings may afford insight into the etiology, such as PVL found on the MRI. However, many of the findings such as cortical atrophy do not imply an etiology. The timing of the insult can be determined in many children. For example, some of the more common etiologies of *prenatal onset* include congenital malformations, intrauterine infection, and stroke. *Perinatal onset* includes hypoxic ischemic encephalopathy and trauma. *Postnatal onset* includes infection, stroke, and trauma. Occasionally, a scan may detect conditions that are surgically treatable that might not be detected by neurologic examination. One retrospective study reported that 22.5% of 120 patients had potentially treatable lesions (hydrocephalus, arteriovenous malformation, subdural hematomas and hygromas, and a vermian tumor) (Kolawole et al. 1989). Rarely will a CT (as well as MRI) detect an abnormality that will suggest a potentially treatable inborn error of metabolism.

Table 21.6 Computed tomography (CT) in children with cerebral palsy (CP)

Reference	Ages (yrs)	Type of CP	% Abn
Wiklund et al. 1991	5–16	H	73
Wiklund et al. 1991	5–16	H	75
Miller & Cala 1989	6–35	A	62
Chen 1981	0.08–7	M	84
Kolawale et al. 1989	1–>10	M	73
Taudorf & Melchior 1984	NA	M	67
Schouman-Claeys et al. 1989	0.6–15	M	63
Cohen & Duffner 1981	0.67–>10	H	87
Molteni et al. 1987	5–16	H	93

Overall yield of finding an abnormal CT scan in children with CP.
M, mixed; H, hemiplegic; A, ataxic.

Table 21.7 Magnetic resonance imaging (MRI) in children with cerebral palsy

Reference	Ages (yrs)	Type of CP	% Abn
Krageloh-Mann et al. 1995	5–17	SQ	91
Yin et al. 2000	0.25–18	M	91
Candy et al. 1993	0.25–2.25	M	77
Okumara 1997 (pt. 2)	1–19	M	78
Cioni et al. 1999	1–18.3	M	100
Jaw et al. 1998	0.33–13	M	95
Sugimoto et al. 1995	0.75–15	M	100
Hayakawa et al. 1996	0.5–6	SD	79
Truwit et al. 1992	0.08–41	M	93
Yamada et al. 1993	NA	M	100
Yokochi et al. 1991a,b	NA	D	68

Mean % abnormal MRI 89%

Metabolic Testing

Metabolic disorders may, on rare occasions, masquerade as CP. Six case series describe 30 children who ultimately developed what appeared to be dyskinetic CP due to glutaric aciduria type 1 (Baric et al. 1998; Hartley et al. 2001; Hauser & Peters 1998; Haworth et al. 1991; Kyllerman et al. 1994; Smith et al. 2001). These children typically develop normally until 5–10 months of age, when they suffer an acute encephalopathy manifested by coma that is followed by dystonia, motor impairment, and macrocephaly (in about 60%). Distinctive MRI and CT findings occur in half the patients and are manifested by frontal and temporal atrophy. Early diagnosis is important, as glutaric aciduria is treatable; early intervention may prevent significant motor and cognitive impairment. Other metabolic disorders presenting with symptoms suggestive of CP also have been reported in small case series and include Lesch-Nyhan syndrome (Mitchell & McInnes 1984), 3-methylglutaconic aciduria (Gibson et al. 1997; Pantaleoni et al. 2000; Straussberg et al. 1998), pyruvate dehydrogenase deficiency (Lissens et al. 1999), argininemia (Prasad et al. 1997; Willis et al. 2000) deficiency, succinic semialdehyde dehydrogenase deficiency (Gibson et al. 1997), and female carriers of ornithine transcarbamylase deficiency (Christodoulou et al. 1993). Other childhood neurologic disorders (e.g., dopa-responsive dystonia, hereditary spastic paraplegia, ataxia telangiectasia) may initially be misdiagnosed as CP because of the slow rate of symptom progression (Swaiman 1999). Clinical or laboratory features of such conditions, and observations that the neurologic symptoms are progressive should suggest that the child does not have CP and mandates the need for further evaluation.

Coagulopathy Testing

Patients with hemiplegic CP frequently have suffered a prenatal or perinatal cerebral infarction. Children, in contrast to adults, often have a coagulopathy, congenital heart disease, or an infectious process as the etiology of stroke (Lynch et al. 2001). Several studies have reported coagulation abnormalities as the etiology of neonatal cerebral infarction (Nelson & Lynch 2004a). These have included factor V Leiden deficiency, the presence of anticardiolipin or antiphospholipid antibodies, and protein C or S deficiency. The studies have also described the relation between neonatal cerebral infarction, coagulopathies, and a later diagnosis of hemiplegic CP. There is no evidence that babies with an in utero stroke benefit from anticoagulation. Further, no data answers the question of whether, if a coagulopathy is identified as possibly being causally related to the motor disability, future siblings will be at risk.

Pearls and Perils

Associated problems

- Hemiplegic patients with CP commonly have a smaller hand and somewhat smaller foot compared with the normal side. This is not the result of disuse but rather the result of the lack of a trophic factor.
- Such hands not only will be small but also will have sensory loss. One can unequivocally state that the hand will be a helping hand and but not good at skilled acts.
- Therapists may be unrealistically enthusiastic about making this hand "normal" with an aggressive program.
- Hemiplegic patients may have homonymous hemianopsia. Identification of this problem is important so that one can give advice regarding appropriate classroom seating.

Associated problems

Problems commonly associated with a diagnosis of CP are listed in Table 21.8.

Epilepsy

Approximately 43% (range 35–62%) of children with CP develop epilepsy (Table 21.9). One prospective study compared patients with CP and epilepsy to those with epilepsy alone. Children with CP had a higher incidence of epilepsy with onset within the first year of age (47% versus 10%), history of neonatal seizures (19% versus 3%), status epilepticus (16% versus 1.7%), need for polytherapy (25% versus 3%), and treatment with second-line antiepileptic drugs (31% versus 6.7%). They also had a lower incidence of generalized seizures (28% versus 59%) and of remaining seizure free (37% versus 90%) (Kwong et al. 1998). Factors associated with a seizure-free period of 1 year or more in epileptic children with CP include normal intelligence, single seizure type, monotherapy, and spastic diplegia. Similar findings have been observed by other investigators in the studies listed in Table 21.8 and are summarized in the review by Wallace (Wallace 2001). Children with CP who have abnormal neuroimaging studies are more likely to have epilepsy. Data from the studies listed in Table 21.8 indicate that children with spastic quadriplegia (50–94%) or hemiplegia (30%) have a higher incidence of epilepsy than patients with diplegia or ataxic CP (16–27%) (Cohen & Duffner 1981). In patients with dyskinetic CP, it may occasionally be difficult to differentiate partial complex seizures from dyskinetic movements. Even though a higher incidence of epilepsy occurs in CP, an electroencephalogram (EEG) is not recommended as part of the routine evaluation of a child with this diagnosis (Ashwal et al. 2004).

Mental retardation

In general, there is some, but no absolute relation between the type of CP and severity of cognitive impairment. Chil-

Table 21.8 Associated conditions in children with cerebral palsy

Reference	% Mental retardation	%Visual defects	Speech-language disorders	% Hearing impaired
Zafeiriou et al. 1999	40	39	54	15
Murphy et al. 1993	65	10	NA	4
von Wendt et al. 1985	70	19	NA	7
Kolawale et al. 1989	66	15	59	14
Total	52	28	38	12

NA, not available

Table 21.9 Prevalence of epilepsy in children with cerebral palsy

References	Types of CP	% Patients with epilepsy
Murphy et al. 1993	M	46
von Wendt et al. 1985	M	48
Miller & Cala 1989	A	59
Zafeiriou et al. 1999	M	36
Hadjipanayis 1997	M	42
Al-Sulaiman et al. 2001	M	54
Chambers et al. 1999	M	36
Bruck et al. 2001	M	62
Cioni et al. 1999	M	35
Kwong et al. 1998	M	38
Kaushik et al. 1997	M	56
Taudorf & Melchior1984	M	35
Cohen & Duffner 1981	H	58
Total		43

NA, not available; M, mixed; H, hemiplegic, A, ataxic; SQ, spastic quadriplegia.

dren with spastic quadriplegia, as opposed to dyskinetic quadriplegia, have greater degrees of mental impairment than children with spastic hemiplegia (Fennell & Dikel 2001). Further, motor deficits of children with spastic CP appear to correlate with the severity of cognitive deficits in contrast to those children with dyskinetic CP, in whom this relation is lacking. Laterality of hemiplegia may also be a contributing factor; those children with right hemiplegia may be more likely to have impaired language function due to left hemisphere injury (Aram & Eisele 1994), although this remains controversial (Trauner et al. 1996). A strong association also exists between greater intellectual impairment in children with CP and the presence of epilepsy, an abnormal EEG, or an abnormal neuroimaging study (Wallace 2001).

Ophthalmologic impairments

Visual impairments and disorders of ocular motility are common (28%) in children with CP (Table 21.8). There is an increased presence of strabismus, amblyopia, nystagmus, optic atrophy, and refractive errors (American Academy of Pediatrics Committee on Practice and Ambulatory Medicine 1996; Schenk-Rootlieb et al. 1992). Children whose CP is due to PVL are also more likely to have visual perceptual problems. Children with these MRI findings should not only be screened for visual problems, but also for visual perceptual deficits.

Speech and language disorders

Because of bilateral corticobulbar dysfunction in many CP syndromes, anarthric or dysarthric speech and other impairments related to oral-motor dysfunction are common. Because their impaired mobility can cause limited interaction with individuals in the environment, children with CP might not be able to develop the linguistic skills necessary to develop more complex speech patterns (Uvebrant & Carlsson 1994). Language (as opposed to speech) deficits in CP go hand in hand with verbal intellectual limitations associated with mental retardation (Falkman et al. 2002). Oral-motor problems including feeding difficulties (Reilly et al. 1996; Sullivan et al. 2000), swallowing dysfunction (Clarke & Hoops 1980), and drooling (Blasco & Allaire 1992) may lead to potential serious impacts on nutrition and growth (Stallings et al. 1993), oral health (Pope & Curzon 1991), respiration (Shaw 1996), and self-esteem.

Hearing impairment

Hearing impairment occurs in approximately 12% of children with CP (Table 21.8). This occurs more commonly if the etiology of CP is related to very low birth weight, kernicterus, neonatal meningitis, or severe hypoxic–ischemic insults. Children with CP who have mental retardation or abnormal neuroimaging studies are at greater risk for hearing impairment. Of concern are recent studies from the Center for Disease Control that almost half the children found to have severe congenital hearing loss (with or without CP) in the greater Atlanta area were not recognized until almost 3 years of age (Van Naarden et al. 1999). Established guidelines for neonatal audiometric screening have been published (American Academy Pediatrics 2000).

Common health problems

There are few data regarding the occurrence of common health problems in children with CP. For example, the frequency of pneumonia, urinary tract infections, and otitis media is unknown. On the other hand, three health problems have been studied in detail, namely drooling, nutrition, and incontinence.

Drooling

The significance of drooling should not be underestimated and should be openly discussed with the parents as part of the routine care of children with CP. This problem may be responsible for severe skin irritations, but of greater significance is its unpleasant cosmetic effect (Dunn et al. 1987; Rapp 1980; Sochaniwskyj et al. 1986). Many studies have shown that drooling is secondary to swallowing difficulties rather than to hypersalivation (Senner et al. 2004). The treatment of this problem is difficult (Blasco 2002). Medication has been helpful but the side effects are significant. Surgical intervention, including reposition of the salivary ducts and dividing the cordi-tympani has sometimes been effective. Finally, botulinum toxin therapy has been helpful (Suskind & Tilton 2002; Van der Burg et al. 2006).

Nutrition

Poor nutrition is associated with significant health problems in children with CP (Patrick et al. 1986; Shapiro et al. 1986; Waterman et al. 1992). Oromotor deficits, in about one-third of cases, are responsible for the problem. Medical treatment has been modest at best (Rogers 2004). The use of gastrostomy, on the other hand, has led to significant improvement in height and weight. The outcome of such intervention can potentially cause problems if the child becomes overweight. There is no evidence that improving nutrition status will improve the child's function (Calis et al. 2007).

Bladder dysfunction

Bladder dysfunction, but not urinary tact infections, is a third health problem. In a review of 50 patients with CP (both children and adults) referred to a urologic service, 28% complained of enuresis, 26% complained of stress incontinence, 18% complained of urgency, and 6% noted dribbling (McNeal et al. 1983). More than 36% of the patients had more than one symptom. Pathologic urodynamic dysfunction is more common in the nonambulatory patient with CP (Bross et al. 2007). Bladder and bowel control occurs at a later age compared to matched siblings (Ozturk et al. 2006). Are the bladder difficulties related to lack of sphincter control? Are the problems more prevalent in patients who are retarded? Is it a more frequent problem for children whose primary deficit is spasticity or dyskinesia? Future studies are also needed in this area. For the present, clinical awareness and surveillance should lead to recognition of problems of practical importance to the patient and family.

Other health conditions

Constipation

Constipation is a problem that must be monitored by the physician. Presumably, this problem occurs as a result of the patient's inability to control the abdominal muscles that provide the propulsion for the stool. Symptomatic treatment must be provided.

Secondary sexual characteristics

A survey of 207 patients with CP has shown that those patients who are barely or nonambulatory (GMCS 3, 4, or 5) begin puberty earlier but end later when compared to the able-bodied population (Worley et al. 2002). In addition, menarche occurs later in girls with CP.

Pain

Painful hips in children with CP is a very common phenomenon (Hodgkinson et al. 2001). Only since the early 2000s has generalized pain in children with CP been appreciated and studied. It is difficult to assess pain in children with CP, as many of the patients have limited or no communication skills and some of the patients are cognitively challenged (Nolan et al. 2000). Scales that can be used to determine the presence or absence of pain, both by the patient and by the caretaker, have been developed (Hadden & von Baeyer 2002). Using a questionnaire that was found to be valid and reliable, two-thirds of the parents felt that their children experienced pain for at least several days during the month prior to the completion of the questionnaire. Unfortunately, there is no data as to how to manage pain in children with CP who are nonverbal. Whether the pain is secondary to spasms, positional discomfort, or other causes is still unknown.

Treatment

General treatment principles

Prior to discussing specific treatment programs, some general principles should be stated:

Pearls and Perils

Treatment

- None of the various occupational or physical therapy programs has ever been validated or clearly shown to be more efficacious than other comparable programs. Empirically, they seem to be extremely helpful, and clearly provide emotional benefit for patients and families.
- Early-intervention programs to enhance motor and cognitive development in the physically handicapped population have not been shown to be beneficial, as opposed to early-intervention programs for the environmentally deprived population (for example, Head Start). On the other hand, the need to foster compensatory abilities early on and to provide emotional support must be considered when one is developing a program.
- The goals of any specific treatment program must be carefully outlined. Orthopedic intervention is not necessarily intended to change function dramatically. Rather, the goal of a specific procedure might be limited to better positioning.

1. Long-term treatment objectives must be defined to the extent possible, taking into consideration not only the patient's motor deficits, but also the associated problems including cognitive abilities, social skills, emotional status, vocational potential, and, most important, the availability of family support.
2. The effects of the patient's growth and development on his problem, with and without the proposed treatment, should be evaluated (for example, change in muscle tone, development of contractures).
3. Valid alternatives, which look at risk–benefit ratios and humane/ethical dilemmas, and which might include nontreatment, should be considered.

Because the manifestations of CP vary from patient to patient, treatment programs must be individualized. A team of knowledgeable individuals with different expertise best accomplishes the treatment of a child with CP. A typical team includes a physician trained in the evaluation and treatment of developmentally disabled children. The diagnosis must be established, progressive disease must be considered and excluded, and, if possible, specific genetic syndromes identified. A knowledgeable orthopedist is another physician member of the team. Contracture, subluxed or dislocated hips, and scoliosis are deformities that can interfere with function and comfort. Nonphysician members of the team usually include a physical therapist, occupational therapist, orthotist, speech/language pathologist, and a clinical nurse specialist. Many programs have found that a psychologist, social worker, and educator can play vital roles.

Treatment principles for the infancy and toddler ages

The diagnosis of CP in most patients is established during the first 2 years of life. At that time, the patient should become involved in a physical or occupational therapy program or both. A variety of therapy programs are available, none of which have proved to be more efficacious than others. The complexity of motor relationships, the inconsistent correlation of pathology with function, the lack of correlation of therapy with functional outcomes, and the lack of a careful analysis of the natural course of disease are explanations for this situation (Goldberg 1991). The first therapeutic programs developed included passive range of motion exercises (to prevent contracture) and bracing (to prevent the abnormal muscles from interfering with normal muscle function) (Weiss & Betts 1967). In the late 1950s and early 1960s, the Bobaths developed a program now known as neurodevelopmental treatment (NDT), which was aimed at inhibiting the primitive reflexes and facilitating normal movement by active patient participation (Bobath 1967). Variations of this form of therapy have been advocated during the past 15 years, although attempts to validate any one treatment program have been unsuccessful (Palmer et al. 1988; Palmer et al. 1990). Early intervention programs that provide not only specific "hands-on" therapy but also psychological support are thought to be beneficial, although there is no evidence that they enhance the child's development (Binder & Eng 1989; Palmer et al. 1990). Even this concept has been questioned in a study of parent satisfaction with an infant stimulation program for CP.

The psychological impact of rearing a disabled child can be devastating. This subject has been the focus of several studies. A study addressing the issue of psychological stress in mothers whose children are disabled concluded that the specific diagnosis did not cause as much stress as expected among mothers; however, the dependency of the disabled child on the mother for help in accomplishing activities of daily living was significantly correlated with maternal stress (Breslau et al. 1982). Recent studies have corroborated these early findings (Raina et al. 2005). This study found that the intactness of the immediate family is more helpful than the extended family including neighbors. Further, behavior of the child with CP and the extent of the physical demands (level 5 patients compared to level 1 patients) was significantly correlated with both the physical and emotional health of the primary caregiver, who was usually the mother. There is no specific data regarding the siblings.

Treatment principles for the school age and adolescence age groups

As the child with CP approaches school age, the goals of the therapy programs begin to shift from enhancing motor development and minimizing contracture toward helping the child cope with the expectations of the classroom. Sitting properly and moving about the environment (including the use of a wheelchair) are gross motor needs that may require physical therapy (Nwaobi et al. 1983). Use of the small muscles for fine motor function such as writing, cutting, and other activities may need to be enhanced. Most important is a therapy program to help the child communicate, either with speech or communication devices. Dressing, feeding, toileting, and other activities of daily living (ADLs) are important needs that should be incorporated into the educational/"treatment" program. The occupational therapist is usually the person to work with the patient toward these ends.

Treatment Options

Motor deficits can be analyzed in four distinct ways:

Pearls and Perils

- Evaluation of the patient after a diagnosis has been made based on History and Physical examination:
  - Obtain magnetic resonance imaging (MRI), rather than a computed tomography (CT) scan when the etiology is not obvious.
  - Metabolic and genetic testing is not indicated unless atypical features are present, such as dysmorphic findings on physical examination or the history suggests intermittent changes such as dyskinetic movements.
  - Consider testing for a coagulopathy if the child has a hemiplegia. However, it is very unclear if the presence of positive findings will alter the management of the patient or change the advice about the risk for future children.

1. *Loss of selective motor control and dependence on primitive reflex patterns for ambulation.* A remedy does not exist that can significantly alter selective motor loss, such as lack of control of lower extremity muscles. Physical and occupational therapy programs can provide help. The primary goals of a physical therapy program are to minimize the impairment, reduce the disability, and optimize function. Various schools of therapy promote programs that superficially vary greatly, but nevertheless have certain principles in common, including development of sequence learning, normalization of tone, training of normal movement patterns, inhibition of abnormal patterns, and prevention of deformity.
2. *Abnormal muscle tone that is strongly influenced by body posture and/or position and/or movement.*
   - *Oral medications.* The use of oral medication for the management of abnormal tone has been disappointing. For spasticity, dantrolene, baclofen, diazepam, and tizanidine have been used. Medications for the dyskinesias, including dystonia, athetosis, and hemiballismus, have been equally disappointing (Pranzatelli 1996).
   - *Botulinum toxin.* Botulinum toxin A therapy (Botox) is approved by the U.S. Food and Drug Administration (FDA) for strabismus, hemifacial spasm, cervical dystonia, severe primary axillary hyperhydrosis, and for cosmesis. Extensive literature shows that Botox is effective for children and adults who have spasticity and/or dystonia. A combination of muscle weakening and strengthening of the agonist muscle minimizes or prevents contracture development with bone growth. This type of intervention is used when a limited number of muscles are causing deformities, such as spasticity of the gastrocnemius muscle causing a toe-heel gait or hamstring spasticity being responsible for a crouch gait. Recovery of the muscle tone occurs because of the sprouting of the nerve terminals, a process which peaks at approximately 60 days (Cosgrove et al. 1994). Botox use in the upper extremity spasticity has been shown to improve cosmesis and function (Fehlings et al. 2000; Yang et al. 2003). Although the evidence is not conclusive, nevertheless this procedure is commonly performed and, in this author's experience, has been very effective.
   - *Selective dorsal rhizotomy.* Selective dorsal rhizotomy (SDR) involves the cutting of approximately 50% of the dorsal roots, thereby decreasing the muscle tone in the lower extremities (Abbott 1996). As a result of the decrease in the muscle tone, discomfort or pain will be alleviated, and sitting posture and/or gait will improve. The ideal candidate is a child who has normal or near normal strength in the lower extremities, who has not developed fixed contractures, and whose alteration of tone will lead to the desired improvements in function. Combining the data from three separate studies that compared physical therapy with SDR plus physical therapy revealed a direct relationship between percentage of dorsal root tissue transected and functional improvement. The combination of SDR and physical therapy is efficacious in reducing spasticity in children with spastic diplegia and has a small positive effect on gross motor function (McLaughlin et al. 2002).
   - *Intrathecal baclofen infusion.* Baclofen, a γ-aminobutyric acid (GABA) agonist, administered intrathecally via an implanted pump (intrathecal baclofen; ITB) has been helpful to patients whose muscle tone is more generalized and whose muscle tone is interfering with function (Albright 1996). As baclofen dose not cross the blood–brain barrier very effectively, large oral doses must be used to achieve success, compared

to administering baclofen intrathecally. Invariably, the patient on oral medication becomes lethargic. Candidates for this intervention can be divided into two groups. Group 1 is the patient whose gait is adversely affected by muscle tone and who have some underlying muscle weakness. Selective dorsal rhizotomy is contraindicated in these patients, as the procedure will cause additional muscle weakness, possibly causing an ambulatory patient to become nonambulatory. A second group of patients are those whose generalized tone interferes with activities such as hygiene, transferring from a chair to a bed, or simply maintaining a safe upright position. Although the complication rate, including infection and baclofen withdrawal symptoms, occurring as a result of catheter breakage or leakage is about 50%, parent satisfaction is extremely high with this type of intervention. Once the complication is corrected, over 90% of the parents/caretakers/patients request that the pump be reimplanted or the catheter replaced (Albright & Ferson 2006; Gooch et al. 2004).

- *Other treatment modalities.* Transcutaneous electrical stimulation as advocated by Pape and colleagues consists of a low-level electric stimulus to the nonspastic antagonist muscles for prolonged periods of time, while the patient is sleeping (Pape et al. 1993). The theory is that this treatment will strengthen the stimulated muscles, which in turn will overcome the effect of the spastic muscles, thereby improving the patient's function. Research is lacking to support the theoretical basis of this treatment. Most of the information about the success of this type of intervention is anecdotal.

3. *Imbalance between muscle agonists and antagonists.* Static contracture of muscle related to spasticity is a common problem for which surgical lengthening of the musculotendinous unit is frequently performed. Fixed muscle contractures are almost never seen in patients with pure dyskinesias. When they do occur, surgical intervention is considered, but with extreme caution. Rang and associates and Bleck have both argued cogently that the overall result is much better if all contracted muscles are lengthened simultaneously rather than staging the procedures (Bleck 1987; Rang 1986). Not only does accomplishing all surgery during the course of a single procedure lessen morbidity, but by simultaneously balancing all major lower extremity joints, much better function is possible. In many centers for CP, gait analysis is felt to be necessary for objective pre- and postoperative evaluations (Gage 1994). Gait analysis is a method by which the walking pattern of an individual is examined in detail. It is based on the gait cycle, which is the basic unit of walking.
4. *Impaired body balance mechanisms.* The child with CP invariably has some degree of balance abnormalities. In spastic diplegia, posterior balance is affected most severely. A child with only disturbances in posterior equilibrium is usually able to walk without the use of external aids. If anterior balance is also affected, crutches are necessary for ambulation. Children with deficiencies in lateral equilibrium usually require a walker or, if the lateral equilibrium reactions are severely deficient, may be unable to walk independently. The deficiencies in equilibrium are related to an irreparable neurologic lesion and are lifelong.

Prevention

Can CP be prevented? With the advent of immunizations, early recognition of hyperbilirubinemia, folic acid supplementation, avoidance of toxins like mercury, and the addition of iodine to the diet, the incidence of CP has decreased—at least in developing countries. On the other hand, the prevalence of CP in developed countries has basically remained stable over the last 50 years (Nelson 2003).

Perinatal stroke in the fetus is usually associated with childhood hemiplegic CP. Infants vulnerable to this problem include those with an inherited or acquired thrombophilia, placental thrombosis, infection, or the use of intravenous catheters; these same risk factors apply to the mothers of these infants. Despite the recognition of these risk factors, preventative measures have not been effective (Lanska & Kryscio 2000; Ros et al. 2002). Intrauterine exposure to infection, such as chorioamnionitis, has also been associated with CP. Randomized control studies have not shown that CP associated with this problem can be prevented. Multiple pregnancies have been associated with CP for reasons that are not well established (Grether et al. 1998). Finally, IVF has been associated with twin pregnancies, increased risk of CP, and fetal loss (Hvidtjorn et al. 2006).

Except for prematurity, birth asphyxia is the most common risk factor for the development of CP. Electronic fetal monitoring has not led to a decrease in the prevalence of CP. Further, the number of caesarian sections based on electronic monitoring has increased; the false-positive rate has been shown to be approximately 99.8% (Nelson et al. 1996). As concluded by Nelson, despite the risk factors and the assumption that early delivery might prevent CP, there is little evidence at present to suggest that CP can be prevented.

In a review of intraventricular hemorrhage and the use of phenobarbital to prevent this phenomenon, Kuban and colleagues noted that the incidence of CP in those mothers who were toxemic and had received magnesium sulfate was less than a comparable group (Kuban et al. 1992). Nelson found that only 7.1% of mothers receiving magnesium sulfate gave birth to babies who developed CP, as opposed to 30 % who did not receive magnesium sulfate (Nelson & Grether 1995). However, the hypothesized association with the use of magnesium sulfate in mothers who have preeclampsia and a decrease in instances of CP has not been borne out by randomized controlled trials (Crowther et al. 2003; Doyle et al. 2007).

Prognosis

When the diagnosis of CP is first established in a nonambulatory child, the first question asked is "Will my child walk?" Criteria for predicting independent walking have been developed (Bleck 1975). If, by the age of 1 year the patient still has persistent primitive reflexes and the protective reflexes have not developed, it is unlikely that the child will ever ambulate independently. Further, if the child has severe dyskinesias, or falls into the dysequilibrium category, ambulation will not be achieved. In addition to the Bleck criteria, the GMFCS at 2 years of age is predictive (Wood & Rosenbaum 2000). A retrospective review of more than 5,000 study subjects, of which 2,300 were evaluated at age 6, found that only 10% of children not yet walking at age 2 were able to walk independently by age 7; an additional 17% of this cohort could walk with some support, such as a walker. The authors concluded that the most useful factors for predicting future ambulation were motor milestones at age 2 (Wu et al. 2004). Those children who were not rolling by age 2 years demonstrated the lowest probability of achieving ambulation of more than 20 feet; incidentally, they also had the highest mortality rate. Finally, even though CP is a result of a nonprogressive central nervous system lesion, the child who is a marginal ambulator, upon entering the early teens, may lose walking ability because of contractures, excess weight gain, or lack of motivation.

As the child matures, changes in muscle tone and function may occur, which might raise concerns about the diagnosis. For example, the hypotonic infant and toddler commonly develops spasticity or athetoid movement. Not only may the muscle tone change, but the disability may lessen or disappear entirely. An analysis of the data from the National Collaborative Perinatal Project (completed in 1973) showed that 118 of 229 children diagnosed as having mild CP at age 1 showed no motor disability at age 7. However, as a group, they had a higher incidence of learning difficulties and afebrile seizures compared to the general population. Obviously, even the child who improves over time is at risk for CP-associated problems (Nelson & Ellenberg 1982).

Pearls and Perils

Prognosis

- On reaching the early teens, marginally ambulatory children may stop walking because of contractures, excessive weight gain, or lack of motivation. This does not necessarily mean that the patient has a progressive disease.
- Quadriplegic patients with epilepsy at best are mildly cognitively impaired.
- Muscle tone in some patients will change over the years. Hypotonic patients may eventually become ataxic or might develop dyskinesias. Hypotonic boys should always have a uric acid test to rule out Lesch-Nyhan disease.
- Some children with the diagnosis of cerebral palsy (CP) at age 1 year will not have significant motor disabilities at age 7 years. However, such children have a higher incidence of learning disabilities.
- Communication is much more important than ambulation or even having self-help skills.
- Do not think that all patients with CP who cannot speak are retarded. This specifically applies to the patient with choreoathetosis.
- A change for the worse in muscle tone or functional status does not necessarily mean that the patient has a progressive disease.

To answer concerns about the life expectancy of patients with CP, an analysis of a cohort of individuals with CP born between 1940 and 1950 concluded that of individuals who survive until age 20 years, almost 85% would survive until age 50, versus a comparable estimate for the general population of 96% (Hemming et al. 2006). Even of those who died, very few of the deaths could be directly attributed to CP. Life expectancy in severe CP has also been studied (Hutton & Pharoah 2006). The combination of cognitive impairment with an IQ of less than 50, inability to ever walk, inability to feed or dress, severe vision disability, and hearing disability are associated with early mortality.

Because CP is commonly associated with mental retardation, parents also express concerns about the child's cognitive development. Data from the analyses of large series help address this issue. The quadriplegic patient who has epilepsy almost certainly will be, at best, educable mentally retarded. Of patients with dysequilibrium syndrome, 90% are also retarded. CT and MRI studies also offer prognostic insights into cognitive development. Lesion size, degree of motor disability, and EEG abnormalities in one study was found to correlate with cognitive impairment. However, location of the lesion was not predictive (Cohen & Duffner 1981).

In most patients, a prognosis about intellectual development must be deferred pending the development of language, because this skill is correlated with intellectual development. Therefore, in questionable situations, a prognosis cannot and should not be rendered until after age 2 years. Furthermore, in the athetoid patient who might have a severe dysarthria, a prognosis about intelligence should be postponed until school age. An examiner experienced with the severely disabled, dyskinetic population should perform the evaluation, as the patient may be a poor examinee because of the motor disability and the scores might thus be misleading.

Finally, the examiner must be able to discuss issues of lifestyle with the parents. Communication is the most important skill required by a human being. Without this ability, even with a normal intellect, the child will have difficulty making his wants known, thus limiting his ability to participate in family activities, peer activities, and other social interactions. However, technical advances being made now and expected in the future allow a more positive outlook for even the most severely disabled patient with CP.

Prognosis about vocation

Earlier studies regarding the vocational status of individuals with CP indicated that employability is related to cognitive skills, self-care, independency, severity of the physical disability, educational level attained, and mobility in the community. Ninety-seven students with CP in the San Francisco, California area, between the ages of 7 and 16, were evaluated in the 1960s and 1970s, and predictions were made as to their future employability. In 1983, 60 of the 76 individuals over age 18 years were contacted (O'Grady et al. 1985). At the time of the survey, only 17 were employed, although 39 had been employed at some time. Employment was related to the severity of the disability and the cognitive skills of the patient. A positive correlation was found between employment and mildness of CP; that is, an individual with normal or near normal intelligence and minimal physical disability was more likely to be employed. Further, unemployment was correlated with those individuals who had severe physical disabilities and/or were retarded. An accurate prediction for patients with CP who were in the middle range of intelligence, severity of handicap, and self-help abilities was unreliable. For those individuals who did better than predicted, family support and personal determination were felt to be paramount in their ability to attain their specific status. Further, the development of technology helped at least one individual who was predicted to be unemployable, but was working as an office computer assistant. Other positive factors identified in the present investigation as being important to vocational status were an integrated education and a community-based assessment program.

An analysis from the Danish CP registry compared the employability of patients with CP born between 1965 and 1978 with a controlled cohort (Michelsen et al. 2005). They reviewed the educational and employment prospects of such individuals. Thirty-three percent of the individuals with CP compared to 77% of the controlled population had an education beyond the lower secondary school. Twenty-nine percent were competitively employed versus 82% of the controls. The hemiplegic CP patients had the highest rate of employment, as one would anticipate. One has to conclude from this recent study, as well as those in the past, that employability is not related solely to the individual's disability, but rather to other factors including family support, educational programs, technology, and community-based programs.

Conclusion

Cerebral palsy is a term used to describe a patient who has a nonprogressive brain lesion leading to a motoric deficit. A degenerative disease is suspected if the patient loses function that cannot be explained by a change in muscle tone, contracture development, or a change in body size. Associated problems including seizures, mental retardation, language disorder, speech deficits, and strabismus must be evaluated and treated appropriately. There are many causes of CP, including genetic diseases and embryologic abnormalities. Most often, a specific cause cannot be identified. However, risk factors can be identified in about 30% of cases. Risk factors alert the clinician to anticipate the presence of CP in a patient; they should be considered separate from causation.

Cerebral palsy is an acceptable term as long as it is used appropriately and as long as the issues associated with this term are carefully explained to parents. Cerebral palsy

Consider Consultation When...

- The diagnosis of cerebral palsy (CP) is in question.
- The child has the hypotonic form of CP.
- The etiology of the child's motor deficit is unclear.
- The patient is losing motor skills.
- There is a family history of similar problems.

ranges in severity from minimal limitations, requiring no treatment, to total care and intensive treatment. The public commonly associates those who require "total care" with the term "cerebral palsy." Consequently, the diagnosis must be carefully articulated to the parents, emphasizing the various degrees of impairment. If one anticipates a treatment program including physical therapy and potential orthopedic intervention, the term is appropriate and should be used.

Annotated bibliography

Abbott R. Sensory rhizotomy for the treatment of childhood spasticity. [review]. *J Child Neurol* 1996;11(Suppl 1):S36–S42.

Albright AL. Intrathecal baclofen in cerebral palsy movement disorders. [review]. *J Child Neurol* 1996;11(Suppl 1):S29–S35.

Ashwal S, Russman BS, et al. Practice parameter: Diagnostic assessment of the child with cerebral palsy. *Neurology* 2004;62:851–863.

A committee of child neurologists and developmental pediatricians produced this article. The recommendations for diagnostic evaluation of the child with CP are based on a review of the evidence from articles published in peer-reviewed journals.

Nelson KB, Ellenberg JH. Children who "outgrew" cerebral palsy. *Pediatrics* 1982;69:529–536.

This article is still the classic. Children diagnosed as having CP may improve from the age 1 to age 7, so that the child's motor skills are not a major problem and rehabilitation programs for the motor disability are unnecessary.

Russman BS, Tilton A, Gormley ME, Jr. Cerebral palsy: A rational approach to a treatment protocol, and the role of botulinum toxin in treatment. [review]. *Muscle Nerve Suppl* 1997;6:S181–S193.

These three articles provide information about the current use of tone management protocols for the child with CP whose abnormal muscle tone is interfering with function or quality of life.

CHAPTER 22

Disorders of Motor Execution II: Higher-order Motor Deficits

Ruthmary K. Deuel and Amy C. Rauchway

Outline

- Clumsiness
- Dyspraxia
- Material-specific dyspraxias

Higher-order motor deficits are those motor performance abnormalities that are not caused by paralysis or spasticity. This chapter describes different higher-order motor disorders that manifest through clumsiness and/or inadequate performance of sequential motor acts. Children's motor development and performance may be severely handicapped by such deficits. Thus, for the child's sake, these disorders must be recognized. Such deficits were first found and described in adults with acquired brain damage (Liepmann 1900). They were not recognized in children until the 1920s (Orton 1925), most likely due to the fact that no obvious alteration in strength, tone, coordination, or sensation accompany them (DeRenzi et al. 1968, 1980; Geschwind & Damasio 1985; Liepmann 1900, 1908; Vaivre-Douret 2007). In children, higher-order motor execution deficits are defined as "failure to learn or perform voluntary motor acts with an age-appropriate efficiency, despite adequate strength, sensation, attention and volition" (David et al. 1981).

The true incidence of such higher-order motor deficits (a term currently used to cover all of them is *developmental coordination disorder* [DCD], ICD-9-CM 315.4) is not known, but estimates range from 2% to 12% of first graders in regular schools (Dewey & Wilson 2002; Gubbay 1975; Iloeje 1987; McHale & Cermak 1992; Nichols 1987). Thus, disorders of cerebral function that result only in clumsiness and dyspraxia, without paralysis or spasticity, are common and probably similar in incidence to specific learning disorders with which they are often associated (Deuel 1992; Johnston et al. 1981; Nichols 1987). This general definition may be made much more specific in relation to the three major types of higher-order motor deficit: clumsiness, motor dyspraxia, and material-specific dyspraxia.

Even well-evaluated movement assessment batteries for children (Croce 2001) may not be constructed to distinguish among the different types of higher-order motor deficits. Although literature firmly supports a high incidence of disorders of higher-order motor execution among groups of children with cognitive and attention disorders (Denckla & Rudel 1978; Pyfer & Castelman 1972), there is no support for the view that disorders of motor execution are inevitably linked to them in individual children (Deuel & Doar 1992; Deuel & Robinson 1987; Nichols 1987).

When attention and cognitive disorders are found in conjunction with higher-order motor deficits, it is fitting for the physician to consider whether the motor deficits are actually primary (leading to the major therapeutic effort being directed toward the motor deficits), whether the two are "comorbidities" (leading to major treatment efforts for both), or whether the neuropsychiatric disorder is primary, as in Asperger's syndrome (Green et al. 2002; Myers et al. 2007; Schmitz et al. 2003), again leading to appropriate treatment emphasis. Detecting higher-order execution deficits may be difficult for the physician, as the chief complaint most often suggests a cognitive or attention disorder. When evaluating the presenting illness there may be no mention made of motor difficulties. Nonetheless, a careful developmental history reveals very delayed or even unfulfilled milestones for certain specific gross and/or fine motor acts throughout preschool years. A history of chronic fine motor delays reassures that the problem is *not* acquired.

A basic neurologic examination will not show clumsiness, apraxia, and material-specific dyspraxia. Items

Key Clinical Questions

- *A 7-year-old girl with known Trisomy 21 is brought by her mother, who believes the girl has been misplaced in a class for the severe–moderately retarded. On history, fine motor skills were markedly delayed, while gross motor and language skills were more modestly delayed. On examination, she is attentive and talkative; has mild hypotonia, excellent strength, no adventitious movements, and very slow finger tapping; and after rapidly orally spelling it for you, labors slowly to print the four letters of her first name. What further testing would you request to substantiate your diagnosis of clumsiness? What remedial modalities will you recommend?*
  A Wisc-III IQ test showed Verbal IQ of 78 and Performance IQ of 51. Occupational therapists provided adaptive equipment and training in self-help skills, thus enabling the child to maintain her self-esteem and make good progress in a program for the mildly retarded.
- *A 12-year-old sixth-grade star soccer goalie was seen after he was barred from sports because of failing grades in history, English, and social studies. He commented that he missed his older sister, his longtime "homework monitor," who had just started college in a distant city. His entire past medical history (except onset of speech at about 2 years) was normal, as was his physical and neurologic examination and his drawing, but not writing sample (see Figure 22.1). What specific disorder of motor execution can you designate? What further diagnostic evaluation would you do? What remedial measures would you recommend?*
  This child should be given quantitative specific tests of cognition that do not involve written language, as well as standard individual academic achievement tests, and the TOWL (see text). Management may include bypass methodology, such as teaching him to take cryptic class notes, word processing (with spell-check) written assignments, and some tutoring. He should be allowed to return to his soccer team as soon as these remedial measures are in place.
- *An 8-year-old third-grader comes because "She's stopped paying attention to what she is doing." Past medical and developmental history is normal, but in the past few weeks her mother has noted uncharacteristically slow motor activities. She appears very eager to please, and on neurologic examination has mild hypotonia and a slow, ataxic tandem gait with dysmetria and a marked end-excursion tremor of the dominant right hand. What are your differential diagnostic thoughts? What specific test would you request?*
  Since you have found unequivocal signs of right cerebellar dysfunction in a child whose personality is prompting her futile efforts to halt them, a high-resolution magnetic resonance imaging (MRI) with attention to the posterior fossa is first in order. All three common forms of cerebellar tumor are suspect.

deliberately aimed at detecting higher-order deficits must be used. They are most apparent during naturalistic action (Buxbaum et al. 1995), and are best termed "dynamic signs," since they appear during motion. To examine for them, one should employ age-appropriate sequences of motions performed under the examiner's surveillance. These will establish on an objective basis whether a higher-order motor deficit is present (Table 22.1) in the school-age and adolescent child. When motor deficits appear to be of recent onset or progressive, they may be proclaiming significant medication side effects, collagen vascular disorders, or other potentially treatable and/or progressive diseases, such as metachromatic leukodystrophy, subacute sclerosing panencephalitis (Jabbour 1969; Percy et al. 1977), or Rett syndrome (Hagberg et al. 1983). In addition, cerebellar lesions may lead to motor execution deficits. Sydenham chorea, dystonia musculorum deformans, and kinesigenic dystonia are among entities that may need to be considered in the differential diagnostic process.

Although DCD has had a reputation for independence from progressive pathology, recent increases in sensitivity of available measures have altered this rule. Investigation of etiology by magnetic resonance imaging (MRI) and other pertinent tests is warranted at any juncture when a therapist, physician, parent, or teacher notes worsening of motor performance. In general, recent literature supports judicious use of sensitive neuroimaging and electroencephalographic (EEG) investigations in children with motor execution deficits (Menkes 2006).

Once the issue of etiology is settled, the major reason to define and treat higher-order motor deficits is their propensity to cause severe long-term educational and social handicaps (Gubbay 1975, 1985; Knuckey & Gubbay

Table 22.1 Neurologic evaluation

- Gross motor milestones: Walked independently (10–15 months), climbed stairs by self (14–24 months), rode big wheel or trike (2–3 years), rode bicycle (4–6 years)
- Fine motor milestones: Held cup (10–14 months), drew (3–4 years), buttons and snaps (3–4 years), prints name (4–6 years), ties shoes (4–6 years)
- Direct examination
- Gaits: Walking, running, skipping, tandem, hopping on one foot, climbing stairs
- Upper extremity: Finger-tapping, wrist-turning, button-pressing, finger-nose-finger, copying, drawing, writing
- Dyspraxia: Imitation of nonsense gestures, pantomime to command, use of actual objects
- Tests with age-standardized normative values: Purdue Peg Board, Kaufman ABC hand movements, Spatial memory PANESS (Larson, 2007)

1983; Segal et al. 2002; Vaivre-Douret 2007). This happens through various intermediary mechanisms, starting with the effects on self-esteem of being always behind peers in motor performance.

When a higher-order deficit is found and is chronically handicapping, long-term remedial management is in order. Individually tailored management can be very helpful in restoring self-esteem and functional ability. Even in children with cerebral palsy and other disorders of primary motility who, as often happens, suffer additionally from higher-order motor dysfunction (Crothers & Paine 1959; Frei 1986), analyzing all motor deficits with the goal of determining the specific handicapping potential of each deficit for that individual child is recommended. This is particularly true for children with primary neuropsychiatric disorders such as Asperger's syndrome and autistic spectrum disorders (Green et al. 2002; Myers et al. 2007; Schmitz et al. 2003).

Developmental coordination disorder may be considered an umbrella term. As such, it has the deficit of leaving the therapist, parent, or teacher to discover on their own the individual child's specific treatment needs. The separate headings—clumsiness, dyspraxia, and material-specific dyspraxia—allow treatment to be optimally directed from the outset, although even within these fairly specific categories, individuation must be maintained.

Clumsiness

A child with clumsiness suffers from slowness and imprecision in completion of very simple (single-phase) acts, such as flexing a finger or rotating the wrist and forearm. In the past, this developmental motor disability has been considered together with the pure dyspraxias (Ford 1960; Gubbay 1975; Iloeje 1987) but is separable from it on empirical grounds (David et al. 1981; Deuel 1992; Poeck 1986).

The main point of differentiating clumsiness from pure dyspraxia is that speed and dexterity are affected in clumsiness (Table 22.2). The deficits observed in the purely clumsy child fulfill the criteria of Liepmann's (1908) limb-kinetic apraxia or Kleist's (1934) melokinetic apraxia. These authors described a decrement in dexterity and speed of movements without strength or tone changes in adult stroke victims. The purely clumsy child similarly exhibits slow and inaccurate fine and/or gross motor performance in the face of an otherwise normal neurologic examination.

Fortunately, items such as finger tapping and wrist supination and pronation are part of the standard examination, so direct recognition of clumsiness is more likely than recognition of pure motor dyspraxia (described in the next section). Even so, if direct resistive strength of finger muscles is not also tested, the slowness may be misinterpreted as weakness.

Table 22.2 Clumsiness

Discriminating features

- Slow completion of single-phase movements of single joints, in the absence of weakness, spasticity, or spontaneous adventitious movements

Consistent features

- Finger or foot tapping, or both, too slow for age
- Outcome of movement sequences improved when there are no time constraints

Variable features

- Association with dyspraxia
- Association with adventitious movements
- May affect facial, pedal, or axial motion separately

Pearls and Perils

Clumsiness

- Slow, fine finger movements due to clumsiness are sometimes mistaken for distal weakness.
- A direct test of flexor and extensor finger strength will determine the correct designation.
- Clumsiness is a primary cause of school failure in the early grades, preventing adequate academic achievement because mechanical demands are heavy and intellectual ones are light. Clumsiness is very conducive to low self-esteem, starting very early in development. This early secondary low self-esteem mediates depression, continued failure, and thus failure in areas that have no motor requirements whatsoever.
- Some clumsy individuals can improve their performance with guidance from a specific modality of sensory input. For example, the musically gifted clumsy child may be a superb performer on the flute even though she cannot tie her shoes. It is important to evaluate a range of motor performances.
- Clumsiness is not a soft sign of cognitive or attention disorders, although it is statistically associated with both (Denckla & Rudel 1978; Dewey et al. 2002; Nichols 1987). In fact some believe that it is one of several possible causes of attention-deficit/hyperactivity disorder (ADHD).
- Often a simple explanation to parents and teachers of the mechanical difficulties at the root of the child's slow and labored performances will change these authorities' attitudes and demands to a great extent, allowing a marked increase in the child's self-esteem and improved performance through improved motivation.

A quantifiable assessment of fine motor skills, the Physical and Neurological Assessment of Subtle Signs (PANESS) instrument has been normed by age and gender. The method of administration and normative values has been published (Larson et al. 2007).

The neurologic examination (see Chapter 4) enables differentiation of clumsiness, not only from weakness and spasticity, but also from synkinesis, movement disorders elicited by motor acts, and tremor. Each brings its own differential diagnosis, prognosis, and treatment.

Synkinesis is unwilled activity (involuntary movement) of voluntary musculature that occurs during the course of a voluntary action (Fog & Fog 1963; Rasmussen 1993; Wolff et al. 1983). It has been confirmed that the amount of effort required for the voluntary (commanded) activity predicates mirror synkinesis in normal children (Todor & Lazarus 1986). Thus, to find true excess mirror synkinesis, avoid tasks that require strenuous effort. A patient suffering from extreme mirror movements produces them in simple, nonstrenuous, everyday unimanual activities, such as turning a door handle. The incidence of mirror movements is much less (2%) than that of higher-order motor deficits in general (Nichols 1987). Clumsy children very often exhibit mirror movements. The above-mentioned finding concerning interaction between degree of exertion and occurrence of mirror movements may explain their occurrence in clumsy children, who have to exert a large amount of effort to accomplish simple motor acts. Developmentally determined mirror movements diminish with increasing age (Wolff et al. 1983). For persistent and handicapping mirror movements, an effective treatment is not known, but it may be helpful to deliberately engage the hand not involved in the voluntary action with grasping or pressing a surface. Some children spontaneously use this maneuver.

Tremor (involuntary oscillations of a body part occurring at rest or during willed action) has several types. *Intention tremor*, when the oscillation increases as the limb in motion nears its target, is generally a sign of cerebellar disease. To test for it, use the finger-to-nose and the heel-to-shin test of the neurologic examination and observe for it during the tandem gait test and during writing, drawing, and picking up small objects. In every child with intention tremor, particularly if signs of ataxia are present, a lesion of the cerebellum or its brainstem connections must be considered.

Action tremor, on the other hand, occurs throughout the limb movement but not when the limb is at rest. Action tremor, often benign in etiology (for example, benign familial tremor), may severely restrict fine motor performance.

To help a clumsy child, the limits and influence of that particular child's motor disability should first be defined. Most pediatric occupational therapy facilities are able to quantify, using age-normed tests, clumsiness in young children for whom the current major effective remedy is a combination of "bypass" and practice. However, self-esteem usually remains an issue despite therapy, and caretakers need to take an active role in alleviating the child's performance anxieties and poor self-image. The reduction of mechanical impediments to speedy production in required activities (a so-called *bypass method*) is often used (e.g., Velcro flap shoes instead of laced shoes, zippers instead of buttons, snapped rather than buckled belts).

Although practice improves the child's performance of a given act, stress may lead to disintegration of the performance. Thus, under stress (as when dressing for school), certain amounts of help may be granted, but when the child is in a more relaxed situation (as when undressing for bed), this additional help can be withdrawn.

It is important to realize that purely clumsy (as opposed to other types of DCD) children's performance problem is just mechanical. The brain's "motor program" is appropriate to the goal of the action. Only speed and precision of execution are deficient.

As for prognosis, severe clumsiness is unlikely to be fully resolved by maturity (Hollander et al. 1996; Knuckey & Gubbay 1983). However, enough dexterity to allow survival in a society of people who are more adroit is usually achieved. A general rule is that if the child can learn to overcome or circumvent mechanical blocks and thus avoid the deficit in self-esteem created by the performance deficit, clumsiness will not be a severe handicap in the adult life of a normally intelligent individual (Ford 1960).

Dyspraxia

Dyspraxia (called *apraxia* when acquired in adulthood) is defined as the inability to perform developmentally appropriate sequences of voluntary movements in the face of preserved power, coordination, dexterity, sensation, and cooperation. Individual fine and gross movements are often dexterous and well-aimed (Table 22.3). However, depending on the type of activity required, an incorrect sequence of individual movements is produced, sometimes with additions of unrequired movements (parapraxes) (Poeck 1986), with the spatial requirements of the sequence violated, or both. Thus the final product of what looks like a quick, dexterous complex movement may be completely ineffectual; for example, the rapid manipulation of shoelaces with no resulting tie.

Failure to complete complex voluntary acts without observed clumsiness or slowness may be the reason why motor dyspraxia is generally unrecognized as a source of defective actions. Motor deficit is seldom suspected, even by experienced professionals. Because primary motility (strength, coordination, and dexterity) is preserved, a

Table 22.3 Dyspraxia

Discriminating features
- Inability to perform developmentally appropriate sequences of voluntary movements in the face of preserved volition, power, speed, coordination for single motions, and sensation

Consistent features
- Abnormal outcome of rapidly performed movement sequences
- Ability to choose the correct sequence when alternatives are modeled
- Extra or inappropriate movements (parapraxis)

Variable features
- Association with clumsiness
- May affect manual, pedal, axial, facial, or orobuccal motions separately, or occasionally, all of these

basic neurologic examination does not reveal the dyspraxic deficit. Although neurodevelopmental examinations for DCD may contain items that are affected by dyspraxia, dyspraxia per se, not contaminated by clumsiness, may not be recognized (Rosenblum 2006).

Unrecognized dyspraxic deficits often lead the child to be labeled as lazy, oppositional, or unintelligent, with adverse effects on self-esteem, motivation, and conduct. Any of a wide array of school and behavioral problems may be the presenting complaint for the dyspraxic child. However, if a detailed account of motor development is obtained, the history will indicate a motor abnormality. Dyspraxic children are usually delayed in dressing and grooming themselves independently and have specific problems with buttoning, snapping, zippering, donning coats and boots, tying shoes, and manipulating combs, toothbrushes, and scissors. They are often unwilling even to attempt coloring, carpentry, sewing, and cooking. This may happen despite the fact that gross motor (sitting, walking, climbing stairs, and playing soccer, for example) milestones were normal.

The etiologies of dyspraxia are diverse. Adults with apraxia after stroke usually have damage to cerebral gray matter. It may follow a stroke in childhood (Crothers & Paine 1959), and it may be one of the first signs of a degenerative disease. One family's children presented with marked oromotor dyspraxia, severe impairment of linguistic and grammatical skills, and abnormalities in the basal ganglia on MRI, that have been attributed to a point mutation in the FOXP2 gene (Lai et al. 2001).

Although dyspraxia is said to occur in mental retardation, perhaps if a developmental quotient of praxic ability could be reliably determined, it would be commensurate with the intelligence quotient (IQ) in most mentally retarded children, as it is in normal children (Deuel & Doar 1992). Dyspraxia is also frequent in frank cerebral palsy (Frei 1986) as an additional deficit. In most

Pearls and Perils

Dyspraxia

- The best screening test for dyspraxia is an accurate, detailed history of motor development, followed by observation of age-appropriate motor sequences.
- On a general-purpose neurologic examination of school-aged children, the item most prone to be disturbed in manual dyspraxia is the finger-to-nose test (for the child it is a new, nonsense motor sequence)
- To ascertain dyspraxia definitively, a standard manual dyspraxia battery may readily be administered in conjunction with the neurologic examination.
- Facial dyspraxia is often seen in the developmental language disorder called verbal apraxia, or dilapidated speech (Aram & Horwitz 1983), and oral-buccal dyspraxia is a constant finding. The finding of facial dyspraxia can help differentiate this diagnostic entity from other speech and language disorders and point the way to appropriate therapy.
- Parents and teachers generally do not recognize a "motor" deficit in the motor dyspraxic child, but, as with the clumsy child, complain of the child's laziness, sloppiness, or avoidance of tasks. Dyspraxia is not systematically ascertained on the general-purpose neurologic examination, nor is it discriminated specifically in most neurodevelopmental examinations designed to detect DCD.
- The secondary developmental effects of dyspraxia, diminished self-esteem and avoidance of motor sequencing tasks, may be much more handicapping than the motor deficit per se. The secondary effects may remain long after the child has developed effectual praxis.
- Speech pathologists may understand the term dyspraxia to refer only to dyspraxia of speech.

dyspraxia that is associated with learning and attention problems, the etiology is obscure. It seems likely that involvement of the association cortex in some fashion underlies such functional deficits (Deuel 1977), but direct evidence is not available. Functional imaging studies that could elucidate these facets have yet to be carried out, and those studies that have recently addressed physiologic aspects of motor abnormalities (Estil et al. 2002; Johnston et al. 2002; Wilson et al. 2002) have involved the lumped DCD, without separating different types of dyspraxia from pure clumsiness.

Because gross morphologic pathology is not found in the vast majority of children with either dyspraxia or clumsiness, variations in information processing at the neuronal system interaction level, related to genetic and epigenetic factors, may be the cause. To test for subtypes of dyspraxia, it is best to conduct a complete neurologic examination that includes several kinds of patient-performed tasks, including pantomiming of actions, imitating actions of the examiner, and using actual familiar objects (DeRenzi et al. 1980). Such tasks should demand of the child age-appropriate complex voluntary motor activity, and be separated as to whether they demand pantomime, imitation, or use of actual objects skills. Items N115–N 149 of the Preschool and School-Age Pediatric and Neurologic Examination Scoring Form (Deuel & Rauchway 2005) incorporate all three types of tasks and is a useful screening test for dyspraxia.

Possible items for pantomime testing in younger children are asking the child to blow a kiss or wave goodbye. For older children, items from the adult apraxia examination are valid (e.g., pantomime pouring water from a pitcher into a glass, batting a baseball, or brushing teeth). The child should also be able to recognize any act he was unable to perform from among three examiner-performed actions. Choosing the correct one demonstrates the child's recognition of the act and understanding of the command.

Effective completion of a complex act by a dyspraxic child, unlike completion by a clumsy child, does not improve with extended periods of time allowed for completion. This facet of the child's performance can help differentiate clumsiness from dyspraxia, although some children demonstrate both difficulties.

There are no psychometric-style tests for dyspraxia. However, the KABC–II (Kaufman & Kaufman 2004) test for ages 3–18 has a hand-movement copying subtest that does at least test sequential manual abilities. The just cited Deuel & Rauchway (2005) instrument does provide tests aimed at separating the three types of dyspraxia.

The management of dyspraxia depends on its handicapping significance for, and the age of, the child displaying it. Simple recognition of the apraxic deficit, and counseling of the child and parents that it is due to a specific motor problem (and not carelessness, laziness, or other voluntary oppositional personality traits) may be very helpful in removing an unnecessary stigma from the child. If the dyspraxia is idiopathic or the result of static brain damage, further management should include a combination of practice of absolutely needed motor sequences and bypass of the complex motor acts when possible.

Dyspraxia is most likely to be handicapping and obvious when the child is learning a new complex motor sequence. One 10-year-old child was introduced to throwing darts when at a social gathering. At each attempt, she threw the dart backward, with incremental embarrassment to her parents. The incident caused them to seek medical consultation for mental retardation in their child, whose full scale (WISC-R) IQ was 110. Apraxic children, placed in unfamiliar situations that require unfamiliar acts, are often not able to devise new or effective motor sequences. Embarrassing motor inefficiencies cannot be completely avoided by dyspraxic children, but learning to use conscious strategies, such as verbal self-cuing, can help, particularly in the older child. The child can develop a system of conscious self-questioning: "How are the other kids in line ahead of me doing this?" "Which hand comes first, which part of the object is the front/the left/the right?" Such questions may help the older apraxic child consciously control motor sequencing.

The child should be made aware of situations in which the apraxic deficit will surface. She should be encouraged to understand that the problem is motor output, not intelligence. This will shore up self-esteem which, in turn, empowers her to seek innovative ways to fulfill academic requirements. Teachers, parents, and therapists should help her to avoid excessive motor demands.

Because it has rarely been evaluated separately from clumsiness, both incidence and prognosis of the idiopathic dyspraxias are unclear. In most cases they seem to improve with age.

Material-specific dyspraxias

Material-specific dyspraxias are the most circumscribed higher-order motor deficits. They cannot be detected unless the specific material with which there is difficulty is presented during testing. The most commonly recognized material-specific dyspraxia is linguistic (or dyslexic) dys-

Pearls and Perils

Dysgraphia

- Highly abbreviated handwritten output or downright refusal to complete written assignments in the verbally advanced or normal child suggests isolated dysgraphia as a cause.
- In dysgraphia, scores on individual IQ tests, such as the Wechsler Intelligence Scale for Children, are generally normal on all subtests except the coding subtest.
- Neat but very slow writing characterizes dysgraphic children. Slow output leads to paucity of written output.
- The first-grade child who writes letters backward should not be declared dyslexic or dysgraphic. It is important to test writing speed in the child whose school performance is under consideration.
- It is important to test for oral spelling in a child who always fails written spelling. Otherwise, an incorrect attribution to a linguistically based abnormality rather than to a simple motor abnormality or to a spatial disorder may be made.

graphia. In linguistic dysgraphia, the child cannot orally spell or write words correctly, but may be able to draw quite well, presenting a true material-specific (verbal material) dysgraphia. When affected children make written letters and words very poorly, spell incorrectly in both written and oral attempts, and truncate written assignments but read fluently and with good comprehension, they are clearly different from dyslexics (see Chapter 28), who have the written language disorder described, plus an inability to read. Far from 100% of children with dysgraphia have severe dyslexia, whereas some form of dysgraphia does appear in 100% of severely dyslexic children (Deuel 1981).

The material specificity of the disorder is certainly best exemplified by the dyslexic child with dysgraphia, because many such dyslexic children have excellent fine and gross motor abilities when tested on material other than written expression of letters, words, and sentences. Motor execution deteriorates not only from drawing to writing but also as words become more difficult to spell. An example is seen in Figure 22.1, in which a writing sample may be compared with the same child's drawing of a band.

Clumsy children may also be called dysgraphic, but in them the defect is not material-specific, because oral spelling is normal, and they show evidence of clumsiness when they draw or perform any fine motor activity. Written productions are sparse from both dysgraphic and clumsy children.

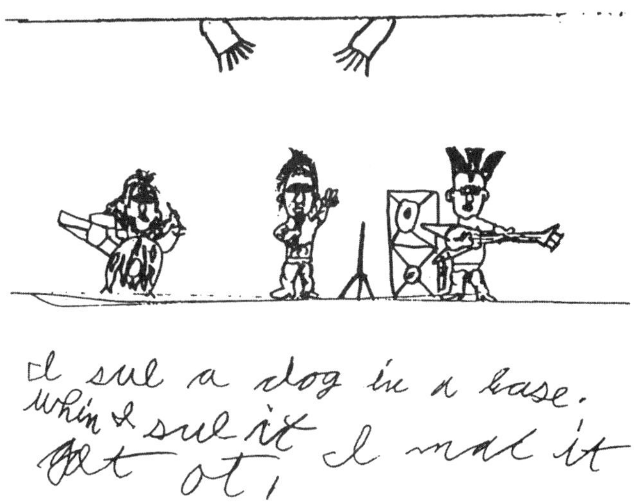

Figure 22.1 A cartoon (produced in about 5 minutes) after the request to "draw me a picture and write a paragraph." The text says, "I saw a dog in a case. When I saw it, I made it get out." This paragraph required about 7 minutes to compose and write out. The writer was a 12-year-old sixth-grade student with a performance IQ of 112. Adapted with permission from Deuel R. Developmental dysgraphia and motor skills disorders. *J Child Neurol* 1995; 10(Suppl 1):S6–S8.

To evaluate dysgraphia, a pertinent history is important and a review of written schoolwork is helpful. One should observe production of written words, sentences, or paragraphs, depending on the subject's educational status. Copying of a grade-appropriate sample should also be evaluated. To determine if spelling deficits are related to writing, as in the clumsy child with poor writing, the child should be asked to spell words aloud. When giving these tasks, it is important to remember that letter reversals are common in early childhood and do not per se indicate dyslexia or clumsiness. Psychologists often employ the Test of Written Language (TOWL-3; Hammill & Larson 1996), which has age-appropriate norms to determine if there is an abnormality and its extent.

Constructional dyspraxia is the second kind of material-specific dyspraxia. It may be related to poor right hemisphere or interhemispheric communication (Makuuchi et al. 2003). Poor spatial intuition with resultant great difficulty drawing and constructing three-dimensional models are its hallmarks. Some children with this disorder may also present poor social and organization skills, such as the right hemisphere deficit syndrome (Voeller 1995). Spatial recognition deficits can lead to getting lost in various indoor and outdoor venues, a great drawback to a new teenage driver. Constructional dyspraxia can be differentiated from clumsiness and from dysgraphia by normal oral spelling and drawings that are more severely disordered than writings. Testing for constructional dyspraxia should include drawing age-appropriate shapes and figures, in addition to writing and spelling exercises for dysgraphia. More formal tests include the Bender Gestalt test (Bender 1946; Lacks 1999) and the Benton test of visual memory (Benton 1974; Walsh & Bruce 1990).

The management of material-specific dyspraxias is various. Dysgraphia can be severely handicapping scholastically, and its treatment with bypass methodologies (for example, dictation of essays) is well known to most educators. Word processors with spell-check are very helpful, presumably because the motor demands of keyboarding are less than those of handwriting.

Constructional dyspraxia is easier to bypass than dysgraphia. Electronic media can not only help check

Consider Consultation When…

- A child has a significantly unusual walking or running gait.
- A child is consistently the last to finish a race.
- A child exhibits significant fine or gross motor deficits on physical therapy, occupational therapy, or psychoeducational testing.

spelling, but can also help drawing, while the constructionally dyspraxic driver can use on-board navigators to find his way around.

Conclusion

Higher-order motor deficits are an important source of school failure and low self-esteem. This source is often completely unsuspected before the child encounters an informed clinician. This chapter can only briefly discuss the modes of presentation of such disorders, their differential diagnoses, ways to make a positive diagnosis, as well as outlining principles of remediation for the specific subtypes. The clinician's awareness of these issues remains the most valuable resource for the patient.

Annotated bibliography

Deuel RK, Doar BP. Developmental manual dyspraxia: a lesson in mind and brain. *J Child Neurol* 1992;7:(S1):99–103.

A study of 164 school children 5–12 years of age given an apraxia battery and WISC-R IQ tests. Twenty-four of the children had dyspraxia according to their battery performance. Within this subgroup, there was no correlation between WISC full-scale IQ and severity of dyspraxia. In contrast, there was a positive correlation between motor performance on the apraxia battery and full-scale IQ in the entire 164-member group, again suggesting that specific cognitive and motor dysfunctions are best segregated and quantified before treatment is recommended.

Gubbay SS. Clumsiness. In: Fredriks JAM, ed. *Handbook of clinical neurology*, vol. 46. *Neurobehavioral disorders*. Amsterdam: Elsevier North Holland; 1985:159–167.

This chapter includes a great deal about the general dilemma of a child with higher-order motor deficits. However, in common with much more recent writings, it fails to differentiate the various forms of these motor execution disorders.

Larson J, Mostofsky SH, Goldberg MC, et al. Effects of gender and age on motor exam in developing children. *Dev Neuropsychol* 2007;32(1):543–562.

Method for administering PANESS and normative scores by age and gender.

Leiguarda RC, Marsden CD. Limb apraxias: Higher-order disorders of sensorimotor integration. *Brain* 2000;126:860–879.

A thoughtful analysis of brain functional and anatomic studies in human adults with the three classic forms of apraxia, correlated with results from monkey neurophysiologic studies that raises the notion that a conceptual system (failure of which would lead to ideational apraxia) and a production system (failure of which would lead to ideo-motor and limb-kinetic apraxia) may be separable entities. This analysis depends on the relatively recent concept of multiple parallel-distributed pathways being used in concert to effect action.

Liepmann H. *Drei Aufsatze aus dem Apraxiegebiet*. Berlin: Karger, 1908.

This is a thoughtful synoptic text that reviews the general concept of apraxia as a higher-order motor execution deficit. It describes and coherently classifies forms of apraxia commonly seen after focal cerebral lesions in adults. It presents tests to differentiate the various types and describes parapraxis (extra movements sometimes inhibitory to task completion). It outlines a very modern concept: that many brain areas initiate movement depending upon the type and purpose of the action.

Wilson PH. Practitioner review: Approaches to assessment and treatment of children with DCD: An evaluative review. *J Child Psychol Psychiatry* 2005;46:8:806–823.

This is a "DCD-oriented" version of examination and treatment. As such, it does not specifically separate the different forms of higher-order motor deficits. However, it does emphasize the important role of the individual child's specific needs.

CHAPTER 23

Disorders of Cognitive Function in the Preschooler

Ruth D. Nass and Gail Ross

Outline

- Developmental language disorders
- Autistic spectrum disorders
- Developmental coordination disorders
- Visuospatial disabilities
- Attention deficit hyperactivity disorder

Developmental language disorders

A developmental language disorder (DLD) is diagnosed when a child with normal intelligence and hearing fails to develop language in an age-appropriate fashion (Table 23.1). Most children have good receptive language by age 2 years, along with a 50- to 100-word (or more) vocabulary and some two-word phrases. Lack of well-developed expressive language by age 3 years is definitely abnormal. However, the large degree of individual variability in the rate of language acquisition (Verhoeven & van Balkom 2003) makes it difficult at times to distinguish DLD from initial idiosyncratic delay with eventual catch-up and normal language. This variability, as well as the range of screening instruments, accounts, at least in part, for the wide range (1–25%) in the reported prevalence of DLD in preschool children (Nelson et al. 2006). Erring on the side of overdiagnosis in the young child and initiating therapy is probably better than underdiagnosis.

Risk factors for DLD include low birth weight or prematurity, parental mental retardation, and a family history of developmental language disorders (National Collaborative Perinatal Project, Lassman et al. 1980). The effect of decreased hearing is debated (Moeller et al. 2007a,b). Family studies indicate both hereditary and environmental influences (Choudhury & Benasich 2003; Spinath et al. 2004; Viding et al. 2004). A number of gene loci have been implicated (SLI Consortium 2002). In the three-generation KE family, half the members are affected with a severe speech and language disorder that is transmitted as an autosomal dominant monogenic trait, the FOXP2 forkhead-domain gene (Vargha-Khadem et al. 2005).

Diagnosis

Table 23.2 lists warning signs that suggest DLD during the first 3 years. However, a DLD diagnosis based on milestones achieved at age 2 years may not be reliable (Bishop et al. 2003). In one study, only about 40% of children retained the diagnosis at ages 3 and 4 years (Dale et al. 2003). In another study only one-quarter of children diagnosed with a DLD as preschoolers still had a DLD at school age, while more than half of the original cohort turned out to have IQs too low to diagnose DLD. Ten percent were normal (Webster et al. 2004). Another basis for diagnosis is a large discrepancy between nonverbal intelligence and language capabilities. In one study, children clinically designated as having a developmental language disorder were identified only 40–60% of the time, using variations of the Stanford Binet IQ–Test of Language Development discrepancy score. A nonverbal IQ-specific language test performance discrepancy criterion of 1 standard deviation (i.e., Wechsler Performance IQ versus the Peabody Picture Vocabulary Test, Token Test, Rapid Automatized Naming, Sentences Repetition subtest of the Comprehensive Evaluation of Language Function) identified 34% of very-low-birth-weight 7-year-olds and 45% of controls as having a developmental language disorder. A 2 standard deviation discrepancy yielded 14% and 19% frequency in the two groups, respectively (Aram et al. 1992). Thus, both under- and overdiagnosis occurs. The best criteria are still debated (Nelson et al. 2006).

Table 23.1 Developmental language disorders

Discriminating features
- Language deficit

Consistent features
- Problems with comprehension and/or production

Variable features
- Mental retardation
- Social problems
- Pragmatics difficulty

Subtypes of developmental language disorders

Depending on subtype, DLDs vary in their characteristic features, etiology, prognosis, and treatment response (Table 23.3). The subtypes listed focus on psycholinguistic features and are named for the areas that are most problematic (Table 23.4) (Rapin 1996).

Articulation and expressive fluency disorders

Pure articulation disorders

Most children (70%) speak intelligibly by age 2 years. Unintelligible speech is the exception at age 3 years (15%). However, almost 50% of children at age 4 years still have articulation difficulties. A common problem is defective use of "th" or "r." At kindergarten entry, one-third of children still have minor to mild articulation defects, but speech is unintelligible in fewer than 5% (Morley 1965).

Stuttering and cluttering

Stuttering is a disorder in the rhythms of speech. The speaker knows what to say, but is unable to say it because of an involuntary, repetitive prolongation or cessation of a sound. Some degree of dysfluency is common as language skills evolve during the preschool years. However, stuttering, in contrast to developmental dysfluency, is probably a linguistic disorder as well as a motor planning problem (Logan 2003). Neurologic explanations for stuttering include anomalous dominance and abnormalities of interhemispheric connections (Foundas et al. 2001) and abnormalities of basal ganglia timing cues (Alm 2004). Stuttering is often familial. Stuttering occurs more frequently in children with other DLDs and with mental retardation (Gordon 2002). *Cluttering*, as seen in fragile X syndrome, is characterized by incomplete sentences and short outbursts of two- to three-word phrases, along with echolalia, palilalia (compulsive repetition reiterated with increasing rapidity and decreasing volume), perseveration, poor articulation, and stuttering.

Pearls and Perils

Developmental Language Disorders (DLDs)

- If in any doubt, assess hearing. Missing a hearing loss is missing a potentially treatable cause of DLD.
- In spite of individual variability, failure to develop normal expressive language skills by age 3 years is pathologic.
- Between 18 months and 3 years, those children with both expressive and receptive delays are more likely to ultimately be diagnosed with a developmental language disorder than those with only expressive delays, who may catch up. Erring on the side of overdiagnosis in the young child with transient institution of unnecessary therapy is better than underdiagnosis.
- An electroencephalogram (EEG) is a useful screening procedure in children with DLDs, because treatment of an underlying paroxysmal disorder may improve language function.
- Failure to develop intelligible speech by age 6 years is a poor prognostic sign in verbal dyspraxia.
- DLDs often diminish, but the basic deficit affects language-related academic skills, particularly reading. Suggesting to the parents that they are merely an element of immaturity is generally inaccurate. Expectant assessment should be performed if there is any hint of reading readiness difficulties.
- Regression of articulation skills during stress and excitement is common during the preschool years. Articulation in the office may be less adept than is actually the case.
- Beware of the child whose conversation is fluent but lacking in content. His parents may be the most resistant to accepting the diagnosis of DLD.
- The child with developmental language problems is at risk for emotional difficulties and should be monitored for possible intervention.
- The child who appears to "talk to talk" rather than to communicate and whose head is large ought to be assessed for hydrocephalus, in view of the frequency of the cocktail party syndrome in this disorder.

Key Clinical Questions

- Is the child's language normal, including his prosody and pragmatics?
- Is the child socially engaged in the usual circumstances?
- Is the child over-focused and very poor at transitions?

Phonological programming disorder

Children with a phonological programming disorder (PPD) have fluent speech, and mean length of utterance

Table 23.2 Warning signs of a developmental language disorder

- Limitations in expressive language
- Has feeding problems related to sucking, swallowing, and chewing
- Fails to vocalize to social stimuli and fails to vocalize two syllables at 8 months
- Produces few or no creative utterances of three words or more by age 3
- Limitations in vocabulary
- Has small repertoire of words understood or used and acquires new words slowly or with difficulty
- Limitations in comprehending language
- Relies too much on contextual cues to understand language
- Limitations in social interaction
- Rarely interacts socially, except to have needs met
- Limitations in play
- Has not developed symbolic, imaginative play by age 3
- Does not play interactively with peers
- Limitations in learning speech
- Expressive speech contains numerous articulation errors or is unintelligible to unfamiliar listeners
- Limitations in using strategies for language learning
- Uses unusual or inappropriate strategies for age level, e.g., overuses imitation (echolalia), does not imitate verbalizations of others (dyspraxia), does not use questions for learning ("why" questions)
- Limitations in attention for language activities
- Shows little interest in book reading, talking, or communicating with peers

Source: Modified with permission from Nelson NW. Childhood language disorders in context: Infancy through adolescence. New York: Macmillan, 1993; and Hall N. Developmental language disorders. *Semin Pediatr Neurol* 1997;4:77–85.

Consider Consultation When...

- Table 23.2 warning signs are present; a consultation with a speech and language pathologist is indicated.

(MLU) approaches normal. Despite initially poor intelligibility, serviceable speech is expected. Language comprehension is relatively preserved. Most such children show delayed rather than deviant phonology, and improve during elementary school. Phonological programming disorder may be a severe articulation problem or a mild form of verbal dyspraxia (Shriberg 1994). The fact that children with a PPD have more difficulty learning manual signs than controls supports an association with dyspraxia (Bishop 2002a). A pre-remediation paired associate learning task may help select the best remediation method for each child (Pearce et al. 1987). An adult aphasia equivalent does not exist.

Verbal dyspraxia

The speech of children with verbal dyspraxia (Nevo et al. 2001), also called *dilapidated speech* (Critchley 1970; Ferry et al. 1975), is extremely dysfluent. Utterances are short and laboriously produced. Phonology is impaired and includes inconsistent omissions, substitutions, and distortions of speech sounds. Syntactic skills are difficult to assess in the face of dysfluency. Language comprehension is relatively preserved. Many require long-term speech and language therapy. Children with verbal dyspraxia who do not develop intelligible speech by age 6 years are unlikely to acquire it. Children with DLD appear to be at increased risk for developmental coordination disorders (Gaines & Missiuna 2007). The presence of

Table 23.3 Subtypes of developmental language disorders

	Verbal auditory agnosia	Phonological syntactic	Verbal dyspraxia	Phonological programming	Semantic pragmatic	Lexical syntactic
Comprehension – receptive						
Phonology	↓	↓				
Syntax	↓↓	↓				
Semantics	↓↓	?			↓↓	↓
Production – expressive						
Semantics (lexical)	↓↓	↓			↓↓	Nl or ↓
Syntax	↓↓	↓	?	?		↓
Phonology	↓↓	↓	↓	↓		
Fluency	↓↓	↓	Nl or ↓	Nl or ↓	Nl or ↓ or ↓	↓
Pragmatics	Nl or ↓	Nl or ↓			↓↓	↓

Nl, normal.
Modified with permission from Rapin I. *Preschool children with inadequate communication*. London: MacKeith Press, 1996.

Table 23.4 Glossary of linguistic terms

Functors	The small words of the language like prepositions, conjunctions, etc. These are also called closed-class words because they are limited in number.
Lexicon	The words in a language, the dictionary of word meanings.
Mean length of utterance	Number of morphemes per utterance.
Morpheme	The smallest meaningful unit in a language occurring either in a word or as a word. A compound word like "compounding" is made up of three morphemes, com*pound*ing. Prefixes, suffixes, and inflected endings like *ed, *s, and *ly are also morphemes.
Phoneme	A distinct sound unit in a language. In English there are 46: 9 vowels and 37 consonants.
Phonology	The rules a speaker follows when combining speech sounds.
Pragmatics	The communicative intent of speech rather than its content; e.g., asking a question at the right time and in the right way.
Prosody	The melody of language, the tone of voice used to ask questions, for example, or show emotion.
Semantics	The meaning of words, their definition.
Syntax	The grammar of a language, the acceptable relationship between words in a sentence.

a more diffuse disorder of praxis has significant therapeutic implications, because children with verbal dyspraxia may depend on signing and writing skills for communication (Shriberg et al. 1997). Although often accompanied by additional neurologic symptoms, verbal dyspraxia most resembles the adult aphasia called aphemia.

Disorders of receptive and expressive language

Phonological syntactic syndrome

Phonological syntactic syndrome (also called mixed receptive expressive disorder, expressive disorder, and nonspecific formulation-repetition deficit) is probably the most common DLD (Korkman & Hakkinen-Rihu 1994; Rvachew et al. 2003; Wilson & Risucci 1986). The phonological disturbances consist of omissions, substitutions, and distortions of consonants and consonant clusters in all word positions. The production of unpredictable and unrecognizable sounds makes speech impossible to understand. The syntactic impairment consists of a lack of functors (e.g., the, a, -ed) and an absence of appropriately inflected endings. Grammatical forms are atypical, not just delayed: "baby cry" versus "the baby is cry" (Bishop et al. 2000). Telegraphic speech is common. The presence or absence of difficulties in other language areas is variable. Overall, comprehension is relatively spared. Semantic skills tend to be intact. Repetition, pragmatics, and prosody may be normal. Autistic children with this DLD subtype produce a significant amount of jargon. Neurologic dysfunction is also frequent in this developmental language disorder subtype. This DLD most resembles Broca aphasia in adults.

Verbal auditory agnosia

Despite intact hearing, meaningful language is not understood by children with verbal auditory agnosia (VAA) (also called generalized low performance and global dysfunction). Verbal auditory agnosia may occur on a developmental basis, and as an acquired disorder, the Landau-Kleffner syndrome (Hirsch et al. 2006; Tuchman 1997). Verbal auditory agnosia is common in low-functioning children with autism. The outcome from the developmental form of VAA is generally poor. The outcome from the acquired disorder is somewhat better, with approximately one-third of children having a good outcome. Verbal auditory agnosia is seen in adults with acquired bitemporal lesions.

Higher-order language disorders

Semantic pragmatic syndrome

Children with the semantic pragmatic syndrome (also called repetition strength and comprehension deficit, language without cognition, and cocktail party syndrome) are fluent speakers, even verbose. Vocabulary is generally large and somewhat formal. Parents are often encouraged by the child's sizable vocabulary only to find later that the verbosity did not indicate superior cognitive abilities. Many children do not have meaningful conversations. They talk to talk. Pragmatic skills are lacking. Children with semantic pragmatic syndrome often have abnormal prosody; their speech has a monotonous, mechanical, or sing-song quality. Comprehension may be impaired. Phonological and syntactic skills are generally intact (Rapin 1996). Semantic pragmatic syndrome is often seen in higher-functioning autistic children (Bishop 2002b). Repetition strength in the setting of fluent speech with impaired comprehension characterizes the adult aphasia syndrome of transcortical sensory aphasia. Difficulties with prosody and pragmatics suggest right-hemisphere dysfunction.

Lexical syntactic syndrome

The lexical syntactic syndrome is relatively common, occurring in approximately 15% of children with DLD (Wolfus et al. 1980). Speech is generally dysfluent, even to the point of stuttering, because of word-finding difficulties and poor syntactic skills, with many hesitancies and false starts. Both literal and semantic paraphasias are common. Syntax is immature, not deviant. Phonology is spared, and therefore speech is intelligible. Repetition is generally better than spontaneous speech. In conversation, idiom use is better than spontaneous speech. Pragmatics may be impaired, particularly when this syndrome occurs in autistic children. Comprehension is generally acceptable, although comprehension that requires processing highly complex syntactic utterances may be deficient. No clear counterpart for the lexical syntactic syndrome exists among the acquired aphasias of adulthood.

Outcome of developmental language disorders

The occurrence of a DLD, even when it appears to resolve, may affect later social emotional adjustment, educational achievement, and vocational choices. Short- and long-term behavioral, social-emotional, and psychiatric problems are associated with early language problems and may even be DLD type-specific (Rescorla et al. 2007; Van Daal et al. 2007). In school-age children with speech and language problems, the frequency of attention deficit hyperactivity disorder (ADHD) ranges from 30% to 49%, and the frequency of behavioral and emotional problems ranges from 10% to 50% (Beitchman et al. 2001; Toppelberg & Shapiro 2000). The biggest differentiating factor between those with and without a psychiatric diagnosis is the degree of language deficit. In the National Collaborative Perinatal Project (Lassman et al. 1980), children with receptive and expressive language problems at age 3 years were at significantly increased risk for one of the three study-defined "minimal brain dysfunction" syndromes—hyperkinesis, soft signs, learning disabilities—at age 7 years (Nichols & Chen 1981). In preschool children with DLD, nonverbal intelligence is the best single predictor of overall long-term outcome, and severity of language problems is the best predictor of later language skills. Preschool language skills are the best single predictor of later reading ability and disability (Carroll & Snowling 2004; Schlaggar & McCandliss 2007; Snowling et al. 2000). Even children with good receptive skills who speak late may be at risk for continuing subtle language difficulties and later reading and language-based academic difficulties (Rescorla 2002), including writing (Bishop & Clarkson 2003). Thus, both screening and follow-up studies of children with DLD are important. Persisting, although often subtle, language problems in adolescence and beyond have been reported in as many as 90% (Conti-Ramsden et al. 2001; Rescorla 2002). Communication problems, again often subtle, may continue into adult life in 50–70% (Young et al. 2002).

Workup

The workup of the child with a developmental language disorder must include an assessment of hearing and overall level of cognitive functioning. An electroencephalogram (EEG), including a sleep record, may occasionally be useful in children with isolated language delay to exclude subclinical seizures (McVicar et al. 2005). Major risk factors for epilepsy and epileptiform EEGs are mental retardation, cerebral palsy, language regression, and the VAA language disorder subtype. Perisylvian abnormalities associated with language disorders have been reported, particularly in verbal dyspraxia and the phonological syntactic syndromes. Complete opercular agenesis has been reported in association with suprabulbar palsy (Worster-Drought syndrome). Polymicrogyria has also been reported in the perisylvian region. Patients with the most extensive disease have the greatest language impairments, whereas those with posterior parietal polymicrogyria have milder symptoms (Alarcon et al. 2002; Guerreiro et al. 2002; Nevo et al. 2001). Callosal size may be decreased in some children with DLD (Preis et al. 2000). Semantic pragmatic syndrome has been reported in patients with agenesis of the corpus callosum and with hydrocephalus, which supports a possible localization in the subcortex and its connections or a disconnection effect. Most recently, decreased white matter density in a left-sided fronto-temporal network was been reported in children with developmental language disorder, supporting an overlap between motor and language networks (Jancke et al. 2007). Some children and adults with DLD (as well as relatives of DLD probands) do not have the typical planum temporale and frontal cortex asymmetry patterns (De Fosse et al. 2004; Herbert et al. 2005). The absence of the typical planum asymmetry may be the result of aberrant neurogenesis, which leads to reduced cell development in the perisylvian regions or atypical patterns of cell death (Herbert et al. 2005; Semrud-Clikeman 1997). An extra sulcus in the inferior frontal gyrus was statistically associated with a history of DLD (Clark & Plante 1998) in a group of 41 neurologically normal adults. Rare reports document right-hemisphere abnormalities in the DLD child suggestive of a right-hemisphere contribution to language acquisition (Plante et al. 2001). This is corroborated by the finding of developmental language disorders in children with both left and right congenital strokes (Stiles et al. 2007). In the KE family (discussed earlier), the caudate nucleus and inferior frontal gyrus are reduced in size bilaterally, while the left frontal opercular region (pars triangularis and anterior insular cortex) and the putamen bilaterally have a greater volume of gray matter (Vargha-Khadem et al. 2005). Functional imaging shows more posterior and more bilateral activation in the family members with the *FOXP2* mutation (Liegeois et al. 2003). An insufficient dosage of critical forkhead transcription factors during embryogenesis may lead to maldevelopment of brain speech and language regions of the brain (MacDermot et al. 2005). Metabolic imaging suggests abnormalities in the left temporal region, and may vary by DLD subtype. Some children with DLD may be right-hemisphere language dominant (Bernat & Altman 2003). Despite these research results, there is no reason to image the typical DLD child in clinical practice, unless focal abnormalities are suspected from the history, such as a nonfamilial, early-declaring left-hander or on examination.

Treatment

Whether intensive early therapy changes the long-term outcome to an appreciable degree remains to be determined (Nelson et al. 2007). Treatment of language-disordered preschool children varies according to the kind of language impairment as well as its degree of severity (Dunn 1997; Bishop et al. 2006). Children with a moderate to severe language impairment, who suffer associated social, cognitive, and behavioral difficulties, are best treated in a therapeutic nursery. Mildly impaired children can often do well in a regular nursery program combined with individual speech-language therapy.

Autistic spectrum disorders

The triad of impaired verbal and nonverbal communication skills, impaired sociability, and restricted activities and interests, all of early onset, are diagnostic of the autistic spectrum disorders (ASD) (Table 23.5) (American Psychiatric Association, DSM–IV-TR 2000; Nass & Leventhal 2004). The presence or absence of social disabilities distinguishes DLD from ASD. IQ, language, and social normalcy distinguish nonautistic mental retardation (NAMR) from DLD and ASD (Figure 23.1). The range of disabilities seen among children in the autistic spectrum is considerable (Constantino et al. 2005). Asperger's syndrome may represent the high-functioning end of the ASDs rather than a separate disorder (Cederland et al. 2008; Frith 2004). Paralinguistic rather than linguistic problems are characteristic (Bishop 2002b). The reported frequency of ASD has ranged from 0.4 to 70.0 per 10,000 children, depending on how the disorder is defined (Honda et al. 2005); however, the best current estimate is approximately 6 per 1,000 (Baird et al. 2006; Centers for Disease Control 2006; Johnson et al. 2007). A Canadian study, estimating an overall rate of 6.5 per 1,000, found the rates to be 2.2 per 1,000 for autistic disorder, 1.0 for Asperger's syndrome, and 3.3 for PDD-NOS (Fombonne et al. 2004). The reported increase in frequency of the ASDs most likely reflects an increasing awareness of the different possible manifestations of the disorder (Fombonne & Tidmarsh 2003), rather than a true increase in the incidence of ASDs.

Table 23.5 Autistic spectrum disorders

Discriminating features
▶ Sociability deficit
▶ Language disability
▶ Need for sameness
Consistent features
▶ Play impairment
▶ Stereotypic behaviors
Variable features
▶ Mental ability

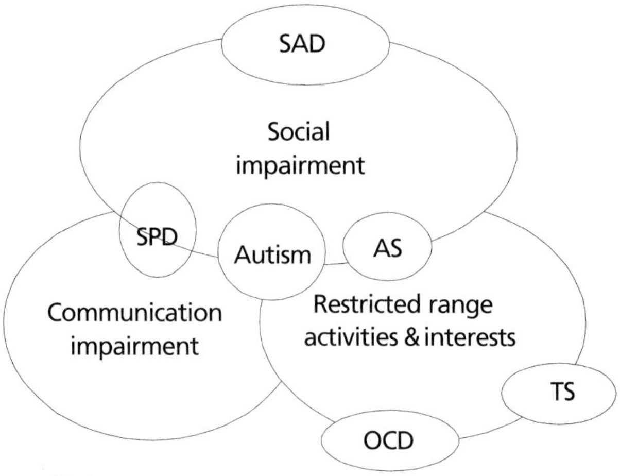

Figure 23.1 Venn diagram showing the overlap of all three symptom areas in autism, of two areas in Asperger syndrome (AS), and of disorders involving a single symptom often reported in autistic spectrum disorders (ASD) families. TS, Tourette syndrome; OCD, obsessive-compulsive disorder; AS, Asperger syndrome; SAD, social anxiety disorder; SPD, semantic pragmatic disorder. Modified with permission from Nass R, Leventhal F.: Autistic spectrum disorders. In: Rizzo M, Eslinger P, eds. *Principles and practice of behavioral neurology and neuropsychology*. New York: Saunders, 2004.

A hereditary basis is supported in many cases by (a) a high concordance in monozygotic twins (90%), (b) an approximately 5–10% increased risk for dizygotic twins and siblings, (c) a broader autistic phenotype in the families of probands (Dawson et al. 2007), and (d) an association with a number of genetic disorders (Autism Genome Project Consortium 2007; Gillberg & Coleman 2000; Mazzocco & Ross 2007). The dramatically diminished risk in relatives who share 50% versus 100% of their DNA is most consistent with an oligogenic inheritance pattern, where more than two and as many as 100 genetic variants may contribute to susceptibility to developing autism. Each gene may make a different contribution to the disorder, with gene A more important for the development of repetitive stereotyped behaviors and gene B more important for language acquisition (Veenstra-Vanderweele & Cook 2003). Both fragile X chromosome disorder and the Rett syndrome mutation can present

Pearls and Perils

Autistic Spectrum Disorders (ASDs)

- Social deficits, rather than language deficits, may be key to defining the autistic spectrum disorders.
- If there is no language by age 5–6 years, language development is unlikely and the probable outcome is poor.
- Some children with autism may have subtle seizures and may benefit from anticonvulsants. If in any doubt, obtain an electroencephalogram (EEG). Video-EEG monitoring is superior to routine monitoring.
- Fragile X syndrome is one of the most common known causes of autism. Obtain fragile X DNA. The Rett mutation can also manifest in an atypical form as an ASD. A fluorescence in situ hybridization (FISH) for a maternal deletion of 15q11–13 and studies looking for sub telomeric deletions may be appropriate in families planning for more children to help to make a prenatal diagnosis on future siblings.
- Look for extrapyramidal signs in autistic children as a reflection of dopaminergic dysfunction.
- The child with an ASD mistakenly thought to have attention deficit hyperactivity disorder (ADHD) may become worse on stimulants, but he may also improve.
- Children with autism may respond to selective serotonin reuptake inhibitors (SSRIs), but higher doses may cause significant agitation or aggressiveness
- Early diagnosis is possible and important. Early and intensive intervention may make a significant difference.
- Although intellectual level is not a defining characteristic of the ASDs, it is an important predictor of long-term outcome.
- Look carefully at peer relations and language prosody and pragmatics in the child with attention and over focus issues, he may actually have Asperger syndrome and not ADHD.
- Tuberous sclerosis is a common cause of autism. A careful examination of the skin is mandatory in all children with ASDs.

with an autistic spectrum phenotype. However, the most common currently known specific genetic causes of autism appear to be the maternally inherited duplication of chromosome 15q11–13 (diagnosed by FISH), accounting for 1–3% of cases (Veenstra-Vanderweele & Cook 2003) and the TSC2 mutation causing tuberous sclerosis complex (Nass & Crino 2008).

Diagnosis

A number of different assessment tools, including parent questionnaires, parent interviews, and direct assessments are available for use in the office by specialists in pediatric neurology, psychiatry, neurodevelopmental disabilities, and psychology to evaluate for the three key features (de Bildt et al. 2004; Johnson & Scott 2007). Office screening using the Modified Checklist for Autism in Toddlers (M-CHAT; Robins et al. 2001) and the Social Communication Questionnaire are reasonable choices (Rutter et al. 2003). The Autism Diagnostic Observation Scale (ADOS) and the Autism Diagnostic Interview (ADI) are generally considered the gold standard for diagnosis, particularly for research studies, but are not usually necessary for making a clinical diagnosis (Gotham et al. 2007; Le Couteur et al. 2003).

Specific clinical features

Intelligence and cognition

The presence of language and social deficits defines ASD, not the IQ level (Figure 23.1). It was previously estimated that 70–85% of children with ASD have mental retardation, although more recent estimates are somewhat lower and range from 30–60% (Chakrabart & Fombonne, 2005). IQ is a key predictor of long-term outcome in autism, especially when the IQ is less than 50 (Stevens et al. 2000). Those with higher IQ generally fare better. Although IQ generally remains constant over time, in some instances it does decline; adolescents with Asperger's syndrome are the most common example (Cederland et al. 2008).

Some consider the core cognitive deficit of ASD to be an inability to grasp other people's thoughts; a failure to develop a theory of mind. "Mindblindness" manifests differently at different stages of development Others have suggested that the metacognitive basis of autism is an abnormality of executive functioning—the ability to problem solve, shift sets, and plan to reach a goal. A third theory postulates the underlying basis as a failure of central coherence, the capacity to integrate information and see the gestalt (Frith 2003).

Language

Verbal and nonverbal communication difficulties are a cardinal feature of ASD. The extent of the language deficit generally parallels IQ. In lower-functioning ASD children, language, if present, is echolalic; repetitive and stereotyped phrases are common. Some children fail to process language and, despite normal hearing, can appear deaf (VAA). Phonological syntactic and lexical syntactic language disorders are also seen in relatively low-functioning and relatively higher-functioning ASD children, respectively. The highest-functioning children often have semantic and pragmatic deficits (Bishop & Norbury 2002). They talk too much; in essence they talk to talk. Such children are often extremely literal and concrete. Prosody is frequently impaired, as evidenced by mechanical, excessively rapid, monotonic, high-pitched, or poorly modulated speech. Still other children have the phonologic syntactic syndrome. Joint attention in the toddler and preschooler also predicts language outcome (Anderson et al. 2007). Language skills at age 5–6 years are predictive of long-term prognosis. Children with conversational language will do significantly better than children who have little or no language at school age.

Abnormalities of play are generally considered part of the autistic child's communication disorder, although some have suggested that it is a reflection of their repetitive behaviors (Honey et al. 2007). The range of early play includes repetitive stereotypic and indiscriminate sensory use of objects (mouthing, rubbing, etc.); purely functional object use and imitation; mechanical play with puzzles and the like; limited interactive play with adults like running, catching, and tickling games; and activities involving their circumscribed areas of interest (e.g., board games, computers, electronic games, or high-level word and number tasks). These activities may provide pleasure. Pretend play is often rudimentary even in higher-functioning children (Waterhouse et al. 1996). As with language, joint attention is a predictor of pretend play development (Rutherford et al. 2007).

Social skills

Social dysfunction is a hallmark of the ASDs and a predictor of outcome as measured by joint attention (Sullivan et al. 2007). The aloof child most resembles the classic notion of autism. They tend to have low intelligence, poor verbal and nonverbal communication skills, and little symbolic play. Passive children are generally somewhat higher functioning overall. They do not make social approaches, but will accept them when made by others. They engage in some pretend play and join in games, but take a passive role. Children who are interactive but odd make social approaches, but do so in a peculiar way. They tend to talk at other people, and their persistence may become annoying. Pragmatic language skills are impaired. Many persons on the autistic spectrum are relatively unaware of their social ineptitude except to the extent that others tease them (Waterhouse et al. 1996). However, some are quite self-conscious. Books written by high-functioning people with ASD highlight the different levels of awareness and concern (Grandin 1995; Willey 1999). Some people with Asperger's syndrome have dubbed other people "neurotypicals."

Recent research has focused on the autistic child's lack of interest in the human face, manifest both in atypical ways of scanning it in social situations and by differences in the brain areas involved in the perception of facial emotion. The face is at the epicenter of social cognition. Difficulties in the domain of social cognition are considered by some the critical feature of the ASD (Hadjikhani et al. 2007).

Restricted range of behaviors, interests, and activities

A restricted range of behaviors, interests, and activities is the third cardinal feature of autism. In lower-functioning children, repetitive, stereotyped behaviors consist of activities like twirling, rocking, flapping, licking, and opening and closing doors. Abnormal sensory reactivity is common in ASD children (Rogers et al. 2003) and may underlie some stereotypies. Overlap and comorbidity with tic disorders and obsessive-compulsive disorders are seen in higher-functioning children (Nass & Leventhal 2004; Zandt et al. 2007). Many of these children have marked difficulties with transitions. Often they don't attend to others because they are in their own world. But, they can also have difficulty transitioning because they are over-focused on something. Some individuals with exceptional artistic, musical, or mathematical talents, as well as idiot savants, may meet criteria for a diagnosis of an ASD or Asperger's disorder. Some of these children grow up to be single-minded, perhaps peculiar, nonsocial chess or mathematics geniuses.

Natural history and outcome

Considering autism as a spectrum disorder, it is not surprising that the natural history of autism shows great variability. The diagnosis is often suspected by 12–18 months or even earlier (Zwaigenbaum et al. 2007). Review of videotapes of first birthday parities have been reliably used to demonstrate ASD in hindsight. At-risk siblings can be diagnosed as early as 6 months by using eye tracking to evaluate their interest in their mother's mouth versus eyes (Merin et al. 2007). As many as one-third of autistic children appear to regress between the ages of 1 and 3 years and are at higher risk for poor outcome (Bernabei et al. 2007; Lord et al. 2004; Rogers 2004). Diagnoses at age 2 years may not hold up at age 4 in as many as 30% (Turner & Stone 2007). Early motor deficits appear to predict persistence of the diagnosis (Sutera et al. 2007). Nonverbal cognitive ability at age 2 was generally the strongest predictor of age 5 language, whereas at age 3, communication scores were a stronger predictor of age 5 language for children with autism. Early joint attention as well as vocal and motor imitation skills were more impaired in children who did not develop language by age 5 (but had relatively strong nonverbal cognitive skills) than in children who did develop language by 5 (Thurm et al. 2007). Scholastic success at school age is best predicted by overall intelligence and by language facility. Nonverbal learning disabilities, ADHD, tics, Tourette syndrome, or obsessive-compulsive disorder may become the more accurate middle school-age diagnosis During adolescence, about one-third of high-functioning patients improve and as many as one-third deteriorate (Cederland & Gillberg 2006). Onset of seizures (Canitano 2007) or mood disorders, especially depression, usually underlie adolescent decline. About two-thirds of adults have limited independence, and almost one-half require institutionalization. Fair to good adult outcomes are reported in 15–30%, but only about 5% become competitively employed, lead independent lives, marry, and raise families. Psychiatric problems are common even in this group. As our view of this disorder as a spectrum evolves, the percentage with better outcomes will probably increase. Some odd adults, including family members who share phenotypic characteristics with an autistic proband, may go undiagnosed in childhood and adolescence, and even function in the mainstream. Some adults with ASD are highly productive and original in their work (Baghdadli et al. 2007). Indeed, the broader autistic phenotype seen in families of an autistic proband exemplifies this (Dawson et al. 2007).

Evaluation and etiology

Diagnosis is based on the presence of the three cardinal features (Allen et al. 2007; Johnson & Scott 2007). The standard neurologic examination is generally normal. The skin must be carefully examined for evidence of tuberous sclerosis, the most common diagnosable disease associated with autism (Bolton 2004). The extent of metabolic and genetic workup depends on the clinical suspicions and the relevance to family counseling (Autism Genome Consortium 2007). Many medical disorders can be associated with an ASD phenotype (Table 23.6).

Formal audiological assessment is required to exclude a hearing impairment. An EEG, including a sleep record or overnight video-EEG monitoring, may be appropriate to exclude subclinical seizures, especially when language comprehension is impaired or developmental regression has occurred (McVicar et al. 2005). Mild to severe epilepsy, partial and generalized, occurs in up to one-third of patients with autism by early adulthood. Infancy (infantile spasms) and puberty are particularly vulnerable periods (Saemundsen et al. 2007). Those who are retarded are at higher risk, but epilepsy occurs in high-functioning children as well.

Autism appears to be a disorder of the association cortex, both of neurons and their projections. In particular, it is a disorder of connectivity, which appears, from current evidence, to primarily involve intrahemispheric connectivity. The focus of connectivity studies thus far has been on white matter, but alterations in functional magnetic resonance imaging (fMRI) activation suggest that intracortical connectivity is also likely to be disturbed (Minshew & Williams 2007).

Table 23.6 Disorders associated with autistic symptoms: Double disorders

Congenital malformations
- Unilateral cerebellar hypoplasia
- Hydrocephalus
- Microcephaly
- Moebius syndrome

Metabolic
- Addison disease
- Adenylosuccinate lyase deficiency
- Adrenoleukodystrophy
- Celiac disease
- Histidinemia
- Hurler syndrome
- Hyperthyroidism
- Hyperuricosuria
- Hypothyroidism
- Lactic acidosis
- Lipidosis
- Mucopolysaccharidosis
- Peroxisomal disorders
- Phenylketonuria

Syndromes
- Angelman
- Anorexia nervosa
- CHARGE association
- Cohen
- Cornelia de Lange
- Dandy-Walker
- De Lange
- Duchenne muscular dystrophy
- Ehlers-Danlos
- Goldenhar
- Hypomelanosis of Ito
- Joubert
- Kleine-Levin
- Lujan-Fryns
- Mobius
- Neurofibromatosis
- Noonan
- Oculocutaneous albinism
- Rett complex
- Smith-Magenis
- Steinert myotonic dystrophy
- Tuberous sclerosis
- Velo-cardio-facial
- Williams

Chromosomal
- Trisomy 21
- 18q-, XYY, XXX
- Fragile X
- Marker chromosome syndrome
- Sex chromosome abnormalities

Epilepsy
- Infantile spasms
- Landau-Kleffner variant

Vascular Infection
- Meningitis
- Herpes encephalitis
- Congenital Infections: rubella, herpes, CMV, toxoplasmosis

Trauma Toxins
- Fetal alcohol syndrome
- Fetal cocaine syndrome
- Fetal thalidomide

Modified with permission Gillberg C, Coleman M. *The biology of autistic syndromes*, 3rd ed. London: MacKeith Press, 2000.

Key Clinical Questions

- Is the child's language normal, including his prosody and pragmatics?
- Is the child socially engaged in the usual circumstances?
- Is the child over-focused and very poor at transitions?

Structural MRI studies document an increase in total brain volume in autism due to both increased total cerebral white matter and total cortical gray matter, which may explain the high rate of macrocephaly. Neither the corpus callosum nor internal capsule are enlarged, indeed the former may be reduced in size. By contrast, white matter volume is increased throughout, with a frontal predominance (Herbert et al. 2004). These findings suggest overgrowth of short- and medium-range intrahemispheric corticocortical connections with no detectable involvement of interhemispheric connections or connections between cortex and subcortical structures (Minshew & Williams 2007). At the microscopic level, minicolumns have been reported to be increased in number and narrower in width, with reduced neuropil space, and with smaller neuron cell bodies and nucleoli (Casanova et al. 2006). This may manifest as a disturbance of cortical inhibition (Minshew & Williams 2007). Imaging data show abnormalities in the cerebellum. cingulate gyrus, hippocampus, and amygdala (Allen et al. 2004; De Fosse et al. 2004; Herbert et al. 2005; Tsatsanis et al. 2003). Many metabolic imaging studies reveal hypometabolism in frontal and temporal regions. Recent functional imaging studies suggest abnormalities along the pathway responsible for processing emotional faces (Hadjikhani et al. 2007) and performing theory of mind tasks. Some researchers suggest that deficits in language, imitation, and empathy are due to abnormal functioning of mirror neuron systems (Dapretto et al. 2006; Rizzolatti et al. 2002). Brain imaging is generally unproductive in routine clinical practice.

Consider Consultation When...

- Aggressiveness, anxiety, or mood changes dramatically. A psychiatric consultation is indicated.
- The child is significantly disrupting family life and is dangerous to himself or others.
- There are new prolonged lapses or episodes of staring, in which case video-encephalographic monitoring may be appropriate.

However, a recent meta-analysis of imaging in children with developmental delay, including autism, does demonstrate that MRI may show abnormalities in as many as one-third, especially when the neurologic examination is abnormal (Shevell et al. 2003).

Treatment

Early intervention offers the best opportunity for mitigating the developmental abnormalities in ASD and related developmental disorders. In many states, children under 3 years of age with developmental delay are eligible for state-financed early intervention programs. Toddlers and preschool children with a diagnosis of ASD should receive special education services in a therapeutic nursery or in a home-based behavioral modification program. Several university centers throughout the United States (i.e., TEACCH, University of North Carolina or Young Autism Program, UCLA) have programs specifically for ASD children (Handleman & Harris 2001; Myers & Johnson 2007). Treatment of Asperger syndrome often focuses around the use of social groups and interest groups. Medication treatment can be useful and may be necessary (Table 23.7).

Developmental coordination disorders

Diagnosis

A developmental coordination disorder (DCD) is defined by motor coordination difficulties that are markedly inappropriate for age and IQ and that cause significant interference with academic achievement or activities of daily living (American Psychiatric Association, 2000; Dyck et al. 2004; Gubbay 1980; Magalhaes et al. 2006) (Table 23.8). The reported frequency in various studies and age groups ranges from 1% to 10%; the frequency tends to drop as children get older (Hadders-Algra 2002). In one large population study of 7-year-old children, moderate coordination disturbances occurred in 9% and severe disturbances in 5% (Kadesjö & Gillberg 1999). There is a clear male preponderance, and DCD is associated with ADHD symptoms about half the time (Landgren et al. 2000). Gillberg (2003) has described a disorder of attention, motor coordination, and perceptual problems (DAMP) occurring in as many as 1–2% in a severe form and 3–6% in milder versions among preschool and early elementary school age children. Children with DCD also have high rates of oppositional defiant disorder (ODD), which is generally a comorbidity of the ADHD. Asperger's syndrome and social skill difficulties have been reported in children with isolated DCD and in those with both DCD and ADHD (Cummins et al. 2007; Kadesjö & Gillberg 1999). Developmental coordination disorder

Table 23.7 Medications for autism

Hyperactivity and inattention	Psychostimulants (methylphenidate; amphetamine); clonidine (Catapres), guanfacine (Tenex), atomoxetine (Strattera)
Obsessive-compulsive behaviors	Tricyclics: Clomipramine (Anafranil)
	SSRIs: Fluoxetine (Prozac), sertraline (Zoloft), paroxetine (Paxil), fluvoxamine (Luvox)
	Atypical neuroleptics: Risperidone (Risperdal), olanzapine (Zyprexa), ziprasidone (Geodon), aripiprazole (Abilify)
	Glutaminergic: Rilutek, cycloserine
Mood and mood stabilizers	SSRIs, bupropion (Wellbutrin), venlafaxine (Effexor), valproate (Depakote), carbamazepine (Tegretol), gabapentin (Neurontin), topiramate (Topamax), lamotrigine (Lamictal)
Aggressive and impulsive behaviors	Mood stabilizers: Carbamazepine (Tegretol), oxcarbazepine (Trileptal), divalproex sodium (Depakote), gabapentin (Neurontin), topiramate (Topamax), lithium
	A-Agonists: Clonidine, guanfacine
	B-Blockers: Propranolol (Inderal)
	Anxiolytics: Buspirone (BuSpar)
	Cholinergic, nicotinics: Galantamine
Tics/stereotypies	Clonidine, clonazepam (Klonopin), pimozide (Orap), haloperidol (Haldol), risperidone, baclofen (Lioresal)
Self-mutilation	Naloxone (Narcan), propranolol, fluoxetine, clomipramine, lithium
Psychosis	Neuroleptics: Haloperidol decanoate (Haldol), risperidone (Risperdal), chlorpromazine (Thorazine), olanzapine (Zyprexa), ziprasidone (Geodon), quetiapine (Seroquel), aripiprazole (Abilify), clozapine (Clozaril)
Seizures	Divalproex sodium (Depakote) and other antiepileptic medications, adrenocorticotropic hormone (ACTH)
Sleep problems	Clonidine (Catapres), melatonin, antihistamines

alone and in combination with ADHD shows a strong correlation with DLDs, school difficulties, and later reading problems (Gillberg 2003). Developmental coordination disorder also co-occurs relatively frequently with visuoperceptual problems (Drummond et al. 2005).

Low socioeconomic class, familial motor clumsiness, prenatal factors (particularly maternal smoking during pregnancy), and neonatal problems (10% with complicated neonatal courses and 7% with normal neonatal courses) (Hadders-Algra 2002) appear to be risk factors for DCD and DAMP (Gillberg 2003). In the National Collaborative Perinatal Project (Nichols & Chen 1981), familial retardation and mental illness were risk factors for DCD and DAMP, as were a number of pregnancy complications and chorioamnionitis.

Table 23.8 Developmental coordination disorders

Discriminating features
- Gross and/or fine motor difficulties

Consistent features
- None

Variable features
- Hyperactivity
- Neurologic soft signs
- Visuomotor and spatial perception difficulties

Several discrete types of developmental coordination disorders occur (Magalhaes et al. 2006), and more than one may occur in the same child (Macnab et al. 2001): clumsiness, dyspraxia, dysgraphia, adventitious movements, and anomalous dominance or handedness. Clumsiness is defined as a slowness and/or inefficiency in performing elementary fine motor and sometimes gross motor movements (Gubbay 1980). Children with developmental dyspraxia have difficulty with motor learning and motor execution. Dyspraxia can be a generalized deficit or a material-specific deficit (Deuel 1995). It can occur alone, in association with clumsiness, and/or in combination with other learning disabilities. Dysgraphia (difficulty with writing) can be a primary disturbance, a manifestation of clumsiness or dyspraxia, or be secondary to dyslexia occurring as a manifestation of a higher-order cognitive disorder. Adventitious movements (e.g., synkinesis, chorea, tremor, and tic) may occur normally on a developmental basis and are designated developmental soft signs when they persist beyond the age when they

Pearls and Perils

Developmental Coordination Disorders (DCDs)

- Children with DCD are at risk for behavioral problems, attention deficit hyperactivity disorder (ADHD), and oppositional defiant disorder (ODD) at school age.
- Children with DCD are at risk for a variety of learning difficulties.
- Children with DCD are at risk for social difficulties.
- Monitor the academic and emotional development of children with DCD.
- Classic dyspraxic syndromes occur in preschoolers, but it is necessary to look specifically for them.

ought normally to cease. With regard to handedness, most ultimately right-handed children declare handedness after 1 year of age and before age 5 years. Strong dominance when established before age 1 year should raise concern that handedness is pathologic and indicates disturbed use of the other hand. The percentage of right-handed children, and probably the strength of handedness, increases through age 5 years. Eventually, more than 90% of children are right-handed. Most right-handers are strongly right-handed, whereas most left-handers are ambidextrous. Dexterity in left-handed and right-handed people is equal.

Evaluation and etiology

Developmental coordination disorders, because of their heterogeneity, can only be fully evaluated using a battery that taps the gamut of motor skills (Ayres 2003; Miller 2003; Wilson 2005). In one study (Geuze et al. 2001), about 75% of children who were judged to have DCD by a team of specialists (physiatrist, occupational therapist, and physical therapist), performed below the 15th percentile on a comprehensive motor battery. The remaining 25% had handwriting problems or low muscle tone issues not measured by the particular battery used. Adventitious movements are generally assessed separately. Synkinesia is best elicited by finger tapping, finger sequencing, and stressed gait testing. Choreiform movements are best elicited by having the child stand with eyes closed, tongue out, and pronated arms extended with fingers spread.

Key Clinical Questions

- Do your child's motor coordination difficulties interfere with academic achievement or activities of daily living?

Consider Consultation When...

- The child's pencil grip or handwriting is delayed, or when the child is frustrated by his graphomotor difficulties; consultation with an occupational therapist is indicated.
- Motor coordination difficulties are markedly inappropriate for age and IQ and cause significant interference with academic achievement or activities of daily living.

Some investigators suggest that children with DCDs have difficulty internally representing the visuospatial coordinates of intended movements. Such a deficit implicates parietal lobe dysfunction in DCD since it is involved in processing feed-forward information from downstream motor areas by comparing it with local visuospatial representations that specify the coordinates of the prospective actions (Wilson et al. 2004). Others (Smits-Engelsman et al. 2003) suggest that children with DCD/LD rely more on feedback during movement execution and have difficulty switching to a feed-forward or open-loop strategy. They base this on the fining that on a writing task children with DCD handled the discrete task, but made significantly more errors on the cyclic task.

Treatment

Children with significant DCD may benefit from process-oriented occupational therapy, motor imagery intervention, and perceptual motor training (Gemignani et al. 2004; Wilson et al. 2002). Computers can facilitate output for those with poor graphomotor skills. Sometimes children with DCD require a scribe in the classroom.

Visuospatial disabilities

Diagnosis

Visuospatial disabilities (VSDs) involving perceptual, organizational, memory, imagery, and/or motor functions occur in isolation and in the context of nonverbal learning disabilities when children reach school age (Drummond et al. 2005) (Table 23.9). Spatial difficulties are usually apparent on traditional IQ testing as a large discrepancy between the verbal and performance IQ subtest scores, which occurs because several performance IQ subtests measure visual spatial and perceptual processing. Although the literature on visuomotor and spatial disabilities in the preschool age child is rather scanty, the importance of visuomotor and spatial skills to future ac-

Key Clinical Questions

- Can the child draw a person with the age-appropriate number of body parts?
- Can the child draw spontaneously, and on request, age-appropriate shapes?

ademic achievement is attested to by the predictive power of visuomotor tasks (Beery & Buktenica 2003), which require the child to copy geometric shapes, for academic achievement in reading and math throughout the elementary grades (Weeks & Ewer-Jones 1991). Data from the National Collaborative Perinatal Project (NCPP) (Nichols & Chen 1981) document that a low score on a block sort task (which required matching blocks by color, size, and shape) or a poor copy of a circle (about 5%) at age 4 years increased the risk of hyperactivity and abnormal neurologic signs at age 7 years. By contrast, hyperactivity and abnormal neurologic signs, as well as learning disabilities, were infrequent in high-scoring block sorters. Children who could not copy a cross (about 30%) were at increased risk for both learning disabilities and neurologic soft signs. The 25% of the cohort failing a maze task were at increased risk for all three syndromes. By contrast, only about 10% of the 4-year-olds were able to copy a square (mostly girls) and those children were at decreased risk for all three syndromes.

Evaluation and etiology

Difficulties in the visuospatial domain that are suggested by a large verbal performance IQ discrepancy can be corroborated by specific neuropsychologic measures of design copy and memory, picture memory, and mental rotation ability. Visuospatial abilities are easily assessed in the office by the simply administered "draw a person test" and drawing shapes to request or copying them.

Right hemisphere dysfunction as the etiology of visuospatial and motor deficits in the preschooler is suggested by the documentation of, for example, difficulties creating spatial arrays during toy play and poor copying and drawing skills in preschoolers with congenital right hemisphere strokes (Stiles et al. 2007). Despite normal gross motor functioning and intelligence, premature children are more likely to exhibit deficits in visuomotor functioning than full-term children. Like term infants in the NCPP (Nichols & Chen 1981), children born prematurely and who perform less well on a standard figure copy task (Beery & Buktenica 2003) at 3–4 years old are more likely to have learning disabilities at school age (Caravale et al. 2005; Ross et al. 1996). Theoretically, the white matter damage in preterms may affect the right hemisphere white matter more than the left (Gimenez et al. 2006; Isaacs et al. 2004; Nosarti et al. 2002; Westrup et al. 2004). Visuospatial difficulties are also hallmark deficits in such genetically divergent syndromes as Turner syndrome, William syndrome, velo-cardio-facial syndrome, and neurofibromatosis, each of which probably predominantly involves right hemisphere dysfunction (Mazzocco & Ross 2007).

Table 23.9 Visuospatial dysfunction

Discriminating features
- Visuomotor and spatial perception difficulties

Consistent features
- None

Variable features
- Hyperactivity
- Neurologic soft signs
- Developmental coordination disorders

Pearls and Perils

Visuospatial Disabilities (VSDs)

- Preschoolers who are even mildly delayed in visuoperceptual development are at risk for later learning disabilities.
- Preschoolers who are even mildly delayed in visuoperceptual development are at risk for hyperactivity and neurologic soft signs. Some of these children will merit a diagnosis of Gillberg disorder of attention, motor, and perception (DAMP).
- Difficulties in visuomotor integration are relatively common in the preterm child and may stem from perinatal white matter injury.
- Children who show perceptual delays are at increased risk for hyperactivity and neurologic soft sign syndromes. Do not dub it maturational too quickly.
- Preterms and other children with early spatial deficits need to be monitored for nonverbal learning issues when they reach school age.

Treatment

Visuospatial disabilities may seriously impair the child's perception of the world. Ordinarily simple tasks, like navigating the playground at school, become difficult. Visuospatial misperceptions may lead to serious social errors. Successful perceptual training programs for preschoolers have been described (Tanguay & Thompson 2002), although long-term follow-up studies documenting their effectiveness have

Consider Consultation When...

- The child is notably delayed, especially if there are associated graphomotor difficulties and a failure to perform perceptual tasks age appropriately. A consultation with an occupational therapist should be sought.

not been reported. In general, the treatment of VSD emphasizes the use of verbal strategies to compensate in demanding visuospatial solutions.

Attention deficit hyperactivity disorder

Attention deficit hyperactivity disorder is characterized by a persistent pattern of inattention and/or hyperactivity-impulsivity that is more frequent and severe than is generally observed in children of the same age (Table 23.10). In about one-half of the children with ADHD, onset occurs prior to 4 years of age (Posner et al. 2007). The estimated frequency of ADHD in children between 2 and 5 years has varied widely from as low as 2% to as high as 18%, with the most recent U.S. estimates at 7% (Bloom & Cohen, 2007; Polancyk et al. 2007). Like older children, preschool males are more likely than females to have ADHD (3:1). But the diagnosis of ADHD at 4–6 years of age has predictive validity for both sexes. Both girls and boys with ADHD were more likely to have symptoms of conduct disorder, major depression, and anxiety in adolescence than same-sex comparison children (Lahey et al. 2007).

Attention deficit hyperactivity disorder symptoms are quite common in normal preschoolers. Approximately one-third of "ADHD behaviors" are frequently noted in early childhood. Hyperactive-impulsive symptoms are more common in preschoolers than inattentive behavior (Smidts & Oosterlaan 2007). Indeed, inattentive behavior in preschoolers may actually be indicative of other psychopathology. Because some degree of hyperactivity, impulsivity, and inattention is common in preschool children, an accurate diagnosis of ADHD can be difficult. Since teachers and parents do not always agree about the presence of symptoms, it is important to get ratings from multiple informants prior to making a diagnosis (Murray et al. 2007). Furthermore, a number of studies suggest that ADHD symptoms are often transient, lasting only 3–6 months. For example, in one prospective study of 224 children followed from birth to kindergarten school entry, 41% of the preschoolers were found by parents, teachers, or the researchers to have some attentional difficulties (Palfrey et al. 1985). In 5%, the attentional issues were significant and persisted at least into elementary school; but an additional 8% had significant problems that abated before school age. Another study found that even among those with severe and persistent enough symptoms to be diagnosed with ADHD, only one-half still met criteria for the diagnosis in elementary school. Therefore, a duration of symptoms of 12 months (rather than the 6 months suggested for school-age children) has been proposed as a more appropriate criterion for the diagnosis of ADHD in preschoolers (Barkley 1998). A number of studies do document a strong correlation between a diagnosis of ADHD during the preschool period and at school age (Campbell 1990; McGee et al. 1991; Richman et al. 1982). Preschool internalizing (anxiety and mood) and externalizing (hyperactivity and conduct) problems have been found to be predictive of their DSM-IV counterparts 8 years later (Mesman & Koot 2001).

Table 23.10 Attention deficit hyperactivity disorder

Discriminating features
- No major psychopathology
- Hyperactivity

Consistent features
- Difficulty with sustained attention
- Distractibility
- Impulsivity

Variable features
- Intense responsiveness to stimulation
- Stimulus-seeking behaviors

Diagnosis

Preschool children with ADHD are characteristically very hyperactive (Kadesjö et al. 2001; Palfrey 1985). Clinical observations of children diagnosed with ADHD demonstrate marked difficulties and/or difficulties in multiple domains of behavior (Kadesjö et al. 2001). Only 6% had no problems during clinical observation. Behavioral comorbidities are common in preschoolers with ADHD. In one recent study (Posner et al. 2007), approximately 70% of preschoolers with moderate to severe ADHD had co-

Key Clinical Questions

- Does your child have difficulty sustaining attention?
- Is your child easily distracted?
- Is your child often "on the go"?
- Does your child run/climb about excessively?
- Does your child not follow through on instructions?
- Does your child have difficulty remaining seated?

Pearls and Perils

Attention Deficit Hyperactivity Disorder (ADHD)

- ADHD is a developmental disorder with onset prior to 7 years of age, but the peak onset actually occurs during the preschool period.
- ADHD in the preschool years is more likely to pose behavior management rather than learning difficulties.
- The critical time to detect and intervene for ADHD is during years 3–4, when concerns about attention and manageability peak.
- Unusually high activity level is a hallmark of ADHD during the preschool period.
- Inattentive ADHD is relatively uncommon and should raise concerns about the accuracy of the diagnosis.
- ADHD during the preschool years is often associated with comorbid disorders.
- Parent and teacher behavior rating forms are best means of diagnosing ADHD in the preschool child, but age-appropriate scales should be used.
- Parent training programs are effective interventions for preschool children with ADHD and are the first line of treatment.
- Stimulant therapy should be considered when the child has not responded to behavior therapy, the family is unable to implement behavior therapy, or the child has severe symptoms of ADHD that are not sufficiently reduced through behavior therapy.
- Stimulants may have less efficacy and more side effects in the preschooler.
- A high percentage of children who will have ADHD at school age can be diagnosed during the preschool years.
- ADHD has a marked hereditary component, but environmental factors play a role.
- Complete disappearance of preschool ADHD symptoms do occur.
- IQ, academic, and behavioral standing of ADHD children may lag throughout childhood.

morbid disorders. Oppositional defiant and communication and anxiety disorders predominated. Developmental coordination disorders are also rather common in young children with ADHD (Gillberg 2003).

Parent and caregiver rating scales are the most accurate means of diagnosing ADHD during the preschool years (Achenbach & Rescorla 2000; Behar 1977; Conners 2008; Sprafkin et al. 2002), although teachers and parents do not always show concordance regarding ADHD symptoms (Murray et al. 2007). Six DSM ADHD symptoms may discriminate preschool children with ADHD from controls better than the remaining 12 items. The symptoms were (1) difficulty sustaining attention, (2) easily distracted, (3) often "on the go," (4) runs/climbs about excessively, (5) does not follow through on instructions, and (6) difficulty remaining seated (Speltz et al. 1999). Impulsivity symptoms were not frequently endorsed, possibly because the examples and wording of the DSM apply more clearly to older children. Scales designed specifically for preschoolers are favored over traditional DSM-based scales.

Questions more relevant to diagnosing ADHD in the preschooler are shown in Table 23.11. Cognitive performance on measures that are useful for corroborating the diagnosis in the older child may be less helpful in discriminating between ADHD and normal preschool children. For example, preschoolers do not differ from controls on intelligence tests or on tests of attention and impulse control (Campbell et al. 1984) such as Matching Familiar Figures, Embedded Figures (Coates 1972), and Draw-A-Line Slowly (Maccoby & Hagen 1965). Measures of executive function may be the most reliable (Mahone et al. 2007; Youngwirth et al. 2007).

Etiology and associated factors

Attention deficit hyperactivity disorder has a significant genetic component, particularly among males. About 30% of parents and 20% of siblings of children with ADHD also have the disorder. Twin studies yield a model that

Table 23.11 Characteristics of the preschool child with attention deficit hyperactivity disorder

- Rushes through tasks paying little attention to details
- Has difficulty paying attention to tasks or play activities
- Does not seem to listen
- Shifts from one activity to another
- Has difficulties organizing activities
- Avoids doing tasks that require mental effort
- Loses things
- Is easily distracted
- Is forgetful
- Fidgets or squirms
- Has difficulty remaining seated
- Runs about or climbs on things when asked not to
- Has difficulty playing quietly
- Is always on the go
- Talks excessively
- Blurts out answers before the question is complete
- Has difficulty awaiting his turn
- Interrupts people or disrupts group activities

0–3 scale.
Modified with permission from Gadow KD, Sprafkin J. *Early childhood inventory-4 screening manual.* Stony Brook, NY: Checkmate Plus, 2000.

includes genetic dominance (48%), additive genetic factors (30%), and unique environmental factors (22%) (Hudziak et al. 2005) Candidate genes for ADHD include *DRD5*, *SLC6A3*, *HTR1B*, *SNAP25*, and DRD4 (Johansson, 2007). One recent study suggests that a variant in DRD5 may affect age at onset for ADHD (Lasky-Su et al. 2007). The *DRD4* seven-repeat allele, which is widely associated with a diagnosis of ADHD, and may be associated with better clinical outcome, is associated with cortical thinning in regions important in attentional control. Interestingly, this regional thinning is most apparent in childhood and largely resolves during adolescence (Shaw et al. 2007).

A number of nongenetic conditions may play a role in the etiology of ADHD including perinatal factors, such as fetal alcohol and drug exposure, smoking during pregnancy, chorioamnionitis and prematurity; sequelae of early childhood illnesses, such as encephalitis and meningitis; head trauma; and environmental toxins (Braun et al. 2006; Langley et al. 2007; Neuman et al. 2007), as well as psychosocial factors like lower social class and family discord (Nichols & Chen 1981). Risk factors in the preschool child for hyperactivity at age 7 years found in the NCPP included hyperactivity and fine motor coordination problems.

Attention deficit hyperactivity disorder is a neurobiologic disorder. In general, studies suggest that ADHD is characterized by specific learning and cognitive deficits due to abnormalities in dopamine-rich prefrontal circuitry. In addition to prefrontal cortical areas, the basal ganglia, cerebellum, and parietal cortex have been implicated by imaging studies (Kelly et al. 2007). These regions are part of unique circuits that project both to and from the prefrontal cortex, thus providing a means for signaling prefrontal regions when top-down control of behavior needs to be imposed. Ineffective signaling of control systems by any one of these regions can lead to poor regulation of behavior. Likewise, intact signaling but inefficient top-down control could result in poor regulation of behavior (Casey et al. 2007; Swanson et al. 2007). Functional imaging results are consistent with this theoretical model (Kelly et al. 2007).

Outcome

As discussed previously, preschool ADHD may or may not persist into elementary school and beyond. When it does, comorbid behavior problems often persist, as well as language and perceptual motor difficulties (Gillberg 2003). Studies indicate that both the presence of ADHD in the preschool period and its persistence into elementary school may correlate with poor school achievement later (DuPaul et al. 2001; Nichols & Chen 1981).

Consider Consultation When...

- ADHD is accompanied by significant oppositional behavior, anxiety, or mood issues. A consultation with a behavior modification expert would be indicated.
- Inattentive ADHD is the presenting complaint. A psychiatric consultation is appropriate.

Treatment

The preschool period presents parents with special problems in child management and is associated with high levels of parental stress and low confidence in parenting skills. Early identification of children with ADHD and prompt intervention are important in minimizing the deleterious effects of this disorder on the child's later academic achievement, personal relationships with peers and family members, self-esteem, and behavior. Behavior management strategies are always indicated at home and nursery school as the first line of treatment for preschool aged children. Training parents and teachers in behavioral management skills can modify noncompliant behaviors in preschoolers (Sonuga-Barke et al. 2001).

Stimulant medications are used to treat preschool children. Reports from the Preschool ADHD Treatment Study (PATS) support the safety and efficacy of short-acting Ritalin in a group of 147 3–5.5-year-olds. (Greenhill et al. 2006). Ritalin given at 2.5–7.5 three times a day reduced symptoms in preschoolers, although the effect size was smaller than in older children. This could have been due to the low dose required by the study protocol or to differences between the effects of stimulants on preschoolers compared with older children. Preschoolers appeared to have more side effects. Thirty percent of parents reported emotional outbursts, sleep difficulties, decreased appetite, and/or weight loss. Eleven percent ultimately discontinued medications despite benefit (Wigal et al. 2006). Secondary data from the study demonstrated pharmacogenetic effects in which particular genotypes were associated with specific side effects (McGough et al. 2006). α-Agonists like clonidine and guanfacine have also been used with some success in the preschool child, particularly in those with marked hyperactivity and conduct disorders. Overall, preschool children tend to have a less robust response to treatment and a higher side-effect burden, perhaps because of their high rates of comorbidity—particularly mood and anxiety disorders—leading to more complex cases (Wilens et al. 2002a,b). Given these issues, making an accurate diagnosis is all the more important.

Annotated bibliography

Developmental language disorders

Bishop DVM, Leonard LB, eds. *Speech and language impairments in children: causes, characteristics, intervention and outcome*. Hove, UK: Psychology Press, 2000.

Aram DM, Morris R, Hall NE. The validity of discrepancy criteria for identifying children with developmental language disorders. *J Learn Disabil* 1992;25:549.

Nelson, H, Nygren, P, Walker, M, Panoscha, R. Screening for speech and language delay in preschool children: Systematic evidence review for the US Preventive Services Task Force. *Pediatrics* 2006;117:e298-e319.

Rescorla L, Achenbach TM. Use of the language development survey (LDS) in a national probability sample of children 18 to 35 months old. *J Speech Lang Hearing Res* 2002;45:733–743.

Rapin I. *Preschool children with inadequate communication.* London: MacKeith Press, 1996.

Verhoeven L, van Balkom B, eds. *Classification of developmental language disorders.* New Jersey: Lawrence Erlbaum, 2003.

Good reviews of the general definition and nosology of the DLDs.

Lassman FM, Fisch RO, Vetter DK, LaBenz ES. *Early correlates of speech, language and hearing.* Littleton MA: PSG Publishing, 1980.

Nichols P, Chen T. *Minimal brain dysfunction.* New Jersey: Lawrence Erlbaum, 1981.

These volumes provide data on language development and risk factors for maldevelopment from the National Perinatal Collaborative Project.

MacDermot KD, Bonora E, Sykes N, et al. Identification of FOXP2 truncation as a novel cause of developmental speech and language deficits. *Am J Hum Genet* 2005;76(6):1074–1080.

Smith SD. Genes, language development, and language disorders. *Mental Retard Dev Dis Res Rev* 2007;13(1):96–105.

Two good reviews of the genetics of the DLDs.

Tuchman RF. Acquired epileptiform aphasia. *Semin Pediatr Neurol* 1997;4:95–101.

Hirsch E, Valenti MP, Rudolf G, et al. Landau-Kleffner syndrome is not an eponymic badge of ignorance. *Epilepsy Res* 2006;70(Suppl 1):S239–247.

Key references on verbal auditory agnosia in isolation as a DLD and in association with epilepsy as Landau-Kleffner syndrome.

Bishop DVM. Exploring borderlands of autistic disorder and specific language impairment: A study using standardised diagnostic instruments. *J Child Psychol Psychiatry* 2002b;43: 917–929.

A key reference on the semantic pragmatic syndrome.

Korkman M, Hakkinen-Rihu P. A new classification of DLD. *Brain Lang* 1994;47:96–104.

Bishop DVM, Bright P, James C, et al. Grammatical SLI: A distinct subtype of developmental language impairment? *Applied Psycholinguist* 2000;21:159–181.

Wolfus B, Moscovitch M, Kinsbourne M. Subgroups of developmental language disorders. *Brain Lang* 1980;9:152–171.

Wilson B, Risucci D. A model for clinical quantitative classification of the DLDs. *Brain Lang* 1986;27:281–309.

Good theoretical reviews of the syntactic deficits in the DLDs, manifesting in isolation and as phonologic syntactic syndrome and lexical syntactic syndrome.

Alm PA. Stuttering and the basal ganglia circuits: A critical review of possible relations. *J Commun Disord* 2004;37:325–369.

Gordon N. Stuttering: incidence and causes. *Dev Med Child Neurol* 2002;44:278–281.

Good reviews about stuttering and its pathophysiology.

Bishop DV, Maybery M, Wong D, et al. Are phonological processing deficits part of the broad autism phenotype? *Am J Med Genetics B (Neuropsychiatric Genetics)* 2004;128(1): 54–60.

Bishop DVM. Motor immaturity and specific speech and language impairment: Evidence for a common genetic basis. *Am J Med Genet Neuropsychiatr Genet* 2002a;114:56–63.

These studies address the diagnosis and treatment of the phonological programming disorder.

Critchley M. *Aphasiology*. London: Edward Arnold, 1970.

Ferry P, Hall S, Hicks J. Dilapidated speech: Developmental verbal apraxia. *Dev Med Child Neurol* 1975;17:749–756.

Morley ME. *The development and disorders of speech in childhood*, 2nd ed. Baltimore MD: Williams &Wilkins, 1965.

Nevo Y, Segev Y, Gelman Y, et al. Worster-Drought and congenital perisylvian syndromes: A continuum. *Pediatr Neurol* 2001;24:153–155.

Visscher C, Houwen, S, Scherder EJA, et al. Motor profile of children with developmental speech and language disorders. *Pediatrics* 2007;120:e158–163.

Both classic and more recent works on articulation and verbal dyspraxia.

Bernat B, Altman N. Speech delay in children: A functional MR imaging study. *Radiology* 2003;229:651–658.

Friederici AD. The neural basis of language development and its impairment. *Neuron* 2006;52(6):941–952.

Herbert MR, Kenet T. Brain abnormalities in language disorders and in autism. *Pediatric Clin N Am* 2007;54(3):563–583, vii.

Jancke L, Siegenthaler TH, Preis S, Steinmetz H. Decreased white-matter density in a left-sided fronto-temporal network in children with developmental language disorder: Evidence for anatomical anomalies in a motor-language network. *Brain Lang* 2007;102(1):91–98.

Saletti V, Bulgheroni S, D'Incerti L, et al. Verbal and gestural communication in children with bilateral perisylvian polymicrogyria. *J Child Neurol* 2007;22(9):1090–1098.

Vargha-Khadem F, Gadian D, Copp A, Mishkin M. FOXP2 and the neuroanatomy of speech and language. *Nat Rev Neurosci* 2005;6:131–139

Recent papers pertaining to pathophysiology of DLD.

Bishop DVM, Price TS, Dale PS, Plomin R. Outcomes of early language delay II: Etiology of transient and persistent language delay. *J Speech Lang Hear Res* 2003;46:561–575.

Clegg J, Hollis C, Mawhood L, Rutter M. Developmental language disorders: A followup in later adult life. Cognitive, language and psychosocial outcomes. *J Child Psychol Psychiatry* 2005;46:128–149.

Dale PS, Price TS, Bishop DVM, Plomin R. Outcomes of early language delay I: Predicting persistent and transient delay at 3 and 4 years. *J Speech Lang Hearing Res* 2003;46:544–560.

Lyytinen P, Eklund K, Lyytinen H. Language development and literacy skills in late-talking toddlers with and without familial risk for dyslexia. *Ann Dyslexia* 2005;55(2): 166–192.

Snowling MJ, Bishop DV, Stothard SE, et al. Psychosocial outcomes at 15 years of children with a preschool history of speech-language impairment. *J Child Psychol Psychiatry* 2006;47(8):759–765.

Good papers on follow-up and outcome.

Dunn M. Remediation of children with DLD. *Semin Pediatr Neurol* 1997;4:135–142.

Bishop DV, Adams CV, Rosen S. Resistance of grammatical impairment to computerized comprehension training in children with specific and non-specific language impairments. *Intern J Lang Commun Dis* 2006;41(1):19–40.

These papers speak to techniques and efficacy of treatment.

Autistic spectrum disorders

Chakrabart S, Fombonne E. Pervasive developmental disorder in preschool children: Confirmation of high prevalence. *Am J Psychiatry* 2005;162:1133–1141.

Frith U. *Autism: Explaining the enigma.* Oxford, UK: Blackwell Publishers, 2003.

Gillberg C, Coleman M. *The biology of autistic syndromes*, 3rd ed. London: MacKeith Press. 2000.

Volkmar F, Pauls D. Autism. *Lancet* 2003;362:1133–1139.

Rapin I, Tuchman R. *Autism: A neurological disorder of early brain development.* International Review of Child Neurology Series (ICNA). London: MacKeith Press, 2006.

Waterhouse L, Morris R, Allen D et al. Diagnosis and classification in autism. *J Autism Dev Disord* 1996;26:59–86.

Good general references— classic and current—about autism and its prevalence.

Frith U. Emmanuel Miller lecture: Confusions and controversies about Asperger syndrome. *J Child Psychol Psychiatry* 2004;45:672–686.

Gillberg C. *A guide to Asperger disorder.* New York: Cambridge University Press, 2002.

Two excellent books that specifically discuss Asperger syndrome.

Clifford S, Young R, Williamson P. Assessing the early characteristics of autistic disorder using video analysis. *J Autism Dev Dis* 2007;37(2):301–313.

Zwaigenbaum L, Thurm A, Stone W, et al. Studying the emergence of autism spectrum disorders in high-risk infants: Methodological and practical issues. *J Autism Dev Dis* 2007; 37(3):466–480.

These papers discuss early diagnosis.

Autism Genome Project Consortium. *Nature Genetics*. 2007; 39(3):319–328.

This is the most up-to-date review of the genetics of ASDs.

Allen G, Muller R-A, Courchesne E. Cerebellar function in autism. *Biol Psychiatry* 2004;56:269–278.

Canitano R. Epilepsy in autism spectrum disorders. *Eur Child Adolesc Psychiatry* 2007;16(1):61–66.

Hadjikhani N, Joseph RM, Snyder J, Tager-Flusberg H. Abnormal activation of the social brain during face perception in autism. *Human Brain Mapping* 2007;28(5):441–449.

Keller TA, Kana RK, Just MA. A developmental study of the structural integrity of white matter in autism. *Neuroreport* 2007;18(1):23–27.

Minshew N, Williams D. The new neurobiology of autism: Cortex, connectivity, and neuronal organization. *Arch Neurol* 2007;64(7):945–950.

Good reviews of the pathophysiology of autism.

Shattuck PT, Grosse SD. Issues related to the diagnosis and treatment of autism spectrum disorders. *Mental Retard Dev Dis Res Rev* 2007;13(2):129–135.

Shevell M, Ashwal S, Donley D et al. Practice parameter: Evaluation of the child with global developmental delay. *Neurology* 2003;60:367–380.

These papers include practice parameters with suggested workups for children with delay and on the autistic spectrum.

Baghdadli A, Picot M-C, Michelon C, et al. What happens to children with PDD when they grow up? Prospective follow-up of 219 children from preschool age to mid-childhood. *Acta Psychiatrica Scand* 2007;115(5):403–412.

Bernabei P, Cerquiglini A, Cortesi F, D'Ardia C. Regression versus no regression in the autistic disorder: Developmental trajectories. *J Autism Dev Dis* 2007;37(3):580–588.

Turner LM, Stone WL. Variability in outcome for children with an ASD diagnosis at age 2. *J Child Psychol Psychiatry* 2007; 48(8):793–802.

These references are about outcome.

Towbin KE. Strategies for pharmacologic treatment of high functioning autism and Asperger syndrome. *Child Adolesc Psychiatr Clin North Am* 2003;12:23–45.

A good review about medication management.

Handleman J, Harris S. *Preschool education programs for children with autism.* Austin TX: Pro-Ed, 2001.

Myers SM, Johnson CP. American Academy of Pediatrics Council on children with disabilities. Management of children with autism spectrum disorders. *Pediatrics* 2007;120(5): 1162–1182.

Two good reviews of behavioral treatment.

Developmental Coordination Disorders

Gubbay L. *The clumsy child.* Philadelphia: Saunders, 1980.

A classic on the subject.

Wilson PH. Practitioner review: Approaches to assessment and treatment of children with DCD. An evaluative review. *J Child Psychol Psychiatry* 2005;46(8):806–823.

Gillberg C. Disorders of attention, perception and motor function. *Arch Dis Child* 2003;88:904–910.

Good general reviews.

Wilson P, Thomas P, Maruff P. Motor imagery training ameliorates motor clumsiness in children. *J Child Neurol* 2002; 27:491–499.

Some innovative therapies for developmental coordination disorders are available.

Visuospatial disorders

Stiles J, Reilly J, Levine S, Nass R. Prenatal stroke: Effects and outcomes. In: Yeats KO, Ris MD, Taylor G, Pennington B, eds. *Pediatric neuropsychology: Research, theory, and practice.* New York: Guilford Press, 2007.

This reference is about visuospatial skills in a population with congenital strokes; those with right hemisphere injury are at particular risk.

Caravale B, Tozzi C, Albino G, Vicari, S. Cognitive development in low risk preterm infants at 3-4 years of life. *Arch Dis Child* (Fetal Neonatal Edition) 2000;90(6):F474–479.

A recent reference about cognitive function in preterms, another group at particular risk for visuospatial difficulties.

Mazzocco M, Ross J. *Neurogenetic developmental disorders*. Cambridge, MA: MIT Press, 2007.
About specific neurogenetic disorders. Visuospatial deficits are common in this population.

Attention deficit hyperactivity disorder

Murray D, Kollins S, Hardy K, et al. Parent versus teacher ratings of attention-deficit/hyperactivity disorder symptoms in the Preschoolers with Attention-Deficit/Hyperactivity Disorder Treatment Study (PATS). *J Child Adolesc Psychopharmacol* 2007;17(5):605–620.
A good review about diagnosis in the preschool period.

Wilens T, Biederman J, Brown S, et al. Patterns of psychopathology and dysfunction in clinically referred preschoolers. *Dev Behav Pediatr* 2002;23:S31–36.
A good review of comorbidities in preschool ADHD.

Sprafkin J, Volpe R, Gadow K, et al. A DSM-IV–referenced screening instrument for preschool children: The Early Childhood Inventory-4. *J Am Acad Child Adolesc Psychiatry* 2002;41:604–612.
Good discussions of diagnostic criteria in the preschool child.

Johansson S, Halleland H, Halmoy A, et al. Genetic analyses of dopamine related genes in adult ADHD patients suggest an association with the DRD5-microsatellite repeat, but not with DRD4 or SLC6A3 VNTRs. *Am J Med Genet B, Neuropsychiat Genet* 2007;1010–1015.
A good recent review of genetics.

Kelly AM, Margulies DS, Castellanos FX. Recent advances in structural and functional brain imaging studies of attention-deficit/hyperactivity disorder. *Curr Psychiatry Rep* 2007; 9(5):401–407.
A good general review of imaging findings in ADHD.

McGough J, McCracken J, Swanson J, et al. Pharmacogenetics of methylphenidate response in preschoolers with ADHD. *J Am Acad Child Adolesc Psychiatry* 2006;45(11):1314–1322.

Greenhill L, Kollins S, Swanson J, et al. Efficacy and safety of immediate release methylphenidate treatment for preschoolers with ADHD. PATS study. *J Am Acad Child Adolesc Psychiatry* 2006;45(11):1284–1293.
Good summaries of stimulant treatment for preschoolers.

CHAPTER 24

Learning Disabilities

Max Wiznitzer and Debora L. Scheffel

Outline

- Dyslexia (reading disability)
- Dyscalculia (mathematics disability)
- Dysgraphia (writing disability)
- Dysphasia (oral language disability)
- Nonverbal learning disability
- Epidemiology
- Neurobiology
- Evaluation
- Treatment
- Prognosis

Learning disabilities are disorders of higher cognitive functions, present from birth or early childhood, neurologically based, and impact on the ability to learn or process information in one or more specific areas rather than a global intellectual impairment. Individuals with learning disabilities may present to the child neurologist with a question of developmental delays, poor school performance, or behavioral problems. Also, for children who are already being followed for chromosomal/genetic disorders, consequences of prematurity, attention deficit hyperactivity disorder (ADHD), traumatic brain injury (TBI), or epilepsy, learning disabilities can later become evident.

This population of children has been described in educational, psychological, and medical communities by a number of terms, including d*evelopmentally learning disabled*, *minimal brain dysfunction syndrome*, *developmental aphasia*, *dysgraphia*, *dyscalculia*, and *dyslexia*. These terms diverge based on their relative orientation toward the etiology or behavioral manifestations of the disorder.

In 1963, the term *learning disability* was formally introduced. At that time this term referred to disorders in development of language, speech, reading, and associated communication skills needed for social interaction. This definition has been the source of debate and revision since its introduction. The federal definition is based on guidelines developed after passage of Public Law 94–142 (IDEA 97) and the operational definition from 1968:

> A severe discrepancy between achievement and intellectual ability in one or more of these areas: (a) oral expression, (b) listening comprehension, (c) written expression, (d) basic reading skills, (e) reading comprehension, (f) mathematics calculation, or (g) mathematics reasoning. The child may not be identified as having a specific learning disability if the discrepancy between ability and achievement is primarily the result of: (a) a visual, hearing, or motor handicap; (b) mental retardation; (c) emotional disturbance; or (d) environmental, cultural, or economic disadvantage.

A consensus statement of the National Joint Committee on Learning Disabilities, composed of representatives from major professional organizations dealing with this subject, expanded the definition by adding length of occurrence and coexistence with other conditions, thereby defining learning disabilities as:

- Manifested by significant difficulties in the acquisition and use of listening, speaking, reading, writing, reasoning, or mathematical abilities
- Intrinsic to the individual, presumably caused by central nervous system (CNS) dysfunction, and sometimes occurring over a person's entire life span
- Occurring, in some cases, concomitantly with other handicapping conditions (for example, sensory impairment, mental retardation, or serious

emotional disturbance) or extrinsic influences (such as cultural differences or insufficient or inappropriate instruction), but not resulting from those conditions or influences

This legislative definition is primarily aimed at addressing societal needs by authorizing programs and mandating services. Definitions more operational in character are used for research purposes and, at the state level, for identification. Implementing the definition requires specifying how the diagnosis is made and determining the relationship between average intellectual competence and a learning disorder. Definitions for this purpose use any of at least four methods to arrive at a diagnosis: (a) deviation from grade level, (b) expectancy formulas, (c) simple standard score differences, and (d) standard regression analysis (Berninger & Abbott 1994). Based on deviation from grade level, a learning-disabled child might be identified by demonstrating achievement at a predetermined point below expected grade level. Expectancy formulas use IQ to adjust expected level of achievement based on potential ability; the difference between expected and observed achievement needed to define a learning disability is arbitrary. Using a standard score difference approach, the age- or grade-corrected standard score for achievement is subtracted from the IQ standard score. The cutoff criterion for amount of discrepancy is arbitrary. The regression discrepancy model takes into account measurement error, effects of regression toward the mean, and correlations between ability and achievement measures (Reynolds 1984).

The validity of all of these assessment methods has been criticized. The result of this has been a movement toward changing the Individuals with Disabilities Education Act during the 2004 Reauthorization. The new law will probably recommend portfolio assessment, authentic observation, and comparison of daily performance in natural environments to determine eligibility of services. Exactly how this will be done and decisions made will be determined once the legal language has been translated and regulations are written. In addition, some studies conclude that there is a spectrum of function, rather than a bimodal distribution, in skills such as reading, so that children at the lower end of the continuum will be identified as "learning disabled" with no clear cut-off between dyslexic and typically reading children (Beichtman et al. 1998; Fletcher et al. 1999; Gottesman & Kelly 2000; Levine 1999; Shaywitz & Shaywitz 1999). Incorporating this information and the new regulations into daily practice will be a challenge for special education providers in the next few years.

In addition to complex identification issues, learning-disabled children comprise a heterogeneous group. Research has attempted to identify homogeneous subgroups within the larger population. All have core dysfunction in one or a combination of the following processes (Gottesman & Kelly 2000; Levine 1999):

- *Memory*. Skills in this area are needed to follow directions, to retain information while solving problems, reading or transferring thoughts to paper (active working), to consistently study and remember information for tests (long-term consolidation), and to remember facts in a timely fashion (long-term retrieval). Dysfunction can be visual or auditory in nature.
- *Language*. Difficulties can occur in expressive, receptive, or processing skills and affect the various components of language: phonology (decoding and encoding the core sounds of language), syntax (the grammar and organization of sentences), semantics (meaning of vocabulary and sentences/communication), and pragmatics (the nonverbal communication and social aspects of language, e.g., gestures and facial expression). Dysfunction can be manifest as poor pronunciation and immature grammar, problems decoding written language, or difficulties following complex directions, retaining written language, detailing ideas in writing, and/or distinguishing homonyms or learning sequences.
- *Visuospatial skills*. Academic skills require the ability to discriminate shapes (which affects letter and number recognition), differentiate between foreground and background (to attend to relevant details), understand form constancy, and develop a sense of direction and right–left discrimination (for sports participation and daily organization). Difficulties in this area rarely cause a significant learning disability, but may aggravate other areas of dysfunction.
- *Temporal sequencing*. These abilities address core skills such as correctly following multistep directions and the daily classroom schedule, learning to tell time and the understanding of serial order in writing, reading, and mathematics. Deficiencies can affect learning the concept of mathematical computation, development of good organizational skills (including time management), following concepts in written language, and performing in music class.
- *Higher-order cognition*. Thinking skills show a maturational process throughout the school years. This includes developments in concept acquisition (the grouping of ideas into defined categories with a gradual shift towards more abstract concepts), problem solving skills, the use of critical thinking and brainstorming, and an appreciation for rules in learning. Problems in this area can result in difficulties understanding the core rules of mathematics and the relationships in computational strategies, learning how to estimate or to formulate new ideas

in writing, developing analytic skills, or recognizing patterns in learning (such as capitalization of proper names or countries).

- *Motor skills*. Coordination of fine and gross motor skills is essential for adequate school performance. The child needs to master abilities ranging from dressing, cutting, and copying to appropriate pen/pencil grasp, letter formation (print and cursive), and speed of writing and computer keyboard use. Difficulties in this area can impact on a variety of core academic skills such as writing and performance in physical education, art, and musical instrument use.
- *Social ability*. Social skills are essential to navigate the daily life in schools. Individuals should be able to initiate and maintain social interactions, problem-solve in challenging situations, and terminate an interaction. Difficulties in this area can affect one's ability to request help, develop friendships, and enjoy the school experience.

In addition to these areas, adequate attention is essential. This is a skill that affects all areas of functioning. Dysfunction can be subtle and task-specific (such as visual or auditory processing) or so significant that it meets criteria for ADHD (inattention, hyperactivity, impulsivity). Although attentional dysfunction represents a behavioral rather than an academic deficiency, its impact can potentiate underlying learning disabilities or mimic a primary academic deficiency.

Each individual presents his own profile of strengths and weakness in these areas. Given the individuality of each case, it is often difficult to determine a specific etiology, intervention, or prognosis.

There are five main types of learning disabilities.

Table 24.1 Reading disorders (dyslexia)

Discriminating features

- At least average verbal or nonverbal intellectual potential
- Significant discrepancy between intellectual potential and performance on measures of reading

Consistent features

- Not a unitary disorder; heterogeneous population demonstrates a variety of levels of functioning in facets of reading performance
- Deficient functioning in any one or combination of reading silently or orally, individual words in context; decoding, comprehension or rate

Variable features

- Occur concomitantly with other handicapping conditions or extrinsic influences but are not primarily attributed to either
- Deficient performance in skills representing either disrupted visual processes (for example, poor sight vocabulary, reversals), disrupted lexical or semantic access (for example, poor reading comprehension), disrupted phonemic processes (for example, poor decoding of multisyllabic words), or combinations thereof
- Often occur concomitantly with oral language and written language disorders
- Familial history of learning disorder
- Indications of neurologic pathology

Dyslexia (reading disability)

It is estimated that, of all children with learning disabilities, 80% present with dyslexia, a reading disability (Table 24.1). Due to differences of opinion in how dyslexia is assessed and determined, dyslexia may be even more prevalent (Shaywitz 2003). Using the 2003 definition, the International Dyslexia Association defines dyslexia as:

> [A] specific learning disability that is neurobiological in origin. It is characterized by difficulties with accurate and/or fluent word recognition and by poor spelling and decoding abilities. These difficulties typically result from a deficit in the phonological component of language that is often unexpected in relation to other cognitive abilities and the provision of effective classroom instruction. Secondary consequences may include problems in reading comprehension and reduced reading experience that can impede growth of vocabulary and background knowledge. (Lyon et al. 2007)

In the past, attempts were made to differentiate dyslexia into subtypes, such as surface dyslexia (greater difficulty decoding irregular words), deep or phonologic dyslexia (difficulty reading regular words and nonwords), and dyseidetic dyslexia (difficulty recognizing letters and their meaning). Neurophysiologic and neuroimaging studies have supported the conclusion that dyslexia is primarily an inability to decode written language due to impairment in phonologic (or phonemic) awareness (knowledge that words can be broken down into smaller units of sound). Three areas of the brain are required to effectively read: the anterior region, temporoparietal region, and the occipitotemporal region (Pugh et al. 2000). It is hypothesized that repeated reading of a word transfers it from the anterior area, through the parieto-temporal area, and to the occipito-temporal area. As a reader becomes more sophisticated and experienced, the occipito-temporal area is relied on more heavily and the anterior area becomes less active. However, dyslexic readers increase their reliance on the anterior area as they mature. This limits the reader to attempting word analysis without recall of word form and transfer of letters into sounds, thereby limiting fluency and impeding reading speed and comprehension (Booth 2001; Lyon et al. 2007; Pugh et al. 2000; Shaywitz 2003; Shaywitz & Shaywitz 2004).

A small number of individuals with dyslexia may have difficulties with the spatial skills needed for letter recognition, sequencing, or with comprehension of written language due to inadequate sight vocabulary or recall of earlier text. These skills are localized in the occipito-temporal area.

The gap in reading skills increases as the nonimpaired reader becomes more adept in word recognition and automaticity. Because of these difficulties, affected individuals may actively avoid any task that requires sustained reading, leading to a further worsening in ability from lack of practice. Since school and life performance usually demands an adequate ability to read, this block in phonologic analysis interferes with the ability to understand written text and limits learning and job opportunities.

Dyscalculia (mathematics disability)

Mathematics skills appear to be innate. Elementary abilities, such as counting, one-to-one correspondence, quantities, and volumes, are usually present by kindergarten age. Later milestones include writing three-digit numbers, addition and subtraction by age 8 years, and aptitude in multiplication and division by age 10–12 years. Failure to achieve these milestones without more global cognitive impairment defines dyscalculia. Onset by age 6 years is manifested as problems with simple addition and basic math facts. In 10-year-olds, the dysfunction includes difficulties with retrieval of learned information (such as multiplication tables and simple addition and subtraction), with manipulating money, and with following the appropriate sequence for calculation (Table 24.2).

Table 24.2 Disorders of mathematical functioning (dyscalculia)

Discriminating features
- At least average verbal or nonverbal intellectual potential
- Significant discrepancy between intellectual potential and performance on measures of mathematics achievement

Consistent features
- Not a unitary disorder; heterogeneous population demonstrating a variety of levels of functioning in facets of mathematical performance
- Deficient functioning in any one or combination of performing written and oral mathematic calculations or comprehension and application of mathematic concepts

Variable features
- Occur concomitantly with other handicapping conditions or extrinsic influences but are not primarily attributed to either
- Deficient performance in skills representing either language-based disorder (for example, poor comprehension of instructional vocabulary), disrupted visual-nonverbal processing (for example, inaccurate reading of operations signs), or a combination thereof
- May be associated with poor eye-hand coordination, poor tactile form recognition, finger agnosia, cognitive inflexibility, gross motor incoordination, and poor socioemotional adjustment, if the disorders are not language-based

Those with developmental disorders in math represent a heterogeneous group due to the complexity of processing necessary to reason mathematically or calculate (Geary 1993). A number of studies investigating subtypes of mathematical disabilities have suggested that at least three types may be identified: those with visual-perceptual deficits; those with linguistic deficits, including reading; and those with deficits in both areas (Spreen & Haaf 1986). Those with visual-perceptual deficits only exhibit visual-spatial orientation difficulties (e.g., right–left orientation problems), general psychomotor incoordination (e.g., problems characteristic of dysgraphia), and impaired tactile discrimination (e.g., finger agnosia). This pattern of abilities and deficits appears to be compatible with relatively deficient right hemisphere systems. Mechanical math errors associated with visual-perceptual deficits include difficulty aligning numbers for calculation or conceptualizing mathematical values related to relative size or distance, directionality (i.e., proceeding from right to left when the problem is arranged vertically and left to right when the problem is arranged horizontally), of operational signs or numbers, inattention to the significance of sequence (e.g., 574/547), missing or adding a step in calculation of multistep problems, and difficulties writing numbers. Those with linguistic deficits may present with both math and reading/spelling deficits. Features include difficulty understanding the words used to describe operations or word meanings in application problems, difficulty recalling the auditory equivalents of numerical symbols that affect oral problem solving and oral number fact drills, difficulty remembering steps in multistep problems, and avoidance of problems that require reading printed words (Geary 2004; Johnson & Myklebust 1967). These characteristics are representative of relatively deficient left hemisphere systems. Strang and Rourke (1985) have found that the majority of children who experience difficulties in arithmetic calculation have deficiencies in one or more linguistic abilities.

In addition to the mathematical disorders due to visual-perceptual, linguistic, or mixed deficits, some posit a fourth subgroup differentiated by specific deficits in nonverbal symbolic representation and quantitative thinking (Geary 1993; Johnson & Myklebust 1967). Individuals within this subgroup evidencing disorders of nonverbal thinking may demonstrate inability to estimate calculation outcomes, count meaningfully (i.e., establish one-to-on correspondence), grasp the meaning of process signs, interpret graphs or maps, follow a sequence of logical steps toward problem solutions, monitor performance, shift set (as when two separate operations are required to solve a problem), and control impulsivity in problem-solving strategies (Moses 1984; Pellegrino & Goldman 1987).

Researchers have traditionally devoted comparatively little attention to mathematical abilities of individuals with learning disabilities as compared with performance in other areas (Pellegrino & Goldman 1987). Carpenter's (1985) survey of elementary and secondary school learning disabilities teachers indicated that the average student with learning disorders spends one-third of his time in special education on instruction in mathematics. Comorbidity of reading and mathematics disabilities is well documented (Kulak 1993), such that many children diagnosed early as reading disabled will eventually display deficiencies in mathematics learning as well (Light & DeFries 1995).

Dysgraphia (writing disability)

The majority of individuals with learning disabilities have communicative difficulties in the acquisition and use of written language (Adelman & Vogel 1991). The written form of language is the most sophisticated and complex type of communication. It requires a level of abstraction not equaled in oral language since it is removed in time and space from its intended audience. Whereas oral speech is generally acquired spontaneously, the ability to communicate in writing is a result of conscious effort and explicit instruction. Writing requires the intention to communicate, formulation of the message, retrieval of auditory and corresponding graphic language symbols, sequencing of the content, and planning and execution of the graphomotor sequences necessary for writing. (Gaddes & Edgell 1994) (Table 24.3).

Table 24.3 Writing disorders (dysgraphia)

Discriminating features
- At least average verbal or nonverbal intellectual potential
- Significant discrepancy between intellectual potential and performance on measures of writing

Consistent features
- Not a unitary disorder; demonstrating a variety of levels of functioning in facets of writing performance
- Deficient functioning in any one or combination of motor control or planning affecting legibility, spelling, syntax and grammaticality, word retrieval, ideation, or formulation

Variable features
- Occur concomitantly with other handicapping conditions or extrinsic influences but are not primarily attributed to either
- Deficient performance in skills representing either disrupted visuomotor, auditory and verbal (for example, syntax or dysphonetic spelling errors), visual and verbal (for example, over-phoneticized spellings, capitalization omissions), or combined processing deficits
- May occur concomitantly with reading and oral language disorders

Problems with writing occur at several levels (Berninger et al. 2006). Children with underlying motor difficulties (dyspraxia) can have problems with the mechanical aspects of putting words on paper with a writing instrument. An inability to adequately copy and, therefore, correctly make letter shapes and connections can also interfere with this motor component. Higher-order language- and memory-based impairments can lead to problems recalling and writing appropriate names, adequately sequencing or remembering the core components of written paragraphs, attending to the mechanical or conceptual aspects of writing, overcoming inherent problems due to an underlying developmental language disorder, or implementing abstraction skills. Difficulty with spelling is frequently associated with dyslexia or an underlying developmental language disorder (Basso & Marangolo 2000; Blondis 1999; Cotelli et al. 2003; Gubbay & deKlerk 1995; Hamstra-Bletz & Blote 1993; Levine 1999; Mather 2003, Miozzo & De Bastiani 2002; Shaywitz 2004).

Dysphasia (oral language disability)

Of all the problems experienced by children with disorders of higher cortical function, those with oral language impairments may be the most prevalent (Wiig & Semel 1984). It is estimated that 90% of youths classified as learning disabled have oral language disorders (Gough et al. 1992; Liberman et al. 1984; Vellutino 1991). Normal language acquisition requires that a child learn to hear and discriminate different phonemes, recognize the subtle auditory speech cues that occur in temporal sequence, master the motor skills of articulation, and relate language ability to experiences needed to understand its meaning (Gaddes & Edgell 1994) (Table 24.4).

Developmental dysphasia includes disorders related to understanding and receiving linguistic information and using language for meaningful communication. Children with impaired receptive language may have deficits at different levels of language ability. Problems in aural processing may result in inconsistent or absent response to language, frustration, difficulty with attention and self-control, echolalic verbalizations, and/or inability to follow verbal directions. Difficulty with abstract concepts

Table 24.4 Language disorders (dysphasia)

Discriminating features
- At least average verbal or nonverbal intellectual potential
- Significant discrepancy between intellectual potential and performance on measures of oral language functioning

Consistent features
- Not a unitary disorder; heterogeneous population demonstrates a variety of levels of functioning in facets of receptive and expressive language
- Occur concomitantly with disorders in other verbal symbol systems such as reading, writing, and math applications
- Deficient functioning in any one or combination of auditory discrimination, memory, comprehension, temporal sequencing, syntax, grammaticality, word retrieval, pragmatics, or formulation

Variable features
- Occur concomitantly with other handicapping conditions or extrinsic influences but are not primarily attributed to either
- Deficient performance in skills representing either a receptive, expressive, or global language disorder
- Delayed language acquisition
- Indications of neurologic pathology
- Familial history of learning disorder

such as *before/after*, *few/many*, and *all/except* is characteristic. Because oral language is based on intentional meaning, perceiving the nuances of inferred meaning is often problematic. Understanding the significance of meta-linguistic elements, such as prosody, may also be impaired (Stark et al. 1991).

Most children with difficulty in understanding language also have expressive language disorders. Impaired expressive language and limited syntax may be present when receptive understanding is limited. Children can have expressive disorders related to auditory-motor execution of speech; word retrieval; sequencing sounds in words, words in sentences, or sentences in text; analyzing oral language into component parts (i.e., words into sounds, syllables, or sentences into words); and/or syntax. Dysfunction can also involve higher-order skills in semantics, oral formulation and organization of ideas, and pragmatics (Curtiss & Tallal 1985; Johnston & Kamhi 1984; Leonard 1989; Vogel 1983). Deficient performance may be observed in finding the desired word to express an idea, naming the days of the week, counting in sequence, or naming items in a common category. Sound reversals or substitutions (e.g., *binglejells/jinglebells*) and generally poor oral fluency (owing to word retrieval difficulty or difficulty planning and organizing expression) often occur. Deficits in oral language development, such as sound discrimination, sequencing, and understanding of abstract linguistic concepts, often affect other language-related functions and limit general academic achievement. Oral reading performance, reading comprehension, spelling, written expression, and arithmetic reasoning may be affected (Kamhi & Catts 1989; Stanovich 1991).

Nonverbal learning disability

The syndrome of nonverbal learning disability (NLD or right hemisphere learning disability) has been conceptualized as the association of impairments in social/interpersonal skills, visuospatial and directionality abilities, fine and gross motor coordination, and academic dysfunction in reading comprehension, arithmetic, and subjects requiring abstract and problem solving skills (Table 24.5). Manifestations include problems in social interaction, adjusting to unexpected transitions, activity level (increased or decreased), manipulation of objects (scissors, dressing), handwriting, concept formation, complex problem solving, reading comprehension, and arithmetic. As a result of these deficits, a child's social imperception may limit her social growth and significantly affect reasoning and adaptive behavior. Thus, nonverbal learning disabilities may have more profound negative effects than verbal disabilities since they distort fundamental life experience (Badian 1996; Semrud-Clikeman & Hynd 1991). In social situations, individuals with a nonverbal learning disability are unable to readily interpret novel information and, therefore, tend to respond in scripted, matter-of-fact verbal responses. Rote memorization of verbal information is a

Table 24.5 Disorders of nonverbal functioning

Discriminating features
- At least average verbal intellectual potential
- Significant discrepancy between intellectual potential and performance on measures of nonverbal functioning

Consistent features
- Not a unitary disorder, heterogeneous population demonstrating a variety of levels of functioning on nonverbal tasks
- Occur concomitantly with relative proficiency in rote verbal capacities necessary for aspects of reading and spelling performance

Variable features
- Occur concomitantly with other handicapping conditions or extrinsic influences but are not primarily attributable to either
- Deficits in tactile perception, psychomotor coordination, and visuospatial and organizational functioning
- Deficits in aspects of complex language functioning (that is, understanding inference and humor, figurative language, language pragmatics)
- Deficits in social perception, judgment, and social interaction
- Psychiatric complications including depression

Pearls and Perils

- Disorders of higher cortical function are more prevalent in children with genetic syndromes and acquired conditions that directly impact on brain development. Individuals with these disorders require close monitoring and heightened vigilance and awareness to ensure early identification of learning difficulties.
- Evidence supports the impression that a neuropathologic underpinning exists for disorders of higher cerebral function in children. This should be clearly communicated to parents, affected individuals, and educational personnel to avoid inappropriate conclusions of laziness or poor effort as reasons for poor performance.
- Testing instruments used to identify intellectual potential and patterns of achievement or processing performance are imprecise and potentially influenced by many factors. The way in which a child achieves the score is more significant than the score itself. Therefore, caution in interpretation of raw data is necessary.
- Cultural and stylistic differences must be considered when interpreting the test or school performance of children from minority populations.
- It is important to remember that tests, such as those of memory or perception, are related to skills such as reading and mathematics by theoretical assumptions. These theories can change over time. Therefore, the physician, psychologist, and allied educational personnel must be aware of the way in which this relationship is represented, especially to individuals who are not familiar with the theoretical basis of test conclusions.
- Effective intervention should be developmentally appropriate and based on proven theoretical constructs and evaluation results. Use of predetermined rote remedial treatments that are not based on the child's specific areas of strength and weakness and required needs can compromise generalization and transfer of learning.
- It is important to understand the impact of disorders of higher cortical function on the child's school, home, and social environments.
- Identification of common comorbid conditions, such as attention deficit hyperactivity disorder, dyspraxia, and social skills impairment, is needed for the development of appropriate educational interventions and the understanding of the impact of disorders of higher cortical function on the child's daily functioning.
- The pursuit of alternative therapies by families of children with disorders of higher cortical function should be done in conjunction with implementation of proven interventions. This will provide the child with the greatest opportunity for earliest intervention and maximal achievement.

strength that often masks their difficulty in understanding concepts (Matte & Bolaski 1998).

Epidemiology

The prevalence of learning disabilities is about 10–20% and depends on the diagnostic criteria, assessment tools, and population sample being used. For example, the United States Department of Education estimate of 5% only identifies those children receiving special education services and classified as having a learning disability.

Dyslexia is reported to be the most common learning disability, present in about 40–80% of those with the diagnosis of learning disability, and has a prevalence of 5–17%. Although early studies suggested a male predominance, more recent research reports nearly equal male–female distribution. Dyscalculia occurs in about 3–6% of the population with either no gender or greater female predominance. Prevalence estimates range from 6% to 26% of those identified as learning disabled; Fletcher and Loveland (1986) estimated that 18% of their population evidenced specific deficits in mathematics, whereas McLeod and Armstrong (1982) reported 26% of their population experienced selective impairments in mathematics. Problems with written expression are estimated in 2–8% of school-aged children, more so in boys. Dyspraxia is reported in 5–15% of children (Beitchman et al. 1998; Shapiro 2001; Shaywitz & Shaywitz 1999; Shelav et al. 2000).

More than one learning disorder can occur in the same individual. Language-based disorders such as dyslexia, dysgraphia, and higher-order written language dysfunction can co-occur and may be preceded in the preschool years by a developmental language disorder. Dyslexia and dyscalculia can coexist and result in worsened performance in testing compared to either disorder alone. The combination of dyscalculia, dysgraphia, finger anomia, and right–left confusion has been labeled *developmental Gerstman syndrome*, although no structural abnormality of the angular gyrus of the dominant parietal lobe is usually present, unlike in the acquired adult form. Co-occurrence of learning disability with ADHD has been categorized in the past as minimal brain dysfunction (ADHD, perceptual-motor problems, and language-based learning disability) and, more recently, as dysfunction of attention, motor function, and perception (DAMP) (Beitchman et al. 1998; Blondis 1999; Fletcher et al. 1999; Levine 1999; Shaywitz & Shaywitz 1999; Surresh & Sebastian 2000).

Neurobiology

Learning disabilities are clearly linked to various syndromes. Language-based learning disability is more prevalent than expected in disorders having an extra sex chromosome, such as 47,XXX, Klinefelter syndrome and 47,XYY. Girls with Turner syndrome can have dyscalculia, dysgraphia, and social skills deficits. Learning disability is higher in prevalence in neurofibromatosis, Tourette syndrome, treated phenylketonuria (more so in mathematics), and fragile X syndrome (with relative visuospatial and executive function weaknesses). Children with William syndrome have relative strengths in expressive language with atypical word choices on naming tasks and relative deficits in semantics and grammar that are masked by their good verbal memory. However, they have significant problems with visuospatial skills involving the ability to perceive parts and reconstruct items. Anatomically, they have relatively smaller occipital and posterior parietal areas in addition to microcephaly. Children with velo-cardio-facial syndrome have an average IQ of 70 (typical range 50–100) with emergence of a learning disability at or after second grade, when educational demands shift to greater need for concept formation rather than rote memorization. They have relative deficits in visuospatial, perceptual motor, mathematics, and nonverbal reasoning (problem solving, abstraction and planning) skills that persist through adulthood. Individuals with periventricular nodular heterotopia (PNH), a disorder of neuronal migration, have a discrepancy between reading skills and intelligence similar to that seen in patients with developmental dyslexia (Beitchman et al. 1998; Bruandet et al. 2004; Chang et al. 2005; Molko et al. 2003; Rivera et al. 2002).

Conditions occurring after birth that have a higher risk of learning disability include prematurity and low birth weight, meningitis and encephalitis, TBI, stroke, lead poisoning, and pediatric epilepsy (Gaddes & Edgell 1994). Significant prematurity typically results in children with normal intelligence, learning disabilities, and attention deficits. The degree and nature of cognitive dysfunction after CNS infection and head trauma is dependent on the severity of the initial condition and the localization of anatomic lesions/brain dysfunction. Stroke is associated with delays in language development, especially in the preschool years. Verbal IQ may be higher than performance IQ, with potential problems in attention, memory, and visuospatial skills (Nass 1997). Language-based learning disability is more common in those with concomitant epilepsy (Doose et al. 1996). Lead poisoning can be associated with executive function problems and language-based learning disability, reflecting the purported anatomic dysfunction in frontal lobes and deep gray nuclei (Finkelstein et al. 1998). Known environmental factors in at-risk populations include low socioeconomic status, limited exposure to educational opportunities and home-based language stimulation, and impaired nutritional status (Beitchman et al. 1998; Grigorenko 2001; Shapiro 2001; Shaywitz & Shaywitz 1999). In educational settings, the identification of a TBI, epilepsy, or other physical causes of learning difficulties will often be labeled a physical disability rather than a learning disability.

Despite the large number of potential causative conditions, the most likely reasons for learning disabilities are familial and genetic predispositions. Dyslexia is the most studied learning disability. Twin studies have shown a higher concordance rate for dyslexia in identical compared to dizygotic twins. Studies have consistently shown the familial patterns in dyslexia. If a family member has a reading disability, a higher than expected probability exists that other relatives will also have reading problems. This risk increases in proportion to the nearness of the relationship (i.e., higher for a sibling than a cousin). The mode of transmission is uncertain, although polygenic or dominant inheritance is most likely. Linkages to loci on chromosomes 1, 2, 3, 6, 13, 15, and 18 have been established, some suggesting an association with specific components of the reading process (phonological, awareness, automatic reading, and memory). A candidate gene, *DYX1C1*, on chromosome 15 has been reported. How this genetic predisposition interacts with potential environmental factors is still inadequately defined (Francks et al. 2002; Grigorenko 2001; Taipale et al. 2003).

The biologic tendency for learning disabilities appears to manifest as abnormalities in brain anatomy. Pathologic studies have demonstrated a lack of asymmetry of the planum temporale (posterior portion of the superior temporal lobe), microscopic ectopias and dysplasia in both frontal and left language areas, and minicolumnar abnormalities. Volumetric magnetic resonance imaging (MRI) studies have been equivocal in confirming the lack of planum temporale asymmetry, although differences from control subjects in other anatomic areas, such as the basal ganglia, frontal language region, and parietal lobe, have been reported. This lack of concordance between studies may be explained by measurement techniques and specific characteristics of the test subjects (Casanova et al. 2002; Grigorenko 2001; Habib 2000).

Functional studies of reading dysfunction using electrophysiologic techniques such as electroencephalographic (EEG) activity and event-related potentials have shown that dyslexic individuals fail to differentiate between meaningful compared to meaningless reading stimuli. However, localization of the area of dysfunction using electrophysiology is limited (although magnetoencephalography has been helpful). Functional neuroimaging has revolutionized the examination of reading ability by using positron emission tomography (PET) and fMRI techniques. Studies using these techniques have resulted in identification of brain areas activated by reading. In the left hemisphere there is a posterior reading system with ventral and dorsal components. The dorsal part (the angular and supramarginal gyri of the parietal lobe and posterior portion of the superior temporal gyrus) is thought to mediate phonologic analysis. The ventral portion, located in the lateral extra-striate and inferior occipital-temporal region, is related to memory-based word identification. The left hemispheric anterior system is located around the Broca area in the inferior frontal lobe and is involved in silent reading, naming, and phonemic articulatory processing (Grigorenko 2001; Habib 2000; Pugh et al. 2000; Shaywitz 2004).

The prevailing theory about the functional disruption in dyslexia is based on the need for appropriate processing of phonologic and lexical–semantic features of words. Dysfunction of the dorsal component of the posterior circuits leads to failure to adequately phonologically decode the written word and may be caused by the anatomic abnormalities described in neuropathologic studies. The dysfunction does not allow transference of processed information to the ventral component. Therefore, the individual is unable to develop fast and automated "sight word" reading ability. As a consequence, the dyslexic reader tries to compensate by relying more on the anterior circuit and by activating the right hemispheric areas homologous to the posterior circuitry. This results in a reliance on covert pronunciation as a means of phonologic decoding (inferior frontal region–based) and nonphonologic visuosemantic pattern recognition (right posterior hemisphere–based), both less efficient in developing mature and functional reading skills. Whether the initial dysfunction has a selective effect on one cognitive process or results in disruption of all processes in the area of the initial abnormality is still debated (Grigorenko 2001; Habib 2000; McCandliss & Noble 2003; Shaywitz & Shaywitz 1999; Shaywitz & Shaywitz 2005).

Several other theories exist (Habib 2000). The "magnosystem" theory is based on the concept of a visual processing deficit. Children with dyslexia process visual information more slowly than their peers and have problems with letter confusion. The underlying dysfunction involves the visual processing of information by sustained (parvosystem) and transient (magnosystem) visual channels. Usually, the sustained channel inhibits the transient channel and allows processing of the written word without interference from preceding words. Failure of this inhibition results in dyslexia. There is anatomic and electrophysiological evidence for this theory, although not all studies are confirmatory.

The temporal-processing theory states that reading problems are caused by deficits in the brain's ability to process the rate and temporal features of stimuli. This could cause problems processing transient auditory stimuli, such as consonants, and result in difficulties with rapid processing skills in reading, such as letter order and sight word perception, and a generalized dysfunction in temporal order skills. Electrophysiologic studies have demonstrated problems in analyzing temporal sound features in individuals with developmental dyslexia. Children with developmental language disorder have been shown to have impairment in processing rapidly changing auditory stimuli, such as consonant-vowel syllables (Tallal 2000). However, this finding has not been consistently corroborated for visually based language (reading). Finally, individuals with dyslexia have problems with motor skills, time awareness, calendar sequencing, and temporal distance. These observations have been used to support this theory and to extend the sphere of dysfunction to spelling and mathematics.

The cerebellar deficit hypothesis claims that a general impairment exists in the ability to automatically perform skills. This leads to an inability to develop fluency in reading and other skills, such as motor coordination, spelling, and writing. The core deficit resides within the cerebellum (Nicolson et al. 2001).

The biologic basis of other learning disabilities is less well defined. Investigations into normal mathematics skills suggest involvement of anterior and posterior areas in cerebral hemispheres, including simple multiplication in the left parietal cortex, arithmetic in both prefrontal and inferior frontal cortices, and number size/relations in both parietal lobes. Only a limited number of studies have examined individuals with dyscalculia. Functional studies localized dysfunction to the parietal regions. Volumetric MRI studies in prematurely born children with dyscalculia demonstrated less gray matter in an area of the left parietal lobe. Problems with motor coordination may be due to cerebellar deficits, although the research in this area is sparse and does not exclude dysfunction in other areas such as the peri-rolandic region and basal ganglia (Bruandet et al. 2004; Isaacs 2001; Shalev et al. 2000; Shalev & Gross-Tsur 2001).

Evaluation

Frequently, the physician is the first professional approached by the family with concerns regarding developmental functioning. The goals of the assessment should include recognition of learning problems, referral for appropriate academic testing, monitoring of intervention methods and their impact, and identification of comorbid conditions.

A complete and detailed history is essential in the diagnosis of learning disabilities. Information about prenatal and perinatal events as well as developmental milestones can identify risk factors (Table 24.6). Review of available school records and teacher reports can contribute important information.

The medical examination can help identify underlying syndromes (such as neurofibromatosis or fragile X syndrome) that can be associated with learning disabilities. Screening of hearing and vision is important. However, a

Table 24.6 Medical history: clues of underlying learning disabilities

Family history

- Prematurity
- Underlying syndrome
- Past central nervous system insult
- Development
  - Developmental language disorder
  - Difficulty learning alphabet letters/number symbols
  - Problem with letter-sound association
- Present skills
  - Isolated academic difficulty (reading, math)
  - Slow and dysfluent reading
  - Impaired spelling
  - Inability to learn rote math skills
  - Poor school performance with normal development

Table 24.7 Motor milestones

Skill	Age (years)
Stand on one foot	3
Draw a circle	3
Draw a cross	3.5
Throw a ball	4
Button	4
Draw a square	4.5
Cut with scissors	5
Print name	5
Hop (repetitive)	5
Draw a triangle	5.5
Skip	6
Catch a thrown ball	6
Finger identification	8
Rapid finger apposition	9
Absent mirror movements	11
Necker cube	12

child may pass the screening but still have a hearing or visual impairment that the screening was not sensitive enough to detect. For instance, a child may have difficulty hearing only when background noise is present. In a screening, this would not be evident, as all background noise is blocked out during the evaluation; however, in the classroom this would place the child at a severe disadvantage as there is often a constant background noise of peers and classroom materials. The neurologic examination can identify associated conditions such as dyspraxia (developmental coordination disorder) that can aggravate learning problems. This requires knowledge of milestones for gross and fine motor skills that can be assessed during the examination (Table 24.7). Motor skills mature over time, with overflow and mirror movements common in preschool and early school-age children. However, the persistence of choreiform movements with arm extension and arm posturing with heel and toe walking, or the failure to develop mature trunk and extremity movements with gait (walk, run, skip) by middle school and adolescence may indicate the presence of immature neural integration and inherent clumsiness. Commonly used assessment scales include the Bruininks-Oseretsky Test of Motor Proficiency Scale, the Henderson Test of Motor Performance, the Test of Visuomotor Integration, and the Physical and Neurological Examination for Soft Signs (PANESS) (Blondis 1999; Denckla 1985).

Although the physician's office is not usually the place for extensive psychoeducational testing, screening for potential learning problems can be done. The child can be evaluated for ability to identify letters and numbers; demonstrate letter–sound relationships; read simple words, sentences, or paragraphs; write basic text, like names or dictated sentences; and show skills in mathematical calculation. These screening methods are not a replacement for the formal psychoeducational assessment that is mandatory for the identification of learning disabilities.

Comorbid conditions can aggravate or mimic learning disabilities. Therefore, the assessment should screen for features of ADHD, anxiety disorders, depression, and social skills deficits. Ongoing monitoring is necessary since learning problems can result in poor self-esteem, school avoidance, or social regression, especially during adolescence, with worsening academic performance or inappropriate classroom placement. Psychiatric consultation may be advisable.

Medical testing is usually not necessary in most children with learning disabilities. Electroencephalogram and neuroimaging should only be ordered if history or findings on examination suggest a structural brain abnormality or seizures. Epileptiform activity is sometimes present on the EEG of individuals with learning disabilities and may be secondary to the structural abnormalities causing the disability rather than to the cognitive effects of epileptiform activity. Therefore, its significance is uncertain. Treatment clearly depends on the facts of the clin-

Key Clinical Questions

- Are there other family members who have had:
  - Attention disorders? Reading difficulty?
  - Poor handwriting? or Experienced academic difficulties?
- Are there other family members who have taken medication for any attention disorders?

ical scenario. Similarly, clinical indications, not solely the presence of learning disabilities, should be the basis for ordering chromosomal analysis or metabolic testing. Research tools, such as PET scan, functional MRI, magnetoencephalography, or specialized electrophysiologic testing, have no role in the clinical evaluation. Educational assessment can assist in providing insights into an individual's strengths and learning style.

The physician should be part of a multidisciplinary team, including a psychologist/neuropsychologist, speech and language therapist, teachers, occupational therapist, physical therapist, and social worker. These specialists are necessary for the formal assessment of intelligence, academic achievement, language, and motor abilities that can identify learning disabilities and their comorbid disorders. The extent of the evaluation should be tailored to the concerns and needs of the individual child. The psychoeducational evaluation is most often completed through the local school system (an entitlement under the Individuals with Disabilities Education Improvement Act, IDEA), although concerns about school personnel bias, waiting lists, and funding limitations lead many parents to seek an evaluation outside the school system.

Treatment

Intervention is a long-term program requiring the input and cooperation of the child, family, school personnel, outside consultants, therapists, and physicians. The child and family need to become educated about the diagnosis and its impact. Learning the facts about learning disabilities and the entitlements provided by the IDEA (Office of Special Education Rehabilitative Services) is essential when planning for intervention. IDEA provides for modifications and accommodations in daily instruction and testing (both state and local), specialized instruction, and fundamentally, a free and appropriate education. Knowing the law and the medical implications of a learning disability can assist in making the individual an "informed consumer" and strong advocate for needed intervention and instruction. The family should know how to request a multidisciplinary evaluation and how to develop an individualized educational plan (IEP), including participation on the IEP team. Referral to local and national parent and consumer organizations helps establish a local network and support system. These include International Dyslexia Society (http://www.interdys.org), Learning Disabilities Association of America (http://www.ldanatl.org), All Kinds of Minds (http://www.allkindsofminds.org), the Center for Law and Education (http://www.cleweb.org), the National Information Center for Children and Youth with Disabilities (http://www.nichcy.org), and National Center for Learning Disabilities (http://www.ncld.org). In short, "knowledge is power."

Most academic interventions will occur within the school setting. Public schools are required by law to provide support services to any student who qualifies under the guidelines outlined in IDEA. A number of laws guide the education of all students. The newest comprehensive policy is No Child Left Behind (NCLB). A portion of this law specifically addresses the selection of intervention programs and limits schools to utilizing only scientifically based practices. Exactly which practices meet these requirements is still being debated as the regulations are implemented in the schools. Treatments that are based on existing theories of dyslexia are supported by brain imaging research (Aylward et al. 2003; Kujala et al. 2001; Temple et al. 2003). Functional MRI (fMRI) studies show improved activation from normal reading associated areas that mirrors the clinical improvement in reading ability and is not based on a specific type of intervention. However, since the clinical study populations have been small, study results have been marginal or not necessarily transferable to the real-world environment, and reproduction of results has not always been successful; further validation is required before these techniques are widely implemented or meet the requirements of NCLB. Most programs that focus on phonemic awareness and phonics, such as Wilson, have been shown to be effective by cognitive neuroscience and educational research. These programs provide direct instruction in using phonemes to determine words, recall the word quickly, and provide meaning. For more information on scientifically based practices, refer to the Council for Excellence in Government (http://www.excelgov.org), Doing What Works (http://dww.ed.gov), or the NCLB website (http://www.nclb.gov).

Law, policy, regulations, and neuroscience are the foundation for the chosen intervention. However, the key to an intervention's success is the child and the professionals supporting that child. Teachers, special education teachers, occupational therapists, physical therapists, speech and language therapists, psychologists, social workers, parents, and therapists for specific interventions or programs work together to create a cohesive environment to support the needs of the child while building on strengths. The teacher and special education support personnel work on the basics of reading, writing, and math skills. This includes using exercises for helping the student learn techniques such as phonologic awareness and decoding or mathematical computation. Occupational therapists can help improve motor skills in writing and daily living activities such as dressing and eating. Adaptive physical education can improve gross motor coordination. Speech and language therapists can improve a child's speech and language processing. Social skills training can strengthen the individual's ability to interact with peers and adults. Coordination of treatments is necessary for each intervention to be most effective. Regular communication between home, school, and outside therapists should be established early in the process. This does not necessarily mean a face-to-face meeting. Technology such as phone conferences, e-mail, and interactive webpages or chat rooms can be utilized. The result of this communication will be a list of accommodations or modifications that will ensure success and learning.

Accommodations are slight changes to the environment. These may include multiplication tables, calculators, word processors, preferential seating, assignments given in small pieces or steps, and extended time. There are three types of modifications: process, product, and content. Process refers to how a student will learn the content. Pre-written notes, small chunks of lecture at a time or videotaped lecture, and standing versus sitting are all examples of modified process. Product refers to what the student does to give evidence of knowledge. The most common product is a test or paper. For a student with dysgraphia, an oral report may provide a better measure of what the student has learned. Finally, content can be modified. The Revolutionary War may be difficult for a student with dysphasia or a nonverbal learning disability to conceptualize. However, a paper on why they think a school rule is unfair may help the student understand the basic premise and make a connection that is elaborated and abstracted as the student's level of educational sophistication increases. Modifications and accommodations can be provided throughout a student's education. Some universities and colleges also provide support for students with learning disabilities.

Periodic reevaluation of the effectiveness of any chosen treatment on a regular basis and implementation of needed program changes is important. The affective needs of the individual should also be regularly evaluated. The stresses of learning disabilities can have an impact on the individual and family members, resulting in poor self-esteem, acquisition of bad habits, depression, and, in some cases, family disruption such as divorce. Counseling can help address these issues, provide advice on behavior management strategies, and teach coping skills to deal with stressors. Utilization of an individual's strengths is another way to support self-esteem and self-concept. Furthermore, by utilizing a child's aptitude, an instructional intervention can be designed that will then remediate learning deficits when a cognitive impairment is absent.

With the introduction of NCLB and the reauthorization of IDEA (2004), the requirement to address the needs of all students has now been federally mandated. Response to intervention (RTI) is a model designed to support students with a focus on early identification and intervention, thereby reducing the time and expense inherent in the typical identification systems. Response to intervention models are dynamic and base identification on the assessment of ability changes over time. By tying multiple assessment measures to targeted intervention, the construct of unexpected underachievement can be operationalized on the basis that adequate progress, as a response to instruction that is effective with most individuals (Fuchs & Fuchs 1998; Gresham 2002), has not occurred. Individuals who do not show progressive growth from increasingly intense instruction should be further evaluated as having a learning disability. The National Research Council's most recent report (Donavon & Cross 2002), along with various other publications addressing learning disability identification (Bradley et al. 2002; President's Commission on Excellence in Special Education 2002), specify that one strong predictor of a learning disability is that the individual does not respond to appropriate instruction and high-quality intervention.

Response to intervention has foundational roots in the public health models of disease prevention, which led to the development of more comprehensive intervention practices (Vaughn et al. In press). These models were originally designed to avert behavior problems in the educational setting (Donavon & Cross 2002). Response to intervention is a process, not a single approach or model; therefore, considerable variation exists in the design and implementation process. The primary goal is to enhance educational opportunities for all children, not simply to identify students as learning disabled or requiring special education. Effective implementation incorporates three essential components: (a) reliable and valid measures that are sensitive to intervention and allow for multiple administrations over time (Stecker et al. 2005); (b) authenticated intervention protocols for targeted outcomes (Vaughn et al. 2003a), and (c) incorporates a school-level model that delineates a system for screening, intervention, and placement (Vaughn et al. In press).

Response to intervention models do not represent new classification categories for learning disabilities, but rather evaluate the discrepancy between unexpected underachievement and assessment of learning and development over time (Flecher et al. 2003). The process of discrepancy classification is fraught with a host of issues comparable to the more traditional normative classification systems and continues to be moderately subjective. The decision process requires a definition of the academic skills/abilities to be evaluated and the criteria for expected progress over time based on multiple assessments administered at periodic intervals. Consequently, unexpected underachievement is quantified on the basis of a discrepant response to the delivery of effective instruction measured by multiple assessments. With this foundation, identification entails stipulating criteria for categorizing individuals into subsets based on whether or not they responded to the delivered intervention.

The evidence from both research and school-based implementations indicate that RTI models can enhance student outcomes and reduce rates of referrals to special education (Burns et al. 2005; VanDerHeyden & Burns 2005). Essential to RTI is a fundamental adjustment to the identification process. By focusing on early identification and utilization of successive measures, the RTI identification method shifts from the traditional model of comparing two different abilities (ability to ability comparison) utilizing one measure at a single point in time to evaluating individual ability as it responds to intervention (ability to change) over time. Furthermore, by utilizing multiple measures, a more accurate estimation of growth can be determined on an individualized basis. Therefore, RTI models have the promise of incorporating functional outcomes, which are tied to intervention response and incorporate more meaningful criteria into the identification and intervention process. Another treatment option that has shown promising outcomes is the use of pharmaceutical therapies. Although medication has no significant effect on learning disabilities, it can lessen dysfunction by reducing the impact of comorbid conditions. Attention deficit hyperactivity disorder, depression, and anxiety can be effectively treated with multimodal interventions that include the judicious use of medication. Claims of the efficacy of treatments using vitamins and minerals, elimination diets, vision training, special eyeglasses, and electrophysiologic retraining continue to be made. At this time, these have little, if any, research to support their use. The physician should be knowledgeable about these claims and should be able to answer family questions.

Consider Consultation When...

- Initial psychoeducational testing does not identify the reason for the child's underachievement.
- There are discrepancies in the findings of different evaluations.
- Present educational intervention has not successfully narrowed the discrepancy between achievement and potential.
- A concern exists about the appropriateness of service delivery for the child.
- The school is not fulfilling its legal obligation to provide a free and appropriate public education that meets the child's needs and fosters the achievement of his maximum potential in a least restrictive placement.
- Features of significant psychiatric disorders, such as anxiety or depression, are identified.
- Medical conditions or their treatment adversely affect the child's educational abilities.
- A disorder of higher cortical function is identified after years of adequate educational performance. Alternative causes for a deterioration in academic ability, such as epilepsy, brain tumor, stroke, or degenerative or neuropsychiatric disorders, must be considered.
- Poor academic performance is present in children who are at higher risk for disorders of higher cortical function.

Prognosis

Outcome studies in learning disabilities suggest that these are chronic and persistent disorders. The majority of individuals with dyslexia continue to be poor readers and do not catch up to their peers in reading abilities. Moderate-severe dyslexia and a lower socioeconomic status appear to be predictors of a less-than-optimal outcome. Positive influences include positive self-esteem and appropriate decisions on future goals and work choices. However, vocational placement is at a lower level than expected for intellectual level (Sanchez & Coppel 2000; Shaywitz et al. 1999; Shaywitz 2004).

Functional MRI studies have shown improved activation closer to normal controls in left hemispheric reading areas and in the right hemisphere for those who respond to intervention. In young adults with a history of dyslexia, fMRI demonstrated underactivation of posterior reading areas by compensated, but not fluent, readers, and different activation patterns by those with continued impairment (Shaywitz et al. 2003).

Follow-up information on individuals with dyscalculia is limited. Short-term improvement has been reported during the early school years. Adolescent outcomes of individuals who were symptomatic at age 10–11 years were poor, with 95% still scoring in the lowest 25% of their grade. Predictors of poor outcome included the severity of the dyscalculia and a positive family history. Those with nonverbal learning disabilities may also have difficulties in adulthood; this was also dependent on the severity of the childhood disorder (Dugbartey 2000; Shalev et al. 2005).

Psychiatric problems can occur during adolescence and adulthood. There is an increased rate of delinquency, depression, anxiety, and impaired social/interpersonal skills. Occupational placement is adversely influenced by a lower percentage of individuals who attend and graduate college, the severity and type of childhood learning disability, the individual's level of self-esteem, and the presence of comorbid psychiatric disorders. However, even if the learning disability limits job opportunities, most individuals achieve gainful employment and independent living (Beitchman et al. 1998).

With early intervention and coordinated services, the prognosis for children with learning disabilities can be positive. Continuing research will increase the likelihood that individuals with learning disabilities will have a successful future.

Annotated bibliography

Gaddes W, Edgell D. *Learning disabilities and brain function.* New York: Springer-Verlag, 1994.

The authors begin their volume by presenting information about the brain and learning and behavior, and relate this information to perceptual disorders, sensorimotor pathways in learning, attention, language, and learning disorders in academic areas. Clinical cases and associated treatment suggestions are also illustrative.

Johnson D, Myklebust H. *Learning disabilities: Educational principles and practices*. New York: Grune & Stratton, 1967.
A classic in the field of learning disabilities, this volume contains a series of informative chapters on the characteristics and treatment of childhood disorders of higher cognitive functioning. Chapters are organized according to areas of dysfunction, and an explicit attempt is made to relate underlying deficits in processing to behavioral manifestations in reading, arithmetic, and other areas of underachievement, as well as to associated treatments useful for educators.

Lyon GR, ed. *Frames of reference for the assessment of learning disabilities*. Baltimore: Brookes, 1994.
This volume provides a current understanding of assessment in learning disabilities in attention, executive function, oral language, and academic areas, and brings insight to a number of controversial issues related to assessment, such as the use of discrepancy formulas and measuring change over time.

Obrzut J, Hynd G, eds. *Neuropsychological foundations of learning disabilities*. San Diego: Academic Press, 1994.
This volume represents a scholarly treatment of the field of learning disabilities, including neurologic and genetic etiologic evidence, neuropsychological models of learning disabilities, treatments suggestions, and case studies.

Rourke BP, Fisk JL, Strang JD. *The neuropsychological assessment of children: A treatment-oriented approach*. New York: Guilford, 1986.
This volume presents a coherent treatment-oriented framework for evaluating and discussing assessment issues and provides detailed case studies that illustrate this framework, as well as major assessment and intervention issues in childhood neuropsychology. The strength of the text is in its use of illustrative case studies and attention to treatment issues, which are often neglected in favor of assessment issues.

Wong B, ed. *Learning about learning disabilities*. San Diego: Academic Press, 1991.
Wong's edited volume presents a varied treatment of learning disabilities including historical and research aspects of the field, and assessment and instructional issues from a number of perspectives and across the lifespan.

SECTION 3

COMMON PEDIATRIC NEUROLOGIC PROBLEMS

Barbara Olson

CHAPTER 25

Coma and Other States of Altered Awareness in Children

Stavros M. Hadjiloizou and James J. Riviello, Jr.

Outline

Coma, the extreme state of altered awareness with total unawareness of self and environment, is a medical emergency indicating a significant central nervous system (CNS) insult. Its pathophysiology involves either bilateral cortical dysfunction, brainstem dysfunction, or diffuse (metabolic) dysfunction.

The goals of coma therapy are: (a) adhere to the principles of neuroresuscitation, the A, B, and Cs; (b) immediately identify signs of intracranial pathology: herniation, increased intracranial pressure (ICP), or a focal neurologic examination; (c) identify and specifically treat the underlying cause; (d) determine prognosis; and (e) plan appropriate long-term therapy. We emphasize important aspects of the history, physical examination, and neurologic examination in the evaluation and treatment of coma.

Terminology

Consciousness is defined as the state of awareness of one's self and environment. Coma is the extreme state of altered awareness, without spontaneous eye opening, verbalization, or purposeful response to external stimulation of any type. However, gradations in the continuum of altered consciousness between full consciousness and coma are defined by the degree of stimulation needed to achieve purposeful responses. Imprecise and ambiguous terminology is used for these. Consciousness may also be heightened, as in delirium. The common terms used to differentiate these are described, although, to avoid confusion, it is best to describe the actual mental state and responses evoked by stimuli.

Delirium is a heightened mental state, characterized by disorientation, irritability, fearful responses, and sensory misperception. Hallucinations, usually visual, as well as delusions may occur. *Confusion* is a state of impaired ability to think and reason clearly, resulting in difficulty with orientation, simple cognitive processing, and acquisition of new memory. Confusion may occur in a depressed or activated mental state.

Gradations exist in depressed states. *Drowsiness* is a light sleep-like state with easy arousals and brief periods of alertness. *Obtundation* describes a patient who appears to be asleep when not stimulated. *Stupor* is a state in which the patient does not respond to verbal commands but can be aroused to some degree by vigorous, painful, or noxious stimulation.

The anatomic and physiologic basis of consciousness

Both wakefulness (arousal) and awareness are fundamental to maintain consciousness. The awake state requires the integrity of the reticular activating system (RAS), located in the upper brainstem and thalamus. The regions of the reticular formation extend from the rostral brainstem (midbrain and upper pontine tegmentum) to the lower thalamus (Moruzzi & Magoun 1949). The hypothalamus is also important for consciousness. Awareness, a higher cognitive function, is the combination of cognition and affect and is determined by the cerebral hemispheres. Integral consciousness requires an intact RAS, cerebral hemispheres, and healthy projections between the two systems.

Unconsciousness may be physiologic during sleep: a stimulus returns the person to normal consciousness. Coma and other alterations of consciousness result from three primary causes, occurring separately or in combination: (a) diffuse or multifocal bilateral cerebral dysfunction, (b) substantial damage to the RAS, or (c) impaired communication between these two regions. Diffuse dysfunction may occur with metabolic causes (i.e., drugs or toxins). The level of overall depression of consciousness is proportionate to the degree of cortical dysfunction. Unilateral cortical lesions should not impair arousal function unless there is secondary compression or compromise of the other hemisphere or reticular structures, as sometimes occurs with herniation syndromes. Small cortical lesions confined to one or both cerebral hemispheres or small portions of the RAS do not typically affect consciousness.

Key Clinical Questions

- What is the tempo of coma development?
- What is the patient's baseline function level?
- Is there history of trauma (including nonaccidental)?
- Is there evidence of meningitis?
- Is there history of seizures or status epilepticus?
- Is there history or evidence of substance abuse or toxicity?
- What is the patient's past medical history (e.g., diabetes)?
- Are there focal findings on neurologic examination?
- Are there signs of increased intracranial pressure or herniation on neurologic examination?

Coma etiology: A pathophysiologic approach

After stabilization, the clinician must immediately decide whether coma has a surgical cause, such as a structural brain lesion with necessary emergency neurosurgical intervention, or a medical cause (diffuse encephalopathic process caused by meningitis, seizures, or a metabolic reason).

Coma is typically divided into traumatic and nontraumatic causes. The basic mechanisms for coma are divided into two broad categories: structural lesions (usually more focal, may include trauma) or metabolic disorders (diffuse and symmetric). Structural lesions are further divided into supratentorial (hemispheric) and infratentorial (brainstem). Diffuse axonal injury is also considered in the structural group, occurring typically following trauma.

Focal neurologic signs are suggestive of a structural etiology, although may occasionally occur with diffuse or metabolic disorders. Supratentorial structural lesions that are bilateral can cause secondary damage to the RAS (e.g., herniation). Unilateral cerebral hemisphere lesions cause focal neurologic signs but usually not coma. Examples of structural lesions include trauma, subdural or epidural hematomas, tumors, stroke, and hydrocephalus. Nonaccidental trauma should be specifically considered in the infant. Congenital malformations should be excluded as a cause of hydrocephalus in the infant.

Infratentorial lesions may directly damage the RAS and may be relatively small in size. Examples include brainstem infarctions, hemorrhage, or tumors. Due to the anatomic proximity of the cerebellum, its lesions may cause secondary brainstem compression (such as cerebellar tumors in children or cerebellar hemorrhage in adults).

Metabolic etiologies cause the majority of cases in children and usually cause diffuse brain dysfunction, with a nonfocal examination. Examples of common pediatric primary neurologic causes include seizures (nonconvulsive status epilepticus or postictal state) and meningoencephalitis. Examples of systemic metabolic derangement that secondarily affect the CNS include accidental and intentional ingestions of drugs and toxins, systemic infections, anoxia, and metabolic disease. Inborn errors of metabolism and intussusception should be specifically considered in the infant. Of note, focality may be seen at times with some metabolic disorders like hyperglycemia, hypoglycemia, hyper- or hypocalcemia, hepatic encephalopathy, uremia, and some toxic ingestions. Subarachnoid hemorrhage, even if not metabolic in origin, may also be included in this category as it affects the brain in a more diffuse manner.

Herniation syndromes

The intracranial contents (brain, cerebrospinal fluid [CSF], blood) have a fixed volume (V) because of the bony confines of the skull. The volume of a lesion must also be included in the intracranial (IC) volume. This relation is shown by the Monro-Kellie equation (Stern 1963):

$$V_{IC} = V_{brain} + V_{CSF} + V_{blood} + V_{lesion}, \text{ (if present)}$$

The ICP is determined by the volume of these constituents. Within a fixed space, if the volume of any one component increases, there must be a compensatory decrease in the volume of other components, or the pressure will rise. This relationship is described by the volume-pressure curve. Brain tissue needs perfusion, which is dependent on a greater inflow than outflow pressure: if outflow pressure increases above inflow pressure, there will be no perfusion. The inflow pressure is related to the mean arterial pressure (MAP), and the outflow pressure is related to the intracranial and cerebral venous pressures. Compensation may occur for volume increases in one component; initially the CSF may shift into the spinal subarachnoid spaces, or the lesion might compress venous or interstitial structures.

The intracranial cavity is further divided by dural projections into smaller compartments; the tentorium separates the anterior and posterior fossae and the falx separates the two cerebral hemispheres. *Herniation* is the shifting of brain tissue—due to a pressure effect—from its normal position into a different compartment, resulting in neuronal compression, with resultant ischemia and hypoxemia. To compensate for initial increases in the ICP, the MAP will increase, thereby promoting perfusion. Within certain limits of the MAP, there is a constant delivery of blood to brain tissue; this is called *cerebral autoregulation*. However, when a certain MAP is reached, then an increase in CBF occurs. Ultimately, this increased blood pressure may further increase the ICP.

Different herniation syndromes have been described according to the direction of tissue displacement and/or dura in-folding involvement. A practical approach (Figure 25.1) is to divide herniation into vertical and horizontal. Coma associated with herniation was classically considered secondary to the vertical displacement of brain compartments. In a study (Ropper 1986) of altered awareness with a unilateral hemisphere mass, early alterations in awareness were associated with horizontal, rather than vertical displacement. Horizontal displacement of the pineal body of 0–3 mm from the midline was associated with alertness, 3–4 mm with drowsiness, 6–8 mm with stupor, and 8–13 mm with coma. Vertical herniation (downward/descending or upward/ascending) may be transtentorial (through the tentorial opening) or foraminal (through the foramen magnum). Two transtentorial syndromes have been described: the syndrome of central transtentorial herniation and the syndrome of lateral mass (uncal or hippocampal) transtentorial herniation. Horizontal herniation occurs when the cingulate gyrus shifts under the falx (transfalcial) and across the midline. Transcranial herniation refers to displacement of brain tissue after an open head injury.

Central transtentorial herniation syndrome is the result of increased supratentorial pressure, which secondarily causes caudal displacement of the diencephalon through the tentorial notch. Depending on the degree of pressure, there is a rostrocaudal progression of brainstem involvement, which is reflected by the clinical findings. The RAS involvement results in alteration of consciousness; and small but reactive pupils, at least initially, result from sympathetic hypothalamic output damage.

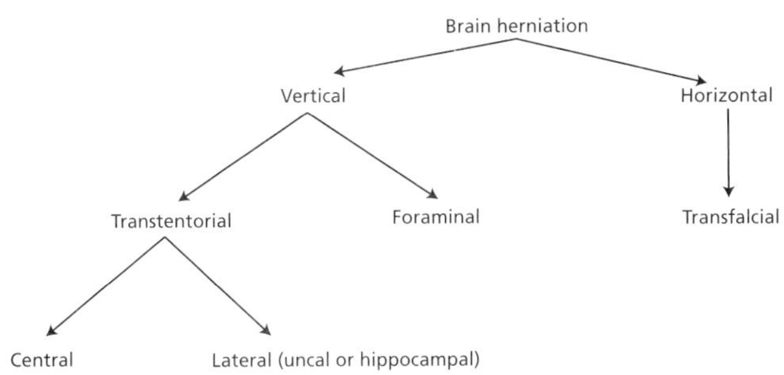

Figure 25.1 Different types of brain herniation.

Pearls and Perils

- Describe the actual mental state—avoid ambiguous terms. Describe the responses evoked by various stimuli.
- Keep fundamental anatomy and physiology in mind. Coma results from bilateral cortical and/or brainstem dysfunction, or diffuse (metabolic) dysfunction.
- During the initial evaluation and treatment, adhere to the fundamental principles of resuscitation, regardless of etiology.
- After stabilization, immediately decide whether focal signs suggestive of a structural process or signs of increased intracranial pressure (ICP) exist and if emergency neurosurgical consultation is needed.
- Remember: Papilledema may be absent even with documented increased ICP. If you have evidence of increased ICP, don't be reassured by its absence as it may take several hours to develop.
- Order a head CT scan as soon as the patient is stabilized:
  - In the presence of focal signs
  - Prior to a lumbar puncture when concerned about increased ICP.
- Do not delay antibiotic therapy while awaiting results or head CT scan, if meningitis is strongly suspected.
- Retrieve the tempo (evolution) of coma onset whenever possible; it will provide important clues about the underlying pathology.
- A detailed general physical examination is invaluable, especially when the history is not available; always exclude trauma, including nonaccidental.
- Localization clues:
  - The brainstem nuclei are in close proximity to structures involved in regulation of consciousness.
  - Ocular movement and pupillary function abnormalities are of critical importance.
- The most important factors to determine the outcome and prognosis are the underlying etiology and the duration of the comatose state.
- Somatosensory evoked potentials (SSEPs) have high positive predictive value for outcome.

Lateral mass (uncal or parahippocampal) transtentorial herniation syndrome is the result of lateral extracerebral or temporal lobe masses pushing the mesial temporal lobe (uncus anteriorly, parahippocampal gyrus posteriorly) between the ipsilateral aspect of the midbrain and the free edge of the tentorium (Brazis 2002). This results in compression of the third cranial nerve with subsequent dilatation of the ipsilateral pupil, and a contralateral hemiparesis. It is vital to recognize this stage promptly and intervene before occlusion of the posterior cerebral artery occurs, which may cause infarction. Altered consciousness is usually the result of lateral compression of the midbrain against the opposite tentorial edge by the displaced parahippocampal gyrus. The Kernohan notch sign ("false localizing sign") may be found occasionally and refers to hemiparesis and a Babinski response ipsilateral to the original lesion, as a result of compression of the opposite cerebral peduncle.

Upward transtentorial herniation may occur with a cerebellar mass lesion that may displace the cerebellum through the tentorial notch. This is most likely to happen in patients with ventriculostomy. Decerebrate posturing occurs with initially reactive and miotic pupils, progressing to anisocoria and pupillary dilatation.

Foraminal herniation occurs usually with downward displacement of the cerebellar tonsils into the foramen magnum (called *coning*) and secondary obstructive hydrocephalus. Compression of the medulla may produce apnea.

Transfalcial herniation occurs through compression of one hemisphere by the other anteriorly. This is inconsistently related to alertness, although very large anterior displacements may have caused stupor in some patients (Ropper 1986).

Approach to diagnosis

History

The time period over which coma develops provides clues about the underlying disease. Coma usually presents in one of three ways: a predictable progression of an underlying illness (e.g., widespread malignancy), an unpredictable event on a known medical background (e.g., cardiac arrhythmia), or a totally unexpected event (e.g., trauma, intoxication). Knowledge about specific preexisting conditions may provide clues for particular diagnostic considerations (Table 25.1).

General physical examination

A thorough systematic physical examination is important, especially when no history is available (an unresponsive patient). Table 25.2 lists useful findings in the physical that may help make a diagnosis.

Table 25.1 Useful historical hints related to particular diagnostic entities

Condition	Consider
Recent trauma	Hematoma or brain injury
Recent infection	Sepsis or meningitis
Headaches or personality change	Increased intracranial pressure (ICP)
Seizure disorder	Status epilepticus or postictal state
Medications or potential toxins	Ingestion (purposeful or accidental)
Metabolic disorder, i.e. diabetes	Hypo- or hyperglycemic coma
Cardiac disease	Arrhythmias or cardiac arrest
Pulmonary disease	Central nervous system infections, increased ICP

Neurologic examination

The neurologic examination is the cornerstone of localization in the comatose patient (Fisher 1969) and helps identify the underlying pathogenesis. It is important to examine the following (Riviello 1988):

- *Mental status (coma scales)*. Determination of level is important. An objective determination of the level of altered awareness is needed, especially when multiple caregivers assess a response to therapy or for prognosis, since interobserver variability occurs when describing the various states of altered awareness (lethargy to coma). The Glasgow Coma Scale (GCS) (Teasdale & Jennett 1974) is one objective measure (Table 25.3), using motor and verbal responses, which may not all be appropriate for infants and younger children. Although modified for children (Hahn et al. 1988), it is not appropriate for those younger than 2 years of age, has high interrater reliability, and is difficult to apply when intubated (Table 25.4). The CHOP infant face scale (Table 25.5) was developed for children younger than 2 years of age (Durham et al. 2000); this is also referred to as the Infant Face Scale (IFS), since it relies on the infant's crying and facial expressions. It differs from other scales by reliance on objective behavioral observations and assesses cortical and brainstem function; it parallels the GCS in scoring, but is based on infant behaviors and can be applied to the intubated child. In their prospective study, the interrater reliability was almost perfect when applied to infants, and when compared to the GCS, the GCS interrater reliability was fair.

Table 25.2 Physical examination findings related to particular diagnostic entities

Finding	Consider
Skin	
Ecchymoses	Trauma, child abuse, bleeding disorder
Petechiae	Meningococcal disease, Rocky Mountain spotted fever, bleeding disorder
Cyanosis	Inadequate oxygenation (cardiac or pulmonary disease)
Excessive sweating or pallor	Hypoglycemia or shock
Decreased skin turgor	Dehydration
Head	
Battle sign ("raccoon eyes")	Basilar skull fracture or bleeding disorder
Fundi	
Papilledema	Increased intracranial pressure (ICP)
Retinal hemorrhages	Child abuse, e.g., whiplash shaken infant syndrome
Ears	
Otitis	Meningitis or venous sinus thrombosis
Hemotympanum or otorrhea	Basilar skull fracture
Nose	
Rhinorrhea	Basilar skull fracture
Mouth	
Intraoral laceration	Trauma, seizure, stroke
Oral smell	Metabolic disorder, e.g., fruity with DKA; ethanol, etc.
Neck	
Nuchal rigidity	Meningitis, subarachnoid hemorrhage
Chest	
Respiratory distress	Airway obstruction or pneumonia
Heart	
Murmur or dysrhythmia	Embolism, brain abscess, endocarditis
Abdomen	
Hepatosplenomegaly	Liver disease
Tenderness	Perforation or trauma

- *Pupils (size, shape, reactivity)*. A preserved pupillary reaction to light implies a metabolic rather than structural etiology, since pupillary pathways are relatively resistant to metabolic insults. The pupils may be small, but generally symmetric and reactive pupils signify an intact midbrain. Unreactive pupils signify midbrain dysfunction (usually structural in etiology). A unilaterally dilated and unresponsive pupil indicates ipsilateral third nerve compression, usually related to uncal herniation of the temporal lobe associated with a contralateral hemiplegia. Midposition dilated pupils imply structural damage to the midbrain and may be seen with central herniation. However, several ingestions (atropine, scopolamine) may lead to unreactive large pupils. Small pupils may be seen with narcotic, barbiturate ingestions or with pontine lesions.
- *Oculomotor movements (normal, asymmetric, or absent)*. Conjugate gaze requires intact cranial nerves III, IV, and VI and their connections via the medial longitudinal fasciculus (MLF). Asymmetrical oculomotor responses usually imply a structural brainstem lesion rather than a metabolic lesion (however, phenytoin and carbamazepine may cause oculomotor dysfunc-

Table 25.3 The Glasgow Coma Scale

Activity	Best response	Score
Eye opening	Spontaneous	4
	To verbal stimuli	3
	To pain	2
	None	1
Verbal	Oriented	5
	Confused	4
	Inappropriate words	3
	Nonspecific sounds	2
	None	1
Motor	Follows commands	6
	Localizes pain	5
	Withdraws in response to pain	4
	Flexion in response to pain	3
	Extension in response to pain	2
	None	1

Table 25.4 Modified Coma Score for Infants

Activity	Best response	Score
Eye opening	Spontaneous	4
	To speech	3
	To pain	2
	None	1
Verbal	Coos, babbles	5
	Irritable cries	4
	Cries to pain	3
	Moans to pain	2
	None	1
Motor movements	Normal spontaneous	6
	Withdraws to touch	5
	Withdraws to pain	4
	Abnormal flexion	3
	Abnormal extension	2
	None	1

Table 25.5 The CHOP infant coma scale (infant face scale)

Activity	Score
Eye opening	
Spontaneous	4
Verbal stimulation to touch	3
Painful stimulation	2
None	1
Motor	
Spontaneous normal movements	6
Spontaneous normal movements, reduced in frequency or excursion; hypoactive	5
Nonspecific movement to deep pain only (trapezius pinch)	4
Abnormal rhythmic spontaneous movements: seizure-like activity	3
Extension, either spontaneous, or to painful stimuli	2
Flaccid	1
Verbal/face	
Cries spontaneously or with handling, or to minor pain, alternating with periods of quiet wakefulness	5
Cries spontaneously, or with handling, or to minor pain, alternating with sleep only	4
Cries to deep pain only (trapezius pinch)	3
Grimaces only to pain	2
No facial expression to pain	1

tion). Tonic conjugate deviation implies either a unilateral hemisphere or brainstem lesion, although seizure activity may also cause tonic deviation. Both a destructive lesion and a focal seizure can be accompanied by a hemiparesis. In a destructive lesion, the eyes deviate away from the side of the hemiparesis and a focal seizure, an "irritative lesion," causes eye deviation to the contralateral side (i.e., the eyes look toward the hemiparesis). In the unconscious patient, two main reflexes are used to test extraocular function. The oculocephalic ("doll's eyes") reflex is elicited by holding the eyelids open and turning the head briskly to each side. When the response is normal, the eyes shift to left when the head is turned right and vice versa. If a low brainstem lesion is present, the eyes will move along with the head mimicking oculoparesis. This reflex should not be performed in a patient with suspected spinal cord injury. The oculovestibular reflex (cold caloric) is elicited by elevating the head 30 degrees and inserting a small catheter into the external auditory canal, near the tympanic membrane. The eyes are held open while ice water is flushed into the ear. The normal response in an unconscious patient is nystagmus with the slow component toward the ear being irrigated and the fast component away from the irrigated side (the reverse is true in conscious patients). In patients with a unilateral MLF lesion, the eye will deviate only on the unaffected side while those with low brainstem lesions will not move either eye in response to this maneuver.

- *Motor responses to pain (normal, decorticate, decerebrate, or flaccid).* With a mild insult, the patient has purposeful withdrawal to noxious stimuli. Hemiplegia suggests either a cortical or brainstem lesion. Hyperreflexia and the Babinski (plantar extensor) sign classically signify an upper motor neuron lesion. Hyporeflexia may be seen in metabolic or toxic (ingestion) disorders or with acute structural lesions. With more severe brain impairment, two typical reflex responses to painful stimuli are described. Decorticate posturing (adduction of the arm at the shoulder with elbow flexion and leg extension) usually suggests contralateral hemispheric or diencephalic damage. Decerebrate posturing (arm extension, adduction, and internal rotation along with leg extension) usually implies more severe brain damage and may be suggestive of upper brainstem involvement, including downward herniation, as well as a metabolic insult (hypoglycemia, hepatic encephalopathy, or severe anoxia). Flaccid posturing is an ominous sign and indicates compression of the medulla, a terminal event.
- *Respiratory patterns.* Different processes may damage the respiratory centers in the brainstem and give rise to particular abnormal respiratory patterns. Cheyne-Stokes respiration (hyperpnea in a crescendo and decrescendo pattern followed by an apneic phase) was described in diffuse rather than focal processes (i.e., metabolic insults). Central neurogenic hyperventilation (a sustained, rapid, and deep respiratory pattern) is suggestive of midbrain or pontine lesions. Apneustic breathing (deep inspiration followed by a pause) is consistent with damage to the pons. Ataxic (irregular) breathing, which may progress to apnea, results from medullar damage, in which the respiratory centers responsible for the normal rhythm of breathing are located.

Initial evaluation and emergency management

Immediate stabilization is needed, with adherence to the A, B, and Cs (Table 25.6), regardless of etiology, followed by identifying and specifically treating the underlying

Table 25.6 Priorities during the initial evaluation and stabilization of the comatose patient

	Assure	Exclude	Consider
Airway	Patency	Obstruction (posterior displacement of the soft tissues; e.g., tongue, mucous, or foreign bodies)	Oropharyngeal or nasopharyngeal airway or intubation
Breathing	Oxygenation	Apnea (primary or secondary causes) Ingestions	Oxygen Positive pressure ventilation
Circulation	Blood pressure and heart rate	Shock (hemorrhagic, septic, cardiac) and dehydration	IV access
Dextrose	Normoglycemia	Hypoglycemia	Glucose IV (with thiamine in malnourished patients)
Temperature	Normothermia	Severe infection; e.g., meningitis or sepsis	Lumbar puncture Antibiotics IV
Intracranial pressure (ICP)	Normal ICP	Herniation (Focal exam?)	Computed tomography brain Hyperventilation Hyperosmolar agents Neurosurgical intervention?
Antidotes		Overdose Intoxication	Specific antidotes; e.g., naloxone for opiates or nonspecific elimination procedures (activate charcoal, gastric lavage, catharsis, dialysis, etc.)
Seizures		Status epilepticus or postictal state	Electroencephalogram

cause. The neurologic assessment must immediately identify (a) signs of increased ICP, or focality, both suggestive of a structural (mass) lesion or brain herniation, in which emergency neurosurgical intervention may be critical; (b) evidence of meningitis, encephalitis, or other systemic infections; (c) a severe metabolic derangement, including intoxication; and (d) seizures as the cause of altered awareness. Again, it is important to identify disorders that have specific treatment.

Initial lab workup

Table 25.7 summarizes investigations that should be considered during the initial evaluation of a patient with altered consciousness that may help identify particular coma etiologies.

Differential diagnosis

Other conditions cause altered awareness conditions, but are not coma.

- *Vegetative state (VS).* This consists of wakefulness with complete unawareness, which may evolve when recovering from coma, and results from a relatively intact brainstem combined with severe bihemispheric damage and partial or complete preservation of hypothalamic and brainstem functions. It is generally preferred to avoid the term "permanent vegetative state" and rather describe the exact duration and cause of this condition (Ashwal & Cranford 2002). Three main patterns of pathology are described (Zeman 1997): (a) diffuse axonal injury, (b) extensive laminar necrosis of the cerebral cortex, and (c) occasionally thalamic necrosis. Distinguishing features from coma include spontaneous eye opening and the presence of sleep–wake cycles. This state may persist for years and until death. Most common acute causes are head trauma (diffuse axonal injury) and hypoxic–ischemic encephalopathy. Three factors clearly influencing prognosis are: age, etiology, and time already spent in the vegetative state. The outlook is better in children and after TBI, and worse with longer durations.
- *Minimally conscious state.* This condition has severely altered consciousness with minimal and inconsistent, but clearly visible, evidence of consciousness (Giacino et al. 1997). Diagnostic criteria distinguishing the minimally conscious state from the VS include: (a) ability to follow simple commands, (b) gestural or verbal "yes/no" responses (regardless of accuracy), (c)

Table 25.7 Initial investigations in the comatose patient

	Classification No.	Name
Blood	Encephalopathies • Metabolic (including SIADH) • Toxic, or • Drug-induced	Electrolytes, glucose, calcium, phosphorus, osmolarity, blood urea nitrogen and creatinine, ammonia and liver enzymes Arterial blood gas Toxicologic analysis Blood cultures
Urine	Same	Toxicologic analysis Urine cultures
Cerebrospinal fluid (CSF)	Meningitis Encephalitis Subarachnoid hemorrhage Increased intracranial pressure	Glucose, protein, white and red blood cells as well as CSF cultures (bacterial and viral) Look for xanthochromia Opening pressure
Electrocardiogram	Cardiovascular integrity	Cardiac monitoring
Neuroimaging	Hydrocephalus, various intracranial hemorrhages,	CT, MRI
Electrophysiology	Nonconvulsive status epilepticus Herpes encephalitis and subacute sclerosing periencephalitis	Electroencephalogram

intelligible verbalization, and (d) purposeful behavior (Giacino et al. 2002). Common causes include perinatal or genetic conditions, as well as acquired brain injuries (Strauss et al. 2000). This state may become permanent 12 months after TBI and 3 months after nontraumatic injury (Ashwal 2003).

- *"Locked-in" syndrome (LIS).* This de-efferented condition is rare in children. It consists of quadriplegia, paralysis of lower cranial nerves (inability to speak and swallow), and bilateral paresis of horizontal gaze. It is usually the result of corticospinal and corticobulbar pathway interruption due to lesions at the base of the pons. The two hemispheres are intact retaining consciousness and cognition. The patient is awake with eye opening and sleep–wake cycles, but movement and communication are markedly impaired. Attention should be paid to the vertical eye movements, which remain intact. Other possible causes include tumors and central pontine myelinolysis. Early recovery of lateral eye movements has been suggested as a favorable prognostic sign (Yang et al. 1989).
- *Akinetic mutism.* This is a lack of responsiveness with apparently preserved vigilance (Ackermann & Ziegler 1995). The patient shows slow or nearly absent body movements and loss of speech, particularly when nonstimulated, although remains aware of self and environment. This results from reduced motor activation following damage to (a) the bilateral frontal lobes (Mega & Cohenour 1997), (b) the diencephalomesencephalic reticular formation, (c) the globus pallidus, and d) the hypothalamus. Common causes include anoxia, head trauma, infarctions, acute hydrocephalus (Lin & Wang 1997), and tumors.

Outcome and prognosis

As with neurologic diseases in general, etiology is a very important determinant of prognosis. For nontraumatic coma, Wong and Forsyth (2001) reported infection in 37.9%, followed by intoxication in 10.3%, epilepsy in 9.6%, congenital causes in 8.2%, accident (smoke inhalation, strangulation, burns, and drowning) in 6.7%, others in 7.8%, and an unknown causes in 14.5%. The clinical presentations, either CNS-specific (altered level of consciousness, convulsion, headache, irritability, photophobia, and behavioral change), organ-specific (rash, UTI, cutaneous hemorrhage, sore throat), and systemic (vomiting, nausea, fever, lethargy, poor feeding, shortness of breath, pallor, cyanosis, respiratory arrest, poor weight gain, limb weakness) were age-dependant. Systemic presentations occurred more frequently in infants whereas CNS specific presentations were frequent in children older than 5 years. The overall mortality was 127 in 278 (45.6%); there were 59 prehospital deaths.

The duration of coma is also prognostic (Bates & Caronna 1977): severe disability or the vegetative state, occurred in 25% of those comatose for greater than 6 hours, and in 79% of those comatose after a week. Regaining an independent existence was more likely in those who by day 1 could obey commands or move limbs appropriately to noxious stimuli, had normal motor tone, had normal responses to oculocephalic or oculocaloric testing, or had orienting eye movements. In a larger follow-up study (Levy et al. 1981), only one of 120 patients lacking two of corneal, pupillary, and oculovestibular responses ever regained independent function. In a study of serial neurologic examinations (Levy et al. 1985), at the initial examination 52 out of 210 patients had absent pupillary light responses, and none of these recovered independent daily function. Out of 27 patients who had pupillary light reflexes, spontaneous or conjugate eye movements, or motor responses to pain, 11 of those (41%) regained independence.

How to follow the patient

The clinical examination

The comatose patient is followed by sequential neurologic examinations, important for determining therapeutic responses and prognosis. Objective scales are preferred: the GCS, the modified scale for children, or the CHOP Coma Scale. Two other scales, the Pediatric Risk of Mortality (PRISM) Score (Balakrishnan et al. 1992) and the Acute Physiology and Chronic Health (APACHE) Scale (Knaus et al. 1989), have prognostic value at presentation. The PRISM III score has 17 physiologic variables (Pollack 1996). Those most predictive of mortality are minimum systolic blood pressure, abnormal pupillary light reflexes, and stupor or coma. The APACHE scale uses 12 routine physiologic measurements, age, and previous health status. These include temperature, mean arterial blood pressure, and GCS.

Neurophysiology

Neurophysiology is used to monitor patients and provide prognostic information. No matter the cause, an invariant electroencephalographic (EEG) background, without reactivity, carries a poor prognosis. Invariant backgrounds include electrocerebral inactivity, burst-suppression or suppression-burst, or low-voltage invariant. Postanoxic myoclonus carries a poor prognosis.

No specific patterns are seen on EEG in pediatric coma (Fois & Malandrini 1983). Diffuse slowing occurred with infectious, postictal, metabolic, and posttraumatic etiologies. Mixed fast and slow activity occurred with intoxications, especially benzodiazepines, barbiturates, and alcohol. Intracerebral hemorrhages had focal slowing associated with generalized slow activity, and in trauma, generalized slowing with focal attenuation occurred. A poor prognosis was seen with extreme slowing or electrocerebral inactivity.

In near drowning, a poor prognosis is associated with a loss of β rhythms, diffuse δ activity, often with admixed α or β activity (α–δ and β–δ pattern), poor sleep–waking differentiation, abnormal reactivity, biphasic sharp waves, and either an invariant or burst-suppression EEG background (Cheliout-Heraut et al. 1991; Janati & Erba 1982). Cerebral edema and decerebration were associated with attenuation or disappearance of fast frequencies and reactivity to painful stimuli, or slow and biphasic sharp waves. In severe head injury, patients with electrocerebral inactivity died. Reactivity of the EEG to external stimulation was associated with a favorable outcome (Hutchinson 1991).

Periodic findings, such as paroxysmal lateralizing epileptiform discharges (PLEDs) suggest herpes simplex virus (HSV), although PLEDs occur in many infectious disorders. Periodic EEG patterns are also seen with subacute sclerosing periencephalitis (SSPE), or triphasic waves may be seen in metabolic encephalopathies. Also, nonconvulsive status epilepticus (NCSE) may account for unexplained coma (Towne et al. 2000).

Evoked potentials (EP) have prognostic value and are used as confirmatory studies for brain death. The EP waveform may be preserved in metabolic or "therapeutic" comas (for example, pentobarbital therapy for increased ICP). Wave II of the brainstem auditory evoked potential (BAEP) may be present in brain death.

Visual evoked potentials (VEPs) have had less predictive value than either auditory evoked potentials (AEPs) or somatosensory evoked potentials (SSEPs) (Taylor & Farrell 1989). In a study of SSEPs in 73 comatose

Consider Consultation When…

- Neurology:
  - Unexplained change in mental status
  - Focal neurologic signs on examination
  - Suspected increased intracranial pressure (ICP) or meningitis
  - Suspected nonconvulsive status epilepticus
  - Determination of outcome and prognosis is needed
  - Determination of brain death
- Neurosurgery:
  - History of, or suspected, head or neck trauma
  - Focal neurologic signs on examination
  - Suspected increased ICP or signs of herniation (clinically or on neuroimaging)
  - Suspected intracranial space-occupied process (e.g., tumor or hemorrhage)
- Intensive care unit:
  - Close monitoring and support of vital functions are needed
  - Certain disorders are best managed in the ICU, such as refractory status epilepticus

children upon admission to the pediatric intensive care unit (PICU) (De Meirleir & Taylor 1987), 50 children had a GCS of less than 7 upon admission, only 3 had normal SSEPs, and in the 27 patients who died, none had a normal SSEP. The SSEP was not altered by etiology. SSEPs have also demonstrated predictive value in TBI in children (Beca 1995; Carter 1999).

In a prospective study (Mandel 2002) of coma outcome in 57 children with HIE, the PPV of a poor outcome was 100% with a discontinuous EEG and either spikes or epileptiform activity on EEG; the PPV was 100% for the bilateral absence of the N20 wave on the SSEP. Electroencephalogram and computed axial tomography (CAT/CT) scan together on admission help predict outcome (Singhi 2005).

Neuroradiology

Neuroimaging includes CAT/CT scan, magnetic resonance imaging (MRI), magnetic resonance spectroscopy (MRS), magnetic resonance angiography (MRA), MRI with diffusion-weighted imaging (DWI), and conventional angiography. CAT scan is readily available and shows most lesions that demand immediate attention such as hydrocephalus, tumor, or hemorrhage. It well visualizes the signs of herniation, especially encroachment of the suprasellar and interpeduncular cisterns. Late findings include obstructive hydrocephalus and posterior cerebral artery infarction.

MRI is more sensitive than CAT scan, but is difficult to obtain on an emergency basis and may place the child at a greater risk because of the longer acquisition time. Other studies that can be done with MRI include MRA and MRS. MRI with DWI better images acute ischemia. MRS can measure brain metabolic activity, such as N-acetyl-aspartate, choline, and lactic acid. An elevation of lactate may have prognostic value in various etiologies: perinatal asphyxia, near-drowning, and head injury. In a study of MRI in children with hypoxic–ischemic coma, a strong correlation existed between the first MRI score and neurologic outcome (Dubowitz et al. 1998). However, patients with definite abnormal findings could have a good outcome.

Brain death

Brain death occurs in up to 2% of PICU admissions (Martinot et al. 1995). Caution is urged in making this diagnosis in the newborn. Various criteria for brain death have been employed according to the report of the American Academy of Pediatrics Special Task Force for the Determination of Brain Death in Children (Table 25.8). These include the clinical examination, focusing on both cortical and brainstem functions, done over repeat times, and various confirmatory tests. The latter include EEG,

Table 25.8 Guidelines of the Task Force for the Determination of Brain Death in Children

History

- Determination of cause of death is necessary to ensure the absence of treatable or reversible conditions

Physical examination

- Coma and apnea must coexist
- Absence of brainstem function:
  - Midposition or fully dilated pupils
  - Absence of spontaneous eye movements (induced by oculocaloric/oculovestibular testing)
  - Absence of movement of facial and oropharyngeal muscles (include corneal, gag, cough, sucking, and rooting reflexes)
  - Absence of respiratory movements using standardized testing for apnea
- Absence of hypothermia or hypotension
- Flaccid tone and absence of spontaneous or induced movements (spinal cord reflex withdrawal not included)
- Examination should be consistent with brain death throughout the observation and testing period

Age-dependent observation period

Age	Hours between two examinations	Recommended number of EEGs
7 days–2 months	48	2
2 months–1 year	24	2
More than 1 year	12	Optional

Table 25.9 Minimum technical standards for electroencephalogram (EEG) recording in suspected brain death

- Minimum number of scalp electrodes: eight (8)
- Interelectrode impedances: 100–10,000 ohms
- The integrity of the entire recording system should be tested.
- Interelectrode distances at least 10 cm
- Sensitivity: Must be increased from 7 μV/mm to at least 2 μV/mm for at least 30 minutes of the recording with inclusion of the appropriate calibrations
- Filter settings: Appropriate for the assessment of electrocerebral silence (ECS)
- Additional monitoring techniques should be employed when necessary (e.g., to exclude artifactual activity).
- There should be no EEG reactivity to intense somatosensory, auditory, or visual stimuli.
- Recording should be made only by a qualified technologist.
- A repeat EEG should be performed if there is doubt about ECS.

evoked potentials, radionuclide brain scanning, and angiography, either conventional four-vessel angiography, or CAT scan angiography. The presence of apnea is crucial for the diagnosis of brain death, and specific apnea testing can be done (Riviello et al. 1988).

The EEG, used as a confirmatory test, shows electrocerebral inactivity but must be done under specific circumstance: no hypothermia, cardiovascular instability, hypotension, hypoxemia, metabolic disturbances, intoxication, or electrolyte disturbances, and with specific minimal technical requirements (Table 25.9).

Other confirmatory studies typically done include brain scan showing no intracranial blood flow or CAT scan angiography showing no filling of intracranial arteries.

Annotated bibliography

American Academy of Pediatrics Task Force on Brain Death in Children. Report of a special task force: guidelines for the determination of brain death in children. *Pediatrics* 1987; 80:298–300.
This paper separates the diagnosis of brain death in children from brain death in adults.

American Electroencephalographic Society. Guideline three: Minimum technical standards for EEG recording in suspected cerebral death. *J Clin Neurophysiol* 1994;11:10–13.
Highlights the importance of adhering to rigorous EEG technical standards when using EEG to confirm brain death.

Bates D, Caronna JJ, Cartlidge NE et al. A prospective study of nontraumatic coma: Methods and results in 310 patients. *Ann Neurol* 1977;2:211–220.
Important study that delineated prognostic factors in nontraumatic coma.

Booth CM, Boone RH, Tomlinson G, Detsky AS. Is this patient dead, vegetative, or severely neurologically impaired? Assessing outcome for comatose survivors of cardiac arrest. *JAMA* 2004; 291:870–879.

Brazis PW, Masdeu JC, Biller J. *Localization in clinical neurology*, 4th ed. Philadelphia: Lippincott Williams & Wilkins, 2002.
Comprehensive source of neurologic localization that includes detailed analysis of neurologic findings in coma.

DeLorenzo RJ, Waterhouse EJ, Towne AR, et al. Persistent nonconvulsive status epilepticus after the control of convulsive status epilepticus. *Epilepsia* 1998;39:833–840.
Describes the incidence of nonconvulsive status epilepticus after the control of overt convulsive movements.

Fisher CM. The neurological examination of the comatose patient. *Acta Neurol Scand* 1969;45(Suppl 36):1–56.
A landmark paper for the examination.

Giacino JT, Ashwal S, Xhilds N, et al. The minimally conscious state: Definition and diagnostic criteria. *Neurology* 2002;58: 349–353.
This paper defines the newly characterized "minimally conscious state," and helps differentiate it from other states of altered awareness.

Kirkham FJ, Newton CRJC, Whitehouse W. Pediatric coma scales. *Dev Med Child Neuro* 2008;50:267–274.
British Paediatric Neurology Association recommends the modified child's Glasgow Coma Scale.

Moruzzi G, Magoun HW. Brain-stem reticular formation and activation of the EEG. *EEG Clin Neurophysiol* 1949;1:455–473.
Classic paper on the pathophysiology of consciousness exploring animal models.

Plum F, Posner J. *The diagnosis of stupor and coma*, 3rd ed. Oxford: Oxford University Press, 1982.
The classic textbook on coma.

Ropper AH. Lateral displacement of the brain and level of consciousness in patients with an acute hemispheral mass. *N Engl J Med* 1986;314:953–958.
This paper defines the significance of horizontal (rather than vertical) displacement in altered awareness.

Teasdale G, Jennett B. Assessment of coma and impaired consciousness. A practical scale. *Lancet* 1974;2:81–84.
Describes the Glasgow Coma Scale.

Towne AR, Waterhouse EJ, Boggs JG, et al. Prevalence of nonconvulsive status epilepticus in comatose patients. *Neurology* 2000;54:340–345.
Identifies the incidence of undetected status epilepticus as a cause of coma.

Wong CP, Forsyth RJ. Incidence, aetiology, and outcome of nontraumatic coma: A population based study. *Arch Dis Child* 2001;84:193–199.
The only population-based study of nontraumatic pediatric coma.

Ropper AH, Bolton CF. Coma and impaired consciousness: A clinical perspective. In: *An extensive text of acute and critical care medical neurology*. New York: McGraw-Hill, 1998.
In addition to its excellent pathophysiology, this textbook addresses many clinical aspects of the management of coma and altered awareness.

CHAPTER 26

Headaches

Andrew D. Hershey

Outline

- Headache diagnosis
- Primary headache disorders
- Secondary headache disorders
- Epidemiology
- Headache disability
- Headache evaluation
- Treatment of headache disorders

Headache is a frequent problem for many adults and children. Historically, it has been recognized as early as 6000 B.C. in ancient Sumerian writings. This ancient problem persists, frequently unrecognized in adults and children, as a significant health problem. Estimates are as high as 40–70% of the population having some form of headache, with 25% of 5-year-olds and up to 75% of 15-year-olds having complained of significant headaches (Bille 1962). This makes headache one of the most frequent health conditions for children. The diagnosis, however, is often overlooked because of the patient's inability to recognize headache as a true disease or the physician's inability to appreciate the impact on the child. The first potential step in identifying this illness is asking the patient about headaches and then making the proper diagnosis.

Headache diagnosis

Owing to the common nature of headache, patients often have a preconceived, often incorrect, diagnosis of the cause of their headaches. Many recent studies demonstrated that adults are more likely to diagnose their headaches as sinus headaches or tension-type headaches when, in fact, up to 90% of these "sinus headaches" are actually migraines.

The initial step is making the proper diagnosis. The International Headache Society has developed a classification scheme that has been revised based on further understanding and scientific testing of the original criteria; this classification scheme is found in the *International Classification of Headache Disorders*, 2nd edition (ICHD-II) (2004). This scheme serves to aid in diagnosis and divides headaches into either primary or secondary disorders (Tables 26.1 and 26.2). The primary headache disorders are those in which the headache is the sole manifestation of the disease, whereas secondary headache disorders are those headaches directly due to other causes.

One significant change in the ICHD-II requires that the headache be directly *attributed* to the secondary cause, as opposed to only *associated* with a secondary cause; this change in wording emphasizes the fact that the secondary headaches must have a direct cause and effect both in time and anatomic structure. Furthermore, when the secondary cause is treated, it should be expected that the headaches will resolve. Secondary causes are usually obvious, rarely contributing to recurrent headaches. Secondary causes, however, can exacerbate primary headaches, and the treatment of the secondary cause only returns the headaches to the previous level. The primary headache disorders, however, make up a most significant cause of recurrent headache disorders.

Primary headache disorders

Primary headache disorders are divided into four major groups: migraine headaches, tension-type headaches, trigeminal autonomic cephalalgias including cluster headaches, and other primary headache disorders. Migraine is the most common disabling primary headache

Table 26.1 Common headache syndromes

Type	Discriminating features	Consistent features	Variable features	Consider referral when
Primary				
Migraine	Unilateral; paroxysmal	Throbbing, accompanied by nausea, vomiting, photophobia	Supraorbital/parietal temporal location	Focality consistent, stable neurologic deficit
Secondary				
Tumor	Signs of increased intracranial pressure, progressive neurologic deficit	Constant but worse in the morning; severity progressive	Waxing and waning	Tumor suspected
Trauma	None	History of trauma	Site of trauma or 'contrecoup'	Symptoms progressive or hematoma suspected
Infection	Meningismus	Other evidence of infection	Steady character; photophobia, hyperacusis	Infection warrants
Vascular	Explosive onset	Throbbing character	Focality, meningismus, fundal hemorrhages, focal neurologic deficit	Vascular lesion suspected
Toxic	None	Systemic toxicity	Steady character, vomiting, neuropathy	Toxin not easily dealt with

disorder in children, accounting for 90% or more of recurrent episodic headaches (Hershey et al. 2001a). Although ICHD-I was often criticized for its lack of sensitivity and specificity for diagnosing children's and adolescent's headaches, the ICHD-II tries to answer some of these problems (Hershey et al. 2005).

For children, the most common type of migraine is migraine without aura. The ICHD-II criteria require this to be a recurrent headache disorder with attacks lasting 4–72 hours untreated. The patient must have at least five attacks. The headaches must have at least two characteristics including unilateral location, pulsatile quality, moderate or severe pain intensity and aggravation with or causing avoidance of physical activity. The headaches must also have the associated symptoms of nausea and/or vomiting, or photophobia and phonophobia; all secondary causes must be ruled out.

Allowances to the criteria recognize that children may have shorter headaches, and a 1–72 hour time range is allowed with documentation if under 2 hours. It was also noted that pain is more commonly bilateral in location, with a frontotemporal location being the most common. If occipital pain is present, further evaluation may be necessary. Photophobia and phonophobia may need to be inferred based upon the child's activities and parental observations.

Migraine without aura makes up approximately 80–90% of childhood migraine. The remaining 10–20% is migraine with aura or migraine with aura variants. The aura must have either a fully reversible visual alteration, sensory alteration, or dysphasic speech. The symptoms must be either homonomous visual symptoms or unilateral sensory symptoms. The single aura must increase over 5 minutes or consist of two successive auras in more than 5 minutes, but not last longer than 60 minutes. The most typical type of aura is photopsias (flashing of lights) and is frequently bilateral. Rare subtypes of migraines include cyclical vomiting syndrome and recurrent abdominal pain (abdominal migraines). Both of these may be a gastrointestinal manifestation of the periodic syndromes associated with childhood migraines. In addition, benign paroxysmal vertigo of childhood is thought to be a migraine variant.

One migraine subtype that has become increasingly recognized in adult tertiary headache centers as well as pediatric headache centers is chronic daily headache (CDH). In ICHD-II a diagnosis of chronic migraine has been added to incorporate this observation. Chronic migraine is defined as having 15 or more headache days per month for more than 3 months with symptoms consistent with the diagnosis of migraine without aura. In the largest pediatric study on CDH, the majority of headaches did have migrainous features and could be further subdivided into daily intermittent, daily continuous, and frequent, but not daily headaches (Hershey et al. 2001a).

Key Clinical Questions

- Is the headache primary or secondary?
- Is the neurologic examination normal?
- Does the patient understand and agree with the three-level treatment approach?

Table 26.2 Headache diagnosis

Primary headaches	Secondary headaches	Cranial neuralgias, central and primary facial pain, and other headaches
Migraine	Headache attributed to:	Cranial neuralgias and central causes of facial pain
Migraine with aura	Head and/or neck trauma	Other headache, cranial neuralgia, central or primary facial pain
Migraine without aura	Cranial or cervical vascular disorder	
Tension-type headache	Nonvascular intracranial disorder	
Infrequent episodic	A substance or its withdrawal	
Episodic	Infection	
Chronic	Disorder of homoeostasis	
Cluster headache and other trigeminal autonomic cephalalgias	Disorder of cranium, neck, eyes, ears, nose, sinuses, teeth, mouth or other facial or cranial structures	
Other primary headache	Psychiatric disorder	

International Classification of Headache Disorders, 2nd ed.

Tension-type headache makes up 10% of the recurrent headache disorders for children. It can be divided into either infrequent episodic tension-type headaches, frequent episodic tension-type headaches, or chronic tension-type headaches associated with or without pericranial muscle tenderness. Tension-type headaches can be thought of as the opposite of migraines. They are defined as lasting from 30 minutes to 7 days or must have at least two characteristic features: bilateral location, a pressing or tightening but not pulsatile quality, mild to moderate intensity, and not aggravated by routine physical activity. There should be no nausea or vomiting, and only photophobia or phonophobia is allowed. One distinguishing feature is the absence of vomiting in tension-type headaches. When children vomit with their headaches, diagnosis of migraine is more likely.

Pearls and Perils

- Headaches are very common in children.
- Migraines are the most prevalent cause of recurrent, disabling headaches.
- Use of standardized criteria (ICHD-II) is essential for proper diagnosis.
- Headaches are:
  - Primary if no other cause is identified;
  - Secondary if directly related to another cause.
- An abnormal neurologic examination is highly associated with significant abnormalities on neuroimaging.
- Treatment involves several equally important approaches:
  - Acute therapy (at headache onset)
    - Avoid medication overuse
    - Rescue therapy is considered
  - Preventative therapy
    - Pain frequency and disability is lowered
  - Biobehavioral therapy
    - Develop lifelong healthy habits

Two separate models have been developed to explain the relationship between migraine and tension-type headaches. One is the continuum model, in which migraine with aura is viewed as the most extreme form and infrequent tension-type headache is the mildest with a continuum between these two headache types (Cady et al. 2002). This is in contrast to the spectrum model (Lipton et al. 2000). This model suggests that migraines and tension-type headaches are two distinct headache types. A patient with migraine can have a full spectrum of headaches ranging from very mild headaches (which may be interpreted as tension-type headache, but are actually mild migraines) to more severe migraines. The patient with pure tension-type headache only has tension-type headaches and never has migrainous features.

In children, the other primary headache disorders include trigeminal autonomic cephalalgia, including cluster-type headaches and paroxysmal hemicrania, although these are rarely seen. There are also rare other primary headache disorders that are outside the scope of this chapter.

Secondary headache disorders

The concern of a secondary headache disorder is often what brings the headaches to attention. Secondary headaches should be thought of as a headache being caused by another etiology. Eight subtypes of secondary headache disorders are defined by the ICHD-II (Table 26.1):

1. *Traumatic headache.* This headache type is due to head and neck trauma, including both acute posttraumatic, chronic posttraumatic, and whiplash headaches. One caveat in traumatic headache disorders is that the head trauma may induce a migraine-like headache. Retrospective history is then essential, as it may reveal a history of recurrent headaches prior to the head trauma. Acute posttraumatic headache occurs immediately after head trauma (within 7 days), but resolves within 3 months. Chronic posttraumatic headache also starts within 7 days, but persists longer than 3 months. Head trauma, however, is very common in children. Our experience at Cincinnati Children's Headache Center has demonstrated that of 1,000 headache patients, 120 reported a head trauma, and only 20 of these headaches could be directly attributed to the head trauma itself.
2. *Vascular headache.* Headache attributed to cranial or cervical vascular disorders is seen less commonly in children. These include headaches related to stroke, nontraumatic intracranial hemorrhage, vascular malformations, and arthritis. This includes cerebrovascular accident associated with the headache and (the "worst headache of my life") subarachnoid hemorrhage. These headaches require acute assessment of the underlying intracranial hemorrhage. Aneurysms and intracranial bleeding are much less frequent in children than in adults, but must be considered due to the severe consequences.
3. *Nonvascular, intracranial disorder headaches.* These headaches include idiopathic intracranial hypertension, intracranial hypertension due to other causes, low cerebral blood pressure, noninfectious inflammatory diseases, and intracranial neoplasm. A rapid increase in headache symptoms may be due to an increased intracranial pressure (ICP), either due to the increase in cerebrospinal fluid or due to a mass effect. Idiopathic intracranial hypertension frequently occurs in obese adolescents, girls more so than boys, and most often is associated with papilledema, although case reports have noted increased intracranial hypertension without papilledema. When papilledema is detected, a cause of the intracranial hypertension must be evaluated. This evaluation includes a detailed medical history including medications (e.g., high levels of vitamin A have been noted to be associated with intracranial hypertension), clotting disorder symptoms for venous thrombosis, and changes consistent with a mass effect. Imaging studies should be obtained prior to documenting the increased ICP with a lumbar puncture. The American Academy of Neurology and Child Neurology Society practice parameters state that neoplasms were most often associated with an abnormal neurologic examination (Lewis et al. 2002a).
4. *Substance abuse or withdrawal headaches.* Some medications and food components have been suggested as triggers to headaches, however this is anecdotally based with little evidence to support a triggering mechanism for most of these compounds. Medication overuse headaches, formally known as *analgesic rebound headaches*, however, are being seen with increasing frequency. Studies indicate that anywhere from 60% to 100% of chronic daily headaches are due to overusing analgesics, including over-the-counter analgesics (Katsarava et al. 2001; Tepper & Dodick 2002; Vasconcellos et al. 1998). A detailed history of the analgesic use including nonprescribed analgesics is essential for recognizing this disorder, as proper treatment involves the withdrawal of all analgesics.
5. *Infection-related headache.* These headaches are usually straightforward and occur in direct association with infectious symptoms. A detailed analysis in the emergency department is essential to evaluate and treat symptoms of meningoencephalitis.
6. *Headaches due to disorders of homeostasis.* This headache type rarely occurs in children and a further detailed description of this type can be reviewed in the ICHD-II criteria.
7. *Headaches or facial pain attributed to disorders of the cranium, neck, eyes, ears, nose, sinuses, teeth, mouth, or other facial or cranial structures.* This type of headache is one of the most frequently overdiagnosed. This type includes headaches attributed to refractory errors and is diagnosed by resolution of the head and eye pain within 7 days of visual correction. Many times, however, patients will see an ophthalmologist for their episodic headache disorders, with a temporary response, but then the headache recurs due to a missed diagnosis of their migraines. Even more common is the misdiagnosis of "sinus headaches." Several studies have demonstrated that up to 90% of adults who believe they have sinus headaches or have been diagnosed with sinus headaches actually have migraines (Cady & Schreiber 2002). To diagnose sinus headaches by the ICHD-II criteria, the headaches must be clearly associated with

proven disease in the sinuses, either by nasal endoscopy, computed tomography (CT), magnetic resonance imaging (MRI), or laboratory evidence. Headache and facial pain should develop simultaneously and resolve simultaneously with effective treatment.

8. *Headache due to psychiatric disorders*. These were included in ICHD-II to establish criteria for further scientific research into headache etiologies and psychiatric association.

The ICHD-II criteria also include two categories for the diagnosis of cranial neuralgias and facial pain and their relationship to headache.

Epidemiology

Epidemiology studies have demonstrated that the most common recurrent headache brought to medical attention is migraine, especially in children. Up to 10.6% of children ages 5–15 years old complain of recurrent headaches that are migraines (Abu-Arafeh & Russell 1994). In the 15–19 age group the estimates are as high as 28% in girls and 15% in boys (Split & Neuman 1999). Of special note in the older age group was the observation that a significant number of these children will suffer from status migrainosus or a migraine that lasts longer than 72 hours. This frequency of headache makes headache and migraine one of the most common disorders of childhood.

Headache disability

Not only is migraine very common, but it has also been noted to cause significant disability in children and adults. In adults, several studies have demonstrated that migraines can cause as much impact on the quality of life as other chronic conditions including arthritis, diabetes, and hypertension (Osterhaus et al. 1994). Similarly, in children, the quality of life may be impacted by migraines at a level similar to juvenile rheumatoid arthritis and diabetes (Powers et al. 2002). Successful treatment can improve this impact on quality of life.

An additional area in which migraine impacts a patient is disease-specific disability. Disability is defined as loss of function due to a disease. The Migraine Disability Assessment (MIDAS) was developed for measuring disability in adults (Stewart et al. 2001). PedMIDAS was subsequently developed for assessing migraine disability in children (Hershey et al. 2001b). Not only were children shown to have significant disability due to migraine and recurrent headache, but it was also shown that successful treatment would resolve this disability. Using MIDAS for adults or PedMIDAS for children is a simple tool that can be used in a clinical office to track the headache treatment progress, with eventual outcome measurement.

Headache evaluation

Headache evaluation requires a detailed medical and headache history with a thorough general pediatric and neurologic examination. Additionally a comprehensive headache examination may be included. The history and examination should be detailed enough to rule out secondary causes for headaches. If there is suspicion of a secondary cause, further evaluation is indicated. Recent practice parameters have been developed by the American Academy of Neurology in association with the Child Neurology Society and the American Academy of Pediatrics for the evaluation, assessment, and treatment of childhood headaches (Lewis et al. 2002a). Many of these mirror the National Headache Consortium Guideline that was developed for the management of adult headaches (Silberstein & Rosenberg 2000).

The first step in evaluating a child with headache is obtaining a detailed history, including both a general medical history and a headache-specific history. The purpose of the general medical history, which includes the review of systems and past medical history, is to identify any potential causes of the headaches leading to a secondary headache disorder. A recent history of trauma, infection, or other acute health changes needs to be clearly identified.

The headache history entails several components, as well as the contribution of the family history and psychosocial interactions. A timeline of headache development can identify many of the features of the headache. First is the often difficult identification of a possible prodrome, the clear recognition that a headache is going to occur. It is distinct from the aura and has been described as a heightened sensitivity to surroundings with the development of food cravings. This development of food cravings is thought to be the basis of the incorrect identification of dietary triggers. Possible triggering mechanisms, however, should be investigated. The most common triggering mechanisms that have been identified in adolescents are skipping meals or inadequate sleep. In the adolescent girls, the identification of a menstrual association may also be important for long-term management.

The presence or absence of aura is also a key component of the headache assessment. Aura is a fully reversible neurologic dysfunction. The most common form is visual, the second most common is sensory, and the third is dysphagia. Historically, the presence of an aura suggested the need for further evaluation in a child, including possible neuroimaging and an electroencephalogram (EEG). However, further review has questioned the usefulness of either of these techniques if the pattern is consistent to cause headaches, and the neurologic examination is normal between headache attacks (Lewis et al. 2002a).

Characterization of the headache includes identifying the location of the onset, quality, and quantity of the pain; duration of the headache; effects on activity; and identification of associated symptoms. A migraine is more typically unilateral in adults, but bifrontal in a child. A face pain scale or a 10-point pain scale is used for quantification of the pain. Children frequently have difficulty describing the quality of the pain. The examiner must be careful not to lead the child. Having the child physically demonstrate what the pain feels like or drawing pictures is often useful in assisting with this assessment. Duration may be difficult to assess due to the child's sleeping with a headache. In this regard, the time of sleep is included as part of the headache duration. The effects on physical activity may also be ascertained, both in terms of whether physical activity is altered due to the headache, as well as whether physical activity exacerbates the headache symptoms.

Headache-associated symptoms include the nausea, vomiting, and light and sound sensitivity typical of migraines. Additional associated symptoms can include sensitivity to smell, lightheadedness, vertiginous symptoms, weakness (both perceived and actual), confusion, and difficulty thinking.

Disability due to the headache should also be included. For adults, this can be assessed with MIDAS, and for the younger patient, with PedMIDAS.

Additional headache assessments that may be useful include pattern recognition of the time of day, time of week, time of month, or association with particular events. In adolescent and pubertal girls, a monthly pattern may be ascertained.

The family history assessment is especially important in migraine. Other family members are often unaware of their diagnosis; an additional evaluation of one or both parents, as well as siblings, may reveal multiple family members with migraine or other primary headache disorders.

Social history assessment may reveal particular psychosocial stressors. An assessment of school function may indicate a fall-off in school function due to either school absences or the presence of frequent headaches while in school.

The next step in assessing a child with headaches is a thorough general and neurologic examination. A selective comprehensive headache examination may identify additional particular headache features. For adult headache sufferers, the most sensitive test is the neurologic examination. A thorough and detailed neurologic examination is essential for children as well. This includes a funduscopic evaluation to look for papilledema and lack of venous pulsations, which are suggestive of increased ICP. An asymmetric or abnormal neurologic examination warrants further evaluation.

The comprehensive headache examination may also be considered when evaluating the headache patient. This has been described elsewhere, but in general is a detailed assessment of head and neck structures that may be involved in headache etiology (Linder & Winner 2001). This examination includes an assessment of neck suppleness including pericranial and temporal muscle tightness, lymphadenopathy, temporomandibular joint disease, identification of point tenderness, examination of the ears and the orbits, and a test of neck sublimation including specific testing of the C1–C2 joint as well as the C2–C3 joint. This can be assessed by moving the head in a forward positioning and flexing to different angle degrees. One test that has been considered useful in the assessment of headache patients for sinus disease is the Muller sign. In this test, the patient is asked to pinch their nose, blow against this closed nose to increase the sinus pressure for a count of 5 seconds and then cough. This creates a positive pressure in the sinuses, followed by a rapid decompression. When sinus disease is present, this causes pain over the involved sinus, whereas if sinus disease is not present no pain is elicited. Caution must be used in doing this procedure when there is an ongoing headache, as it may be misinterpreted as sinus disease if the headache itself worsens. In the setting of increased ICP, ICP is also increased by this same maneuver. A variation of this maneuver involves light pressure on the jugular veins during this same procedure. If this causes increased headache over the cranium, the possibility of increased ICP must be considered.

When a secondary cause of headaches has been clearly identified, specific laboratory and/or neuroimaging testing is indicated. For the diagnosis of secondary headache disorders, the headache must be directly attributed to this secondary cause. Often, this attribution cannot be made until the secondary cause has been treated and the headache symptoms have been resolved. For a primary headache disorder, no specific testing has been identified as useful. Recently published practice parameters for childhood headaches show that, for primary headache disorders, the most sensitive assessment is the neurologic examination. Neuroimaging abnormalities were found in 16% of children with primary headache disorders; the most medically and surgically significant ones all were associated with abnormalities of the neurologic examination. An EEG assessment was done in the past, but only proved useful for the auras where a suspicion of a seizure with secondary headache was clearly identified. Blood and chemical testing has not clearly been identified as useful unless indicated to rule out a secondary cause.

Treatment of headache disorders

Treatment of secondary headache involves the treatment of the underlying cause. In many instances, however, the headache is a primary headache and a secondary cause has been erroneously implicated. When the headache persists after effective treatment of the presumed secondary cause, then a primary headache must be reconsidered.

For primary headache disorders in children, the most frequently needed treatment is for migraine. Treatment can be divided into three components: acute treatment, prophylactic treatment, and biobehavioral treatment (Table 26.3).

Acute treatment

The first component is acute therapy. Acute therapy is the treatment to utilize at the onset of each episodic headache. Key in this treatment is a reliance on the child to recognize the onset of the headache and to notify parents, teachers, or caregivers. It is important to use effective doses of a migraine proven medication while avoiding medication overuse. It is also essential to educate the patient and parents about this treatment strategy, as well as to define an effective goal. Furthermore, the National Headache Consortium's recommended goal is for rapid treatment with quick return to functioning without significant sedation or loss of functioning due to the treatment. Although no specific medications have been approved for the use of childhood headache and migraine, several studies have shown the effectiveness of these medications. These can be roughly divided into two groups for outpatient therapy: nonsteroidal anti-inflammatory drugs (NSAIDs) and triptans (5-HT-1_{BD} serotonin agonist).

The NSAIDs, in particular ibuprofen, have been shown in several studies to be effective in childhood headache (Hämäläinen et al. 1997; Lewis et al. 2002b) and have been proven effective for adult migraine. Early administration, with the child catching the headache at the onset, adequate dosing (7.5–10 mg/kg/dose), and limiting the use to not more than two to three times per week to avoid medication overuse headaches are important treatment considerations. For children in whom this is ineffective, other NSAIDs, including naproxen sodium and aspirin, may be considered, although the use of aspirin in children under age 15 may have the potential risk of the development of Reye syndrome.

For patients in whom NSAIDs are ineffective or for more severe headaches, triptans may be employed. Two strategies have been described for using triptans for migraine. In the stratified care model, patients use NSAIDs for mild to moderate headaches, and reserve triptan use for their severe headaches. For most children, this determination is very difficult. In the rescue therapy model, the patients use an NSAID as primary headache treatment. When they recognize an unresponsive headache or a conversion to a severe headache, a triptan is used for rescue therapy.

A detailed description of these individual triptans and their uses is beyond the scope of this chapter. Triptans are 5-HT-1BD receptor agonists with both a vascular

Table 25.3 Headache treatment

	Multidisciplinary treatment	
Acute treatment	**Prophylactic treatment**	**Biobehavioral treatment**
NSAIDS	Antidepressants	Healthy habits
Aspirin	Amitriptyline	Adequate hydration
Ibuprofen	Imipramine	Regular sleep
Naproxen sodium	Antiepileptic	Regular nutrition
Triptans	Divalproate	Regular exercise
Almotriptan	Gabapentin	Biofeedback-assisted relaxation therapy
Eletriptan	Topiramate	
Frovatriptan	Antiserotonergic	
Naratriptan	Cyproheptadine	
Rizatriptan	Methylsergide	
Sumatriptan	β-Blockers	
Zolmitriptan	Atenolol	
Dihydroergotamine	Propranolol	
Dopamine antagonist	Timolol	
Prochlorperazine		
Metoclopramide		
Combined treatments (such as aspirin + caffeine)		

component and a central effect that has been implicated in the development of central sensitization and allodynia (Burstein & Cutrer 2000). The development of allodynia stresses the importance of early recognition and treatment. Although several of these agents have been tested in children and adolescents, none are currently approved for their use. Several studies have shown their effectiveness, although due to design problems and a high placebo effect, statistical significance has not been reached for the primary end-point of these studies.

The NSAIDs and triptans appear to have a synergistic effect in the treatment of moderate to severe headaches (Smith et al. 2005). Using this multi-mechanism technique, NSAIDs are used for mild to moderate headaches; then NSAIDs can be combined with a triptan for moderate to severe migraine. Caution must be observed not to overuse either the NSAIDs or the triptans.

When outpatient therapy is not effective, emergency department or inpatient therapy may be necessary. Dopamine antagonists, including prochlorperazine and metoclopramide, have been historically shown to be effective, although essentially only in intravenous (IV) formulations. Prochlorperazine's usefulness in childhood headaches has been shown to yield a good response in an open-labeled study (Kabbouche et al. 2001). An adequate dose for prochlorperazine appears to be 0.15 mg/kg IV dose, while for metoclopramide a higher dose of 0.25 mg/kg may be required. The goal of emergency room treatment should be complete cessation of the headache attack. This may be assisted with IV hydration due to the vascular dilatory effect of a migraine attack. If headache freedom is not completely reached, additional IV therapy in an inpatient setting may be required. Additional emergency department treatment that may be considered (although of limited tested value in children and adolescents), includes IV valproic acid, which has been shown to be effective in adult migraine sufferers.

In the inpatient setting, one of the most useful medications is dihydroergotamine. It may be associated with significant nausea and vomiting that can be minimized with premedication with antiemetics (Linder 1994). Additional therapies that have been utilized for inpatient therapy include steroid treatment, IV magnesium infusions, and recurrent divalproate infusions.

Prophylactic treatment

For patients with frequent headaches and disability, preventative treatment is indicated. No preventative therapies have been specifically recommended for childhood headache disorders. For adults, there have been several U.S. Food and Drug Administration (FDA)-approved options, including topiramate, divalproate, methysergide, propranolol, and timolol.

Prophylactic agents can be divided into antiepileptic medications, antidepressant medications (specifically the tricyclic antidepressants), β-blockers, and antiserotonergic agents (cyproheptadine or methylsergide). Specific uses of these agents can be reviewed elsewhere. The general guidelines are to educate the patients about the goals of therapy (typically to reduce headache frequency to one to two times per month or less, and to reduce disability to allow functioning at a normal level). To achieve these goals, adequate doses must be utilized, increasing the dose to a level slowly to minimize side effects, as well as to increase the overall effectiveness. Once an adequate dose has been achieved, the medication must be sustained for a long enough period to observe a treatment effect, typically at least 2–3 months. If the goal of treatment has not been obtained at this point, a second prophylactic agent may need to be considered. Once sustained response has been achieved for 4–6 months, withdrawal of the medicine should be attempted. If this is unsuccessful, the preventative treatment can be restarted. Once a 4–6-month sustained period of headache response has been obtained, a weaning should again be attempted.

Choosing the preventative therapy may be guided by identification of comorbid conditions. For comorbid depression, a tricyclic antidepressant may be useful; if a patient has seizures, an antiepileptic may treat both conditions. Two of the antiepileptics used for headache prevention have weight effects, with the divalproate having a chance of increased weight (which can assist with people who are especially thin), whereas topiramate may have a weight loss effect (which may assist with obesity). Side effects of medications must be carefully considered. In particular, the β-blockers are associated with increased depressive symptoms and asthma attacks, thus limiting their usefulness.

Biobehavioral treatment

The third component of treatment is biobehavioral treatment. Biobehavioral treatment is essentially managing the day-to-day habits of the child while assisting with reducing triggering events. This can be a combination of lifestyle adjustments, as well as biofeedback-assisted relaxation therapy and psychological intervention. Multidisciplinary headache centers often combine these services to assist in the global management of the patient. Particular lifestyle adjustments that are useful include adequate fluid hydration with limited caffeine intake, adequate exercise on a regular basis, eating a regular healthy diet, and a regular adequate sleep schedule. Adequate hydration corresponds to the vascular dilation and plasma extravasation hypothesis of migraine pathogenesis. Exercise may assist with improving vascular tone both in the cerebral vasculature, and diffusely throughout the body, minimizing the vascular stretch as a triggering phenomenon for migraines. Skipping meals has been shown to be a common trigger for adolescent migraines. Several nutrients

Consider Consultation When...

- Abnormalities in the history or neurologic examination are evident.
- Acute therapy is not effective (including both primary and rescue strategies).
- An adequate dose and time of prophylactic therapy has been unsuccessful.

have been shown to assist with migraine prevention, and a balanced diet rich in green vegetables should help provide this balanced nutritional support. Sleep deprivation and altered sleep schedules have frequently been demonstrated to be a migraine trigger. This has been noted as a jet lag phenomenon in people with migraine, as well as a frequent trigger in childhood headaches when the sleep schedule is altered from the weekend to the week days.

Biofeedback-assisted relaxation therapy may also be beneficial (Daly et al. 1983). Single-session treatment has been shown to be effective and maintained over time in children (Powers & Hershey 2002). The overall use of biofeedback-assisted relaxation therapy is discussed in greater detail elsewhere (Powers & Hershey 2002).

In summary, the management of childhood headache first involves the recognition of the primary versus secondary nature of the headache. For recurrent episodic headaches, primary headaches are most likely to be migraine. A thorough history and a physical, neurologic, and comprehensive headache examination helps identify any possible secondary headache disorders that require further investigation. Once the diagnosis of primary headache disorders and migraine has been established, then a treatment program needs to be initiated that involves a plan for treating acute headache attacks, preventing future headache attacks, and maintaining a balanced lifestyle. Additional investigative work is often not needed, but should be directed by the history and physical, and in particular by the neurologic examination. Referral to headache specialty care may be necessary when initial treatments fail, or when significant disability or comorbid conditions exist.

Annotated bibliography

Cephalalgia 2004;24:1–160.
A comprehensive criteria set for all headache disorders, divided into primary and secondary disorders.

Cady RK, Schreiber CP. Sinus headache or migraine? Considerations in making a differential diagnosis. *Neurology* 2002; 58:S10–14.
Points out the high overdiagnosis of sinus headache and the importance of the use of standardized criteria.

Lewis DW, Ashwal S, Dahl G, et al. Practice parameter: Evaluation of children and adolescents with recurrent headaches. Report of the Quality Standards Subcommittee of the American Academy of Neurology and the Practice Committee of the Child Neurology Society. *Neurology* 2002a;59:490–498.
Outlines the current evidence for the evaluation of children with headache.

Powers SW, Patton SR, Hommel KA, Hershey AD. Quality of life in childhood migraines: Clinical impact and comparison to other chronic illnesses. *Pediatrics* 2003;112:e1–e5.
Demonstrates the significant impact of headaches in a child's life.

CHAPTER 27

Febrile Seizures

Deborah G. Hirtz and Karin B. Nelson

Outline

Febrile seizures are the most common convulsive disorder of early childhood, occurring in approximately 2–5% of young children in the United States.

> A febrile seizure is defined as an event in infancy or childhood, usually occurring between three months and five years of age, associated with fever but without evidence of intracranial infection or defined cause. Seizures with fever in children who have suffered a previous afebrile seizure are excluded. Febrile seizures are to be distinguished from epilepsy, which is characterized by recurrent afebrile seizures. (Consensus Statement 1981).

Young children may experience seizures during a febrile illness caused by such disorders as meningitis, dehydration, or toxic encephalopathy. These are not considered to be febrile seizures and do not have the same prognosis because the underlying illness may cause central nervous system damage.

Febrile seizures are often categorized into two subgroups: simple febrile seizures, which are brief and generalized, and complex febrile seizures, which are prolonged, focal, or multiple (more than one seizure in 24 hours) or followed by neurologic deficit. A family history of febrile or nonfebrile seizures or preexisting neurologic abnormality may accompany seizures in either of these categories (Table 27.1).

Clinical presentation

Febrile seizures tend to occur early in the course of the febrile illness, sometimes as the first sign the child is ill. Although a rapid rise of the fever has been thought to be important, it is actually the height of the temperature that is associated with the occurrence of a febrile seizure (Berg 1993). The fever is usually at least 38°C. The age of the child is usually between 3 months and 5 years (Table 27.2). The most common seizure type is tonic–clonic, but other seizure types may also occur. The duration is usually less than 15 minutes; in one large study, less than 8% of febrile seizures were longer than 15 minutes (Nelson & Ellenberg 1976), and in another study 13% were longer than 10 minutes and 5% were longer than 30 minutes in duration (Berg & Shinnar 1996).

Most of the febrile illnesses associated with febrile seizures are due to infections, such otitis media, tonsillitis, or upper respiratory infections. Human herpes virus 6 (HHV6) infection can be implicated in many cases; in 416 children younger than 3 years of age with febrile seizures, 24% were infected with HHV6 and of 902 children with HHV6 infection and fever, 16.5% had a seizure (Millichap & Millichap 2006). Influenza A virus is a frequent cause of febrile seizures in the Netherlands (van Zeijl et al. 2004) and China (Chung & Wong 2007), but is not as frequent a cause in the United States and other parts of Europe.

Some serious and potentially fatal conditions, not febrile seizures by definition, can present as seizures with fever but require prompt and specific treatment. The possibility of bacterial meningitis should always be considered, particularly if the child is too young to exhibit

Table 27.1 Febrile seizures: definitions

	Simple	Complex
Duration	<15 minutes	May be ≥15 minutes
Type	Generalized	May be generalized or focal
Number during one illness	One	May be multiple
Followed by transient neurologic deficit	Never	Possible
Family history of febrile seizures	Possible	Possible
Family history of afebrile seizures	Possible	Possible
Preexisting neurologic abnormality	Possible	Possible

Table 27.2 Febrile seizures

Discriminating features
- Seizures in the presence of fever

Consistent features
- Absence of previous afebrile seizure
- Absence of central nervous system infection

Variable features
- Usually age 3 months to 5 years
- Focal or generalized
- May be multiple within one illness
- Usually brief, may be prolonged (≥15 minutes)
- Family history of febrile or afebrile seizures

typical symptoms such as meningismus. Viral meningitis or encephalitis may also present with seizures and fever, as may hypernatremic dehydration owing to gastrointestinal infection, acute toxic encephalopathy, or cerebrovascular accidents of infancy.

Children with preexisting epilepsy or brain damage may have their seizure thresholds lowered by fever. If a child has previously had one or more nonfebrile seizures, a seizure occurring with fever should be treated as an epileptic seizure and not as a febrile convulsion.

Epidemiology

In the United States, South America, and Western Europe, between 2% and 5% of all children experience convulsions with febrile illness before age 5 years (Shinnar & Glauser 2002). Febrile seizures are reported to be about twice as common in certain Asian countries as in Europe and America (Tsuboi 1984).

The first febrile seizure was complex in approximately 20–35% of all cases reported in three large studies (Berg & Shinnar 1996a; Nelson & Ellenberg 1976; Verity et al. 1985a,b). Two-thirds of the children had only a single febrile seizure, and about 10% had three or more seizures (Annegers et al. 1990; Berg et al. 1997; Nelson & Ellenberg 1976; Offringa et al. 1992; Verity et al. 1985a,b), and the seizure lasted 30 minutes or longer in 5% (Berg & Shinnar 1996b). Thirteen percent of all initial febrile seizures lasted 10 minutes or longer.

In about half of the children with febrile convulsions, the onset is in the second year of life. About 90% begin by 3 years. The average age of onset is 18–22 months. Febrile seizures are more common in males. In 24% there is a family history of febrile seizures, and 4% have a family history of epilepsy (Offringa 1994).

Mechanisms

Inflammatory cytokines associated with fever such as interleukin (IL)-1β have been postulated to be involved in the pathogenesis of febrile seizures (Matsuo et al. 2006; Virta et al. 2002). Reports of gene polymorphisms involved in cytokine production have not been replicated in other studies (Haspolat et al. 2005; Tomoum et al. 2007). One theory supported by data from the rat model is that fever is accompanied by compensatory hyperventilation, causing alkalosis and an increase in brain pH. In the developing rat model, behavioral seizures and electroencephalographic (EEG) changes were induced by hyperventilation and alkalosis (Schuchmann et al. 2006). A rise in brain temperature alone could possibly be causative for febrile seizures, but whether this actually has a direct role remains unclear (Dubé et al. 2007).

Genetics

Febrile convulsions are more frequently found among family members of children with febrile convulsions than in the general population (Hauser et al. 1985). A history of febrile seizures in a first-degree relative was a significant risk factor for a first febrile seizure (Berg et al. 1995). Younger siblings of the child with febrile convulsions have a 10–20% risk of having febrile convulsions. If both parents and a previous child have had febrile convulsions, the risk for another sibling may be increased to as high as one in three (Baraitser 1983).

Although it is well accepted that familial factors, probably genetic, cause a predisposition to febrile seizures, the pattern of heredity is not known. Genetic susceptibility may allow the fever to promote neuronal excitability and thus a seizure. It is clear that the hereditary factors are complex, involving variations in a number of susceptibility genes (Abou-Khalil et al. 2007; Nakayama & Arinami 2006). Six susceptibility loci have been identified (FEB 1–6). In addition, genetic loci have been identified for specific genetic syndromes within the clinical spectrum of febrile

> **Pearls and Perils**
>
> **Febrile Seizures**
>
> - Most children with febrile seizures do extremely well. The closer the clinical picture to the typical case, the more ensured is a good prognosis.
> - The earlier the age at which the first febrile convulsion occurs, the more likely are recurrences.
> - There is no increase in risk of intellectual deficit owing to the occurrence of febrile seizures.
> - The number of febrile seizure recurrences does not directly relate to the risk of later epilepsy.
> - Intermittent administration of phenobarbital at the time of fever only is not effective in preventing recurrences.
> - Diagnostic laboratory tests should never be routine but should be justified by the specific clinical setting.
> - The risk for later epilepsy after febrile seizures is relatively increased but still low when:
>   - There is neurologic or developmental abnormality before any seizures. There is a history of seizures without fever in a parent or sibling. The first febrile seizure is focal, is multiple, or lasts longer than 15 minutes.

seizures such as *generalized epilepsy with febrile seizures plus* (GEFS+), which usually begins with febrile seizures that may continue into late childhood and be accompanied by afebrile tonic–clonic or other forms of seizures, such as absence, myoclonic, or tonic. Genes encoding voltage-gated sodium channels and ligand-gated ion channel subunits, and γ-aminobutyric acid (GABA) receptors have been identified in GEFS+; these include *SCN1B*, *SCN1A*, *SCN2A*, *GABRG2*, and other loci (Audenaert et al. 2006; Nagao et al. 2005). A more severe subset, severe myoclonic epilepsy of infancy (SMEI) or Dravet syndrome (Dravet et al. 1992), occurs in infants who have been developing normally until about age 6 months, when febrile seizures develop, often as status or hemiclonic seizures, followed by increasingly more seizures including myoclonic types that become refractory to therapy and are accompanied by intellectual deterioration. Approximately 80% of children with SMEI have mutations in the sodium channel 1 subunit gene *SCN1A* (Scheffer et al. 2005).

Progress now being made in genotyping for mutations in children with afebrile seizures will allow for better diagnoses and prognoses, and genetic counseling, but the ultimate goal is to use these findings to advance effective prevention and treatments.

Recurrence

About one-third of children who experience a single febrile seizure will experience a second. Of those who have a second, half will have two or more subsequent recurrences. About 9% of children with febrile seizures will have three or more. Approximately three-fourths of recurrences take place within 1 year, and 90% within 2 years.

The earlier the age at which the first febrile convulsion occurs, the greater the chance that there will be additional convulsions (Table 27.3, Pavilidou et al. 2007). A family history of febrile or afebrile convulsions, or both, also has been associated with an increased recurrence rate (Berg et al. 1997; El-Radhi 1998), and number of febrile episodes and a positive family history for febrile seizures were identified as significant as risk factors for recurrence (Rantala & Uhari 1994).

If the initial seizure is complex, the risk of a recurrence being complex is not increased. If the initial febrile seizure is brief, prolonged recurrence is very unlikely (only 1.4% in the National NINDS Collaborative Perinatal Project [NCPP]). If the initial seizure is prolonged, a recurrence is no more likely to happen, but if it does, it is more likely to be prolonged than if the first seizure was brief (Berg et al. 1995; Offringa et al. 1994).

Epilepsy

Most population-based studies estimate that between 2% and 10% of children with febrile seizures go on to develop epilepsy (Annegers et al. 1987; Berg & Shinnar 1996b; Ellenberg & Nelson 1980; Verity & Golding 1991; Vestergaard et al. 2007). Other reports from selected populations of children with febrile seizures tend to cite a much higher rate of development of epilepsy than those from large population-based studies. Risk factors for epilepsy identified from large cohort studies include abnormal neurodevelopment, a family history of epilepsy, complex febrile seizures, and short duration of fever (<1 hour) before the seizure (Nelson & Ellenberg 1976; Shinnar & Glauser 2002). With no risk factors, the rate of epilepsy is essentially no different than for children without febrile seizures (Annegers et al. 1987; Nelson & Ellenberg 1976). A higher number of febrile seizure recurrences does not appear to influence the prognosis adversely with regard to later epilepsy or intellectual function. Risk factors

Table 27.3 Likelihood of recurrence by age at first febrile seizure

Age at first febrile seizure	Proportion with at least one recurrence
≤1 year	1:2
≤2 years	1:3
≤3 years	1:4
≤4 years	1:5

are more important than number of recurrences in predicting later epilepsy.

About 34% of the children with febrile seizures had one risk factor; of these, 3% later experienced at least one afebrile seizure. An increase in the rate of later epilepsy appeared in those children with two or more risk factors; 13% later had one or more afebrile seizures. In a Danish cohort, 7% of children with febrile seizures developed epilepsy by age 23; the risk factors were a family history of epilepsy, cerebral palsy, or low 5-minute Apgar score (<7) (Vestergaard et al. 2007).

A neurologic abnormality occurring in the child before any seizure tends to be an important factor increasing the risk of epilepsy (Addy 1986). In the NCPP, prolonged convulsions were followed by epilepsy in 1.4% of children with no prior neurologic abnormality and in 9% of children who were neurologically abnormal. The risk of epilepsy after a first complex convulsion was 10% in a neurologically abnormal child, but was not significantly increased in normal children (1.7% vs. 1.1%) (Nelson & Ellenberg 1978). Of the features of complex febrile convulsions, the most important in prediction of later epilepsy is partial or focal seizure type.

Sofijanov and associates (1983) found that all types of epilepsy were seen in patients with prior febrile convulsions. Camfield and colleagues (1994) reported that febrile seizures preceded 15% of childhood-onset epilepsy, more often among those with generalized tonic–clonic seizures. A positive family history of epilepsy is a risk factor for development of generalized but not partial epilepsy, and the development of partial epilepsy is associated with the risk factors developmental delay and prolonged or focal febrile seizures (Birca et al. 2005).

Partial complex seizures

Only a very small percentage of children with febrile seizures develop complex partial seizures, and a causal relationship has not been proven (Camfield et al. 1994). A statistical association exists between both prolonged and focal febrile seizures and intractable temporal lobe epilepsy (Dubé et al. 2007). However, population-based studies and prospective studies do not confirm that mesial temporal lobe epilepsy is caused by prolonged or atypical febrile seizures in childhood (Annegers et al. 1987; Berg & Shinnar 1996a,b; Nelson & Ellenberg 1978; Verity et al. 1993; Verity et al. 1985a,b).

Prolonged experimental seizures in a rat pup model led to partial seizures in one-third of adult animals and to epileptiform discharges in most of the other adults (Dubé et al. 2006). No evidence from human studies can distinguish between a causal effect of febrile seizures and an independent effect of preexisting factors on both febrile seizures and epilepsy. Twelve children with prolonged febrile seizures showed hippocampal volume abnormalities compared to controls, correlating with length of seizures, suggesting possible causation (Natsuma et al. 2007). This is not supported by another recent clinical study in which 23 children were studied by diffusion-weighted imaging within 5 days of a prolonged (>30 minute) febrile seizure. Early vasogenic edema was seen in those investigated within 2 days, but was resolved in those imaged at 3–5 days. Age-dependent decrease in the apparent diffusion coefficient (ADC) was seen in controls, but not in the children with prolonged febrile seizures. This data was considered by the authors to be consistent with a preexisting hippocampal abnormality that may dispose children to having a prolonged febrile seizure (Scott et al. 2006).

Neurologic outcome

Children who have febrile seizures generally show no difference from controls in cognitive abilities and school performance (Ellenberg & Nelson 1978; Ross et al. 1980; Verity et al. 1985a,b). With regard to motor handicap following febrile seizures, two large prospective series have not found any apparent association with febrile seizures (Nelson & Ellenberg 1978; Verity et al. 1985a,b, 1993). A study from Taiwan in which 6-year-old children with a history of febrile convulsions were compared to controls showed no disadvantage and even a trend towards better performance on achievement tests (Chang et al. 2000).

In a population-based study from Denmark, there was a weak association between childhood febrile seizures and schizophrenia at age 23, which could be due to shared etiologic factors or confounding unmeasured factors (Vestergaard et al. 2005).

Management

Acute management

In most cases, a child with a febrile seizure is not brought to medical attention until after the seizure has ended. But an actively convulsing febrile child may present to an emergency room or doctor's office. In that case, the airway must be kept clear, proper oxygenation maintained, intravenous (IV) access established, and medication administered to stop the convulsion. Either lorazepm (.05–0.1 mg/kg) infused slowly over 2–5 minutes, or diazepam (0.2–0.3 mg/kg to a maximum of 10 mg given at a maximum rate of 1 mg/min IV) is usually the first drug used. Intramuscular midazolam (0.1–0.2 mg/kg) may be used or rectal diazepam in a dose of 0.5 mg/kg if an IV line cannot be readily established. It is important to be alert for, and prepared to deal with, respiratory depression, particularly if other anticonvulsant drugs have been previously administered.

When the child is seen following a febrile convulsion and is no longer convulsing, the most important task is to identify whether there is an underlying illness that may require treatment. A medical history should include a review of the patient's developmental progress and a family history of febrile and afebrile seizures. If this was not the first episode, details of previous seizures should be noted. Particular attention should be paid to the level of consciousness, the presence of meningismus or a tense or bulging fontanel, measurement of head circumference, and muscle strength, tone, and symmetry.

Lumbar puncture

The most urgent diagnostic decision is whether or not a lumbar puncture (LP) should be performed to rule out meningitis. In the younger child, classic meningeal signs may not be present and the index of suspicion should be very high; this is especially true for infants younger than 1 year of age. The American Academy of Pediatrics (1996) has recommended that in the case of a single febrile seizure, an LP should be performed in all children younger than 1 year of age, and considered between 12 and 18 months, but is not necessary in the absence of clinical indications over 18 months. For children with complex febrile convulsions, recommendations have not been published.

Joffe and associates (1983) reviewed the records of 241 children of ages 6 months to 6 years who were seen for a first episode of seizure and found five items in the history and physical examination that identified all of the 13 children with meningitis and would have spared 62% of those without meningitis from LP. The findings were a physician visit within 48 hours before the seizure, the occurrence of convulsions on arrival at the emergency room, a focal seizure, and suspicious findings on physical or neurologic examination (for example, rash or petechiae, cyanosis, hypotension, respiratory distress, stiff neck, increased tone, lack of responsiveness, or tense fontanel). However, use of these criteria is only recommended if a careful history and physical examination have been performed and if close follow-up for children not receiving LP is available. Should increased intracranial pressure be suspected clinically, the decision to perform an LP must be made by an experienced physician, who will weigh the risk in delaying a diagnosis of meningitis against the risk of LP.

Other studies

The search for a cause for the fever should begin with a careful examination. Laboratory evaluation in cases of febrile seizure should be guided by specific clinical indications (Table 27.4).

Diagnostic tests performed in children presenting with febrile seizures should be clinically indicated, because physicians are under pressure to reduce unnecessary expenditures and because the yield from these tests, if routinely used, is negligible. Electrolytes, blood glucose, blood urea nitrogen, calcium, and phosphorus should be evaluated when a specific indication exists, such as the presence of vomiting, diarrhea, or a history consistent with possible hypoglycemia.

Table 27.4 Evaluation after febrile convulsions

- Workup of fever:
  - History
  - Physical examination
  - Blood culture
  - Throat culture
  - Chest x-ray study
  - Urinalysis
  - Urine culture
  - Complete blood count
  - Lumbar puncture
- As clinically indicated, measurement of
  - Electrolytes
  - Blood urea nitrogen
  - Calcium
  - Phosphorus
  - Glucose
  - Toxins
- If there are focal abnormalities, a history of trauma, or a specific neurologic deficit present following the seizure:
  - CT scan or magnetic resonance imaging
  - EEG

A computed tomographic (CT) or magnetic resonance imaging (MRI) scan is indicated only if there is a history of significant head trauma or progressive neurologic changes, neurologic abnormalities present after the seizure is over, or specific clinical features suggesting possible acute focal pathology. Even if the first febrile seizure is complex, intracranial pathologic conditions that require emergency surgical or medical intervention are very rare (Teng et al. 2006). Non-urgent MRI should be considered in children with additional findings such as abnormal head size, developmental delay, and focal or persistent motor signs (Sadleir & Schaffer 2007).

Although there may be a higher incidence of EEG abnormalities in children with febrile seizures, the EEG has not been shown to be helpful in diagnosis or predicting recurrences or the risk for later epilepsy (Stores 1991). An EEG performed within 1 week of a febrile seizure usually is normal (Maytal et al. 2000) although up to one-third may have occipital slowing. The incidence of paroxysmal abnormalities increases with age (Sofijanov et al. 1992).

Hospitalization

Whenever possible, children presenting with a febrile seizure should be kept in an emergency room holding area for up to several hours and then reevaluated. Hospitalization can usually be avoided. The majority of children will have improved after a short time. If they are alert, and the etiology of the fever is clear, they can be sent home, provided that follow-up care can be ensured. It is not possible to predict which children with febrile seizures will have a second seizure during the same febrile illness (Green & MacFaul 1985).

Parental counseling

The parents of a child with a first febrile convulsion are likely to be extremely upset and in a state of panic. When a seizure is first witnessed, parents often think the child is dead or dying (Hansen et al. 1984). They may pick up and shake the child, bang him on the back, try to insert fingers or an object between the teeth, or desperately attempt mouth-to-mouth resuscitation. These actions may actually endanger a convulsing child. Parents will need instructions on management of possible recurrences, which may occur either during the same illness or later on. Information and instructions in a written format are helpful. The following points must be stressed:

- Although the seizure may have been frightening to witness, the child will not have suffered brain damage as a result of the fit, and the likelihood of future epilepsy is very small.
- There is a risk of another convulsion when the child has another febrile illness, as well as a small risk of another convulsion within 24 hours.
- If a febrile seizure recurs, parents must be told to stay calm, to place the child on his side or stomach with the face downward on a protected surface, and not force anything between the teeth. It is very important that parents observe the child, note any focal features (especially at onset), and time the duration of the seizure. If the seizure lasts longer than 10 minutes, then the child should be brought to the nearest medical facility by car or ambulance.

It is reasonable to avoid high fevers when possible in a child who has experienced a febrile seizure, so parents should be instructed in temperature taking and fever management. However, it has not been shown that using antipyretics will lower the risk of a febrile convulsion (Camfield et al. 1980).

It should be stressed that, in general, children with febrile seizures do very well. Physicians can feel comfortable in reassuring parents that children do not die because of febrile convulsions; in large cohort studies, no deaths were reported. Parents' views should be considered in any decision regarding medication, and if medication is prescribed, a full discussion of the goals, risks, benefits, and side effects is needed.

Questions regarding the advisability of continuation of routine childhood immunizations may arise, because most routine immunizations are scheduled at the age of susceptibility to febrile seizures. Seizures following childhood immunizations generally have the characteristics and benign outcome of febrile seizures (Hirtz et al. 1983). There may be an increase in febrile but not afebrile seizures following diphtheria-pertussis-tetanus immunization (Griffin et al. 1990; Walker et al. 1988). In each child the advantages of the protection offered by the vaccine must be weighed against the possible complications of immunization, and the advisability of immunization with pertussis should be reevaluated at each subsequent medical visit. The risks and benefits of immunization should be discussed fully with parents and a record made of the discussion, whatever the conclusion.

Long-term management

Although antipyretics reduce fever, they cannot be relied on to prevent febrile seizures. Often, a febrile seizure may be the first sign that the child is feverish. Nevertheless, it is important to make certain that parents are aware of proper dosage and administration of antipyretics and that they try to reduce their child's fever to promote the comfort of the child and prevent dehydration.

No convincing evidence suggests that treating children with febrile seizures with anticonvulsant therapy can prevent the development of epilepsy (Hirata et al. 1985). Studies showing a reduction in risk of recurrence have not demonstrated an effect on the risk of developing later epilepsy (Knudsen et al. 1996; Rosman et al. 1993 a,b; Shinnar & Berg 1996; Wolf & Forsythe 1989).

A number of series have reported that continuous daily treatment with phenobarbital or valproate decreases the risk of recurrent febrile seizures (Lee & Melchior 1981; Mamelle et al. 1984; Wolf et al. 1977). Other British trials of treatment with phenobarbital and pooled analyses of valproate (Newton 1988), did not show significant reduction in recurrence seizures with either agent. Two randomized trials (Farwell et al. 1990; McKinlay & Newton 1989), which examined selected populations of children with febrile seizures at increased risk of subsequent seizures and analyzed according to intention to treat, do not demonstrate efficacy for phenobarbital (in the former) or valproate for the chronic treatment of febrile seizures.

Barbiturates may pose a risk to cognitive and behavioral function in children. In a randomized clinical trial designed to address this question, mean IQ was 7 points lower in children with early, complex, or repeated febrile seizures who were randomly assigned to treatment for 2 years with phenobarbital, as compared with children given a placebo (Farwell et al. 1990). There was no difference in the occurrence of subsequent seizures between the group assigned to phenobarbital and the group assigned to the placebo. The incidence of side effects was very low in studies of sodium valproate. However, rare but life-threatening complications of pancreatitis and acute liver failure have been reported. Less serious complications include weight gain, gastrointestinal dysfunction, and hair loss. Its use in children for prevention of febrile seizures is generally unwarranted.

Intermittent oral and rectal diazepam have been used successfully for febrile seizure prophylaxis (O'Dell et al. 2005). When rectal administration of diazepam at the onset of illness was compared with daily phenobarbital, febrile seizure recurrences were less frequent with diazepam, even though, in a few cases, parents did not recognize illness was present until the seizure occurred (Thorn 1981). Diazepam administered rectally was given every 12 hours for fever (38.5°C) and was effective in preventing recurrences. However, some mild transient sedation was seen in one-third of the children (Knudsen 1985).

Oral diazepam has been used at the onset of fever (Dianese 1979; Minagawa et al. 1985). Rosman and others (1993a) showed a 44% reduction in risk of febrile seizure recurrence with oral diazepam (1 mg/kg/day given every 8 hours) administered when the child is febrile. There were fairly frequent moderate side effects of lethargy or ataxia, which decreased when dosage was reduced. The primary concern of this treatment is the possibility of sedation of a sick child that may mask underlying serious illness. Home treatment with rectal diazepam once a seizure begins is designed to prevent the convulsion from being prolonged. Rectal diazepam reduced the recurrence rate of febrile seizures in a randomized trial (Pavilidou 2007), given as .33 mg/kg every 8 hours on the first day of fever and every 12 hours on the second day at a maximum of 7.5 mg per dose. Febrile seizure recurrences were reduced by 45% in the highest-risk treated group. Side effects of somnolence and irritability were mild and transient. For the rare situation in which prophylactic treatment is appropriate, such as when the child has recurrent prolonged seizures or is geographically isolated from medical treatment, either prophylactic oral diazepam at the time of febrile illness or rectal diazepam gel to be administered in the event of a seizure are at present the best treatment options available (Camfield et al. 1989; Morton et al. 1997).

Conclusion

Although febrile seizures may be frightening to witness, the child who has one or several will usually do well. Parental reassurance and counseling form the cornerstone of management of the child with febrile seizures. Treatment has not been shown to prevent development of epilepsy. Few children need be placed on treatment to prevent recurrences. Potential risks of anticonvulsant therapy must be weighed against its benefits. Further investigations of new therapies are needed before we can be assured that they are both safe and efficacious. Fortunately, the great majority of children with febrile seizures will have a good outcome whatever management strategy the physician and family choose.

Consider Consultation When…

- A child has more than two or three febrile convulsions.
- A child has a preexisting neurodevelopmental abnormality.
- A febrile convulsion is prolonged, for example, lasting more than 30 minutes.

Annotated bibliography

Addy DP. Nosology of febrile convulsions. *Arch Dis Child* 1986;61:318–320.

A discussion of factors that have an impact on the prognosis of the child with afebrile seizures. The evidence resulting from the major studies is very well presented and summarized, and logical conclusions are drawn. Where questions remain, they are well defined.

Berg AT, Shinnar S, Hauser WA, et al. A prospective study of recurrent febrile seizures. *N Engl J Med* 1992;327:1122–1128.

This study presents the factors affecting risk of febrile seizure recurrence in 347 children with a first febrile seizure. The recurrence rate was greater for a shorter duration of fever and lower temperature before the seizure.

Farwell JR, Lee YJ, Hirtz DG, et al. Phenobarbital for febrile seizures: Effects on intelligence and seizure recurrence. *N Engl J Med* 1990;322:364–369.

This article reports the results of a randomized, double-blind, placebo-controlled study to investigate the side effects of phenobarbital for prevention of febrile seizures. An adverse effect on intellectual function was seen.

Verity C, Butler NR, Golding J. Febrile convulsions in a national cohort following up from birth. I. Prevalence and recurrence in the first five years of life. *Br Med J* 1985;290:1307–1310.

Verity C, Butler NR, Golding J. Febrile convulsions in a national cohort following up from birth. II. Medical history and intellectual ability at 5 years of age. *Br Med J* 1985;290:1311–1314.

This study gives the results of follow-up of about 16,000 neonatal survivors born in 1 week in Britain in 1970. Children with febrile convulsions were compared with their peers at 5 years. This study is in good agreement with the results of the previous large American studies but unfortunately also repeats some of their weaknesses, such as lack of reporting for treatment.

Shinnar S, Glauser TA. Febrile seizures. *J Child Neurol* 2002;17:544–552.

A current review of the epidemiology, evaluation, and management of febrile seizures.

CHAPTER 28

The Child with Attention Deficit Hyperactivity Disorder

Kevin M. Antshel, Michelle M. Macias, and Russell A. Barkley

Outline

- Signs and symptoms
- Etiology
- Workup and diagnosis
- Treatment
- Prognosis

Attention deficit hyperactivity disorder (ADHD) is perhaps the most common neurobehavioral disorder. It is characterized by developmentally inappropriate degrees of inattention, impulsiveness, and/or hyperactivity that most often arise in early to middle childhood, result in impairment across multiple domains of daily life activities, and remain relatively persistent over time. The prevalence was once estimated to be 3–5% of school-age children (American Psychiatric Association 2001), but current studies that include the more recently recognized inattentive-only subtype place the figure closer to 7–8% of school-age children (Barbaresi et al. 2002) and 4–5% of adults (Kessler et al. 2006). Prevalence clearly varies as a function of age, male gender, chronic health problems, family dysfunction, low socioeconomic status, presence of a developmental impairment, and urban living (Lavigne et al. 1996). The disorder is found in all countries surveyed, with rates similar to if not higher than those found in North America (Barkley 2005a,b; Polanczyk et al. 2007). Differences across ethnic groups within the North America are sometimes found but seem to be more a function of social class than ethnicity (Bloom & Cohen, 2007). Although diagnosed as a categorical disorder, ADHD may actually represent an extreme end along a normal continuum for the traits of attention, inhibition, and the regulation of motor activity (Levy et al. 1997).

The current edition of the American Psychiatric Association's *Diagnostic and Statistical Manual of Mental Disorders* (DSM-IV) sets forth the diagnostic criteria to be used in diagnosis. These symptoms are classified under three categories: inattention, impulsivity, and hyperactivity. Developmentally inappropriate levels of *inattention* are signaled by six or more of the following symptoms that have persisted for at least 6 months:

1. Often fails to give close attention to details or makes careless mistakes in schoolwork, work, or other activities
2. Often has difficulty sustaining attention in tasks or play activities
3. Often does not seem to listen when spoken to directly
4. Often does not follow through on instructions, and fails to finish schoolwork, chores, or duties in the workplace (not due to oppositional behavior or failure to understand instructions)
5. Often has difficulty organizing tasks and activities
6. Often avoids, dislikes, or is reluctant to engage in tasks that require sustained mental effort (such as schoolwork or homework)
7. Often loses things necessary for tasks or activities (e.g., toys, school assignments, pencils, books, or tools)
8. Is often easily distracted by extraneous stimuli
9. Is often forgetful in daily activities

To diagnose *hyperactive-impulsive* behavior, developmentally inappropriate levels of six or more of the following symptoms must likewise be present for 6 months:

1. Often fidgets with hands or feet or squirms in seat

Key Clinical Questions

- *Are the symptoms of inattention, overactivity, and poor impulse control clinically significant and developmentally inappropriate for age?*
  Distinguishes normal variation in age-typical behavior from clinical levels of severity.
- *Are at least two or more domains of major life activity impaired by these symptoms?*
  Ensures true disorder is present from simply elevated levels of normal temperament.
- *Are there other disorders coexistent with ADHD, such as oppositional or conduct disorder, major depression, anxiety, or learning disorders?*
  Affects future risks of impairment, types of treatment, and/or response to treatment.
- *Does the parent have ADHD?*
  May help distinguish familial-genetic forms of disorder from acquired ones; presence adversely impacts delivery of treatment services to child if parental disorder remains untreated.

2. Often leaves seat in classroom or in other situations in which remaining seated is expected
3. Often runs about or climbs excessively in situations in which it is inappropriate (in adolescents or adults, this may be limited to subjective feelings of restlessness)
4. Often has difficulty playing or engaging in leisure activities quietly
5. Is often "on the go" or often acts as if "driven by a motor"
6. Often talks excessively
7. Often blurts out answers before the questions have been completed
8. Often has difficulty awaiting turn
9. Often interrupts or intrudes on others (e.g., butts into conversations or games)

Other diagnostic criteria include the presence of some inattention or hyperactive-impulsive symptoms prior to age 7 years and in two or more settings (e.g., home and school), with these symptoms resulting in impairment in major life activities (family, school, peers, community) and not being easily attributable to other mental disorders. The inclusion of the age of onset of 7 years has been challenged (Barkley & Biederman 1997) as without scientific foundation and can probably be ignored in favor of the more general criterion that the disorder develops during childhood (e.g., onset before puberty). Other disorders may coexist (are comorbid) with ADHD. The most frequent of these are listed in Table 28.1.

Table 28.1 Attention deficit hyperactivity disorder

Discriminating features

- Difficulties with sustained attention, persistence, and resistance to distraction and/or
- Difficulties with impulse control, regulating activity level, and self-regulation

Consistent features

- For combined and hyperactive-impulsive types:
  - Difficulties with concentration, forgetfulness, disorganization, procrastination
  - Excessively talkative, blurts out comments thoughtlessly
  - Can't wait for things in line or for taking turns; impatient
  - Busy, on the go, fidgety, restless
- Or (for predominantly inattentive type):
  - Passive, sluggish, lethargic, or hypoactive
  - Daydreams, spacey, easily confused, stares, "in a fog"

Variable features

- Specific learning disability (20–70%)
- Specific language disorder (15–60%)
- Oppositional defiant disorder (45–65%)
- Conduct disorder (25–45%)
- Dysthymia or major depression (20–30%)
- Anxiety disorder (10–30%)
- Childhood bipolar disorder (3–10%)
- Poor peer relations (50–70%)
- Developmental coordination disorder (50%+)
- Poor educational performance (70–90%+), grade retention (25–50%), or suspension/expulsion (15–30%)

Adapted from Barkley RA, Murphy KR. *Attention deficit hyperactivity disorder: A clinical workbook*, 3rd ed. New York: Guilford 2005.

The syndrome of attention difficulties, impulsive behavior, distractibility, and overactivity has been known for many years (see Barkley 2005a,b for a historical summary). Numerous attempts have been made at definition and nomenclature, including Strauss syndrome, minimal brain dysfunction or damage, hyperkinetic child syndrome (or hyperkinesis), and attention deficit disorder with and without hyperactivity. Currently, the disorder is labeled *attention deficit hyperactivity disorder* with the subtype of the disorder further specified (predominantly inattentive, predominantly hyperactive-impulsive, or combined type) (American Psychiatric Association [APA] 2001).

Despite the prevalence of the hyperactive syndrome and its description in the medical literature since the turn of the century (Still 1902), its existence as a clinical entity has been questioned continually, particularly in the popular media. Some social critics believe that the term has been used as a wastebasket diagnosis for children who present with a variety of socially unacceptable behaviors, or that the diagnosis is too often used to excuse aggressive, disruptive, or poorly disciplined children. However,

Pearls and Perils

Attention Deficit Hyperactivity Disorder (ADHD)

- You are only as good as your Rolodex or personal data assistant. It is critical that clinicians maintain an extensive file of potential referral agencies and professionals to whom families of children with ADHD can be directed for the myriad additional, nonmedical services they are likely to require (parent training, special educational services, tutoring, counseling, parent support groups, residential treatment, substance abuse treatments, vocational assessments, as well as treatments for parents, etc.).
- Base the diagnosis on several sources of information rather than relying exclusively on office behavior or parental report alone. Teacher information, reports from other caregivers, past records including report cards, prior evaluations, etc., are indispensable in providing a multi-source evaluation. Each source has its limitations that can be partially corrected by other sources.
- There is no set age at which one can initiate or terminate medication treatment. Although children 5 years of age and older arguably respond better than preschool children, some preschoolers require and can benefit from medication. If needed and effective, medications can be continued into adulthood.
- Avoid the diagnosis of ADHD in children younger than age 3 years as there may not be sufficient history of persistent symptoms on which to confidently render a diagnosis. Moreover, mental disorders at this age often have yet to differentiate themselves and thus what may become ADHD, oppositional defiant disorder (ODD)/conduct disorder (CD), childhood bipolar illness (CBI), or even autistic spectrum disorders often cannot be discerned from each other at this age. Below this age, consider using the term "at risk for" or "probable" ADHD, and follow the case for further development of symptoms before giving a confident diagnosis.
- Watch for and query parents about parental psychopathology including ADHD, depression, anxiety disorders, substance use disorders, or marital discord, among others. When present, these can result in a worse prognosis for the child, greater risk for comorbid disorders such as ODD or CD, poorer compliance with treatment recommendations, and consequently less effective intervention for the child. As many as 25% of parents may require treatment for their own conditions.
- Be attuned to the possibilities of child physical abuse and posttraumatic stress disorder (PTSD), particularly when comorbid ODD and CBI are present, or when genetically unrelated adults reside in the home. The child with ADHD, especially when these other parental disorders are comorbid, can be exceptionally stressful for caregivers, particularly when the caregiver is compromised by psychopathology. The threshold for eliciting physical abuse from others in these instances may be lower than usual.
- When titrating medications, always obtain information directly from the school staff rather than rely exclusively on parental filtering of such information. This can be repeated quarterly as part of routine monitoring of the child's medication.
- Not all children who are inattentive have ADHD. Children with anxiety, depression, sleep disorders, otitis media, autistic spectrum disorders, PTSD, and the learning disabilities (LDs), among others, can all have periodic difficulties with attention as part of the presenting complaints. Hence knowledge of and careful attention to differential diagnosis is paramount in the evaluation of children with ADHD.
- Medications may diminish irritating and disruptive behaviors in a child sufficiently so that he is no longer an overt problem. Take care that other less obvious disorders or impairments are not overlooked (educational underachievement, LDs, PTSD, etc.).

numerous professionals who have worked with or studied children with ADHD have mounted a plethora of evidence to show that ADHD symptomatology constitutes a cluster distinct from those of other disorders, is associated with specific neuroimaging and genetic findings, comprises a distinct and persistent developmental course with numerous risks for various harms, and responds to various treatment approaches (Barkley 2002; Barkley 2005a,b).

There is near universal agreement that more boys than girls qualify for the diagnosis, with an average ratio of 3:1 in community samples, which increases to as much as 5:1 to 9:1 in tertiary care or specialty clinics (APA 2001; Szatmari 1992). The reason for this gender difference is not clear, although it may be partly due to multifactorial neurologic and genetic factors for which males are more at risk than females. Higher sex ratios in specialty clinics may also be partly due to factors related to referral bias, such as greater aggression and conduct problems among males.

Signs and symptoms

The primary symptoms that distinguish children with ADHD from others are their significant difficulties with inhibition (including hyperactivity) and/or their inability to attend to tasks for an age-appropriate period of time while resisting distractions (APA 2001; Barkley 2005a,b). For some children, this may occur in most situations, including those with high-interest activities. But for most children with ADHD, however, these difficulties with attention and inhibition are manifested primarily in settings requiring self-restraint, persistence, and a high level of concentration to relatively uninteresting activities. This can be viewed as an exaggeration of the normal response to having to study or work on a project that demands sustained attention and resistance to interference. These difficulties obviously have a major impact on classroom functioning and may result in limited learning, disruption of class activities, poor work completion, impaired peer interactions, and increased conflict with teachers.

Distractibility is a major component of the difficulties with attention difficulty foreseen in children with ADHD. This inability to inhibit responding to task-irrelevant events or information leads the child to frequently and inappropriately attend to sights, sounds, and movements within range of vision or hearing. In the classroom, a teacher who finds that the child is unable to remember what has been said or leaves most work assignments unfinished may label the child as lazy or unmotivated. At home, the parent who finds the son or daughter diverted from a requested task is understandably upset and may interpret the behavior as frank disobedience. In community settings such as stores, restaurants, or church, observers may interpret the child's hyperactive, restless, inattentive, and otherwise challenging behavior as a result of poor parenting and lack of proper discipline.

Another common symptom in most children with ADHD (except the inattentive type) is impulsivity or poor behavioral inhibition (Barkley 1999; Nigg 2001). This is often associated with excessive talking, touching of nearby objects, exploration of nearby areas, difficulties waiting, and poor delayed gratification. Teachers describe a child who blurts out comments without much reflection; prepares papers or takes tests too quickly, carelessly, and inaccurately; and talks out inappropriately in class. Problems with taking turns, sharing, cooperation, and following rules are also commonplace.

Excessive motor activity is sometimes the symptom that prompts parents to seek professional assistance, especially in younger children (Posner et al. 2007). A mother may report a history of a baby overactive since birth, but more commonly the excessive activity is first noticed when the child is a toddler or preschooler (2–4 years of age) (Smidts & Oosterlan 2007). At this age, the child's waking hours may be a whirlwind of activity, constantly climbing on or jumping off things, with excessive movement, as if driven by a motor. At this age, children with ADHD may put themselves in dangerous situations through lack of forethought resulting in caretakers being constantly vigilant for the safety of the child, siblings, or possessions.

Up to 30–50% of children diagnosed with ADHD have minimal problems with hyperactivity. This group is subtyped as having the predominantly inattentive form of ADHD. A large minority manifests a sluggish cognitive tempo, show passive and sometimes withdrawn behavior, may stare and daydream more than others, and are often withdrawn or reticent in social interactions (Hartman et al. 2004; McBurnett et al. 2001; Milich et al. 2001). It is not yet clear whether this represents a qualitatively different subtype of ADHD or an entirely separate disorder of attention (Todd et al. 2004). Regardless, such children are unlikely to show impulsive or hyperactive behavior, have less comorbid oppositional defiant or conduct disorders, may not respond as well to stimulant medications, yet may be more responsive to social skills training (Carlson & Mann, 2002; Milich et al. 2001).

In the preschool years, a child's inhibition, activity level, or attention span is more easily compared with that of other children. Preschool teachers point out that the children with ADHD cannot stay with a task, sit for a story, sustain attention to some assigned activity, or complete a task as well as other children of the same age (Murray et al. 2007). These children cannot sit still for snacks, circle time, or other sedentary activities and thereby demand a considerable amount of staff attention, supervision, and engagement.

It is in elementary school, however, that the child's inattention, impulsiveness, or hyperactivity tends to be most troublesome. Prior dismissals of the child's excess energy, activity, or zeal as "just normal boy behavior" or as an immaturity to be outgrown are now a real impediment to the ability to adjust to and learn in the classroom. This often earns the child negative teacher attention, peer rejection, and a greater than normal amount of punishment. The hours spent in the classroom are the time when a child's behavior is most expected to conform to that of others of the same age, and walking around in the classroom, disturbing other children, playing the class clown, or otherwise getting into trouble are poorly tolerated. At home, this is the child who has trouble sitting through meals, and who while watching a TV program, may be in and out of the room constantly, moving about or doing somersaults or headstands in front of the screen, antagonizing a sibling, or throwing toys about the room.

As the child enters middle childhood, he often is more able to control the gross motor movements such as running about or climbing on objects, but still may be noted to be fidgety, to be restless while seated, to change positions frequently, to play with objects constantly, and to talk excessively (Hurtig et al. 2007; Weiss & Hechtman 1993). Excessive talking is often evident in settings requiring restraint or quiet behavior, such as in church, in movie theaters, while others are talking, or in the classroom.

The majority of normal children seem to acquire appropriate social skills such as reciprocity, sharing, turn taking, recognition of ownership, and empathy by a combination of instinct and learning. In contrast, the child with ADHD is often self-centered, demanding, selfish, disruptive, and with little regard for the effect of his behavior on others. They may often view themselves as more competent in tasks or activities than they actually are in reality, may be more boastful of their talents, and are less attentive to the emotional behavior of others and other social cues (Hoza et al. 2000). Signs of peer displeasure or rejection may appear within minutes of joining a new play group (Mrug et al. 2007). By elementary school, the social isolation may be further compounded by peer teasing or other provocation, and by fourth grade, most ADHD children have very few close friendships. These mutual experiences among ADHD or other socially rejected children may lead them to seek out each others' companionship and thus sow the seeds for a deviant peer group that may even encourage antisocial behavior.

In addition to the difficulties in school that may result from the symptoms of ADHD, children with the disorder are more likely to have learning disabilities, language delays, and developmental coordination disorders. These disorders are separate primary conditions that require distinct interventions apart from those introduced for the management of ADHD. Although many ADHD children may seem like ideal candidates for grade retention to address their apparent behavioral and academic immaturity, research shows that school retention results in no benefits and multiple harms (Pagani et al. 2001).

Although gross and fine motor milestones may be met early by some children with ADHD, more often motor milestones are met behind schedule, consistent with developmental coordination disorder (Kadesjo & Gillberg 1998). Such children may be clumsy in the gym or during sports; show less physical fitness, stamina, and endurance; and have poor graphomotor skills.

Many parents complain of discipline problems with their ADHD children, with as many as 45–65% or more meeting criteria for oppositional defiant disorder (ODD), with frequent temper outbursts. Stubborn, defiant, and otherwise resistant behavior is the norm, and aggressive and destructive behavior may appear. Research suggests that as many as half of these oppositional children will progress to early-onset conduct disorder such as lying, stealing, fighting, and otherwise violating the rights of others (Barkley et al. 1990; van Lier et al. 2007; Weiss & Hechtman 1993).

A smaller but still significant proportion of ADHD children (20–30%) may eventually develop signs of major depression (Brown 2001; Pliszka et al. 2000). These are the children most characterized by low self-esteem, statements of self-hatred, apparent demoralization, social withdrawal, and sometimes suicidal ideation. Although less apparent in childhood, these problems may become more obvious by adolescence, particularly in teens with ADHD and conduct disorder. Repeated family stress, economic disadvantage, and exposure to physical or emotional trauma is more common among such children, potentially triggering events for their otherwise genetic vulnerability toward depression. Of considerable interest is the research suggesting that a history of major depressive disorder before age 13 is a powerful predictor of the syndromic persistence of ADHD into adolescence (Hurtig et al. 2007). Anxiety disorders may also be seen in a minority of ADHD children (10–30%), and individuals with the predominantly inattentive type of ADHD arguably may be more prone to comorbid anxiety disorders (Carlson & Mann, 2002; Milich et al. 2001).

Controversy abounds on the overlap of ADHD with childhood bipolar disorder (Sachs et al. 2000; Spencer et al. 2001). This may represent a one-way comorbidity, in that having ADHD may not elevate risk for bipolar disorder whereas childhood bipolar illness (CBI) may be commonly associated with ADHD (up to 97%). The differential between ADHD and CBI can often be quite difficult and is compounded by the lack of consensus for CBI diagnostic criteria. However, differential diagnosis of CBI from ADHD is often predicated not only on symptom presentation and severity, but also a family history of bipolar disorder in the former but rarely the latter disorder. Convergent symptoms include hyperactivity, impulsivity, distractibility, disorganization, and conduct problems. Childhood bipolar disorder shows frequent, severe, and capricious mood swings having little to do with rational environmental precipitants, whereas ADHD children often show poor emotional self-control to routine emotionally provocative events. Clearly more research is needed on CBI and its defining features, as well as its overlap with ADHD.

Etiology

Significant advances in the understanding of the neurobiology of ADHD have taken place over the last decade using central nervous system (CNS) neuroimaging, molecular genetics, family genetic studies, and neuropharmacology. The etiology of ADHD most likely involves multiple potential biologic causes possibly interacting with psychosocial ones (Connor 2002; Sonuga-Barke & Sergeant 2005). Neuropharmacologic studies support a central dopamine/norepinephrine dysregulation etiology for ADHD. The proposed model involves dysregulation in the primarily noradrenergic inhibitory influence of prefrontal cortical activity on primarily dopaminergic subcortical CNS structures.

ADHD is now viewed as largely a genetic neurobiologic disorder having striking levels of heritability rivaling some physical traits, such as height, and exceeding most psychological traits, such as intelligence or personality (Faraone et al. 2005; Levy & Hay 2001). Family, adoption, and twin studies have investigated the genetic component to ADHD. These studies show that the ability to inherit ADHD ranges from 0.6 to almost 1 (average 0.76), indicating ADHD is one of the most heritable disorders. Significant advances in the molecular genetics of ADHD have also been made. Researchers have focused on genes in the dopamine pathway, as the pathophysiology of ADHD has implicated dopaminergic dysfunction. The dopamine transporter (*DAT1*) gene (Todd et al. 2005) and the D4 receptor (*DRD4*) gene on chromosome 11 (Barkley et al. 2006) have been implicated in ADHD but inconsistent results have been found (Levy & Hay 2001). Large-scale molecular genetic studies are needed to more completely investigate the genetic heterogeneity of ADHD.

In a minority of cases, risk factors including pregnancy complications; fetal exposure to alcohol, cocaine, and tobacco; premature birth; low birth weight and/or associated minor hemorrhagic CNS lesions; pre-, peri-, or postnatal hypoxia; CNS infection; head trauma; CNS cancers or leukemia or their treatments (radiation or chemotherapy); or significantly elevated lead levels during the first 3 years of life may be contributory to the disorder. Males may be somewhat more likely to have ADHD secondary to acquired disturbances of CNS development, but it is increasingly clear that the majority of both sexes can derive their ADHD entirely from genetic contributions. However, etiology may be difficult to establish and may not be especially pertinent to treatment planning. Acquired cases may arguably be somewhat less responsive to stimulant medications (Greenhill & Osmon 2002). The clinician should allay parental feelings of guilt over having socially induced the disorder through poor child rearing, as there is no convincing evidence that ADHD can arise through purely social origins. Some conditions may exacerbate the disorder, such as treatment with some anticonvulsants (e.g., phenobarbital, phenytoin), limited sleep, excessive ingestion of food dyes or preservatives, bouts of otitis media, and even recurring mild closed head trauma from some routine sports (soccer, football).

Workup and diagnosis

Both the American Academy of Child and Adolescent Psychiatry (AACAP 2007) and the American Academy of Pediatrics (AAP 2000, 2001) have established guidelines for the assessment and treatment of ADHD. The consensus is that laboratory testing is unhelpful in the diagnosis of ADHD. No neurologic, genetic, neuropsychological, or behavioral tests have sufficient positive and negative predictive power to accurately classify ADHD cases with sufficient success to recommend them for clinical diagnosis (Barkley 2005a,b). This is not to say that groups of ADHD children cannot be differentiated from groups of control children in studies comparing them on these various parameters (Tannock 1999), but clinicians do not compare group means using modern statistics. They classify individual cases and, for such purposes, current tests have proven grossly inadequate (Gordon & Barkley 1998).

Like all other psychiatric disorders and many medical ones, clinical diagnosis is based largely on careful history taking, use of structured interviews containing DSM-IV criteria for ADHD and related disorders, and the expert knowledge of the clinician in the differential diagnosis among childhood mental disorders. Paramount in the evaluative process is the time to listen to parental concerns; probe for details concerning nature, onset, and course; elaborate the specific impairments resulting from these concerns; and place them within the larger framework of the clinical taxonomy of mental disorders. The clinical interview is then supplemented by the use of parent and teacher behavior rating scales to assess developmental deviance of symptoms, screening of intelligence and academic achievement skills by standardized testing, brief observation of the child during unstructured and structured activities, contact with school personnel concerning classroom functioning, and compilation of prior school and mental health records available on the child.

Other sources of information essential for the diagnostic process are behavioral rating scales or checklists on which normative data are available. These include "broad-band" questionnaires, such as the Behavioral Assessment System for Children–2nd edition (Kamphaus & Reynolds 2005) or Child Behavior Checklist (Achenbach 2001) for screening the major dimensions of childhood psychopathology (e.g., anxiety, depression, attention, hyperactivity, aggression, etc.). "Narrow-band" questionnaires specifically evaluate the symptoms of ADHD as set forth in DSM-IV. Rating scales can reliably, validly, and efficiently measure DSM-IV-based ADHD symptoms. Some examples of instruments demonstrating appropriate psychometric properties with a strong normative base include the ADHD Rating Scale IV (DuPaul et al. 1998) and the Conners Rating Scales–Revised (Conners 1997). Reports of prior assessments are important to obtain, and written permission should be obtained from parents to communicate with school personnel concerning the child's school behavior and performance. Telephone contact with school staff can then be initiated.

Medical assessment involves taking a thorough medical history, including probing for the potential etiologic factors previously mentioned. When taking the medical history, it is useful to know not only of major trauma but also minor trauma and whether this is a child who has sustained more than his share of cuts, bumps, scrapes, or broken bones. The child with ADHD's impulsiveness, lack of judgment, inattention, hyperactivity, and poor motor coordination often earns preferred customer status at the local emergency room (Barkley et al. 2002; Rowe et al. 2004). Accidental poison ingestions are more common in children with ADHD, warranting anticipatory guidance regarding aggressive childproofing of the home from these substances and from dangerous objects such as power tools and firearms. Children with ADHD may be more prone to physical abuse by virtue of the stress they may impose on already compromised caretakers (Ford et al. 2000). The risk for such abuse may be even more elevated in those children with comorbid ODD or comorbid CBI.

Developmental history frequently identifies an onset of disorder between 3 and 8 years, although it may be somewhat later for those children manifesting the predominantly inattentive type (Applegate et al. 1997; Barkley & Biederman 1997). Earlier onset may be arguably associated with more severe disorder and higher risk for school failure or psychiatric comorbidity. Infancy may be uneventful, although a significant minority of ADHD children are described as having been difficult or colicky babies. Once locomotor behavior emerges, however, the hyperactive and combined subtypes of ADHD children are likely to be identified by caregivers as excessively active. Developmental milestones may be met at normal ages in many ADHD children, but a significant subset (50%+) may show developmental coordination disorder or language disorders. If not evident beforehand, impairment due to ADHD symptoms is frequently present within the first few years of elementary school. The presence of other children in the home obviously has some bearing on the parents' ability to identify when the ADHD child became noticeably different from normal behavioral standards.

In a large number of cases (15–40%), family history reveals at least one other immediate family member as having ADHD or symptoms sufficient to warrant that diagnosis (Biederman et al. 1996; Faraone et al. 2000). Up to 35% of siblings may have ADHD, whereas 15–20% of mothers and 15–30% of fathers may fulfill criteria for ADHD as adults. If the parent has a diagnosis of ADHD, the risk to offspring may be as high as 52–54% (Barkley 2005a,b). Gentle probing may be needed to unearth educational or behavioral problems in the parents' history. Questioning parents about their own educational attainment, adjustment problems in school, poor grades on report cards, grade retention, and any extra assistance received at school often produce a surprising number of positive endorsements. Physicians are sometimes reluctant to inquire about the occurrence of mental health problems such as depression, alcoholism, other substance dependencies, or sociopathy in family members. However, if the questioning is conducted sensitively in the context of completing a family medical history, it seldom causes offense and can provide significant information in view of the elevated risk of such disorders among biologic family members.

The examination of the child should include a complete physical examination, formal neurologic examination, and an extended neurodevelopmental assessment. In the course of the physical examination, height, weight, and head circumference should be measured and plotted on standardized graphs. Hearing and vision should be screened, and blood pressure should be measured. Findings on the history and physical examination suggestive of medical conditions, including hyper- or hypothyroidism, lead exposure, anemia, or other chronic illness, need to be evaluated. Certain medical conditions warrant closer consideration of medication management in ADHD. For instance, stimulants are primarily central-acting sympathomimetic amines, but may have peripheral effects. Therefore, the presence of hypertension is not a contraindication to stimulant medication usage, but needs to be closely monitored and treated appropriately.

On the neurologic examination the examiner must look for subtle signs of previous CNS insult or progressive neurologic conditions. Abnormalities of muscle tone or a difference in strength, tone, or deep tendon reflex responses between the two sides previously may have gone unnoticed. Nystagmus, ataxia, tremor, decreased visual field, or fundal abnormalities also should be noted and investigated.

The extended neurologic examination provides a systematic approach for describing the progression of higher neurologic function in the areas of motor coordination, visuoperceptual skills, language skills, and global cognitive function through the school-age years. Test items have been developed in an attempt to find a clinical window allowing identification of more specific areas of functional deficit. Formal testing is possibly most useful as a means for observing the child over a period of time and while engaged in a variety of tasks. Often the behavioral symptoms prompting the appointment are evident only if the child is seen for a more extended period. If the appointment is the standard 10-minute physical examination, many parents have been frustrated to find that their child demonstrates none of the "referral" behaviors. If the physician then declares the child to be normal and in no need of treatment, parents are forced to seek help and support elsewhere.

When the examiner sits with the child at a table for paper and pencil tasks, fidgety and distractible behavior may become more apparent (Barkley et al. 2000). Useful activities for this part of the examination are spontaneous or directed handwriting and form copying. Handwriting allows observation of pencil grasp, as well as facility of execution and the finished product. Form copying allows the examiner to assess the child's visuoperceptual skills.

Solving a few math problems at the child's current grade level demonstrates how she may tackle schoolwork. In all tasks, the examiner has an opportunity to see how the child organizes the work on the page, whether she monitors and self-corrects, whether her approach to the task is impulsive, and how well she is able to maintain attention on the work. Once again, the absence of behavioral difficulties or symptoms of ADHD is not evidence against the diagnosis of the disorder, as many ADHD children function well in such one-to-one encounters. However, evidence suggests that behavioral problems that do occur in this context are reasonably predictive of similar such problems in the school setting (Barkley et al. 2000; Campbell 1990).

Whether the physician wishes to include one of the standardized reading tests or screening for receptive and expressive language abilities depends on other testing already performed or planned by other professionals, as well as the interest of the individual clinician and his training in conducting such tests. Clinical or school psychologists may be requested to assist with such evaluations when a more thorough assessment of psychoeducational functioning seems in order.

A number of specific tests have been devised to provide objective measures of a subject's vigilance and impulse control, such as the Gordon Diagnostic System, Conners Continuous Performance Test, or the Test of Variables of Attention, among others (Gordon & Barkley 1998). Research suggests that these tests are not especially accurate at classifying children as ADHD, as the 20–50% false-negative rate is too high and thus the clinician would incorrectly "rule out" the disorder. Although the presence of abnormal scores on such tests indicates the presence of a disorder in as many as 90% of children who perform poorly, such scores cannot indicate the specific disorder present. Moreover, the ecological validity of these tests is low, thus precluding the ability to predict from the test scores how the child will function in more natural settings, such as home and school (Barkley 2005a,b). These tests are therefore not recommended for routine diagnostic evaluations of children with ADHD, although they may be used in clinics specializing in ADHD as part of research or drug trials. More useful information is likely to be obtained from the parent and teacher rating scales discussed earlier. These ratings can also be supplemented with more specific ratings of executive functioning from these sources using the Behavior Rating Inventory of Executive Functioning (BRIEF) (Gioia et al. 2000) or Brown Attention-Deficit Disorder Scales for Children and Adolescents (BADDES) scales (Brown 2001).

Laboratory tests such as blood or urine panels, electroencephalogram (EEG), and neuroimaging scans are seldom of help in making the diagnosis of ADHD. As a rule, they should be undertaken only if there is a clinical indication by the history or physical examination. An EEG can be obtained when there is suspicion of a seizure disorder (e.g., absence spells), but is otherwise unnecessary. Other tests that may be helpful in specific cases include a complete blood count, lead level, blood glucose, and thyroid studies.

Treatment

The evaluation is the first step of intervention; a proper diagnosis is central to an effective treatment plan. As previously stated, the AACAP (AACAP 2007) and the AAP (AAP 2001) have established guidelines for the treatment of ADHD. Treatment for ADHD in children typically involves three components: parent and child education and support, classroom accommodations, and medication. As described earlier, the child with ADHD presents with problems in several areas of adaptive functioning (home, school, community, peers, etc.) and often with additional comorbidity for other disorders (ODD, depression, learning disabilities, etc.). All of these problems and settings must be considered when formulating a treatment plan. The initial explanation and discussion of the disorder is in itself very helpful and therapeutic. A child who has been putting forth his best effort to obey directions, finish his work, and remember facts but is constantly chastised for being lazy and disobedient can be very relieved to know that someone believes that he is trying and understands his difficulties. He needs to hear that he is not "dumb," "retarded," or "stupid," as classmates may have concluded. For the parent, who may have been told on the one hand that there is nothing wrong with the child, or that he will grow out of it, or on the other hand, that the fault lies with their poor child-rearing practices and lack of adequate disciplinary measures, a description of the syndrome can help dispel years of guilt and frustration. At the same time, the physician must convey the message that freedom from blame does not relieve the child or his parent from the responsibility of managing the problem as best as they can.

For most children with ADHD, individual psychotherapy is *not* indicated, unless there is evidence of a reactive form of depression, posttraumatic stress disorder (PTSD), or some other emotional upheaval occurring as a consequence or correlate of family or other forms of stress, trauma, or disruption. This is not to say that the child and family cannot benefit from some counseling about the disorder and its management. It is to say that traditional forms of play therapy, psychotherapy, or some other psychodynamically or psychoanalytically founded therapy has no scientific evidence of efficacy for ADHD at this time.

Group treatment with other children may seem sensible at first blush, given the significant social problems experienced by most children with ADHD. However, research indicates that group social skills training is of little benefit to children with the combined type of ADHD (Antshel & Remer 2003). The greatest hope for improving the efficacy of such treatment is to incorporate parents and teachers into the training program to try to generalize the skills being conveyed in the treatment group to more natural settings. Even then, evidence for effectiveness is scant. In contrast, recent studies indicate that the inattentive subtype, especially those manifesting the sluggish cognitive tempo noted earlier, may benefit from this treatment approach. Such children are more passive and possibly anxious in social settings and may respond better to social skills initiatives. Caution is warranted in placing the ADHD child into any social skills group, as evidence is mounting that putting nonaggressive ADHD children in with more aggressive peers may increase aggression or other forms of antisocial conduct (Antshel & Remer 2003).

Substantial evidence exists to show that training parents in child behavior management skills can be of significant benefit in the reduction of parent–child conflict and improvement in child success within the home (Anastopoulos et al. 1993; MTA Group 1999). Such an intervention does not ameliorate the symptoms of ADHD, given their substantial neurogenetic origins. Instead, it reduces oppositional, defiant, and noncompliant behavior through improvement in parental reinforcement, and disciplinary tactics and instruction giving, among other skills. Such training can occur in groups. Often, a first step in the parent training intervention is to gather a detailed accounting of behavioral problems including when and in what situations misbehaviors occur. It is also useful to record how parents and other adults react to the behaviors and what subsequent interactions take place as a result of those reactions. In sum, what are the social contingencies that might be cueing, exacerbating, or sustaining inappropriate behavior, if any? (See Barkley 2005a,b for more information.) What disciplinary methods are used in the home now and in the past, and what formalized help have parents sought and obtained for managing the problems? Both parents need to be involved if both have contact with the child. At the very least, the nonattending parent must be supportive of the one attending training if the transfer of skills from the group to the home setting is to be enhanced. If others regularly care for the child, they may also be involved in the training, so that the child experiences consistency across the routine caregivers in his life. Family therapy or training is maximally effective with preschool or elementary school-aged children and may decline sharply in effectiveness after 12–14 years of age. Thereafter, interventions will need to be added that address influences outside the family, such as peers, school, and others. Other forms of family therapy can be used when there are interactional issues needing attention, as in marital discord, parenting stress, or parent–ADHD teen conflict.

The school setting frequently requires adjustment to meet the special needs of the child with ADHD (DuPaul & Stoner 2003). As ADHD is included within the Individuals with Disabilities in Education Act (IDEA) as well as Section 504 of the Rehabilitation Act of 1973, many children with ADHD are eligible for free educational evaluations through their school districts and, in many cases, access to a variety of special educational services and 504 accommodations. A child can be eligible for 504 accommodations (classroom and curriculum modifications and adaptations) if it can be demonstrated that the child's ADHD adversely affects his learning. Under the IDEA, ADHD may be considered under the specific category of "Other Health Impaired," and special education and related services can be provided. Simply having an ADHD diagnosis does not qualify the child in either the ADA or IDEA; the link between ADHD and adverse learning outcomes must be demonstrated for the child to qualify.

School interventions often include alterations to the curriculum and work load to better mesh with the limited attention, persistence, and disorganization of the child with ADHD; special educational services (push-in or mainstreaming assistance to regular teachers, pull-out services to focus on more individualized child training, self-contained classes, etc.); increases in sources of positive reinforcement for work productivity; occasional use of immediate and systematic negative consequences for disruptive or inappropriate behavior; implementation of a daily school behavior report card (the ratings of which are linked to a home token economy); peer-tutoring or other innovative approaches to using peer influence to achieve classroom goals; and more frequent communication with parents. In short, greater accountability of the child to teachers and others including more immediate, frequent, and salient feedback for performance, and increased structuring of the classroom environment and teaching materials have all been shown to benefit the child with ADHD in school. The presence of learning disabilities in 20–50% or more of children with ADHD necessitates additional services to address the specific academic domain of disability (reading, math, spelling, language, handwriting, etc.).

The mainstay of treatment for many children with ADHD is medication, frequently psychostimulants. Space precludes a detailed consideration of the various medications that may benefit children with ADHD, and the physician should consult more detailed texts on pediatric psychopharmacology (Green, 2007; Werry & Aman 1999) or the specific chapters in Barkley (2005) dealing with medications for ADHD. Four classes of medication appear to be useful for management of ADHD, these being: psychostimulants (methylphenidate, amphetamines), noradrenergic reuptake inhibitors (atomoxetine), tricyclic antidepressants, and antihypertensive medications (clonidine, guanfacine). The patient's response to stimulant medication should not be used as a diagnostic tool, given that normal children may also show modest benefits from such medication.

Stimulants have been used to treat ADHD children since 1937. They are the best-studied medications for the management of ADHD, showing efficacy in 75% or more of ADHD children, and possibly more if all stimulant classes are tested in sequence during the drug trial. The general benefits and side effects of stimulants are shown in Table 28.2. Beneficial effects are substantial, with 50–60% of children with ADHD being normalized in their behavior during active medication therapy, and another 20% or more improved but not normalized. The response rate for children younger than 5 years of age may be less robust, and side effects may be somewhat greater. A large-scale multisite trial of stimulants in preschoolers sponsored by the National Institute of Mental Health, the multicenter Preschool ADHD Treatment Study (PATS) (Greenhill et al. 2006), suggested that methylphenidate was efficacious relative to placebo; however, effect sizes (0.4–0.8) were generally less than observed in the school-aged population and with more adverse effects (Wigal et al. 2006).

The side effects of stimulants are fairly benign, short-lived, dose-related, and often managed through dose or timing adjustments, or by switching to a different delivery system or stimulant. Initial concerns about growth were overrated, with more recent studies suggesting a relatively limited impact on weight of 1–4 pounds during the first year of treatment with little or no impact thereafter. Effects on height are arguable and may be in the range of 1–2 mm during the initial year of treatment, again with little evidence for any ongoing growth prevention thereafter (MTA Group 2004). However, the fact that a few children may have more significant growth problems on stimulants warrants periodic monitoring and plotting of growth parameters on published standardized growth charts.

The two most commonly used stimulant categories for management of ADHD are methylphenidate (Ritalin, Ritalin SR, Ritalin LA, Concerta, Metadate CD, Methylin, Daytrana) and the amphetamines (Dexedrine, Adderall, Adderall XR). Two newer stimulant categories are dexmethylphenidate (Focalin, Focalin XR) and lisdexamfetamine (Vyvanse). These are well-studied medications and highly effective for the management of most cases of ADHD. Recent years have witnessed the development of once-daily delivery systems for methylphenidate and related medications (Concerta, Metadate CD, Ritalin LA, Daytrana, Focalin XR) and the amphetamines (Adderall XR, Vyvanse) such that children may not require any administration of medication while in school. This is a remarkable accomplishment for clinical practice in view of the understandable resistance of children to be singled out at school for dosing, with its associated stigma (the short

Table 28.2 Effects, side effects, and common public misconceptions of stimulants

Behavioral effects

- Increased concentration and persistence
- Decreased impulsivity and hyperactivity
- Increased work productivity (and accuracy)
- Better emotional control
- Decreased aggression and defiance/ODD/CD
- Improved compliance and rule-following
- Better working memory and internalized language
- Improved handwriting and motor coordination
- Improved self-esteem
- Decreased punishment from others
- Improved peer acceptance and interactions
- Better awareness of game in sports

Side effects

- Insomnia and loss of appetite (50%+)
- Headaches and stomach aches (20–40%)
- Irritability, prone to crying (<10%)
- Nervous habits and mannerisms (<10%)
- Tics (<3%) and Tourette syndrome (rare)
- Mild weight loss (mean = 0.5–1.8 kg; transient)
- Minimal long-term effects on height (1–2 mm in first year)
- Increased heart rate (3–10 b.p.m.), blood pressure (1.5–14 mm Hg)
- Monitor higher risk African American males
- <3% stimulant psychosis
- 5% discontinuation due to adverse events
- No discernible long-term adverse consequences to date
- Pemoline requires frequent monitoring of liver enzymes.

Common public misconceptions

- Stimulants are addictive when used as prescribed.
  - No. To be abused, they must be inhaled or injected.
- Stimulants are overprescribed.
  - Only 2–3% are on medication vs. the 7+% prevalence of ADHD.
- Stimulants create aggressive, assaultive behavior.
  - No. Stimulants decrease aggression and antisocial actions.
- Stimulants increase the risk of seizures.
  - No. This occurs only at very, very high doses.
- Stimulants cause Tourette syndrome.
  - No. Although they can increase tics in 30%; they decrease tics in 35%.
- Stimulants create a greater risk of later substance abuse.
  - No. Fourteen studies find no such result; a few also found decreased risk if treatment continued through teens (Barkley et al. 2003; Wilens et al. 2003).
- Stimulants don't improve academic achievement.
  - Not if one means academic knowledge; no pill contains knowledge. However, stimulants improve work productivity (often dramatically); and have less but some effect on accuracy. They improve classroom conduct and rule-following, and improve peer interactions. Their use can result in improved grades (due to more completed assignments) and result in reduced punishment from teachers and peers.

time course of earlier preparations necessitated multiple daily dosing). These compounds provide 8–12 hours of therapeutic benefit.

These medications appear to increase brain inhibitory mechanisms while providing the child with greater concentration, persistence, and resistance to distractions. Methylphenidate is now known to act primarily by blocking the dopamine and norepinephrine reuptake transporters, while the amphetamines have a greater impact on the production and release of dopamine into the extracellular space (and some arguable secondary effects on the transport and inhibition of dopamine metabolism via monoamine oxidase). Both medications result in increased intrasynaptic availability of dopamine and norepinephrine, allowing for greater action on postsynaptic binding sites. The evidence on the safety and efficacy of the stimulants is abundant (Greenhill & Osmon 2002). When prescribed appropriately and monitored carefully, these medications are safe and effective, with no evidence currently available suggesting any long-term consequences from years of medication use.

The effects of the immediate-release preparations of the stimulants are evident with 15–30 minutes of ingestion, seem to peak in 2–4 hours, and typically dissipate in 3–5 hours. The once-daily extended release preparations result in a considerable extension of this time course, such that behavioral effects may last for 8–12 hours, depending on the delivery system.

When prescribing stimulants for a child with ADHD, a number of factors must be considered. Whether the patient should take the medication only on school days or 7 days a week and vacation time depends on whether the benefit is mainly in improved classroom performance or needs to include better behavior in nonschool settings. Where weight gain and height issues have been demonstrated to be problematic during stimulant therapy, drug holidays may be indicated. Otherwise, the settings in which impairment exists should determine the schedule and amount of dosing for the vast majority of cases. At least once per year, medication should be discontinued for a period of up to 1 week when the schedule is stable and teachers have had occasion to become familiar with this child on medication (usually by end of October of the new school year) so as to provide informed feedback on efficacy and continued need for medication. Medication discontinuation can be considered when the child does just as well without as with it; this can result after several years of maturational improvement and/or additional classroom and home accommodations. There is considerable individual variation in this regard, with some able to stop in elementary school while others require continued treatment into adulthood. Monitoring of growth, heart rate, blood pressure, as well as clinical effectiveness and side effects should be done several times per year of treatment (every 3–4 months).

Atomoxetine (Strattera) is a nonstimulant approved for management of ADHD. Atomoxetine is an exclusive noradrenergic reuptake inhibitor and is the first drug indicated for ADHD that is not a Schedule II controlled substance. It has a low potential for abuse, making it more convenient than the stimulants for sampling, prescribing, and titrating. Available evidence suggests equal efficacy with immediate-release methylphenidate yet with fewer side effects (less insomnia, better morning behavior). As with the stimulants, treatment can be dispensed either once or twice daily. Over 75% of children show a positive response, and this response has been maintained for up to 2 years in longitudinal research. Studies indicate that atomoxetine reduces ADHD, ODD, aggression, and depression; increases school productivity; improves social behavior and self-esteem; benefits parent–child relations; and may improve enuresis where present. Interestingly, "morning after dose" behavior is also improved, perhaps owing to greater sleep the previous evening. Side effects include: sedation (10–20+%), decreased appetite (14–22%), nausea (12%), dizziness (6%), increased blood pressure (2 mm Hg diastolic, 3 mm Hg systolic), increased heart rate of 8 b.p.m., temporary weight loss (0.5–2.3 kg), and liver function test abnormalities. Full effects of atomoxetine can take up to 3 weeks, so families should be cautioned to be patient in evaluating drug response.

If the clinician wishes to evaluate drug response to the stimulants in more detail, he can conduct a double-blind placebo-controlled trial, alternating doses of medication with placebo on a weekly basis and collecting parent and teacher ratings of ADHD symptoms and side effects each week. The assistance of a pharmacist in preparing the placebo will be required; our own trials utilize lactose powder placed in gelatin capsules with a comparable capsule used to house the comparison medication and dose.

Pearls and Perils

Attention Deficit Hyperactivity Disorder (ADHD)

- ADHD symptoms should result in obvious, not subtle, impairments in important daily activities.
- Comorbid behavior and mood disorders, as well as learning disabilities and language disorders, are common.
- ADHD symptoms are not because of mental retardation.
- A visual inspection of the child's handwriting before and after successful medication use frequently reveals a noticeable improvement in legibility.
- Complete medication coverage must be seriously considered for ADHD teenagers who drive after school hours.

Key Clinical Questions

- *Are the symptoms of inattention, overactivity, and poor impulse control clinically significant and developmentally inappropriate for age?*
  Distinguishes normal variation in age-typical behavior from clinical levels of severity.
- *Are at least two or more domains of major life activity impaired by these symptoms?*
  Ensures true disorder is present from simply elevated levels of normal temperament.
- *Are there other disorders coexistent with ADHD, such as oppositional or conduct disorder, major depression, anxiety, or learning disorders?*
  Affects future risks of impairment, types of treatment, and/or response to treatment.
- *Does the parent have ADHD?*
  May help distinguish familial-genetic forms of disorder from acquired ones; presence adversely impacts delivery of treatment services to child if parental disorder remains untreated.

Other medications that are not U.S. Food and Drug Administration (FDA) approved for the treatment of ADHD but may be helpful in the management of ADHD in children in whom the stimulants or atomoxetine are ineffective include bupropion (primarily a noradrenergic reuptake inhibitor) and the tricyclic antidepressants (TCAs), which also probably work by blocking norepinephrine reuptake (Barkley 2005a,b; Green 2007; Werry & Aman 1999). The TCAs are declining in use due to the availability of the safer noradrenergic agents such as atomoxetine and bupropion. The TCAs require cardiac monitoring both before and during treatment, may be prone to habituation in some cases, and often manifest greater side effects than do atomoxetine or bupropion. The serotonergically mediated antidepressants (SSRIs), such as fluoxetine, as well as the modern anxiolytics are not effective for the management of ADHD symptoms, but may be needed for treating cases involving comorbid depression or anxiety.

Clonidine and guanfacine are α-noradrenergic agonists that have some effectiveness for the management of hyperactive-impulsive ADHD symptomatology. They are also considered "off-label" for treatment of ADHD, as they have not been specifically approved by the FDA for treatment of ADHD. They work in part by decreasing arousal via noradrenergic inhibition at the level of the locus coeruleus. Such medications should be considered second- or third-line because of greater concerns regarding their safety with children, their markedly longer phase for titration, and their potential need for monitoring of cardiac functioning, as well as the frequent sedation that may occur during the titration and even maintenance stages of management relative to stimulants and atomoxetine. These antihypertensive agents may be indicated when the child demonstrates a failed response to stimulants and atomoxetine, or has significant problems with serious aggressive or destructive/explosive behavior, severe hyperactivity, or tic disorders that have been shown to be exacerbated in a stimulant trial. Dosing for clonidine is typically between 0.25 and 0.3 mg/day given three or four times per day in divided doses. Parents must be forewarned not to alter the dose or its scheduling or to skip doses due to the potential for invoking rebound hypertension. A summary table concerning medications for ADHD is shown in Table 28.3.

When a problem affects as many children as does ADHD, parents search far and wide for treatments and cures. Not surprisingly, a number of controversial treatment methods have been proposed. Because their proponents are generally more available and willing to promote their (often farfetched) theories in the popular media than are busy clinicians who follow a scientist-practitioner model or than legitimate clinical researchers, these "alternative" therapies often achieve considerable publicity. Of the complementary and alternative treatments, only the removal of food coloring and sodium benzoate from the diet has empirical support (McCann et al. 2007; Schab & Trinh 2004), albeit with small effect sizes (0.2–0.3). Dietary supplements (typically involving antioxidants, trace elements, minerals, or oils), various allergen therapies, chiropractic manipulations or manual pressure placed on points about the skull, sensory integration therapy, ocular-motor exercises or visual perspective training, electromyogram (EMG) or EEG biofeedback, or social skills training (especially when administered only in clinical settings) have very limited or no empirical support. Parents wishing to try these treatments should be apprised of the lack of scientific evidence in favor of their use and the fact that perceived changes may well result from placebo effects, increased child monitoring, expectancy effects, or (if sufficient time is spent in treatment) maturation.

Prognosis

The outlook for children with ADHD is quite mixed. Although not a life-threatening or completely debilitating disorder, ADHD can result in a rather wide swath of impairments in major life activities (Barkley 2005a,b; Weiss & Hechtman 1993). The disorders likely to be comorbid with ADHD have been discussed earlier, and many can contribute further to impairments in adaptive functioning beyond that produced by ADHD itself. Current research suggests that upwards of 66% of children diagnosed with ADHD (combined type) continue to

Table 28.3 Medications for attention deficit hyperactivity disorder

Class	Generic (brand) name	Daily dosage	Duration	Mechanism of action	Side effects
Stimulants	Methylphenidate Immediate release/ short-acting (Ritalin, Methylin, Methylin) Intermediate-acting (Ritalin SR, Metadate ER, Methylin ER)	Initial: 0.3–5 mg/kg b.i.d. to t.i.d.; can titrate up to ~1 mg/kg/dose	3–5 hr	Primary: blocks reuptake of DA, NE Secondary: release of DA from storage vesicle	Appetite suppression Delay of sleep onset Abdominal pain Headache Rebound irritability Tics (motor, vocal) Jitteriness
		q.d. to b.i.d.	3–8 hr		
	Extended release/long acting (Concerta, Metadate CD, Ritalin LA, Daytrana)	q.d.	8–12 hr		
	Dexmethylphenidate	b.i.d. to t.i.d.:	Same		
	Short acting (Focalin) Extended release/ Long-acting (Focalin XR)	Initial ½IR MPH			
	Amphetamine	b.i.d. to t.i.d.;	4–6 hr	Primary: release of DA	Same
	Immediate release/ short-acting (Dexedrine, DextroStat)	Initial dose ½IR MPH		from storage vesicle Secondary: blocks reuptake of DA, NE	
	Intermediate-acting (Adderall, Dexedrine spansule)	q.d. to b.i.d.	4–8 hr		
	Extended release/ Long-acting (Adderall-XR)	q.d.	10–12 hr		
	Lisdexamfetamine (Vyvanse)	q.d. 10–12 hr	Same	Same	
Antidepressants					
Tricyclics (TCAs)					
	Imipramine (Tofranil) Desipramine (Norpramin) day in divided doses	b.i.d. to t.i.d.; dose 1–4 mg/kg/		Blocks reuptake of NE	Anticholinergic SE Cardiac SE
	Atypicals				
	Bupropion (Wellbutrin; Wellbutrin SR)	b.i.d. to t.i.d. q.d. to b.i.d. 1.5–6 mg/kg/daytic		NE reuptake inhibitor	Seizure threshold, exacerbation
β_2 agonists Clonidine (Catapres, Catapres TTS)	t.i.d. to QID; initial dose 0.05 mg q.d., titrate slowly to max of 0.4 mg TDD			Arousal at locus coeruleus by NE inhibition	Sedation Low BP
	Guanfacine (Tenex)	b.i.d. to t.i.d.; initial dose 0.5 mg q.d.; titrate to max 4 mg TDD			
SNRI	Atomoxetine (Strattera)	q.d. to b.i.d.; initial dose 0.5 mg/kg, increase to max 1.2–1.8 mg/kg			Blocks reuptake of NE in synapse

demonstrate substantial symptoms of disorder (98th percentile) into young adulthood (Barkley et al. 2002), with as many as 80% demonstrating impairment. No longitudinal studies exist of the inattentive type. The remainder is not necessarily normalized by this age but fall short of current diagnostic criteria for full disorder. When followed to adolescence and adulthood, children with ADHD are at greater risk for a variety of adverse outcomes (Table 28.4), including educational failure and/or underachievement, delinquency, substance use disorders, and personality disorders. Most of these risks are associated more with the development of early-onset conduct disorder (before age 12) than with ADHD alone, although educational underachievement, nicotine use, drug-related antisocial activities, and driving problems are attributable to severity of ADHD rather than its comorbid disorders. The eventual outcome of ADHD children has been difficult to predict. Modest evidence suggests that earlier onset, greater severity of disorder, comorbidity (especially for conduct disorder), lower intelligence, parental psychopathology, family discord, and social disadvantage may worsen the prognosis although even children experiencing one or more of these risk factors may function satisfactorily as adults.

A positive response to medication and implementation of behavioral and educational accommodations can bring about a dramatic change in a child's ability to attend, inhibit, persist, be organized and timely, and produce more schoolwork, as well as in his ability to interact more positively and reasonably with others. To date there is no evidence that treatment with medication, behavioral therapy, and/or special education that is limited to a few years of childhood results in any sustained improvement in academic functioning or other major life activities into adulthood. Evidence suggests that continuation of medication treatment into adolescence might result in a reduced risk for substance use disorders and even antisocial behavior. Evidence from longer-term trials (1–3 years) of medication and behavioral-educational accommodations suggests them to be beneficial so long as treatment is sustained.

Despite this rather negative prognosis for the group of children as a whole, one should be as optimistic as possible when evaluating, advising, and following the individual child and family. With appropriate medical treatment, counseling and parent training, school adjustments, and special educational services as needed, as many as half or more of childhood cases can be expected to grow into a satisfactory level of adult functioning. While the same basic temperamental characteristics usually persist, they can take on a more positive aspect in adulthood, where more numerous occupational and social niches exist within which the symptoms of disorder may no longer be as impairing. Thus, the child with ADHD has the potential to be more successful and accepted as an adult than during childhood with its formal

Table 28.4 Developmental risks and adverse outcomes

Educational risks (ADHD vs. control groups)

- More grade retention (25–45% vs. 13%)
- More placed in special educational (25–50%)
- More are suspended (40–60% vs. 19%)
- Greater expulsion rate (10–18% vs. 6%)
- Higher drop-out rate (30–40% vs.9%)
- Lower class ranking (69% vs. 50%)
- Lower GPA (1.7 vs. 2.6)
- Fewer enter college (22% vs. 77%)
- Lower college graduation rate (5% vs. 35%)

Driving risks

- Poorer steering, more false braking, and slower reaction times to significant events
- Rated by self, others, and driving instructors as using fewer safe driving habits
- More likely to drive before legally licensed
- More accidents (and more at faults) (2–3 vs. 0–2)
  - % with 2+ crashes: 40 vs. 6
  - % with 3+ crashes: 26 vs. 9
- More citations (speeding: mean 4–5 vs. 1–2)
- Worse accidents ($4,200–5,000 vs. $1,600–2,200)
  - (% having a crash with injuries: 60 vs.17)
- More suspensions/revocations (mean 2.2 vs. 0.7); (% suspended: 22–24 vs. 4–5)

Sexual risks

- Begin sexual activity earlier (15 vs. 16 years)
- More sexual partners (18.6 vs. 6.5)
- Less time with each partner
- Less likely to employ contraception
- Greater risk of teen pregnancy (38% vs. 4%)
- Ratio for number of births (42:1)
  - 54% do not have custody of offspring
- Higher risk for STDs (16% vs. 4%)

Employment risks

- Enter workforce at unskilled/semiskilled level
- More likely to be fired (55% vs. 23%; mean 1.1 vs. 0.3 jobs)
- Change jobs more often (2.7 vs. 1.3 times over 2–8 years since leaving high school)
- More ADHD/ODD symptoms on the job (as rated by current supervisors)
- Lower work performance ratings (as reported by current supervisors)
- Lower social class (SES) (limited by education)
- By 30s, 35% self-employed

Adapted from Barkley RA. Attention deficit hyperactivity disorder: A handbook for diagnosis and treatment, 3rd ed. New York: Guilford Press, 2005. Barkley RA, Murphy KR. *Attention deficit hyperactivity disorder: A clinical workbook*, 3rd ed. New York: Guilford 2005.

Consider Consultation When...

- A serious psychiatric disorder exists; for instance, major depression, generalized anxiety disorder, childhood bipolar illness, psychosis, autistic spectrum disorders.
- The physical examination reveals localized neurologic findings not previously detected, the history suggests a degenerative course, or the inattention is consistent with absence or petit mal seizures.
- A movement disorder such as tics or Tourette syndrome develops or worsens while taking stimulant medications and does not resolve after discontinuation of the drug.
- The child's behavior escalates such that he is a danger to self or others or is unable to function in the normal school or home environment.
- The most commonly used psychopharmacologic agents (stimulants, atomoxetine) have not proven effective, and the symptoms warrant further trials on other medications.

educational system. The task of professionals working with such a child is to help her reach that point along as smooth a course as possible with periodic interventions as required.

Annotated bibliography

American Academy of Pediatrics. Clinical practice guidelines: Diagnosis and evaluation of the child with attention-deficit/hyperactivity disorder. *Pediatrics* 2000;105:1158–1170.

American Academy of Pediatrics. Clinical practice guideline: Treatment of the school-aged child with attention-deficit/hyperactivity disorder. *Pediatrics* 2001;108:1033–1043.

AACAP Work Group on Quality Issues. Practice parameter for the assessment and treatment of children and adolescents with attention-deficit/hyperactivity disorder. *J Am Acad Child Adolesc Psychiatry* 2007;46(7):894–921.

Barkley RA. *Attention deficit hyperactivity disorder: A handbook for diagnosis and treatment*, 3rd ed. New York: Guilford Press, 2005a.

Barkley RA, Murphy KR. *Attention deficit hyperactivity disorder: A clinical workbook*, 3rd ed. New York: Guilford 2005b.

Barkley RA, Robin AL, Benton CM. *Your defiant teen: 10 steps to resolve conflict and rebuild your relationship*. New York: Guilford, 2008.

DuPaul GJ, Stoner G. *ADHD in the schools: Assessment & intervention strategies*, 2nd ed. New York: Guilford, 2004.

Faraone SV, Biederman J, Spencer TJ, Aleardi M. Comparing the efficacy of medications for ADHD using meta-analysis. *Med Gen Med* 2006;8(4):4.

Gordon M, Antshel K, Faraone S, et al. Symptoms versus impairment: the case for respecting DSM-IV's Criterion D. *J Atten Disord* 2006;9(3):465–475.

Nigg J. *What causes ADHD: Understanding what goes wrong and why*. New York: Guilford, 2006.

Shaw P, Eckstrand K, Sharp W, et al. Attention-deficit/hyperactivity disorder is characterized by a delay in cortical maturation. *Proc Natl Acad Sci* 2007;104:19649–19654.

The ADHD Report, a bimonthly newsletter for clinicians. Edited by Dr Barkley with contributions from leading clinicians and researchers. Guilford Publications, New York.

Websites

ADDA Organization: http://www.add.org
American Academy of Child & Adolescent Psychiatry: http://www.aacap.org
American Academy of Pediatrics: http://www.aap.org
CHADD Organization: http://www.chadd.org
Council for Exceptional Education (CEC): http://www.cec.sped.org
Learning Disabilities Association of America (LDA): http://www.ldanatl.org
National Resource Center on AD/HD: http://www.help4adhd.org
National Information Center for Children and Youth with Disabilities: http://www.nichcy.org

CHAPTER 29

Sleep Disorders

O'Neill F. D'Cruz and Bradley V. Vaughn

Outline

Sleep is an inherent physiologic phenomenon, as well as a marker of biologic integrity and environmental adaptation. Sleep is also a sensitive process that maybe disrupted by a variety of neurologic and systemic disorders, as well as by developmental, behavioral, and environmental factors. This chapter provides a review of the normal sleep–wake cycle and a summary of common pediatric sleep disorders.

The normal sleep–wake cycle

In humans, wakefulness and sleep are noted during any 24-hour period. Sleep, which is often classified as a unitary state, actually consists of periods of non–rapid eye movement (NREM) and rapid eye movement (REM) sleep. NREM sleep is further classified into three stages. Stage N1 and N2 sleep occur at onset of sleep and during transitions between sleep cycles. Stage N3 (slow-wave sleep, SWS) is noted during the early portions of the sleep period. REM sleep propensity increases during the sleep period. The amount of normal sleep, as well as its quality, also changes with age.

Sleep states and stages are identified by distinct electroencephalographic (EEG) characteristics. Stage NI sleep is associated with loss of the posterior dominant rhythm and desynchronized, low-voltage background patterns with prominent frontocentral β activity and vertex sharp waves. Stage N2 is comprised of a well-defined pattern of sleep spindles and K-complexes. Stage N3 is characterized by predominant high-voltage δ activity. NREM sleep is associated with regular respirations and heart rate and moderate muscle tone, and lack of eye and body movements. REM sleep (which is further classified as phasic and tonic REM) is distinguished from NREM sleep by the occurrence of rapid eye movements (hence the name), intermittent brief nonperiodic body movements, variable respiratory and heart rate, low muscle tone and a low-voltage, mixed-frequency EEG pattern.

Periodicity of sleep and sleep stages is noted during the normal sleep–wake cycle. The occurrence of the major sleep period during the 24-hour day defines the sleep phase of the individual. Slow-wave sleep decreases progressively through the night, whereas REM sleep, occurring at 80–90-minute intervals during the sleep period, increases in amount with each successive sleep cycle. A normal sleep period consists of several sleep cycles, depending on the amount of sleep.

Sleep duration and amount vary considerably with age. Nocturnal sleep lasts from 7–9 hours in most adults. Fragmentation of sleep, either occurring naturally with advanced age, or due to sleep disruption, adversely affects the restorative quality of sleep.

The evolution of sleep from infancy to adolescence

Sleep in infancy

During the neonatal period, the sleep–wake cycle consists of short periods of sleep, alternating with wakefulness throughout a 24-hour period. State differentiation is a marker of biologic maturation, and normal newborns demonstrate sustained states of active, quiet, and indeterminate sleep. Indeterminate sleep is gradually replaced by differentiated sleep states during infancy.

Sleep in infants is consolidated into longer nocturnal sleep periods between 6 weeks and 3 months of age. The amount of total sleep during a 24-hour period ranges from 10–19 hours at 3 months. Total sleep duration averages around 14 hours between 6 months and 1 year of age. Daytime sleep decreases from 3.5 hours at 6 months of age to 2.5 hours by 1 year of age. REM sleep in infants occurs at sleep onset and has a shorter period of 50–60 minutes.

Sleep in childhood

Sleep phase is well established in the majority of children by 6 months of age. Daytime naps decrease in duration and number in the preschool years. The number of children taking daytime naps also decreases from over 90% at 1 year of age to around 35% by 4 years of age. Rapid changes in physical, neurodevelopmental, and social milestones during early childhood make this group of children vulnerable to sleep disruption.

School-aged children have excellent biologic sleep parameters, with sustained efficient nocturnal sleep lasting 10–11 hours. Daytime naps are unusual at this age. Hence, sleep complaints during this period are often secondary to environmental or physical causes.

Sleep in adolescence

Adolescence is a period of rapid physical, emotional, and social maturation. Sleep during adolescence reflects the effect of several of these factors. Teenagers experience a physiologic delay in sleep phase (the DSPS, discussed later). Sleep need during adolescence is unchanged from preteen years, and may even increase during periods of rapid growth. Teenagers are most likely to have a multifactorial origin for sleep complaints.

> **Key Clinical Questions**
>
> - *Does the child wake up refreshed and well rested?*
>   Restorative sleep usually makes a significant sleep disorder unlikely.
> - *Does the child function well during the day?*
>   Sleep disorders affect child mood, social and school functioning, and may lead to inappropriate behavior.
> - *Has anybody been injured or hurt, or likely to be so?*
>   Screen for violent nocturnal behavior, seizures, sleepwalking, obstructive sleep apnea syndrome, periodic limb movement disorder, adverse social implications.
> - *Are any other family members affected by sleep complaints, or in a similar way?*
>   Familial predisposition, effect on caregivers.

Sleep disorders

Clinical symptoms of pediatric sleep disorders

The second International Classification of Sleep Disorders (ISCD2) categorizes pediatric sleep disorders in a special section. Symptoms of sleep disorders in children are strikingly different from adults, and hence are likely to be overlooked or misinterpreted. In young children, sleep disturbances may present as poor growth, persistent fussiness or inconsolability, and increased oppositional behavior. School-aged children may exhibit suboptimal academic performance, inattentive or hyperactive behavior, or appear to be daydreaming. Adolescents may fall asleep in class or present with affective symptoms. Poor nocturnal sleep is often a clue to the source of these symptoms in all age groups.

During the sleep period, a variety of clinical symptoms suggest sleep disorders. Sleep apnea, with or without associated effort, may be witnessed by caregivers. Frequent movements in one or more extremities, occurring in a stereotypic or periodic fashion, should raise suspicion of seizures, sleep-related movement disorders, or parasomnias. Any nocturnal event associated with injury warrants further investigation.

Sleep characteristics

Sleep phase

Sleep phase is determined by chronobiologic factors, along with behavioral and environmental influences.

Advanced sleep phase syndrome

Advanced sleep phase syndrome (ASPS) is associated with sleep onset in the early evening hours, followed by early morning awakening. Inability to stay awake during homework may be misinterpreted as sleep deprivation or school avoidance. When allowed to choose their own sleep–wake schedule (e.g., on vacation or weekends) children with ASPS often prefer to wake up earlier, reflecting their chronophysiologic predisposition. If the child awakens earlier than other family members, caregivers may request medications or evaluation for insomnia. If the child is able to function well during the day, there is rarely any need for further evaluation.

Delayed sleep phase syndrome

Delayed sleep phase syndrome (DSPS) is partly related to a physiologic phase delay that becomes evident in the early teen years. Inability to fall asleep until early morning hours is a consistent feature in this disorder. Attempts to induce sleep with the use of sedatives are generally unsuccessful. Since DSPS is also associated with a delay in awakening, the sleep period often extends into the morning hours, and may overlap with the start of the school day. Compensating for sleep deprivation during the school week by sleeping late on weekends introduces a further phase delay. When allowed to sleep on a self-dictated schedule, adolescents with DSPS choose a sleep period that mimics the sleep–wake schedule for "second-shift" workers.

Irregular sleep–wake pattern

The essential characteristic of this disorder is an inability to synchronize the sleep–wake cycle into a consistent diurnal pattern. Sleep is disorganized, without a single, sustained primary sleep period. Multiple sleep periods (at least three) occur throughout the day. Although this pattern is rarely seen in the general population, it is normal in the first few weeks of life. Similar patterns of sleep–wake behavior may occur temporarily during the course of an acute, severe illness, and need to be differentiated from the chronic course reported with this disorder. Persistence of this pattern is likely to have a severe impact on the sleep of caregivers. The pattern is most likely to be seen in children with severe and diffuse cerebral dysfunction, and is reported in severely impaired and institutionalized children.

Sleep amount

Inadequate sleep hygiene

In this disorder, persistent failure to obtain adequate sleep leads to complaints of excessive daytime sleepiness. In children with insufficient sleep, an improvement in symptoms is noted following an increase in the duration of the sleep period. Often, symptoms are related to hectic schedules and resolve when these are modified to allow adequate rest. This disorder should be distinguished from other conditions in which excessive sleepiness is due to sleep disruption or fragmentation, rather than insufficient sleep. In the former, symptoms do not improve with increased sleep duration.

In children with sleep needs that are among the lower percentiles for age, caregivers may be concerned about insufficient sleep. Children with below-normal sleep needs may appear to have insomnia, since their sleep period is much less than time spent in bed. The child with reduced sleep need sleeps consistently and efficiently in a short sleep period, wakes up refreshed, does not take naps, and functions well during the waking period. These features distinguish the short sleeper from other sleep disorders.

Hypersomnia

Narcolepsy

Narcolepsy is a primary disorder of sleep, with four cardinal clinical manifestations: excessive daytime sleepiness (EDS), cataplexy, hypnagogic hallucinations, and sleep paralysis. The disorder has a familial predisposition and a high association with HLA-DQB1*0602. The symptoms of narcolepsy are related to the loss of hypocretin (orexin)-producing neurons in the lateral hypothalamus. Clinical manifestations are due to poor regulation of sleep–wake patterns and dissociation of REM sleep features, with REM intrusion into wakefulness.

Excessive daytime sleepiness is the earliest and most prevalent symptom. Although EDS may be present from early childhood, the diagnosis of narcolepsy is often delayed for several years, unless one or more of the other cardinal manifestations are present in the first decade.

Cataplexy has a high diagnostic value, but symptoms may be infrequent or subtle, especially at the onset of the disorder. During a cataplectic spell, transient weakness occurs due to an abrupt decrease in muscle tone affecting antigravity muscles. Cataplexy may occur spontaneously, but is characteristically provoked by emotional arousal. Consciousness is not affected, although sleep may ensue after the event. There is complete recall for events, and examination during the spell reveals diminished or absent deep tendon reflexes.

Hypnagogic hallucinations and sleep paralysis occur normally in some children, and are less likely to be primary clinical presentations of narcolepsy without associated EDS or cataplexy. Hypnagogic hallucinations may be described as actual events by young children. The child may avoid going to bed, seek parental company, or report the presence of "monsters." Most hallucinations are visual or auditory in nature. Some of these concerns need to be distinguished from normal bedtime conflicts. Sleep paralysis may occur at sleep onset or offset, as REM-related atonia persists during wakefulness. The child appears awake, but lies immobile and unable to move spontaneously in bed. Tactile or other sensory input terminates the event. The child may be distressed if these events occur frequently.

The diagnosis of narcolepsy is confirmed by overnight polysomnography (PSG) and multiple sleep latency tests. Overnight PSG is performed to document sleep efficiency and exclude comorbid sleep disturbances. The multiple sleep latency test (see diagnostic evaluation, later) reveals multiple sleep-onset REM periods, along with an average sleep latency of less than 8 minutes.

In children, symptoms and PSG findings evolve over months to years, and several PSGs may be needed before a diagnosis is established. HLA haplo-typing for DQB1*0602 is suggestive of a genetic predisposition, but not diagnostic for narcolepsy. Patients with narcolepsy-cataplexy have a marked reduction in cerebrospinal fluid (CSF) hypocretin (orexin) levels, and this test is helpful in confirming the diagnosis.

Recurrent hypersomnia

Recurrent hypersomnia is associated with intermittent periods of irresistible sleepiness lasting several days, with symptom-free intervals of weeks to months. Klein-Levin syndrome is a disorder reported predominantly in males, with initial onset during adolescence. During the symptomatic phase, excessive sleepiness is observed, with irritability or aggressive behavior if the child is disturbed. Compulsive eating, sexual disinhibition, and affective symptoms are also noted in some patients. Onset may be spontaneous or in the setting of an intercurrent illness or head trauma. Episodes occur at varying intervals and may decrease in severity or frequency over time. Catamenial hypersomnia, associated with periodic hypersomnia in adolescent girls, occurs in the luteal phase of the menstrual cycle, with resolution at the time of menses. The symptoms are most likely related to hormonal imbalance, since onset is most often noted around menarche. Symptoms resolve over time, with pregnancy, or with use of oral contraceptives.

Pediatric insomnia

Sleep quality

Sleep quality is an important, but often underestimated, component of good sleep. Sleep disorders that produce frequent arousals and sleep state transitions lead to sleep fragmentation and disruption of sleep architecture. Sleep fragmentation, along with reduced efficiency of sleep, results in nonrestorative sleep. Attempts to increase sleep amount do not compensate for poor sleep quality. Two common sleep disorders that have an adverse impact on sleep quality are obstructive sleep apnea syndrome (OSAS) and periodic limb movement disorder (PLMD).

Sleep apnea

Sleep apnea is characterized by sleep-related respiratory disturbance that ranges from increased resistance to airflow during sleep (upper airway resistance syndrome) to reduction (hypopnea) or cessation (sleep apnea) of airflow. The absence of effort during a respiratory event is characteristic of central apnea and distinguishes it from obstructive apnea and hypopnea.

Sleep apnea in childhood is associated with conditions that affect respiratory control during sleep (e.g., congenital central hypoventilation syndrome), craniofacial structural abnormalities (macroglossia, micrognathia), abnormal airway tone (cerebral palsy), or structure (adenotonsillar hypertrophy). Systemic disorders (e.g., sickle cell disease) may be associated with higher risk of complications due to OSAS. Children with neurologic disorders often have a multifactorial etiology to sleep-disordered breathing.

Clinical guidelines are available for diagnosis and management of OSAS in children. A history of snoring, presence of adenotonsillar hypertrophy, and sleep disturbance provides clinical clues to the presence of OSAS. Overnight PSG is the diagnostic study of choice, and adenotonsillectomy is often adequate treatment for uncomplicated OSAS. High-risk patients (with concomitant medical or neurologic disorders) need evaluation by sleep disorder specialists for residual or refractory sleep problems.

Periodic limb movement disorder

Periodic, stereotyped movements of one or more extremities, occurring after sleep onset, that result in insomnia or EDS are classified as PLMD. The disorder has a genetic predisposition and is influenced by age, medical problems (iron deficiency status), and medications (tricyclics, selective serotonin reuptake inhibitors [SSRIs], and withdrawal from sedatives and anticonvulsants). A history of restless legs syndrome is often reported in adult first-degree relatives. Periodic limb movement disorder may also coexist with other primary sleep disorders, including narcolepsy and OSAS. Children with PLMD are noted to have daytime symptoms that are similar to those of attention deficit hyperactivity disorder. Sometimes the soreness or discomfort in the extremities that is related to PLMD is attributed to growing pains.

A diagnosis of PLMD is confirmed by overnight PSG. The accuracy of the study may be increased by utilizing additional electromyogram (EMG) recordings, since the movements show considerable variation in location and frequency between sides and extremities. Severity of PLMD correlates with low serum and CSF ferritin levels. Alteration of dopaminergic transmission is postulated, as iron is a cofactor in dopamine synthesis. Iron supplementation, both in oral or parenteral forms, reduces the severity of the disorder. Dopamine agonists are also used in the treatment of PLMD.

Parasomnias

Parasomnias are classified according to their occurrence in the sleep–wake cycle. Primary parasomnias reflect an age-dependent expression of a familial predisposition. Sleep–wake transition parasomnias include sleep starts (Table 29.1), sleep-talking, nocturnal leg cramps, and rhythmic movement disorder (RMD) (Table 29.2). Arousal from NREM sleep is associated with sleepwalking (Table 29.3), confusional arousals, and sleep terrors (Table 29.4). REM behavior disorder (RBD), nightmares (Table 29.5), and sleep paralysis occur as REM-sleep related events. Enuresis and bruxism (teeth-grinding) are examples of nonstate specific parasomnias.

Table 29.1 Sleep starts

Discriminating features
- Sudden brief contractions of extremities
- Subjective feeling of falling, or sensory experience
- Associated with arousal

Consistent features
- Occurs at sleep onset
- Benign course and outcome

Variable features
- Number and frequency of movements
- Age of occurrence (any age)

Parasomnias may be precipitated in susceptible individuals (secondary parasomnias) by arousals or state transitions due to OSAS and PLMD, with reduction or resolution of symptoms after treatment of the underlying primary sleep disorder. Nocturnal seizures, headaches, dystonic disorders, and acid-reflux disease should also be considered in the differential diagnosis of secondary parasomnias.

Parasomnias are often more distressing to the parent than the child. In such situations, education and reassurance may suffice, since most parasomnias resolve with increasing age. In some instances, however, further evaluation is indicated. In patients with coexisting medical or neurologic disorders, a low threshold for evaluation is appropriate, since the underlying disorders and/or the medical treatment may affect or be influenced by sleep.

Biologic–environmental interactions

Biologic factors

Genetics

Genetic predispositions may be expressed as primary sleep disorders or disorders manifest during sleep. Narcolepsy and PLMDs have a marked familial preponderance. Nocturnal seizure disorders, including benign epilepsy with centrotemporal spikes (benign rolandic epilepsy) and autosomal dominant nocturnal frontal lobe epilepsy, are state-dependent expressions of a genetic tendency. Fatal familial insomnia is associated with sleep disorders at the onset of a neurodegenerative disorder.

Gender

In prepubertal children, there are no significant differences in prevalence of common sleep disorders (including OSAS), although referral patterns may influence frequency of diagnosis. Some parasomnias including enuresis, RMD, and sleep terrors are more common in males, whereas bruxism, somniloquy, and nightmares are equally prevalent in boys and girls.

Table 29.2 Rhythmic movement disorder

Discriminating features
- Stereotyped, rhythmic movements of large muscles
- Involve head and neck, rarely limb muscles
- Body movements (rocking, rolling)

Consistent features
- Occur prior to sleep onset
- Common in infants and children
- Decrease with age

Variable features
- Associated vocalizations
- Age of resolution (persists in autistic children)

Table 29.3 Sleepwalking (somnambulism)

Discriminating features
- Initiated during NREM sleep
- Complex behaviors with walking or wandering during event
- Subsides spontaneously with return to sleep without intervening arousal

Consistent features
- Amnesia for episode

2. Inability to arouse child during event

- Occur during slow wave sleep

Variable features
- Two subtypes—agitated or quiet walkers
- Associated sleep talking during event
- Injury during event
- Response to attempted arousal or redirection during event (agitation or compliance)

Table 29.4 Sleep terrors

Discriminating features
- Occurs during slow-wave sleep (usually first third of sleep period)
- Agitation and screaming during event
- Autonomic arousal during event

Consistent features
- Inconsolable crying
- Tachycardia, tachypnea, diaphoresis, terrified look
- Difficult to arouse
- Amnesia for event

Variable features
- Duration of event
- Degree of agitation and autonomic arousal
- Recall of fragmentary, vivid hallucinations

Table 29.5 Nightmares

Discriminating features
- Occur during REM sleep (usually latter part of sleep period)
- Vivid dream imagery after arousal
- Arousal at end of event

Consistent features
- Associated with REM sleep
- Element of fright or anxiety with dream
- Arousal (spontaneous or provoked) at end of event
- Recall of event

Variable features
- Duration and content of dream
- Amount of emotional agitation with event

Growth phase

Maturation of the sleep–wake cycle and consolidation of sleep state features occurs gradually over several months to years in healthy children. Abnormal psychomotor development affects sleep maturation adversely, leading to persistence of infantile sleep patterns into childhood. Children with coexisting genetic and neurologic disorders often have delayed sleep maturation. In addition, social and language development influences the interaction between caregivers and children. These factors predispose young children with a variety of developmental disorders to sleep disturbances. Prematurity, autistic spectrum disorders, severe mental retardation, and static encephalopathy are associated with a high incidence of sleep disorders. In these children, consolidated sleep may not occur in the first year of life, parasomnias persist well beyond early childhood, and sleep disruption often adversely affects quality of life.

Environmental factors

Transition from wakefulness to sleep, as well as sustained nocturnal sleep, are influenced by a variety of environmental factors. The child's ability to settle down to sleep is a learned behavior that involves disengagement from the caregivers in a secure, comfortable sleep environment. Parenting styles, social and cultural expectations, as well as sleeping arrangements are among the environmental determinants of sleep patterns in children. In otherwise healthy children, environmental influences play a significant role in several pediatric sleep disorders.

Sleep–wake transition

Behavioral insomnia of childhood: Sleep-onset association type. Sleep onset in infants is often facilitated by the parents. Initially, feeding, rocking, and cuddling are common antecedents to onset of sleep. Later, these interventions are replaced with transitional objects (pacifiers, bottles, blankets). The place and setting in which the child falls asleep become environmental reinforcements for transition to sleep. Children who learn to sleep using one or more of these aids develop a sleep-onset association with the facilitatory object, place, or person. They seek the same aids to settle down after nocturnal arousals. The lack of these sleep aids during the night leads to prolonged periods of arousal, during which the child attempts to restore the environment that facilitated onset of sleep. If the sleep-onset association involves parental interaction or a place other than the child's customary sleeping area, parents have to intervene before the child settles down. The frequency and duration of these interventions leads to sleep disruption for the caregivers and is often the reason for seeking medical advice. A new set of nondisruptive sleep-onset associations need to be cultivated for resolution of the sleep-onset association disorder. This process may take several days to weeks.

Behavioral insomnia of childhood: Limit-setting type. Voluntary disengagement from the environment is an initial step before going to sleep. In children, this process requires parental supervision and reinforcement. Children may find ways to postpone bedtimes by making repeated requests for minor interventions. If the caregivers do not reinforce limits consistently, this behavioral pattern delays sleep onset, leading to insufficient sleep for the preschool-aged child. Older children may lack the self-discipline to go to bed at an appropriate time, and adolescents often choose to sleep on an irregular schedule. In all cases, there is no difficulty after sleep onset. Sleep-related complaints resolve after a consistent sleep schedule is enforced.

Socioeconomic factors

A child's sleep environment varies widely based on the socioeconomic status of the family. Among the lower socioeconomic classes, inadequate sleeping areas, lack of electricity, overcrowding, and a noisy environment contribute to the child's sleep difficulties. Conversely, easy access to television, computers, and video-games and numerous social engagements or after-school activities may predispose children in more affluent families to insufficient or disrupted sleep. Consumption of caffeinated beverages, inadequate or inappropriate food intake, and poor sleep hygiene affect sleep in all children.

Stressors

Sleep disorders may be precipitated by extrinsic and intrinsic stressors. Extrinsic stressors affect sleep based on their duration and severity. The impact may be mild and self-limited in some instances (e.g., prior to travel or a test). Changes in school or residential settings produce changes that may last for several weeks to months. Other social stressors, including domestic or societal violence, geopolitical events, and major environmental disasters that affect entire segments of society, may induce long-term changes in children's sleep patterns (posttraumatic stress disorder of childhood). Intrinsic stressors include fever, systemic illness, chronic pain, and medical disorders.

Diagnostic evaluation

A thorough history and physical examination often provide clues to the cause of sleep disorders. A 2–4-week sleep diary provides information about sleep phase and average sleep amount in an individual child. Sleep diaries are diagnostic for sleep phase disorders and may be complemented by actigraphy for objective analysis. Several sleep questionnaires are available to assess probable cause and impact of sleepiness, including Pediatric Sleep Questionnaire (PSQ) and Epworth Sleepiness Scale (ESS). The authors use an acronym, INBED, which outlines a clinical protocol for the evaluation and management of sleep disorders (see Pearls and Perils).

In a child with sleep disruption or excessive daytime sleepiness, additional investigations may be necessary to confirm a suspected diagnosis. Polysomnography is the "gold standard" for diagnostic evaluation of sleep disorders, and is combined with the multiple sleep latency test (MSLT) for objective assessment of daytime sleepiness. Polysomnography provides information about sleep stages and architecture, limb movements, sleep-related respiratory disorders, and nocturnal seizures. Modifications of the technique also allow diagnosis of acid-reflux, effect of interventions to maintain airway patency and oxygenation, and video-review of nocturnal events.

The multiple sleep latency test consists of five naps that are performed 2 hours apart and reviewed for sleep onset latency and occurrence of sleep-onset REM periods. It is a validated measure of daytime sleepiness in older children and adolescents.

Pearls and Perils

INBED Protocol

- I Individual sleep characteristics (FAQ); sleep "Ph"ase, "A"mount and "Q"uality
- N Nature ("B"iologic factors); genetics, gender, growth phase
  Nurture ("E"nvironmental factors); sleep–wake transitions, socioeconomic factors, stressors
  Neither ("D"iagnostic evaluation)
- B Behavioral therapy
- E Environmental therapy
- D Drug therapy

Management

The management of sleep disorders in children is dictated by the primary source of the sleep disturbance. If multiple contributory factors are identified in the genesis of a sleep disorder, one or more of the following approaches may be necessary.

Behavioral therapy

Behavioral therapy is extremely helpful as a primary intervention in several sleep disorders (e.g., sleep-onset association disorder and limit-setting sleep disorder). Behavioral techniques are useful in the treatment of parasomnias (anticipatory awakening in night terrors, reinforcement therapy for enuresis, stress reduction in anxious children). Desensitization therapy preceding the use of face masks to maintain airway patency improves compliance and tolerance of therapy. Family education and counseling is essential in management of sleep disorders that are related to inappropriate parental expectations or interventions.

Environmental therapy

A quiet, comfortable, and secure sleep environment is conducive to restorative sleep. Variations in ambient temperature, humidity, noise, and light act as environmental triggers that produce sleep disruption. Humidifiers and fans may be used as needed, along with removal of noise, light, and sources of distraction. Age-appropriate sleep settings are important in young children, to ensure safety and minimize extrinsic causes of arousals. A supine position during sleep is particularly important in young infants. Time in bed should match sleep need to minimize prolonged sleep latency, repeated arousals, and sleep fragmentation.

Specific environmental interventions may be used in certain sleep disorders. Bright light therapy is used in sleep phase disorders. Chronotherapy is a technique of voluntary, sequential delay of the sleep period, to allow resynchronization of sleep phase with time zone, and is particularly helpful in severely phase-delayed adolescents. Overnight sleep-deprivation also induces phase advance the following day and may be used as a weekend technique for DSPS in selected cases. Positional therapy is helpful in cases of acid-reflux disease or positional apnea.

Drug therapy

A recent survey of community-based pediatricians indicates that prescriptions for sedatives are most commonly used in children with pain or neurodevelopmental disorders (including mental retardation, autism, and ADHD) or during travel. Antihistamines and α-agonists were the

Consider Consultation When...

- Indications for polysomnography:
  - Conventional therapy fails.
  - There is a clinical suspicion of obstructive sleep apnea syndrome or periodic limb movement disorder.
  - Child complains of excessive daytime sleepiness.
  - There is a suspicion of nocturnal seizures.
  - Violent sleep-related behavior occurs.
  - Unusual or atypical parasomnias are present.

most common prescription medications, while melatonin and herbal remedies were utilized as nonprescription alternatives. In children with nocturnal seizures, acid-reflux disease, or asthma, optimization of specific therapy is preferable.

Specific therapy is available for some sleep disorders. Excessive daytime sleepiness is usually treated with stimulant medications, including methylphenidate, dexmethylphenidate, and dextroamphetamine. The use of stimulants is associated with side effects and requires close monitoring. Modafinil, approved for use in narcolepsy in adults, may be useful in selected patients. Cataplexy is treated with tricyclics and SSRIs; in severe cases, sodium oxybate is helpful in treating cataplexy and excessive daytime sleepiness. Iron supplementation is useful in treating PLMD in pediatric patients.

Conclusion

Sleep disorders occur at all ages. An age-appropriate expectation of sleep phase and need coupled with an understanding of common age-specific sleep disorders enables the clinician to evaluate and manage a number of these conditions. The use of a simple protocol (INBED, described earlier) may be helpful in formulating a clinical approach to sleep disorders and making appropriate referrals for diagnostic studies and further evaluation.

Annotated bibliography

Grigg-Damberger M, Gozal D, Marcus CL, et al. The visual scoring of sleep and arousal in infants and children. *J Clin Sleep Med* 2007;3(2):201–240.
Evidence-based review of age-related development of PSG features.

Mason TB, Pack AI. Pediatric parasomnias. *Sleep* 2007;30(2): 141–151.
Update on current knowledge of parasomnias.

American Academy of Sleep Medicine. *International classification of disorders: Diagnostic and coding manual*, 2nd ed. Rochester, MN: American Sleep Disorders Association, 2006.
A comprehensive resource outlining the classification and features of sleep disorders.

Owens JA, Rosen CL, Mindell JA. Medication use in the treatment of pediatric insomnia: Results of a survey of community-based pediatricians. *Pediatrics* 2003;111:628–635.
Survey of clinical practice patterns of use of sedative medications by clinicians.

Iglowstein I, Jenni OG, Molinari L, Largo RH. Sleep duration from infancy to adolescence: Reference values and generational trends. *Pediatrics* 2003;111:302–307.
Prospective study on sleep amount percentiles at various ages from childhood to adolescence.

Clinical Practice Guideline. Diagnosis and management of childhood obstructive sleep apnea syndrome. *Pediatrics* 2002; 109:704–712.
AAP practice guideline with algorithms and treatment recommendations.

Kotagal S, ed. Circadian rhythm disorders in children. *Semin Pediatr Neurol* 2001;51(1):89–115.
Update on sleep and neurologic disorders in children.

Ferber R, Kryger M, eds. *Principles and practice of sleep medicine in the child.* Philadelphia: WB Saunders, 1995.
Textbook of pediatric sleep disorders with multiauthor chapters on the common sleep disorders.

Appendix: A Proposed Approach to Nosology

Ronald B. David

Although the practice of medicine has experienced major technological advances in recent years, nosologic systems (e.g., *International Classification of Diseases – 10* and the *Diagnostic and Statistical Manual – IV* of the American Psychiatric Association) present at times a confusing array of diagnostic possibilities. Many diseases/disorders may even be represented in more than one place in the diagnostic system. Lack of a comprehensive framework leads to diagnostic confusion in the clinical, teaching, and often, in the research setting. Clearly, organization and orderliness are needed to better discriminate between entities. *Webster's International Dictionary* defines *nosology* as the branch of medical science that deals with the orderly classification of diseases. My purpose is to propose such a system. This system will submit a priori that, if a disease/disorder exists, there must also exist features that discriminate it from similar entities. It is clinically derived by expert opinion, categorical and multidimensional. Where the state of the art permits, discriminators have been empirically validated.

Classification issues have historic roots. Hippocrates suggested that "whoever undertakes to speak or write on medicine, should have first laid themselves some hypothesis as to their argument, such as hot or cold or moist or dry or whatever else they choose, thus reducing their subject within a narrow compass." The work of Thomas Sydenham on acute diseases, first published in 1675, is seminal. Sydenham suggested that all diseases can be classified as to a certain definite species, in the same manner as botanists describe their plants. He further suggested that pathologic phenomena should be described in precise detail, in the same way that a portrait painter seeks to capture the likeness of a subject. He noted that particular and constant symptoms should be distinguished from accidental phenomena. John Locke, in describing Sydenham, suggested that he had a poor opinion of those who attempted to look at disease from a chemical point of view. On the other hand, he noted that Sydenham recognized the utility of chemotherapeutics, recognizing, for instance, that certain chemicals could induce vomiting, implying that treatment outcome was not a good basis for classification, but overlooking its potential value as a validator of diagnosis.

Carl Linnaens graduated as a doctor of medicine in 1735. While he is best known for his biological classification system (e.g., phyla, genera, species), his attempt to use this approach for medicine was never widely accepted, principally because of a confusion between the definitions of symptom and disease. Laennec, in 1826, was among the first to link symptoms to pathologic anatomy when he described the pathology of disseminated tuberculosis. In the mid nineteenth century, the pathophysiologic basis of disease came into focus. Methods for counting cells, methods for the measurement of the color of blood, as well as methods for the examination of urine, were developed. In the later nineteenth century, an etiologic approach for the classification of disease became possible with the identification of a specific bacterium as the cause for a specific disease (Koch-Pasteur). This became the first good example of using the best and most robust discriminator, etiology. As the reader can see, there was therefore an evolutionary progression from phenomenologic descriptions to those based on etiology. Each reflected the state of knowledge at that time.

Many disorders in psychiatry and neurology still can be described only phenomenologically. Although seemingly the least robust, phenomenologic validity is attainable. Skinner suggested that a phenomenologically based system should have certain features that make descriptions of specific entities valid. These include *reliability*; that is, agreement across examiners using the same diagnostic methodology; *coverage*, referring to the applicability of the classification domain of the patients for which it was intended; *descriptive validity*, implying homogeneity in characterizing behavioral symptoms, personality characteristics, social history data, and other kinds of information that are used to make a diagnosis; and *predictive validity*, in which a classification system can determine the potential effectiveness of treatment or the natural history of a psychiatric disorder. Although Skinner's conceptual framework was meant to be applied to psychiatric disorders described phenomenologically, it can obviously be generalized. It can also provide a mechanism for a classification system.

Classification in science is important to medicine. A successful and therefore useful classification should be simple and easy to use. Second, it should be organized hierarchically and have the flexibility to reflect the state of the art as it evolves. Last, the goal ideally should be to define the disease/disorder etiologically through the rigorous application of the scientific method. Classification domains in medicine are usually defined according to the following schema:

- *Phenomenologically*, by listing commonly agreed upon observations and distinguishing between entities based on these observations (a good example of this would be the clinical classification of the epilepsies)
- *Anatomically*, by the site of origin of the disorder
- *Pathologically*, by the gross or microscopic pathologic anatomy, revealed by either traditional pathologic study or imaging
- *Pathophysiologically*, by demonstrating altered chemical or electrophysiologic parameters
- *Etiologically*, by cause

Under these general domains, subdomains can be identified (e.g., histopathology versus radiologic pathology). Much of the confusion that arises in diagnosis occurs when the clinician crosses classification domains—for example, the inclusion of an anatomically oriented "temporal lobe seizure" in a phenomenologically based classification system that includes complex partial seizures. It is, therefore, extremely important from both a clinical and a research standpoint that the classification domain to be used should be predetermined, and that contrasting discriminators be comparable (e.g., bacterial meningitides should not be enmeshed with viral meningitides). For a disease/disorder to exist, it must have some feature or features that discriminate between it and similar entities. Discriminating features may have inclusionary as well as exclusionary features. The ideal is to have a single discriminator. This then makes the contrast between a particular entity and similar entities more robust. When more than a single discriminator is involved, this in essence becomes a *criterion-based system*. Although this is obviously less robust, a criterion-based system may simply reflect the state of the art.

Just as there are discriminant features, disease/disorder entities often have consistent as well as variable features. In the current Mosby/Yearbook N*eurology/Psychiatry Access Series*, the series editor has defined consistent features as those that occur 75% of the time and variable features as those that occur less than 75% of the time. These need not be consistent with the discriminator domain; for example, cerebral spinal fluid glucose is consistently low in bacterial tuberculous meningitis. Tables I–III reflect what is believed to be the best way of distinguishing between these and similar entities, again reflecting the state of the art. In this textbook series, contributor experts were asked to identify discriminant, consistent, and variable features. William Nyhan used this model for distinguishing inborn errors of metabolism from one another using pathophysiologic discriminators. Current knowledge permitted the use of only one discriminator (Table I). When the defective gene is identified for each of these disorders, each can then be discriminated from the other based on genotype. This will enhance etiologic discrimination and will more powerfully distinguish similar entities from one another.

Joseph Sirven and Michael Sperling use the same system to classify the epilepsies, but the result is much different (Table II). In this case, discriminators are *phenomenologically based*, again reflecting the state of the art. A phenomenologically based system is probably the most appropriate to use at this state of the art rather than using one that is etiologically derived. Unfortunately, the universal use of this system will probably impede its evolution into an etiologically based system, although usage alone should not preclude developing an etiologically based system. Practicality also plays an important operative function in domain selection. To demonstrate that this system can be applied to other medical diseases/disorders, the reader is referred to Table III. Here valvular stenotic heart disease is classified using this nosologic system.

It should always be acknowledged that classification of science is dynamic, not etched in stone, but clearly necessary so that clear discourse is possible. Medicine needs a clear nosologic framework today, irrespective of how it may have changed.

In summary, to put this system into operation, experts should agree on the following questions.

- Which features discriminate one group of similar diseases/disorders from one another (e.g., enzyme deficiency)?
- Into what classification domain does this fall (e.g., genetic disorder—defective gene, pathophysiologic domain)?
- Can a single discriminator suffice, or are multiple discriminators required, reflective of the state of the art (e.g., in a genetic disorder, a single discriminator is sufficiently robust)?

Table I Nosologic classification

Lesch-Nyhan syndrome

Discriminating features

- Complete deficiency of hypoxanthine-guanine phosphoribosyltransferase

Consistent features

- Hyperuricemia
- Uricosuria
- Mental retardation
- Spastic cerebral palsy
- Choreoathetosis
- Self-mutilation

Variable features

- Convulsions
- Hematuria
- Urinary tract stones
- Urinary tract infections
- Tophi
- Urate nephropathy
- Vomiting

Purine nucleoside phosphorylase deficiency

Discriminating features

- Deficiency of PNP

Consistent features

- Immunodeficiencies
- T-cell depletion
- Infections
- Hypouricemia
- Nucleoside accumulation

Variable features

- Neurologic abnormalities

Phenylketonuria

Discriminating features

- Deficient hepatic phenylalanine
- Elevated plasma phenylalanine
- Depressed plasma tyrosine

Consistent features

- Mental retardation
- Diminished pigment
- Phenylpyruvic aciduria
- Phenyllactic aciduria
- Phenylacetylglutamic aciduria

Variable features

- Vomiting
- Eczematoid rash
- Odd odor
- Restriction fragment length polymorphism

Table I Nosologic classification (continued)

Abnormalities in the metabolism of biopterin

Discriminating features

- Defective activity of dihydropteridine reductase
- Evidence of deficient synthesis of tetrahydrobiopterin

Consistent features

- Hyperphenylalaninemia
- Degenerative neurologic disease
- Convulsions
- Spasticity

Variable features

- Rigidity
- Tremors
- Dystonic movements

Maple syrup urine disease

Discriminating features

- Complete deficiency of branched-chain ketoacid decarboxylase

Consistent features

- Elevated concentrations of leucine, isoleucine and valine
- Positive dinitrophenylhydrazine test of urine
- Branched-chain ketoaciduria

Variable features

- Maple syrup odor to urine
- Mental retardation
- Spasticity
- Opisthotonos
- Coma
- Convulsions
- Hypodense cerebral myelin

Disorders of propionate metabolism

Propionicacidemia

Discriminating features

- Deficiency of propionyl-CoA carboxylase

Consistent features

- Methylcitraturia
- Hydroxypropionaturia
- Propionicacidemia
- Recurrent episodes of ketosis and acidosis, leading to coma and potentially fatal illness
- Osteoporosis
- Vomiting
- Hypotonia
- Anorexia
- Moniliasis

Variable features

- Hyperammonemia
- Anemia
- Hyperglycinemia, hyperglycinuria
- Pathologic fractures
- Mental retardation
- Immunodeficiency
- Abnormal MRI of the basal ganglia

(continued on next page)

Table I Nosologic classification (continued)

Disorders of propionate metabolism
Methylmalonic acidemia
Discriminating features
- Deficiency of methyl malonyl CoA mutase

Consistent features
- As in propionicacidemia, plus failure to thrive

Variable features
- As in propionicacidemia

Disorders of propionate metabolism
Multiple carboxylase deficiency
Discriminating features
- Deficiency of holocarboxylase synthetase
- Deficiency of biotinidase

Consistent features
- As in propionicacidemia, plus
- Alopecia
- Dermatosis
- Lacticacidemia, lactic aciduria
- Deficient leukocyte carboxylases
- Convulsions in biotinidase deficiency
- Sensorineural deafness and visual defects in biotinidase deficiency
- Ataxia in biotinidase deficiency

Variable features
- As in propionicacidemia

Isovalericacidemia
Discriminating features
- Isovaleryl glycinuria
- Deficiency of isovaleryl-CoA dehydrogenase

Consistent features
- Episodes of acute illness
- Ketoacidosis
- Neutropenia, thrombocytopenia

Variable features
- Acrid "sweaty foot" odor
- Mental retardation
- Hyperammonemia
- Anemia
- Ataxia
- Convulsions

Glutaric aciduria
Discriminating features
- Glutaric aciduria

Consistent features
- Spasticity
- Convulsions
- Cerebral degeneration
- Involuntary movements

Variable features
- Metabolic acidosis

Table I Nosologic classification (continued)

3-Hydroxy-3-methylglutaricaciduria
Discriminating features
- 3-Hydroxy-3-methylglutaricaciduria
- 3-Hydroxy-3-methylglutaryl-CoA lyase deficiency

Consistent features
- 3-Methylglutaconicaciduria
- 3-Methylglutaricaciduria
- Hypoketotic hypoglycemia
- Acute overwhelming illness
- Metabolic acidosis
- Lethargy or coma
- Elevated liver function tests
- Convulsions
- Cerebral atrophy

Variable features
- Lacticaciduria
- Lacticacidemia
- Hyperammonemia
- Hypotonia
- Hepatomegaly
- Vomiting
- Elevated liver function tests
- Convulsions
- Cerebral atrophy

4-Hydroxybutyric aciduria
Discriminating features
- Succinic semialdehyde dehydrogenase deficiency

Consistent features
- 4-Hydroxybutyric aciduria
- Convulsions
- Ataxia
- Mental retardation

Variable features
- Hyperactivity
- Somnolence

Nonketotic hyperglycinemia
Discriminating features
- Elevated CSF and plasma glycine ratio

Consistent features
- Hyperglycinemia
- Hyperglycinuria
- Neonatal coma and apnea
- Myoclonic seizures (infantile spasms)
- EEG burst suppression pattern
- Cerebral atrophy

Variable features
- Hypertonia
- Hypotonia
- Increased deep tendon reflexes
- Hiccuping

Table I Nosologic classification (continued)

Homocystinuria

Discriminating features

- Homocystinuria
- Cystathionine synthase deficiency

Consistent features

- Mixed disulfide of cysteine and homocysteine in urine

Variable features

- Hypermethioninemia
- Ectopia lentis
- Mental retardation
- Thromboembolic phenomena
- Failure to thrive
- Genu valgum
- Osteoporosis

Urea cycle disorders

Discriminating features

- OTC deficiency
- CPS deficiency
- Argininosuccinic synthase deficiency
- Argininosuccinase deficiency

Consistent features

- Orotic aciduria in OTC deficiency
- Hyperammonemia in OTC deficiency
- Hyperglutaminemia in OTC deficiency
- Coma
- Citrullinemia
- Citrullinemia and citrullinuria in citrullinemia
- Increased concentrations of argininosuccinate in urine and CSF

Variable features

- Hyperalaninemia
- Hyperaspartic acidemia
- Convulsions
- Mental retardation
- Trichorrhexis nodosa (in argininosuccinic aciduria)

Argininemia

Discriminating features

- Arginase deficiency
- Argininemia

Consistent features

- Spastic diplegia
- Developmental delay
- Hypertonia
- Opisthotonus
- Involuntary movements

Variable features

- Hyperammonemia
- Hepatomegaly
- Abnormal liver function tests
- Convulsions
- EEG abnormalities

Table II The epilepsies

Simple partial seizures

Discriminating features

- No impairment of consciousness
- Stereotyped
- Focal spikes in interictal EEG

Consistent features

- Brief duration
- Paroxysmal
- No impairment of consciousness
- No postictal period

Variable features

- May manifest as abnormal sensations (smells, flashing lights, paresthesias), focal motor activity, or psychic phenomena (déjà vu, fear)
- Associated with a focal structural lesion
- May occur independent of or before a complex partial seizure

Complex partial seizures

Discriminating features

- Consciousness is altered
- Stereotyped
- Focal spikes in interictal EEG

Consistent features

- Approximately 60–180-seconds duration
- Paroxysmal
- Postictal confusion

Variable features

- Presence of aura
- Automatisms
- Autonomic features
- May secondarily generalize to a tonic–clonic seizure
- Associated with focal structural lesion
- May elevate prolactin level

Generalized tonic–clonic seizures

Discriminating features

- Initial tonic phase followed by clonic activity involving all extremities

Consistent features

- Loss of consciousness
- Typically 60 seconds duration
- Postictal period associated with confusion and drowsiness
- Elevation of prolactin

Variable features

- Tongue biting or injury
- Urinary incontinence
- Nonspecific prodrome
- Postictal paralysis

(continued on next page)

Table II The epilepsies (continued)

Absence seizures

Discriminating features

- Very brief duration (5–15 seconds)
- Family history of typical absence seizures
- Response to ethosuximide and valproate

Consistent features

- EEG correlate to typical absence of 3 cycles per second of generalized spike-and-wave; in atypical absence of 1.5–2.5 generalized spike-and-wave
- No aura
- Impaired consciousness
- No postictal state

Variable features

- Automatisms
- Change in body tone
- Precipitation by hyperventilation

Myoclonic seizures

Discriminating features

- Shock-like muscle contractions
- No impairment of consciousness

Consistent features

- Brief duration
- No aura
- No postictal state
- Generalized spike wave in the interictal EEG

Variable features

- Specific muscle groups involved (isolated or whole body; unilateral or bilateral)
- Association with a progressive neurologic syndrome
- Occur spontaneously or may be provoked by sensory stimulation

Mesial temporal lobe epilepsy

Discriminating features

- Unitemporal or bitemporal spikes in the interictal EEG
- Hippocampal sclerosis

Consistent features

- Simple partial and/or complex partial seizures
- Impaired memory

Variable features

- MRI demonstrating hippocampal atrophy or a focal temporal structural lesion
- History of febrile convulsions at an early age
- Psychic or emotional auras

Table II The epilepsies (continued)

Juvenile myoclonic epilepsy

Discriminating features

- Multiple seizure types including myoclonic seizures, absence seizures, and generalized tonic–clonic seizures
- Presence of myoclonus

Consistent features

- Onset at puberty
- Seizures often occur shortly after awakening
- 4–6 Hz generalized polyspike and slow wave on EEG
- Good response to ethosuximide or valproic acid

Variable features

- Concurrent absence seizures
- Seizures precipitated by sleep deprivation
- Normal neurologic examination

Lennox-Gastaut syndrome

Discriminating features

- Triad of (1) mental retardation, (2) generalized slow spike-and-wave on EEG, (3) multiple seizure types—atonic, atypical absence, myoclonic, partial, and tonic–clonic seizures

Consistent features

- Atonic seizures
- Onset before age 8
- Seizures are refractory to treatment
- Poor prognosis

Variable features

- Association with symptomatic early brain insults
- Cryptogenic onset in 30% of cases
- Behavioral disturbances

Psychogenic seizures

Discriminating features

- Gradual onset
- Variability in duration of episodes
- No increase in serum prolactin
- Induced by suggestion

Consistent features

- Normal EEG during seizures and in the interictal state
- Never occur during sleep

Variable features

- Manifestations of episodes (altered responsiveness, motor activity, vocalizations)
- Asynchronous extremity movements
- Minnesota Multiphasic Personality Inventory suggestive of conversion

Table III Valvular stenotic heart disease

Pulmonary stenosis

Discriminating features
- Echocardiographic appearance

Consistent features
- Systolic murmur

Variable features
- EKG changes
- Ejection clicks

Types
- Subpulmonary
- Supravalvular

Aortic stenosis

Discriminating features
- Echocardiographic appearance

Consistent features
- Systolic murmur

Variable features
- EKG changes
- Chest pain
- Ejection clicks

Types
- Supravalvular
- Subaortic (membranous vs. idiopathic hypertropic subaortic stenosis)

Mitral stenosis

Discriminating features
- Echocardiographic appearance

Consistent features
- Diastolic murmur

Variable features
- Opening sound
- Pulmonary edema
- Wheezing (cardiac)

Types
- Suprastenotic ring
- Coarctation

Tricuspid stenosis

Discriminating features
- Echocardiographic appearance

Consistent features
- Diastolic murmur

Variable features
- Hepatomegaly
- Clicks

Types
- Suprastenotic ring
- Coarctation

- If multiple discriminators are needed (i.e., a criterion-based system), are inclusionary as well as exclusionary criteria to be used?
- What consistent and variable features should be used to enhance understanding and more clearly define the entity?
- What should be the relative frequency to distinguish between consistent and variable features?

In conclusion, I propose that, as knowledge permits, medicine should define a discriminator-based system for the classification of diseases and disorders. The use of additional consistent and variable features will further enhance distinctions between diagnostic entities.

Acknowledgments

The author wishes to acknowledge Dr. Robin Morris, Dr. Isabelle Rapin, Dr. Jack Fletcher, and Dr. Barbara Wilson, who fostered the author's interest in nosologic issues, and the National Institute of Neurologic Disease and Stroke, which provided support for the author's desire to apply nosologic perspective to disorders of higher cerebral function in children (Nosology: Higher Cerebral Function in Children) (NINDS 1PO1 NS20489–01A1).

The author also wishes to acknowledge the invaluable assistance of Dr. G. Thomas Albrecht, who prepared the table describing the features of valvular stenotic heart disease, and C. L. Womack, who reviewed the manuscript.

References

Blashfield RK, Draguns JG. Evaluative criteria for psychiatric classification. *J Abnorm Psychol* 1996;83(2):140–150.

Fader K. *Nosography in modern internal medicine*. New York: Paul B. Hoeber, 1922.

King LS. Empiricism and rationalism in the works of Thomas Sydenham. *Bull Hist Med* 1970;44(1).

Nyhan WL. Child and adolescent neurology. In: David RB, ed. *In-born errors of metabolism*. II. Disorders of purine and amino acid metabolism. St. Louis: Mosby/Yearbook, 1998; 359–378.

Riesman D. *Thomas Sydenham, Clinician*. New York: Paul B. Hoeber, 1926;17.

Sirven JI, Sperling MR. The epilepsies. In: Corey-Bloom J, ed. *Adult neurology*. St. Louis: Mosby/Yearbook, 1998.

Bibliography

Chapter 2

Amil-Tison C. A method for neurologic evaluation within the first years of life. *Curr Probl Pediatr* 1976:7(1)1–150.

Amil-Tison C, Grenier A. *Neurobiological assessment during the first year of life*. New York: Oxford University Press, 1986.

Daily DK, Ellison PH. The premie-neuro: A clinical neurological examination of premature infants. *Neonatal Netw* 2005;24(1):15–22.

Drillien CM, Thomson AJ, Burgoyne K. Low birth weight children at early school age: A longitudinal study. *Dev Med Child Neurol* 1980;22(1):26–47.

Ellison P. Neurologic development of the high-risk infant. *Clin Perinatol* 1984;11(1):41–58.

Ellison P. Long-term follow-up studies: The prediction of the neurologic examination in infancy. In: Moss AJ, ed. *Pediatrics update*. New York: Elsevier Biomedical;1984:187–200.

Ellison P. The infant neurological examination. In: Wolraich M, Routh DK, eds. *Advances in developmental and behavioral pediatrics*. London: Jessica Kingsley Publisher Ltd. 1990;9: 75–138.

Ellison P, Browning C, Trostmiller T. Evaluation of tone in infancy: Physical therapist versus pediatric neurologist. *J Calif Perinatal Assoc* 1982;2:63–66.

Ellison P, Browning CA, Larson B, Denny J. Development of a scoring system for the Milani-Comparetti and Gidoni method of assessing neurologic abnormality in infancy. *Phys Ther* 1983;63(9):1414–1423.

Ellison P, Foster M. Developmental pathways through childhood for children treated in a neonatal intensive care unit. *Acta Pediatr* 1992;(Suppl 380)81:1–14.

Ellison P, Horn JL, Browning CA. The construction of an infant neurologic international battery (Infanib) for the assessment of neurologic integrity in infancy. *Phys Ther* 1985;65(9): 1326–1331.

Ellison P, Prasse D, Siewert J, Browning C. The outcome of neurological abnormality in infancy. In: Harel S, Stern S, eds. *The at risk infant*. Baltimore: Brookes;1985:253–260.

Ellison PH. The Infanib: A reliable method for the neuromotor assessment of infants. Tucson: Skill Builders, 1994.

Inder TE, Anderson NJ, Spencer C, et al. White matter injury in the premature infant: A comparison between serial cranial sonographic and MR findings at term. *Am J Neuroradiol* 2003;24(5):805–809.

Ment LR, Vohr B, Allan W, et al. Change in cognitive function over time in very low-birth-weight infants. *JAMA* 2003; 289(6):705–711.

Nelson KB, Ellenberg JH. Children who "outgrew" cerebral palsy. *Pediatrics* 1982;69(5):529–536.

Prechtl HF, Dijkstra J. Neurological diagnosis of cerebral injury in the newborn. In: Ten Berge BS, ed. *Proceedings of the symposium on prenatal care*. Groningen: Noordhoff;1960:222–231.

Sheridan-Pereira M, Ellison PH, Helgeson V. The construction of a scored form of the neonatal neurological examination. *J Dev Behav Pediatr* 1991;12(1):25–30.

Spitzmiller RE, Phillips T, Meinzen-Derr J, Hoath SB. Amplitude-integrated EEG is useful in predicting neurodevelopmental outcome in full-term infants with hypoxic-ischemic encephalopathy: A meta-analysis. *J Child Neurol* 2007; 22(9):1069–1078.

Woodward LJ, Anderson PJ, Austin NC, et al. Neonatal MRI to predict neurodevelopmental outcomes in preterm infants. *N Engl J Med* 2006;355(7):685–694.

Chapter 3

Achenbach TM, Rescorla L. Manual for the preschool child behavior checklist and revised child behavior profile. Burlington, VT: University Associates in Psychiatry, 2000.

Annett M. *Left, right, hand and brain: The right shift theory*. Hillsdale: NJ Erlbaum Associates, 1985.

Beery K, Buktenica N. *Beery developmental test of visual-motor integration*, 4th ed. Lutz FL:. Psychological Assessment Resources, Inc., 2003.

Behar L. The preschool behavior questionnaire. *J Abnorm Child Psychol* 1977;5:265–276.

Blackman J, Levine M, Markowitz M. *Pediatric extended examination at three*. Cambridge, MA: Educators Publishing Service, 1986.

Blondis J, Snow J, Roizen N, et al. Early maturation of motor delayed children at school age. *J Child Neurol* 1993;8:323–329.

Capute AJ, Accardo PJ. The infant neurodevelopmental assessment: A clinical interpretative manual for CAT-CLAMS. *Curr Probl Pediatr* 1996;26:238–257.

Committee on Children with Disabilities, American Academy of Pediatrics. Developmental surveillance and screening of infants and young children. *Pediatrics* 2001;108:192–196.

Conners CK. *Conners' Rating Scales: Revised user's manual.* North Tonawanda, NY: Multi-Health Systems, Inc., 2008.

Connolly K, Stratton P. Developmental changes in associated movements. *Dev Med Child Neurol* 1968;10:49–56.

Coplan J. *The Early Language Milestone Scale*. Austin, TX: PRO-ED, 1987.

Corballis MC. *Human laterality*. New York: Academic Press, 1983.

Denckla MB. Development of motor coordination in normal children. *Dev Med Child Neurol* 1974;16:729–741.

Denckla MB. Development of speed in repetitive and successive finger movements in normal children. *Dev Med Child Neurol* 1973;15:635–645.

Dennis M. Impaired sensory and motor differentiation with callosal agenesis: A lack of callosal inhibition during ontogeny? *Neuropsychologia* 1976;14:455–469.

Dunn LL, Dunn L. *Peabody Picture Vocabulary Test-III*. Circle Pines, MN: AGS Publishing. Phone: 800-328-2560.

Egan D. *Developmental examination of infants and preschool children*. Clinics in Developmental Medicine No. 12. Philadelphia: Lippincott, 1990.

Filipek P, Accardo P, Ashwal S, et al. Practice parameter: Screening and diagnosis of autism: A report of the quality standards subcommittee of the American Academy of Neurology and the Child Neurology Society. *Neurology* 2000;55:468–479.

Frankenburg W, Dodds J. Denver Developmental Screening Test II (DDST-II). Denver, CO, 2002-2005. Phone: (303) 355–4729.

Frankenburg WK, Fandal AW, Thornton SM. Revision of Denver prescreening developmental questionnaire. *J Pediatr* 1987;110:653–658.

Gadow KD, Sprafkin J. *Early childhood inventory, parent and teacher checklists*. Stony Brook, NY: Checkmate Plus, 2002.

Galin D, Diamond R, Herron J. Development of crossed and uncrossed tactile localization of the fingers. *Brain Lang* 1977;4:588–590.

Gillberg C. Children with preschool minor neurological disorders. IV. Behavior and school achievement at age 13 years. *Dev Med Child Neurol* 1988;31:3–24.

Glascoe FP, Byrne KE, Chang B, et al. Accuracy of the Denver-II in developmental screening. *Pediatrics* 1992;89:1221–1225.

Glaser JS. *Neuro-ophthalmology*. New York: Harper & Row, 2000.

Goodenough F, Harris D. *Goodenough-Harris Drawing Tests*. Los Angeles: Western Psychological Services, 1963.

Hoon A, Pulsifer M, Gopalan R, et al. Clinical adaptive test/clinical linguistic auditory milestone scale in early cognitive assessment. *J Pediatr* 1993;123:S1–S8.

Jolles I. *A catalog for the qualitative interpretation of the house-tree-person (H-T-P)*, 11th ed. Los Angeles, CA: Western Psychological Services, 1996.

Kadesjo B, Gillberg C. Developmental coordination disorder in Swedish 7-year-old children. *Journal of the Academy of Child & Adolescent Psychiatry*, 38(7):820–8, 1999.

Kinsbourne M, Hicks R. Functional cerebral space: A model for overflow, transfer and interference effects in human performance: A tutorial review. In: Renquin J, ed. *Attention and performance*. Hillsdale, NJ: Lawrence Erlbaum, 1978.

Kinsbourne M, Warrington EK. The development of finger differentiation. *J Exp Psychol* 1963;15:132–137.

Landgren M, Kjellman B, Gillberg C. Deficits in motor control and perception (DAMP): a simplified school entry examination. [*Research Support, Non-U.S. Gov't*]. *Acta Paediatrica*. 89(3):302–9, 2000.

Lefford A, Birch HG, Green G. The perceptual and cognitive bases for finger localization and selective finger movement in preschool children. *Child Dev* 1974;45:335–343.

Levine M, Schneider E. *Pediatric Exam of Educational Readiness (PEER)*. Cambridge, MA: Educators Publishing Service, 1985.

Levine M. *PEET (Pediatric Extended Examination at Three)*. Cambridge, MA: Educators Publishing Service, 1985.

Levine M. *The Anser System*. Cambridge, MA: Educators Publishing Service, 1996.

Levine MD. *Developmental variation and learning disorders*, 2nd ed. Cambridge, MA: Educators Publishing Service, 1992.

Lewis BA, Aram DM, Horwitz SJ. Language and motor findings in benign megalencephaly. *Percept Mot Skills* 1989;68(3 Pt 2):1051–1054.

Lindgren SD. Finger localization and the prediction of reading disability. *Cortex* 1978;14:87–101.

Meisels S, Marsden D, Wiske MS, Henderson L. *Early Screening Inventory-Revised (ESI-R)*. Ann Arbor, MI: Pearson Education, 1997.

Nass R. Mirror movement asymmetries in congenital hemiparesis: The inhibition hypothesis revisited. *Neurology* 1985; 35:1059–1062.

Nelson K, Eng G. Congenital hypoplasia of the depressor angularis oris muscle: Differentiation from congenital facial palsy. *J Pediatr* 1972;81:16–20.

Nevo Y, Kramer U, Shinnar S, et al. Macrocephaly in children with developmental disabilities. *Pediatr Neurol* 2002;27: 363–368.

Nichols P, Chen T. *Minimal brain dysfunction: A prospective study*. Hillsdale, NJ: Lawrence Erlbaum, 1981.

Njiokikjien C, Driessen M, Kabraken L. Development of supination-pronation movements in normal children. *Hum Neurobiol* 1986;5:199–203.

Roeltgen MG, Tucker DM, Roeltgen DP. Asymmetric lateralized attention in children. *Neurology* 1986;20:413.

Ross G, Lipper E, Auld P. Hand preferences in four-year-old children: Relation to prematurity. *Dev Med Child Neurol* 1987;29:615–622.

Rudel RG, Healey J, Denckla MB. Development of motor coordination by normal left handed children. *Dev Med Child Neurol* 1984;26:104–111.

Schwartz A, Murphy M. Cues for screening language disorders in preschool children. *Pediatrics* 1975;55:717–722.

Shevell M, Ashwal S, Donley D, et al. Practice parameter: Evaluation of the child with global developmental delay: Report of the quality standards subcommittee of the American Academy of Neurology and the practice committee of the child neurology society. *Neurology* 2003;60:367–380.

Smith D. *Recognizable patterns of human malformation*. Philadelphia: Saunders, 2006.

Stromland K, Sjogreen L, Miller M, et al. Mobius sequence: A Swedish multidiscipline study. *Eur J Paediatr Neurol* 2002;6: 35–45.

Sturner RA, Green JA, Funk SG. Preschool Denver Developmental Screening Test as a predictor of later school problems. *J Pediatr* 1985;107:615–721.

Suresh PA, Sebastian S. Developmental Gerstmann's syndrome: A distinct clinical entity of learning disabilities. *Pediatr Neurol* 2000;22:267–278.

Touwen BC, Prechtl HFR. The neurological examination of the child with minor central nervous system dysfunction. London: Spastics International, 1970.

Voress J, Maddox T. *Developmental Assessment of Young Children (DAYC)*. Lutz, FL: Psychological Assessment Resources, Inc., 2003.

Waldrup M, Pedersen F, Bell RQ. Minor physical anomalies and behavior in preschool children. *Child Dev* 1968;39:391–400.

Wolff P, Gunnoe C, Cohen C. Associated movements as a measure of developmental age. *Dev Med Child Neurol* 1983;25: 417–429.

Yakovlev PI, LeCours AR. The myelogenetic cycles of regional maturation of the brain. In: Minkowski A, ed. *Regional development of the brain in early life*. Oxford: Blackwell Scientific, 1967.

Zimmerman I, Steiner V, Pond R. *Preschool language scale*. San Antonio, TX: The Psychological Corporation, 2006.

Chapter 4

Barlow C. "Soft signs" in children with learning disorders. *Am J Dis Child* 1974;128:605–606.

Bellugi U, Lichtenberger L, Jones W, et al. The neurocognitive profile of Williams Syndrome: A complex pattern of strengths and weaknesses. *J Cogn Neurosci* 2000;12(Suppl 1):7–29.

Berg B. Unusual neurocutaneous syndromes. *Neurol Clin North Am* 1985;3:165–178.

Beumer J, 3rd, Trowbridge HO, Silverman S, Jr., Eisenberg E. Childhood hypophosphatasia and the premature loss of teeth: A clinical and laboratory study of seven cases. *Oral Med Oral Pathol* 1973;35:631.

Brindley GS. Cortical blindness and the functions of nongeniculate fibers of the optic tracts. *J Neurol Neurosurg Psychiatr* 1969;32:259–264.

Bryden M. Measuring handedness with questionnaires. *Neuropsychologia* 1977;15:617–624.

Campbell WW. *DeJong's the neurologic examination*, 6th ed. Philadelphia: Lippincott Williams & Wilkins, 2005.

Cassidy SB, Morris CA. Behavioral phenotypes in genetic syndromes: Genetic clues to human behavior. *Adv Pediatr* 2002;49:59–86.

Cogan DG. *Neurology of the ocular muscles*, 2nd ed. Springfield, IL: Charles C Thomas, 1956.

Coplen J. Deafness: Ever heard of it? Delayed recognition of permanent hearing loss. *Pediatrics* 1987;79:206–213.

Damasio A, Geschwind N, Klawans HL. Anatomic localization in clinical neuropsychology. In: Vinken PU, Bruyn GW, eds. *Clinical neuropsychology, handbook of neurology*, Vol. 1(45). Amsterdam: Elsevier/North-Holland;1985:7–22.

David R. *Nosology of disorders of higher cerebral function in childhood*. St. Paul MN: Child Neurology Society, 1981.

David RB, ed. *Child and adolescent neurology*, 2nd ed. Oxford, UK: Blackwell Publishing, 2005.

Denckla MB. Development of motor coordination in normal children. *Dev Med Child Neurol* 1974;16:729–741.

Deuel RK, Doar BP. Testing manual praxis in school-aged children. *Ann Neurol* 1990;28:425.

Deuel RK, Moran CC. Cerebral dominance and cerebral asymmetries on computed tomogram in childhood. *Neurology* 1980;30:934–938.

Deuel RK, Rauchway AC. Preschool and school-age pediatric and neurologic examination scoring form. In: David RB, ed. *Child and adolescent neurology*, 2nd ed. Oxford: Blackwell; 2005:74–80.

Dodge PR, Volpe JJ. Neurologic history and examination. In: Farmer TW, ed. *Pediatric neurology*, 3rd ed. Philadelphia: Harper & Row;1983:1–41.

Fog E, Fog M. Cerebral inhibition examined by associated movements. In: Bax M, MacKeith R, eds. *Clinics in developmental medicine*. London: Heineman;1963:35–47.

Grossman H, Dorst J. The mucopolysaccharidoses. In: Kaufman H, ed. *Progress in pediatric radiology*, Vol. 4. Chicago: Year Book;1973:495–544.

Hall JG, Allanson JE, Gripp KW, Slovotinek AM. *Handbook of physical measurements*, 2nd ed. New York: Oxford University Press, 2007.

Kuczmarski RJ, Ogden CL, Guo SS, et al. 2000 CDC growth charts for the United States: Methods and development. National Center for Health Statistics. *Vital Health Stat* 2002; 11(246).

Menkes JH, Sarnat HB, Maria BL, eds. *Child neurology*, 7th ed. Philadelphia: Lippincott Williams & Wilkins, 2006.

Money J. Specific neuro-cognitive impairments associated with Turner (45,X) and Klinefelter (47XXY) syndromes. *Soc Biol* 1993;40:147–151.

Nellhaus G. Head circumference from birth to eighteen years. Practical composite international and interracial graphs. *Pediatrics* 1968;41:106–114.

Nichols PL, Chen TC. *Minimal brain dysfunction: A prospective study*. Hillsdale, NJ: Lawrence Erlbaum, 1981.

Pennington B, Puck M, Robinson A. Language and cognitive development in 47 XXX females followed since birth. *Behav Genet* 1980;10:31.

Provins K, Cunliffe P. The reliability of some motor performance tests of handedness. *Neuropsychologia* 1972;10:199–206.

Pryor HB. Objective measurement of interpupillary distance. *Pediatrics* 1969;44:973–977.

Ratcliffe SG. Speech and learning disorders in children with sex chromosome abnormalities. *Dev Med Child Neurol* 1982; 24:80–84.

Reitan R. *Manual for administration of neuropsychological test batteries for adults and children*. Tucson, AZ: Neuropsychology Laboratory, 1969.

Robertson J, Shilkofski N. *The Harriet Lane handbook*, 17th ed. Philadelphia: Mosby;2005:244, 248.
Roid G, Miller L. *Leiter International Performance Scale—Revised*. Wood Dale, IL: Stoelting Company, 1996.
Schimke R, McKusick VA, Huang T, Pollack AD. Homocystinuria: Studies of 20 families with 38 affected members. *JAMA* 1965;193:711–716.
Scriver CR, Sly WS, eds. *The metabolic and molecular bases of inherited disease*. New York: McGraw-Hill, 2000.
Slosson R, Nicholson CL, Hibpshman TL. *Slosson Intelligence Test Revised, 3rd ed. (SIT-R3), for children and adults*. East Aurora, NY: Slosson Educational Publications, Inc., 2002.
Slosson R. *Slosson Intelligence Test (SIT-R3) for children and adults*. East Aurora, NY: Slosson Educational Publications, Inc., 1998.
Spriesterbach D, Morris HL, Darley FL. Examination of the speech mechanisms. In: Darley FL, Spriesterbach D, eds. *Diagnostic methods in speech pathology*, 2nd ed. New York: Harper & Row;1978:215–231.
Tanner JM. *Growth at adolescence*, 2nd ed. Oxford: Blackwell Scientific, 1962.
Taylor EM. *Psychological appraisal of children with cerebral defects*. Cambridge, MA: Harvard University press, 1959.
Taylor A, Hamden DG, Arlett CF, et al. Ataxia telangiectasia: A human mutation with abnormal radiation sensitivity. *Nature* 1975;258:427–429.
Thompson HS. Perimetry in neuroophthalmology. In: Frisen L, ed. *Topics in neuroophthalmology*. Baltimore, MD: Williams & Wilkins;1979:3–90.
Traquiar H. *An introduction to clinical perimetry*, 6th ed. London: Kimpton, 1949.
Waber DP. Neuropsychological aspects of Turner's syndrome. *Dev Med Child Neurol* 1979;21:58–70.
Wechsler D. *Wechsler Intelligence Scale for Children, 4th ed. (WISC-IV)*. San Antonio, TX: Psychological Corporation, 2003.
Witelson S. Hemispheric specialization for linguistic and nonlinguistic tactual perception using a dichotomous stimulation technique. *Cortex* 1978;10:3–17.
Wright CM, Booth IW, Buckler JMH, et al. Growth reference charts for use in the United Kingdom. *Arch Dis Child* 2002; 86;11–14.

Chapter 5

Adams DJ, Lueders H. Hyperventilation and 6-hour EEG recording in evaluation of absence seizures. *Neurology* 1981; 31:1175–1177.
Aicardi J. *Epilepsy in children*, 2nd ed. New York: Raven Press; 1994:168.
Aliberti V, Grünewald A, Panayiotopoulos CP, et al. Focal electroencephalographic abnormalities in juvenile myoclonic epilepsy. *Epilepsia* 1994;35:297–301.
Al-Qudah AA, Abu-Sheik S, Tamimi AF. Diagnostic value of short duration outpatient video electroencephalographic monitoring. *Pediatr Neurol* 1999;21(3):622–625.
Andermann F. Clinical features of migraine epilepsy syndromes. In: Andermann F, Lugaresi E, eds. *Migraine and epilepsy*. Boston: Butterworths;1987:3–30.
Aoki Y, Lombroso CT. Prognostic value of electroencephalography in Reye's syndrome. *Neurology* 1973;23:333–343.
Ashwal S, Schneider S. Failure of electroencephalography to diagnose brain death in comatose children. *Ann Neurol* 1979; 6:512–517.
Bauer G. Coma and brain death. In: Niedermeyer E, Lopes da Silva F, eds. *Electroencephalography: Basic principles, clinical applications and related fields*, 2nd ed. Baltimore, MD: Urban & Schwarzenberg;1987:391–404.
Beydoun A, Garofalo EA, Drury I. Generalized spike waves, multiple loci, and clinical course in children with EEG features of benign epilepsy of childhood with centrotemporal spikes. *Epilepsia* 1992;33:1091–1096.
Bickford RG, Butt HR. Hepatic coma: The electroencephalographic pattern. *J Clin Invest* 1955;34:790–799.
Blume WT, David RB, Gomez MR. Generalized sharp and slow wave complexes. Associated clinical features and long-term follow-up. *Brain* 1973;96:289–306.
Blume WT, Girvin JP, Kaufmann JCE. Childhood brain tumors presenting as chronic uncontrolled focal seizure disorders. *Ann Neurol* 1982;12:538–541.
Blume WT, Kaibara M. *Atlas of pediatric electroencephalography*, 2nd ed. New York: Lippincott-Raven Publishers, Philadelphia;1999:154–156.
Blume WT, Young GB, Lemieux JF. EEG morphology of partial epileptic seizures. *Electroencephalogr Clin Neurophysiol* 1984;57:295–302.
Blume WT. *Atlas of pediatric electroencephalography*. New York: Raven Press, 1982.
Bobele GB, Steele K, Leonard J. Determination of brain death in newborns and infants: A comparison of electroencephalograms and radionuclide cerebral perfusion scans. *Ann Neurol* 1993;34:478.
Bridgers SL, Ebersole JS. The clinical utility of ambulatory cassette EEG. *Neurology* 1985;35:166–173.
Browne TR, Penry JK, Dreifuss FE. Responsiveness before, during, and after spike-wave paroxysms. *Neurology* 1974;24: 659–665.
Carbonell J, Carrascosa G, Diersen S, et al. Some electrophysiological observations in a case of deep coma secondary to cardiac arrest. *Electroenceph Clin Neurophysiol* 1963;15: 520–525.
Carmant L, Kramer U, Holmes GL, et al. Differential diagnosis of staring spells in children: A video-EEG study. *Pediatr Neurol* 1996;14:199–202.
Carpay JA, de Weerd AW, Schimsheimer RJ, et al. The diagnostic yield of a second EEG after partial sleep deprivation: A prospective study in children with newly diagnosed seizures. *Epilepsia* 1997;38:595–599.
Chatrian GE, Shaw CM, Leffman H. The significance of periodic lateralized epileptiform discharges in EEG: An electrographic, clinical and pathological study. *Electroenceph Clin Neurophysiol* 1964;17:177–193.
Chen KS, Kuo MF, Wang HS, Huang SC. Periodic lateralized epileptiform discharges of pediatric patients in Taiwan. *Pediatr Neurol* 2003;28:100–103.
Chen LS, Mitchell WG, Horton EJ, Snead OC, 3rd. Clinical utility of video-EEG monitoring. *Pediatr Neurol* 1995;12:220–224.
Cooper GW, Lee SI. Reactive occipital epileptiform activity: Is it benign? *Epilepsia* 1991;32:63–68.

Dalla Bernardina B, Capovilla G, Gattoni MV, et al. Epilepsie myoclonique grave de la première année. *Rev Electroencephalogr Neurophysiol Clin* 1982;12:21–25.

Dravet C, Roger J, Bureau M. Severe myoclonic epilepsy of infants. In: Roger J, Dravet C, Bureau M, et al., eds. *Epilepsy syndromes in infancy, childhood and adolescence*. London: John Libbey;1985:58–67.

Dulac O. Epileptic encephalopathy. *Epilepsia* 2001;42(Suppl 3):23–26.

Ebersole JS, Schomer DL, Ives JR. Ambulatory EEG monitoring. In: Ebersole JS, Pedley TA, eds. *Current practice of clinical electroencephalography*, 3rd ed. Philadelphia: Lippincott Williams & Wilkins;2003:610–638.

Eeg-Olofsson O, Petersen I, Sellden U. The development of the electroencephalogram in normal children from the age of 1 through 15 years. Paroxysmal activity. *Neuropadiatrie* 1971; 2:375–404.

Falconer MA, Taylor DC. Surgical treatment of drug-resistant epilepsy due to mesial temporal sclerosis. *Arch Neurol* 1968; 19:353–361.

Frantzen E, Lennox-Buchthal M, Nygaard A. Longitudinal EEG and clinical study of children with febrile convulsions. *Electroencephalogr Clin Neurophysiol* 1968;24:197–212.

Gambardella A, Palmini A, Andermann F, et al. Usefulness of focal rhythmic discharges on scalp EEG of patients with focal cortical dysplasia and intractable epilepsy. *Electroencephalogr Clin Neurophysiol* 1996;98:243–249.

Garg BP, Patel H, Markand ON. Clinical correlation of periodic lateralized epileptiform discharges in children. *Pediatr Neurol* 1995;12:225–229.

Gastaut H, Broughton R, Roger J, et al. Generalized convulsive seizures without local onset. In: Vinken PJ, Bruyn GW, eds. *Handbook of clinical neurology*. Amsterdam: Elsevier; 1974: 107–129.

Gastaut H, Poirier F, Payan H, et al. H.H.E. syndrome: Hemiconvulsions, hemiplegia, epilepsy. *Epilepsia* 1960;1:418–447.

Gastaut H. Benign epilepsy of childhood with occipital paroxysms. In: Roger J, Dravet C, Bureau M, et al., eds. *Epileptic syndromes in infancy, childhood and adolescence*, 2nd ed. London: John Libbey;1992:201–217.

Genton P, Guerrini R, Dravet C. The Lennox-Gastaut syndrome. In: Meinardi H, ed. *Handbook of clinical neurology*, Vol. 73(29): *The epilepsies, Part II*. Amsterdam: Elsevier; 2000:211–222.

Genton P, Roger J. The progressive myoclonus epilepsies. In: Wyllie E, ed. *The treatment of epilepsy: Principles and practice*. Philadelphia: Lea & Febiger;1993:571–583.

Gibbs FA, Gibbs EL, Lennox WG. Influence of the blood sugar level on the wave and spike formation in petit mal epilepsy. *Arch Neurol Psychiatry* 1939;41:1111–1116.

Gibbs FA, Gibbs EL. *Atlas of electroencephalography, Vol. 3: Neurological and psychiatric disorders*. Reading MA: Addison-Wesley;1964:185–198.

Gloor P, Kalabay O, Giard N. The electroencephalogram in diffuse encephalopathies: Electroencephalographic correlates of grey and white matter lesions. *Brain* 1968;91:779–802.

Gobbi G, Ambrosetto G, Parmeggiani A, et al. The malignant variant of partial epilepsy with occipital spikes in childhood. *Epilepsia* 1991;32(Suppl 1):16–17.

Gross DW, Wiebe S, Blume WT. The periodicity of lateralized epileptiform discharges. *Clin Neurophysiol* 1999;110:1516–1520.

Haga Y, Watanabe K, Negoro T, et al. Do ictal, clinical, and electroencephalographic features predict outcome in West syndrome? *Pediatr Neurol* 1995;13:226–229.

Hirsch E, Marescaux C, Maquet P, et al. Landau-Kleffner syndrome: A clinical and EEG study of five cases. *Epilepsia* 1990;31:756–767.

Hou JW, Wang PJ, Wang TR. Angelman syndrome assessed by neurological and molecular cytogenetic investigations. *Pediatr Neurol* 1997;16:17–22.

Hrachovy RA, Frost JR, Kellaway P. Hypsarrhythmia: Variations on the theme. *Epilepsia* 1984;25:317–325.

Jonkman EJ. Cerebral death and the isoelectric EEG. *Electroenceph Clin Neurophysiol* 1969;27:215.

Klass DW, Westmoreland BF. Nonepileptogenic epileptiform electroencephalographic activity. *Ann Neurol* 1985;18:627–635.

Kramer U, Carmant L, Riviello JJ, et al. Psychogenic seizures: Video telemetry observations in 27 patients. *Pediatr Neurol* 1995;12:39–41.

Laan LA, Vein AA. A Rett patient with a typical Angelman EEG. *Epilepsia* 2002;43:1590–1592.

Lairy GC, Harrison A, Leger EM. Foyers EEG bi-occipitaux asynchrones de pointes chez l'enfant mal voyant et aveugle d'age scolaire. *Rev Neurol* 1964;111:351–353.

Lancman ME, Asconapé JJ, Penry JK. Clinical and EEG asymmetries in juvenile myoclonic epilepsy. *Epilepsia* 1994;35: 302–306.

Lemieux JF, Blume WT. Topographical evolution of spike-wave complexes. *Brain Res* 1986;373:275–287.

Leroy RF, Ebersole JS. An evaluation of ambulatory, cassette EEG monitoring: I. Montage design. *Neurology* 1983;33: 1–7.

Maher J, Ronen GM, Ogunyemi AO, Goulden KJ. Occipital paroxysmal discharges suppressed by eye opening: Variability in clinical and seizure manifestations in childhood. *Epilepsia* 1995;36:52–57.

Niedermeyer E, Naidu S. Degenerative disorders of the central nervous system. In: Niedermeyer E, Lopes da Silva F, eds. *Electroencephalography: Basic principles, clinical applications and related fields*, 2nd ed. Baltimore MD: Urban & Schwarzenberg;1987:317–338.

Niedermeyer E. Epileptic seizure disorders. In: Niedermeyer E, Lopes da Silva F, eds. *Electroencephalography: Basic principles, clinical applications and related fields*. Baltimore, MD: Urban & Schwarzenberg;1987:415–416.

Nordli DR, Jr., Leary LD, De Vivo DC. Progressive pediatric neurological syndromes. In: Ebersole JS, Pedley TA, eds. *Current practice of clinical electroencephalography*, 3rd ed. Philadelphia: Lippincott Williams & Wilkins;2003:483–505.

Ohtahara S, Ishida T, Oka E, et al. On the age-dependent epileptic syndromes: The early infantile encephalopathy with suppression burst. *Brain Dev* 1976;8:270–288.

Olson DM. Success of ambulatory EEG in children. *J Clin Neurophysiol* 2001;18:158–161.

Palmini A, Andermann F, Olivier A, et al. Focal neuronal migration disorders and intractable partial epilepsy: Results of surgical treatment. *Ann Neurol* 1991;30:750–757.

Pampiglione G, Harden A. Neurophysiological identification of a late infantile form of "neuronal lipidosis." *J Neurol Neurosurg Psychiatry* 1973;36:68–74.

Pampiglione G, Harden A. Resuscitation after cardiocirculatory arrest. *Lancet* 1968;1:1261–1265.

Pampiglione G, Harden A. So-called neuronal ceroid lipofuscinosis. Neurophysiological studies in 60 children. *J Neurol Neurosurg Psychiatry* 1977;40:323–330.

Panayiotopoulos CP. Early-onset benign childhood occipital seizure susceptibility syndrome: A syndrome to recognize. *Epilepsia* 1999;40:621–630.

Patry G, Lyagoubi S, Tassinari CA. Subclinical "electrical status epilepticus" induced by sleep in children. *Arch Neurol* 1971; 24:242–252.

Pedley TA, Mendiratta A, Walczak TS. Seizures and epilepsy. In: Ebersole JS, Pedley TA, eds. *Current practise of clinical electroencephalography*, 3rd ed. Philadelphia: Lippincott Williams & Wilkins;2003:506–587.

Pringle CE, Blume WT, Munoz DG, et al. Pathogenesis of mesial temporal sclerosis. *Can J Neurol Sci* 1993;20:184–193.

Raymond AA, Fish DR, Sisodiya SM, et al. Abnormalities of gyration, heterotopias, tuberous sclerosis, focal cortical dysplasia, microdysgenesis, dysembryoplastic neuroepithelial tumour and dysgenesis of the archicortex in epilepsy. Clinical, EEG and neuroimaging features in 100 adult patients. *Brain* 1995;118(Pt 3):629–660.

Reilly EL, Peters JF. Relationship of some varieties of electroencephalographic photosensitivity to clinical convulsive disorders. *Neurology* 1973;23:1050–1057.

Roger J, Genton P, Bureau M, et al. Less common epileptic syndromes. In: Wyllie E, ed. *The treatment of epilepsy: Principles and practice*. Philadelphia: Lea & Febiger; 1993:624–635.

Rubin DI, Patterson MC, Westmoreland BF, Klass DW. Angelman's syndrome: Clinical and electroencephalographic findings. *Electroencephalogr Clin Neurophysiol* 1997;102:299–302.

Saravanan K, Acomb B, Beirne M, Appleton R. An audit of ambulatory cassette EEG monitoring in children. *Seizure* 2001; 10:579–582.

Shinnar S, Kang H, Berg AT, et al. EEG abnormalities in children with a first unprovoked seizure. *Epilepsia* 1994;35:471–476.

Silverman D. Electroencephalographic study of acute head injury in children. *Neurology* 1962;12:273–281.

Smith JMB, Kellaway P. The natural history and clinical correlates of occipital foci in children. In: Kellaway P, Petersen I, eds. *Neurological and electroencephalographic correlative studies in infancy*. New York: Grune & Stratton;1964:230–249.

Sundaram MBM, Blume WT. Triphasic waves: Clinical correlates and morphology. *Can J Neurol Sci* 1987;14:136–140.

Takahashi T. Activation methods. In: Niedermeyer E, Lopes da Silva F, eds. *Electroencephalography: Basic principles, clinical applications and related fields*. Baltimore, MD: Urban & Schwarzenberg;1987:212.

Tassinari CA, Bureau M, Dravet C, et al. Electrical status epilepticus during sleep in children (ESES). In: Sterman MB, Shouse MN, Passouant P, eds. *Sleep and epilepsy*. London: Academic Press;1982:465–479.

Tassinari CA, Bureau-Paillas M, Dalla Bernardina B, et al. La maladie de Lafora. *Rev EEG Neurophysiol* 1978;8:107–122.

Tassinari CA, Daniele O, Dravet C, et al. Sleep polygraphic studies in some epileptic encephalopathies from infancy to adolescence. In: Degen R, Niedermeyer E, eds. *Epilepsy, sleep and sleep deprivation*. Amsterdam: Elsevier;1984:175–189.

Tassinari CA, Rubboli G, Volpi L, et al. Encephalopathy with electrical status epilepticus during slow sleep or ESES syndrome including the acquired aphasia. *Clin Neurophysiol* 2000;111(Suppl 2):S94–S102.

Trauner DA, Haas RH. Electroencephalographic abnormalities in Rett's syndrome. *Ann Neurol* 1985;18:394.

Trojaborg W. Changes of spike foci in children. In: Kellaway P, Petersen I, eds. *Clinical electroencephalography of children*. New York: Grune & Stratton;1968:213–225.

Valente KD, Andrade JQ, Grossmann RM, et al. Angelman syndrome: Difficulties in EEG pattern recognition and possible misinterpretations. *Epilepsia* 2003;44:1051–1063.

Valente KD, Freitas A, Fiore LA, et al. The diagnostic role of short duration outpatient V-EEG monitoring in children. *Pediatr Neurol* 2003;28:285–291.

Veggiotti P, Beccaria F, Guerrini R, et al. Continuous spike-and-wave activity during slow-wave sleep: Syndrome or EEG pattern? *Epilepsia* 1999;40:1593–1601.

Visser SL. Two cases of isoelectric EEGs (apparent exceptions proving the rule). *Electroenceph Clin Neurophysiol* 1969; 27:215.

Weir B. The morphology of the spike-wave complex. *Electroencephalogr Clin Neurophysiol* 1965;19:284–290.

Yoshinaga H, Terasaki T, Ogino T, et al. Incidence of epileptic discharge in various epileptic syndromes. *Pediatr Neurol* 2001;25:38–42.

Young B, Mirsattari S, Ives J. Direct electroencephalographic comparison of Ag-Ag/Cl subdermal wire vs surface electrodes in the intensive care unit. *Muscle Nerve Suppl* 2003; 12:S170.

Chapter 7

Aminoff MJ, ed. *Electrodiagnosis in clinical neurology*, 5th ed. London: Churchill Livingstone, 2005.

Baker RS, Schmeisser ET, Epstein AD. Visual system electrodiagnosis in neurological disease of childhood. *Pediatr Neurol* 1995;12:99–110.

Chiappa KH, ed. *Evoked potentials in clinical medicine*, 3rd ed. Philadelphia: Lippincott-Raven, 1997.

DeMeirleir LJ, Taylor MJ. Prognostic utility of SEPs in comatose children. *Pediatr Neurol* 1987;3:78–82.

Ducati A, Fava E, Motti EDF. Neuronal generators of the visual evoked potentials: Intracerebral recording in awake humans. *EEG Clin Neurol* 1988;71:89–99.

Flores-Guevara R, Renault F, Ostre C, Richard P. Maturation of the electroretinogram in children: Stability of the amplitude ratio a/b. *Electroencephalogr Clin Neurophysiol* 1996; 100:422–427.

Harden A, Adams GGW, Taylor DSI. The electroretinogram. *Arch Dis Child* 1989;64:1080–1087.

Kriss A, Jeffrey B, Taylor D. The electroretinogram in infants and children. *J Clin Neurophysiol* 1992;9:373–393.

Kurtzberg D. Event-related potentials in the evaluation of high-risk infants. *Ann N Y Acad Sci* 1982;388:557–571.

Levin KH, Luders HO, eds. *Comprehensive clinical neurophysiology*. Philadelphia: WB Saunders, 2000.

Willis J, Seales D, Frazier E. Short latency somatosensory evoked potentials in infants. *Electroencephalogr Clin Neurophysiol* 1984;59:366–373.

Chapter 11

Adab N, Kini U, Vinten J, et al. The longer term outcome of children born to mothers with epilepsy. *J Neurol Neurosurg Psychiatry* 2004;75:1575–1583.

Andermann F, Zifkin B. The benign occipital epilepsies of childhood: An overview of the idiopathic syndromes and of the relationship to migraine. *Epilepsia* 1998;39(Suppl 4):S9–S23.

Appleton R, et al. Gabapentin as add-on therapy in children with refractory partial seizures: A 12-week, multicentre, double-blind, placebo-controlled study. Gabapentin Paediatric Study Group. *Epilepsia* 1999;40:1147–1154.

Arzimanoglou A, Guerrini R, Aicardi J. *Aicardi's epilepsy in children*. Philadelphia: Lippincott Williams & Wilkins, 2004a.

Arzimanoglou A, Guerrini R, Aicardi J. Diagnosis and differential diagnosis. In: Arzimanoglou A, Guerrini R, Aicardi J, eds. *Aicardi's epilepsy in children*. Philadelphia: Lippincott WIlliams & Wilkins;2004b:325–341.

Arzimanoglou A, Guerrini R, Aicardi J. General aspects of prognosis. In: Arzimanoglou A, Guerrini R, Aicardi J, eds. *Aicardi's epilepsy in children*. Philadelphia: Lippincott Williams & Wilkins;2004c:342–353.

Austin JK, Caplan R. Behavioral and psychiatric comorbidities in pediatric epilepsy: Toward an integrative model. *Epilepsia* 2007;48:1639–1651.

Ballaban-Gil K, Tuchman R. Epilepsy and epileptiform EEG: Association with autism and language disorders. *Ment Retard Dev Disabil Res Rev* 2000;6:300–308.

Baram TZ, Mitchell WG, Tournay A, et al. High-dose corticotropin (ACTH) versus prednisone for infantile spasms: A prospective, randomized, blinded study. *Pediatrics* 1996;97: 375–379.

Baram TZ, Shinnar S, eds. *Febrile seizures*. New York: Academic Press, 2002.

Bax M. Problems for the child with epilepsy. *Dev Med Child Neurol* 1999;41:723.

Baxter P. Pyridoxine-dependent and pyridoxine-responsive seizures. *Dev Med Child Neurol* 2001;43:416–420.

Ben-Ari Y. Excitatory actions of GABA during development: the nature of the nurture. *Nat Rev Neurosci* 2002;3:728–739.

Ben-Ari Y, Holmes GL. Effects of seizures on developmental processes in the immature brain. *Lancet Neurol* 2006;5: 1055–1063.

Benbadis SR. Epileptic seizures and syndromes. *Neurol Clin* 2001;19:251–270.

Berg AT, Shinnar S, Levy SR, et al. Two-year remission and subsequent relapse in children with newly diagnosed epilepsy. *Epilepsia* 2001;42:1553–1562.

Berkovic SF, Harkin L, McMahon JM, et al. De-novo mutations of the sodium channel gene SCN1A in alleged vaccine encephalopathy: A retrospective study. *Lancet Neurol* 2006;5: 488–492.

Bhatia MS, Sapra S. Pseudoseizures in children: A profile of 50 cases. *Clin Pediatr (Phila)* 2005; 44:617–621.

Bleasel A, Kotogal P. Paroxysmal nonepileptic disorders in children and adolescents. *Semin Neurol* 1995;15:203–217.

Bough KJ, Rho JM. Anticonvulsant mechanisms of the ketogenic diet. *Epilepsia* 2007;48:43–58.

Bourgeois BFD. Temporal lobe epilepsy in infants and children. *Brain Dev* 1998;20:135–141.

Bourgeois BFD. Valproate. In: Pellock JM, Dodson WE, Bourgeois BFD, eds. *Pediatric epilepsy diagnosis and therapy*. New York: Demos;2001:433–446.

Breningstall GN. Breath-holding spells. *Pediatr Neurol* 1996; 14:91–97.

Breningstall GN. Mortality in pediatric epilepsy. *Pediatr Neurol* 2001;25:9–16.

Brodie MJ. Pregabalin as adjunctive therapy for partial seizures. *Epilepsia* 2004;45(Suppl 6):19–27.

Brunson KL, Avishai-Eliner S, Baram TZ. ACTH treatment of infantile spasms: Mechanisms of its effects in modulation of neuronal excitability. *Int Rev Neurobiol* 2002;49:185–197.

Bryant AE, Dreifuss FE. Valproic acid hepatic fatalities: III. US experience since 1986. *Neurology* 1996;46:465–469.

Camfield PR, Camfield CS, Gordon K, Dooley JM. If a first antiepileptic drug fails to control a child's epilepsy, what are the chances of success with the next drug? *J Pediatr* 1997;131:821–824.

Chahine LM, Mikati MA. Benign pediatric localization-related epilepsies. Part 1. Syndromes in infancy. *Epileptic Disord* 2006;8:169–183.

Claassen J, Hirsch LJ, Emerson RG, Mayer SA. Treatment of refractory status epilepticus with pentobarbital, propofol, or midazolam: A systematic review. *Epilepsia* 2002;43:146–153.

Commission on classification and terminology of the international league against epilepsy: Proposal for revised clinical and electroencephalographic classification of epileptic seizures. *Epilepsia* 1981;22:489–501.

Commission on classification and terminology of the international league against epilepsy: Proposal for revised classification of epilepsies and epilepsy syndromes. *Epilepsia* 1989; 30:389–399.

Conry JA. Progressive myoclonic epilepsies. *J Child Neurol* 2002;17(Suppl 1):S80–S84.

Conry JA. Pharmacologic treatment of the catastrophic epilepsies. *Epilepsia* 2004; 45(Suppl 5):12–16.

Cross JH. Epilepsy surgery in childhood. *Epilepsia* 2002; 43(Suppl 3):65–70.

Crunelli V, Leresche N. Childhood absence epilepsy: Genes, channels, neurons, and networks. Nat Rev Neurosci 2002;3:371–382.

Daoud AS, Batieha A, al-Sheyyab M, et al. Effectiveness of iron therapy on breath-holding spells. *J Pediatr* 1997;130:547–550.

DeVivo DC. Metabolic determinants of infant epilepsy. *J Child Neurol* 2002;17(Suppl 3):3S1–3S102.

DeVivo DC, Bohan TP, Coulter DL, et al. L-Carnitine supplementation in childhood epilepsy: Current perspectives. *Epilepsia* 1998;39:1216–1225.

Donner EJ, Smith CR, Snead OC, 3rd. Sudden unexplained death in children with epilepsy. *Neurology* 2001;57:430–434.

Dubé CM, Brewster AL, Richichi C, Zha Q, Baram TZ: Fever, febrile seizures and epilepsy. Trends Neurosci 30:490-496, 2007.

Dulac O. Epileptic encephalopathy. *Epilepsia* 2001;43(Suppl. 3):23–26.

Engel J Jr. A proposed diagnostic scheme for people with epileptic seizures and epilepsy: report of the ILAE task force on classification and terminology. *Epilepsia* 2001;42:796–803.

Engel J Jr., Chair. Report of the ILAE classification core group. *Epilepsia* 2006;47:1558–1568.

Freeman JM, Kossoff EH, Freeman JB. *The ketogenic diet: A treatment for children and others with epilepsy*, 4th ed. New York: Demos Publications, 2007.

Frost JD Jr, Hrachovy RA. Pathogenesis of infantile spasms: a model based on developmental desynchronization. *J Clin Neurophysiol* 2005;22:25–36.

Fukuyama Y. West syndrome and other infantile epileptic encephalopathies. *Brain Dev* 2001;(special issue) 23(7).

Glauser TA, Nigro M, Sachdeo R, et al. Adjunctive therapy with oxcarbazepine in children with partial seizures. The Oxcarbazepine Pediatric Study Group. *Neurology* 2000;54:2237–2244.

Gobbi G, Boni A, Filippini M. The spectrum of idiopathic Rolandic epilepsy syndromes and idiopathic occipital epilepsies: From the benign to the disabling. *Epilepsia* 2006; 47(Suppl 2):62–66.

Gordon N. Episodic dyscontrol syndrome. *Dev Med Child Neurol* 1999;41:786–788.

Gospe SM. Pyridoxine-dependent seizures: Findings from recent studies pose new questions. *Pediatr Neurol* 2002;26:181–185.

Gudmundsson O, Prendergast M, Foreman D, Cowley S. Outcome of pseudoseizures in children and adolescents: A 6-year symptom survival analysis. *Dev Med Child Neurol* 2001;43: 547–551.

Guerrini R. Epilepsy in children. *Lancet* 2006;367:499–524.

Guerrini R, Belmonte A, Genton P. Antiepileptic drug-induced worsening of seizures in children. *Epilepsia* 1998;9(Suppl 3):S2–S30.

Guerrini R, Filippi T. Neuronal migration disorders, genetics, and epileptogenesis. *J Child Neurol* 2005;20:287–299.

Hadjiloizou SM, Bourgeois BFD. Antiepileptic drug treatment in children. *Exp Rev Neurother* 2007;7:179–193.

Hancock E, Cross H. Treatment of Lennox-Gastaut syndrome. Cochrane Database Syst Rev 3: 2003;CD003277.

Hartman AL, Gasior M, Vining EP, Rogawski MA. The neuropharmacology of the ketogenic diet. *Pediatr Neurol* 2007;36:281–292.

Hauser WA. Epidemiology of epilepsy in children. *Neurosurg Clin North Am* 1995;6:419–429.

Hawash KY, Rosman NP. Do partial seizures predict an increased risk of seizure recurrence after antiepilepsy drugs are withdrawn? *J Child Neurol* 2003;18:331–337.

Heck C, Helmers SL, DeGiorgio CM. Vagus nerve stimulation therapy, epilepsy, and device parameters: Scientific basis and recommendations for use. *Neurology* 2002;59(6 Suppl 4):S31–S37.

Henry TR, Heertum RLV. Positron emission tomography and single photon emission computed tomography in epilepsy care. *Semin Nucl Med* 2003;33:88–104.

Hirtz D, Berg A, Bettis D et al. Quality Standards Subcommittee of the American Academy of Neurology; Practice Committee of the Child Neurology Society. Practice parameter: Treatment of the child with a first unprovoked seizure. *Neurology* 2003;60:166–175.

Holmes GL. Epilepsy surgery in children. *Neurology* 2002; 58(Suppl 7):S13–S20.

Holmes GL, Ben-Ari Y. Seizures in the developing brain: Perhaps not so benign after all. *Neuron* 1998;21:1231–1234.

Holmes GL, Stafstrom CE, Tuberous Sclerosis Study Group. Tuberous sclerosis complex and epilepsy: Recent developments and future challenges. *Epilepsia* 2007;48:617–630.

Hyland K, Arnold LA. Value of lumbar puncture in the diagnosis of genetic metabolic encephalopathies. *J Child Neurol* 1999;14(Suppl. 1):S9–S15.

Iannetti P, Spalice A, Perla FM, et al. Visual field constriction in children with epilepsy on vigabatrin treatment. *Pediatrics* 2000;106:838–842.

Jarrar RG, Buchhalter JR. Therapeutics in pediatric epilepsy, part 1: The new antiepileptic drugs and the ketogenic diet. *Mayo Clin Proc* 2003;78:359–370.

Kossoff EH. More fat and fewer seizures: Dietary therapies for epilepsy. *Lancet Neurol* 2004;3:415–420.

Kuzniecky RI, Knowlton RC. Neuroimaging of epilepsy. *Semin Neurol* 2002;22:279–288.

Kwan P, Brodie MJ. Early identification of refractory epilepsy. *N Engl J Med* 2000;342:314–319.

Landau WM, Kleffner FR. Syndrome of acquired aphasia with convulsive disorder in children. *Neurology* 1957;7:523–530.

LaRoche SM. A new look at the second-generation antiepileptic drugs: A decade of experience. *Neurologist* 2007;13:133–139.

Levy RH, et al., eds. *Antiepileptic Drugs*. 5th Philadelphia: Lippincott, Williams & Wilkins, 2002.

Lux AL, Edwards SW, Hancock E, et al. The United Kingdom infantile spasms study (UKISS) comparing hormone treatment with vigabatrin on developmental and epilepsy outcomes to age 14 months: A multicentre randomised trial. *Lancet Neurol* 2005;4:712–717.

Mackay MT, Weiss SK, Adams-Webber T, Ashwal S, et al. Practice parameter: Medical treatment of infantile spasms. *Neurology* 2004;62:1668–1681.

Mackay M, Weiss S, Snead OC, 3rd. Treatment of infantile spasms: An evidence-based approach. *Int Rev Neurobiol* 2002;49:157–184.

Mandelbaum DE, Kugler SL, Wollack JB, Wenger EC. Apparent induction or exacerbation of primary generalized seizures after initiation of oxcarbazepine. *Epilepsia* 2002;43:208.

Maytal J, Shinnar S, Moshe SL, Alvarez LA. Low morbidity and mortality of status epilepticus in children. *Pediatrics* 1989; 83:323–331.

McLean MJ, Gidal BE. Gabapentin dosing in the treatment of epilepsy. *Clin Ther* 2003;25:1382-1406.

McNamara JO, Whitney KD, Andrews PI, et al. Evidence for glutamate receptor autoimmunity in the pathogenesis of Rasmussen encephalitis. *Adv Neurol* 1999;79:543–550.

Messenheimer J. Efficacy and safety of lamotrigine in pediatric patients. *J Child Neurol* 2002;17(Suppl 2):2S34–2S42.

Mitchell WG. Status epilepticus and acute serial seizures in children. *J Child Neurol* 2002;17(Suppl. 1):S36–S43.

Mizrahi EM. Neonatal seizures and neonatal epilepsy syndromes. *Neurol Clin* 2001;19:427–463.

Mizrahi EM, Kellaway P. Characterization and classification of neonatal seizures. *Neurology* 1987;37:1837–1844.

Neubauer BA. The genetics of rolandic epilepsy. *Epileptic Disord* 2002;2(Suppl 1):S67–S68.

Nieuwenhuis L, Nicolai J. The pathophysiological mechanisms of cognitive and behavioral disturbances in children with Landau-Kleffner syndrome or epilepsy with continuous spike-and-waves during slow wave sleep. *Seizure* 2006;15: 249-258.

Noebels JL. The biology of epilepsy genes. *Annu Rev Neurosci* 2003;26:599–625.

Nordli DR. Diagnostic difficulty in infants and children. *J Child Neurol* 2002;17(Suppl. 1):S28–S 35.

Obead M, Mikati MA. Expanding spectrum of paroxysmal events in children: Potential mimickers of epilepsy. *Pediatr Neurol* 2007;37:309–316.

O'Dell C, Shinnar S. Initiation and discontinuation of antiepileptic drugs. *Neurol Clin* 2001;19:289–311.

Otsubo H, Snead OC. Magnetoencephalography and magnetic source imaging in children. *J Child Neurol* 2001;16:227–235.

Panayiotopoulos CP. Panayiotopoulos syndrome: A common and benign childhood epileptic syndrome. Eastleigh, England: John Libbey & Company, Ltd., 2002.

Pellock JM, Faught E, Leppik IE, et al. Felbamate: consensus of current clinical experience. *Epilepsy Res* 2006;71:89–101.

Perucca E. Pharmacological and therapeutic properties of valproate: A summary after 35 years of clinical experience. *CNS Drugs* 2002;16:695–714.

Pitkanen A, Sutula TP. Is epilepsy a progressive disorder? Prospects for new therapeutic approaches in temporal lobe epilepsy. *Lancet Neurol* 2002;1:173–181.

Porter BE, Brooks-Kayal A, Golden JA. Disorders of cortical development and epilepsy. *Arch Neurol* 2002;59:361–365.

Posner E. Pharmacological treatment of childhood absence epilepsy. *Expert Rev Neurother* 2006;6:855–862.

Prensky AL. An approach to the child with paroxysmal phenomena with emphasis on nonepileptic disorders. In: Pellock JM, Dodson WE, Bourgeois BFD, eds. *Pediatric epilepsy diagnosis and therapy*. New York: Demos;2001:97–116.

Raspall-Chaure M, Neville BG, Scott RC. The medical management of the epilepsies in children: conceptual and practical considerations. *Lancet Neurol* 2008;7:57–69.

Rice GM, Hsu DA. Metabolic disorders in pediatric neurology. *Hosp Phys Board Rev Man* 2005;9:2–12.

Riikonen R. Long-term outcome of patients with West syndrome. *Brain Dev* 2001;23:683–687.

Rivera R, Segnini M, Baltodano A, Perez V. Midazolam in the treatment of status epilepticus in children. *Crit Care Med* 1993;21:991–994.

Rosman NP, Donnelly JH, Braun MA. The jittery newborn and infant: A review. *J Dev Behav Pediatr* 1984;5:263–273.

Samaniego EA, Sheth RD. Bone consequences of epilepsy and antiepileptic medications. *Semin Pediatr Neurol* 2007;14: 196–200.

Sankar R, Painter MJ. Neonatal seizures: After all these years we still love what doesn't work. *Neurology* 2005;64:776–777.

Scheffer I, Berkovic S. Generalized epilepsy with febrile seizures plus: A genetic disorder with heterogeneous clinical phenotypes. *Brain* 1997;120:479–490.

Scheffer IE, Berkovic SF. The genetics of human epilepsy. *Trends Pharmacol Sci* 2003;24:428–433.

Scheffer IE, Harkin LA, Dibbens LM, et al. Neonatal epilepsy syndromes and generalized epilepsy with febrile seizures plus (GEFS+). *Epilepsia* 2005;46(Suppl 10):41–47.

Scher MS, Alvin J, Gaus L, et al. Uncoupling of EEG-clinical neonatal seizures after antiepileptic drug use. *Pediatr Neurol* 2003;28:277–280.

Sheth RD, Stafstrom CE, Hsu D. Non-pharmacologic treatment options for epilepsy. *Semin Pediatr Neurol* 2005;12:106–113.

Shields WD. Infantile spasms: Little seizures, BIG consequences. *Epilepsy Curr* 2006;6:63–69.

Shinnar S, Berg AT, O'Dell C, et al. Predictors of multiple seizures in a cohort of children prospectively followed from the time of their first unprovoked seizure. *Ann Neurol* 2000;48:140–147.

Shinnar S, Pellock JM. Update on the epidemiology and prognosis of pediatric epilepsy. *J Child Neurol* 2002;17(Suppl 1):S4–S17.

Sillanpää M, Jalava M, Kaleva O, Shinnar S. Long-term prognosis of seizures with onset in childhood. *N Engl J Med* 1998;338:1715–1722.

Sillanpää M, Shinnar S. Status epilepticus in a population-based cohort with childhood-onset epilepsy in Finland. *Ann Neurol* 2002;52:303–310.

Silverstein FS, Jensen FE. Neonatal seizures. *Ann Neurol* 2007; 62:112–120.

Singh NA, Charlier C, Stauffer D, et al. A novel potassium channel gene, KCNQ2, is mutated in an inherited epilepsy of newborns. *Nature Genet* 1998;18:25–29.

Stafstrom CE. Neonatal seizures. *Pediatr Rev* 1995;16:248–255.

Stafstrom CE. The pathophysiology of epileptic seizures: a primer for pediatricians. *Pediatr Rev* 1998;19:335–344.

Stafstrom CE, Lynch M, Sutula TP. Consequences of epilepsy in the developing brain: Implications for surgical management. *Semin Pediatr Neurol* 2000;7:147–157.

Staley KJ. Wrong-way chloride transport: is it a treatable cause of some intractable seizures? *Epilepsy Curr* 2006;6:124–127.

Stephenson JBP. *Fits and faints*. Oxford: MacKeith Press, 1990.

Stroink H, Brouwer OF, Arts WF, et al. The first unprovoked, untreated seizure in childhood: A hospital based study of the accuracy of the diagnosis, rate of recurrence, and long term outcome after recurrence. Dutch study of epilepsy in childhood. *J Neurol Neurosurg Psychiatry* 1998;64:595–600.

Tassinari CA, Rubboli G, Volpi L, et al. Encephalopathy with electrical status epilepticus during slow sleep or ESES syndrome including the acquired aphasia. *Clin Neurophysiol* 2000;111(Suppl 2):S94–S102.

Tein I. Role of carnitine and fatty acid oxidation and its defects in infantile epilepsy. *J Child Neurol* 2002;17(Suppl 3):3S57–3S83.

Treiman DM. Status epilepticus. In: Wyllie E, ed. *Treatment of epilepsy: Principles and practice*. Philadelphia: Lippincott Williams Wilkins;2001:681–697.

Vining EPG. Clinical efficacy of the ketogenic diet. *Epilepsy Res* 1999;37:181–190.

Welty TE. Juvenile myoclonic epilepsy: Epidemiology, pathophysiology, and management. *Paediatr Drugs* 2006;8:303–310.

Wheless JW, Clark DF, Carpenter D. Treatment of pediatric epilepsy: expert opinion, 2005. *J Child Neurol* 2005; 20(Suppl 1):S1–S60.

Wheless JW, Constantinou JEC. Lennox-Gastaut syndrome. *Pediatr Neurol* 1997;17:203–211.

Wheless JW, Venkataraman V. New formulations of drugs in epilepsy. *Exp Opin Pharmacother* 1999;1:49–60.

Wong M. Advances in the pathophysiology of developmental epilepsies. *Semin Pediatr Neurol* 2005;12:72–87.

Wyllie E, Friedman D, Luders H, et al. Outcome of psychogenic seizures in children and adolescents compared with adults. *Neurology* 1991;41:742–744.

Chapter 12

Abelson JF, Kwan KY, O'Roak BJ, et al. Sequence variants in SLITRK1 are associated with Tourette's syndrome. *Science* 2005;310:317–320.

ACMG/ASHG statement. Laboratory guidelines for Huntington disease genetic testing. The American College of Medical Genetics/American Society of Human Genetics Huntington Disease Genetic Testing Working Group. *Am J Hum Genet* 1998;62:1243–1247.

Albin RL, Young AB, Penny JB. The functional anatomy of basal ganglia disorders. *Trends Neurosci* 1989;12:366–374.

Allen N, Knopp W. Hereditary parkinsonism-dystonia with sustained control by L-dopa and anticholinergic medication. *Adv Neurol* 1976;14:201–213.

Altman AJ, Bachner RL. Favorable prognoses for survival in children with coincident opsomyoclonus and neuroblastoma. *Cancer* 1976;37:846–852.

American Academy of Neurology. Training guidelines for the use of botulinum toxin for the treatment of neurological disorders. *Neurology* 1994;44:2401–2403.

American Academy of Pediatrics Subcommittee on Hyperbilirubinemia. Management of hyperbilirubinemia in the newborn infant 35 or more weeks of gestation. *Pediatrics* 2004;114:297–316.

Antonini A, Leenders KL, Spiegel R, et al. Striatal glucose metabolism and dopamine D2 receptor binding in asymptomatic gene carriers and patients with Huntington's disease. *Brain* 1996;119(Pt 6):2085–2095.

Antunes NL, Khakoo Y, Matthay KK, et al. Antineuronal antibodies in patients with neuroblastoma and paraneoplastic opsoclonus-myoclonus. *J Pediatr Hematol Oncol* 2000;22: 315–320.

Arden F. Idiopathic hypoparathyroidism. *Med J Aust* 1953;2: 217–219.

Arnoldi KA, Tychsen L. Prevalence of intracranial lesions in children initially diagnosed with disconjugate nystagmus (spasmus nutans). *J Pediatr Ophthalmol Strabismus* 1995;32: 296–301.

Aron AM, Freeman JM, Carter S. The natural history of Sydenham's chorea. *Am J Med* 1965;38:83–95.

Atmaca M, Kuloglu M, Tezcan E, Ustundag B. Nizatidine treatment and its relationship with leptin levels in patients with olanzapine-induced weight gain. *Hum Psychopharmacol* 2003;18:457–461.

Ayoub EM, Wannamkaer LW. Streptococcal antibody titers in Sydenham's chorea. *Pediatrics* 1966;38:946–956.

Baloh RW, Jen JC. Genetics of familial episodic vertigo and ataxia. *Ann N Y Acad Sci* 2002;956:338–345.

Barron TF, Younkin DP. Propanolol therapy for shuddering attacks. *Neurology* 1992;42:258–259.

Bergman I, Hirsch RP, Fria TJ, et al. Cause of hearing loss in the high risk premature infant. *J Pediatr* 1985;106:95–101.

Berlin CI, Bordelon J, St John P et al. Reversing click polarity may uncover auditory neuropathy in infants. *Ear Hear* 1998;19:37–47.

Berlin CI, Morlet T, Hood LJ. Auditory neuropathy/dyssynchrony: its diagnosis and management. *Pediatr Clin North Am* 2003;50:331–340, vii–viii.

Beskind DL, Keim SM. Choreoathetotic movement disorder in a boy with Mycoplasma pneumonia encephalitis. *Ann Emerg Med* 1994;23:1375–1378.

Bhatia KP, Soland VL, Bhatt MH, et al. Paroxysmal exercise-induced dystonia: Eight new sporadic cases and a review of the literature. *Mov Disord* 1997;12:1007–1012.

Billard C, Dulac O, Boulloche J, et al. Encephalopathy with calcification of the basal ganglia in children. *Neuropediatrics* 1989;20:12–19.

Bird MT, Palkes HP, Prensky AL. A follow-up study of Sydenham's chorea. *Neurology* 1976;26:601–606.

Bird TD, Carlson CB, Horning M. Ten year follow-up of choreoathetosis: A sporadic case becomes familial. *Epilepsia* 1978;19:129–132.

Blakeley J, Jankovic J. Secondary paroxysmal dyskinesias. *Mov Disord* 2002;17:726–734.

Boecker H, Ceballos-Baumann A, Bartenstein P, et al. Sensory processing in Parkinson's and Huntington's disease: Investigations with 3D H(2)(15)O-PET. *Brain* 1999;122:1651–1665.

Boyd K, Patterson V. Dopa responsive dystonia: a treatable condition misdiagnosed as cerebral palsy. *Br Med J* 1989;298: 1019–1020.

Braveman P, Egerter S, Marchi K, Miller C. Early discharge of newborns and mothers: A critical review of the literature. *Pediatrics* 1995;96:716–726.

Bressman SB, Sabatti C, Raymond D, et al. The DYT1 phenotype and guidelines for diagnostic testing. *Neurology* 2000; 54:1746–1752.

Brinkman RR, Mezei MM, Theilmann J, et al. The likelihood of being affected with Huntington disease by a particular age, for a specific CAG size. *Am J Hum Genet* 1997;60:1202–1210.

Brown AK, Johnson L. Loss of concern about jaundice and the reemergence of kernicterus in full term infants in the era of managed care. In. Fanaroff AA, Klaus M, eds. Yearbook of neonatal and perinatal medicine. St Louis, MO: Mosby Yearbook;1996:xvii–xxviii.

Budman CL, Gayer A, Lesser M, et al. An open-label study of the treatment efficacy of olanzapine for Tourette's syndrome. *J Clin Psychiatry* 2001;62:290–294.

Butler IJ. Movement disorders of children. *Pediatr Clin North Am* 1992;39:727–742.

Byers RK, Dodge PA. Huntington chorea in children. *Neurology* 1967;17:587-596.

Calne DB. Dopa-responsive dystonia. *Ann Neurol* 1994;35: 381–382.

Chisin R, Perlman M, Sohmer, H. Cochlear and brain stem responses in hearing loss following neonatal hyperbilirubinemia. *Ann Otol* 1979;88:352–357.

Chun RWM, Daly RF, Mansheim BJ Jr, Wolcott GJ. Benign familial chorea with onset in childhood. *JAMA* 1973;225: 1603–1607.

Cohen DJ, Leckman JF, Shaywitz B. A physician's guide to diagnosis and treatment of Tourette syndrome. A neurological multiple tic disorder. Bayside, NY: Tourette Syndrome Association, 1984.

Chudnow RS, Mimbela RA, Owen DB, Roach ES. Gabapentin for familial paroxysmal dystonic choreoathetosis. *Neurology* 1997;49:1441–1442.

Church AJ, Cardoso F, Dale RC, et al. Anti-basal ganglia antibodies in acute and persistent Sydenham's chorea. *Neurology* 2002;59:227–231.

Church AJ, Dale RC, Cardoso F, et al. CSF and serum immune parameters in Sydenham's chorea: evidence of an autoimmune syndrome? *J Neuroimmunol* 2003;136:149–153.

Cif L, El Fertit H, Vayssiere N, et al. Treatment of dystonic syndromes by chronic electrical stimulation of the internal globus pallidus. *J Neurosurg Sci* 2003;47:52–55.

Cif L, Valente EM, Hemm S, et al. Deep brain stimulation in myoclonus-dystonia syndrome. *Mov Disord* 2004;19:724–727.

Connolly AM, Dodson WE, Prensky AL, Rust RS. Course and outcome of acute cerebellar ataxia. *Ann Neurol* 1994;35: 673–679.

Connolly AM, Volpe JJ. Clinical features of bilirubin encephalopathy. *Clin Perinatol* 1990;17:371–379.

Connolly AM. Chronic inflammatory demyelinating polyneuropathy in childhood. *Pediatr Neurol* 1997;24:177–182.

Curless RG, Katz DA, Perryman RA, et al. Choreoathetosis after surgery for congenital heart disease. *J Pediatr* 1994; 124:737–739.

Danek A. Geniospasm: Hereditary chin trembling. *Mov Disord* 1993;8:335–338.

Deltenre P, Mansbach AL, Bozet C, et al. Auditory neuropathy: A report on three cases with early onsets and major neonatal illnesses. *Electroencephalogr Clin Neurophysiol* 1997; 104:17–22.

Demirkiran M, Jankovic J. Paroxysmal dyskinesias: Clinical features and classification. *Ann Neurol* 1995;38:571–579.

DiMario FJ. Childhood head tremor. *J Child Neurol* 2000;15: 22–25.

Djousse L, Knowlton B, Hayden M, et al. Interaction of normal and expanded CAG repeat sizes influences age at onset of Huntington disease. *Am J Med Genet* 2003;119A:279–282.

Dooling E, Schoene WC, Richardson EP. Hallervorden-Spatz syndrome. *Arch Neurol* 1974;30:70–83.

Doummar D, Roussat B, Beauvais P, et al. Spasmus nutans: Apropos of 16 cases. *Arch Pediatr* 1998;5:264–268.

El-Youssef M. Wilson disease. *Mayo Clinic Proc* 2003;78:1126–1136.

Erenberg G, Cruse RP, Rothner AD. The natural history of Tourette syndrome: A follow-up study. *Ann Neurol* 1987;22:383–385.

Erickson GR, Chun RWM. Acquired paroxysmal movement disorders. *Pediatr Neurol* 1987;3:226–229.

Fischbeck KH, Layzer RB. Paroxysmal choreoathetosis due to hypoglycemia. *Arch Neurol* 1979;6:453–454.

Fletcher NA, Harding AE, Marsden CD. The relationship between trauma and idiopathic torsion dystonia. *J Neurol Neurosurg Psychiatry* 1991;54:713–717.

Fouad GT, Servidei S, Durcan S, et al. A gene for familial paroxysmal dyskinesia (FPD 1) maps to chromosome 2q. *Am J Human Genet* 1996;59:135–139.

Freeman JM, Aron AM, Collard JE, MacKay MC. The emotional correlates of Sydenham chorea. *Pediatrics* 1965;35: 42–48.

Garg BP. Dystonia musculorum deformans. Implications of therapeutic response to levodopa and carbamazepine. *Arch Neurol* 1982;39:376–377.

Gartner LM, Snyder RN, Chabon RS, Bernstein J. Kernicterus: High incidence in premature infants with low serum bilirubin concentrations. *Pediatrics* 1970;45:906–917.

Garvey MA, Giedd J, Swedo SE. PANDAS: The search for environmental triggers of pediatric neuropsychiatric disorders. Lessons from rheumatic fever. *J Child Neurol* 1998;13:413–423.

Garvey MA, Perlmutter SJ, Allen AJ, et al. A pilot study of penicillin prophylaxis for neuropsychiatric exacerbations triggered by streptococcal infections. *Biol Psychiatry* 1999;45: 1564–1571.

Gatti RA, Berkel I, Boder E et al. Localization of an ataxia-telangectasia gene to chromosome 11q22–23. *Nature* 1989;336:577–580.

Gerrard J. Nuclear jaundice and deafness. *J Laryngol Otol* 1952;66:39–46.

Gilbert DL, Batterson JR, Sethuraman G, Sallee FR. Tic reduction with risperidone versus pimozide in a randomized double-blind, crossover trial. *J Am Acad Child Adolesc Psychiatry* 2004;43:206–214.

Goodenough DJ, Fariello RG, Annis BJ, Chun RWM. Familial and acquired paroxysmal dyskinesias. A proposed classification with delineation of clinical features. *Arch Neurol* 1978;35:827–831.

Gottlob I, Wizov SS, Reinecke RD. Spasmus nutans. A long-term follow-up. *Invest Ophthalmol Vis Sci* 1995;36:2768–2771.

Govaert P, Lequin M, Swarte R, et al. Changes in globus pallidus with (pre)term kernicterus. Pediatrics 2003;112:1256–1263.

Griggs RC, Moxley RT, 3rd, Lafrance RA, McQuillen J. Hereditary paroxysmal ataxia: Response to acetazolamide. *Neurology* 1978;28:1259–1264.

Grimes DA, Han F, Bulman D, et al. Hereditary chin trembling: A new family with exclusion of the chromosome 9q13-q21 locus. *Mov Disord* 2002;17:1390–1392.

Guthrie M. Foreword. In: Phillips DH, ed. *Living with Huntington's disease*. Madison: University of Wisconsin Press, 1982; xi.

Haerer AF, Currier RC, Jackson JF. Hereditary unprogressive chorea of early onset. *N Engl J Med* 1967;276:1220–1224.

Hallervorden J, Spatz H. Eigenartige Erkrankung in extrapyramidalen System mit besonderer Beteiligung des Globus pallidus und der Substantia nigra. *Z Neurol Psychiatr* 1922; 79:254–302.

Hallett M. Physiology of basal ganglia disorders: An overview. *Canadian J Neurol Sci* 1993;20:177–183.

Hansotia P, Cleeland CS, Chun RWM. Juvenile Huntington chorea *Neurology* 1968;18:217–224.

Harper PS. Benign hereditary chorea: Clinical and genetic aspects. *Clin Genet* 1978;13:85–96.

Harris GJ, Codori AM, Lewis RF, et al. Reduced basal ganglia blood flow and volume in pre-symptomatic, gene-tested persons at-risk for Huntington's disease. *Brain* 1999;122(Pt 9):1667–1678.

Harris GJ, Pearlson GD, Peyser CE, et al. Putamen volume reduction on magnetic resonance imaging exceeds caudate changes in mild Huntington's disease. *Ann Neu*rol 1992;31: 69–75.

Hartley LM, Ng SY, Dale RC, et al. Immune mediated chorea encephalopathy syndrome in childhood. *Dev Med Child Neurol* 2002;44:273–277.

Hayflick SJ. Unraveling the Hallervorden-Spatz syndrome: pantothenate kinase-associated neurodegeneration is the name. *Curr Opin Pediatr* 2003;15:572–577.

Haymaker W, Margles C, Pentshew A et al. Pathology of kernicterus and posticteric encephalopathy. In: Swinyeard CA, ed. *Kernicterus and its importance in cerebral palsy.* Springfield, IL: Charles C Thomas; 1961:21–228.

Herd JK, Medhi M, Uzendoski DM, Sadivar VA. Chorea associated with systemic lupus erythematosus: Report of two cases and review of the literature. *Pediatrics* 1978;61:308–315.

Hersch S, Jones R, Koroshetz W, Quaid K. The neurogenetics genie: Testing for the Huntington disease mutation. *Neurology* 1994;44:1369–1373.

Hunt JR./ Progressive atrophy of the globus pallidus. (Primary atrophy of the pallidal system). A system disease of the paralysis agitans type, characterized by atrophy of the motor cells of the corpus striatum. *Brain* 1917;40:58–148.

Huntington Disease Collaborative Research Group: A novel gene containing a trinucleotide repeat that is expanded and unstable on Huntington disease chromosomes. *Cell* 1993;72: 971–983.

Husby G, Rijn IVD, Zabriskie JB, et al. Antibodies reacting with cytoplasm of subthalamic and caudate nuclei neurons in chorea and acute rheumatic fever. *J Exp Med* 1976;144: 1094–1110.

Hyman CB, Keaster J, Hanson V, et al. CNS abnormalities after neonatal hemolytic disease or hyperbilirubinemia. A prospective study of 405 patients. *Am J Dis Child* 1969;117:395–405.

Jarman PR, Bhatia KP, Davie C, et al. Paroxysmal dystonis choreo-athetosis: Clinical features and investigation of pathophysiology in a large family. *Mov Disord* 2000;15: 648–657.

JCAHO issues warning on kernicterus danger. *Hosp Peer Rev* 2001;26:100–101.

Jen J. Familial episodic ataxias and related ion channel disorders. *Curr Treat Options Neurol* 2000;2:429–431.

Jensen KB, Dredge BK, Stefani G, et al. Nova-1 regulates neuron-specific alternative splicing and is essential for neuronal viability. *Neuron* 2000;25:359–371.

Jervis JA. Huntington chorea in childhood. *Arch Neurol* 1963;9:244–256.

Johnson L, Boggs TR. Bilirubin-dependent brain damage: Incidence and indications for treatment. In: Odell GB, Schalffer R, Sionpoulous AP, eds. *Phototherapy in the newborn: An overview.* Washington, DC: National Academy of Sciences;1974:122–149.

Johnson LH, Bhutani VK, Brown AK. System-based approach to management of neonatal jaundice and prevention of kernicterus. *J Pediatr* 2002;140:396–403.

Johnson SL, Hall DM. Post-traumatic tremor in head injured children. *Arch Dis Child* 1992;67:227–228.

Johnston MV, Hoon AH, Jr. Possible mechanisms in infants for selective basal ganglia damage from asphyxia, kernicterus, or mitochondrial encephalopathies. *J Child Neurol* 2000;15: 588–591.

Kernicterus in full-term infants – United States, 1994–1998. *MMWR Morb Mortal Wkly Rep* 2001;50:491–494.

Kienzle GD, Breger RK, Chun RWM, et al. Sydenham chorea: MR manifestations in two cases. *AJNR Am J Neuroradiol* 1991;12:73–76.

Kinsbourne M. Myoclonic encephalopathy of infants. *J Neurol Neurosurg Psychiatr* 1962;25:271–276.

Koller WC, Davenport J. Genetic testing in HD. *Ann Neurol* 1984;16:511–513.

Kuban KC, Leviton A. Cerebral palsy. *N Eng J Med* 1994;330: 188–195.

Kuhl DE, Phelps ME, Markham CH, et al. Cerebral metabolism and atrophy in Huntington's Disease determined by (18)FDG and computed tomographic scan. *Ann Neurol* 1982;12:425–434.

Kurlan R, Behr J, Medved L, Como P. Transient tic disorder and the spectrum of Tourette's syndrome. *Arch Neurol* 1988; 45:1200–1201.

Kurlan R, Behr J, Medved L, Shoulson I. Familial paroxysmal dystonic choreoathetosis: A family study. *Mov Disord* 1987; 2:187–192.

Kurlan R, Shoulson I. Familial dystonic choreoathetosis and response to alternate day oxazepam therapy. *Ann Neurol* 1983;13:456–457.

Kurlan R, Whitmore BA, Irvine C, et al. Tourette's syndrome in a special education population. *Neurology* 1994;44:699–702.

Kurlan R. The PANDAS hypothesis: Losing its bite? *Mov Disord* 2004;19:371–374.

Lagregran J. Children with motor handicaps. *Acta Pediatr Scand Suppl* 1981;289:1–71.

Lance JW. Familial dystonic choreoathetosis and its differentiation from related syndromes. *Ann Neurol* 1977;2:285–293.

Lancman ME, Asconape JJ, Penry JK. Choreiform movements associated with the use of valproate. *Arch Neurol* 1994;51: 702–704.

Leckamn JF, Zhang H, Vitale A et al. Course of tic severity in Tourette syndrome: The first two decades. *Pediatrics* 1998; 102:14–19.

Leli DA, Furlow TW, Jr., Falgout JC. Benign familial chorea: An association with intellectual impairment. *J Neurol Neurosurg Psychiatr* 1984;47:471–474.

Li JL, Hayden MR, Almqvist EW, et al. A genome scan for modifiers of age at onset in Huntington disease: The HD MAPS study. Am J Hum Genet 2003;73:682–687.

Littrup PL, Gebarski SS. MR imaging of Hallervorden-Spatz disease. *J Comput Assist Tomogr* 1985;9:491–493.

Lott I, Kinsbourne M. Myoclonic encephalopathy of infants. *Adv Neurol* 1986;43:127–136.

Lotze T, Jankovic J. Paroxysmal kinesigenic dyskinesias. *Semin Pediatr Neurol* 2003;10:68–79.

Louis ED, Dure LS, Pullman S. Essential tremor in childhood: A series of nineteen cases. *Mov Disord* 2001;16:921–923.

Louis ED. Etiology of essential tremor: Should we be searching for an environmental cause? *Mov Disord* 2001;16:822–829.

MacMillan JC, Morrison PJ, Nevin NC, et al. Identification of an expanded CAG repeat in the Huntington's disease gene (IT15) in a family reported to have benign hereditary chorea. *J Med Genet* 1993;30:1012–1013.

Maisels MJ Newman TB. Jaundice in full-term and near-term babies who leave the hospital within 36 hours. The pediatrician's nemesis. *Clin Perinatol* 1998;25:295–302.

Malamud N. Pathogenesis of kernicterus in the light of its sequelae. Kernicterus and its importance. In: Swinyard CA, ed. *Cerebral palsy*. Springfield, IL: Charles C. Thomas;1961: 230–246.

Markham CH, Knox JW. Observations on Huntington chorea in childhood. *J Pediatr* 1965;67:46–56.

Marsden CD, Obeso JA, Zarranz JJ, Lang AE. The anatomical basis of symptomatic hemidystonia. *Brain* 1985;108:461–483.

Marsden CD. The focal dystonias. *Clin Neuropharm* 1986;9: S49–S60.

Martin WE, Resch JA, Baker AB. Juvenile parkinsonism. *Arch Neurol* 1971;25:494–500.

Matkin ND, Carhart R. Auditory profiles associated with Rh incompatibility. *Arch Otolaryngol* 1966;84:502–513.

Matsuo H, Kamakura K, Saito M, et al. Familial paroxysmal dystonic choreoathetosis: Clinical findings in a large Japanese family and genetic linkage to 2 q. *Arch Neurol* 1999; 56:721–726.

Mayeux R, Fahn S. Paroxysmal dystonic choreoathetosis in a patient with familial ataxia. *Neurology* 1982;32:1184–1186.

McGeer EG, McGeer PL. The dystonias. *Can J Neurol Sci* 1988;15:447–483.

Medlock MD, Cruse RS, Winek SJ, et al. A 10-year experience with post-pump chorea. *Ann Neurol* 1993;34:820–826.

Miguel EC, Shavitt RG, Ferrao YA, et al. How to treat OCD in patients with Tourette syndrome. *J Psychosom Res* 2003;55: 49–57.

Miley CE, Forster FM. Paroxysmal signs and symptoms in multiple sclerosis. *Neurology* 1974;24:458–461.

Montagna P. Nocturnal paroxysmal dystonia and nocturnal wandering. *Neurology* 1992;42(Suppl 6):61–67.

Mount LA, Reback S. Familial paroxysmal choreoathetosis: Preliminary report on a hitherto undescribed clinical syndrome. *Arch Neurol Psychiatr* 1940;44:841–847.

Naeye RL. Amniotic fluid infections, neonatal hyperbilirubinemia and psychomotor impairment. *Pediatrics* 1978;62:497–503.

Naidu S, Narasimhachari N. Sydenham's chorea: A possible presynaptic dopaminergic dysfunction initially. *Ann Neurol* 1980;8:445–447.

Nausieda PA, Bieliauskas LA, Bacon LD, et al. Chronic dopaminergic sensitivity after Sydenham chorea. *Neurology* 1983;33:750–754.

Nausieda PA, Grossman BJ, Koller WC, et al. Sydenham chorea: An update. *Neurology* 1980;30:331–334.

Nausieda PA, Koller WC, Weiner WJ, Klawans HL. Chorea induced by oral contraceptives. *Neurology* 1979;29:1605–1609.

Newman RP, Kinkel WR. Paroxysmal choreoathetosis due to hypoglycemia. *Arch Neurol* 1984;41:341–342.

Nicolson R, Swedo SE, Lenane M, et al. An open trial of plasma exchange in childhood-onset obsessive compulsive disorder without poststreptococcal exacerbations. *J Am Acad Child Adolesc Psychiatry* 2000;39:1313–1315.

Niehaus DJ, Emsley RA, Brink P, Stein DJ. Stereotypes. prevalence and association with compulsive and impulsive symptoms in college students. *Psychopathology* 2000;33:31-5.

Nwaesei CG, Van Aerde J, Boyden M, Perlman M. Changes in auditory brainstem responses in hyperbilirubinemic infants before and after exchange transfusion. *Pediatrics* 1984;74: 800–803.

Nygaard TG, Duvoisin RC. Hereditary dystonia-parkinsonism syndrome of juvenile onset. *Neurology* 1986;36:1424–1428.

Odell GB, Storey GN, Rosenberg LA. Studies in kernicterus III: The saturation of serum proteins with bilirubin during neonatal life and its relationship to brain damage at five years. *J Pediatr* 1970;76:12–21.

Osborne JP, Munson P, Burman D. Huntington chorea: Report of 3 cases and review of literature. *Arch Dis Child* 1982; 57:99–103.

Pahwa R, Lyons KE. Essential tremor: Differential diagnosis and current therapy. *Am J Med* 2003;115:134–142.

Pappert EJ, Goetz CG, Louis ED, et al. Objective assessments of longitudinal outcome in Gilles de la Tourette's syndrome. *Neurology* 2003;61:936–940.

Park RHR, Park MP. St. Vitus' dance: Vital misconceptions by Sydenham and Bruegel. *J R Soc Med* 1990;83:512–515.

Parker HL. Periodic ataxia. *Mayo Clin Proc* 1946;38:642–645.

Paul DL. The genetics of Tourette syndrome. *Curr Psychiatry Rep* 2001;3:152–157.

Paviour DC, Surtees RAH, Lees AJ. Diagnostic considerations in juvenile parkinsonism. *Mov Disord* 2004;19:123–135.

Penn AA, Enzmann DR, Hahn JS, Stevenson DK. Kernicterus in a full term infant. *Pediatrics* 1994;93:1003–1006.

Perlmutter SJ, Leitman SF, Garvey MA, et al. Therapeutic plasma exchange and intravenous immunoglobulin for obsessive-compulsive disorder and tic disorders in childhood. *Lancet* 1999;354:1153–1158.

Perlstein MA. The late clinical syndrome of posticteric encephalopathy. *Pediatr Clin North Am* 1960;7:665–687.

Pranzatelli MR. The neurobiology of opsoclonus-myoclonus syndrome. *Clin Neuropharm* 1992;15:186–228.

Quarrell OWJ, Youngman S, Sarfarazi M, Harper PS. Absence of close linkage between benign hereditary chorea and the locus D4S10. *J Med Genet* 1988;25:191–194.

Rajput AH, Gibb WRG, Zhong XH, et al. Dopa-responsive dystonia: Pathological and biochemical observations in a case. *Ann Neurol* 1994;35:396–402.

Ranen NG, Stine OC, Abbott MH, et al. Anticipation and instability of IT-15 (CAG)n repeats in parent-offspring pairs with Huntington disease. *Am J Hum Genet* 1995;57:593–602.

Roberts EA, Schilsky ML. A practice guideline on Wilson Disease. *Hepatology* 2003;37:1475–1492.

Robertson MM. Diagnosing Tourette syndrome: Is it a common disorder? *J Psychosom Res* 2003;55:3–6.

Robertson WC, Jr., Smith CD. Sydenham's chorea in the age of MRI: A case report and review. *Pediatr Neurol* 2002;27:65–67.

Robinson RO, Thornett CEE. Benign hereditary chorea: Response to steroids. *Dev Med Child Neurol* 1985;27:814–821.

Rosas HD, Koroshetz WJ, Chen YI, et al. Evidence for more widespread cerebral pathology in early HD: An MRI-based morphometric analysis. *Neurology* 2003;60:1615–1620.

Rosen JA. Paroxysmal choreoathetosis associated with perinatal hypoxic encephalopathy. *Arch Neurol* 1964;11:385–387.

Rubin RA, Balow B, Fisch RO. Neonatal serum bilirubin levels related to cognitive development at ages 4 through 7 years. *J Pediatr* 1979;94:601–604.

Sallee FR, Kurlan R, Goetz CG, et al. Ziprasidone treatment of children and adolescents with Tourette's syndrome: A pilot study. *J Am Acad Child Adolesc Psychiatry* 2000;39:292–299.

Sanger TD, Delgado MR, Gaebler-Spira D, et al. Classification and definition of disorders causing hypertonia in childhood. *Pediatrics* 2003;111:e89–97.

Savitsky K, Bar-Shira A, Gilad S, et al. A single ataxia telangiectasia gene with a product similar to PI-3 kinase. *Science* 1995;268:1749–1753.

Sax DS, Menzer L. Computerized tomography in Huntington disease. *Neurology* 1977;27:388.

Schrag A, Lang AE. Psychogenic movement disorders. *Curr Opin Neurol* 2005;18:399–404.

Segawa M, Hosaka A, Miyagawa F, et al. Hereditary progressive dystonia with marked diurnal fluctuation. *Adv Neurol* 1976;14:215–233.

Seidman D, Stevenson DK, Ergaz Z, Gale R. Hospital readmission due to neonatal hyperbilirubinemia. *Pediatrics* 1995;96:727–729.

Sethi KD, Adams RJ, Loring DW, El Gammal T. Hallervorden-Spatz syndrome: clinical and magnetic resonance imaging correlations. *Ann Neurol* 24:692–694.

Shapiro SM, Nakamura H. Bilirubin and the auditory system. *J Perinatol* 2001;21(Suppl 1):S52–55; discussion S59–62.

Shevell M. Hallervorden and history. *N Engl J Med* 2003; 348:3–4.

Shimura H, Hattori N, Kubo S et al. Familial Parkinson disease gene product, parkin, is a ubiquitin-protein ligase. *Nat Genet* 2000;25:302–305.

Singer HS, Brown J, Quaskey S, et al. The treatment of attention-deficit hyperactivity disorder in Tourette's syndrome: A double-blind placebo-controlled study with clonidine and desipramine. *Pediatrics* 1995;95:74–81.

Singer HS, Giuliano JD, Zimmerman AM, Walkup JT. Infection: A stimulus for tic disorders. *Pediatr Neurol* 2000;22: 380–383.

Singer HS. PANDAS and immunomodulatory therapy. *Lancet* 1999;354:1153–1158.

Sleigh G, Lindenbaum R. Benign (nonparoxysmal) familial chorea. Pediatric perspectives. *Arch Dis Child* 1981;56:616–621.

Solomon GE. From tics to Tourette syndrome. *Pediatr Adolesc Med* 1991;1:95–109.

Spacey SD, Valente EM, Wali GM, et al. Genetic and clinical heterogeneity in paroxysmal kinesigenic dyskinesia: Evidence for a third EKD gene. *Mov Disord* 2002;17:717–725.

Spinella GM, Sheridan PH. Research opportunities in dystonia. *Neurology* 1994;44:1177–1179.

Starr A, Picton TW, Sininger Y, et al. Auditory neuropathy. *Brain* 1996;119:741–753.

Stephenson JBP, Graham-Pole J, Ogg L, Cochran AJ. Reactivity to neuroblastoma extracts in childhood cerebellar encephalopathy ("dancing eyes" syndrome). *Lancet* 1976;2:976.

Stumpf DA. Acute ataxia. *Pediatr Rev* 1987;8:303–306.

Stumpf DA. The inherited ataxias. *Pediatr Neurol* 1985;1:129–133.

Swaiman KF, Smith SA, Trock GL, Siddiqui AR. Sea-blue histiocytes, lymphocytic cytosomes, movement disorder and (59)Fe uptake in basal ganglia: Hallervorden-Spatz disease or ceroid storage disease with abnormal isotope scan? *Neurology* 1983;33:301–305.

Swedo SE, Leonard HL, Garvey M, et al. Pediatric autoimmune neuropsychiatric disorders associated with streptococcal infections: Clinical description of the first 50 cases. *Am J Psychiatry* 1998;155:264–271.

Swedo SE. A model for childhood autoimmune neuropsychiatric disorders. *JAMA* 1994;272:1788–1791.

Swift M, Reitnauer PJ, Morrell D, Chase CL. Breast and other cancers in families with ataxia-telangectasia. *N Engl J Med* 1987;316:1289–1294.

Tachi N, Nagata N, Chiba S. Detection of Epstein-Barr virus genome in cerebrospinal fluid from a patient with acquired chorea by the polymerase chain reaction. *J Child Neurol* 1993;8:424–425.

Takahashi H, Ohama E, Suzuki S et al. Familial juvenile parkinsonism. *Neurology* 1994;44:437–441.

Teixeira AL, Jr., Cardoso F, Souza AL, Teixeira MM. Increased serum concentrations of monokine induced by interferon-gamma/CXCL9 and interferon-gamma-inducible protein 10/CXCL-10 in Sydenham's chorea patients. *J Neuroimmunol* 2004;150:157–162.

Temel Y, Visser-Vandewalle V. Surgery in Tourette syndrome. *Mov Disord* 2004;19:3–14.

Terrence CF, Delaney JF, Alberts MC. Computed tomography for Huntington disease. *Neuroradiology* 1977;13:173–175.

Thomas GR, Forbes JR, Roberts EA, et al. The Wilson disease gene. Spectrum of mutations and their consequences. *Nat Genet* 1995;9:210–217.

Tibbles JAR, Camfield PR, Cron CC, Farrell K. Dominant recurrent ataxia and vertigo of childhood. *Pediatr Neurol* 1986;2:35–38.

Tourette Syndrome Study Group. Treatment of ADHD in children with tics: A randomized controlled trial. *Neurology* 2002;58:527–536.

Vanasse M, Bedard P, Andemann F. Shuddering attacks in children: An early clinical manifestation of essential tremor. *Neurology* 1976;26:1027–1030.

Volpe JJ. Bilirubin and brain injury. In: Volpe JJ, ed. *Neurology of the newborn*, 2nd ed. Major problems in clinical pediatrics, Vol. 22. Philadelphia: WB Saunders, 1987;386–408.

Volpe JJ. Bilirubin and brain injury. In: Volpe JJ, ed. *Neurology of the newborn*, 2nd ed. Major problems in clinical pediatrics. Philadelphia: WB Saunders, 1987;336–356.

Wang BJ, Chang YC. Therapeutic blood levels of phenytoin in treatment of paroxysmal choreoathetosis. *Ther Drug Monit* 1985;7:81–82.

Wennberg RP, Ahlfors CE, Bickers R, et al. Abnormal auditory brainstem response in a newborn infant with hyperbilirubinemia: Improvement with exchange transfusion. *J Pediatr* 1982;100:624–626.

Wheeler PG, Weaver DD, Dobyns WB. Benign hereditary chorea. *Peditr Neurol* 1993;9:337–340.

Wilson SAK, Bruce BA. *Neurology*, 2nd ed., Vol. 2. Baltimore: Williams & Wilkins, 1955;709–719.

Yokochi K, Aiba K, Kodama M, Fujimoto S. Magnetic resonance imaging in athetotic cerebral palsied children. *Acta Paedriatr Scand* 1991;80:818–823.

Yokochi M, Narabayashi H, Lizuka R, Nagatsu T. Juvenile parkinsonism: Some clinical, pharmacological, and neuropathological aspects. *Adv Neurol* 1984;40:407–413.

Zupanc ML, Chun RWM, Gilbert-Barness EF. Osmiophilic deposits in cytosomes in Hallervorden-Spatz syndrome. *Pediatr Neurol* 1990;6:349–352.

Chapter 13

American Academy of Pediatrics. In: Pickering LK, Baker CJ, Long SS, McMillian JA, eds. *Red Book: 2006 Report of the Committee on Infectious Diseases*, 27th e. Elk Grove Village, IL: American Academy of Pediatrics;2006:426–433

American Academy of Pediatrics. Meningococcal infection. In: Pickering LK, Baker CJ, Long SS, McMillan JA, eds. *Red Book: 2006 Report of the Committee on Infectious Diseases*, 27th ed. Elk Grove Village, IL: American Academy of Pediatrics;2006:452–460.

Choux M, Genitori L, Lang D, et al. Shunt implantation: Reducing the incidence of shunt infection. *J Neurosurg* 1992; 77:875–880.

Fernandez M, Maylett EH, Noyola DE, Baker CJ. Candidal meningitis in neonates. A 10-year review. *Clin Infect Dis* 2000;31:458–463.

Garcia LS. Classification of human parasites, vectors, and similar organisms. *Clin Infect Dis* 1999;29:734–736.

Ma P, Visvesvara G, Martinez AJ, et al. Naegleria and Acanthamoeba infections. *Rev Infect Dis* 1990;12:490–513.

McAuley J, Boyer KM, Patel D, et al. Early and longitudinal evaluation of treated infants and children and untreated historical patients with congenital toxoplasmosis: The Chicago collaborative treatment trial. *Clin Infect Dis* 1994;18:38–72.

Schuchat A, Robinson K, Wenger JD, et al. Bacterial meningitis in the United States in 1995. *N Engl J Med* 1997;337:970–976.

Schumacher DJ, Tien RD, Lane K. Neuroimaging findings in rare amoebic infections of the CNS. *AJNR Am J Neuroradiol* 1995;16:930–935.

Steere A. Lyme disease. *N Engl J Med* 2001;345:115–125.

Sundell HW, Yan H, Carter CE, et al. Isolation and identification of the group B streptococcal toxin CM101 from infants with sepsis. *J Pediatr* 2000;137:338–344.

Unhanand M, Mustafa MM, McCracken GH, et al. Gram-negative enteric bacillary meningitis: A twenty-one-year experience. *J Pediatr* 1993;122:15–21.

Wong VK, Hitchcock W, Mason WH. Meningococcal infections in children: A review of 100 cases. *Pediatr Infect Dis J* 1989; 8:224–227.

Wong S, Remington JS. Toxoplasmosis in pregnancy. *Clin Infect Dis* 1994;18:853–862.

Chapter 14

Adams RJ, Brambilla DJ, Granger S, et al. Stroke and conversion to high risk in children screened with transcranial Doppler ultrasound during the STOP study. *Blood* 2004;103:3689–3694.

Andrew M, Marzinotto V, Massicotte P, et al. Heparin therapy in pediatric patients. a prospective cohort study. *Pediatr Res* 1994;35:78–83.

Andrew ME, Monagle P, deVeber G, Chan AK. Thromboembolic disease and antithrombotic therapy in newborns. *Hematology* (Am Soc Hematol Educ Program) 2001;358: 358–374.

Armstrong-Wells, J et al., Prevalence and predictors of perinatal hemorrhagic stroke. *Oral abstract, International Stroke Conference, New Orleans*, 2008.

Askalan R, Laughlin S, Mayank S, et al. Chickenpox and stroke in childhood. a study of frequency and causation. *Stroke* 2001;32:1257–1262.

Atluru VL. Spontaneous intracerebral hematomas in juvenile diabetic ketoacidosis. *Pediatr Neurol* 1986;2:167–169.

Barek L, Ledor S, Ledor K. The Klippel-Trenaunay syndrome. a case report and review of the literature. *Mt Sinai J Med* 1982;49:66–70.

Barmada MA., Moossy J, Shuman RM. Cerebral infarcts with arterial occlusion in neonates. *Ann Neurol* 1979;6:495–502.

Boers GH, Smals AG, Trijbels FJ, et al. Heterozygosity for homocystinuria in premature peripheral and cerebral occlusive arterial disease. *N Engl J Med* 1985;313:709–715.

Boushey CJ, Beresford SA, Omenn GS, Motulsky AG. A quantitative assessment of plasma homocysteine as a risk factor for vascular disease. Probable benefits of increasing folic acid intakes. *JAMA* 1995;274:1049–1057.

Bozzao A, Di Paolo A, Mazzoleni C, et al. Diffusion-weighted MR imaging in the early diagnosis of periventricular leukomalacia. *Eur Radiol* 2003;13:1571–1576.

Brawley OW, Cornelius LJ, Edwards LR, et al. National Institutes of Health Consensus Development Conference statement: hydroxyurea treatment for sickle cell disease. *Ann Intern Med*. 2008 Jun 17;148(12):932–8.

Broderick J, Talbot GT, Prenger E, et al. Stroke in children within a major metropolitan area: The surprising importance of intracerebral hemorrhage. *J Child Neurol* 1993;8:250–255.

Broderick JP, Swanson JW. Migraine-related strokes. Clinical profile and prognosis in 20 patients. *Arch Neurol* 1987;44: 868–871.

Burlina AP, Manara R, Calderone M, et al. Diffusion-weighted imaging in the assessment of neurological damage in patients with methylmalonic aciduria. *J Inherit Metab Dis* 2003;26: 417–422.

Camerlingo M, Finazzi G, Casto L, et al. Inherited protein C deficiency and nonhemorrhagic arterial stroke in young adults. *Neurology* 1991;41:1371–1373.

Chabrier S, Buchmuller A. Editorial comment – specificities of the neonatal stroke. *Stroke* 2003;34:2892–2893.

Chasnoff IJ, Bussey ME, Savich R, Stack CM. Perinatal cerebral infarction and maternal cocaine use. *J Pediatr* 1986;108: 456–459.

Clancy R, Malin S, Laraque D, et al. Focal motor seizures heralding stroke in full-term neonates. *Am J Dis Child* 1985; 139:601–606.

Clarke R, Daly L, Robinson K, et al. Hyperhomocysteinemia. an independent risk factor for vascular disease. *N Engl J Med* 1991;324:1149–1155.

Claster S, Vichinsky EP. Managing sickle cell disease. *BMJ* 2003;327:1151–1155.

Cohen M, Levin SE. Significance of intracranial bruits in neonates, infants, and young children. *Arch Dis Child* 1978; 53:592–594.

Counsell SJ, Maalouf EF, Rutherford MA, Edwards AD. Periventricular haemorrhagic infarct in a preterm neonate. *Eur J Paediatr Neurol* 1999;3:25–27.

Counsell SJ, Rutherford MA, Cowan FM, Edwards AD. Magnetic resonance imaging of preterm brain injury. *Arch Dis Child* Fetal Neonatal 88:F269–F274, 2003.

Crutchfield KE, Patronas NJ, Dambrosia JM, et al. Quantitative analysis of cerebral vasculopathy in patients with Fabry disease. *Neurology* 1998;50:1746–1749.

Darlow BA, Cust AE, Donoghue DA. Improved outcomes for very low birthweight infants: Evidence from New Zealand national population based data. *Arch Dis Child Fetal Neonatal Ed* 2003;88:F23–F28.

Dean LM, Taylor GA. The intracranial venous system in infants: Normal and abnormal findings on duplex and color Doppler sonography. *AJR Am J Roentgenol* 1995;164:151–156.

Del CO Jr, Kelly DL Jr, Elster AD, Craven TE. An analysis of the natural history of cavernous angiomas. *J Neurosurg* 1991; 75:702–708.

deVeber G. Risk factors for childhood stroke: Little folks have different strokes! *Ann Neurol* 2003;53:149–150.

deVeber G, Andrew M. Cerebral sinovenous thrombosis in children. *N Engl J Med* 2001;345:417–423.

de Vries LS, Roelants-van Rijn AM, Rademaker KJ, et al. Unilateral parenchymal haemorrhagic infarction in the preterm infant. *Eur J Paediatr Neurol.* 2001;5(4):139–49.

Dixon SD, Bejar R. Echoencephalographic findings in neonates associated with maternal cocaine and methamphetamine use: Incidence and clinical correlates. *J Pediatr* 1989;115:770–778.

Dubowitz LM, Levene MI, Morante A, Palmer P, Dubowitz V. Neurologic signs in neonatal intraventricular hemorrhage: A correlation with real-time ultrasound. *J Pediatr* 1981;99: 127–133.

Earley CJ, Kittner SJ, Feeser BR, et al. Stroke in children and sickle-cell disease: Baltimore-Washington Cooperative Young Stroke Study. *Neurology* 1998;51:169–176.

Elbers J, Benseler SM. Central nervous system vasculitis in children. *Curr Opin Rheumatol.* 2008 Jan;20(1):47–54.

Fanaroff AA, Hack M, Walsh MC. The NICHD neonatal research network: Changes in practice and outcomes during the first 15 years. *Semin Perinatol* 2003;27:281–287.

Flodmark O, Roland EH, Hill A, Whitfield MF. Periventricular leukomalacia: Radiologic diagnosis. *Radiology* 1987;162: 119–124.

Forsyth LL, Liu-DeRyke X, Parker D Jr, Rhoney DH. Role of hypertonic saline for the management of intracranial hypertension after stroke and traumatic brain injury. *Pharmacotherapy*. 2008 Apr;28(4):469–84.

Friede RL. Cerebral infarcts complicating neonatal leptomeningitis. Acute and residual lesions. *Acta Neuropathol (Berl)* 1973;23:245–253.

Fullerton HJ, Chetkovich DM, Wu YW, Smith WS, Johnston SC. Deaths from stroke in US children, 1979 to 1998. *Neurology* 2002;59:34–39.

Fullerton HJ, Wu YW, Zhao S, Johnston SC. Risk of stroke in children: Ethnic and gender disparities. *Neurology* 2003;61: 189–194.

Fullerton HJ, Wu YW, Sidney S, Johnston SC. Risk of recurrent childhood arterial ischemic stroke in a population-based cohort: the importance of cerebrovascular imaging. *Pediatrics*, 2007. 119(3): p. 495-501.

Gabis LV, Yangala R, Lenn NJ. Time lag to diagnosis of stroke in children. *Pediatrics* 2002;110:924–928.

Ganesan V, Prengler M, McShane MA, et al. Investigation of risk factors in children with arterial ischemic stroke. *Ann Neurol* 2003;53:167–173.

Gerszten PC, Adelson PD, Kondziolka D, et al. Seizure outcome in children treated for arteriovenous malformations using gamma knife radiosurgery. *Pediatr Neurosurg* 1996;24:139–144.

Giroud M, Lemesle M, Gouyon JB, et al. Cerebrovascular disease in children under 16 years of age in the city of Dijon, France: A study of incidence and clinical features from 1985 to 1993. *J Clin Epidemiol* 1995;48:1343–1348.

Goddard-Finegold J, Mizrahi EM. Understanding and preventing perinatal, intracerebral, peri- and intraventricular hemorrhage. *J Child Neurol* 1987;2:170–185.

Golomb MR, Dick PT, MacGregor DL, Neonatal arterial ischemic stroke and cerebral venous thrombosis are more commonly diagnosed in boys. *J. Child Neurol* 2004;19:493.

Golomb MR, Garg BP, Saha C, et al. Cerebral palsy after perinatal arterial ischemic stroke. *J Child Neurol.* 2008 Mar;23(3):279–86.

Gordon AL, Ganesan V, Towell A, Kirkham FJ. Functional outcome following stroke in children. *J Child Neurol* 2002;17: 429–434.

Gould DB, Phalan FC, Breedveld GJ, et al., Mutations in Col4a1 cause perinatal cerebral hemorrhage and porencephaly. *Science*, 2005. 308(5725): p. 1167–71.

Gould DB, Phalan FC, van Mil SE, et al., Role of COL4A1 in small-vessel disease and hemorrhagic stroke. *N Engl J Med*, 2006. 354(14): p. 1489–96.

Gould SJ and Howard S., An immunohistochemical study of the germinal layer in the late gestation human fetal brain. *Neuropathol Appl Neurobiol*, 1987.13(6): p. 421–37.

Gould SJ, Howard S, Hope PL, Reynolds EO. Periventricular intraparenchymal cerebral haemorrhage in preterm infants: The role of venous infarction. *J Pathol* 1987;151:197–202.

Govaert P, Matthys E, Zecic A, et al. Perinatal cortical infarction within middle cerebral artery trunks. *Arch Dis Child Fetal Neonatal Ed.* 2000 Jan;82(1):F59–63.

Greenberg J, Massey EW. Cerebral infarction in sickle cell trait. *Ann Neurol* 1985;18:354–355.

Haas RH, Marsden DL, Capistrano-Estrada S, et al. Acute basal ganglia infarction in propionic academia. *J Child Neurol* 1995;10:18–22.

Hardart GE, Hardart MK, Arnold JH. Intracranial hemorrhage in premature neonates treated with extracorporeal membrane oxygenation correlates with conceptional age. *J Pediatr.* 2004 Aug;145(2):184–9.

Heiskanen O, Vilkki J. Intracranial arterial aneurysms in children and adolescents. *Acta Neurochir (Wien)* 1981;59:55–63.

Hogeveen M, Blom HJ, Van Amerongen M, Boogmans B, Van Beynum IM, Van De BM. Hyperhomocysteinemia as risk factor for ischemic and hemorrhagic stroke in newborn infants. *J Pediatr* 2002;141:429–431.

Huda W, Lieberman KA, Chang J, Roskopf ML. Patient size and x-ray technique factors in head computed tomography examinations. I. Radiation doses. *Med Phys* 2004;31:588–594.

Iwata O, Iwata S, Tamura M, et al. Periventricular low intensities on fluid attenuated inversion recovery imaging in the newborn infant. Relationships to the clinical data and long-term outcome. *Pediatr Int* 2004;46:150–157.

Kachaner J, Nouaille JM, Batisse, A. Major cardiomegalies of the newborn. Les cardiomegalies massives du nouveau-ne. *Arch Fr Pediatr* 1977;34:297–322.

Kamper J, Feilberg JN, Jonsbo F, et al. The Danish national study in infants with extremely low gestational age and birthweight (the ETFOL study): Respiratory morbidity and outcome. *Acta Paediatr* 2004;93:225–232.

Kang HS, Kim SK, Cho BK, et al. Single nucleotide polymorphisms of tissue inhibitor of metalloproteinase genes in familial moyamoya disease. *Neurosurgery*. 2006 Jun;58(6):1074–80.

Khamashta MA, Hughes GR. Antiphospholipid antibodies and antiphospholipid syndrome. *Curr Opin Rheumatol* 1995;7:389–394.

Koch TK, Jahnke SE, Edwards MS, Davis SL. Posterior fossa hemorrhage in term newborns. *Pediatr Neurol* 1985;1:96–99.

Koelfen W, Freund M, and Varnholt V, Neonatal stroke involving the middle cerebral artery in term infants: clinical presentation, EEG and imaging studies, and outcome. *Dev Med Child Neurol*, 1995. 37(3): p. 204–12.

Koga Y, Akita Y, Nishioka J, et al. MELAS and L-arginine therapy. *Mitochondrion*. 2007 Feb-Apr;7(1-2):133–9.

Kurnik K, Kosch A, Strater R, et al. Recurrent thromboembolism in infants and children suffering from symptomatic neonatal arterial stroke: A prospective follow-up study. *Stroke* 2003;34:2887–2892.

Lanthier S, Carmant L, David M, Larbrisseau A, de Veber G. Stroke in children: The coexistence of multiple risk factors predicts poor outcome. *Neurology* 2000;54:371–378.

Lanthier S, Lortie A, Michaud J, et al. Isolated angiitis of the CNS in children. *Neurology* 2001;56:837–842.

Larroque B, Marret S, Ancel PY, et al. White matter damage and intraventricular hemorrhage in very preterm infants. the EPIPAGE study. *J Pediatr* 2003;143:477–483.

Laugesaar R, Kolk A, Tomberg T, et al., Acutely and retrospectively diagnosed perinatal stroke: a population-based study. *Stroke*, 2007. 38(8): p. 2234–40.

Lenn NJ. Spinal cord infarction due to minor trauma. *Neurology* 1977;27:999.

Lee J, Croen LA, Backstrand KH, et al., Maternal and infant characteristics associated with perinatal arterial stroke in the infant. *JAMA*, 2005. 293(6): p. 723-9.

Lefèvre N, Dufour D, Gulbis B, et al. Use of hydroxyurea in prevention of stroke in children with sickle cell disease. *Blood*. 2008 Jan 15;111(2):963–4

Looney, CB, Smith JK, Merck LH, et al., Intracranial hemorrhage in asymptomatic neonates: prevalence on MR images and relationship to obstetric and neonatal risk factors. *Radiology*, 2007. 242(2): p. 535–41

Lou HC, Friis-Hansen B. Arterial blood pressure elevations during motor activity and epileptic seizures in the newborn. *Acta Paediatr Scand* 1979;68:803–806.

Lyden P, Lu M, Kwiatkowski T, et al. Thrombolysis in patients with transient neurologic deficits. *Neurology* 2001;57:2125–2128.

McGuinness GA, Smith WL. Head ultrasound screening in premature neonates weighing more than 1,500 g at birth. *Am J Dis Child* 1984;138:817–820.

Ment LR, Allan WC, Makuch RW, Vohr B. Grade 3 to 4 intraventricular hemorrhage and Bayley scores predict outcome. *Pediatrics*. 2005 Dec;116(6):1597–8.

Ment LR, Duncan CC, Ehrenkranz RA. Perinatal cerebral infarction. *Ann Neurol* 1984;16:559–568.

Ment LR, Scott DT, Ehrenkranz RA, Duncan CC. Neurodevelopmental assessment of very low birth weight neonates: Effect of germinal matrix and intraventricular hemorrhage. *Pediatr Neurol* 1985;1:164–168.

Ment LR, Vohr BR, Makuch RW, et al. Prevention of intraventricular hemorrhage by indomethacin in male preterm infants. *J Pediatr*. 2004 Dec;145(6):832–4.

Mercuri E, Rutherford M, Cowan F, et al., Early prognostic indicators of outcome in infants with neonatal cerebral infarction: a clinical, electroencephalogram, and magnetic resonance imaging study. *Pediatrics*, 1999. 103(1): p. 39–46.

Mikati MA, Kramer U, Zupanc ML, Shanahan RJ. Alternating hemiplegia of childhood: Clinical manifestations and long-term outcome. *Pediatr Neurol* 2000;23:134–141.

Molyneux A, Kerr R, Stratton I, et al. International Subarachnoid Aneurysm Trial (ISAT) of neurosurgical clipping versus endovascular coiling in 2143 patients with ruptured intracranial aneurysms. a randomised trial. *Lancet* 2002;360: 1267–1274.

Nagel MA, Cohrs RJ, Mahalingam R, et al. The varicella zoster virus vasculopathies: clinical, CSF, imaging, and virologic features. *Neurology*. 2008 Mar 11;70(11):853–60.

Nanda A, Vannemreddy PS, Polin RS, Willis BK. Intracranial aneurysms and cocaine abuse: Analysis of prognostic indicators. *Neurosurgery* 2000;46:1063–1067.

Nelson KB, Ellenberg JH. Children who 'outgrew' cerebral palsy. *Pediatrics* 1982;69:529–536.

Olson JC, Konkol RJ, Gill JC, et al. Childhood stroke and lupus anticoagulant. *Pediatr Neurol* 1994;10:54–57.

Paneth N, Rudelli R, Monte W, et al. White matter necrosis in very low birth weight infants. neuropathologic and ultrasonographic findings in infants surviving six days or longer. *J Pediatr* 1990;116:975–984.

Papile LA, Munsick-Bruno G, Schaefer A. Relationship of cerebral intraventricular hemorrhage and early childhood neurologic handicaps. *J Pediatr* 1983;103:273–277.

Pavlakis SG, Phillips PC, DiMauro S, et al. Mitochondrial myopathy, encephalopathy, lactic acidosis, and stroke-like episodes: A distinctive clinical syndrome. *Ann Neurol* 1984; 16:481–488.

Pearson E, Lenn NJ, Cail WS. Moyamoya and other causes of stroke in patients with Down syndrome. *Pediatr Neurol* 1985;1:174–179.

Perlman JM, Volpe JJ. Intraventricular hemorrhage in extremely small premature infants. *Am J Dis Child* 1986;140:1122–1124.

Piepgras DG, Sundt TM Jr, Ragoowansi AT, Stevens L. Seizure outcome in patients with surgically treated cerebral arteriovenous malformations. *J Neurosurg* 1993;78:5–11.

Posnikoff J. Spontaneous spinal epidural hematoma of childhood. *J Pediatr* 1968;73:178–183.

Rahemtullah A, Van Cott EM. Hypercoagulation testing in ischemic stroke. *Arch Pathol Lab Med.* 2007 Jun;131(6):890–901.

Rigamonti D, Hadley MN, Drayer BP, et al. Cerebral cavernous malformations. Incidence and familial occurrence. *N Engl J Med* 1998;319:343–347.

Robinson JR, Awad IA, Little JR. Natural history of the cavernous angioma. *J Neurosurg* 1991;75:709–714.

Rossi LN, Penzien JM, Deonna T, Goutieres F, Vassella F. Does migraine-related stroke occur in childhood? *Dev Med Child Neurol* 1990;32:1016–1021.

Rothman SM, Nelson JS. Spinal cord infarction in a patient with sickle cell anemia. *Neurology* 1980;30:1072–1076.

Rousseaux P, Vieillart A, Scherpereel B, et al. [Benign intracranial hypertension (17 cases) and cerebral venous thromboses (49 cases). Comparative study]. Hypertension intracranienne benigne (17 cas) et thromboses veineuses cerebrales (49 cas). Etude comparative. *Neurochirurgie* 1985;31:381–389.

Rumack CM, Manco-Johnson ML, Manco-Johnson MJ, et al. Timing and course of neonatal intracranial hemorrhage using real-time ultrasound. *Radiology* 1985;154:101–105.

Sandberg DI, Lamberti-Pasculli M, Drake JM, et al., Spontaneous intraparenchymal hemorrhage in full-term neonates. *Neurosurgery*, 2001. 48(5): p. 1042–8; discussion 1048–9.

Sarwar M, McCormick WF. Intracerebral venous angioma. Case report and review. *Arch Neurol* 1978;35:323–325.

Schoenberg BS, Mellinger JF, Schoenberg DG. Cerebrovascular disease in infants and children: A study of incidence, clinical features, and survival. *Neurology* 1978;28:763–768.

Shinnar S, Gammon K, Bergman EW Jr, et al. Management of hydrocephalus in infancy: Use of acetazolamide and furosemide to avoid cerebrospinal fluid shunts. *J Pediatr* 1985;107:31–37.

Solomon GE, Hilal SK, Gold AP, Carter S. Natural history of acute hemiplegia of childhood. *Brain* 1970;93:107–120.

Soul JS, Robertson RL, Tzika AA, et al. Time course of changes in diffusion-weighted magnetic resonance imaging in a case of neonatal encephalopathy with defined onset and duration of hypoxic-ischemic insult. *Pediatrics* 2001;108:1211–1214.

Spetzler RF, Hargraves RW, McCormick PW, et al. Relationship of perfusion pressure and size to risk of hemorrhage from arteriovenous malformations. *J Neurosurg* 1992;76:918–923.

Steen RG, Emudianughe T, Hankins GM, et al. Brain imaging findings in pediatric patients with sickle cell disease. *Radiology* 2003;228:216–225.

Stein BM, Wolpert SM. Arteriovenous malformations of the brain. I: Current concepts and treatment. *Arch Neurol* 37:1–5, 1980a.

Stein BM, Wolpert SM. Arteriovenous malformations of the brain. II: Current concepts and treatment. *Arch Neurol* 37: 69–75, 1980b.

Suzuki J, Takaku A. Cerebrovascular 'moyamoya' disease. Disease showing abnormal net-like vessels in base of brain. *Arch Neurol* 1969;20:288–299.

Thorpe ML, Cordato DJ, Morgan MK, Herkes GK. Postoperative seizure outcome in a series of 114 patients with supratentorial arteriovenous malformations. *J Clin Neurosci* 2000; 7:107–111.

Toft PB, Leth H, Peitersen B, Lou HC. Metabolic changes in the striatum after germinal matrix hemorrhage in the preterm infant. *Pediatr Res* 1997;41:309–316.

Tong KA, Ashwal S, Obenaus A, et al. Susceptibility-weighted MR imaging: a review of clinical applications in children. *AJNR Am J Neuroradiol.* 2008 Jan;29(1):9–17.

Trauner DA, Chase C, Walker P, Wulfeck B, et al., Neurologic profiles of infants and children after perinatal stroke. *Pediatr Neurol*, 1993. 9(5): p. 383–6.

Trauner DA. Hemispatial neglect in young children with early unilateral brain damage. *Dev Med Child Neurol* 2003;45: 160–166.

Trauner DA, Nass R, Ballantyne A. Behavioural profiles of children and adolescents after pre- or perinatal unilateral brain damage. *Brain* 2001;124:995–1002.

Volpe JJ. Neurobiology of periventricular leukomalacia in the premature infant. *Pediatr Res* 50:553–562, 2001a.

Volpe JJ. *Neurology of the newborn.* 3rd ed. Philadelphia, Pa: WB. Saunders Co; 1995

Volpe JJ. *Neurology of the newborn*, 4th ed. Philadelphia: W.B. Saunders, 2001b.

Volpe JJ. *Neurology of the newborn*, 5th ed. Philadelphia: Elsevier, 2008.

Wang XY, Noguchi K, Takashima S, et al. Serial diffusion-weighted imaging in a patient with MELAS and presumed cytotoxic oedema. *Neuroradiology* 2003;45:640–643.

Wardlaw JM, Farrall AJ. Diagnosis of stroke on neuroimaging. *BMJ* 2004;328:655–656.

Wilimas J, Goff JR, Anderson HR Jr, et al. Efficacy of transfusion therapy for one to two years in patients with sickle cell disease and cerebrovascular accidents. *J Pediatr* 1980;96: 205–208.

Williams LS, Garg BP, Cohen M, et al. Subtypes of ischemic stroke in children and young adults. *Neurology* 1997;49: 1541–1545.

Wojtacha M, Bazowski P, Mandera M, et al. Cerebral aneurysms in childhood. *Childs Nerv Syst* 2001;17:37–41.

Wood KC, Hsu LL, Gladwin MT. Sickle cell disease vasculopathy: a state of nitric oxide resistance. *Free Radic Biol Med.* 2008 Apr 15;44(8):1506–28.

Wu YW, Escobar GJ, Grether JK, Chorioamnionitis and cerebral palsy in term and near-term infants. *JAMA*, 2003. 290(20): p. 2677–84.

Wu YW, March WM, Croen LA, et al. Perinatal stroke in children with motor impairment: a population-based study. *Pediatrics*, 2004. 114(3): p. 612–9.

Wu YW, Miller SP, Chin K, et al. Multiple risk factors in neonatal sinovenous thrombosis. *Neurology* 2002;59:438–440.

Yasui N, Magarisawa S, Suzuki A, et al. Subarachnoid hemorrhage caused by previously diagnosed, previously unruptured intracranial aneurysms: A retrospective analysis of 25 cases. *Neurosurgery* 1996;39:1096–1100.

Zafeiriou DI, Ikeda H, Anastasiou A, et al. Familial moyamoya disease in a Greek family. *Brain Dev* 2003;25:288–290.

Chapter 15

Åagenes O. Hereditary recurrent cholestasis with lymphedema: Two new families. *Acta Paediatr Scand* 1974;63:465–471.

Acosta PB. Theoretical and practical aspects of dietary treatment of Smith-Lemli-Opitz syndrome. *Int Pediatr* 1995;10: 32–40.

Adinolfi S, Trifuoggi M, Politou AS, et al. A structural approach to understanding the iron-binding properties of phylogenetically different frataxins. *Hum Mol Genet* 2002;11:1865–1877.

Afif Hentati H-X, Deng W-Y, Hung S, et al. Human-tocopherol transfer protein: Gene organization and identification of mutations in patients with familial vitamin E deficiency. Am J Hum Genet 1985;557:A214 (abstract 1236).

Alagille D, Estrada A, Hadchouel M, et al. Syndromatic paucity of intrahepatic bile duct (Alagille's syndrome or arteriohepatic dysplasia): Review of 80 cases. *J Pediatr* 1987;110:195–200.

Allard J, Tila S, Carter A. CT and MR of MELAS syndrome. *AJNR Am J Neuroradiol* 1988;9:1234–1238.

Aminoff M, Carter JE, Chadwick RB, et al. Mutations in CUBN, encoding the intrinsic factor-vitamin B12 receptor, cubilin, cause hereditary megaloblastic anemia 1. *Nat Genet* 1999;21:309–313.

Amir RE, Van den Veyver IB, Wan M, et al. Rett syndrome is caused by mutations in the X-linked MECP2, encoding methyl-CpG-binding protein 2. *Nat Genet* 1999;23:185–188.

Andréasson S, Blennow G, Ehinger B, Strömland K. Full-field electroretinogram in patients with carbohydrate-deficient glycoprotein syndrome. *Am J Ophthalmol* 1991;112:83–86.

Atkin BM, Buist NRM, Utter M, et al. Pyruvate carboxylase deficiency and lactic acidosis in a retarded child without Leigh's disease. *Pediatr Res* 1979;13:109–116.

Baloh R, Yee RD, Boder E. Eye movements in ataxia-telangiectasia. *Neurology* 1978;28:1099–1104.

Barbieri F, Santoro L, Crisci C, et al. Is the sensory neuropathy in ataxia-telangiectasia distinguishable from that in Friedreich's ataxia? *Acta Neuropathol* 1986;69:213–219.

Barkovich AJ, Good WV, Koch TK, Berg BO. Mitochondrial disorders: Analysis of their clinical and imaging characteristics. *AJNR Am J Neuroradiol* 1993;14:1119–1137.

Basel-Vanagaite L, Muncher L, Straussberg R, et al. Mutated nup62 causes autosomal recessive infantile bilateral striatal necrosis. *Ann Neurol* 2006;80:214–222.

Beaudet AL. Aspartoacylase deficiency (Canavan disease). In: Scriver CR, Beaudet AL, Sly WS, Valle D, eds. *The Metabolic and Molecular Bases of Inherited Disease.* New York, NY: McGraw-Hill: 1997;3:4599–4604.

Becker-Catania SG, Chen G, Hwang MJ, et al. Ataxia-telangiectasia: Phenotype/genotype studies of ATM protein expression, mutations, and radiosensitivity. *Mol Genet Metab* 2000;70:122–133.

Beckman DR, Hoganson G, Berlow S, Gilbert E. Pathological findings in 5, 10-methylene tetrahydrofolate reductase deficiency. *Birth Defects* 1987;23:47–64.

Benomar A, Yahyaoui M, Meggouh F, et al. Clinical comparison between AVED patients with 744 del A mutation and Friedreich ataxia with GAA expansion in 15 Moroccan families. *J Neurol Sci* 2002;198:25–29.

Berginer V, Salen G, Shefer S. Cerebrotendinous xanthomatosis. In: Rosenberg RN, Prusiner SB, DiMauro S, eds. *The Molecular and Genetic Basis of Neurological Disease.* Boston, Mass: Butterworth Heinemann Publisher; 1997:1051–1064.

Bernes SM, Bacino C, Prezant TR, et al. Identical mitochondrial DNA deletion in mother with progressive external ophthalmoplegia and son with Pearson-Marrow pancreas syndrome. *J Pediatr* 1993;123:598–602.

Beutler E, Saven A. The misuse of marrow examination in the diagnosis of Gaucher disease. *Blood* 1990;76:646–648.

Beutler E. Gaucher's disease, current concepts. *N Engl J Med* 1991;325:1354–1360.

Bicknese AR, May W, Hickey WF, Depson WE. Early childhood hepatocerebral degeneration misdiagnosed as valproate toxicity. *Ann Neurol* 1992;32:767–775.

Bindoff LA, Desnuelle C, Birch-Machin MA, et al. Multiple defects of the mitochondrial respiratory chain in a mitochondrial encephalopathy (MERRF): A clinical, biochemical and molecular study. *J Neurol Sci* 1991;102:17–24.

Blom TS, Linder MD, Snow K, et al. Defective endocytic trafficking of NPC1 and NPC2 underlying infantile Niemann-Pick type C disease. *Hum Molec Genet* 2003;12:257–272.

Bodian EL. Skin manifestations of Conradi's disease: Chondrodystrophia congenita punctata. *Arch Dermatol* 1966;94: 743–748.

Boespflug-Tanguy O, Mimault C, Melki, et al. Genetic homogeneity of Pelizaeus-Merzbacher disease: Tight linkage to the proteolipid locus in 16 affected families PMP clinical group. *Am J Hum Genet* 1994;55:461–467.

Boles RG, Seashore MR, Mitchell WG, et al. Glucose transporter type 1 deficiency: A study of two cases with video EEG. *Eur J Pediatr* 1999;158:978–983.

Bonsignore M, Tessa A, Di Rosa G et al. Novel CLN1 mutation in two Italian sibs with late infantile neuronal ceroid lipofuscinosis. *Eur J Paediatr Neurol* 2006;10:154–156.

Bourdon A, Minai L, Serre V, et al. Mutation of RRM2B, encoding p53-controlled ribonucleotide reductase (p53R2), causes severe mitochondrial DNA depletion. [Letter.] *Nat Genet* 2007;39:776–780.

Breningstall G, Lockman LA. Massive focal brain swelling as feature of MELAS. *Pediatr Neurol* 1988;4:366–370.

Brenner M, Johnson AB, Boespflug-Tanguy O, et al. Mutations in GFAP, encoding glial fibrillary acid protein, are associated with Alexander disease. *Nat Genet* 2001;27:117–120.

Byrne E, Dennett X, Trounce I, et al. Mitochondrial myoneuropathy with respiratory failure and myoclonic epilepsy. A case report with biochemical studies. *J Neurol Sci* 1985;71: 273–281.

Campistol J, Cusi V, Vernet A, Fernandez-Alvarez E. Dystonia as a presenting sign of subacute necrotizing encephalomyelopathy in infancy. *Eur J Pediatr* 1986;144:589–591.

Carmel R, Watkins D, Goodman SJ, Rosenblatt DS. Hereditary defect of cobalamin metabolism (cblG mutation) prescribing as a neurologic disorder in adulthood. *N Eng J Med* 1988; 318:1738–1741.

Chang Y, Twiss JL, Horoupian DS, et al. Inherited syndrome of infantile olivopontocerebellar atrophy, micronodular cirrhosis, and renal tubular microcysts: Review of the literature and report of an additional case. *Acta Neuropathol* 1993;86: 399–404.

Christensen E, Van Eldere J, Brandt NJ, et al. A new peroxisomal disorder: Di- and trihydroxycholestanaemia due to a presumed trihydroxycholestanoyl-CoA oxidase deficiency. *J Inherit Metab Dis* 1990;13:363–366.

Ciafaloni E, Ricci E, Shanske S, et al. MELAS: Clinical features, biochemistry, and molecular genetics. *Ann Neurol* 1992;3: 391–398.

Clayton PT, Smith I, Harding B, et al. Subacute combined degeneration of the cord, dementia and Parkinsonism due to an inborn error of folate metabolism. *J Neurol Neurosurg Psychiatr* 1986;49:920–927.

Clayton PT. Bile and metabolism in children with hepatobiliary disease. *Int Pediatr* 1995;10:44–50.

Cornford ME, Philippard M, Jacobs B, et al. Neuropathy of Rett syndrome: Case report with neuronal and mitochondrial abnormalities in the brain. *J Child Neurol* 1994;9:424–431.

Cosma MP, Pepe S, Annunziata I, et al. The multiple sulfatase deficiency gene encodes an essential and limiting factor for the activity of sulfatases. *Cell* 2003;113:445–456.

Danks DM, Cartwright E. Menkes kinky hair disease: Further definition of the defect in copper transport. *Science* 1973; 179:1140–1141.

Danks DM. Copper and liver disease. *Eur J Pediatr* 1991;150: 142–148.

Danks DM. The mild form of Menkes disease: Progress report on the original case. *Am J Med Genet* 1988;30:859–964.

De Vivo DC, Burke C, Trifiletti R, et al. Glucose transport protein deficiency: An emerging syndrome with therapeutic implications. *Ann Neurol* 1994;36:491.

De Vivo DC, Garcia-Alvarez M, Ronen G, Trifiletti R. Glucose transport protein deficiency: An emerging syndrome with therapeutic implications. *Int Pediatr* 1995;10:51–56.

De Vivo DC, Trifiletti RR, Jacobson RJ, et al. Defective glucose transport across the blood-brain barrier as a course of persistent hypoglycorrhachia, seizures, and developmental delay. *N Engl J Med* 1991;325:703–709.

Demange P, Gia H, Kalifa G, et al. MR of Kearns-Sayre syndrome. *AJNR Am J Neuroradiol* 1989;10:S91.

Di Mauro S. Mitochondrial encephalopathies. In: Rosenberg RN, Prusiner SB, Di Mauro S, et al., eds. *The metabolic and genetic basis of neurologic disease*. Boston, MA: Butterworth-Heinemann;1993:665–694.

Di Rocco M, Lamba LD, Minniti G, et al. Outcome of thiamine treatment in a child with thiamine-responsive pyruvate dehydrogenase deficiency. *Eur J Pediatr Neurol* 2000;4:115–117.

Dillon MJ, England TM, Gompertz D, et al. Mental retardation, megaloblastic anemia, methylmalonic aciduria, and abnormal homocysteine metabolism due to an inborn error in vitamin B12 metabolism. *Clin Sci Mol Sci* 1974;47:43–61.

DiMauro S, Quinzii CM, Hirano M. Mutations in coenzyme Q19 biosynthetic genes. *J Clin Invest* 2007;117:587–589.

Doerflinger N, Linder C, Ouahchi K, et al. Ataxia with vitamin E deficiency: Refinement of genetic localization and analysis of linkage disequilibrium by using new markers in 14 families. *Am J Hum Genet* 1995;56:1116–1124.

Dotti MI, Mauneschi L, Malandrini A, et al. Mitochondrial dysfunction in Rett syndrome. An ultrastructural and biochemical study. *Brain Dev* 1993;15:103–106.

Duclos F, Rodius F, Wrogemann K et al. The Friedreich ataxia region: characterization of two novel genes and reduction of the critical region to 300 kb. *Hum Mol Genet* 1994;3:909–914.

Dunn HG, Dolman CL. Necrotizing encephalomyelopathy. Report of a case with relapsing polyneuropathy and hyperalonemia and with manifestations resembling Friedreich's ataxia. *Neurology* 1969;19:536.

Dyken P, Krawiecki N. Neurodegenerative diseases of infancy and childhood. *Ann Neurol* 1983;13:351–364.

Dyken PR. Reconsideration of the classification of the neuronal ceroid-lipofuscinoses. *Am J Med Genet* 1988;55:69–84.

Elleder M, Jirasek A, Vik J. Adult neurovisceral lipidosis compatible with Niemann-Pick disease Type C. *Virchows Arch* 1983;401:35–43.

Fang W, Huang CC, Lee CC, et al. Ophthalmoplegic manifestations in MELAS syndrome. *Arch Neurol* 1993;50:977–980.

Fauler J, Tsikas D, Mayatepek E, et al. Impaired degradation of prostaglandins and thromboxane in Zellweger syndrome. *Pediatr Res* 1994;36:449–455.

Feigenbaum A, Moore R, Clarke J, et al. Canavan disease: Carrier-frequency determination in the Ashkenazi Jewish population and development of a novel molecular diagnostic assay. *Am J Med Genet* 2004;124A:142–147.

Fernet M, Gribaa M, Salih MA, et al. Identification and functional consequences of a novel MRE11 mutation affecting 10 Saudi Arabian patients with the ataxia telangiectasia-like disorder. *Hum Mol Genet* 2005;14:307–318.

Figarella-Branger D, Pellissier JF, Scheiner C, et al. Defects of mitochondrial respiratory chain complexes in three pediatric cases with hypotonia and cardiac involvement. *J Neurol Sci* 1992;108:105–113.

Finocchiarro G, Baio G, Micossi P, et al. Glucose metabolism alterations in Friedreich's ataxia. *Ann Neurol* 1985;17:612–614.

Fournier B, Saudubray JM, Benichou B, et al. Large deletion of the peroxisomal acyl CoA oxidase gene in pseudoneonatal adrenoleukodystrophy. *J Clin Invest* 1994;94:526–531.

Frydman M, Jager-Roman E, de Vries L, et al. Alpers progressive infantile neuronal poliodystrophy: An acute neonatal form with findings of fetal akinesia syndrome. *Am J Med Genet* 1993;47:31–36.

Fryer A, Appleton R, Sweeney MG, et al. Mitochondrial DNA 8993 (NARP) mutation presenting with a heterogeneous phenotype including "cerebral palsy." *Arch Dis Child* 1994; 71:419–422.

Fujii T, Okuno T, Ito M, et al. CT, MRI, and autopsy findings in brain of a patient with MELAS. *Pediatr Neurol* 1990;6: 253–256.

Fukuhara N. MERRF: A clinicopathological study. Relationship between myoclonus epilepsies and mitochondrial myopathies. *Rev Neurol (Paris)* 1991;147:476–479.

Fukuhara N. Myoclonus epilepsy and mitochondrial myopathy. In: Scarlato G, Cerri C, eds. *Mitochondrial pathology in muscle disease*. Padua: Piccin Medical Books, 1983.

Furuya H, Kukita Y, Nagano S, et al. Adult onset globoid cell leukodystrophy (Krabbe disease): Analysis of galactosylceramidase cDNA from four Japanese patients. *Hum Genet* 1997;100: 450–456.

Gabreels F, Prick MJ, Trijbels JM, et al. Defects in citric acid cycle and the electron transport chain in progressive poliodystrophy. *Acta Neurol Scand* 1984;70:145–154.

Geoffroy G, Barbeau A, Breton G, et al. Clinical description and roentgenologic evaluation of patients with Friedreich's ataxia. *Can J Neurol Sci* 1976;3:279–286.

Gibson KM, Stellaard F, Hoffmann GF, et al. Bile acid metabolism in three patients with mevalonic aciduria due to mevalonate kinase deficiency. *Clin Chim Acta* 1993;217:217–220.

Goldfischer S, Collins J, Rapin I, et al. Pseudo-Zellweger syndrome: Deficiencies in several peroxisomal oxidative activities. *J Pediatr* 1986;108:25–32.

Goodman WN, Cooper WC, Kessler GB, et al. Ataxia-telangiectasia. A report of 2 cases in siblings presenting a picture of progressive spinal muscular atrophy. *Bull Los Angeles Neurol Soc* 1969;34:1–22.

Goyette P, Sumner JS, Milos R, et al. Human methylenetetrahydrofolate reductase: Isolation of cDNA, mapping, and mutation detection. *Nat Genet* 1994;7:195–200.

Gravel RA, Triggs-Raine BL, Mahuran DJ. Chemistry and genetics of Tay-Sachs disease. *Can J Neurol Sci* 1991;18:419–423.

Gray GF, Green A, Chapman S, et al. Rhizomelic chondrodysplasia punctate: A new variant. *J Inherit Metab Dis* 1992;15: 931–932.

Grunnet ML, Zalmeraitis EL, Russman BS, Barwick MC. Juvenile Leigh's encephalomyelopathy with peripheral neuropathy, myopathy and cardiomyopathy. *J Child Neurol* 1991;6: 153–163.

Hall CA. The neurologic aspects of transcobalamin II deficiency. *Br J Haematol* 1992;80:117–120.

Harding AE, Young EP, Shon F. Adult onset supranuclear ophthalmoplegia, cerebellar ataxia, and neurogenic proximal muscle weakness in a brother and sister: Another hexosaminidase A deficiency syndrome. *J Neurol Neurosurg Psychiatry* 1987;50:687–690.

Harding AR. Friedreich's ataxia: A clinical and genetic study of 90 families with analysis of early diagnosis criteria and intrafamilial clustering of clinical features. *Brain* 1981;104: 589–620.

Hartmann A, Mast H, Choi JH, et al. Treatment of arteriovenous malformations of the brain. *Curr Neurol Neurosci Rep.* 2007 Jan;7(1):28–34.

Harvey JN, Barnett D. Endocrine dysfunction in Kearns-Sayre syndrome. *Clin Endocrinol* 1992;37:97–103.

Heiman-Patterson TD, Bonnilla E, DiMauro S, et al. Cytochrome c oxidase deficiency in a floppy infant. *Neurology* 1982;32:898–901.

Hershkovitz E, Narkis G, Shorer Z, et al. Cerebral X-linked adrenoleukodystrophy in a girl with Xq27-Ter deletion. *Ann Neurol* 2002;52:34–237.

Herzberg NH, van Schooneveld MJ, Bleeker-Wagemakers EM, et al. Kearns-Sayre syndrome with a phenocopy of choroideremia instead of pigmentary retinopathy. *Neurology* 1993; 43:218–220.

Hewer RL. Study of fatal cases of Friedreich's ataxia. *Br Med J* 1968;3:649–652.

Heymans HSA, Oorthuys JWE, Nelck G, et al. Peroxisomal abnormalities in rhizomelic chondrodysplasia punctata. *J Inherit Metab Dis* 1986;9:329–331.

Hirano M, Silvestri G, Blake DM, et al. Mitochondrial neurogastrointestinal encephalomyopathy (MNGIE). *Neurology* 1994;44:721–727.

Hodes ME, Pratt VM, Dlouhy SR. Genetics of Pelizaeus-Merzbacher disease. *Dev Neurosci* 1993;15:383–394.

Hoffmann GF, Charpentier C, Mayatepek E, et al. Clinical and biochemical phenotype in 11 patients with mevalonic aciduria. *Pediatrics* 1993;91:915–920.

Holleran WM, Ziegler SG, Goker-Alpan O, et al. Skin abnormalities as an early predictor of neurologic outcome in Gaucher disease. [Letter.] *Clin Genet* 2006;69:355–357.

Holme E, Larsson NG, Oldfors A, et al. Multiple symmetric lipomas with high levels of mtDNA with the tRNA (LYS) A–G (8344) mutation as the only manifestation of disease in a carrier of myoclonus epilepsy and ragged red fibers (MERRF) syndrome. *Am J Hum Genet* 1993;52:551–556.

Holt IJ, Harding AE, Petty RKH, Morgan-Hughes JA. A new mitochondrial disease associated with mitochondrial DNA heteroplasmy. *Am J Hum Genet* 1990;46:428–433.

Horiguchi Y, Fujii T, Imamura S. Purpuric cutaneous manifestations in mitochondrial encephalomyopathy. *J Dermatol* 1991;18:295–301.

Hors-Cayla MC, Heuertz S, Van Cong N, et al. Confirmation of the assignment of the gene for arylsulfatase-A to chromosome 22 using somatic cell hybrids. *Hum Genet* 1979;49:33.

Hübner C, Hoffmann GF, Charpentier C, et al. Decreased plasma ubiquinone-10 concentration in patients with mevalonate kinase deficiency. *Pediatr Res* 1993;34:129–133.

Hyland K, Surtees RA, Rodeck C, Clayton PT. Aromatic L-amino acid decarboxylase deficiency: Clinical feature, diagnosis, and treatment of a new inborn error of neurotransmitter amine synthesis. *Neurology* 1992;92:1980–1988.

Inui K, Fukushima H, Tsukamoto H, et al. Mitochondrial encephalomyopathies with the mutation of the mitochondrial tRNALEU UUR gene. *J Pediatr* 1992;120:62–66.

Inui K, Kao FT, Fujbayashi S, et al. The gene coding for a sphingolipid activator protein. SAP-1 is on human chromosome 10. *Hum Genet* 1985;69:197–200.

Iwanga K, Mori K, Inove M, et al. Myoclonus epilepsy associated with ragged red fibers. Report of a patient with negative myoclonus. *Clin Neurol* 1992;32:870–873.

Jaeken J. Congenital disorders of glycosylation (CDG): It's all in it! *J Inherit Metab Dis* 2003;26:99–118.

Jansen GA, Hogenhout EM, Ferndusse S, et al. Human phytanoyl-CoA hydroxylase: Resolution of the gene structure and molecular basis of Refsum's disease. *Hum Mol Genet* 2000;9:1195–1200.

Johnson JL, Duran M. Molybdenum cofactor deficiency and isolated sulfite oxidase deficiency. In: Scriver CR, Beaudet AL, Sly WS, ed. *The metabolic and molecular bases of inherited disease*, Vol. II. New York: McGraw-Hill;2001: 3163–3177.

Jun AS, Brown MD, Wallace DC. A mitochondrial DNA mutation of nucleotide 14459 of the NADH dehydrogenase subunit 6 gene associated with maternally inherited Leber hereditary optic neuropathy and dystonia. *Proc Natl Acad Sci USA* 1994;91:6206–6210.

Kaye EM, Doll RF, Natowicz MR, Smith FI. Pelizaeus-Merzbacher disease presenting as spinal muscular atrophy: Clinical and molecular studies. *Ann Neurol* 1994;36:916–919.

Keller-Wood H, Robertson N, Govan GG, et al. Leber's hereditary optic neuropathy mitochondrial DNA mutations in multiple sclerosis. *Ann Neurol* 1994;36:109–112.

Kelly RI, Datta NS, Dobyns WB, et al. Neonatal adrenoleukodystrophy: New cases, biochemical studies, and differentiation from Zellweger and related peroxisomal polydystrophy syndromes. *Am J Med Genet* 1986;33:869–901.

Kendall B. Disorders of lysosomes, peroxisomes, and mitochondria. *AJNR Am J Neuroradiol* 1992;13:621–653.

Kim KS, Kubota S, Kuriyama M, et al. Identification of new mutations in sterol 27-hydroxylase gene in Japanese patients with cerebrotendinous xanthomatosis (CTX). *J Lipid Res* 1994;35:1031–1039.

Kirmani BF, Jacobowitz DM, Kallarakal AT, Namboodiri MA. Aspartoacylase is restricted primarily to myelin synthesizing cells in the CNS: Therapeutic implications for Canavan disease. *Brain Res Mol Brain Res* 2002;107:176–182.

Koga Y, Nonaka I, Kobayashi M et al. Findings in muscle complex I (NADH coenzyme Q reductase) deficiency. *Ann Neurol* 1988; 124: 746–749.

Kollberg G, Moslemi A-R, Darin N. POLG1 mutations associated with progressive encephalopathy in childhood. *J Neuropathol Exp Neurol* 2006;65:758–768.

Krivit W, Aubourg P, Shapiro E, Peters C. Bone marrow transplantation for globoid cell leukodystrophy, adrenoleukodystrophy, metachromatic leukodystrophy, and Hurler syndrome. *Curr Opin Hematol* 1999;6:377–382.

Lagier-Tourenne C, Tazir M, Lopez LC, et al. ADCK3, an ancestral kinase, is mutated in a form of recessive ataxia associated with coenzyme Q(10) deficiency. *Am J Hum Genet* 2008;82:661–672.

Lance JW, Evans WA. Progressive myoclonic epilepsy, nerve deafness, and spinal muscular atrophy. *Clin Exp Neurol* 1984;20:141–151.

Langmade SJ, Gale SE, Frolov A, et al. Pregnane X receptor (PXR) activation: A mechanism for neuroprotection in a mouse model of Niemann-Pick C disease. *Proc Natl Acad Sci USA* 2006;103:13807–13812.

Larsson NG, Andersen I, Home E, et al. Leber's hereditary optic neuropathy and complex I deficiency in muscle. *Ann Neurol* 1991;30:701–708.

Le Ber I, Dubourg O, Benoist J-F, et al. Muscle coenzyme Q10 deficiencies in ataxia with oculomotor apraxia 1. *Neurology* 2007;68:295–297.

Lewis S, Hutchison W, Thyagarajan D, Hans-Henrick D. Clinical and molecular features of adPEO due to mitations in the Twinkle gene. *J Neurol Sci* 2002;201:39–44.

Li M, Pan H, Bao X-H, et al. MECP2 and CDKL5 gene mutation analysis in Chinese patients with Rett syndrome. *J Hum Genet* 2007;52:38–47.

Li R, Johnson AB, Salomons G, et al. Glial fibrillary acid protein mutations in infantile, juvenile and adult forms of Alexander disease. *Ann Neurol* 2005;57:310–326.

Ligtenberg MJ, Kemp S, Sarde C-O, et al. Spectrum of mutations in the gene encoding the adrenoleukodystrophy protein. *Am J Hum Genet* 1995;56:44–50.

Linden H-U, Klein RA, Egge H, et al. Isolation and structural characterization of sialic acid-containing glycopeptides of the O-glycosidic type from the urine of two patients with a hereditary deficiency in N-acetylgalactosaminidase activity. *Biol Chem Hoppe-Seyler* 1989;370:661.

Lopez LC, Schuelke M, Quinzii CM, et al. Leigh syndrome with nephropathy and CoQ10 diphosphate synthase subunit 2 (PDSS2) mutations. *Am J Hum Genet* 2006;79:1125–1129.

Lundberg A, Lilja IG, Lundberg PO, et al. Heredopathia atactica polyneuritiformis (Refsum's disease). Experiences of dietary treatment and plasmapheresis. *Eur Neurol* 1972;8: 308–324.

Maclean WC, Graham GG. Vegetarianism in children. *Am J Dis Child* 1980;134:513–519.

Maertens P, Richardson R, Bastian F, et al. A new type of mitochondrial encephalomyopathy with stroke-like episodes due to cytochrome oxidase deficiency. *J Inherit Metab Dis* 1988;11:186–188.

Mancini J, Philip W, Chabrol B, et al. Mevalonic aciduria in 3 siblings: A new recognizable metabolic encephalopathy. *Pediatr Neurol* 1993;9:243–246.

Maniura-Weber K, Taylor RW, Johnson MA, et al. A novel point mutation in the mitochondrial tRNA (Trp) gene produces a neurogastrointestinal syndrome. *Eur J Hum Genet* 2004;12:509–512.

Martidis A, Yee R, Azzarelli B, Biller J. Neuro-ophthalmic, radiologic, and pathologic manifestations of adult-onset Alexander disease. *Arch Ophthalmol* 1999;117:265–267.

Martinez M, Pineda N, Vidal R, et al. Docosahexanoic acid: A new therapeutic approach to peroxisomal disorder patients: Experience with two cases. *Neurology* 1993;43:1389–1397.

Matsuishi T, Urabe F, Percy AK, et al. Abnormal carbohydrate metabolism in cerebrospinal fluid in Rett syndrome. *J Child Neurol* 1994;9:26–30.

Matsumoto N, Tamura S, Furuki S, et al. Mutations in novel peroxin gene PEX26 that causes peroxisomal-biogenesis disorders of complentation group 8 provide a genotype-phenotype correlation. *Am J Hum Genet* 2003;73:233–246.

Matthews PM, Andermann F, Silver K, et al. Proton MR spectroscopic characterization of differences in regional brain metabolic abnormalities in mitochondrial encephalomyopathies. *Neurology* 1993;43:2484–2490.

Mayatepek E, Hoffmann G, Bremer HJ. Enhanced urinary excretion of leukotriene E4 in patients with mevalonate kinase deficiency. *J Pediatr* 1993;123:96–98.

Mazzei R, Conforti FL, Magariello A et al. A novel mutation in the CLN1 gene in a patient with juvenile neuronal ceroid lipofuscinosis. *J Neurol* 2002;249:1432–1459.

McKelvie PA, Morley JB, Byrne E, Marzuki S. Mitochondrial encephalomyopathies: A correlation between neuropathological findings and defects in mitochondrial DNA. *J Neurol Sci* 1991;102:51–60.

Meek D, Wolfe L, Andermann E, Anderrmann F. Juvenile progressive dystonia: A new phenotype of GM2 gangliosidosis. *Ann Neurol* 1984;15:348–352.

Millat G, Chikh K, Naureckiene S, et al. Niemann-Pick disease type C: Spectrum of HE1 mutations and genotype/phenotype correlations in the NPC2 group. *Am J Hum Genet* 2001;69: 1013–1021.

Miller DM. The kinetics of selective biological transport: Further data on the erythrocyte-monosaccharide transport system. *Biophys J* 1971;11:915–923.

Mollet J, Delahodde A, Serre V, et al. CABC1 gene mutations cause ubiquinone deficiency with cerebellar ataxia and seizures. *Am J Hum Genet* 2008;82:623–630.

Mollet J, Giurgea I, Dallner G, et al. Phenyldiphosphatase, subunit 1 (PDSS1) and OH-benzoate polyprenyltransferase (CoG2) mutations in ubiquinone deficiency and oxidative phosphorylation disorders. *J Clin Invest* 2007;117:765–772.

Moraes CT, Ciacci F, Bonilla E, et al. Two novel pathogenic mitochondrial DNA mutations affecting organelle number and protein synthesis. Is the tRNA (LEU)(UUR) gene on etiologic hot spot? *J Clin Invest* 1983;92:2906–2915.

Moraes CT, Zeviani M, Shon EA, et al. Mitochondrial DNA deletion in a girl with manifestations of Kearns-Sayre and Lowe syndromes: An example of phenotypic mimicry? *Am J Med Genet* 1991;41:301–305.

Mori K, Narahara K, Ninomiya S, et al. Renal and skin involvement in a patient with complete Kearns-Sayre syndrome. *Am J Med Genet* 1991;38:583–587.

Morita M, Takahashi I, Kanai M, et al. Baicalein 5,6,7-trimethyl ether, a flavonoid derivative, stimulates fatty acid -oxidation in skin fibroblasts of X-linked adrenoleukodystrophy. *FEBS Lett* 2007;579:409–414.

Morrell D, Cromartie E, Swift M. Mortality and cancer incidence in 263 patients with ataxia-telangiectasia. *J Natl Cancer Inst* 1986;77:89–92.

Mukherji M, Chien W, Kershaw NJ et al. Structure-function analysis of phytanoyl-CoA 2-hydroxylase mutations causing Refsum's disease. *Hum Mol Genet* 2001; 10:1971–82.

Narkwick MR, Sokol RJ, Beckwith B, et al. Liver involvement in Alpers' disease. *J Pediatr* 1991;119:260–267.

Naviaux RK, Nyhan WL, Barshop BA, et al. Mitochondrial DNA polymerase deficiency and mtDNA depletion in a child with Alpers' syndrome. *Ann Neurol* 1999;45:54.

Naylor EW, Ennis D, Davidson AG, et al. Guanosine triphosphate cyclohydrolase I deficiency: Early diagnosis by routine urine pteridine screening. *Pediatrics* 1987;79:374–378.

Newman NJ, Lott MT, Wallace DC. The clinical characteristics of pedigrees of Leber's hereditary optic neuropathy with 11,778 mutation. *Am J Ophthalmol* 1991;111:750–762.

Nikali K, Suomalainen A, Saharinen J, et al. Infantile onset spinocerebellar ataxia is caused by recessive mutations in mitochondrial proteins twinkle and twinky. *Hum Mol Genet* 2005;14:2981–2990.

Nikoskelainen E, Hoyt WF, Nummelin K. Ophthalmologic findings in Leber's hereditary optic neuropathy. The fundus findings in affected family members. *Arch Ophthalmol* 1983;101:1059–1068.

Nishimura RN, Barranger TA. Neurologic complications of Gaucher's disease, type 3. *Arch Neurol* 1980;37:92–93.

Nishino I, Spinazzola A, Hirano M. Thymidine phosphorylase gene mutations in MNGIE, a human mitochondrial disorder. *Science* 1999;283:689–692.

Ogasahara S, Engel AG, Frens D, Mack D. Muscle coenzyme Q deficiency in familial mitochondrial encephalomyopathy. *Proc. Nat. Acad. Sci. U. S. A.* 1989;86:2379–2382.

Ohashi K, Ishibashi S, Osuga J-I, et al. Novel mutations in the microsomal triglyceride transfer protein gene causing abetalipoproteinemia. *J Lipid Res* 2000;41:1199–1204.

Okada S, McCrea M, O'Brien JS. Sandhoff's disease (GM2 gangliosidosis type II): Clinical, chemical, and enzyme studies in five patients. *Pediatr Res* 1972;6:606–615.

Overweg-Plandsoen WCD, Groener JEM, Wang D, et al. GLUT-1 deficiency without epilepsy: An exceptional case. *J Inherit Metab Dis* 2003;26:559–563.

Park JK, Orvisky E, Tayebi N, et al. Myoclonic epilepsy in Gaucher Disease: Genotype-phenotype insights from a rare patient subgroup. *Pediatr Res* 2003;53:387–398.

Peynet J, Laurent A, De Liege P, et al. Cerebrotendinous xanthomatosis: Treatments with simvastatin, lovastatin and chenodeoxycholic acid in three siblings. *Neurology* 1991;41: 434–436.

Pincus JH. Subacute necrotizing encephalomyelopathy (Leigh's disease): A consideration of clinical features and etiology. *Dev Med Child Neurol* 1972;14:87–101.

Pineda-Trujillo N, Cornejo W, Carrizosa J, et al. A CLN5 mutation causing an atypical neuronal ceroid lipofuscinosis of juvenile onset. *Neurology* 2005;64:740–742.

Plioplys AV, Kasnicka I. L-carnitine as a treatment for Rett syndrome. *South Med J* 1993;86:1411–1412.

Poll-Thé BT, Roels F, Ogier H, et al. A new peroxisomal disorder with enlarged peroxisomes and a specific deficiency of acyl CoA oxidase (pseudo-neonatal adrenoleukodystrophy). *Am J Hum Genet* 1988;42:422–434.

Poll-Thé BT, Saudubray JM, Ogier HAM, et al. Infantile Refsum disease: An inherited peroxisomal disorder. Comparison with Zellweger syndrome and neonatal adrenoleukodystrophy. *Eur J Pediatr* 1987;146:477–483.

Prick MJJ, Gabreëls FJM, Trijbels JMF, et al. Progressive poliodystrophy (Alpers' disease) with a defect in cytochrome aa3 in muscle: A report of two unrelated patients. *Clin Neurol Neurosurg* 1983;85:57–70.

Quinzii C, Naini A, Salviati L, et al. A mutation in para- hydroxybenzoate-polyprenyl transferase (CoQ2) causes primary Coenzyme Q10 deficiency. *Am J Hum Genet* 2006;79: 25–349.

Quinzii CM, Kattah AG, Naini A, et al. Coenzyme Q deficiency and cerebellar ataxia associated with an apraxatin mutation. *Neurology* 2005;6:539–541.

Raas-Rothschild A, Wanders RJA, Mooijer PAW, et al. A PEX6-defective peroxisomal biogenesis disorder with severe phenotype in an infant, versus Mild Phenotype Resembling Usher Syndrome in the affected parents. *Am J Hum Genet* 2002;70:1062–1068.

Raghavan SS, Krussell A, Krussel J, et al. GM2 ganglioside metabolism in hexosaminidase a deficiency status: Determination in situ using labeled GM2 added to fibroblast cultures. *Am J Hum Genet* 1985;37:1071–1082.

Rapin I. Myoclonus in neuronal storage and Lafora disease. *Adv Neurol* 1986;43:65–85.

Reina-San-Martin M, Chen HT, Nussenzweig A, Nussenzweig MC. ATM is required for Recombination between Immunoglobulin Switch Regions. *J Environ Monit* 2004;200: 1103–1110.

Rider JA, Rider DL. Batten disease: Past, present, future. *Am J Med Genet Suppl* 1988;5:21–26.

Robinson BH, MacMillian H, Petrova-Benedict R, Sherwood WG. Variable clinical presentation in patients with defective E1 component of pyruvate dehydrogenase deficiency. *J Pediatr* 1987;111:525–533.

Rodriguez D, Gauthier F, Bertini E, et al. Infantile Alexander disease: Spectrum of GFAP mutations and genotype-phenotype correlation. *Am J Hum Genet* 2001;69:1134–1140.

Roesch K, Curran SP, Tranebjaerg L, Koehler CM. Human deafness dystonia syndrome is caused by a defect in the assembly of the DDP1/TIMM8a-TIMM13 complex. *Hum Mol Genet* 2002;11:447–486.

Roger J, Genton P, Bureau M, Dravet C. Progressive myoclonus epilepsies in childhood and adolescence. In: Roger J, Bureau M, Dravet C, et al., eds. *Epileptic syndromes in infancy, childhood and adolescence*. London: John-Libbey, 1992.

Roscher AA, Hoefler S, Hoeffler G, et al. Genetic and phenotypic heterogeneity of disorders of peroxisomal biogenesis: A complementation study involving cell lines from 19 patients. *Pediatr Res* 1989;26:67.

Rose FC, Bowden AN, Bowden PMA. The heart in Leber's optic atrophy. *Br J Ophthalmol* 1970;54:388–393.

Rosen ES, Harris NL. Weekly clinical exercises: Case 2–1987. *N Engl J Med* 1987;316:91–100.

Rosenblum JL, Keating JP, Prensky AL, Nelson JS. A progressive neurologic syndrome in children with chronic liver disease. *N Eng J Med* 1981;304:503–508.

Rosing HS, Hopkins LC, Wallace DC, et al. Maternally inherited mitochondrial myopathy and myoclonic epilepsy. *Ann Neurol* 1985;17:228–237.

Rötig A, Appelkvist EL, Geromel V, et al. Quinone-responsive multiple respiratory-chain dysfunction due to widespread coenzyme C10 deficiency. *Lancet* 2000;356:392–395.

Rowland LP. Molecular genetics, pseudogenetics and clinical neurology. *Neurology* 1983;33:1179–1195.

Rummelt V, Folberg R, Ionasescu V, et al. Ocular pathology of MELAS syndrome with mitochondrial DNA nucleotide 3243 point mutation. *Ophthalmology* 1993;100:1757–1766.

Rustin P, von Kleist Retzow JC, Chantrel Groussard K, et al. Effect of ibedenone on cardiomyopathy in Friedreich's ataxia: A preliminary study. *Lancet* 1999;354:477–479.

Sacconi S, Salviati L, Nishigaki Y, et al. A functionally dominant mitochondrial DNA mutation. *Hum Mol Genet* 2008; 17(12):1814–1820.

Sakai T, Antoku Y, Goto I. Plasmalogen deficiency in cultured skin fibroblasts from neonatal adrenoleukodystrophy. *Exp Neurol* 1986;94:149–154.

Salih MAM, Ahlsten G, Stalberg E, et al. Friedreich's ataxia in 13 children: Presentation and evolution with neurophysiologic, electrocardiographic, and echocardiographic features. *J Child Neurol* 1990;5:321–326.

Santorelli FM, Shanske S, Jain KD, et al. A T–C mutation at nt 8993 of mitochondrial DNA in a child with Leigh's syndrome. *Neurology* 1994;44:972–974.

Sartoris DJ, Luzzatti L, Weaver DD, et al. Type IX Ehlers Danlos syndrome: A new variant with pathognomonic radiologic features. *Radiology* 1984;152:665.

Sarzi E, Goffart S, Serre V, et al. Twinkle helicase (PEO1) gene mutation causes mitochondrial DNA depletion. *Ann Neurol* 2007;62:579–587.

Satoh M, Ishikawa N, Yoshizawa T, et al. N-isopropyl-p-[123I] iodoamphetamine SPECT in MELAS syndromes: Comparison with CT and MR imaging. *J Comput Assist Tomogr* 1991;15:77–82.

Schafer BL, Bischop RW, Kratunis VJ, et al. Molecular cloning of human mevalonate kinase and identification of a missense mutation in the genetic disease mevalonic aciduria. *J Biol Chem* 1992;267:13229–13238.

Schnabel D, Schröder M, Sandhoff K. Mutation in the sphingolipid activator protein-2 in a patient with a variant of Gaucher disease. *FEBS Lett* 1991;284:57–59.

Schulz A, Mousallem T, Venkataramani M et al. The CLN9 protein, a regulator of dihydroceramide synthase. *J Biol Chem* 2006;281: 2784–2794.

Scott BB, Miller JP, Losowsky MS. Hypobetalipoproteinemia: A variant of the Bassen-Kornzweig syndrome. *Gut* 1979;20: 163–168.

Scriver CR, Clow CL, Kaplan P, Niederwieser A. Hyperphenylalaninemia due to deficiency of 6-pyruvoyl tetrahydropterin synthase: Unusual gene dosage effect in heterozygotes. *Hum Genet* 1987;77:168–171.

Sedwick LA, Burde RM, Hodges FJ. Leigh's subacute necrotizing encephalomyelopathy manifesting as spasmus nutans. *Arch Ophthalmol* 1984;102:1046–1048.

Seil FJ, Schochet SS, Earle KM. Alexander's disease in an adult. *Arch Neurol* 1968;19:494–502.

Seitz RJ, Langes K, Frenzel H, et al. Congenital Leigh's disease: Panencephalomyelopathy and peripheral neuropathy. *Acta Neuropathol* 1984;64:167–171.

Sewell AC. Urinary oligosaccharide excretion in disorders of glycolipid, glycoprotein and glycogen metabolism. A review of screening for differential diagnosis. *Eur J Pediatr* 1980; 134:183–194.

Shahbazian MD, Zoghbi HY. Rett syndrome and MePC2: Linking epigenetics and neuronal function. *Am J Hum Genet* 2002;71:1259–1272.

Shanske AL, Shanske S, Silvestri G, et al. MELAS point mutation with unusual clinical presentation. *Neuromuscul Disord* 1993;3:191–193.

Shapira AHV, Cooper JM, Manneschi L, et al. A mitochondrial encephalomyopathy with specific deficiencies of two respiratory chain polypeptides and a circulating autoantibody to a mitochondrial matrix protein. *Brain* 1990;113:419–432.

Shapira Y, Cederbaum SD, Cancilla PA, et al. Familial poliodystrophy, mitochondrial myopathy, and lactate acidemia. *Neurology* 1975;25:614–626.

Shefer S, Salen G, Batta AK, et al. Reduced 7-dehydrocholesterol reductase activity in Smith-Lemli-Opitz syndrome. *Am J Med Genet* 1994;50:336 (abstract).

Shinnar S, Singer HS. Cobalamin C mutation (methylmalonic aciduria and homocystinuria) in adolescence. *N Engl J Med* 1984;311:451–454.

Shuchi M, Deepti D, Kazuhiro Y, et al. Lafora disease proteins malin and laforin are recruited to aggresomes in response to proteasomal impairment. *Hum Mol Genet* 2007;16:733–762.

Siintola E, Partanen S, Stromme P et al. Cathepsin D deficiency underlies congenital human neuronal ceroid-lipofuscinosis. *Brain* 2006;129:1438–1445.

Siintola E, Topcu M, Aula N et al. The novel neuronal ceroid lipofuscinosis gene MFSD8 encodes a putative lysosomal transporter. *Am J Hum Genet* 2007;81: 136–146.

Silvestri G, Ciafaloni E, Santorelli FM, et al. Clinical features associated with A–G transition at nucleotide 8344 of mtDNA ("MERRF mutation"). *Neurology* 1993;43:1200–1206.

Simon A, Kremer HPH, Wevers RA, et al. Mevalonate kinate deficiency: Evidence for a phenotypic continuum. *Neurology* 2004;62:994–997.

Simonaro CM, Desnick RJ, McGovern MM, et al. The demographics and distribution of type B Niemann-Pick disease: Novel mutations lead to new genotype/phenotype correlations. *Am J Hum Genet* 2002;71:1413–1419.

Singh AK, Dhaunsi GS, Gupta MP, et al. Demonstration of glutathione peroxidase in rat liver peroxisomes and its intraorganellar distribution. *Arch Biochem Biophys* 1994;315: 331–338.

Skjeldal OH, Stokke O, Refsum S. Clinical and biochemical heterogenicity in conditions with phytanic acid accumulation. *J Neurol Sci* 1987;77:87–96.

Skrede S, Björkhem I, Kvittingen EA, et al. Demonstration of 26-hydroxylation of C-27 steroid in human skin fibroblasts and a deficiency of this activity in CTX. *J Clin Invest* 1986; 78:729–735.

Sleat DE, Gin RM, Sohar I, Wisniewski K, et al. Mutational analysis of the defective protease in classic late-infantile neuronal ceroid lipofuscinosis, a neurodegenerative lysosomal storage disorder. *Am J Hum Genet* 1999;64:1511–1523. Note: Erratum: *Am J Hum Genet* 2004;75:1158.

Smith LL, Conerly SL. Ataxia-telangiectasia or Louis-Bar syndrome. *J Am Acad Dermatol* 1985;12:681–696.

Sokol RJ, Butler-Simon N, Heubi JE, et al. Vitamin E deficiency neuropathy in children with fat malabsorption. Studies in cystic fibrosis and chronic cholestasis. *Ann N Y Acad Sci* 1989;570:156–169.

Sokol RJ, Kayden HJ, Bettis DB, et al. Isolated vitamin E deficiency in the absence of fat malabsorption: Familial, and sporadic cases: Characterization and investigation of causes. *J Lab Clin Med* 1988;111:548–559.

Sorbi S, Piacentini S, Fani C, et al. Abnormalities of mitochondrial enzymes in hereditary ataxias. *Acta Neurol Scand* 1989; 80:103–110.

Spiegel R, Bach G, Sury V, et al. A mutation in the saposin A coding region of the prosaposin gene in an infant presenting as Krabbe disease: First report of saposin A deficiency in humans. *Mol Genet Metab* 2005;84:160–166.

Spinazzola A, Viscomi C, Fernandez-Vizarra E, et al. MPV7 encodes an inner mitochondrial membrane protein and is mutated in infantile hepatic mitochondrial DNA depletion. *Nat Genet* 2006;38:570–575.

Springer S, Erlewein R, Naegele T, et al. Alexander disease: Classification revisited and isolation of a neonatal form. *Neuropediatrics* 2000;31:86–92.

Steinfeld R, Reinhardt K, Schreiber K et al. Cathepsin D deficiency is associated with a human neurodegenerative disorder. *Am J Hum Genet* 2006;78:988–998.

Storm W, Fasse M. Laryngeal atresia in an infant with chondrodysplasia punctate, rhizomelic type. *Monatsschr Kinderheilkd* 1991;139:629–631.

Striano P, Specchio N, Biancheri R, et al. Clinical and electrophysiological features of epilepsy in Italian patients with CLN8 mutations. *Epilepsy Behav* 2007;10:187–191.

Suzuki Y, Harada K, Miura Y, et al. Mitochondrial myopathy, encephalopathy, lactic acidosis, and stroke-like episodes (MELAS) decrease in diastolic left ventricular function assessed by electrocardiography. *Pediatr Cardiol* 1993;14:162–166.

Suzuki Y, Shimozawa N, Yajimas S, et al. Novel subtype of peroxisomal acyl CoA oxidase and bifunctional enzyme deficiency with detectable enzyme protein: Identification by means of complementation analysis. *Am J Hum Genet* 1994; 54:36–43.

Tadiboyina VT, Rupar A, Atkison P, et al. Novel mutation in DGUOK in hepatocerebral mitochondrial DNA depletion associated with cystathionuria. *Am J Med Genet* 2005;135A: 289–291.

Takanashi J, Inoue K, Tomita M, et al. Brain N-acetylaspartate is elevated in Pelizaeus-Merzbacher disease with PLP1 duplication. *Neurology* 2002;58:237–241.

Tatuch Y, Christodoulou J, Feigenhaum A, et al. Heteroplasmic mt DNA mutation (T-G) at 8993 can cause Leigh disease when the percentage of abnormal mt DNA is high. *Am J Hum Genet* 1992;50:852–858.

Threlkeld AB, Miller NR, Golnik KC, et al. Ophthalmic involvement in myo-neurogastrointestinal encephalopathy syndrome. *Am J Ophthalmol* 1992;114:322–328.

Thyagarajan D, Shanske S, Vasquez-Memije M, et al. A novel mitochondrial ATPase 6 point mutation in familial bilateral striatal necrosis. *Ann Neurol* 1995;38:468–472.

Tritschler HJ, Andreetta F, Moraes CT, et al. Mitochondrial myopathy of childhood associated with depletion of mitochondrial DNA. *Neurology* 1992;42:209–217.

Tulinius MH, Holme E, Kristiansson B, et al. Mitochondrial encephalomyopathy in childhood. II. Clinical manifestations and syndromes. *J Pediatr* 1991;119:251–259.

Tylki-Szymanska A, Czartoryska B, Vanier M-T, et al. Non-neuronopathic Gaucher disease due to saposin C deficiency. *Clin Genet* 2007;72:538–542.

Uhlenberg B, Schuelke M, Ruschendorf F, et al. Mutations in the gene encoding gap junction protein alpha-12 (connexin 46.6) cause Pelizaeus-Merzbacher-like disease. *Am J Hum Genet* 2004;75:251–260. [Note: Erratum: *Am J Hum Genet* 2004;75:737.]

Uusimaa J, Finnila S, Vainionpaa L, et al. A mutation in mitochondrial DNA-encoded cytochrome c oxidase II gene in a child with Alpers-Huttenlocker-like disease. *Pediatrics* 2002; 111:262–268.

van den Brink DM, Brites P, Haasjes J, et al. Identification of PEX7 as the second gene involved in Refsum disease. *Am J Hum Genet* 2003;72:471–477.

van Diggelen OP, Thobois S, Tilikete C, et al. Adult neuronal ceroid lipofuscinosis with palmitoyl-protein thioesterase deficiency: First adult-onset patients of a childhood disease. *Ann Neurol* 2001;50:269–272.

Van Eldere JR, Parmentier GG, Eyssen JH, et al. Bile acids in peroxisomal disorders. *Eur J Clin Invest* 1987;17:386–390.

Van Goethem G, Luoma P, Rantamaki M, et al. POLG mutations in neurodegenerative disorders with ataxia but no muscle involvement. *Neurology* 2004;63:1251–1257.

Van Heycop Ten Ham MW. Lafora Disease: A form of progressive myoclonus epilepsy. In: Vinken PJ, Bruyn GW, eds. *Handbook of clinical neurology*. New York: North Holland, 1974.

Vance JE. Lipid imbalance in the neurological disorder, Niemann-Pick C disease. *FEBS Lett* 2006;580:5518–5524.

Vanhove GF, Van Veldhoven PP, Fransen M, et al. The CoA esters of 2-methyl-branched chain fatty acids and of the bile acid intermediates di- and tri-hydroxycoprotanoic acids are oxidized by a single peroxisomal branched chain acyl-CoA oxidase in human liver and kidney. *J Biol Chem* 1993;268: 10335–10344.

Velinov M, Zellers N, Styles J, Wisniewski K. Homozygosity for mutation G212A of the gene for aspartoacylase is associated with atypical form of Canavan's disease. [Letter.] *Clin Genet* 2008;73:288–289.

Vellodi A, Bembi B, De Villemeur TB, et al. Management of neuropathic Gaucher disease: A European consensus. *J Inherit Metab Dis* 2001;24:319–327.

Vesa J, Hollston E, Verkruyse LA, et al. Mutations in the palmitoyl protein thioesterase gene causing infantile neuronal ceroid-lipofuscinoses. *Nature* 1995;376:584–587.

Vethamany VG, Welch J, Vethamany SK. Type D Niemann-Pick disease (Nova Scotia variant). *Arch Pathol* 1972;93:537–543.

Vulpe C, Levinson B, Whitney S, et al. Isolation of a candidate gene for Menkes disease and evidence that it encodes a copper-transporting ATPase. *Nat Genet* 1993;3:7–13.

Wakai S, Ishikawa Y, Nagaoka M, et al. Central nervous system involvement and generalized muscular atrophy in occipital horn syndrome: Ehlers Danlos type IX. *J Neurol Sci* 1993; 116:1–5.

Waldmann TA. Immunological abnormalities in ataxia telangiectasia. In: Bridges BA, Harnden DG, eds. *Ataxia-telangiectasia: A cellular and molecular link between cancer, neuropathology, and immune deficiency*. New York: John Wiley and Sons, Inc., 1982.

Wallace DC, Zheng XX, Lott MT, et al. Familial mitochondrial encephalomyopathy (MERRF): Genetic, pathophysiological, and biochemical characterization of a mitochondrial DNA disease. *Cell* 1988;55:601–610.

Wanders RJ, Schrakamp G, van der Bosch H, et al. Pre- and postnatal diagnosis of cerebrohepatorenal (Zellweger) syndrome via a simple method directly demonstrating the presence or absence of peroxisomes in cultured skin fibroblasts, amniocytes, or chorionic villi fibroblasts. *J Inherit Metab Dis* 1986;9(Suppl 2):317.

Wanders RJ, Van Roermund CW, Schori DS, et al. 2-Hydroxyphtanic acid oxidase activity in rat and human liver and its deficiency in the Zellweger syndrome. *Biochim Biophys Acta* 1994;1227:177–182.

Wanders RJA, Dekker C, Povarth VAP, et al. Human alkyl dihydroxy acetone phosphate synthase deficiency: A new peroxisomal disorder. *J Inherit Metab Dis* 1994;17:315–318.

Wang D, Pascual JM, Yang H, et al. Glut-1 deficiency syndrome: Clinical, genetic, and therapeutic aspects. *Ann Neurol* 2005; 57:11–18.

Westman JA, Richardson DC, Rennert OM, Morrow G. Atypical Menkes steely hair disease. *Am J Med Genet* 1988;30: 853–858.

Willems PJ, Van Roy BC, Kleije WJ, et al. Atypical clinical presentation of ataxia telangiectasia. *Am J Med Genet* 1993;45: 777–782.

Williams DW, 3rd, Elster AD, Cox TD. Cranial MR imaging in rhizomelic chondrodysplasia punctata. *AJNR Am J Neuroradiol* 1991;12:363–365.

Wilson J. Leber's hereditary optic atrophy: Some clinical and aetiological considerations. *Brain* 1963;86:347–362.

Winston GP, Jaiser SR. Copper deficient myelopathy and subacute combined degeneration of the spinal cord: Why is the phenotype so similar? *Med Hypotheses* 2008;71:229–236.

Winterthunon S, Ferrari G, He L, et al. Autosomal recessive mitochondrial ataxic syndrome due to mitochondrial polymerase-gamma mutations. *Neurology* 2005;64:1204–1208.

Wisniewski KE, Kida E, Golabek AA, et al. Neuronal ceroid lipofuscinoses: Classification and diagnosis. *Adv Genet* 2001;45:1–34.

Wyatt DT, Noetzel MJ, Hillman RE. Infantile beriberi presenting as sub-acute necrotizing encephalomyopathy. *J Pediatr* 1987;100:888–892.

Xiao Ping Y, Akihiro A, Kunimasa Y, et al. Abetalipoproteinemia caused by maternal isodisomy of chromosome 4q containing an intron 9 splice acceptor mutation in the microsomal triglyceride transfer protein gene. *Arterioscler Thromb Vasc Biol* 1999;19:1950–1955.

Yamashita K, Ideo H, Ohkura T, et al. Sugar chains of serum transferrin from patients with carbohydrate-deficient glycoprotein syndrome. *J Biol Chem* 1993;268:5783–5789.

Yang YM, Ducos R, Rosenberg AJ, et al. Cobalamin malabsorption in three siblings due to an abnormal intrinsic factor that is markedly susceptible to acid hydrolysis. *J Clin Invest* 1985;76:2057–2065.

Zeng BJ, Wang ZH, Ribeiro LA, et al. Identification and characterization of novel mutations of the aspartoacylase gene in non-Jewish patients with Canavan disease. *J Inherit Metab Dis* 2002;25:557–570.

Zeviani M, Nonaka I, Bonilla E, et al. Fatal infantile mitochondrial myopathy and renal dysfunction caused by cytochrome c oxidase deficiency: Immunological studies in a new patient. *Ann Neurol* 1985;17:414–417.

Zoghbi HY, Ballabio A. Pelizaeus-Merzbacher disease. In: Scriver CR, et al., eds. *The metabolic and molecular basis of inherited disease*. New York: McGraw-Hill;1995:4481–4585.

Zupanc ML, Moraes CT, Shanske S, et al. Deletion of mitochondrial DNA in patients with combined features of Kearns-Sayre and MELAS syndrome. *Ann Neurol* 1991;29: 680–683.

Chapter 19

Nadarajah B, Parnavelas JG: Modes of neuronal migration in the developing cerebral cortex. *Nat Neurosci.* 2002;3:423.

Chapter 20

Aravind L, Koonin EV. The fukutin protein family: Predicted enzymes modifying cell-surface molecules. *Curr Biol* 1999;9: R836–R837.

Baker EM, Khorasgani MG, Gardner-Medwin D, et al. Arthrogryposis multiplex congenita and bilateral parietal polymicrogyria in association with the intrauterine death of a twin. *Neuropediatrics* 1996;27:54–56.

Balestri P, Vivarelli R, Grosso S, et al. Malformations of cortical development in neurofibromatosis type 1. *Neurology* 2003;61:1799–1801.

Barkovich AJ, Lindan CE. Congenital cytomegalovirus infection of the brain: Imaging analysis and embryologic considerations. *Am J Neuroradiol* 1994;15:703–715.

Barkovich AJ. *Pediatric neuroimaging*. New York: Raven Press; 1995:668.

Barkovich AJ. Subcortical heterotopia: A distinct clinico-radiographic entity. *Am J Neuroradiol* 1996;17:1315–1322.

Barkovich AJ, Ferriero DM, Barr RM, et al. Microlissencephaly: A heterogeneous malformation of cortical development. *Neuropediatrics* 1998;29:113–119.

Barkovich AJ. *Pediatric neuroimaging*, 3rd ed. Philadelphia: Lippincott Williams & Wilkins;2000:405–406.

Barth PG, Mullaart R, Stam FC, Slooff JL. Familial lissencephaly with extreme neopallial hypoplasia. *Brain Dev* 1982;4:145–151.

Becker AJ, Urbach H, Scheffler B, et al. Focal cortical dysplasia of Taylor's balloon cell type: Mutational analysis of the TSC1 gene indicates a pathogenic relationship to tuberous sclerosis. *Ann Neurol* 2002;52:29–37.

Beltran-Valero de Bernabe D, Currier S, Steinbrecher A, et al. Mutations in the O-mannosyltransferase gene POMT1 give rise to the severe neuronal migration disorder Walker-Warburg syndrome. *Am J Hum Genet* 2002;71:1033–1043.

Beltrán-Valero de Bernabé D, van Bokhoven H, van Beusekom E, et al. A homozygous nonsense mutation in the Fukutin gene causes a Walker-Warburg syndrome phenotype. *J Med Genet* 2003;40:845–848.

Berg MJ, Schifitto G, Powers JM, et al. X-linked female band heterotopia-male lissencephaly syndrome. *Neurology* 1998; 50:1143–1146.

Bolton PF, Park RJ, Higgins JN, et al. Neuro-epileptic determinants of autism spectrum disorders in tuberous sclerosis complex. *Brain* 2002;125(Pt 6):1247–1255.

Bond J, Roberts E, Mochida GH, et al. ASPM is a major determinant of cerebral cortical size. *Nat Genet* 2002;32:316–320.

Bond J, Scott S, Hamphire DJ, et al. Protein-truncating mutations in ASPM cause variable reduction in brain size. *Am J Hum Genet* 2003;73:1170–1177.

Brody BA, Kinney HC, Kloman AS, Gilles FH. Sequence of central nervous system myelination in human infancy. I. An autopsy study of myelination. *J Neuropathol Exp Neurol* 1987; 46:283–301.

Brunelli S, Faiella A, Capra V, et al. Germline mutations in the homeobox gene EMX2 in patients with severe schizencephaly. *Nat Genet* 1996;12:94–96.

Çakmakçi H, Kurul S, Iscan A, Dirik K. Proton magnetic resonance spectroscopy in three subacute sclerosing panencephalitis patients: Correlation with clinical status. *Childs Nerv Syst* 2004;20:216–220.

Cardoso C, Leventer RJ, Ward HL, et al. Refinement of a 400-kb critical region allows genotypic differentiation between isolated lissencephaly, Miller-Dieker syndrome, and other phenotypes secondary to deletions of 17p13.3. *Am J Hum Genet* 2003;72:918–930.

Chang BS, Piao X, Bodell A, et al. Bilateral frontoparietal polymicrogyria: Clinical and radiological features in 10 families with linkage to chromosome 16. *Ann Neurol* 2003;53: 596–606.

Chiron C, Dumans C, Jambaque I, et al. Randomized trial comparing vigabatrin and hydrocortisone in infantile spasms due to tuberous sclerosis. *Epilepsy Res* 1997;26:389–395.

Cotter DR, Honavar M, Everall I. Focal cortical dysplasia: A neuropathological and developmental perspective. *Epilepsy Res* 1999;36:155–164.

Cravioto H, Feigin I. Localized cerebral gliosis with giant neurons histologically resembling tuberous sclerosis. *J Neuropathol Exp Neurol* 1960;19:369–387.

Crino PB, Trojanowski J, Eberwine J. Internexin, MAP1B, and nestin in cortical dysplasia as markers of developmental maturity. *Acta Neuropathol* 1997;93:619–627.

Crino PB, Eberwine J. Cellular and molecular basis of cerebral dysgenesis. *J Neurosci Res* 1997;50:907–916.

Crome L. Infantile cerebral gliosis with giant nerve cells. *J Neurol Neurosurg Psychiatry* 1957;20:117–124.

Denckla MB, Hofman K, Mazzocco MMM, et al. Relationship between T2-weighted hyperintensities (unidentified bright objects) and lower IQs in children with neurofibromatosis-1. *Am J Med Genet* 1996;67:98–102.

Denis D, Chateil JF, Brun M, et al. Schizencephaly: Clinical and imaging features in 30 infantile cases. *Brain Dev* 2000;22: 475–483.

DeRosa M, Secor D, Barson M, et al. Neuropathologic findings in surgically treated hemimegalencephaly: Immunohistochemical, morphometric and ultrastructural study. *Acta Neuropathol* 1992;84:250–260.

Devlin AM, Cross JH, Harkness W, et al. Clinical outcomes of hemispherectomy for epilepsy in childhood and adolescence. *Brain* 2003;126:556–566.

Dobyns WB, Pagon RA, Armstrong D, et al. Diagnostic criteria for Walker–Warburg syndrome. *Am J Med Genet* 1989;32: 195–210.

Dobyns WB, Reiner O, Carrozzo R, Ledbetter DH. Lissencephaly. A human brain malformation associated with deletion of the LIS1 gene located at chromosome 17p13. *JAMA* 1993;270:2838–2842.

Dobyns WB, Truwit CL. Lissencephaly and other malformations of cortical development. *Neuropediatrics* 1995;26:132–147.

Dobyns W, Barkovich A. Microcephaly with simplified gyral pattern (oligogyric microcephaly) and microlissencephaly. *Neuropediatrics* 1999;30:105–106.

Eksioglu YZ, Scheffer IE, Cardenas P, et al. Periventricular heterotopia: An X-linked dominant epilepsy locus causing aberrant cerebral cortical development. *Neuron* 1996;16:77–87.

Elterman RD, Shields WD, Mansfield KA, Nakagawa J. US Infantile Spasms Vigabatrin Study Group. Randomized trial of vigabatrin in patients with infantile spasms. *Neurology* 2001; 57:1416–1421.

Endo T. O-mannosyl glycans in mammals. *Biochim Biophys Acta* 1999;1473:237–246.

Flores-Sarnat L. Hemimegalencephaly: Part 1. Genetic, clinical and imaging aspects. *J Child Neurol* 2002;17:373–384.

Fox JW, Lamperti ED, Eksiogly YZ, et al. Mutations in filamin 1 prevent migration of cerebral cortical neurons in human periventricular heterotopia. *Neuron* 1998;21:1315–1325.

Fox JW, Walsh CA. Periventricular heterotopia and the genetics of neuronal migration in the cerebral cortex. *Am J Hum Genet* 1999;65:19–24.

Galluzzi P, Cerase A, Strambi M, et al. Hemimegalencephaly in tuberous sclerosis complex. *J Child Neurol* 2002;17:677–680.

Gleeson JG, Allen KM, Fox JW, et al. Doublecortin, a brain-specific gene mutated in human X-linked lissencephaly and double cortex syndrome, encodes a putative signaling protein. *Cell* 1998;92:63–72.

Granata T, Farina L, Faiella A, et al. Familial schizencephaly associated with EMX2 mutation. *Neurology* 1997;48:1403–1406.

Greenwood R, Whit K, Tupler L, et al. Brain volume and cognition in children with neurofibromatosis type 1. *Ann Neurol* 2004;56:S93.

Grewal PK, Hewitt JE. Glycosylation defects: A new mechanism for muscular dystrophy? *Hum Mol Genet* 2003;12(Review Issue 2):R259–R264.

Guerreiro MM, Andermann F, Andermann E, et al. Surgical treatment of epilepsy in tuberous sclerosis: Strategies and results in 18 patients. *Neurology* 1998;51:1263–1269.

Guerrini R, Dubeau F, Dulac O, et al. Bilateral parasaggital parietooccipital polymicrogyria and epilepsy. *Ann Neurol* 1997; 41:65–73.

Guerrini R, Barkovich J, Sztriha L, Dobyns WB. Bilateral frontal polymicrogyria. A newly recognized brain malformation syndrome. *Neurology* 2000;54:909–913.

Hancock E, Osborne JP. Vigabatrin in the treatment of infantile spasms in tuberous sclerosis: Literature review. *J Child Neurol* 1999;14:71–74.

Hennel SJ, Ekert PG, Volpe JJ, Inder TE. Insights into the pathogenesis of cerebral lesions in incontinentia pigmenti. *Pediatr Neurol* 2003;29:148–150.

Herman TE, Siegel MJ. Hemimegalencephaly and linear nevus sebaceous syndrome. *J Perinatol* 2001;21:336–338.

Hyman SL, Gill DS, Shores EA, et al. Natural history of cognitive deficits and their relationship to MRI T2-hyperintensities in NF1. *Neurology* 2003;60:1139–1145.

Kobayashi K, Nakahori Y, Mizuno K, et al. Founder-haplotype analysis in Fukuyama-type congenital muscular dystrophy (FCMD). *Hum Genet* 1998;103:323–327.

Kornack DR, Rakic P. Changes in cell-cycle kinetics during the development and evolution of primate neocortex. *Proc Natl Acad Sci USA* 1998;95:1242–1246.

Kroon AA, Amit BJ, Barth PG, Hennekam RCM. Lissencephaly with extreme cerebral and cerebellar hypoplasia. A magnetic resonance imaging study. *Neuropediatrics* 1996;27:273–276.

Kuzniecky RI, Andermann F, Guerrini R. The congenital bilateral perisylvian syndrome: Study of 31 patients. The CPBS Multicenter Collaborative Study. *Lancet* 1993;341:608–612.

Kwiatkowski DJ, Zhang H, Bandura JL, et al. A mouse model of TSC1 reveals sex-dependent lethality from liver hemangiomas, and up-regulation of p70S6 kinase activity in Tsc1 null cells. *Hum Mol Genet* 2002;11:525–534.

Lacaze E, Kieffer V, Streri A, et al. Neuropsychological outcome in children with optic pathway tumours when first-line treatment is chemotherapy. *Br J Cancer* 2003;89:2038–2044.

Liang JS, Lee WT, Peng SS, et al. Agyria-pachygyria: Clinical, neuroimaging, and neurophysiologic correlations. *Pediatr Neurol* 2002;27:171–176.

Lynch TM, Gutmann DH. Neurofibromatosis 1. *Neurol Clin* 2002;20:841–865.

Matsumoto N, Leventer RJ, Kuc JA, et al. Mutation analysis of the DCX gene and genotype/phenotype correlation in subcortical band heterotopia. *Eur J Hum Genet* 2001;9: 5–12.

MacCollin M, Mautner VF. The diagnosis and management of neurofibromatosis 2 in childhood. *Semin Pediatr Neurol* 1998;5:243–252.

McComb R, Schaefer B, Olney A, Hattie B. Cerebro-cerebellar lissencephaly, congenital heart defects and other congenital anomalies in male sibs: A new syndrome. Presented at the 23rd Annual March of Dimes Clinical Genetics Conference on Developmental and Genetic Disorders of the Central Nervous System. Vancouver, BC, Canada, 1991.

Miller PD, Pollack IF, Pang D, Albright AL. Comparison of simultaneous versus delayed ventriculoperitoneal shunt insertion in children undergoing myelomeningocele repair. *J Child Neurol* 1996;11:370–372.

Nabbout R. A risk-benefit assessment of treatments for infantile spasms. *Drug Saf* 2001;24:813–828.

Narayanan V. Tuberous sclerosis complex: Genetics to pathogenesis. *Pediatr Neurol* 2003;29:404–409.

North K, Yuille D, Cocks N, Hutchins P. Cognitive function and academic performance in children with neurofibromatosis type 1. *Dev Med Child Neurol* 1995;37:427–436.

O'Callaghan FJ, Harris T, Joinson C, et al. The relation of infantile spasms, tubers, and intelligence in tuberous sclerosis complex. *Arch Dis Child* 2003;89:530–533.

Packard AM, Miller VS, Delgado MR. Schizencephaly: Correlations of clinical and radiologic features. *Neurology* 1997; 48:1427–1434.

Piao X, Basel-Vanagaite L, Straussberg R, et al. An autosomal recessive form of bilateral frontoparietal polymicrogyria maps to chromosome 16q12.2–21. *Am J Hum Genet* 2002; 70:1028–1033.

Plawner LL, Delgado MR, Miller VS, et al. Neuroanatomy of holoprosencephaly as predictor of function: beyond the face predicting the brain. *Neurology* 2002;59:1058–1066.

Powell HW, Hart PE, Sisodiya SM. Epilepsy and perisylvian polymicrogyria in a patient with Kabuki syndrome. *Dev Med Child Neurol* 2003;45:841–843.

Rakic P. A small step for the cell, a giant leap for mankind: A hypothesis of neocortical expansion during evolution. *Trends Neurosci* 1995;18:838–888.

Rakic P. Specification of cerebral cortical areas. *Science* 1988; 241:170–176.

Reiner O, Carrozzo R, Shen Y, et al. Isolation of a Miller-Dieker lissencephaly gene containing G protein beta-subunit-like repeats. *Nature* 1993;364:717–721.

Roach ES, Smith M, Huttenlocher P, et al. Diagnostic criteria: Tuberous sclerosis complex. Report of the diagnostic criteria committee of the national tuberous sclerosis association. *J Child Neurol* 1992;7:221–224.

Robain O. Introduction to the pathology of cerebral cortical dysplasia. In: Guerrini R, Anderman F, Camapicchi R, et al., eds. *Dysplasias of cerebral cortex and epilepsy*. Philadelphia: Lippincott-Raven;1996:1–9.

Santavuori P, Somer H, Sainio K, et al. Muscle-eye-brain disease (MEB). *Brain Dev* 1989;11:147–153.

Sasaki M, Hashimoto T, Shimada M, et al. Nation-wide survey on hemimegalencephaly in Japan. *No To Hattatsu* 2000;32: 255–260.

Sheen VL, Dixon PH, Fox JW, et al. Mutations in the X-linked Filamin A gene cause periventricular nodular heterotopia in males as well as in females. *Hum Mol Genet* 2001;10:1775–1783.

Sheen VL, Feng Y, Graham D, et al. Filamin A and Filamin B are co-expressed within neurons during periods of neuronal migration and can physically interact. *Hum Mol Genet* 2002; 11:2845–2854.

Silan F, Yoshioka M, Kobayashi K, et al. A new mutation of the fukutin gene in a non-Japanese patient. *Ann Neurol* 2003; 53:392–396.

Taniguchi K, Kobayashi K, Saito K, et al. Worldwide distribution and broader clinical spectrum of muscle-eye-brain disease. *Hum Mol Genet* 2003;12:527–534.

Taylor DC, Falconer MA, Bruton CJ, Corsellis JAN. Focal dysplasia of the cerebral cortex in epilepsy. *J Neurol Neurosurg Psychiatry* 1971;34:369–387.

Thakur S, Singh R, Pradhan M, Phadke SR. Spectrum of holoprosencephaly. *Indian J Pediatr* 2004;71:593–597.

Toda T, Kobayashi K, Kondo-Iida E, et al. The Fukuyama congenital muscular dystrophy story. *Neuromuscul Disord* 2000;10:153–159.

Toda T, Segawa M, Nomura Y, et al. Localization of a gene for Fukuyama type congenital muscular dystrophy to chromosome 9q31–33. *Nat Genet* 1993;5:283–286.

Tow SL, Chandela S, Miller NR, Avellino AM. Long-term outcome in children with gliomas of the anterior visual pathway. *Pediatr Neurol* 2003;28:262–270.

Urbach H, Scheffler B, Heinrichsmeier T, et al. Focal cortical dysplasia of Taylor's balloon cell type: A clinicopathological entity with characteristic neuroimaging and histopathological features, and favorable postsurgical outcome. *Epilepsia* 2002;43:33–40.

Verlinsky Y, Rechitsky S, Verlinsky O, et al. Preimplantation diagnosis for neurofibromatosis. *Reprod Biomed Online* 2002; 4:218–222.

Villard L, Naguyenk, Cardoso C, et al. A locus for bilateral perisylvian polymicrogyria maps to Xq28. *Am J Hum Genet* 2002;70:1003–1008.

Volpe JJ. Perinatal brain injury: From pathogenesis to neuroprotection. *Ment Retard Dev Disabil Res Rev* 2001;7:56–64.

Walsh DS, Adzick NS, Sutton LN, Johnson MP. The rationale for in utero repair of myelomeningocele. *Fetal Diagn Ther* 2001;16:312–322.

Woo CLF, Chuang SH, Becker LE, et al. Radiologic-pathologic correlation in focal cortical dysplasia and hemimegalencephaly in 18 children. *Pediatr Neurol* 2001;25:295–303.

Yakolev PI, Wadsworth RC. Schizencephalies: A study of the congenital clefts in the cerebral mantle. I. Clefts with fused lips. *J Neuropath Exp Neurol* 1946;5:116–130.

Yamanouchi H, Zhang W, Jay V, Becker LE. Enhanced expression of microtubule-associated protein 2 in large neurons of cortical dysplasia. *Ann Neurol* 1996;39:57–61.

Yen IH, Khourg MJ, Erickson JD, et al. The changing epidemiology of neural tube defects. United States, 1968–1989. *Am J Dis Child* 1992;146:857–861.

Yoshida A, Kobayashi K, Manya H, et al. Muscular dystrophy and neuronal migration disorder caused by mutations in a glycosyltransferase, POMGnT1. *Dev Cell* 2001;1:717–724.

Potter CJ, Huang H, Xu T. Drosophila Tsc1 functions with Tsc2 to antagonize insulin signaling in regulating cell growth, cell proliferation, and organ size. *Cell* 2001;105:357–368.

Gao X, Zhang Y, Arrazola P, et al. Tsc tumour suppressor proteins antagonize amino-acid 150;TOR signalling. *Nat Cell Biol* 2002;4:699–704.

Inoki K, Corradetti MN, Guan KL. Dysregulation of the TSC-mTOR pathway in human disease. *Nat Genet* 2005;37:19–24.

Franz DN, Leonard J, Tudor C, et al. Rapamycin causes regression of astrocytomas in tuberous sclerosis complex. *Ann Neurol* 2006;59:490–498.

Tietjen I, Bodell A, Apse K, et al. Comprehensive EMX2 genotyping of a large schizencephaly case series. *Am J Med Genet* 2007;143A:1313–1316.

Roll P, Rudolf G, Pereira S, et al. SRPX2 mutations in disorders of language cortex and cognition. *Hum Molec Genet* 2006; 15:1195–1207.

Smahi A, Courtois G, Vabres P, et al. Genomic rearrangement in NEMO impairs NF-kappaB activation and is a cause of incontinentia pigmenti. The International Incontinentia Pigmenti (IP) Consortium. *Nature* 2000;405(6785):466–472.

Pacheco TR, Levy M, Collyer JC, et al. Incontinentia pigmenti in male patients. *J Am Acad Dermatol* 2006;55(2):251–255. Epub 2006 May 15.

Chapter 21

Abbott R. Sensory rhizotomy for the treatment of childhood spasticity. *J Child Neurol* 1996;11(Suppl l):S36–S42.

Albright AL. Intrathecal baclofen in cerebral palsy movement disorders. *J Child Neurol* 1996;11(Suppl 1):S29–S35.

Albright AL, Ferson SS. Intrathecal baclofen therapy in children. *Neurosurg Focus* 2006;21(2):E3.

American Academy of Pediatrics Committee on Practice and Ambulatory Medicine. Eye examination and vision screening in infants. *Pediatrics* 1996;98:153–157.

American Academy Pediatrics. Year 2000 position statement: Principles and guidelines for early hearing detection and intervention programs. *Pediatrics* 2000;106:798–817.

Aram DM, Eisele JA. Limits to a left hemisphere explanation for specific language impairment. *J Speech Hear Res* 1994; 37:824–830.

Ashwal S, Russman BSBP, Miller G, et al. Parameter: Diagnostic assessment of the child with cerebral palsy. *Neurology* 2004;62:851–863.

Back SA. Recent advances in human perinatal white matter injury. *Prog Brain Res* 2001;132:131–147.

Baric I, Zschocke J, Christensen E, et al. Diagnosis and management of glutaric aciduria type I. J Inherit Metab Dis 1998; 21:326–340.

Barkovich AJ, Kuzniecky RI, Jackson GD, et al. Classification system for malformations of cortical development: Update 2001. *Neurology* 2001;57(12):2168–2178.

Bax MC. Terminology and classification of cerebral palsy *Dev Med Child Neurol* 1964;11:295–297.

Beckung E, Hagberg G. Correlation between ICIDH handicap code and gross motor function classification system in children with cerebral palsy. *Dev Med Child Neurol* 2000;42: 669–673.

Binder H, Eng GD. Rehabilitation management of children with spastic diplegic cerebral palsy. *Arch Phys Med Rehab* 1989;70:482–489.

Blair E, Watson L. Epidemiology of cerebral palsy. *Semin Fetal Neonat Med* 2006;11(2):117–125.

Blasco PA, Allaire JH. Drooling in the developmentally disabled: Management practices and recommendations. Consortium on Drooling. *Dev Med Child Neurol* 1992;34: 849–862.

Blasco PA. Management of drooling: 10 years after the Consortium on Drooling, 1990. *Dev Med Child Neurol* 2002; 44(11):778–781.

Bleck EE. Locomotor prognosis in cerebral palsy. *Dev Med Child Neurol* 1975;17:18–25.

Bleck EE. *Orthopedic management in cerebral palsy*. Oxford: MacKeith Press, 1987.

Bobath B. The very early treatment of cerebral palsy. *Dev Med Child Neurol* 1967;9:373–390.

Boyd R, Graham HK. Objective measurement of clinical findings in the use of botulinum toxin A for the management of children with cerebral palsy. *Eur J Neurol* 1999;6(Suppl 4): S23–S36.

Boyle CA, Yeargin-Allsopp M, Doernberg NS, et al. Prevalence of selected developmental disabilities in children 3–10 years of age: The metropolitan Atlanta developmental disabilities surveillance program, 1991. *MMWR CDC Surveill Summ* 1996;45:1–14.

Breslau N, Staruch KS, Mortimer EA, Jr. Psychological distress in mothers of disabled children. *Am J Dis Child* 1982;136: 682–686.

Bross S, Honeck P, Kwon ST, et al. Correlation between motor function and lower urinary tract dysfunction in patients with infantile cerebral palsy. *Neurourol Urodyn* 2007;26(2):222–227.

Brun A, Kyllerman M. Clinical, pathogenetic and neuropathological correlates in dystonic cerebral palsy. *Eur J Pediatr* 1979;131:93–104.

Calis EAC, Olieman JF, Rieken R, Penning V. Impact of malnutrition on gastrointestinal disorders and gross motor abilities in children with cerebral palsy. *Brain Dev* 2007;29:534.

Candy EJ, Hoon AH, Capute AJ, Bryan RN. MRI in motor delay: Important adjunct to classification of cerebral palsy. *Pediatr Neurol* 1993;9:421–429.

Chambers HG, Weinstein CH, Mubarak SJ, et al. The effect of valproic acid on blood loss in patients with cerebral palsy. *J Pediatr Orthoped* 1999;19:792–795.

Chen YH. Correlations between computerized tomography of the head and motor developmental disturbances of children with cerebral palsy. *Nippon Seikeigeka Gakkai Zasshi* 1981; 55:85–99.

Christodoulou J, Qureshi IA, McInnes RR, Clarke JT. Ornithine transcarbamylase deficiency presenting with strokelike episodes. *J Pediatr* 1993;122:423–425.

Cioni G, Sales B, Paolicelli PB, et al. MRI and clinical characteristics of children with hemiplegic cerebral palsy. *Neuropediatrics* 1999;30:249–255.

Clarke WM, Hoops HR. Predictive measures of speech proficiency in cerebral palsied speakers. *J Commun Disord* 1980; 13:385–394.

Cohen ME, Duffner PK. Prognostic indicators in hemiparetic cerebral palsy. *Ann Neurol* 1981;9:353–357.

Cosgrove AP, Corry IS, Graham HK. Botulinum toxin in the management of the lower limb in cerebral palsy. *Dev Med Child Neurol* 1994;36:386–396.

Crowther CA, Hiller JE, Doyle LW, Haslam RR. Australasian collaborative trial of magnesium Sulphate ACTOMg SO: Effect of magnesium sulfate given for neuroprotection before preterm birth: A randomized controlled trial. *JAMA* 2003; 290:2669–2676.

Doyle LW, Crowther CA, Middleton P, Marret S. Magnesium sulphate for women at risk of preterm birth for neuroprotection of the fetus. *Cochrane Database Syst Rev* 2007; (3):CD004661.

Dunn KW, Cunningham CE, Backman JE. Self-control and reinforcement in the management of a cerebral-palsied adolescent's drooling. *Dev Med Child Neurol* 1987;29:305–310.

Eliasson AC, Krumlinde-Sundholm L, Rosblad B, et al. The Manual Ability Classification System (MACS) for children with cerebral palsy: Scale development and evidence of validity and reliability. *Dev Med Child Neurol* 2006;48(7): 549–554.

Falkman KW, Sandberg AD, Hjelmquist E. Preferred communication modes: Prelinguistic and linguistic communication in non-speaking preschool children with cerebral palsy. *Int J Lang Commun Disord* 2002;37:59–68.

Fehlings D, Rang M, Glazier J, Steele C. An evaluation of botulinum-A toxin injections to improve upper extremity function in children with hemiplegic cerebral palsy. *J Pediatr* 2000;137(3):331–337.

Fennell EB, Dikel TN. Cognitive and neuropsychological functioning in children with cerebral palsy.[erratum appears in *J Child Neurol* 2001;16(3):225]. *J Child Neurol* 2001;16:58–63.

Fisher RL, Russman BS. Genetic syndromes associated with cerebral palsy. *Clin Orthopaed Rel Res* 1974;99:2–11.

Freud S. *Infantile cerebral paralysis*. Miami: University Miami Press, 1968.

Gage JR. The role of gait analysis in the treatment of cerebral palsy. *J Pediatr Orthoped* 1994;14:701–702.

Gibson KM, Christensen E, Jakobs C, et al. The clinical phenotype of succinic semialdehyde dehydrogenase deficiency (4-hydroxybutyric aciduria): Case reports of 23 new patients. *Pediatrics* 1997;99:567–574.

Goldberg MJ. Measuring outcomes in cerebral palsy. *J Pediatr Orthoped* 1991;11:682–685.

Gooch JL, Oberg WA, Grams B, et al. Care provider assessment of intrathecal baclofen in children. *Dev Med Child Neurol* 2004;46(8):548–552.

Graham HK, Harvey A, Rodda J, et al. The Functional Mobility Scale (FMS). *J Pediatr Orthoped* 2004;24(5):514–520.

Grether JK, Cummins SK, Nelson KB. The California Cerebral Palsy Project. *Paediatr Perinat Epidemiol* 1992;6:339–351.

Grether JK, Hoogstrate J, Selvin S, Nelson KB. Magnesium sulfate tocolysis and risk of neonatal death. *Am J Obstetr Gynecol* 1998;178(1 Pt 1):1–6.

Hadden KL, von Baeyer CL. Pain in children with cerebral palsy: Common triggers and expressive behaviors. *Pain* 2002;99(1–2):281–288.

Hadjipanayis A, Hadjichristodoulou C, Youroukos S. Epilepsy in patients with cerebral palsy [comment]. *Dev Med Child Neurol* 1997;39:659–663.

Hagberg B, Hagberg G, Beckung E, Uvebrant P. Changing panorama of cerebral palsy in Sweden. VIII. Prevalence and origin in the birth year period 1991–1994. *Acta Paediatr* 2001;90:271–277.

Hartley LM, Mrcp B, Khwaja OS, et al. Glutaric aciduria type 1 and nonaccidental head injury [comment]. *Pediatrics* 2001;107:174–175.

Hauser SE, Peters H. Glutaric aciduria type 1: An underdiagnosed cause of encephalopathy and dystonia-dyskinesia syndrome in children. *J Paediatr Child Health* 1998;34:302–304.

Haworth JC, Booth FA, Chudley AE, et al. Phenotypic variability in glutaric aciduria type I: Report of fourteen cases in five Canadian Indian kindreds. *J Pediatr* 1991;118:52–58.

Hayakawa K, Kanda T, Hashimoto K, et al. MR imaging of spastic diplegia. The importance of corpus callosum. *Acta Radiol* 1996;37:830–836.

Hemming K, Hutton JL, Pharoah PO. Long-term survival for a cohort of adults with cerebral palsy. *Dev Med Child Neurol* 2006;48(2):90–95.

Himmelmann K, Hagberg G, Beckung E, et al. The changing panorama of cerebral palsy in Sweden. IX. Prevalence and origin in the birth-year period 1995–1998. *Acta Paediatr* 2005;94(3):287–294.

Hodgkinson I, Jindrich ML, Duhaut P, et al. Hip pain in 234 non-ambulatory adolescents and young adults with cerebral palsy: A cross-sectional multicentre study. *Dev Med Child Neurol* 2001;43(12):806–808.

Hughes I, Newton R. Genetic aspects of cerebral palsy [comment]. *Dev Med Child Neurol* 1992;34:80–86.

Hutton JL, Pharoah PO. Life expectancy in severe cerebral palsy. *Arch Dis Child* 2006;91(3):254–258.

Hvidtjorn D, Grove J, Schendel DE, et al. Cerebral palsy among children born after in vitro fertilization: The role of preterm delivery: A population-based, cohort study. *Pediatr* 2006; 118(2):475–482.

Jaw TS, Jong YJ, Sheu RS, et al. Etiology, timing of insult, and neuropathology of cerebral palsy evaluated with magnetic resonance imaging. *J Formos Med Assoc* 1998;97:239–246.

Kaushik A, Agarwal RP, et al. Association of cerebral palsy with epilepsy. *J Indian Med Assoc* 1997;95:552–554.

Kolawole TM, Patel PJ, Mahdi AH. Computed tomographic (CT) scans in cerebral palsy (CP). *Pediatr Radiol* 1989;20: 23–27.

Krageloh-Mann I, Petersen D, Hagberg G, et al. Bilateral spastic cerebral palsy: MRI pathology and origin. Analysis from a representative series of 56 cases [comment]. *Dev Med Child Neurol* 1995;37:379–397.

Kuban KC, Leviton A, Pagano M, et al. Maternal toxemia is associated with reduced incidence of germinal matrix hemorrhage in premature babies. *J Child Neurol* 1992;7:70–76.

Kwong KL, Wong SN, So KT. Epilepsy in children with cerebral palsy. *Pediatr Neurol* 1998;19:31–36.

Kyllerman M, Bager B, Bensch J, et al. Dyskinetic cerebral palsy. I. Clinical categories, associated neurological abnormalities and incidences. *Acta Paediatr Scand* 1982;71:543–550.

Kyllerman M, Skjeldal OH, Lundberg M, et al. Dystonia and dyskinesia in glutaric aciduria type I: Clinical heterogeneity and therapeutic considerations. *Mov Disord* 1994;9:22–30.

Kyllerman M. Dyskinetic cerebral palsy. II. Pathogenetic risk factors and intra-uterine growth. *Acta Paediatr Scand* 1982; 71:551–558.

Lance JW. The control of muscle tone, reflexes, and movement: Robert Wartenberg Lecture. *Neurology* 1980;30:1303–1313.

Lanska DJ, Kryscio RJ. Risk factors for peripartum and postpartum stroke and intracranial venous thrombosis. *Stroke* 2000;31(6):1274–1282.

Lissens W, Vreken P, Barth PG, et al. Cerebral palsy and pyruvate dehydrogenase deficiency: Identification of two new mutations in the E1alpha gene. *Eur J Pediatr* 1999;158:853–857.

Lynch JK, Nelson KB, Curry CJ, Grether JK. Cerebrovascular disorders in children with the factor V Leiden mutation. *J Child Neurol* 2001;16:735–744.

Mandelbaum DD, Paneth N. Pediatric neurology: Cerebral palsy. In: De Vivo DC, Percy AK, eds. *Continuum* 2000;6: 8–30.

McLaughlin J, Bjornson K, Temkin N, et al. Selective dorsal rhizotomy: Meta-analysis of three randomized controlled trials. *Dev Med Child Neurol* 2002;44(1):17–25.

McNeal DM, Hawtrey CE, Wolraich ML, Mapel JR. Symptomatic neurogenic bladder in a cerebral-palsied population. *Dev Med Child Neurol* 1983;25:612–616.

Ment LR, Bada HS, Barnes P, et al. Practice parameter: Neuroimaging of the neonate: Report of the quality standards subcommittee of the American Academy of Neurology and the practice committee of the child neurology society. *Neurology* 2002;58:1726–1738.

Michelsen SI, Uldall P, Kejs AM, Madsen M. Education and employment prospects in cerebral palsy. *Dev Med Child Neurol* 2005;47(8):511–517

Miller G, Cala LA. Ataxic cerebral palsy: Clinico-radiologic correlations. *Neuropediatrics* 1989;20:84–89.

Minear WL. A Classification of cerebral palsy. *Pediatrics* 1956; 18:841.

Mitchell G, McInnes RR. Differential diagnosis of cerebral palsy: Lesch-Nyhan syndrome without self-mutilation. *Can Med Assoc J* 1984;130:1323–1324.

Molteni B, Oleari G, Fedrizzi E, Bracchi M. Relation between CT patterns, clinical findings and etiological factors in children born at term, affected by congenital hemiparesis. *Neuropediatrics* 1987;18:75–80.

Murphy CC, Yeargin-Allsopp M, Decoufle P, Drews CD. Prevalence of cerebral palsy among ten-year-old children in metropolitan Atlanta, 1985 through 1987. *J Pediatr* 1993;123: S13–S20.

Mutch L, Alberman E, Hagberg B, et al. Cerebral palsy epidemiology: Where are we now and where are we going? *Dev Med Child Neurol* 1992;34(6):547–551.

Nelson KB, Ellenberg JH. Antecedents of cerebral palsy. I. Univariate analysis of risks. *Am J Dis Child* 1985;139:1031–1038.

Nelson KB, Grether JK. Can magnesium sulfate reduce the risk of cerebral palsy in very low birthweight infants? *Pediatrics* 1995;95:263–269.

Nelson KB, Lynch JK. Stroke in newborn infants. *Lancet Neurol* 2004;3(3):150–158.

Nelson KB. Can we prevent cerebral palsy? *N Engl J Med* 2003; 349(18):1765–1769.

Nelson KB, Dambrosia JM, Ting TY, Grether JK. Uncertain value of electronic fetal monitoring in predicting cerebral palsy. *N Engl J Med* 1996;334(10):613–618.

Nolan J, Chalkiadis GA, Low J, et al. Anaesthesia and pain management in cerebral palsy. *Anaesthesia* 2000;55(1):32–41.

Nwaobi OM, Brubaker CE, Cusick B, Sussman MD. Electromyographic investigation of extensor activity in cerebral-palsied children in different seating positions. *Dev Med Child Neurol* 1983;25:175–183.

O'Grady RS, Nishimura DM, Kohn JG, Bruvold WH. Vocational predictions compared with present vocational status of 60 young adults with cerebral palsy. *Dev Med Child Neurol* 1985;27:775–784.

O'Shea M, Savitz DA, Hage ML, Feinstein KA. Prenatal events and the risk of subependymal/intraventricular haemorrhage in very low birthweight neonates. *Paediatr Perinat Epidemiol* 1992;6:352–362.

Okumura A, Kato T, Kuno K, et al. MRI findings in patients with spastic cerebral palsy. II: Correlation with type of cerebral palsy. *Dev Med Child Neurol* 1997;39:369–372.

Ozturk M, Oktem F, Kisioglu N, et al. Bladder and bowel control in children with cerebral palsy: Case-control study. *Croat Med J* 2006;47(2):264–270.

Palisano R, Rosenbaum P, Walter S, et al. Development and reliability of a system to classify gross motor function in children with cerebral palsy. *Dev Med Child Neurol* 1997;39: 214–223.

Palmer FB, Shapiro BK, Allen MC, et al. Infant stimulation curriculum for infants with cerebral palsy: Effects on infant temperament, parent-infant interaction, and home environment. *Pediatrics* 1990;85(3 Pt 2):411–415.

Palmer FB, Shapiro BK, Wachtel RC, et al. The effects of physical therapy on cerebral palsy. A controlled trial in infants with spastic diplegia. *N Engl J Med* 1988;318:803–808.

Pantaleoni C, D'Arrigo S, D'Incerti L, et al. A case of 3-methylglutaconic aciduria misdiagnosed as cerebral palsy. *Pediatr Neurol* 2000;23:442–444.

Pape KE, Kirsch SE, Galil A, et al. Neuromuscular approach to the motor deficits of cerebral palsy: A pilot study. *J Pediatr Orthoped* 1993;13:628–633.

Patrick J, Boland M, Stoski D, Murray GE. Rapid correction of wasting in children with cerebral palsy. *Dev Med Child Neurol* 1986;28:734–739.

Pope JE, Curzon ME. The dental status of cerebral palsied children. *Pediatr Dent* 1991;13:156–162.

Pranzatelli MR. Oral pharmacotherapy for the movement disorders of cerebral palsy. *J Child Neurol* 1996;11:S22.

Prasad AN, Breen JC, Ampola MG, Rosman NP. Argininemia: A treatable genetic cause of progressive spastic diplegia simulating cerebral palsy: Case reports and literature review. *J Child Neurol* 1997;12:301–309.

Raina P, O'Donnell M, Rosenbaum P, et al. The health and well-being of caregivers of children with cerebral palsy. *Pediatrics* 2005;115(6):E626–E636.

Rang MSRGI. Cerebral palsy. In: Lovell WR, ed. *Pediatric orthopedics*. Philadelphia: Lippincott Co., 1986.

Rapp D. Drool control: Long-term follow-up. *Dev Med Child Neurol* 1980;22:448–453.

Reilly S, Skuse D, Poblete X. Prevalence of feeding problems and oral motor dysfunction in children with cerebral palsy: A community survey. *J Pediatr* 1996;129:877–882.

Rogers B. Feeding method and health outcomes of children with cerebral palsy. *J Pediatr* 2004;145(2 Suppl):S28–S32.

Ros HS, Lichtenstein P, Bellocco R, et al. Pulmonary embolism and stroke in relation to pregnancy: How can high-risk women be identified? *Am J Obstetr Gynecol* 2002;186(2): 198–203.

Rosenbaum P, Paneth N, Leviton A, et al. A report: The definition and classification of cerebral palsy April 2006.[erratum appears in *Dev Med Child Neurol Suppl* 2007;49(6):480. *Dev Med Child Neurol Suppl* 2007;109:8–14.

Rosenbloom L. Dyskinetic cerebral palsy and birth asphyxia [comment]. *Dev Med Child Neurol* 1994;36:285–289.

Sanger TD, Delgado MR, Gaebler-Spira D, et al. Classification and definition of disorders causing hypertonia in childhood. *Pediatr* 2003;111(1):E89–E97.

Sanner G, Hagberg B. 188 cases of non-progressive ataxic syndromes in childhood. Aspects of aetiology and classification. *Neuropadiatrie* 1974;5:224–235.

Schenk-Rootlieb AJ, van Nieuwenhuizen O, van der Graaf Y, et al. The prevalence of cerebral visual disturbance in children with cerebral palsy. *Dev Med Child Neurol* 1992;34: 473–480.

Senner JE, Logemann J, Zecker S, Gaebler-Spira D. Drooling, saliva production, and swallowing in cerebral palsy. *Dev Med Child Neurol* 2004;46(12):801–806.

Shapiro BK, Green P, Krick J, et al. Growth of severely impaired children: Neurological versus nutritional factors. *Dev Med Child Neurol* 1986;28:729–733.

Shaw BNJ. The respiratory consequences of neurological deficit. In: Sullivan RL, ed. *Feeding the Disabled Child.* New York: Cambridge University Press;1996:40–46.

Smith WE, Millington DS, Koeberl DD, Lesser PS. Glutaric acidemia, type I, missed by newborn screening in an infant with dystonia following promethazine administration. *Pediatrics* 2001;107:1184–1187.

Sochaniwskyj AE, Koheil RM, Bablich K, et al. Oral motor functioning, frequency of swallowing and drooling in normal children and in children with cerebral palsy. *Arch Phys Med Rehab* 1986;67:866–874.

Stallings VA, Charney EB, Davies JC, Cronk CE. Nutritional status and growth of children with diplegic or hemiplegic cerebral palsy. *Dev Med Child Neurol* 1993;35:997–1006.

Straussberg R, Brand N, Gadoth N. 3-Methyl glutaconic aciduria in Iraqi Jewish children may be misdiagnosed as cerebral palsy. *Neuropediatrics* 1998;29:54–56.

Sugimoto T, Woo M, Nishida N, et al. When do brain abnormalities in cerebral palsy occur? An MRI study [comment]. *Dev Med Child Neurol* 1995;37:285–292.

Sullivan PB, Lambert B, Rose M, et al. Prevalence and severity of feeding and nutritional problems in children with neurological impairment: Oxford Feeding Study [comment]. *Dev Med Child Neurol* 2000;42:674–680.

Suskind DL, Tilton A. Clinical study of botulinum-A toxin in the treatment of sialorrhea in children with cerebral palsy. *Laryngoscope* 2002;112:73–81.

Swaiman KF. Cerebral palsy. In: Swaiman AS, ed., CV. *Pediatric neurology.* St Louis: Mosby;1999:312–324.

Taudorf K, Melchior JC, Pedersen H. CT findings in spastic cerebral palsy. Clinical, aetiological and prognostic aspects. *Neuropediatrics* 1984;15:120–124.

Trauner DA, Ballantyne A, Friedland S, Chase C. Disorders of affective and linguistic prosody in children after early unilateral brain damage. *Ann Neurol* 1996;39:361–367.

Truwit CL, Barkovich AJ, Koch TK, Ferriero DM. Cerebral palsy: MR findings in 40 patients [comment]. *AJNR Am J Neuroradiol* 1992;13(1):67–78.

Uvebrant P, Carlsson G. Speech in children with cerebral palsy [comment]. *Acta Paediatr* 1994;83:779.

Van der Burg JJ, Jongerius PH, Van Hulst K, et al. Drooling in children with cerebral palsy: Effect of salivary flow reduction on daily life and care. *Dev Med Child Neurol* 2006; 48(2):103–107.

Van Naarden K, Decoufle P, Caldwell K. Prevalence and characteristics of children with serious hearing impairment in metropolitan Atlanta, 1991–1993 [comment]. *Pediatrics* 1999;103:570–575.

von Wendt L, Rantakallio P, Saukkonen AL, et al. Cerebral palsy and additional handicaps in a 1-year birth cohort from northern Finland: A prospective follow-up study to the age of 14 years. *Ann Clin Res* 1985;17:156–161.

Wallace SJ. Epilepsy in cerebral palsy. *Dev Med Child Neurol* 2001;43:713–717.

Waterman ET, Koltai PJ, Downey JC, Cacace AT. Swallowing disorders in a population of children with cerebral palsy. *Int J Pediatr Otorhinolaryngol* 1992;24:63–71.

Weiss H, Betts HB. Methods of rehabilitation in children with neuromuscular disorders. *Pediatr Clin North Am* 1967;14: 1009–1016.

Wiklund LM, Uvebrant P, Flodmark O. Computed tomography as an adjunct in etiological analysis of hemiplegic cerebral palsy; II: Children born at term. *Neuropediatrics* 1991;22: 121–128.

Wiklund LM, Uvebrant P. Hemiplegic cerebral palsy: Correlation between CT morphology and clinical findings. *Dev Med Child Neurol* 1991;33:512–523.

Willis TA, Davidson J, Gray RG, et al. Cytochrome oxidase deficiency presenting as birth asphyxia. *Dev Med Child Neurol* 2000;42:414–417.

Wood E, Rosenbaum P. The gross motor function classification system for cerebral palsy: A study of reliability and stability over time. *Dev Med Child Neurol* 2000;42:292–296.

Worley G, Houlihan CM, Herman-Giddens ME, et al. Secondary sexual characteristics in children with cerebral palsy and moderate to severe motor impairment: A cross-sectional survey. *Pediatrics* 2002;110:897–902.

Wu YW, Day SM, Strauss DJ, Shavelle RM. Prognosis for ambulation in cerebral palsy: A population-based study. *Pediatrics* 2004;114(5):1264–1271.

Yamada K, Itoh M, Fueki N, et al. The cranial MRI in severe cerebral palsy: A comparative study with clinical data. [Japanese]. *No to Hattatsu. [Brain Dev]* 1993;25:435–441.

Yang TF, Fu CP, Kao NT, et al. Effect of botulinum toxin type A on cerebral palsy with upper limb spasticity. *Am J Phys Med Rehab* 2003;82(4):284–289.

Yin R, Reddihough D, Ditchfield M, Collins K. Magnetic resonance imaging findings in cerebral palsy. *J Paediatr Child Health* 2000;36:139–144.

Yokochi K, Aiba K, Horie M, et al. Magnetic resonance imaging in children with spastic diplegia: Correlation with the severity of their motor and mental abnormality. *Dev Med Child Neurol* 1991;33:18–25.

Yokochi K, Aiba K, Kodama M, Fujimoto S. Magnetic resonance imaging in athetotic cerebral palsied children. *Acta Paediatr Scand* 1991;80:818–823.

Zafeiriou DI, Kontopoulos EE, Tsikoulas I. Characteristics and prognosis of epilepsy in children with cerebral palsy. *J Child Neurol* 1999;14:289–294.

Chapter 22

Aram DM, Horwitz SU. Sequential and non-speech praxic abilities in developmental verbal apraxia. *Dev Med Child Neurol* 1983;25:197–206.

Bender L. Visual Motor Gestalt Test. New York: American Orthopsychiatric Association, 1946.

Benton AL. The revised visual retention test. New York: Psychological Corporation, 1974.

Buxbaum LJ, et al. Naturalistic action and praxis in callosal apraxia. *Neurocase* 1995;1:3–17.

Croce R, Horvat M, McCarthy E. Reliability and concurrent validity of the movement assessment battery (MAB-C) for children. *Percept Mot Skills* 2001;93:275–280.

Crothers B, Paine ES. The natural history of cerebral palsy. Cambridge, MA: Harvard University Press, 1959.

David R, et al. Proposed nosology of disorders of higher cerebral function in children. Minneapolis, MN: Task Force on Nosology Child Neurology Society, 1981.

Denckla MB, Rudel RG. Anomalies of motor development in hyperactive boys. *Ann Neurol* 1978;3:231–233.

Denckla MB. Revised neurological examination for subtle signs. *Psychopharm Bull* 1985;21:773–800.

DeRenzi E, Motti F, Nichelli P. Imitation of gestures. A quantitative approach to ideomotor apraxia. *Arch Neurol* 1980;37: 6–10.

DeRenzi E, Pieczuro A, Vignolo LA. Ideational apraxia: A quantitative study. *Neuropsychologia* 1968;6:41–52.

Deuel RK, Rauchway AC. The neurological examination of the school age and adolescent child. In: David, RB ed., *Child and adolescent neurology*, 2nd ed. St Louis: Mosby, 2005.

Deuel RK, Robinson DJ. Developmental motor signs. In: Tupper DE, ed. *Soft neurological signs*. New York: Grune & Stratton, 987:95–129.

Deuel RK. Loss of motor habits after cortical lesions. *Neuropsychologica* 1977;15:205–215.

Deuel RK. Minimal brain dysfunction: Hyperkinesis, learning disabilities, attention deficit disorder. *J Pediatr* 1981;98:912–915.

Deuel RK. Motor skill disorders. In: Hooper S, Hynd G, Mattison R, eds. *Developmental disorders: Diagnostic criteria and clinical assessment*. Hillsdale, NJ: Earlbaum, 1992:239–281.

Dewey D, Kaplan BJ, Crawford SG, Wilson BN. Developmental coordination disorder: Associated problems in attention, learning, and psychosocial adjustment. *Human Mov Sci* 2002;21:905–918.

Dewey D, Wilson BN. Developmental coordination disorder: What is it? *Phys Occup Ther Pediatr* 2001;20:5–27.

Estil LB, Ingvaldsen RP, Whiting HTA. Spatial and temporal constraints on performance in children with motor coordination problems. *Exp Brain Res* 2002;147:153–161.

Fog E, Fog M. Cerebral inhibition examined by associated movements. *Clin Dev Med* 1963;10:52–57.

Ford F. *Diseases of the nervous system in infancy, childhood and adolescence*. Springfield, IL: Charles C Thomas, 1960.

Frei H. Die "ungeschickte" Kind: Differential Diagnose und therapieindikationen. *Schweiz Med Wochenschr* 1986;116: 294–299.

Geschwind N, Damasio A. Apraxia. In: Fredriks AM, ed. *Handbook of clinical neurology*, Vol. 45: Clinical neuropsychology. Amsterdam: Elsevier/North Holland, 1985:7–22.

Green D, Baird G, Barnett AL, Henderson L. The severity and nature of motor impairment in Asperger's Syndrome: A comparison with specific developmental disorder of motor function. *J Child Psychol Psychiatry* 2002;43:655–668.

Gubbay SS. The clumsy child: A study of developmental apraxia and agnostic ataxia. Philadelphia: WB Saunders, 1975.

Hagberg B, Aicardi J, Dias K, Ramos O. A progressive syndrome of autism, dementia, ataxia and loss of purposeful hand use in girls: Rett's syndrome. *Ann Neurol* 1983;14: 471–479.

Hammill DD, Larson SC. *The test of written language*, 3rd ed. (TOWL-3). Austin, TX: ProEd, 1996.

Hollander E, Weiller F, Cohen L, et al. Neurological soft signs in social phobia. *Neuropsychiatry Neuropsychol Behav Neurol* 1996;9:182–185.

Iloeji SO. Developmental apraxia among Nigerian children in Enugu, Nigeria. *Dev Med Child Neurol* 1987;29:502–507.

Jabbour J. Subacute sclerosing panencephalitis: A multidisciplinary study of eight cases. *JAMA* 1969;207:2248–2254.

Johnston LM, Burns YR, Brauer SG, Richardson CA. Differences in postural control and movement performance during goal directed reaching in children with developmental coordination disorder. *Hum Mov Sci* 2002;21:583–601.

Johnston R, Stark RE, Mellits ED, Tallal P. Neurological status of language impaired and normal children. *Ann Neurol* 1981;10:159–165.

Kaufman AS and Kaufman N. Manual. *Kaufman Assessment Battery for Children* 2nd ed. (KABC II). Shoreview, MN, 2004, American Guidance Service.

Kleist K. *Gehirnpathology*. Leipzig: Barth, 1934.

Knuckey NW, Gubbay SS. Clumsy children: A prognostic study. *Aust Paediatr J* 1983;19:9–13.

Lacks F. *Bender-Gestalt screening for brain dysfunction*, 2nd ed. New York: Wiley, 1999.

Lai CS, Fisher SE, Hurst JA, et al. A novel forkhead-domain gene is mutated in a severe speech and language disorder. *Nature* 2001;413:519–523.

Liepmann H. Das Krankheitsbild der Apraxie. *Monographie Monatsschr Psychiatr Neurol (Berlin)* 1900;8:15–44, 102–132, 182–197.

MaKuuchi M, Kaminaga T, Sugishita M. Both parietal lobes are involved in drawing: An fMRI study and implications for constructional apraxia. *Brain Res Cogn Brain Res* 2003;16: 338–347.

McHale K, Cermak SA. Fine motor activities in elementary school: Preliminary findings and provisional implications for children with fine motor problems. *Am J Occup Ther* 1992; 46:898–903.

Menkes JH, Sarnat HB, Maria BL, editors. *Child Neurology*, 7th ed. Philadelphia, 2006, Lippincott Williams & Wilkins.

Myers SM, Johnson CP, and the Council on Children with Disabilities. Management of children with autism spectrum disorders. *Pediatrics* 2007;120:1162–1182.

Nichols PL. Minimal brain dysfunction and soft signs: The Collaborative Perinatal Project. In: Tupper DE, ed. *Soft neurological signs*. New York: Grune & Stratton, 1987:179–199.

Orton ST. "Word blindness" in school children. *Arch Neurol Psychiatry* 1925;14:581–615.

Percy A, Kaback MM, Herndon RM. Metachromatic leukodystrophy: A comparison of early and late onset forms. *Neurology* 1977;27:933–944.

Poeck K. The clinical examination for motor apraxia. *Neuropsychologia* 1986;24:129–143.

Pyfer JL, Castelman BR. Characteristic motor development of children with learning disabilities. *Percept Motor Skills* 1972;35:291–296.

Rasmussen P. Persistent mirror movements: A clinical study of 17 children, adolescents and young adults. *Dev Med Child Neurol* 1993;82:699–707.

Rosenblum, S. The development and standardization of the Children Activity Scales (ChAS-PT) for the early identification of children with Developmental Coordination Disorders. *Child: Care, Health, and Development* 2006;32:619–632.

Schmitz C, Martineau J, Barthelemy C, Assaiante C. Motor control and children with autism: Deficit of anticipatory function? *Neurosci Lett* 2003;348:17–20.

Segal R, Mandich A, Polatajko H, Cook JV. Stigma and its management: A pilot study of parental perceptions of the experiences of children with developmental coordination disorder. *Am J Occup Ther* 2002;56:422–428.

Todor JI, Lazarus JA. Exertion level and the intensity of associated movements. *Dev Med Child Neurol* 1986;28:205–212.

Vaivre-Douret L. Non-verbal learning disabilities: Developmental dyspraxia. *Arch Pediatr* 2007;14:1334–1339.

Voeller K. Clinical neurologic aspects of the right-hemisphere deficit syndrome. *J Child Neurol* 1995;10:S16–22.

Walsh W, Bruce E, Betz N. *Tests and assessment*, 2nd ed. Englewood Cliffs NJ: Prentice Hall, 1990.

Wilson PH, Thomas PR, Maruff P. Motor imagery training ameliorates motor clumsiness in children. *J Child Neurol* 2002; 17:491–498.

Wolff H, Gunnoe CE, Cohen C. Associated movements as a measure of developmental age. *Dev Med Child Neurol* 1983; 25:417–429.

Chapter 23

Achenbach TM, Rescorla L. *Manual for the preschool child behavior checklist and revised child behavior profile*. Burlington VT: University Associates in Psychiatry, 2000.

Alarcon M, Cantor RM, Liu J, et al., Autism Genetic Research Exchange Consortium. Evidence for a language quantitative trait locus on chromosome 7q in multiplex autism families. *Am J Hum Genet* 2002;70:60–71.

Allen CW, Silove N, Williams K, Hutchins P. Validity of the social communication questionnaire in assessing risk of autism in preschool children with developmental problems. *J Autism Dev Dis* 2007;37(7):1272–1278.

American Psychiatric Association. *Diagnostic and statistical manual of mental disorders*, 4th ed. DSM-IV TR text revised. Washington, DC: Author, 2000.

Anderson AJ. Sensory Integration and Praxis Tests (SIPT). Los Angeles: Western Psychological Services, 2003.

Anderson, DK, Lord C, Risi S, DiLavore PS, Shulman C, Thurm A, Welch K, Picles A. Patterns of growth in verbal abilities among children with autism spectrum disorder. *Journal of Consulting & Clinical Psychology*. 75(4):594–604, 2007.

Barkley RA. *Attention-deficit hyperactivity disorder: A handbook for diagnosis and treatment*, 2nd ed. New York: Guilford Press, 1998.

Beery K, Buktenica N. *Beery Developmental Test of Visual-Motor Integration*, 4th ed. Lutz, FL: Psychological Assessment Resources, Inc., 2003.

Behar, L. The preschool behavior questionnaire. *J Abnorm Child Psychol* 1977;5:265–276.

Beitchman JH, Wilson B, Johnson CJ, et al. Fourteen-year follow-up of speech/language-impaired and control children. psychiatric outcome. *J Am Acad Child Adolesc Psychiatry* 2001;40:75–82.

Bernat B, Altman N. Speech delay in children: A functional MR imaging study. *Radiology* 2003;229:651–658.

Bishop D, Norbury C. Exploring the borderlands of autistic disorder and specific language impairment: A study using standardized instruments. *J Child Psychol Psychiatry* 2002;43: 917–929.

Bishop DVM, Clarkson B. Written language as a window into residual language deficits: A study of children with persistent and residual speech and language impairments. *Cortex* 2003; 39:215–237.

Bloom B, Cohen RA. Summary health statistics for U.S. children: National Health Interview Survey 2006. *Vital Health Stat* 2007;10(234):1–79.

Bolton P. Neuroepileptic correlates of autistic symptomology in tuberous sclerosis. *Ment Retard Dev Disabil* 2004;10:126–131.

Braun JM, Kahn RS, Froehlich T, et al. Exposures to environmental toxicants and attention deficit hyperactivity disorder in U.S. children.*Environ Health Perspect* 2006;114(12): 1904–1909.

Campbell SB, Breaux A, Ewing L, Szumowski E. A one year follow-up study of patient referred hyperactive preschool children. *J Am Acad Child Psychiatry* 1984;23:243–249.

Campbell SB. *Behavior problems in preschoolers: Clinical and developmental issues*. New York: Guilford Press, 1990.

Carroll JM, Snowling MJ. Language and phonological skills in children at high risk of reading difficulties. *J Child Psych Psychiatry* 2004;45(3):631–640.

Casanova MF, van Kooten IAJ, Switala AE, et al. Minicolumnar abnormalities in autism. *Acta Neuropathol (Berl)* 2006; 112(3):287–303.

Casey BJ, Nigg JT, Durston S. New potential leads in the biology and treatment of attention deficit-hyperactivity disorder. *Curr Opin Neurol* 2007;20(2):119–124.

Cederlund M, Hagberg B, Billstedt E, Gillbeg IC, Gillberg C. Asperger syndrome and autism: a comparative longitudinal follow-up study more than 5 years after original diagnosis. *Journal of Autism & Developmental Disorders*. 38(1):72–85, 2008.

Centers for Disease Control. Parental report of diagnosed autism in children aged 4–

Choudhury N, Benasich AA. A family aggregation study: The influence of family history and other risk factors on language development. *J Speech Lang Hearing Res* 2003;46(2):261–272.

Clark M, Plante E. Morphology of the inferior frontal gyrus in developmentally language-disordered adults. *Brain Lang* 1998;61:288–303.

Coates SW. *Preschool embedded figures test*. Palo Alto, CA: Consulting Psychologists Press, 1972.

Conners CK. Conners' rating scales-revised user's manual – 3. North Tonawanda, NY: Multi-Health Systems Inc., 2008.

Constantino J. Social Responsiveness Scale (SRS). Los Angeles: Western Psychological Services, 2005.

Conti-Ramsden G, Botting N, Simkin Z, Knox E. Follow-up of children attending infant language units: outcomes at 11 years of age. *Int J Lang Commun Disord* 2001;36:207–219.

Cummins A, Piek JP, Dyck MJ. Motor coordination, empathy, and social behaviour in school-aged children. *Dev Med Child Neurol* 2007;47:437–442.

Dapretto M, Davies MS, Pfeifer JH, et al. Understanding emotions in others: mirror neuron dysfunction in children with autism spectrum disorders. *Nature Neurosci* 2006;9(1):28–30.

Dawson G. Quantitative assessment of autism symptom-related traits in probands and parents: Broader Phenotype Autism Symptom Scale. *J Autism Dev Dis* 2007;37(3):523–536.

De Bildt A, Systema S, Ketelaars C, et al. Interrelationship between ADOS-G, ADI-R, and the DSM-IV-TR classification in children and adolescents with mental retardation. *J Autism Dev Dis* 2004;34:129–137.

De Fosse L, Hodge S, Makris N, et al. Language association cortex asymmetry in autism and specific language impairment. *Ann Neurol* 2004;56:757–766.

Deuel RK. Developmental dysgraphia and motor skills disorders. *J Child Neurol* 1995;10(Suppl 1):S1–8.

Drummond CR, Ahmad SA, Rourke BP. Rules for the classification of younger children with nonverbal learning disabilities and basic phonological processing disabilities. *Arch Clin Neuropsychol* 2005;20(2):171–182.

DuPaul GJ, McGoey KE, Eckert TL, VanBrakle J. Preschool children with attention-deficit/hyperactivity disorder: Impairments in behavioral, social, and school functioning. *J Am Acad Child Adolesc Psychiatry* 2001;40:508–515.

Dyck MJ, Hay D, Anderson M, et al. Is the discrepancy criterion for defining development coordination disorders valid? *Child Psychol Psychiatry* 2004;45: 979–995.

Fombonne E, Zakarian R, Bennett A, et al. Pervasive developmental disorders: A case-control study. *Lancet* 2004;364: 963–969.

Fombonne E, Tidmarsh L. Epidemiologic data on Asperger disorder. *Child Adolesc Psychiatric Clin North Am* 2003;12:15–21.

Foundas AL, Bollich AM, Corey DM, et al. Anomalous anatomy of speech-language areas in adults with persistent developmental stuttering. *Neurology* 2001;57:207–215.

Gadow KD, Sprafkin J. *Early childhood inventory-4 screening manual*. Stony Brook, NY: Checkmate Plus, 2000.

Gaines R. Missiuna C. Early identification: Are speech/language-impaired toddlers at increased risk for developmental coordination disorder? *Child Care Health Dev* 2007;33(3): 325–332.

Gemignani A, Di Stephano M, Sebastiani L, et al. *Archives Italiennes de Biologie* 2004;142:1–9.

Gemignani A, DiStefano M, Sebastiani L, Ghelarducci B, Jeannerod M, Guazzelli M, Massarelli R. Influence of mental motor imagery on the execution of a finger-to-thumb opposition task. *Italiennes de Biologie*. 142(1)1–9, 2004.

Geuze R, Jongmans M, Schoemaker M, Smits-Engelsmand B. Clinical and research diagnostic criteria for developmental coordination disorder: A review and discussion. *Hum Mov Sci* 2001;20:7–47.

Gimenez M, Junque C, Narberhaus A, et al. White matter volume and concentration reductions in adolescents with history of very preterm birth: A voxel-based morphometry study. *Neuroimage* 2006;32(4):1485–1498.

Gotham K, Risi S, Pickles A, Lord C. The Autism Diagnostic Observation Schedule: Revised algorithms for improved diagnostic validity. *J Autism Dev Dis* 2007;37(4):613–627.

Grandin T. *Thinking in pictures*. New York: Vintage Press, 1995.

Guerreiro MM, Hage SR, Guimaraes CA, et al. Developmental language disorder associated with polymicrogyria. *Neurology* 2002;59:245–250.

Hadders-Algra M. The distinct forms of minor neurologic dysfunction: Perspectives emerging from a review of the data of the Groningen Perinatal Project. *Dev Med Child Neurol* 2002;44:561–571.

Hall N. Developmental language disorders. *Semin Pediatr Neurol* 1997;4:77–85.

Handleman J, Harris S. *Preschool education programs for children with autism*. Austin TX: Pro-Ed, 2001.

Herbert MR, Ziegler DA, Deutsch CK, et al. Brain asymmetries in autism and developmental language disorders: A nested whole brain analysis. *Brain* 2005;128:213–226.

Herbert MR, Ziegler DA, Makris N, et al. Localization of white matter volume increase in autism and developmental language disorder. *Ann Neurol* 2004;55(4):530–540.

Honda H, Shimizu Y, Imai M, Nitto Y. Cumulative incidence of childhood autism: A total population study of better accuracy and precision. *Dev Med Child Neurol* 2005;47:10–18.

Honey E, Leekam S, Turner M, McConachie H. Repetitive behaviour and play in typically developing children and children with autism spectrum disorders. *J Autism Dev Dis* 2007;37(6):1107–1115.

Hudziak JJ, Derks EM, Althoff RR, et al. The genetic and environmental contributions to attention deficit hyperactivity disorder as measured by the Conners' Rating Scales—Revised. *Am J Psychiatry* 2005;162(9):1614–1620.

Isaacs EB, Edmonds CJ, Chong WK, et al. Brain morphometry and IQ measurements in preterm children. *Brain* 2004; 127:2595–2607.

Johnson CP, Scott MM, Council on children with disabilities. Identification and evaluation of children with autism spectrum disorders. *Pediatrics* 2007;120:1183–1215.

Kadesjo B, Gillberg C. Developmental coordination disorder in Swedish 7–year-old children. *Am Acad Child Adolesc Psychiatry* 1999;38:820–828.

Kadesjö C, Kadesjö B, Hägglöf B, Gillberg C. ADHD in Swedish 3– to 7–year-old children. *J Am Acad Child Adolesc Psychiatry* 2001;40:101–1028.

Lahey BB, Hartung C, Loney J, et al. Are there sex differences in the predictive validity of DSM-IV ADHD among younger children? *J Clin Child Adolesce Psychol* 2007;36(2):113–126.

Landgren M, Kjellman B, Gillberg C. Deficits in attention, motor control and perception (DAMP): A simplified school entry examination. *Acta Paediatr* 2000;89:302–309.

Langley K, Holmans PA, van den Bree MBM, Thapar A Effects of low birth weight, maternal smoking in pregnancy and social class on the phenotypic manifestation of attention deficit hyperactivity disorder and associated antisocial behaviour: Investigation in a clinical sample. *BMC Psychiatry* 2007;7:26.

Lasky-Su J, Biederman J, Laird N, et al. Evidence for an association of the dopamine D5 receptor gene on age at onset of attention deficit hyperactivity disorder. *Ann Hum Genetics* 2007;71(Pt 5):648–659.

Le Couteur A, Lord C, Rutter M. The Autism Diagnostic Interview-Revised (ADI-R). Los Angeles:, Western Psychological Services, 2003.

Liegeios F, Baldeweg T, Connelly A, et al. Language fMRI abnormalities associated with FOXP2 gene mutation. *Nat Neurosci* 2003;11:1230–1236.

Logan KJ. The effect of syntactic structure upon speech initiation times of stuttering and nonstuttering speakers. *J Fluency Disord* 2003;28:17–35.

Lord C, Shulman C, DiLavore P. Regression and word loss in ASD. *J Child Psychol Psychiatry* 2004;45:936–955.

Maccoby E, Hagen JW. Effect of distortion upon central vs. incidental recall: Developmental trends. *J Exp Child Psychol* 1965;2:280–289.

Macnab JJ, Miller L, Polatajkoc H. The search for subtypes of developmental coordination disorder: Is cluster analysis the answer? *Hum Mov Sci* 2001;20:49–72.

Magalhaes L, Missiuna C, Wong S. Terminology used in research reports of developmental coordination disorders. *Dev Med Child Neurol* 2006;48: 937–941.

Mahone EM, Hoffman J. Behavior ratings of executive function among preschoolers with ADHD. *Clin Neuropsychol* 2007; 21:569–586.

McGee R, Partridge F, Williams SB, Silva PA. A twelve year follow-up of preschool hyperactive children. *J Am Acad Child Psychiatry* 1991;30:224–232.

McVicar KA, Ballaban-Gil K, Rapin I, et al. Epileptiform EEG abnormalities in children with language regression. Neurology 2005;65(1):129–131.

Merin N, Young GS, Ozonoff S, Rogers SJ. Subgroup of 6–month-old infants at-risk for autism from comparison infants. *J Autism Dev Dis* 2007;37(1):108–121.

Mesman J, Koot H. Early preschool predictors of preadolescent internalizing and externalizing DSM-IV diagnoses. *Am Acad Child Adolesc Psychiatry* 2001;40:1029–1036.

Miller L. Miller Assessment for Preschoolers (MAP). Los Angeles: Western Psychological Services, 2003.

Moeller MP, Hoover B, Putman C, et al. Vocalizations of infants with hearing loss compared with infants with normal hearing: Part I–phonetic development. Ear Hearing 2007b;28(5): 605–627.

Nass R, Crino P. TSC. A tale of two genes. *Neurology* 2008; 18;70(12):904–905.

Nass R, Leventhal F. Autistic spectrum disorders. In: Rizzo M, Eslinger P, eds. *Principles and practice of behavioral neurology and neuropsychology*. New York: Saunders, 2004.

Nelson NW. *Childhood Language disorders in context: Infancy through adolescence*. New York: Macmillan, 1993.

Neuman RJ, Lobos E, Reich W, Henderson CA, Sun, L. Prenatal smoking exposure and dopaminergic genotypes interact to cause a severe ADHD subtype. *Biological Psychiatry*. 61(12):1320–1328, 2007.

Nosarti C, Al-Asady M, Frangou S, et al. Adolescents who were born very preterm have decreased brain volumes. *Brain* 2002;125:1616–1623.

Palfrey J, Levin M, Walker D, Sullivan M. The emergence of attention deficit disorder in early childhood. *J Behav Dev Pediatr* 1985;6:339–348.

Pearce PS, Darwish HZ, Gaines BH. Visual symbol and manual sign learning by children with phonologic programming deficit syndrome. *Dev Med Child Neurol* 1987;29:743–750.

Plante E, Boliek C, Mahendra N, et al. Right hemisphere contribution to developmental language disorder: Neuroanatomical and behavioral evidence. *J Commun Disord* 2001;34:415–436.

Polancyk G, de Lima HS, Horta BL, et al. The worldwide prevalence of ADHD: A systematic review and meta regression analysis. *Am J Psychiatry* 2007;164;942–948.

Posner K, Melvin GA, Murray DW, et al. Clinical presentation of attention-deficit/hyperactivity disorder in preschool children. *Psychophamacol* 2007;17(5):547–562.

Preis S, Steinmetz H, Knorr U, Jancke L. Corpus callosum size in children with developmental language disorder. *Cogn Brain Res* 2000;10:37–44.

Rescorla L. Ross GS. McClure S. Language delay and behavioral/emotional problems in toddlers: findings from two developmental clinics. *J Speech Lang Hearing Res* 2007;50(4): 1063–1078.

Rescorla L. Language and reading outcomes to age 9 in late-talking toddlers. *J Speech Lang Hearing Res* 2002;45:360–371.

Richman N, Stevenson J, Graham PJ. *Preschool to school: A behavioural study*. London: Academic Press, 1982.

Rizzolatti G, Fadiga L, Fogassi L, Gallese V. From mirror neurons to imitation: Facts and speculations. In: Meltzoff A, Prinz W, eds. *The imitative mind: Development, evolution and brain bases*. Cambridge: Cambridge University Press, 2002:247–290.

Robins D, Fein D, Barton M, Green J. The modified checklist for toddlers. *J Autism Dev Disord* 2001;31:131–144.

Rogers S, Hepburn S, Wehner F. Parents reports of sensory symptoms in toddlers with autism and those with other developmental disorders. *J Autism Dev Disord* 2003;33:631–642.

Rogers S. Developmental regression in ASD. *Ment Retard Dev Disabil* 2004;10:139–143.

Ross G, Lipper E, Auld PAM. Cognitive abilities and early precursors of learning disabilities in very-low-birthweight children with normal intelligence and normal neurological status. *Int J Behav Dev* 1996;19:563–580.

Rutherford MD, Young GS, Hepburn S, Rogers SJ. A longitudinal study of pretend play in autism. *J Autism Dev Dis* 2007;37(6):1024–1039.

Rutter M, Bailey A, Lord C. Social Communication Questionnaire (SCQ). Los Angeles: Western Psychological Services 2003.

Rvachew S, Ohberg A, Grawburg M, Heyding J. Phonological awareness and phonemic perception in 4-year-old children with delayed expressive phonology skills. *Am J Speech Lang Pathol* 2003;12(4):463–471.

Saemundsen E, Ludvigsson P, Hilmarsdottir I, et al. Autism spectrum disorders in children with seizures in the first year of life: A population-based study. *Epilepsia* 2007;48(9): 1724–1730.

Schlaggar B, McCandliss B. Development of neural systems for reading. *Ann Rev Neurosci* 2007;30:475–503.

Semrud Clikeman M. Evidence from imaging on the relationship between brain structure and developmental language disorders. *Semin Pediatr Neurol* 1997;4:117–124.

Shaw P, Gornick M, Lerch J, et al. Polymorphisms of the dopamine D4 receptor, clinical outcome, and cortical structure in attention-deficit/hyperactivity disorder. *Arch Gen Psychiatry* 2007;64(8):921–931.

Shriberg L. Five subtypes of developmental phonological disorders. *Clin Commun Disord* 1994;4:38–53.

Shriberg LD, Aram DM, Kwiatkowski J. Developmental apraxia of speech: I. Descriptive and theoretical perspectives. *J Speech Lang Hearing Res* 1997;40:273–285.

SLI Consortium. A genome wide scan identifies two novel loci involved in specific language impairment. *Am J Hum Genet* 2002;70:384–398.

Smidts D, Oosterlaan J. How common are symptoms of ADHD in typically developing preschoolers? A study on prevalence rates and prenatal/demographic risk factors. *Cortex* 2007; 43(6):710–717.

Smits-Engelsman BCM, Wilson PH, Westenberg Y, Duysens J. Fine motor deficiencies in children with developmental coordination disorder and learning disabilities: An underlying open-loop control deficit. *Hum Mov Sci* 2003;22(4–5):495–513.

Snowling MJ, Bishop DVM, Stothard SE. Is pre-school language impairment a risk factor for dyslexia in adolescence? *J Child Psychol Psychiatry* 2000;41:587–600.

Sonuga-Barke E, Daley D, Thompson M, et al. Parent-based therapies for preschool attention-deficit/hyperactivity disorder: A randomized, controlled trial with a community sample. *J Am Acad Child Adolesc Psychiatry* 2001;40:402–408.

Speltz ML, McClellan J, DeKlyen M, Jones K. Preschool boys with oppositional defiant disorder: Clinical presentation and diagnostic change. *J Am Acad Child Adolesc Psychiatry* 1999; 38:838–845.

Spinath FM, Price TS, Dale PS, Plomin R. The genetic and environmental origins of language disability and ability. *Child Dev* 2004;75:445–454.

Stevens MC, Fein DA, Dunn M, et al. Subgroups of children with autism by cluster analysis: A longitudinal examination. *J Am Acad Child Adolesc Psychiatry* 2000;39:346–352.

Sullivan M, Finelli J, Marvin A, et al. Response to joint attention in toddlers at risk for autism spectrum disorder: A prospective study. *J Autism Dev Dis* 2007;37(1):37–48.

Sutera S, Pandey J, Esser EL, et al. Predictors of optimal outcome in toddlers diagnosed with autism spectrum disorders. *J Autism Dev Dis* 2007;37(1):98–107.

Swanson JM, Kinsbourne M, Nigg J, et al. Etiologic subtypes of attention-deficit/hyperactivity disorder: brain imaging, molecular genetic and environmental factors and the dopamine hypothesis. *Neuropsychol Rev* 2007;17(1):39–59.

Tanguay P, Thompson S. *Nonverbal learning disabilities at school: Educating students with Nld, Asperger syndrome and related conditions*. Jessica Kingsley publishers, London: UK, 2002.

Thurm A, Lord C, Lee LC, Newschaffer C. Predictors of language acquisition in preschool children with autism spectrum disorders. *J Autism Dev Dis* 2007;37(9):1721–1734.

Toppelberg C, Shapiro T. Language disorders: A 10-year research update review. *J Am Acad Child Adolesc Psychiatry* 2000;39:143–152.

Tsatsanis KD, Rourke BP, Klin A, et al. Reduced thalamic volume in high-functioning individuals with autism. *Biol Psychiatry* 2003;53:121–129.

Van Daal J, Verhoeven L, van Balkom H. Behavioral problems in children with language impairment. *J Child Psychol Psychiatry* 2007;48:1139–1147.

Veenstra-Vanderweele J, Cook E. Genetics of childhood disorders: XLVI. Autism, Part 5: Genetics of autism. *J Am Acad Child Adolesc Psychiatry* 2003;42:116–118.

Viding E, Spinath F, Price T, et al. Genetic and environmental influence on language impairment in 4-year-old same-sex and opposite-sex twins. *J Child Psychol Psychiatry* 2004;45: 315–320.

Webster R, Majnemer A, Platt R, Shavell M. The predictive value of a preschool diagnosis of developmental language impairment. *Neurology* 2004;63,2327–2331.

Weeks ZR, Ewer-Jones B. Assessment of perceptual-motor and fine motor functioning. In: Bracken BA, ed. *The psychoeducational assessment of preschool children*, 2nd ed. Boston: Allyn and Bacon, 1991:259–283.

Westrup B, Bohm B, Lagercrantz H, Stjernqvist K. Preschool outcome in children born very prematurely and cared for according to the Newborn Individualized Developmental Care and Assessment Program (NIDCAP). *Acta Paediatrica* 2004;93(4):498–507.

Wigal T, Greenhill L, Chuang S, et al. Safety and tolerability of methylphenidate in preschool children with ADHD. *J Am Acad Child Adolesc Psychiatry* 2006;45(11):1294–1303.

Wilens TE, Biederman J, Brown S, et al. Psychiatric comorbidity and functioning in clinically referred preschool children and school-age youths with ADHD. *J Am Acad Child Adolesc Psychiatry* 2002b;41:262–268.

Willey L. *Pretending to be normal*. London: Jessica Kingsley Publishers, 1999.

Wilson PH, Maruff P, Butson M, et al. Internal representation of movement in children with developmental coordination disorder: A mental rotation task. *Dev Med Child Neurol* 2004;46(11):754–759.

Young AR, Beitchman JH, Johnson C, et al. Young adult academic outcomes in a longitudinal sample of early identified language impaired and control children. *J Child Psychol Psychiatry* 2002;43:635–645.

Youngwirth S, Harvey E, Gates E, et al. Neuropsychological abilities of preschool-aged children who display hyperactivity and/or oppositional-defiant behavior problems. *Child Neuropsychol* 2007;13(5):422–443.

Zandt F, Prior M, Kyrios M. Repetitive behaviour in children with high functioning autism and obsessive compulsive disorder. *J Autism Dev Dis* 2007;37(2):251–259.

Chapter 24

Adelman PB, Vogel SA. The learning-disabled-adult. In: Wong B, ed. *Learning about learning disabilities*. San Diego: Academic Press, 1998: 564–594.

Aylward EH, Richards TL, Berninger VW, et al. Instructional treatment associated with changes in brain activation in children with dyslexia. *Neurology* 2003;61:212–219.

Badian N. Nonverbal disorders of learning: The reverse of dyslexia? *Ann Dyslexia* 1996;36:253–269.

Basso A, Marangolo P. Cognitive neuropsychological rehabilitation: The emperor's new clothes? *Neuropsychol Rehabil* 2000;10:219–229.

Beitchman JH, Cantwell DP, Forness SR, et al. Practice parameters for the assessment and treatment of children and adolescents with language and learning disorders. *J Am Acad Child Adolesc Psychiatry* 1998;37(10 Suppl):46S–62S.

Berninger V, Abbot R. Redefining learning disabilities. In: Lyon GR, ed. *Frames of reference for the assessment of learning disabilities*. Baltimore: Brookes, 1994:163–183.

Berninger VW, Abbott RD, Jones J, et al. Early development of language by hand: Composing, reading, listening and speaking connections; three letter-writing modes; and fast mapping in spelling. *Dev Neuropsychol* 2006;29:61–92.

Blondis TA. Motor disorders and attention-deficit/hyperactivity disorder. *Pediatr Clin North Am* 1999;46:899–913.

Booth JR, Burman DD. Development and disorders of neurocognitive systems for oral language and reading. *Learning Disabil Q* 2001;24:205–215.

Bradley R, Danielson L, Hallahan DP, eds. *Identification of learning disabilities: Research to practice*. Mahwah, NJ: Erlbaum, 2002.

Bruandet M, Molko N, Cohen L, Dehaene S. A cognitive characterization of dyscalculia in Turner syndrome. *Neuropsychologia* 2004;42:288–298.

Burns MK, Appleton JJ, Stenhouwer JD. Meta-analytic review of responsiveness-to-intervention research: Examining field-based and research-implemented models. *J Psychoedu Assess* 2005;23:381–394.

Carpenter RL. Mathematics instruction in resource rooms: Instruction time and teacher competence. *Learning Disabil Q* 1985;8:95–100.

Casanova MF, Buxhoeveden DP, Cohen M, et al. Minicolumnar pathology in dyslexia. *Ann Neurol* 2002;52:108–110.

Chang BS, Ly J, Appignani B, et al. Reading impairment in the neuronal migration disorder of periventricular nodular heterotopia. *Neurology* 2005;64(5):799–803.

Cotelli M, Abutalebi J, Zorzi M, Cappa SF. Vowels in the buffer: A case study of acquired dysgraphia with selective vowel substitutions. *Cogn Neuropsychol* 2003;20:99–114.

Curtiss S, Tallal P. On the question of subgroups in language impaired children: A first report. Paper presented at the Tenth Annual Boston University Conference of Language Development, Boston, MA, 1985.

Denckla MB. Revised physical and neurologic examination for subtle signs. *Psychopharmacol Bull* 1985;21:773–800.

Donavon MS, Cross CT. *Minority students in special and gifted education*. Washington, DC: National Academy Press, 2002.

Doose H, Neubauer B, Carlsson G. Children with benign focal sharp waves in the EEG—developmental disorders and epilepsy. *Neuropediatrics* 1996;27:227–241.

Dugbartey AT. Nonverbal learning disability: Adult outcomes. *Semin Clin Neuropsychiatry* 2000;5:198–204.

Finkelstein Y, Markowitz ME, Rosen JF. Low-level lead-induced neurotoxicity in children: An update on central nervous system effects. *Brain Res Rev* 1998;27:168–176.

Fletcher JM, Loveland KA. Neuropsychology of arithmetic disabilities in children. *Focus Learning Problems Mathematics* 1986;8:23–40.

Fletcher JM, Shaywitz SE, Shaywitz BA. Comorbidity of learning and attention disorders: Separate but equal. *Pediatr Clin North Am* 1999;46:885–897.

Francks C, MacPhie IL, Monaco AP. The genetic basis of dyslexia. *Lancet Neurol* 2002;1:483 –490.

Fuchs LS, Fuchs D. Treatment validity: A simplifying concept for reconceptualizing the identification of learning disabilities. *Learning Disabil Res Pract* 1998;4:204–219.

Geary DC. Mathematical disabilities: Cognitive, neuropsychological, and genetic components. *Psychol Bull* 1993;114: 345–362.

Geary DC. Mathematical and learning disabilities. *J Learning Disabil* 2004;37:4–15.

Gottesman RL, Kelly MS. Helping children with learning disabilities toward a brighter adulthood. *Contemp Pediatr* 2000; 17:42–61.

Gough PB, Ehri LC, Treman R, eds. *Reading acquisition*. Hillsdale: Lawrence Erlbaum, 1992.

Gresham FM. Response to treatment. In Bradley R, Danielson L, Hallahan D, eds. *Identification of learning disabilities: Research to practice*. Mahwah, NJ: Erlbaum, 2002:467–519.

Grigorenko EL. Developmental dyslexia: An update on genes, brains, and environments. *J Child Psychol Psychiatry* 2001; 42:91–125.

Gubbay SS, de Klerk NH. A study and review of developmental dysgraphia in relation to acquired dysgraphia. *Brain Dev* 1995;17:1–8.

Habib M. The neurological basis of developmental dyslexia: An overview and working hypothesis. *Brain* 2399;2000;123: 237.

Hamstra-Bletz L, Blote AW. A longitudinal study on dysgraphic handwriting in primary school. J *Learn Disabil* 1993;26: 689–700.

Isaacs EB, Edmonds CJ, Lucas A, Gadian DG. Calculation difficulties in children of very low birthweight: A neural correlate. *Brain* 2001;124:1701–1707.

Johnston JR, Kamhi AG. Syntactic and semantic aspects of the utterances of language impaired children: The same can be less. *Merrill Palmer Quarterly* 1984;30:65–85.

Kujala T, Karma K, Ceponiene R, et al. Plastic neural changes and reading improvement caused by audiovisual training in reading-impaired children. *Proc Nat Acad Sci* 2001;98: 10509–10514.

Kulak AG. Parallels between math and reading disability: Common issues and approaches. *J Learn Disabil* 1993;26:666–673.

Leonard LB. Language learnability and specific language impairment in children. *Applied Psycholinguistics* 1989;10: 179–202.

Levine MD. Neurodevelopmental variation and dysfunction among school-aged children. In: Liberman RG, Moore SP, Hutchinson EC, eds. What's the difference between language impaired and learning disabled children? Paper presented at the meeting of the American Speech-Language-Hearing Association, San Francisco, CA, 1984.

Light JG, DeFries JC. Comorbidity of reading and mathematics disabilities: Genetic and environmental etiologies. *J Learn Disabil* 1995;28:96–106.

Mather DS. Dyslexia and dysgraphia: More than written language difficulties in common. *J Learn Disabil* 2003; 36(4). Retrieved July 6, 2004 from http://0–web17.epnet.com.source.unco.edu.

Matte RR, Bolaski JA. Nonverbal learning disabilities: An overview. *Intervention School Clin* 1998;34:39–43.

McCandliss BD, Noble KG. The development of reading impairment: A cognitive neuroscience model. *Ment Retard Dev Disabil Res Rev* 2003;9:196–205.

McLeod T, Armstrong S. Learning disabilities in mathematics-skills deficits and remedial approaches at the intermediate and secondary level. *Learn Disabil Q* 1982;5:305–311.

Miozzo M, De Bastiani P. The organization of letter-form representations in written spelling: Evidence from acquired dysgraphia. *Brain Lang* 2002;80:366–393.

Molko N, Cachia A, Riviere D. Functional and structural alterations of the intraparietal sulcus in a developmental dyscalculia of genetic origin. *Neuron* 2003;40:847–858.

Moses J. Neurological analysis of calculation deficits. *Focus Learning Problems Mathematics* 1984;6:1–12.

Nass R. Language development in children with congenital strokes. *Semin Pediatr Neurol* 1997;4:109–116.

Nicolson RI, Fawcett AJ, Dean P. Developmental dyslexia: The cerebellar deficit hypothesis. *Trends Neurosci* 2001;24:508–511.

Pellegrino J, Goldman S. Information processing and elementary mathematics. *J Learn Disabil* 1987;20:23–32.

President's Commission on Excellence in Special Education. *A new era: Revitalizing special education for children and their families*. Washington, DC: U.S. Department of Education, 2002.

Pugh KR, Mencl WE, Jenner AR, et al. Functional neuroimaging studies of reading and reading disability (developmental dyslexia). *Ment Retard Dev Disabil Res Rev* 2000;6:207–213.

Reynolds CR. Critical measurement issues in learning disabilities. *J Special Education* 1984;18:451–476.

Rivera SM, Menon V, White CD, et al. Functional brain activation during arithmetic processing in females with Fragile X syndrome is related to FMR1 protein expression. *Hum Brain Mapp* 2002;16:206–218.

Sanchez PN, Coppel D. Adult outcomes of verbal learning disability. *Semin Clin Neuropsychiatry* 2000;5:205–209.

Semrud-Clinkman M, Hynd G. Specific nonverbal and social skills deficits in children with learning disabilities. In: Obrzut J, Hynd G, eds. *Neuropsychological foundations of learning disabilities*. San Diego: Academic Press, 1991.

Shalev RS, Auerbach J, Manor O, Gross-Tsur V. Developmental dyscalculia: Prevalence and prognosis. *Eur Child Adolesc Psychiatry* 2000;9(Suppl 2):58–64.

Shalev RS, Gross-Tsur V. Developmental dyscalculia. *Pediatr Neurol* 2001;24:337–342.

Shapiro BK. Specific reading disability: A multiplanar view. *Mental Retard Dev Disabil Res Rev* 2001;7:13–20.

Shaywitz SE, Fletcher JM, Holahan JM, et al. Persistence of dyslexia. the Connecticut longitudinal study at adolescence. *Pediatrics* 1999;104:1351–1359.

Shaywitz SE, Shaywitz BA, Fulbright RK, et al. Neural systems for compensation and persistence. young adult outcome of childhood reading disability. *Biol Psychiatry* 54:25, 2003

Shaywitz SE, Shaywitz BA. Dyslexia. In: Swaiman KE, Ashwal S, eds. *Pediatric neurology: Principles & practice*, 3rd ed. St Louis: Mosby, 1999:576–584.

Shaywitz SE, Shaywitz BA. Reading disability and the brain. *Educational Leadership* 2004;61:6–12.

Shaywitz, S. Overcoming dyslexia: A new and complete science-based program for reading problems at any level. New York: Alfred A. Knopf, 2003.

Spreen O, Haaf RG. Empirically derived learning disability subtypes: A replication attempt and longitudinal patterns over fifteen years. *J Learn Disabil* 1986;19:170–180.

Stanovich KE. Cognitive science meets beginning reading. *Psychol Sci* 1991;2:77–81.

Stark R, Montgomery JW, Windsor J. Specific speech and language disorders. In: Obrzut J, Hynd G, eds. *Neuropsychological foundations of learning disabilities*. San Diego: Academic Press, 1991.

Stecker PM, Fuchs LS, Fuchs D. Using curriculum-based measurement to improve student achievement: review of research. *Psychology in the schools* 2005;42,795–819.

Strang J, Rourke B. Arithmetic disability subtypes: The neuropsychological significance of specific arithmetical impairment in childhood. In: Rourke B, ed. *Neuropsychology of learning disabilities: Essentials of subtype analysis*. New York: Guilford, 1985:167–183.

Taipale M, Kaminen N, Nopola-Hemmi J, et al. A candidate gene for developmental dyslexia encodes a nuclear tetratricopeptide repeat domain protein dynamically regulated in brain. *Proc Nat Acad Sci USA* 2003;100:11553–11558.

Tallal P. The science of literacy: from the laboratory to the classroom. *Proc Natl Acad Sci USA* 2000;97:2402–2404.

Temple E, Deutsch GK, Poldrack RA, et al. Neural deficits in children with dyslexia ameliorated by behavioral remediation. Evidence from functional MRI. *Proc Nat Acad Sci* 2003;100:2860–2865.

VanDerHeyden AM, Burns MK. Using curriculum-based assessment and curriculum-based measurement to guide elementary mathematics instruction: Effect on individual and group accountability scores. *Assessment Effective Intervention*, 2005;30:15–31.

Vaughn S, Linan-Thompson S, Hickman P. Response to retreatment as a means of identifying students with reading/ learning disabilities. *Exceptional Chidren* 2003a;69:391–409.

Vaughn SR, Wanzek J, Woodruf AL, Linan-Thompson S. A three tier model for preventing reading difficulties and early identification of students with reading disabilities. In: Haager DH, Vaughn SR, Kligner JK, eds. *Validated reading practices for three tiers of intervention*. Baltimore: Brookes, in press.

Vellutino F. Introduction to three studies on reading acquisition: Convergent findings on theoretical foundations of code oriented versus whole language approaches to reading instruction. *J Educ Psychol* 1991;83:437–443.

Vogel S. Quantitative analysis of morphological ability in learning disabled and achieving children. *J Learn Disabil* 1983; 23:44–52.

Wiig EH, Semel EM. *Language assessment and intervention for the learning disabled*. Columbus, OH: Charles E. Merrill, 1984.

Chapter 25

Ackermann H, Ziegler W. Akinetic mutism – a review of the literature. *Fortschr Neurol Psychiatr* 1995;63:59–67.

American Academy of Pediatrics Task Force on Brain Death in Children. Report of a special task force: Guidelines for the determination of brain death in children. *Pediatrics* 1987;80: 298–300.

Ashwal S. Medical aspects of the minimally conscious state in children. *Brain Dev* 2003;25:535–45.

Ashwal S, Cranford R. The minimally conscious state in children. *Semin Pediatr Neurol 2002*;9:19–34.

Balakrishnan G, Aitchison T, Hallworth D, Morton NS. Prospective evaluation of the Paediatric Risk of Mortality (PRISM) score. *Arch Dis Child* 1992;67:196–200.

Beca J, Cox PN. Somatosensory evoked potentials for prediction of outcome in acute severe brain injury. *J Pediatr* 1995; 126:44–49.

Carter BG, Taylor A, Butt W. Severe brain injury in children: Long-term outcome and its prediction using somatosensory evoked potentials (SEPs). *Intensive Care Med* 1999;25:722–728.

Cheliout-Heraut F, Sale-Franque F, Hubert P, Bataille J. Cerebral anoxia in near-drowning of children. The prognostic value of EEG. *Neurophysiol Clin* 1991;21:121–32.

De Meirleir LJ, Taylor MJ. Prognostic utility of SEPs in comatose children. *Pediatr Neurol* 1987;3:78–82.

Dubowitz DJ, Bluml S, Arcinue E, Dietrich RB. MR of hypoxic encephalopathy in children after near drowning: Correlation with quantitative proton MR spectroscopy and clinical outcome. *AJNR Am J Neuroradiol* 1998;19:1617–1627.

Durham SR, Clancy RR, Leuthardt E, et al. CHOP Infant Coma Scale ("Infant Face Scale"): A novel coma scale for children less than two years of age. *J Neurotrauma* 2000;17:729–737.

Fois A, Malandrini F. Electroencephalographic findings in pediatric cases of coma. *Clin Electroencephalogr* 1983;14:207–213.

Giacino JT. Disorders of consciousness: Differential diagnosis and neuropathologic features. *Semin Neurol* 1997;17:105–111.

Hahn YS, Chyung C, Chyung NC, et al. Head injuries in children under 36 months of age. Demography and outcome. *Childs Nerv Syst* 1988;(1):34–40.

Hutchinson DO, Frith RW, Shaw NA, et al. A comparison between electroencephalography and somatosensory evoked potentials for outcome prediction following severe head injury. *Electroencephalogr Clin Neurophysiol* 1991;78:228–233.

Janati A, Erba G. Electroencephalographic correlates of near-drowning encephalopathy in children. *Electroencephalogr Clin Neurophysiol* 1982;53:182–191.

Knaus W, Wagner D, Draper E. APACHE III study design: Analytic plan for evaluation of severity and outcome in intensive care unit patients. Development of APACHE. *Crit Care Med* 1989;17(12 Pt 2):S81–185.

Levy DE, Bates D, Caronna JJ, et al. Prognosis in nontraumatic coma. *Ann Intern Med* 1981;94:293–301.

Levy DE, Caronna JJ, Singer BH, et al. Predicting outcome from hypoxic-ischemic coma. *JAMA* 1985;253:1420–1426.

Lin KL, Wang HS, Chou ML, Rui TN. Role of cavum septum pellucidum in akinetic mutism of hydrocephalic children. *Pediatr Neurol* 1997;16:156–159.

Mandel R, Martinot A, Delepoulle F, et al. Prediction of outcome after hypoxic-ischemic encephalopathy. a prospective clinical and electrophysiologic study. *J Pediatr* 2002;141:45–50.

Martinot A, Lejeune C, Hue V, et al. Modality and causes of 259 deaths in a pediatric intensive care unit. *Arch Pediatr* 1995;2:735–741.

Mega MS, Cohenour RC. Akinetic mutism: Disconnection of frontal-subcortical circuits. *Neuropsychiatry Neuropsychol Behav Neurol* 1997;10:254–259.

Pollack MM, Patel KM, Ruttimann UE. PRISM III: An updated pediatric risk of mortality score. *Crit Care Med* 1996;24:743–752.

Riviello JJ. Coma. In: Selbst SM, Torrey SB, eds. *Pediatric emergency medicine for the house officer*. Baltimore: Williams and Wilkins, 1988:57–67.

Riviello JJ, Sapin JI, Brown LW, et al. Hypoxemia and hemodynamic changes during the hypercarbia stimulation test. *Pediatr Neurol* 1988;4:213–218.

Singhi PD, Bansal A, Ramesh S, Khandelwal N, Singhi SC. Predictive value of electroencephalography and computed tomography in childhood non-traumatic coma. *Indian J Pediatr* 2005;72:475–479.

Stern WE. Intracranial fluid dynamics: The relationship of intracranial pressure to the Monroe-Kellie doctrine and the reliability of pressure assessment. *J R Coll Surg Edinb* 1963;168:18–36.

Strauss DJ, Ashwal S, Day SM, Shavelle RM. Life expectancy of children in vegetative and minimally conscious states. *Pediatr Neurol* 2000;23:312–319.

Taylor MJ, Farrell EJ. Comparison of the prognostic utility of VEPs and SEPs in comatose children. *Pediatr Neurol* 1989;5:145–150.

Yang CC, Lieberman JS, Hong CZ. Early smooth horizontal eye movement: A favorable prognostic sign in patients with locked-in syndrome. *Arch Phys Med Rehabil* 1989;70:230–232.

Zeman A. Persistent vegetative state. *Lancet* 1997;350:795–799.

Chapter 26

Abu-Arafeh I, Russell G. Prevalence of headache and migraine in schoolchildren. *Br Med J* 1994;309:765–769.

Bille B. Migraine in school children. A study of the incidence and short-term prognosis, and a clinical psychological and electroencephalographic comparison between children with migraine and matched controls. *Acta Paediatr* 1962;51:1–151.

Burstein R, Cutrer FM, Yarnitsky D. The development of cutaneous allodynia during a migraine attack clinical evidence for the sequential recruitment of spinal and supraspinal nociceptive neurons in migraine. *Brain* 2000;123:1703–1709.

Cady R, Schreiber C, Farmer K, Sheftell, F. Primary headaches: A convergence hypothesis. *Headache* 2002;42:204–216.

Daly E, Donn P, Galliher M, Zimmerman J. Biofeedback applications to migraine and tension headaches: A double-blinded outcome study. *Biofeedback Self Regul* 1983;8:135–152.

Hämäläinen ML, Hoppu K, Valkeila E, Santavuori P. Ibuprofen or acetaminophen for the acute treatment of migraine in children: A double-blind, randomized, placebo-controlled, crossover study. *Neurology* 1997;48:103–107.

Hershey AD, Powers SW, Bentti A-L, et al. Characterization of chronic daily headaches in children in a multidisciplinary headache center. *Neurology* 2001a;56:1032–1037.

Hershey AD, Powers SW, Vockell ALB, et al. PedMIDAS: Development of a questionnaire to assess disability of migraines in children. *Neurology* 2001b;57:2034–2039.

Hershey AD, Winner P, Kabbouche MA, et al. Use of the ICHD-II criteria in the diagnosis of pediatric migraine. *Headache* 2005;45:1288–1297.

Kabbouche M, Vockell ALB, LeCates SL, et al. Tolerability and effectiveness of prochlorperazine for intractable migraine in children. *Pediatrics* 2001;107:e62.

Katsarava Z, Fritsche G, Muessig M, et al. Clinical features of withdrawal headache following overuse of triptans and other headache drugs. *Neurology* 2001;57:1694–1698.

Lewis DW, Kellstein D, Dahl G, et al. Children's ibuprofen suspension for the acute treatment of pediatric migraine. Headache 42:780–786, 2002b.

Linder SL. Treatment of childhood headache with dihydroergotamine mesylate. *Headache* 1994;34:578–580.

Linder SL, Winner P. Pediatric headache. *Med Clin North Am* 2001;85:1037–1053.

Lipton RB, Stewart WF, Cady R, et al. 2000 Wolfe Award. Sumatriptan for the range of headaches in migraine sufferers: Results of the Spectrum Study. *Headache* 2000;40:783–791.

Osterhaus JT, Townsend RJ, Gandek B, Ware JE, Jr. Measuring the functional status and well-being of patients with migraine headache. *Headache* 1994;34:337–343.

Powers SW, Hershey AD. In: Maria BL, ed. Current management in child neurology. Hamilton, Ontario: Decker, 2002; 83–85.

Powers SW, Patton SR, Hommel KA, Hershey AD. Quality of life in childhood migraines: clinical impact and comparison to other chronic illnesses. *Pediatrics* 2003 Jul;112(1 Pt1):e1–5.

Silberstein SD, Rosenberg J. Multispecialty consensus on diagnosis and treatment of headache. *Neurology* 2000;54:1553.

Smith TR, Sunshine A, Stark SR, et al. Sumatriptan and naproxen sodium for the acute treatment of migraine. *Headache* 2005;45(8):983–991.

Split W, Neuman W. Epidemiology of migraine among students from randomly selected secondary schools in Lodz. *Headache* 1999;39:494–501.

Stewart WF, Lipton RB, Dowson AJ, Sawyer J. Development and testing of the Migraine Disability Assessment (MIDAS) Questionnaire to assess headache-related disability. Neurology 2001;56:S20–28.

Tepper SJ, Dodick DW. Debate: Analgesic overuse is a cause, not consequence of daily headache. Analgesic overuse is a cause of chronic daily headache. *Headache* 2002;42:543–554.

Vasconcellos E, Pina-Garza JE, Millan EJ, Warner JS. Analgesic rebound headache in children and adolescents. *J Child Neurol* 1998;13:443–447.

Chapter 27

Abou-Khalil B, Krie L, Lazenby BG, Harris PA, et al. Familial genetic predisposition, epilepsy localization and antecedent febrile seizures. *Epilepsy Research* 2007; 73:104–110.

American Academy of Pediatrics Provisional Committee on Quality Improvement. Practice parameter: The neurodiagnostic evaluation of the child with a simple febrile seizure. *Pediatrics* 1996;97:769–775.

Annegers JF, Blakely SA, Hauser WA, Kurland LT. Recurrence of febrile convulsions in a population-based cohort. *Epilepsy Res* 1990;66:1009–1012.

Annegers JF, Hauser WA, Shirts SB, Kurland LT. Factors prognostic of unprovoked seizures after febrile convulsions. *N Engl J Med* 1987;316:493–498.

Baraitser M. Relevance of a family history of seizures. *Arch Dis Child* 1983;58:404–405.

Berg AT, Shinnar S, Darefsky AS, et al. Predictors of recurrence febrile seizures. *Arch Pediatr Adolesc Med* 1997;151:371–378.

Berg AT, Shinnar S, Shapiro ED, et al. Risk factors for a first febrile seizure: A matched case-control study. *Epilepsia* 1995; 36:334–341.

Berg AT, Shinnar S. Complex febrile seizures. *Epilepsia* 1996a; 37:126–133.

Berg AT, Shinnar S. Unprovoked seizures in children with febrile seizures: Short term outcome. *Neurology* 1996b;47:562–568.

Berg AT. Are febrile seizures provoked by a rapid rise in temperature? *Am J Dis Child* 1993;147:1101–1103.

Birca A, Guy N, Fortier I, et al. Genetic influence on the clinical characteristiss and outcomes of febrile seizures—retrospective study. *Euro I Pediatric Neurology* 2005;9,339–345.

Camfield CS, Camfield PR, Smith E, Dooley JM. Home use of rectal diazepam to prevent status epilepticus in children with convulsive disorders. *J Child Neurol* 1989;4:125–126.

Camfield P, Camfield C, Gordon K, Dooley J. What types of epilepsy are preceded by febrile seizures? A population-based study of children. *Dev Med Child Neurol* 1994; 36:887–892.

Camfield PR, Camfield CS, Shapiro S, et al. The first febrile seizure antipyretic instruction plus either phenobarbital or placebo to prevent recurrences. *J Pediatr* 1980;97:16–21.

Chang YC, Guo NW, Huang CC, et al. Neurocognitive attention and behavior outcome of school-age children with a history of febrile convulsions: A population study. *Epilepsia* 2000;41:412–420.

Chung B, Wong V. Relationship between five common viruses and febrile seizure in children. *Arch Dis Child* 2007;92:589–593.

Consensus Statement on Febrile Seizures. In: Nelson KB, Ellenberg JH, eds. *Febrile seizures*. New York: Raven Press, 1981:301.

Dianese G. Prophylactic diazepam in febrile convulsions. *Arch Dis Child* 1979;54:244–245.

Dravet C, Bureau M, Guerrini R, et al., eds. *Epileptic syndromes in infancy, childhood and adolescence*, 2nd ed. London: Lohn-Libbey, 1992:75–78.

Dubé C, Richichi C, Bender RA, et al. Temporal lobe epilepsy after experimental prolonged febrile seizures: Prospective analysis. *Brain* 2006;129:911–922.

Dubé CM, Brewster AL, Richichi C, et al. Fever, febrile seizures and epilepsy. *Trends in Neurosci* 2007;30:490–495.

Ellenberg JH, Nelson KB. Febrile seizures and later intellectual performance. *Arch Neurol* 1978;35:17–21.

Ellenberg JH, Nelson KB. Sample selection and the natural history of disease—studies of febrile seizures. *JAMA* 1980;243: 1337–1340.

El-Rahdi AS. Lower degree of fever at initial febrile convulsion is associated with increased risk of subsequent convulsion. *Eur J Paediatr Neurol* 1998;2:91–96.

Green AL, MacFaul R. Duration of admission for febrile convulsions? *Arch Dis Child* 1985;60:1182–1184.

Griffin MR, Ray WA, Mortimer EA, et al. Risk of seizures and encephalopathy after immunization with the diphtheria-tetanus-pertussis vaccine. *JAMA* 1990;263:1641–1645.

Hansen A, Abitbol V, Ibsen KK, et al. Conditions for children and their parents in hospitals. III. Parents' reactions in connection with admission of the child with the diagnosis of the first febrile seizure. *Ugeskr Laeg* 1984;146:689–691.

Haspolat S, Baysal Y, Duman O, et al. Interleukin-α, interleukin-β and interleukin-1Ra polymorphisms in febrile seizures. *J Child Neurol* 2005;20:565–568.

Hauser WA, Annefers JF, Anderson VE, Kurland LT. The risk of seizure disorders among relatives of children with febrile convulsions. *Neurology* 1985;35:1268–1273.

Hirata Y, et al. Epilepsy following febrile convulsions. *Brain Dev* 1985;7:1–75.

Hirtz DG, Nelson KB, Ellenberg JH. Seizures following childhood immunizations. *J Pediatr* 1983;102:14–18.

Joffe A, McCormick M, De Angeles C. Which children with febrile seizures need lumbar puncture? *Am J Dis Child* 1983; 137:1153–1156.

Knudsen FU, Paerragaard A, Andersen R, Andresen J. Long-term outcome of prophylaxis for febrile convulsions. *Arch Dis Child* 1996;74:13–18.

Knudsen FU. PC risk after first febrile seizures and effect of short term diazepam prophylaxis. *Arch Dis Child* 1985;60: 1045–1049.

Lee K, Melchior JC. Sodium valproate versus phenobarbital in the prophylactic treatment of febrile seizures in childhood. *Eur J Pediatr* 1981;137:151–153.

Mamelle N, Mamelle JC, Plasse JC, et al. Prevention of recurrent febrile convulsions – A randomized therapeutic assay: Sodium valproate, phenobarbital and placebo. *Neuropediatrics* 1984;15:37–42.

Matsuo M, Sasaki K, Ichimaru T, et al. Increased IL-β production from dsRNA-stimulated leukocytes in febrile seizures. *Pediat Neurol* 2005;35:102–106.

Maytal J, Steale R, Evator L, et al. The value of early postictal EEG in children with febrile seizures. *Epilepsia* 2000;41: 219–221.

McKinlay I, Newton R. Intention to treat febrile seizures with rectal diazepam, valproate, or phenobarbitone. *Dev Med Child Neurol* 1989;31:617–625.

Millichap JG, Millichap JJ. Role of viral infections in the etiology of febrile seizures. *Ped Neurol* 2006; 35:3 165–172.

Minagawa K, Mizuno S, Shirai H, Miura H. [A pharmacokinetic study on the effectiveness of intermittent oral seizure in the prevention of recurrent febrile convulsions.] *No To Hattatsu* 1985;17:162–167.

Morton LD, Rizkallah E, Pellock JM. New drug therapy for acute seizure management. *Semin Pediatr Neurol* 1997;4:51–63.

Nagao Y, Mazaki-Miyazakie E, Okamura N, et al. A family of generalized epilepsy with febrile seizures plus type 2–a new missense mutation of SCN1A found in the pedigree of several patients with complex febrile seizures. *Epilepsy Res* 2005;63:151–156.

Nakayama J, Arinami J. Molecular genetics of febrile seizures. *Epilepsy Res* 2006;S190–S198.

Natsumo J, Bernaconi N, Miyauchi M, et al. Hippocampal volumes and diffusion-weighted image findings in children with prolonged febrile seizures. *Acta Neurol Scand* 2007; 115(Suppl 186): 25–28.

Nelson KB, Ellenberg JH. Predictors of epilepsy in children who have experienced febrile seizures. *N Engl J Med* 1976;295: 1029–1033.

Nelson KB, Ellenberg JH. Prognosis in children with febrile seizures. *Pediatrics* 1978;61:720–727.

Newton RW. Randomized controlled trials of phenobarbitone and valproate in febrile convulsions. *Arch Dis Child* 1988; 63:1189–1191.

O'Dell C, Shinnar S, Ballaban-Gil KR, et al. Rectal diazepam gel in the home management of seizures in children. *Pediatric Neurol* 2005;33:3 166–172.

Offringa M, Bussuyt PM, Lubsen J. Seizure recurrence after a febrile seizure: A multivariate approach. *Dev Med Child Neurol* 1992;34:15–24.

Offringa M. Bossuyt PM, Lubsen J, et al. Risk factors for seizure recurrence in children with febrile seizures. A pooled analysis of individual patient data from five studies. *J Pediatr* 1994;124:574–84.

Pavilidou E, Tzitiridou M, Kontopoulos E, Panteliadis CP. Which factors determine febrile seizure recurrence: A prospective. *Brain Dev* 2008;30:7–13.

Rantala H, Uhari M. Risk factors for recurrences of febrile convulsions. *Acta Neurol Scand* 1994;90:207–210.

Rosman NP, Colton T, Labazzo J, et al. A controlled trial of diazepam administered during febrile illnesses to prevent recurrence of febrile seizures. *N Engl J Med* 1993a;329:79–84.

Ross EM, Peckham CS, West PB, Butler NR. Epilepsy in childhood. Findings from the National Child Development Study. *Br Med J* 1980;280:207–210.

Sadleir LG, Scheffer IE. Febrile seizures. *BMJ* 2007;334: 307–311.

Scheffer IE, Harkin LA, Dibbens LM, et al. Neonatal epilepsy syndromes and generalized epilepsy with febrile seizures plus (GEFS+). *Eplipsia* 2005;46(Suppl 10):41–47.

Schuchmann S, et al. Experimental febrile seizures are precipitated by a hyperthermia-induced respiratory alkalosis. *Nat Med* 2006;12:817–823.

Scott RC, King MD, Gadian DG, et al. Prolonged febrile seizures are associated with hippocampal vasogenic edema and developmental changes. *Epilepsia* 2006;47(9):1493–1495.

Shinnar S, Berg AT. Does antiepileptic drug therapy prevent the development of "chronic" epilepsy? *Epilepsia* 1996;37:701–708.

Sofijanov N, Emoto S, Kuturec M, et al. Febrile seizures: Clinical characteristics and initial EEG. *Epilepsia* 1992;33:52–57.

Sofijanov N, Sadikario A, Dukovski M, Kuturec M. Febrile convulsions and later development of epilepsy. *Am J Dis Child* 1983;137:123–126.

Stores G. When does an EEG contribute to the management of febrile seizures? *Arch Dis Child* 1991;66:554–557.

Teng D, Dayan P, Tyler S, et al. Risk of intracranial pathologic conditions requiring emergency intervention after a first complex febrile seizure episode among children. *Pediatrics* 2006;117:304–308.

Thorn I. Prevention of recurrence febrile seizures: Intermittent prophylaxis with diazepam compared with continuous treatment with phenobarbital. In: Nelson KB, Ellenberg, et al., eds. *Febrile seizures*. New York: Raven Press, 1981:119–126.

Tomoum H, Badawy NM, Mostafa AA, Harb MY. Plasma Interleukin-β levels in children with febrile seizures. *J Child Neurol* 2007;22:689–692.

Tsuboi T. Epidemiology of febrile and afebrile convulsions in children in Japan. *Neurology* 1984;54:175–181.

Van Zeijl JH, Mullaart RA, Borm GF, Galama JMD. Recurrence of febrile seizures in the respiratory season is associated with Influenza A. *J Pediatr* 2004;145:800–804.

Verity CM, Golding J. Risk of epilepsy after febrile convulsions: A national cohort study. *Br Med J* 1991;303:1373–1376.

Verity CM, Ross EM, Golding J. Outcome of childhood status epilepticus and lengthy febrile convulsions: Findings of a national cohort study. *Br Med J* 1993;307:225–228.

Vestergaard M, Pedersen CB, Sidenius P, et al. The long-term risk of epilepsy after febrile seizures in Susceptible subgroups. *Am J Epidemol* 2007;1–8.

Vestergaard M, Pederson CB, Christensen J., et al. Febrile seizures and risk of schizophrenia. *Schizophrenia Research* 2005;73:344–349.

Virta M, Hurme M, Helminen M. Increased frequency of interleukin-1beta (-511) allele 2 in febrile seizures. *Pediatr Neurol* 2002;26:192–196.

Walker AM, Jick H, Perera DR, et al. Neurologic events following diphtheria-tetanus-pertussis immunization. *Pediatrics* 1988;81:345–349.

Wolf SM, Carr A, Davis DC, et al. The value of phenobarbital in the child who has had a single febrile seizure. A controlled, prospective study. *Pediatrics* 1977;59:378–385.

Wolf SM, Forsythe A. Epilepsy and mental retardation following febrile seizures in childhood. *Acta Paediatr Scand* 1989; 78:291–295.

Chapter 28

Achenbach TM. Manual for the revised child behavior profile and child behavior checklist. Burlington, VT:2001.

American Psychiatric Association. *Diagnostic and statistical manual for mental disorders*, 4th ed. Washington, DC: American Psychiatric Association, 2001.

Anastopoulos AD, Shelton TL, DuPaul GJ, Guevremont DC. Parent training for attention-deficit hyperactivity disorder: Its impact on parent functioning. *J Abnorm Child Psychology* 1993;21:581–596.

Antshel KM, Remer R. Social skills training in children with attention deficit hyperactivity disorder. A randomized-controlled clinical trial. *J Clin Child Adolesc Psychol* 2003; 32(1):152–165.

Applegate B, Lahey BB, Hart EL, et al. Validity of the age-of-onset criterion for ADHD. A report of the DSM-IV field trials. *J Am Acad Child Adolesc Psychiatry* 1997;36:1211–1221.

Barbaresi WJ, Katusic SK, Colligan RC, et al. How common is attention-deficit/hyperactivity disorder? Incidence in a population-based birth cohort in Rochester, Minn. *Arch Pediatr Adolesc Med* 2002;156,217–224.

Barkley RA, Biederman J. Towards a broader definition of the age of onset criterion for attention deficit hyperactivity disorder. *J Am Acad Child Adolesc Psychiatry* 1997;36:1204–1210.

Barkley RA, Fischer M, Edelbrock CS, Smallish L. The adolescent outcome of hyperactive children diagnosed by research criteria: I. An 8 year prospective follow-up study. *J Am Acad Child Adolesc Psychiatry* 1990;29:546–557.

Barkley RA, Fischer M, Smallish L, Fletcher K. Persistence of attention deficit hyperactivity disorder into adulthood as a function of reporting source and definition of disorder. *J Abnorm Psychol* 2002;111:279–289.

Barkley RA, Shelton TL, Crosswait C, et al. Early psycho-educational intervention for children with disruptive behavior: Preliminary post-treatment outcome. *J Child Psychol Psychiatry* 2000;41:319–332.

Barkley RA, Smith KM, Fischer M, Navia B. An examination of the behavioral and neuropsychological correlates of three ADHD candidate gene polymorphisms (DRD4 7+, DBH TaqI A2, and DAT1 40 bp VNTR) in hyperactive and normal children followed to adulthood. *Am J Med Genet B Neuropsychiatr Genet* 2006 5;141(5):487–498.

candidate gene polymorphisms (DRD4 7+, DBH TaqI A2, and DAT1 40 bp VNTR) in hyperactive and normal children followed to adulthood. *Am J Med Genet B Neuropsychiatr Genet* 2006 5;141(5):487–498.

Barkley RA. Response inhibition in attention deficit hyperactivity disorder. *Ment Retard Dev Disabil Res Rev* 1999;5: 177–184.

Barkley RA. The international consensus statement on ADHD. *Clin Child Fam Psychol Rev* 2002;5:89–111.

Biederman J, Faraone S, Milberger S, et al. Predictors of persistence and remission of ADHD into adolescence. Results from a four-year prospective follow-up study. *J Am Acad Child Adolesc Psychiatry* 1996;35:343–351.

Bloom B, Cohen RA. Summary health statistics for U.S. children. National Health Interview Survey, 2006. *Vital Health Stat* 2007;10(234):1–79.

Brown TE. Brown attention-deficit disorder scales for children and adolescents. San Antonio, TX: Psychological Corporation, 2001.

Campbell SB. Behavior problems in preschool children. New York: Guilford Press, 1990.

Carlson CL, Mann M. Sluggish cognitive tempo predicts a different pattern of impairment in the attention deficit hyperactivity disorder, predominantly inattentive type. *J Clin Child Adolesc Psychol* 2002;31(1):123–129.

Conners C. Conners' rating scales-revised technical manual. North Tonawanda, NY: Multi-Health Systems, 1997.

Connor DF. Preschool attention deficit hyperactivity disorder: A review of prevalence, diagnosis, neurobiology, and stimulant treatment. *J Dev Behav Pediatr* 2002;23:S1–S2.

DuPaul GJ, Barkley RA, Connor DF. Stimulants. In: Barkley RA, ed. *Attention deficit hyperactivity disorder: A handbook for diagnosis and treatment.* New York: Guilford, 1998:510–551.

Faraone SV, Biederman J, Mick E, et al. Family study of girls with attention deficit hyperactivity disorder. *Am J Psychiatry* 2000;157(7):1077–1083.

Faraone SV, Perlis RH, Doyle AE, et al. Molecular genetics of attention-deficit/hyperactivity disorder. *Biol Psychiatry* 2005; 57(11):1313–1323.

Ford JD, Racusin R, Ellis CG, et al. Child maltreatment, other trauma exposure, and posttraumatic symptomatology among children with oppositional defiant and attention deficit hyperactivity disorders. *Child Maltreat* 2000;5(3): 205–217.

Gioia GA, Isquith PK, Guy StC, Kenworthy L. Behavior Rating Inventory of Executive Function (BRIEF). Odessa, FL: Psychological Assessment Resources, 2000.

Gordon M, Barkley RA. Psychological tests. In: Barkley RA, ed. *Attention deficit hyperactivity disorder: A handbook for diagnosis and treatment*, 2nd ed. New York: Guilford, 1998.

Green WH. *Child & adolescent clinical psychopharmacology*, 4th ed. Philadelphia: Wolters Kluwer/Lippincott Williams & Wilkins, 2007.

Greenhill L, Kollins S, Abikoff H, et al. Efficacy and safety of immediate-release methylphenidate treatment for preschoolers with ADHD. *J Am Acad Child Adolesc Psychiatry* 2006; 45(11):1284–1293.

Greenhill L, Osmon B. Ritalin: Research, theory, and action. New York: Mary Ann Liebert, 2002.

Hartman CA, Willcutt EG, Rhee SH, Pennington BF. The relation between sluggish cognitive tempo and DSM-IV ADHD. *J Abnorm Child Psychol* 2004;32(5):491–503.

Hoza B, Waschbusch DA, Pelham WE, et al. Attention-deficit/hyperactivity disordered and control boys' responses to social success and failure. *Child Dev* 2000;71(2):432–46.

Hurtig T, Ebeling H, Taanila A, et al. ADHD symptoms and subtypes. relationship between childhood and adolescent symptoms. *J Am Acad Child Adolesc Psychiatry* 2007; 46(12):1605–1613.

Kadesjő B, Gillberg C. Attention deficits and clumsiness in Swedish 7-year-old children. *Dev Med Child Neuro* 1998 40(12):796–804.

Kamphaus R, Reynolds C. *The behavioral assessment system for children,* 2nd ed. Circle Pines, MN: American Guidance Service, 2005.

Kessler RC, Adler L, Barkley R, et al. The prevalence and correlates of adult ADHD in the United States. results from the National Comorbidity Survey Replication. *Am J Psychiatry* 2006;163(4):716–723.

Lavigne JV, Gibbons RD, Christoffel K, et al. Prevalence rates and correlates of psychiatric disorders among preschool children. *J Am Acad Child Adolesc Psychiatry* 1996;35:204–214.

Levy F, Hay D. Attention, genes, and ADHD. Philadelphia, PA: Brunner-Routledge, 2001.

Levy F, Hay DA, McStephen M, et al. Attention-deficit hyperactivity disorder: A category or a continuum? Genetic analysis of a large-scale twin study. *J Am Acad Child Adolesc Psychiatry* 1997;36:737–744.

McBurnett K, Pfiffner LJ, Frick PJ. Symptom properties as a function of ADHD type. an argument for continued study of sluggish cognitive tempo. *J Abnorm Child Psychol* 2001; 29(3):207–213.

McCann D, Barrett A, Cooper A, et al. Food additives and hyperactive behaviour in 3–year-old and 8/9–year-old children in the community. a randomised, double-blinded, placebo-controlled trial. *Lancet* 2007;370(9598):1560–1567.

Milich R, Ballentine AC, Lynam D. ADHD combined type and ADHD predominantly inattentive type are distinct and unrelated disorders. *Clin Psychol* 2001;8:463–488.

Mrug S, Hoza B, Pelham WE, et al. Behavior and peer status in children with ADHD. Continuity and change. *J Atten Disord* 2007;10(4):359–371.

MTA Cooperative Group. National Institute of Mental Health Multimodal Treatment Study of ADHD follow-up. 24-month outcomes of treatment strategies for attention-deficit/hyperactivity disorder. *Pediatrics* 2004;113(4):754–761.

MTA Cooperative Group. A 14-month randomized clinical trial of treatment strategies for attention deficit hyperactivity disorder (ADHD). *Arch Gen Psychiatry* 1999;56:1073–1086.

Murray DW, Kollins SH, Hardy KK, et al. Parent versus teacher ratings of attention-deficit/hyperactivity disorder symptoms in the Preschoolers with Attention-Deficit/Hyperactivity Disorder Treatment Study (PATS). *J Child Adolesc Psychopharmacol* 2007;17(5):605–620.

Nigg JT. Is ADHD an inhibitory disorder? *Psychol Bull* 2001; 125:571–596.

Pagani L, Tremblay R, Vitaro F, et al. Effects of grade retention on academic performance and behavioral development. *Dev Psychopathol* 2001;13:297–315.

Pliszka S, et al. Comorbidity in attention deficit hyperactivity disorder. New York: Guilford, 2000.

Polanczyk G, de Lima MS, Horta BL, et al. The worldwide prevalence of ADHD. a systematic review and meta regression analysis. *Am J Psychiatry* 2007;164(6):942–948.

Posner K, Melvin GA, Murray DW, et al. Clinical presentation of attention-deficit/hyperactivity disorder in preschool children. The Preschoolers with Attention-Deficit/Hyperactivity Disorder Treatment Study (PATS). *J Child Adolesc Psychopharmacol* 2007;17(5):547–562.

Rowe R, Maughan B, Goodman R. Childhood psychiatric disorder and unintentional injury. findings from a national cohort study. *J Pediatr Psychol* 2004;29(2):119–130.

Sachs GS, Baldassano CF, Truman CJ, Guille C. Comorbidity of attention deficit hyperactivity disorder with early- and late-onset bipolar disorder. *Am J Psychiatry* 2000; 157(3): 466–468.

Schab DW, Trinh NH. Do artificial food colors promote hyperactivity in children with hyperactive syndromes? A meta-analysis of double-blind placebo-controlled trials. *J Dev Behav Pediatr* 2004;25(6):423–434.

Smidts DP, Oosterlaan J. How common are symptoms of ADHD in typically developing preschoolers? A study on prevalence rates and prenatal/demographic risk factors. *Cortex* 2007;43(6):710–717.

Sonuga-Barke EJ, Sergeant J. The neuroscience of ADHD. multidisciplinary perspectives on a complex developmental disorder. *Dev Sci* 2005;8(2):103–104.

Spencer T, Wilens T, Biederman J, et al. Attention-deficit/hyperactivity disorder with mood disorders. In: Brown TE, ed. Attention deficit disorders and comorbidities in children, adolescents, and adults. Washington, DC: American Psychiatric Press, 2000:79–128.

Spencer TJ, Biederman J, Wozniak J, Faraone SV, Wilens TE, Mick E. Parsing pediatric bipolar disorder from its associated comorbidity with the disruptive behavior disorders. *Biol Psychiatry* 2001:49(12):1062–1070.

Still GF. Some abnormal psychical conditions in children. *Lancet* 1902;1:1008–1012, 1077–1082, 1163–1168.

Szatmari P. The epidemiology of attention-deficit hyperactivity disorders. In: Weiss G, ed. *Child and adolescent psychiatric clinics of North America: Attention-deficit hyperactivity disorder*. Philadelphia: Saunders, 1992:361–372.

Tannock R. Attention deficit hyperactivity disorder: Advances in cognitive, neurobiological, and genetic research. *J Child Psychol Psychiatry* 1998;39:65–100.

Todd RD, Huang H, Smalley SL, et al. Collaborative analysis of DRD4 and DAT genotypes in population-defined ADHD subtypes. *J Child Psychol Psychiatry*. 2005;46(10):1067–1073.

Todd RD, Rasmussen ER, Wood C, et al. Should sluggish cognitive tempo symptoms be included in the diagnosis of attention-deficit/hyperactivity disorder? *J Am Acad Child Adolesc Psychiatry*. 2004;43(5):588–597.

van Lier PA, van der Ende J, Koot HM, Verhulst FC. Which better predicts conduct problems? The relationship of trajectories of conduct problems with ODD and ADHD symptoms from childhood into adolescence. *J Child Psychol Psychiatry* 2007;48(6):601–608.

Weiss G, Hechtman L. *Hyperactive children grown up*, 2nd ed. New York: Guilford Press, 1993.

Werry J, Aman M. *Practitioners guide to psychoactive drugs with children and adolescents*, 2nd ed. New York: Plenum, 1999.

Wigal T, Greenhill L, Chuang S, et al. Safety and tolerability of methylphenidate in preschool children with ADHD. *J Am Acad Child Adolesc Psychiatry* 2006;45(11):1294–1303.

Index

Note: Page numbers followed by an italicized *t* refer to tables in the indicated page; page numbers followed by a bold-face **f** refer to figures on the indicated page.